MOSBY'S
DENTAL DRUG REFERENCE

TENTH EDITION

MOSBY'S
DENTAL
DRUG
REFERENCE
TENTH EDITION

Editor-in-Chief
Arthur H. Jeske, PhD
Professor
Department of Restorative Dentistry and Biomaterials
University of Texas School of Dentistry at Houston
Houston, Texas

ELSEVIER
MOSBY

ELSEVIER
MOSBY

3251 Riverport Lane
St. Louis, Missouri 63043

MOSBY'S DENTAL DRUG REFERENCE, TENTH EDITION

ISBN: 978-0-323-07960-0
ISSN: 2211-5625

Notices

Knowledge and best practice in this field are constantly changing. As new research and experience broaden our understanding, changes in research methods, professional practices, or medical treatment may become necessary.

Practitioners and researchers must always rely on their own experience and knowledge in evaluating and using any information, methods, compounds, or experiments described herein. In using such information or methods they should be mindful of their own safety and the safety of others, including parties for whom they have a professional responsibility.

With respect to any drug or pharmaceutical products identified, readers are advised to check the most current information provided (i) on procedures featured or (ii) by the manufacturer of each product to be administered, to verify the recommended dose or formula, the method and duration of administration, and contraindications. It is the responsibility of practitioners, relying on their own experience and knowledge of their patients, to make diagnoses, to determine dosages and the best treatment for each individual patient, and to take all appropriate safety precautions.

To the fullest extent of the law, neither the Publisher nor the authors, contributors, or editors, assume any liability for any injury and/or damage to persons or property as a matter of products liability, negligence or otherwise, or from any use or operation of any methods, products, instructions, or ideas contained in the material herein.

ISBN: 978-0-323-07960-0

Vice President and Publisher: Linda Duncan
Executive Editor: John Dolan
Developmental Editor: Joslyn Dumas
Publishing Services Manager: Pat Joiner-Myers
Project Manager: Marlene Weeks
Designer: Maggie Reid

Printed in the United States of America

Last digit is the print number: 9 8 7 6 5 4 3 2 1

Drug Monograph Content Contributors and Reviewers

Catherine Ulbricht, PharmD, MBA
Senior Attending Pharmacist
Massachusetts General Hospital
Co-founder, Natural Standard Research Collaboration
Cambridge, Massachusetts

Catherine M. Flaitz, DDS, MS
Professor
Departments of Diagnostic Sciences and Pediatric Dentistry
University of Texas School of Dentistry at Houston
Houston, Texas

Marshal Shlafer, PhD
Professor
Department of Pharmacology
Director
Undergraduate Medical Pharmacology Education
University of Michigan School of Medicine
Ann Arbor, Michigan

Ruth Fearing Tornwall, RDH, MS
Associate Professor
Department of Allied Health Sciences
Lamar Institute of Technology
Beaumont, Texas

Preface

This tenth edition of *Mosby's Dental Drug Reference* continues Mosby-Elsevier's tradition of providing comprehensive and current information on prescription drugs and recommendations for the care of the dental patients who take them. As in past editions, new individual drugs, as well as new drug classes, are included in this concise reference book, which is designed to address the need of oral health care practitioners and educators for readily accessible and up-to-date drug information and guidance for the dental management of medically compromised patients. The tenth edition incorporates many significant improvements, including:

1. *A revised and updated section on the Therapeutic Management of Common Oral Lesions.*
2. *A revised and updated section on Medically Compromised Patients, addressing the most recent antibiotic prophylaxis guidelines for patients at risk of infective endocarditis and for patients with total joint replacements, as well as a summary of monoclonal antibody therapy.*
3. *Revised and updated monographs on cardiovascular drugs.*
4. *The relocation of the section on Herbal and Nonherbal Remedies to a more comprehensive database within the Evolve Online Learning Resources.*
5. *Practice-oriented precautions, dental considerations, and recommended medical consultations for every drug entry, and essential drug facts that are placed directly in the context of the dentist's and dental hygienist's care.*
6. *Highlights of serious adverse reactions and contraindications.* In each drug entry, the book calls attention to dangerous or life-threatening reactions so that you can identify them easily and deal with them promptly.
7. *Specialized dental care guidelines, including the most recent recommendations for the prevention of infective endocarditis.* Suggested protocols for the treatment of medically compromised patients and the therapeutic management of common oral lesions are also included.
8. *Combination drug guide.* Detailed index of combination drugs arranged by trade name.
9. *Comprehensive appendices.* Eleven ready-reference appendices give you easy access to additional vital drug-related information and detailed sections concerning anesthetics, controlled substances, disorders and conditions, pregnancy and pediatrics, and sample prescriptions for drugs more commonly prescribed in dental practice.

A detailed guide to *Mosby's Dental Drug Reference,* Tenth Edition:

Mosby's Dental Drug Reference provides essential drug information in a user-friendly format. The bulk of this handbook contains an alphabetical listing of drug entries by generic name. Drug entries include the following:

Generic and Brand Names. Drug entries begin with the generic drug name, followed by its pronunciation and its U.S., Canadian, and Australian brand names.

Category and Schedule. This section lists the drug's pregnancy risk category and, when appropriate, its controlled substance schedule or over-the-counter (OTC) status.

Mechanism of Action. This section clearly and concisely describes the drug's mechanism of action and therapeutic effects.

Pharmacokinetics. Under this heading, a quick-reference chart outlines the drug's route, onset, peak, and duration, when known. This information is followed by a brief description of the drug's absorption, distribution, metabolism, excretion, and half-life.

Indications and Dosages. Here, you'll find the approved indications and routes, along with age-appropriate dosage information and, for selected agents, dosage adjustments for preexisting conditions, such as liver or kidney disease.

Precautions/Contraindications. Using a practice-oriented format and written specifically for dentistry, this section presents precautions and considerations for each drug entry. Each entry lists conditions in which use of the generic drug is contraindicated.

Interactions. For drugs, herbal supplements, and food, this section supplies vital information about adverse interactions of the medical drug with drugs prescribed in dentistry.

Adverse Effects. Unlike other handbooks that mix more common adverse effects with rare, minor ones in a long, undifferentiated list, this book ranks side effects by frequency of occurrence, indicating expected, frequent, occasional, and rare.

Serious Reactions. Because serious adverse reactions can be life-threatening emergencies that require prompt intervention, this section highlights them separately from other side effects for easy identification.

Mosby's Dental Drug Reference, **Tenth Edition,** is an easy-to-use source of current drug information for a wide spectrum of dental care providers. When it comes to providing quality patient care, all members of the dental team can rely on the tenth edition of *Mosby's Dental Drug Reference* for current, dentally relevant information, presented in an easy-to-use format. As you use the book, please keep in mind the following:

• The majority of the monographs are descriptions of drugs utilized on an outpatient basis and, therefore, more likely to be encountered in dental practice. Vaccines, biologicals, and medications used only intraoperatively in hospitalized patients are generally not included, and the reader is referred to other resources for this information.

• The Evolve website (http://evolve.elsevier.com/dental/drug/) can be consulted for updates and new information pertinent to this text.

• Several important "Dental Considerations" are relevant to all of the drugs described in the monographs, including:

1. The use of a prescription medication indicates the presence of a medical condition that is being managed by one or more physicians. The physical status of the patient and his or her ability to tolerate dental treatment must be determined.

2. In collaboration with the treating physician(s), the physician, not the dentist, should guide all decisions related to changes in the use of prescription drugs for medical conditions.

3. Vital signs and/or other assessments should be determined at every dental treatment visit, as appropriate and as indicated; many drugs used for systemic conditions result in adverse oral conditions, such as xerostomia. Strict attention must be paid to the prevention of negative outcomes of

these conditions, particularly caries and periodontal disease; education of the patient and the patient's family about his or her medications should be reinforced by the dental team, particularly as it relates to the prevention of oral complications of medication use.

4. This text does not constitute advice about the dental management of specific patients, each of whom must be evaluated individually using all pertinent diagnostic information, and the monographs contained in this book do not constitute full prescribing information for the drugs.

In the production of the book, we have endeavored to make it as current and relevant as possible, while emphasizing the busy oral health care provider's need for rapid access and dentally relevant information. On behalf of the Editor-in-Chief and Mosby, a sincere debt of gratitude is owed to our reviewers, Catherine M. Flaitz, DDS, MS, University of Texas School of Dentistry at Houston; Marshal Shlafer, PhD, University of Michigan School of Medicine; and Ruth Fearing Tornwall, RDH, MS, Lamar Institute of Technology, and to our monograph content contributor, Catherine Ulbricht, PharmD, MBA, Natural Standard Research Collaboration, for their expertise and contributions. Finally, this work is respectfully dedicated to Drs. Raymond P. Ahlquist, Gerald O. Carrier, Alfred E. Ciarlone, Louis P. Gangarosa, Sr., James L. Matheny, and Armand M. Karow, and their faculty colleagues at the Medical College of Georgia, whose passion for pharmacology and its significance to all health care professions will continue to inspire generations of teachers of the discipline.

Contents

Therapeutic Management of Common Oral Lesions, 1

Medically Compromised Patients, 29

Individual Drug Monographs, 55

Appendices
A. Abbreviations, 1397
B. Anesthetics, 1405
C. Combination Drugs by Trade Name, 1414
D. Controlled Substances Classes, 1421
E. Disorders and Conditions, 1422
F. Drugs Associated with Dry Mouth, 1426
G. Drugs That Affect Taste, 1430
H. Complementary and Alternative Medications and Dietary
   Supplements — **for Appendix H and more information on
   Complementary and Alternative Medications, see the
   Companion CD-ROM and the Evolve site.**
 I. Pregnancy and Pediatrics, 1434
J. Preventing Medication Errors and Improving
   Medication Safety, 1439
K. Oral Contraceptives, 1442

Generic and Trade Name Index, 1445

MOSBY'S
DENTAL
DRUG
REFERENCE

TENTH EDITION

This is a summary of the etiologic factors, clinical description, currently accepted therapeutic management, and patient education for the more common oral conditions. Some of the recommended treatments have been investigated more thoroughly than others, but all have been reported to be of clinical value. Many oral conditions described here have no cure, but are managed by a variety of treatment modalities for the purpose of relieving discomfort, shortening their clinical duration and frequency, and minimizing recurrences. The ultimate goal is to provide the individual with some control over the severity of their condition, thereby improving their quality of life.

Clinicians are reminded that an accurate diagnosis is imperative for clinical success. Every effort should be made to determine the diagnosis before initiating treatment. It is critical to confirm that an individual does not have a serious infection, an underlying systemic disease, or a potentially malignant or malignant lesion. When signs, symptoms, microscopic diagnosis, and other laboratory evidence elude a definitive diagnosis, empirical treatment may be initiated and evaluated on a therapeutic, trial basis. Although empiric treatment may be of short-term benefit to the patient, certain drugs may mask or alleviate some of the disease features. Therefore, it is also important to make appropriate and timely referrals in order to obtain a definitive diagnosis when dealing with a persistent oral condition so that the management approach is not masking an underlying condition or to evaluate the individual for drug protocols that are beyond the expertise of the clinician.

In addition to the diagnosis, patient management should be governed by the natural history of the oral condition and whether a palliative, supportive, or curative treatment exists. Referrals of patients should be made when the patients' problems are beyond the scope of the clinician, including the use of more aggressive drug protocols for improved outcome. Furthermore, when healing of a lesion or an anticipated response to treatment is not achieved within an expected period of time, a biopsy or other laboratory studies are recommended.

All drugs require a prescription unless identified as over-the-counter (OTC) drugs. Please note that in recent years, the Food and Drug Administration (FDA) has been active in allowing OTC status for drugs formerly available by prescription only. Be sure to check the dosages of the newly released OTC drugs because they usually are of a different strength than those available by prescription. In addition, these OTC drugs or supplements may contain ingredients, preservatives, and dyes that may cause irritating-to-life-threatening adverse effects, due to relatively minor formulary changes. As with any recommended therapeutic agent, patients should be advised of potential side effects and drug interactions.

SUPPORTIVE CARE

Management of oral mucosal conditions may require topical and systemic interventions. Therapy should address patient nutrition and hydration, oral discomfort, oral hygiene, management of secondary infection, and local control of the disease process. Depending on the extent, severity, and location of oral lesions, consideration should be given to obtaining a consultation from a dentist who specializes in oral medicine, oral and maxillofacial pathology, or oral and maxillofacial surgery. When a question arises involving a medical condition, a physician should be consulted.

Temporary, symptomatic relief of painful conditions can be provided with topical preparations, such as 2% viscous lidocaine hydrochloride or OTC products containing less potent aesthetics in gel, ointment, liquid, spray, and lozenge forms. Topical anesthetics can be used as a rinse in adults to cover a wide surface area, but should be applied with a cotton-tipped applicator or other soft applicator in a young child or adult who is unable to expectorate, in order to limit the amount of medication that is swallowed. Swallowing these topical anesthetics is not recommended because it may interfere with the patient's gag reflex and increase the risk for choking, aspiration, and drug toxicity. Symptomatic relief also can be obtained by mixing equal parts of diphenhydramine hydrochloride elixir and magnesium hydroxide/aluminum hydroxide. Children's formula diphenhydramine hydrochloride elixir does not contain alcohol. Sucralfate suspension also can be used before meals. The diphenhydramine mixture and the sucralfate coat the ulcerated lesions and may allow the patient to eat more comfortably. For specific details, refer to "Herpes Simplex, Topical Anesthetics and Coating Agents."

Meticulous oral hygiene is important in patients who have multiple areas of erosion or ulceration. Mucosal lesions contacting bacterial biofilm on the dentition are more likely to become secondarily infected. Patients should be seen by the dentist or dental hygienist for scaling and root planing, under local anesthesia, when necessary, in all cases in which oral hygiene is suboptimal. Patients must be encouraged to brush and floss their teeth after meals in a gentle yet efficient manner. This may be enhanced by placing a soft toothbrush under hot water to further soften the bristles. The use of fluoride toothpaste is strongly encouraged and some patients with widespread mucosal lesions prefer toothpastes that are not highly flavored and do not contain foaming, whitening, and anti-tartar agents.

HERPES SIMPLEX INFECTION

Common viral infection causes two types of disease patterns: a primary or acute infection and a secondary or recurrent infection.

Primary Herpetic
Gingivostomatitis

Etiology:
A transmissible infection with herpes simplex virus, usually type I or, less commonly, type II.

Clinical description:
Clear-yellowish vesicles develop intraorally and extraorally. These vesicles rupture rapidly and coalesce to form shallow, irregular, painful ulcers. The symptomatic lesions are

widespread but the gingivae are affected primarily and are erythematous, enlarged, hemorrhagic, and ulcerated. The patient may have systemic signs and symptoms including anterior cervical lymphadenopathy, fever, anorexia, and malaise. Adults may develop pharyngotonsillitis that is characterized by vesiculo-ulcerative lesions, severe sore throat, and difficulty swallowing. Usually it is self-limiting, with healing in 7–14 days.

Rationale for treatment:
Early treatment to promote healing, relieve symptoms, prevent secondary infection, and support general health are goals. Supportive therapy includes plenty of fluids, protein, vitamin and mineral food supplements, and rest. Systemic acyclovir is effective when administered in the first 48 hr of symptoms. Topical steroids should be avoided because they tend to permit spread of the viral infection on mucous membranes, particularly ocular membranes. Nutritional liquid supplements, pain, and fever control may be needed. Patients should be cautioned to avoid touching the herpetic lesions and then touching the eyes, genitals, or other body areas because of the possibility of self-inoculation.

Topical Anesthetics and Coating Agents

Rx
Diphenhydramine hydrochloride oral solution 12.5 mg/5 ml mixed with aluminum hydroxide, magnesium hydroxide oral suspension.
Compound to a 1:1 mixture by volume.
Disp. 200 ml
Sig. Rinse with 1–2 teaspoons (5–10 ml) every 2 to 4 hr for 1 min; swish and spit out.

Although these medications are OTC, it is recommended that a pharmacist compound this oral suspension. Examples of aluminum hydroxide, magnesium hydroxide oral suspension are Maalox and Mylanta—they are common OTC brands and are available in a number of flavors. Children younger than 6 yr should not swallow this oral suspension.

Rx
Diphenhydramine hydrochloride liquid 12.5 mg/5 ml lidocaine viscous 2% oral solution/aluminum hydroxide, magnesium hydroxide oral suspension. Compound to a 1:1:1 mixture by volume.
Disp. 200 ml
Sig. Rinse with 1–2 teaspoons (5–10 ml) every 4 hr for 1 min and spit out excess. Shake well before use and store suspension at room temperature.

Compounded by pharmacy and stable for approximately 60 days. Do not use 2% lidocaine hydrochloride in children who cannot expectorate because of potential for aspiration.

Rx
Carafate, generic (sucralfate) suspension 1 g/10 ml
Disp. 200 ml
Sig. Rinse with 1 teaspoon (5 ml) 4 times a day. Rinse for 1 min and spit out excess.

In children younger than 6 yr, who cannot expectorate, the amount should be limited to 0.5 g, four times a day (2 g/day) in case the suspension is swallowed. Safety and efficacy has not been established in children.

Rx
Children's Benadryl Allergy Liquid, others (diphenhydramine hydrochloride) oral solution 12.5 mg/5 ml (OTC)
Disp. 8 oz bottle

Sig. Rinse with 1 teaspoon (5 ml) for 2 min every 2–4 hr and spit out excess.

If swallowed, for adolescents and adults, the maximum amount is 300 mg in 24 hr. For children 6–12 yr, the maximum is 150 mg in 24 hr. Children younger than 6 yr should not swallow this drug.

Rx
Sucrets (dyclonine HCl) throat lozenges (OTC)
Disp. 1 package
Sig. Slowly dissolve one lozenge in mouth every 2 hr as needed for pain. Do not take more than 10 lozenges a day.

The strength of dyclonine HCl ranges from 3 mg (maximum strength) to 1.2 mg for children's formula.

Systemic Antiviral Therapy
Acyclovir and valacyclovir may relieve and decrease the duration of symptoms, but the medications must be initiated at the earliest signs and symptoms for maximum effectiveness.

Rx
Zovirax, generic (acyclovir) capsules 400 mg
Disp. 30 (or 50) capsules
Sig. Take 1 capsule 3 to 5 times a day for 10 days or until lesions resolve.

The Centers for Disease Control and Prevention (CDC) recommends this dosage for severe cases of stomatitis or pharyngitis. Current FDA-approved indication is that systemic acyclovir be used to treat oral herpes only in immunocompromised patients.

Rx
Valtrex, generic (valacyclovir) tablet 1 g
Disp. 20 tablets
Sig. Take 1 tablet twice daily for 10 days.

The protocol is based on the CDC's recommended dosage for primary genital herpes in the immunocompetent patient. The drug should be taken within the first 48 hr of the initial signs and symptoms.

Recurrent (Orofacial) Herpes Simplex Infection
Etiology:
There is reactivation of the latent virus that resides within the sensory ganglion of the trigeminal nerve. Precipitating factors include fever, stress, exposure to sunlight, trauma, and hormonal alterations.

Clinical description:
Intraoral presentation consists of single or small clusters of vesicles that quickly rupture, forming painful ulcers. The lesions usually occur on the keratinized tissue of the hard palate and attached gingiva.

Labial presentation consists of clusters of vesicles on the vermilion border of the lips that rupture within hours and then crust.

Rationale for treatment:
Treatment should be initiated as early as possible in the prodromal stage, with the goal of reducing the duration and symptoms of the lesion. Oral and topical antiviral treatment, prophylactically and therapeutically, can be considered when frequent recurrent herpetic episodes (greater than 6 episodes a year) interfere with daily function and nutrition.

Prevention
Rx
Suncreen lip balm, SPF 30 (OTC)
Disp. 1 tube
Sig. Apply to susceptible area 1 hr before sun exposure and every hour thereafter.

There are several lip balms or gels that are available that contain an SPF of 30 or higher. Several of these agents contain sensitizers that may result in irritation of the lips and surrounding skin. For maximum protection, concurrent use of a sunscreen on the face and other sun-exposed areas is recommended. A wide-brimmed hat or visor is also recommended when excessive sunlight exposure is a triggering factor. Sharing of these lipsticks should be strongly discouraged because of the potential risk of infection in a susceptible individual.

Topical Antiviral Agents

Topical antiviral medications are most effective when initiated in the early stages of lesion formation. Patients should be instructed to gently apply the medication to the affected site or where the prodromal symptoms are noted. Aggressively rubbing the affected site is not recommended because it can cause tissue trauma and the spread of the infection. In order to prevent autoinoculation of the virus to the fingers or other sites, the topical agent should be placed on the lesion using a cotton-tipped applicator, and hands should be thoroughly washed.

Rx
Denavir (penciclovir) cream 1%
Disp. 2-g tube
Sig. Dab on lesion every 2 hr while awake, for 4 days, beginning when symptoms first occur.

Rx
Zovirax (acyclovir) cream 5%
Disp. 2- or 5-g tube
Sig. Dab on lesion 5 times a day during waking hours for 4 days, beginning when symptoms first occur.

Rx
Xerese (acyclovir 5%; hydrocortisone 1%) cream
Disp. 5-g tube

Sig. Dab on lesion 5 times a day during waking hours for 5 days, beginning when symptoms first occur.

This topical agent reduces the likelihood of ulcerative lesions developing.

Rx
Abreva (docosanol) cream 10% (OTC)
Disp. 2-g tube
Sig. Dab on lesion 5 times a day during waking hours for 4 days, beginning when symptoms first occur.

Systemic Antiviral Therapy

Systemic antiviral medications are most effective when initiated in the prodrome or early stages of lesion development. The duration of treatment is convenient because the medication is only taken for 1 day. Studies have evaluated the effectiveness of systemic antiviral medications for herpes labialis, but not intraoral lesions.

Rx
Valtrex, generic (valacyclovir) tablets 1 g
Disp. 4 tablets
Sig. Take 2 tablets twice daily, 12 hr apart, when symptoms first occur.

The CDC recommends 1 g PO every 12 hr for 5–10 days for immunocompromised individuals.

Rx
Famvir, generic (famciclovir) tablets 500 mg
Disp. 3 tablets
Sig. Take 3 tablets as a single dose at the first sign or symptom of the infection.

The CDC recommends 500 mg PO twice daily for 5–10 days for immunocompromised individuals.

Rx
Zovirax, generic (acyclovir) capsules 400 mg
Disp. 15 capsules

Sig. Take 1 capsule 3 times a day for 5 days.

The CDC recommends this dosing schedule for immunocompetent individuals. If the patient is HIV-positive, then the duration of use is increased.

HERPES ZOSTER (SHINGLES)
Etiology:

Herpes zoster represents the reactivation of latent varicella-zoster virus following a previous infection with chickenpox. Precipitating factors include immunosuppressive and cytotoxic drugs, therapeutic radiation, old age, alcohol abuse, malignancies, and trauma, including dental treatment.

Clinical description:

The classic signs and symptoms include painful segmental eruption of small vesicles that later rupture to form punctate or confluent ulcers or crusts. Fever, headache, lymphadenopathy, and referred pain may precede or accompany the lesions. When the head and neck area is involved, one or more of the branches of the trigeminal nerve are affected.

Rationale for treatment:

Prompt initiation of antiviral therapy is recommended to reduce duration and symptoms of the lesions. Patients older than 60 yr are especially prone to developing postherpetic neuralgia. Systemic antiviral medications are most effective if initiated within 48 hr of lesion formation. The treatment of acute herpes zoster with famciclovir significantly decreases the incidence and duration of postherpetic neuralgia. Recently, the herpes zoster virus vaccine, Zostavax, a live, attenuated vaccine, has been developed for the prevention of this infection in adults who are 60 yr or older. Length of treatment with these antiviral agents increases when herpes zoster develops in HIV-infected individuals.

Rx
Famvir, generic (famciclovir) tablets 500 mg
Disp. 21 tablets
Sig. Take 1 tablet every 8 hr for 7 days.

Rx
Zovirax, generic (acyclovir) tablets 800 mg
Disp. 50 capsules
Sig. Take 1 tablet every 4 hr, 5 times a day for 7–10 days.

Rx
Valtrex, generic (valacyclovir) tablets 1 g
Disp. 21 tablets
Sig. Take 1 tablet 3 times a day for 7 days.

RECURRENT APHTHOUS STOMATITIS
Etiology:

An altered local immune response is the predisposing factor. Patients with frequent recurrences should be screened for diseases such as anemia, allergies, vitamin deficiency, inflammatory bowel disease, and immunosuppression. Precipitating factors include stress, trauma, salivary gland hypofunction, certain medications, allergies, endocrine alterations, smoking cessation, dietary components, including cheese, chocolate, cow's milk, gluten, nuts, strawberries, and acidic foods and juices. Inspect the oral cavity closely for sources of trauma.

Clinical description:

Minor aphthous ulcerations (canker sores) are the most common clinical variation. These lesions are smaller than 1 cm, shallow, round to oval, and painful. They are covered by a cream-colored membrane and surrounded by an erythematous halo. They usually occur on nonkeratinized (moveable) oral mucosa and usually heal in 7 to 14 days without scarring.

Major aphthous ulcerations are larger lesions that range from 1 to 3 cm in size and very painful. These ulcerations are not only larger in size but may be deep with irregular borders. They are often multiple and persistent, taking 2 to 6 wk and longer to heal. Mucosal scarring may be extensive. These ulcerations may mimic other persistent diseases, such as deep mycotic infection, granulomatous diseases, or malignant lesions.

Herpetiform aphthous ulcerations appear as crops of small, shallow, painful lesions. They usually occur on nonkeratinized oral mucosa, but any mucosal surface may be involved. These ulcerations typically heal within 7 to 10 days, but closely spaced recurrences are common. Because multiple small ulcers develop suddenly, these lesions resemble recurrent intraoral herpes simplex, clinically.

Rationale for treatment:
Treatment options involve mucosal barriers, topical anesthetics, cauterization, laser therapy, topical or systemic corticosteroids, and immunosuppressant or combination therapy, when indicated. Treatment should be initiated as early as possible in the course of lesions. Identification and elimination of precipitating factors may minimize recurrent episodes. Medications such as mycophenolate mofetil, pentoxifylline, colchicine, and thalidomide are used to treat patients with severe, persistent, recurrent aphthous ulcers, but should not be routinely used. Placing a dissolvable or bioerodible mucosal patch over a topical steroid may prolong tissue contact of the medication and make the patient more comfortable. Multiple topical over-the-counter anesthetics or protective bioadhesive agents are available for patient comfort.

Topical Steroids
Prolonged use of topical steroids (longer than 2 wk of continuous use) may result in mucosal atrophy and secondary candidiasis and may increase the potential for systemic absorption. It may be necessary to prescribe antifungal therapy with steroids use in some patients.

For Mild-to-Moderate Cases:

Rx
Triamcinolone acetonide in dental paste 0.1%
Disp. 5-g tube
Sig. Coat the lesion with a thin film after each meal and at bedtime.

Rx
Dexamethasone oral solution or elixir 0.5 mg/5 ml
Disp. 240 ml
Sig. Rinse with 1 teaspoon (5 ml) for 2 min four times a day and expectorate. Do not eat or drink for 30 min after rinsing.

Rx
Fluocinonide 0.05% gel
Disp. 15-g tube
Sig. Apply a thin layer to the ulcer after meals and at bedtime.

Discontinue use of topical steroids when lesions become asymptomatic.

Other topical steroid preparations (cream, gel, rinse, ointment) are available. In general, creams are not used intraorally because of very poor mucosal adherence. Many topical steroids come with a warning that they are for external use only. However, several of these agents have been used successfully for managing

recurrent aphthous ulcerations.
Examples of some of the topical
steroid medications are listed below
according to potency.
Super-High Potency:
   Betamethasone dipropionate
      (augmented) 0.05%, gel,
      ointment
   Clobetasol propionate 0.05%, gel,
      ointment
   Halobetasol propionate 0.05%,
      ointment
High Potency:
   Betamethasone dipropionate
      0.05%, gel, ointment
   Fluocinonide 0.05%, gel,
      ointment
   Dexamethasone 0.5 mg/5 ml oral
      solution, elixir
   Desoximetasone 0.05%, gel;
      0.25% ointment
Medium Potency:
   Betamethasone valerate 0.1%,
      ointment
   Triamcinolone acetonide 0.1%,
      ointment
Low Potency:
   Alclometasone dipropionate
      0.05%, ointment
   Hydrocortisone acetate 1%, gel,
      ointment
Oral candidiasis may develop from
topical steroid use and, therefore,
periodic monitoring for a candidal
infection is recommended.
Prophylactic antifungal therapy
should be initiated in patients with a
history of fungal infections during
previous steroid administration (see
"Candidiasis")

**Systemic Steroids and
Immunosuppressants for Severe
Cases**
Rx
Dexamethasone (Decadron) elixir
0.5 mg/5 ml
Disp. 320 ml
Sig. As directed in writing, not to
exceed 2 continuous wk.

**Directions for using
dexamethasone oral solution:**
Rinse for 1 min, four times daily,
after meals and before bedtime. Do
not drink or eat for 30 min after
rinsing.
1. For 3 days, rinse with 1
   tablespoon (15 ml) times a day
   and swallow. Then,
2. For 3 days, rinse with 1
   teaspoonful (5 ml) 4 times a day
   and swallow. Then
3. For 3 days, rinse with 1
   teaspoonful (5 ml) 4 times a day
   and swallow every other time.
   Then
4. Rinse with 1 teaspoonful (5 ml)
   4 times a day and expectorate.
   Discontinue medication when
   mouth becomes comfortable.
Rx
Prednisone tablets 5 mg
Disp. 40 tablets
Sig. Take 5 tablets in the morning
for 5 days, then 5 tablets in the
morning every other day until
asymptomatic.
For Very Severe Cases
Rx
Prednisone tablets 10 mg
Disp. 26 tablets
Sig. Take 4 tablets in the morning
for 5 days, then decrease by 1 tablet
on each successive day.
   Therapy with medications,
such as systemic steroids,
immunosuppressants, and
immunomodulators are presented
to inform the clinician that such
modalities have been reported
effective for patients suffering from
severe, persistent, recurrent aphthous
stomatitis. Medications such as
azathioprine, pentoxifylline,
levamisole, colchicine, dapsone, and
thalidomide are used to treat patients
with severe, persistent recurrent
aphthous stomatitis, but should not
be routinely used because of the

potential for serious adverse effects. Close collaboration with the patient's physician is recommended when these medications are prescribed.

CANDIDIASIS

Etiology:

Candida albicans and other species are opportunistic fungal organisms that tend to proliferate with the use of broad-spectrum antibiotics, corticosteroids, medications that reduce salivary output, and cytotoxic agents. Conditions that contribute to candidiasis include xerostomia, poorly controlled diabetes mellitus, anemia, poor oral hygiene, prolonged use of prosthetic appliances, and suppression of the immune system (i.e., AIDS or the side effects of some medications). It is important to determine the predisposing factors prior to initiating therapy.

Clinical description:

The disease is characterized by soft, white, slightly elevated plaques that usually can be wiped away, leaving an erythematous area (pseudomembranous form). Candidiasis also may appear as generalized erythematous, sensitive areas (atrophic or erythematous form) or as confluent white areas that are adherent (hyperplastic form). Angular cheilitis, which is also described in this chapter, is frequently associated with this oral disease (see "Angular Cheilitis").

Rationale for treatment:

The goal of treatment is to reestablish a normal balance of oral flora and improve oral hygiene. The disinfection of all removable prostheses with antifungal denture-soaking solutions and the application of antifungal agents on the tissue-contacting surfaces are necessary to eliminate a potential source of fungal infection.

Medication for the management of oral candidal infection should be continued for 48 hr after the disappearance of clinical signs to prevent immediate recurrence. It is also important that salivary flow be evaluated and managed to prevent recurrences (see "Xerostomia").

Topical Antifungal Agents

Rx

Nystatin oral suspension 100,000 units/ml

Disp. 280 ml

Sig. Rinse with 1 teaspoon (5 ml) 4 times a day. Rinse for 2 min and expectorate or swallow.

    Nystatin suspension has a high sugar content; therefore, good oral hygiene should be reinforced. A few drops of nystatin oral suspension can be added to the water used for soaking acrylic prostheses.

Rx

Oravig (miconazole) buccal tablets 50 mg

Disp. 14 tablets

Sig. Place one tablet above the upper front teeth once daily for 14 days. Alternate sides that you place the tablet.

Rx

Clotrimazole lozenge 10 mg

Disp. 70 lozenges

Sig. Let 1 troche dissolve in mouth 4–5 times a day for 14 days.

Rx

Nystatin vaginal tablet 100,000 units

Disp. 56 tablets

Sig. Let tablet dissolve in mouth 4 times a day for 14 days. Do not rinse for 30 min after use.

    If concern exists about sugar content of the clotrimazole lozenges, vaginal tablets can be substituted.

    In general, lozenges may not be well tolerated when a patient has a dry mouth because of the inability to dissolve this dosage form. Consider a course of systemic antifungal therapy in these cases.

Rx
Nystatin ointment 100,000 units/g
Disp. 15-g tube
Sig. Apply a thin coat to inner surface of prosthesis and to the affected area after each meal.

Rx
Nystatin topical powder 100,000 units/g
Disp. 15 g
Sig. Apply a thin layer under the prosthesis after each meal.

Rx
Ketoconazole topical cream 2%
Disp. 15-g tube
Sig. Apply a thin coat to inner surface of prosthesis and to the affected area after each meal.

Rx
Clotrimazole topical cream 1%
Disp. 15-g tube
Sig. Apply a thin coat to inner surface of prosthesis and to the affected area after each meal.
This product may be obtained over-the-counter.

Rx
Miconazole nitrate cream 2%
Disp. 15-g tube
Sig. Apply a thin coat to inner surface of prosthesis and to the affected area after each meal.
This product may be obtained over-the-counter.

Systemic Antifungal Agents
When topical therapy is not practical or is ineffective, ketoconazole and fluconazole are effective, well-tolerated, systemic drugs for mucocutaneous candidiasis. They should be used with caution in patients with impaired liver function (i.e., with history of alcoholism or hepatitis) and in patients taking drugs metabolized by the cytochrome P450 isoenzyme. Liver

function tests should be performed periodically and/or monitored by the patient's physician when ketoconazole is prescribed for an extended period of time. Several important drug interactions have been reported with ketoconazole.

Rx
Ketoconazole tablets 200 mg
Disp. 14 tablets
Sig. Take 1 tablet a day with a meal or orange juice. Do not take with buffered medications or with gastric acid blockers.

Rx
Fluconazole tablets 100 mg
Disp. 15 tablets
Sig. Take 2 tablets stat, then 1 tablet a day until complete.

Systemic Antifungal Agents for Refractory Oropharyngeal Candidiasis

Rx
Itraconazole oral solution 10 mg/1 ml
Disp. 150 ml
Sig. Rinse and swallow 2 teaspoons (10 ml) 2 times a day for 14 days.
This antifungal medication is for those patients who are unresponsive or refractory to fluconazole tablets. Serious adverse heart and drug reactions have been associated with itraconazole.

ANGULAR CHEILITIS
Etiology:
Fissured lesions in the corners of the mouth are caused by a mixed infection of the microorganisms *C. albicans, Staphylococcus,* and *Streptococcus.* Predisposing factors include excessive licking, drooling, a decrease in intermaxillary space, anemia, vitamin deficiency, immunosuppression, and an extension of oral infections.

Clinical description:
The commissures may appear wrinkled, red, fissured, cracked, or crusted. Scarring may develop in persistent cases. Recurrences are common if the underlying problem is not managed.

Rationale for treatment:
Identification and correction of predisposing factors, elimination of the primary and secondary infections, and decrease of inflammation are the management approaches. Recurrences are common.

Rx
Nystatin/triamcinolone acetonide ointment 100,000 units/g 0.1%
Disp. 15-g tube
Sig. Apply to lips after each meal and at bedtime. Use for no longer that 2 wk.

This is the preferred topical agent when secondary candidal infection is suspected. Concomitant intraoral antifungal treatment may be indicated.

Rx
Ketoconazole cream 2%
Disp. 15-g tube
Sig. Apply a small dab to corners of mouth after meals and before bedtime. Use for 2 wk and re-evaluate.

This topical agent is used when secondary candidal infection is suspected. Concomitant intraoral antifungal treatment may be indicated.

Rx
Hydrocortisone-iodoquinol 1%-1% cream
Disp. 15-g tube
Sig. Apply small dab to the corners of mouth after meals and bed bedtime. Use for 2 wk and re-evaluate.

This topical agent is used when secondary bacterial and candidal infections are suspected.

Rx
Clotrimazole cream 1%
Disp. 1 tube
Sig. Apply small dab to corner of mouth after meals and before bedtime. Use for 2 wk and re-evaluate.

This product may be obtained over-the-counter.

Rx
Miconazole nitrate antifungal cream 2%
Disp. 1 tube
Sig. Apply small dab to corner of mouth after meals and before bedtime. Use for 2 wk and re-evaluate.

This product may be obtained over-the-counter.

Rx
Bacitracin zinc 500 U; Polymyxin B 10,000 U ointment 2% (OTC)
Disp. 1 tube
Sig. Apply small dab to corner of mouth after meals and before bedtime. Use for 1 wk and re-evaluate.

This OTC topical antibacterial agent may be associated with allergic reactions because of its frequent use for skin irritation.

ACTINIC (SOLAR) CHEILITIS
Etiology:
This precancerous lesion is caused by prolonged exposure to sunlight that results in irreversible degenerative changes in the vermilion of the lips, especially the lower lip.

Clinical description:
The normal appearance of the vermilion border with regular vertical fissuring of a smooth surface is replaced by a white plaque or an irregular scaly surface

that may exhibit periodic erythema and ulceration. There is often an indistinct margin between the perioral skin and lip vermilion.

Rationale for treatment:
Prevention of the solar-induced changes is recommended. For maximum protection, concurrent use of sunscreen should be used on the face and other sun-exposed areas. If exposure to the ultraviolet light in the sun's rays is allowed to continue, the degenerative changes may progress to a malignancy. Sunscreens with a sun protection factor (SPF) of 30 or higher and protection from both UVA and UVB should be recommended.

Rx
Several OTC sunscreen preparations for the lips are available. For those patients who are allergic to paraaminobenzoic acid (PABA), PABA-free sunscreens should be recommended. For patients with a history of lip cancer, a zinc oxide product should be used. Regular and repeated use of these products is critical for sun protection.

GEOGRAPHIC TONGUE (BENIGN MIGRATORY GLOSSITIS; ERYTHEMA MIGRANS)

Etiology:
Although a common condition, the etiology of geographic tongue is unknown. Although not supported by large epidemiologic studies, this tongue condition has been associated with atopic conditions and pustular psoriasis.

Clinical description:
Geographic tongue is a benign inflammatory condition caused by desquamation of superficial keratin and filiform papillae. It is characterized by both red, denuded, oval to irregularly shaped patches

that are surrounded by a slightly raised white border. The primary site of involvement is the dorsal and ventrolateral tongue but other oral mucosal sites may be affected. The pattern of these lesions frequently changes and ranges from solitary to multiple affected areas.

Rationale for treatment:
Generally, no treatment is necessary because most patients are asymptomatic. When symptoms are present, they may be associated with acidic or spicy foods and beverages. In addition, tender lesions may be associated with secondary candidal infection. Although there is no well-documented treatment for this condition, symptoms can be improved temporally with topical anesthetics or coating agents. For persistent and tender lesions, topical steroids, especially in combination with topical antifungal agents, are the treatment of choice. Patients should be informed that this condition does not suggest a more serious disease and is not contagious. In most cases, a biopsy is not indicated because of the pathognomonic clinical appearance. However, solitary lesions of the lateral tongue that do not resolve should be biopsied to exclude epithelial dysplasia or squamous cell carcinoma.

Rx
Nystatin/triamcinolone acetonide ointment 100,000 units/g 0.1%
Disp. 15-g tube
Sig. Apply to affected area after each meal and at bedtime.

Rx
Lotrisone (clotrimazole/ betamethasone dipropionate) cream 1%–0.05%
Disp. 15-g tube
Sig. Apply to affected area after each meal and at bedtime.

Rx

Fluocinonide gel 0.05%
Disp. 15-g tube
Sig. Apply to affected areas after
meals and at bedtime.

If there is a secondary candidal
infection, the symptoms may worsen
with a topical steroid.

Rx

Betamethasone valerate ointment
0.1%
Disp. 15-g tube
Sig. Apply to affected areas after
meals and at bedtime.

If there is a secondary candidal
infection, the symptoms may worsen
with a topical steroid.

XEROSTOMIA (REDUCED SALIVARY FLOW AND DRY MOUTH)

Etiology:

Acute or chronic salivary flow
alterations or xerostomia may result
from drug therapy, mechanical
blockage, dehydration, emotional
stress, bacterial infection of the
salivary glands, local surgery,
avitaminosis, diabetes, anemia,
connective tissue diseases, Sjögren's
syndrome, radiation therapy, viral
infections, and congenital disorders.

Clinical description:

The saliva may be ropey with a film
forming over the teeth. The tissues
may be dry, pale or red, and
atrophic. The tongue may be devoid
of papillae, atrophic, fissured, and
inflamed. Multiple carious lesions
may be present, especially at the
gingival margin and on exposed root
surfaces. The quantity and quality of
saliva may be altered.

Rationale for treatment:

Salivary stimulation or replacement
therapy is important to keep the
mouth moistened and comfortable
and for the prevention of caries,
candidal infection, and

traumatically-induced mucosal
lesions. For patients with removable
prosthetic appliances, the application
of an artificial saliva or oral lubricant
gel to the tissue contact surface of the
prosthesis reduces frictional trauma.

Saliva Substitutes

Rx

Sodium carboxymethylcellulose
0.5% aqueous solution (OTC)
Disp. 8 fl oz
Sig. Use as a rinse as frequently as
needed. Solution may be prepared
by the pharmacist.

Sipping on plain water or
crushed ice is often used with some
success in patients with dry mouth.

There are several OTC saliva
substitutes and oral moisturizing
gels that are commercially available
and patients may need to evaluate
which product best meets their
specific needs and preferences.
Relief from oral dryness and
accompanying discomfort can be
achieved conservatively by the
following:

• Sipping water frequently all day
long
• Letting ice melt in the mouth
• Restricting caffeine intake
• Avoiding mouth rinses, drinks, and
medications containing alcohol
• Avoiding tobacco products
• Humidifying the sleeping area
• Coating the lips (see "Chapped/
Cracked Lips")

Saliva Stimulants

The use of sugar-free gum, candy, or
mints is a conservative method to
temporarily stimulate salivary flow
in patients with medication-induced
xerostomia or with salivary gland
dysfunction. Patients should be
cautioned against using products
that contain sugar or have a low pH.

Rx

Salagen, generic (pilocarpine HCl)
tablets 5 mg

Disp. 90 tablets
Sig. Take 1 tablet 3 times a day,
30 min prior to meals.

Dosage may be titrated to 2
tablets (10 mg) 3 times a day. An
alternative is 1 tablet (5 mg) 4 times
a day.

Rx
Evoxac (cevimeline HCl) capsules
30 mg
Disp. 90 capsules
Sig. Take 1 capsule 3 times a day.

Some patients benefit from
taking 1 capsule 4 times a day.

Rx
Urecholine, generic (bethanechol
chloride) tablets 25 mg
Disp. 90 tablets
Sig. Take 1 tablet 3 to 5 times a day.

Not FDA-approved for this
indication.

Cholinergic drugs should be
prescribed in consultation with the
patient's physician because of the
side effects. The pilocarpine and
cevimeline dosage should be
adjusted to increase saliva while
minimizing the adverse side effects
(sweating, stomach upset, etc.).
Patients should be warned that there
is a wide range of sensitivity and
that the adverse side effects may
outweigh the benefit of increased
salivation. If this occurs, then the
cholinergic drug should be
discontinued.

Caries Prevention
Rx
PreviDent, others (neutral NaF)
1.1% gel
Disp. 1 tube
Sig. Place 1-inch ribbon on a
toothbrush; brush teeth for 2 min
daily and expectorate. Avoid rinsing
or eating for 30 min following
application.

As an alternative, place a 1-inch
ribbon in a custom tray; apply for
5–10 min daily.

Rx
PreviDent 5000 Plus, generic
(neutral NaF) 1.1% dental cream
Disp. 1 tube
Sig. Place 1-inch ribbon on a
toothbrush; brush teeth for 2 min
twice daily and expectorate. Avoid
rinsing or eating for 30 min
following application.

In general, the use of stannous
fluoride gels is not recommended
because of the high acidity and
lower fluoride concentration of
1000 ppm, in contrast to the sodium
fluoride gels that have a neutral pH
and contain 5000 ppm. Also,
stannous fluoride gels may etch
ceramic and glass ionomer
restorations and cause extrinsic tooth
staining.

Note that FDA regulations have
limited the size of bottles of fluoride
because of toxicity, if ingested by
infants. Because most preparations
do not come in childproof bottles,
the sizes of topical fluoride
preparations vary; 24 ml is
approximately a 2-wk supply for
application to a full dentition in
custom carriers.

Reduced salivary flow provides
an excellent environment for
overgrowth of *C. albicans*. The
patient is likely to require treatment
for candidiasis, along with treatment
for dry mouth (see "Candidiasis").
In a dry oral environment, plaque
control becomes more difficult.
Scrupulous oral hygiene is essential
to prevent dental and periodontal
disease.

LICHEN PLANUS
Etiology:
Lichen planus is an immunologically
mediated, chronic, mucocutaneous
disorder. Although many cases
develop without a known cause,
some lesions are triggered by

emotional stress, hypersensitivity to drugs, dental products, foods, and a genetic predilection.

Clinical description:

Lichen planus varies in clinical appearance. Oral forms of this disorder include lacy white lines representing Wickham's striae (reticular), an erythematous form (atrophic), and an ulcerating form that often is accompanied by striae peripheral to the ulceration (erosive). The lesions are commonly found on the buccal mucosa, gingiva, and tongue, but they can be found on the lips and palate. Lichen planus lesions are chronic and also may affect the skin. The dental and medical literature remains controversial as to whether lichen planus undergoes malignant transformation. Therefore, any persistent or refractory lesion should be biopsied to establish a diagnosis and to rule out a malignancy.

Rationale for treatment:

Since this is a chronic disease, management of the disease focuses on providing oral comfort, if the lesions are symptomatic. Systemic and local relief with antiinflammatory and immunosuppressant agents is indicated. Identification of any dietary component, dental product, or medication (lichenoid drug reaction) should be undertaken to ensure against a hypersensitivity reaction. Treatment or prevention of a secondary fungal infection with a systemic antifungal agent also should be considered.

Therapies with steroids and immunomodulating drugs are presented to inform the clinician that such modalities are available. Because of the potential for side effects, close collaboration with the patient's physician is recommended

when these medications are prescribed. These modalities are beyond the scope of the clinical experience of general dentists, and referral to a dental specialist or to an appropriate physician is recommended.

Topical Steroids

Prolonged use of topical steroids (for a period longer than 2 wk of continuous use) may result in mucosal atrophy and secondary candidiasis and may increase the potential for systemic absorption. The prescribing of antifungal therapy with steroids may be necessary. Therapy with topical steroids, once the lichen planus is under control, should be tapered to alternate day therapy or less depending on control of the disease and the tendency for recurrence.

Rx

Fluocinonide gel 0.05%
Disp. 30-g tube
Sig. Coat the lesion with a thin film after each meal and at bedtime.

Rx

Dexamethasone elixir, solution 0.5 mg/5 ml
Disp. 240 ml
Sig. Rinse with 1 teaspoon (5 ml) for 2 min 4 times a day and expectorate. Discontinue when lesions become asymptomatic.

Other topical steroid preparations (cream, gel, rinse, ointment) are available. In general, creams are not used intraorally because of very poor mucosal adherence. These topical steroids come with a warning that they are for external use only. However, several of these agents have been used successfully for managing lichen planus. Examples of some of the topical steroid medications are listed below according to potency.

Except when lichen planus occurs on the lips, low-potency topical steroids are generally not effective for intraoral lesions.

Super-High Potency:

Betamethasone dipropionate (augmented) 0.05%, gel, ointment

Clobetasol propionate 0.05%, gel, ointment

Halobetasol propionate 0.05%, ointment

High Potency:

Betamethasone dipropionate 0.05%, gel, ointment

Fluocinonide 0.05%, gel, ointment

Dexamethasone 0.5 mg/5 ml oral solution, elixir

Desoximetasone 0.05%, gel; 0.25% ointment

Medium Potency:

Betamethasone valerate 0.1%, ointment

Triamcinolone acetonide 0.1%, ointment

Low Potency:

Alclometasone dipropionate 0.05%, ointment

Hydrocortisone acetate 1%, gel, ointment

Prolonged use of topical steroids may result in mucosal atrophy and secondary candidiasis and increase the potential for systemic absorption. It may be necessary to prescribe antifungal therapy with topical steroids. The oral cavity should be monitored for emergence of fungal infection in patients who are placed on therapy. Prophylactic antifungal therapy should be initiated in patients with a history of fungal infection with previous steroid administration (see "Candidiasis"). Therapy with topical steroids, once the lichen planus is under control, should be tapered to alternate-day therapy or less

depending on disease control and tendency to recur.

Systemic Steroids and Immunosuppressants for Severe Cases

Rx
Dexamethasone elixir or solution 0.5 mg/5 ml
Disp. 320 ml
Sig. As directed in writing not to exceed 2 continuous wks.
1. For 3 days, rinse with 1 tablespoonful (15 ml) 4 times a day and swallow. Then,
2. For 3 days rinse with 1 teaspoonful (5 ml) 4 times a day and swallow. Then,
3. For 3 days, rinse with 1 teaspoonful (5 ml) 4 times a day and swallow every other time. Then,
4. Rinse with 1 teaspoonful (5 ml) 4 times a day and expectorate.

Rx
Prednisone tablets 10 mg
Disp. 26 tablets
Sig. Take 4 tablets in the morning for 5 days, then decrease by 1 tablet on each successive day.

Rx
Prednisone tablets 5 mg
Disp. 40 tablets
Sig. Take 5 tablets in the morning for 5 days, then 5 tablets in the morning every other day until gone.

If oral discomfort recurs, the patient should return to the clinician for reevaluation.

Rx
Protopic (tacrolimus) ointment 0.1%
Disp. 30-g tube
Sig. Apply to the affected sites twice daily. Use for 2 wk and re-evaluate.

Rx
Protopic (tacrolimus) ointment 0.03%
Disp. 30-g tube
Sig. Apply to the affected sites twice daily. Use for 2 wk and re-evaluate.

Many studies suggest that oral lichen planus has an intrinsic property predisposing to malignant transformation. However, the etiology is complex, with interaction among genetic, infectious agents, environmental, and lifestyle factors. Prospective studies have demonstrated that lichen planus patients have a slightly increased risk to develop oral squamous cell carcinoma. All patients exhibiting lichen planus, intraorally, particularly those who have had the ulcerative form, should receive periodic follow-up.

Therapy with medications such as systemic steroids, immunosuppressants, and immunomodulators is presented to inform the clinician that such modalities have been reported effective for patients suffering from erosive lichen planus. Medications such as azathioprine, mycophenolate mofetil, tacrolimus hydroxychloroquine sulfate, acitretin, and cyclosporine are used to treat patients with severe persistent erosive lichen planus, but should not be routinely used because of the potential for side effects. Close collaboration with the patient's physician is recommended when these medications are prescribed.

Topical tacrolimus has been associated with neoplastic disease, such as lymphoma and skin cancers, and, therefore, should not be used indiscriminately for long periods of time. This medication is indicated for patients who cannot tolerate or are refractory to topical or systemic steroid therapy.

In addition, periodic scaling and professional dental cleanings every 3 to 4 months, are important for controlling this chronic disease

when the gingival tissues are affected. Patients with gingival involvement are at increased risk for gingival recession and periodontitis.

PEMPHIGUS VULGARIS AND MUCOUS MEMBRANE PEMPHIGOID

Pemphigus vulgaris and mucous membrane pemphigoid are relatively uncommon lesions. They should be suspected when chronic, multiple oral ulcerations and a history of oral and skin blisters exist. Often, they may occur only in the mouth. Diagnosis is based on history and on microscopic and immunofluorescence studies of a biopsied sample adjacent to a lesion.

Etiology:
Both of these chronic mucocutaneous diseases are autoimmune disorders with autoantibodies against antigens appearing in different areas of the surface epithelium or lining mucosa. In pemphigus vulgaris, the antigens are within the epithelium (desmosomes), whereas in pemphigoid, the antigens are located at the base of the epithelium in the hemidesmosomes.

Clinical description:
In pemphigus vulgaris, the lesion may stay in one location for a long period of time with small placid bullae. The bullae may rupture, leaving areas of ulceration. Approximately 80%–90% of patients have oral lesions. The oral manifestations are the first signs of the disease in approximately two-thirds of patients. All parts of the mouth may be involved. The bullae rupture almost immediately in the mouth, but may stay intact for some time on the skin. One of the classic signs, the Nikolsky sign (blister formation induced with

gentle rubbing of an affected mucosal site), is positive in pemphigus, but is not pathognomonic, because it is also positive in other disorders. Because the vesicles or bullae are intraepithelial, they often are filled with clear fluid. Microscopically, Tzanck cells or acantholytic cells are observed within the spinous cell layer of the epithelium.

In pemphigoid, the cleavage or split is beneath the epithelium, resulting in bullae that are often blood filled. Mucous membrane pemphigoid is usually limited to the oral cavity, but some patients have ocular lesions (symblepharon) that must be evaluated by an ophthalmologist. The gingiva is the most common oral site involved. Pemphigoid may appear clinically as a red, nonulcerated or ulcerated gingival lesions with a positive Nikolsky sign.

Rationale for treatment:
Because both pemphigus and pemphigoid are autoimmune disorders, the primary treatment is topical or systemic steroids or other immunomodulating drugs. Custom trays can be used to localize topical steroid medications on the gingival tissues (occlusive therapy). Because they can resemble other ulcerative-bullous diseases, a biopsy is necessary for a definitive diagnosis. Specimens should be submitted for light microscopic and immunofluorescence studies. Because of the potentially serious nature of these diseases, referral to a specialist in oral medicine, dermatology, and ophthalmology must be considered. When eye lesions are present, an ophthalmologist must be consulted immediately to prevent blindness.

Therapy with medications such as systemic steroids, immunosuppressants, and immunomodulators are presented to inform the clinician that such modalities have been reported effective for patients suffering from vesiculobullous disorders such as pemphigus vulgaris and mucous membrane pemphigoid. Therapies such as dapsone, methotrexate, mycophenolate mofetil, cyclosporine, or niacinamide with tetracycline are used to treat patients with vesiculobullous disorders such as pemphigus vulgaris and mucous membrane pemphigoid, but they should not be routinely used because of the potential for serious adverse effects. Close collaboration with the patient's physician is recommended when these medications are prescribed.

Rx:
Topical and Systemic Steroids (See Lichen Planus)

ORAL ERYTHEMA MULTIFORME

Etiology:
Oral erythema multiforme is a blistering and ulcerative mucocutaneous disease that is immunologically mediated. It can occur at any age. Drug reactions to medications such as penicillin and sulfonamides may play a role in some cases. In a few patients who develop oral erythema multiforme, a herpetic infection occurs immediately before the onset of clinical signs. Other infectious diseases have also been implicated.

Clinical description:
Signs of oral erythema multiforme include "blood-crusted" lips, "targetoid" or "bull's-eye" skin lesions, and a nonspecific mucosal erythema, ulceration, and necrosis. The name multiforme is used

because its appearance may take different forms. A severe form of erythema multiforme is called Stevens-Johnson syndrome, or erythema multiforme major. Erythema multiforme, as a skin disease, occurs most frequently because of an allergic reaction.

Rationale for treatment:

Treatment is primarily directed at patient comfort, using topical anesthetics and coating agents. Because of the possible relationship of oral erythema multiforme with herpes simplex virus, suppressive antiviral therapy may be indicated to prevent lesion recurrences. Patients should be questioned carefully about a previous history of recurrent herpetic infections and prodromal symptoms that might have preceded the onset of erythema multiforme. It is also important to take a thorough drug history to determine if that is the cause.

Topical Anesthetics and
Coating Agents

Rx

Diphenhydramine hydrochloride oral solution 12.5 mg/5 ml mixed with aluminum hydroxide, magnesium hydroxide oral suspension

Compound to a 1:1 mixture by volume

Disp. 200 ml

Sig. Rinse with 1–2 teaspoons (5–10 ml) every 2 to 4 hr for 1 min; swish and spit out.

Although these medications are OTC, it is recommended that a pharmacist compound this oral suspension. Examples of aluminum hydroxide, magnesium hydroxide oral suspension are Maalox and Mylanta—they are common OTC brands and are available in a number of flavors. Children younger than 6 yr should not swallow this oral suspension.

Rx

Diphenhydramine hydrochloride liquid 12.5 mg/5 ml/lidocaine viscous 2% oral solution/aluminum hydroxide, magnesium hydroxide oral suspension

Compound to a 1:1:1 mixture by volume.

Disp. 200 ml

Sig. Shake well before use. Rinse with 1–2 teaspoons (5–10 ml) every 3–4 hr for 1 min and spit out excess. Store suspension at room temperature.

It is compounded by pharmacy and stable for approximately 60 days. Do not use 2% lidocaine hydrochloride in children who cannot expectorate because of potential for aspiration or swallowing.

Rx

Carafate, generic (sucralfate) suspension 1 g/10 ml

Disp. 200 ml

Sig. Rinse with 1 teaspoon (5 ml) 4 times a day. Rinse for 1 min and spit out excess.

In children younger than 6 yr, who cannot expectorate, the amount should be limited to 0.5 g, four times a day (2 g/day) in case the suspension is swallowed. Safety and efficacy has not been established in children.

Rx

Children's Benadryl Allergy Liquid, others, (diphenhydramine hydrochloride) oral solution 12.5 mg/5 ml (OTC)

Disp. 8 oz bottle

Sig. Rinse with 1 teaspoon (5 ml) for 2 min every 2–4 hr and spit out excess.

If swallowed, for adolescents and adults, the maximum amount is 300 mg in 24 hr. For children 6–12 yr, the maximum is 150 mg in 24 hr. Children younger than 6 yr should not swallow this drug.

Rx
Sucrets (dyclonine HCl) throat lozenges (OTC)
Disp. 1 package
Sig. Slowly dissolve one lozenge in mouth every 2 hr as needed for pain. Do not take more than 10 lozenges a day.

The strength of dyclonine HCl ranges from 3 mg (maximum strength) to 1.2 mg for children's formula.

Suppressive Antiviral Therapy
Rx
Zovirax, generic (acyclovir) tablets 400 mg
Disp. 60 tablets
Sig. Take 1 tablet 2 times daily. Take drug for up to 12 months and re-evaluate.
Rx
Valtrex, generic (valacyclovir) tablets 1 g
Disp. 30 tablets
Sig. Take 1 tablet a day. Take drug for up to 12 months and re-evaluate.

Because of the long-term use of these antiviral agents, patients may be best monitored by a dental specialist or physician.

DENTURE SORE MOUTH
Etiology:
Discomfort under oral prosthetic appliances may result from combinations of candidal infections, poor denture hygiene, an occlusal syndrome, overextension, or excessive movement of the appliance. This condition may be erroneously attributed to an allergy to denture material, which is a rare occurrence. This condition may represent a pressure neuropathy due to advanced atrophy of the alveolar bone and trauma to the nerves emanating from the mental foramen and the incisive foramen. The retention and fit of the denture should be idealized, and mechanical irritation should be ruled out.
Clinical description:
The tissue covered by the appliance, especially if the appliance is made of acrylic, is erythematous and smooth or granular. It may be either asymptomatic or associated with a burning sensation.
Rationale for treatment:
Therapy is directed toward controlling all possible causes and improving oral comfort. If therapy is ineffective, consider underlying systemic conditions such as diabetes mellitus and poor nutrition.
Treatment:
1. Institute appropriate antifungal medication (see "Candidiasis");
2. Improve oral and appliance hygiene. The patient may have to leave the appliance out for extended periods of time and should be instructed to leave the denture out overnight. The appliance should be soaked in a commercially available denture cleanser or soaked in a 1% sodium hypochlorite solution (1 teaspoon of sodium hypochlorite in a denture cup of water) for 15 min and thoroughly rinsed for at least 2 min under running water;
3. Reline, rebase, or construct a new appliance;
4. Apply an artificial saliva or oral lubricant gel to the tissue contact surface of the denture to reduce frictional trauma.

If all the above actions fail to control symptoms, a biopsy or short trial of topical steroid therapy can be used to rule out contact mucositis (an allergic reaction to denture materials). If a therapeutic trial fails to resolve the condition, a biopsy should be performed to establish the diagnosis.

BURNING MOUTH SYNDROME
Etiology:
Burning mouth syndrome is a common dysesthesia that has been associated with a variety of local and systemic factors. Current literature supports a neurogenic cause with psychological component. However, other conditions, such as xerostomia, candidiasis, referred pain from the tongue musculature, chronic infections, gastrointestinal reflux disease, medications, blood dyscrasias, nutritional deficiencies, hormonal imbalances, and allergic and inflammatory disorders, must also be considered.

Clinical description:
Burning mouth syndrome is characterized by persistent tenderness of usually the tongue, followed by the lips and anterior hard palate in the absence of clinical signs.

Rationale for treatment:
If an underlying local or systemic cause is not identified, then treatment approaches focus on reducing discomfort. Either topical anesthetics or mood-altering drugs are prescribed.

Treatment:
It is important to reassure the patient that this disorder is not infectious and does not progress to a malignant condition. On the basis of the history, physical evaluation, and specific laboratory studies, it is important to exclude all local and systemic causes. Minimal blood studies should include complete blood count and differential, fasting glucose, iron, ferritin, folic acid, and vitamin B_{12} levels, and thyroid profile (TSH, T3, T4).

Rx
Benadryl Children's Allergy (diphenhydramine) solution 12.5 mg/5 ml (OTC)
Disp. 1 bottle
Sig. Rinse with 1–2 teaspoons (5–10 ml) for 2 min before each meal and spit out.

When the burning mouth is considered psychogenic or idiopathic, a tricyclic antidepressant or benzodiazepine in low doses exhibits the properties of analgesia and sedation and frequently is successful in reducing or eliminating the symptoms after several weeks or months. The dosage is adjusted according to patient reaction and clinical symptoms. The following systemic therapies for burning mouth disorder are best managed by appropriate specialists or the patient's physician, due to the protracted nature of this therapy.

Rx
Clonazepam orally disintegrating tablets 0.25 mg
Disp. 60 tablets
Sig. Take 1 tablet nightly, then adjust dose after 7 days.

This therapy probably is best managed by an appropriate specialist or the patient's physician at this time. Due to the sedative affects, patients may wish to take this medication only at night and increase the dosage to 2 tablets (0.50 mg). Other patients experience more improvement when they take 1–2 tablets 3 times a day.

Rx
Amitriptyline tablets 25 mg
Disp. 50 tablets
Sig. Take 1 tablet at bedtime for 1 wk, then increase to 2 tablets every night for the next week. Increase to 3 tablets every night after 2 wk and maintain at that dosage or titrate as appropriate.

Rx
Chlordiazepoxide capsules 5 mg
Disp. 50 capsules

Sig. Take 1 capsule 3 times a day, then adjust after 1 wk to 2 capsules 3 times a day as appropriate.

Rx

Xanax, generic (alprazolam) tablets 0.25 mg

Disp. 50 tablets

Sig. Take 1 tablet 3 times a day.

The rationale for use of tricyclic antidepressants and other psychotropic drugs should be thoroughly explained to the patient, and the patient's physician should be consulted. These medications have a potential for addiction and dependence.

Rx

Tabasco sauce (capsaicin) (OTC)

Disp. 1 bottle

Sig. Place one part Tabasco sauce in 2 to 4 parts of water. Rinse with 1 teaspoon (5 ml) 4 times a day and expectorate.

Rx

Zostrix, generic (capsaicin) cream 0.025% (OTC)

Disp. 1 tube

Sig. Apply sparingly to affected site(s) 4 times a day.

Wash hands after each application and do not use near the eyes.

Topical capsaicin may produce a burning sensation in some individuals. An increase in discomfort for a 2- to 3-wk period should be anticipated.

CHAPPED OR CRACKED LIPS (EXFOLIATIVE CHEILITIS)

Etiology:

Chapped lips are due to increased keratinization with subsequent desquamation of the vermilion border that is often secondarily inflamed. Repeatedly licking, picking, and biting the lips are aggravating factors. Other causes include eczema, contact allergies, xerostomia, and secondary candidal infection.

Clinical description:

The surface of the vermilion is rough, scaly, and peeling and may be ulcerated with bleeding and crusting. In severe and chronic cases, the lips are tender, slightly swollen, and deep fissures and scarring may be detected.

Rationale for treatment:

An interrupted and chronically inflamed surface is at increased risk for scarring and secondary infection. Eliminating the cause, especially if the chapped lips are due to a factitial habit or contact allergy, is important. A protective lip emollient, a topical antiinflammatory agent with or without antimicrobial agents, aids in the healing of the lips, but recurrences are common.

Rx

Aquaphor Healing Ointment, others (OTC)

Disp. 1 tube

Sig. Apply to lips after each meal and at bedtime.

Avoid flavored products because they tend to promote increased licking of the lips. Although medicated products may be soothing initially, they should not be used because they can cause increased drying of the lips. Some patients respond better to lanolin cream or ointment than petroleum-based products.

Rx

Nystatin/triamcinolone acetonide ointment 100,000 units/g 0.1%

Disp. 15-g tube

Sig. Apply to lips after each meal and at bedtime. Use for no longer that 2 wk.

Rx

Triamcinolone acetonide ointment 0.1%

Disp. 15-g tube

Sig. Apply to lips after each meal and at bedtime. Use for no longer that 2 wk.

Rx

Betamethasone valerate ointment 0.1%

Disp. 15-g tube

Sig. Apply to lips after each meal and at bedtime. Use for no longer than 2 wk.

Prolonged use of corticosteroids can result in thinning of the tissue, so their use should be closely monitored and for a limited period of time. For maintenance, the frequent application of lip care products that are hypoallergenic should be suggested. Avoid products with desiccants, such as phenols and alcohols and those with flavoring agents. In severe cases with swelling of the lips, systemic antibiotics may be needed, along with topical agents.

DRUG-INDUCED GINGIVAL OVERGROWTH

Etiology:

Certain drugs, such as phenytoin sodium, calcium channel blocking agents (nifedipine, diltiazem, verapamil, amlodipine and others), and cyclosporine therapy are known to predispose some individuals to persistent gingival enlargement. Chronic hyperplastic gingivitis, gingival fibromatosis, and granulomatous gingivitis should be ruled out by clinical history, family history, biopsy, and other indicated laboratory tests.

Clinical description:

The gingival tissues, especially in the anterior region, are firm, stippled, nontender, and enlarged. Depending on the degree of inflammation, the gingival tissues vary from normal in color to dark red and hemorrhagic. Especially in drug-induced examples, the

enlargements originate in the interdental papillae.

Rationale for treatment:

Local factors, such as plaque and calculus accumulation, contribute to secondary inflammation and the hyperplastic process. This further interferes with plaque control. Specific drugs tend to deplete serum folic acid levels, which result in compromised tissue integrity.

Treatment:

Management approaches consists of (1) meticulous plaque control; (2) gingivectomy or other gingival surgery when indicated; (3) when possible, replace the causative drug with an equivalent substitute; and (4) test for serum folate level and supplement folic acid, if necessary. Use of folic acid rinse, topical antimicrobial mouth rinse, and systemic antibiotics may be effective in some cases. Specifically, metronidazole and azithromycin have been successful in resolving some cases.

Rx

Folic acid oral rinse 1 mg/ml

Disp. 16 oz

Sig. Rinse with 1 teaspoonful (5 ml) for 2 min twice a day and expectorate.

Rx

Peridex, PerioGard, generics (chlorhexidine gluconate) oral rinse 0.12%

Disp. 16 oz

Sig. Rinse with 15 ml twice daily for 30 seconds and expectorate. Rinse after breakfast and before bedtime.

TASTE DISORDERS

Etiology:

Taste acuity may be affected by medications and by neurologic and physiologic changes. Clinical examination and diagnostic procedures may identify potential causes such as nasal and sinus disease, viral infection, oral candidiasis, neoplasia, malnutrition, metabolic disorders, trauma, illicit drug use, autoimmune diseases affecting salivary glands, and radiation sequelae. In addition, individuals with anxiety disorders and depression may complain about changes in taste. Laboratory tests for trace elements may be necessary to identify any existing deficiencies.

Rationale for treatment:
A reduction in salivary flow may concentrate the electrolytes in the saliva, resulting in a salty or metallic taste (see "Xerostomia"). Numerous medications have dysgeusia as a reported side effect. Antibiotics, antihypertensives, antifungals, and antiretrovirals are examples of classes of drugs that have been implicated. Rarely, a deficiency of zinc has been associated with a loss of taste and smell sensation. To prevent deficiency, the current recommended dietary allowance for zinc is 10 mg for men and 12 mg for women. Additional zinc supplementation should be reserved for individuals with true deficiency states and in consultation with the physician.

To Ensure Dietary Allowance for Zinc

Rx
Z-BEC tablets (OTC)
Disp. 60 tablets
Sig. Take 1 tablet daily with food or after meals.

This supplement also contains vitamin B complex, vitamin C, and Vitamin E, along with zinc.

For Zinc Deficiency in Patients with Proven Zinc Deficiency

Rx
Zinc sulfate capsules 220 mg (OTC)
Disp. 100 capsules
Sig. Take 1 capsule with food or after meals once a day for 1 month.

Rx
Zinc acetate capsules 50 mg (OTC)
Disp. 100 capsules
Sig. Take 1 capsule a day with food or after meals for 1 month.

Rx
Zinc gluconate tablets 50 mg (OTC)
Disp. 100 capsules
Sig. Take 1 capsule a day with food or after meals for 1 month.

MANAGEMENT OF PATIENTS RECEIVING ANTINEOPLASTIC AGENTS AND RADIATION THERAPY

Etiology:
Cancer chemotherapy and radiation to the head and neck cause direct and indirect effects on the oral tissues. Chemotherapy results in direct cytotoxic effects that may result in mucositis and ulceration of the mucosa. In addition, there are indirect effects of myelosuppression resulting in anemia, thrombocytopenia, and leucopenia. Both local and disseminated infection may develop including fungal, viral, and bacterial infections. Besides odontogenic and periodontal infections, candidal and recurrent herpes simplex infections are among the most common infections in the mouth. Bleeding problems, especially due to decreased platelets, may result in mucosal and gingival bleeding. The use of intravenous bisphosphonates may increase the risk for osteonecrosis of the jaws. The effects of radiation treatment directly affect the targeted tissues. When the head and neck is the targeted site, mucositis, taste alterations, salivary gland hypofunction, dysphagia,

osteoradionecrosis, trismus, periodontal disease, and dental caries are potential complications.

Clinical description:

Due to the wide range of potential complications, the oral findings are diverse in appearance. The more common findings include red, inflamed, and/or ulcerated mucosa and chapped lips. The saliva may be viscous or absent.

Rationale for treatment:

The treatment of these patients is symptomatic and supportive. It should be aimed at patient comfort and education, maintenance of proper nutrition and oral hygiene, and prevention of opportunistic infection. Frequent monitoring and close cooperation with the patient's physician are important. In order to prevent potentially serious oral complication, all patients who undergo chemotherapy and/or radiation therapy should have a thorough oral evaluation to eliminate any source of infection. In patients who will receive radiation treatment to the head and neck region, oral surgical procedures should be performed 14 days prior to the treatment for optimal healing. Oral hygiene is of paramount importance prior to, during, and after radiation treatment.

The oral discomfort may be relieved by periodically using neutral or saline mouth rinses and topical anesthetics and coating agents. Artificial saliva and mouth moisturizing gels aid in reducing oral dryness. Antifungal and antiviral agents are needed to manage specific infections. The use of fluorides is recommended for caries control and root sensitivity. In some patients, chlorhexidine rinses help control plaque when oral hygiene is poor.

Mouth Rinses (See "Xerostomia")

Rx

Alkaline saline (salt/bicarbonate) mouth rinse

Disp. Mix ¼ teaspoon each of salt and baking soda in 16 oz glass of water.

Sig. Rinse for 1 min with copious amounts at least 5 times a day and spit out.

If too irritating, may switch to ½ teaspoon baking soda in 16 oz of water.

Rx

Caphosol (calcium phosphate) solution

Disp. 60 ampules

Sig. Mix 2 ampules in a clean glass and swirl contents of glass to mix. Rinse and gargle with ½ of the solution for 1 min and expectorate. Repeat with the remaining solution. Do not eat or drink for 15 min after use. Use up to 4 times a day.

This solution may be helpful for patients with both dry mouth and mucositis.

Gingivitis Control

Rx

Peridex, PerioGard, generic (chlorhexidine gluconate) rinse 0.12%

Disp. 16 oz

Sig. Rinse with ½ oz (15 ml) twice a day for 1 min and spit out. Avoid rinsing or eating for 30 min following treatment. Rinse after breakfast and at bedtime.

In xerostomic patients, chlorhexidine rinse should be used concurrently with artificial saliva to provide the needed protein-binding agent for efficacy and substantivity. Because of the alcohol content, this rinse may be too irritating to use. A pharmacy can compound an alcohol-free, 2% aqueous solution. It is important to note that both toothpaste and nystatin reduce the effectiveness of chlorhexidine rinse, so it is important to allow 30 min before using these agents.

Caries Control (See "Xerostomia")

Rx

PreviDent, others (neutral NaF) gel 1.1%

Disp. 24 ml

Sig. Place a thin ribbon in custom trays. After inserting trays in the mouth, bite on them to create a pumping action. Keep in the mouth for 5–10 min and spit out excess. Avoid rinsing or eating for 30 min after treatment.

An alternative is to brush on NaF gel twice daily for 2 min and spit out excess. Both of these techniques should be supplemented with conventional 1100 ppm sodium fluoride toothpaste twice daily.

The use of SnF2 gels such as Gel-Kam is not recommended because of the high acidity and lower fluoride concentration of 1000 ppm, in contrast to the NaF gels that have a neutral pH and contain 5000 ppm.

Topical Anesthetics

Rx

Lidocaine hydrochloride viscous solution 2%

Disp. 200 ml

Sig. Rinse with 2–3 teaspoons (10–15 ml) every 3–4 hr for 1 min; swish and spit out.

Do not use 2% lidocaine hydrochloride in children or adults who cannot expectorate because of potential for aspiration or swallowing.

Rx

Diphenhydramine hydrochloride oral solution 12.5 mg/5 ml mixed with aluminum hydroxide, magnesium hydroxide oral suspension

Compound to a 1:1 mixture by volume

Disp. 200 ml

Sig. Rinse with 1–2 teaspoons (5–10 ml) every 2–4 hr for 1 min; swish and spit out.

Although these medications are OTC, it is recommended that a pharmacist compound this oral suspension.

Rx

Diphenhydramine hydrochloride liquid 12.5 mg/5 ml/lidocaine viscous 2% oral solution/aluminum hydroxide, magnesium hydroxide oral suspension.

Compound to a 1:1:1 mixture by volume

Disp. 200 ml

Sig. Shake well before use. Rinse with 1–2 teaspoons (5–10 ml) every 4 hr for 1 min and spit out excess. Store suspension at room temperature.

It is compounded by pharmacy and is stable for approximately 60 days. Do not use 2% lidocaine hydrochloride in children or adults who cannot expectorate because of potential for aspiration or swallowing.

Rx

Children's Benadryl Allergy Liquid, others, (diphenhydramine hydrochloride) oral solution 12.5 mg/5 ml (OTC)

Disp. 8 oz bottle

Sig. Rinse with 1–2 teaspoons (5–10 ml) for 2 min every 2–4 hr and spit out excess.

If swallowed, for adolescents and adults, the maximum amount is 300 mg in 24 hr. For children 6–12 yr, the maximum is 150 mg in 24 hr. Children younger than 6 yr should not swallow this drug.

Rx

Sucrets (dyclonine HCl) throat lozenges (OTC)

Disp. 1 package

Sig. Slowly dissolve one lozenge in mouth every 2 hr as needed for pain. Do not take more than 10 lozenges a day.

The strength of dyclonine HCl ranges from 3 mg (maximum strength) to 1.2 mg for children's formula.

In general, when topical anesthetics are used, patients should be warned about a reduced gag reflex and the need for caution while eating and drinking to avoid possible airway compromise. Allergies are rare but may occur.

Antifungal Agents
(See "Candidiasis")

Saliva Stimulants
(See "Xerostomia")

Bibliography

Neville BW, Damm DD, Allen CM, Bouquot JE, editors: *Oral and maxillofacial pathology*, ed 3, St. Louis, 2009, Saunders, Elsevier.

Rankin KV, Jones DL, Redding SW, editors: *Oral health in cancer therapy. A guide for health care professional*, ed 3, Dallas, TX, 2008, Dental Oncology Education Program.

Siegel MA, Silverman S Jr, Sollecito TP, editors: *American Academy of Oral Medicine clinician's guide. Treatment of common oral conditions*, ed 6, Hamilton, Ontario, 2006, BC Decker.

PREVENTION OF INFECTIVE ENDOCARDITIS

In 2007, the American Heart Association (AHA) updated its recommendations for antibiotic prophylaxis prior to dental procedures to prevent infective endocarditis (Wilson W et al., 2007). These guidelines recommend antibiotic prophylaxis only in patients with cardiac conditions that are associated with the highest risk of adverse outcomes from infective endocarditis, including (1) patients with a **prosthetic heart valve,** (2) patients who have **previously had infective endocarditis,** (3) patients with **congenital heart disease** (unrepaired cyanotic heart disease; completely repaired congenital heart defects with prosthetic material or device, whether placed by surgery or catheter intervention, during the first 6 mo after the procedure; or repaired congenital heart disease with residual defects at the site or adjacent to the site of a prosthetic patch or prosthetic device), and (4) **cardiac transplant recipients** who develop cardiac **valvulopathy.** The list of dental procedures for which prophylaxis is recommended has been expanded and now includes *all dental procedures* that involve manipulation of gingival tissue or the periapical region of teeth or perforation of the oral mucosa (except for routine anesthetic injections through noninfected tissue, taking dental radiographs, placement of removable prosthodontic or orthodontic appliances, adjustment of orthodontic appliances, placement of orthodontic brackets, shedding of deciduous teeth, and bleeding from trauma to the lips or oral mucosa).

The antibiotic regimens recommended for prophylaxis in patients at risk of adverse outcomes of infective endocarditis are to be administered as a *single dose* and *30 min to 1 hr before the dental procedure:*

Oral: Amoxicillin 2 g (children 50 mg/kg)

Patients unable to take/absorb oral medications:
• Ampicillin 2 g IM or IV (children 50 mg/kg IM or IV) OR
• Cefazolin or Ceftriaxone 1 g IM or IV (children 50 mg/kg IM or IV)

Patients allergic to penicillins or ampicillin—oral:
• Cephalexin 2 g (children 50 mg/kg) or
• Clindamycin 600 mg orally (children 20 mg/kg) OR
• Azithromycin or clarithromycin 500 mg (children 15 mg/kg)

Patients allergic to penicillins or ampicillin and unable to take/absorb oral medications:
• Cefazolin or Ceftriaxone 1 g IM or IV (children 50 mg/kg IM or IV) OR
• Clindamycin 600 mg IM or IV (children 20 mg/kg IM or IV)

If the antibiotic was *inadvertently* not administered prior to the procedure, the antibiotic dosage should be administered within 2 hr after the procedure. Practitioners should be cautious of coincidental infective endocarditis in patients at risk who present with a fever or other signs and symptoms of a systemic infection. Patients should also be monitored following the dental procedure for such signs and symptoms, which may be the initial indicators of infective endocarditis. In patients receiving anticoagulant therapy, intramuscular (IM) injections should be avoided and preference given to the oral route of administration if possible.

NONVALVULAR CARDIOVASCULAR DEVICE-RELATED INFECTIONS

In 2011, the AHA updated guidelines regarding the use of antibiotic prophylaxis for patients with cardiovascular implantable electronic devices undergoing dental, respiratory, GI, or GU procedures. A previous (2003) statement addressed devices such as pacemakers, defibrillators, total artificial hearts, ventriculoatrial shunts, patent ductus arteriosus occlusion devices (plugs, umbrellas, buttons, discs, embolization coils), atrial septal defect and ventricular septal defect closure devices (Bard clamshell occluders, discs, buttons, double umbrellas), conduits, patches, peripheral vascular stents, vascular grafts (including hemodialysis), coronary artery stents, and vena caval filters.

Other Surgically Implanted Prosthetic Devices

At this time, there are no guidelines formally promulgated by any professional organizations for antibiotic prophylaxis prior to dental procedures in patients with noncardiac, nonorthopedic implanted devices, such as breast implants. The dental practitioner should consult the patient's physician in cases involving such devices in whom implant infection may be a concern as a result of dental procedures and, with the informed consent of the patient, make a decision regarding the use of antibiotic prophylaxis.

ORTHOPEDIC DEVICES: SCREWS, PLATES, PINS, AND PROSTHETIC JOINTS

In 2009, the American Academy of Orthopedic Surgeons (AAOS) revised its advisory statement on antibiotic prophylaxis for dental patients with total joint replacements. Antibiotic prophylaxis was not indicated for patients with plates or pins. Antibiotic prophylaxis is now recommended for most patients with total joint replacements. The statement no longer allows for exclusion from coverage of patients with prosthetic joints implanted longer than 2 years, and suggests that prophylaxis be considered for patients who may be at "high risk" for hematogenous infection, including patients with inflammatory arthropathies, immunosuppression, type 1 diabetes mellitus, joint replacement within 2 years, previous prosthetic joint infection (PJI), malnourishment, or hemophilia. (Of note, there is no evidence that even these "higher-risk" patients are at increased risk from dentally induced bacteremias. In fact, the microbiology of PJI in these "higher-risk" patients is the same as for other patients with PJI. A more appropriate interpretation is that these patients are at increased risk for PJI from the usual sources, such as wound contamination and acute infection from distant sites.)

The advisory statement also makes clear that the final decision as to whether to provide antibiotic prophylaxis lies with the dentist, who must weigh perceived potential benefits against the risks. The advisory statement provides the following suggested antibiotic regimens:

Amoxicillin 2 g orally, 1 hr before dental procedure

Cephalexin 2 g orally, 1 hr before dental procedure

Cephradine, 2 g orally, 1 hr before dental procedure

* Note that clindamycin and macrolide antibiotics (azithromycin,

clarithromycin) are not included in the current ADA/AAOS guidelines. In patients with allergy to penicillin or cephalosporins, it is recommended that these alternative drugs (included in the AHA infective endocarditis guidelines) be used, until further guidelines are issue by the AAOS.

ADRENAL INSUFFICIENCY (PRIMARY AND SECONDARY): PREVENTION OF ADRENAL CRISIS

Patients with primary (Addison's disease) or secondary (exogenous corticosteroid induced) adrenal insufficiency may be at risk for adrenal crisis during or following surgical procedures performed in dentistry. Adrenal crisis is a medical emergency that requires prompt intervention to save the patient's life. In order to prevent adrenal crisis, supplemental steroids in rather large doses have been recommended since the mid 1950s for patients with adrenal insufficiency. Adrenal crisis is a rare event in dentistry, especially in patients with secondary adrenal insufficiency. Four factors appear to be associated with the risk for adrenal crisis: (1) magnitude of surgery, (2) general anesthesia, (3) health status and stability of the patient, and (4) degree of pain control.

The most significant acute adverse outcome of adrenal insufficiency is adrenal crisis. This event can occur when a patient with adrenal insufficiency, most commonly Addison's disease, is challenged by stress (e.g., illness, infection, or surgery) and in response is unable to synthesize adequate amounts of cortisol and aldosterone. This potentially life-threatening emergency usually evolves slowly over a few hours and then is manifested by severe exacerbation of the condition,

including profuse sweating, hypotension, weak pulse, cyanosis, nausea, vomiting, weakness, headache, dehydration, fever, sunken eyes, dyspnea, myalgias, arthralgia, hyponatremia, and eosinophilia. If not treated rapidly, the patient may develop hypothermia, severe hypotension, hypoglycemia, confusion, and circulatory collapse that can culminate in death.

Four factors appear to contribute to the risk of adrenal crisis during the perioperative period of oral surgery: (1) magnitude of surgery, (2) general anesthesia, (3) overall health of the patient (e.g., stable vs. ongoing infection), and (4) degree of pain control.

Negligible Risk: Nonsurgical Dental Procedures

The vast majority of patients with adrenal insufficiency can undergo routine, nonsurgical dental treatment *without* the need for supplemental glucocorticoids. This is supported by the fact that routine, nonsurgical dental procedures do not stimulate cortisol production at levels comparable to those occurring during oral surgery, and local anesthesia blocks neural stress pathways required for adrenocorticotropic hormone (ACTH) secretion. This guideline does not advocate dental treatment on patients whose adrenal insufficiency is uncontrolled or undiagnosed. However, stable patients with adrenal insufficiency and those with a history of steroid use in whom glucocorticoid medication was discontinued prior to surgery have withstood general surgical procedures without developing adrenal crisis.

Low-Risk Regimen

For minor oral and periodontal surgery (e.g., a few simple extractions, soft tissue surgery), evidence suggests that adrenal insufficiency is prevented when circulating levels of glucocorticoids are approximately 25 mg hydrocortisone equivalent per day. This is equivalent to a dose of approximately 5 mg prednisone. The clinician should confirm that the patient has taken the recommended amount of steroid within 2 hr of the surgical procedure and schedule the surgery in the morning when normal cortisol levels are highest. Stress-reduction measures should be implemented. Benefits can be gained from use of (1) oral, inhalation, or intravenous sedation, which provides stress reduction; (2) intravenous fluids (i.e., 5% dextrose), which can prevent hypovolemia and hypoglycemia; (3) long-acting local anesthetics; and (4) adequate postoperative analgesics.

Moderate-Risk to Major-Risk Regimen

Patients with adrenocortical suppression undergoing major oral surgery are at increased risk for adrenal crisis when compared with minor surgery. Major surgical procedures are more stressful than minor surgical procedures. They increase the demand for cortisol because of postoperative pain. Blood loss is greater, thus increasing the risk for hypovolemia and hypotension.

For major oral surgical stress (multiple extractions, quadrant periodontal surgery, extraction of bony impactions, osseous surgery, osteotomy, bone resections, cancer surgery), surgical procedures involving use of general anesthesia, procedures lasting more than 1 hr, or procedures associated with significant blood loss, the glucocorticoid target is approximately 50–100 mg/day

hydrocortisone equivalent for the day of surgery and at least 1 postoperative day. Higher doses may be necessary if excessive bleeding or complications are encountered. Patients should take their normal steroid dose prior to the procedure and be provided supplemental intravenous hydrocortisone intraoperatively to achieve a total of 100 mg. Hospitalization should be considered for these patients because blood pressure can be more closely monitored postoperatively in this setting. Hydrocortisone 25 mg usually is prescribed every 8 hr following surgery for 24–48 hr, depending on the procedure and anticipated level of postoperative pain.

Following the recommendations listed will further minimize the risk of adrenal crisis associated with surgical stress in adrenally insufficient individuals:

• Define the risk for adrenal insufficiency with a thorough medical history and clinical examination. Patients with a past or present history of tuberculosis or HIV infection are at increased risk for adrenal insufficiency because opportunistic infectious agents can attack the adrenal glands.
• Ensure that adrenally insufficient patients take their glucocorticoid prior to a stressful surgery.
• Schedule surgery in the morning when cortisol levels normally are highest.
• Provide proper stress reduction because anxiety can increase cortisol demand.
• Minor surgeries require minimal steroid coverage. The patient's customary daily dose usually is sufficient.
• Major surgeries and those procedures lasting more than

1 hr or requiring use of general anesthesia should be performed in a hospital with steroid supplementation.

• Use of nitrous oxide-oxygen or intravenous or oral benzodiazepine sedation is helpful, as plasma cortisol levels are not reduced by these agents.

• Avoid outpatient general anesthesia, as general anesthesia increases glucocorticoid demand. Also, avoid use of barbiturates, which increase the metabolism of cortisol and reduce blood levels of cortisol.

SUMMARY OF NEED FOR SUPPLEMENTATION

Negligible-Risk Category

Nonsurgical dental procedures
  Regimen: No supplementation required

Low-Risk Category

Minor oral surgery
Few simple extractions, biopsy
Minor periodontal surgery
  Regimen: Target 25 mg hydrocortisone equivalent (5 mg prednisone), day of surgery

Moderate-Risk to Major-Risk Category

Major oral surgery
Multiple extractions
Quadrant periodontal surgery
Extraction of bony impactions
Osseous surgery
Osteotomy
Bone resections
Cancer surgery
Surgical procedures involving use of general anesthesia
Procedures lasting more than 1 hr
Procedures associated with significant blood loss
  Regimen: Target glucocorticoid is approximately 50–100 mg/day hydrocortisone equivalent, day
  of surgery and at least 1 postoperative day

CONTROL OF BLEEDING IN PATIENTS ON ANTICOAGULANT THERAPY

Oral Anticoagulants

In patients taking oral anticoagulant drugs (e.g., warfarin, Coumadin®) to prevent thromboembolic complications (e.g., stroke), the dentist should consult the patient's physician regarding the patient's reason for taking the drug and determine the level of anticoagulation reported as the international normalized ratio (INR). In most patients, the therapeutic range of the INR is approximately 2.5 to 3.5, whereas some patients may be maintained at higher levels (e.g., up to 4.5). The AMA and the ADA suggest an INR value of 2 to 3 before a surgical procedure is attempted. Local measures should be used to control bleeding if it occurs.

In patients with INR >3.5, the dentist should consult with the patient's physician regarding possible reduction of the anticoagulant dosage before surgery. Minor surgery usually can be performed safely in patients with an INR up to 3.5.

In general, treating these patients without reducing the anticoagulant dose poses a less significant risk than stopping the anticoagulant. The current literature does not support stopping or reducing the dose of the drug, which would increase the risk for thrombotic events. If the physician recommends an alteration of anticoagulant dosage, he or she should manage the adjustment of anticoagulant dosage. At least 3–4 days must pass before the effect of the reduced dosage will be reflected in a decreased INR. The INR value should be checked on the scheduled day of surgery to be certain that the desired reduction of anticoagulation effect has occurred.

If acute infection is present, surgery should be delayed until the infection has been treated. When the patient is free of acute infection and the INR is 3.5 or lower, routine surgery can be performed. The procedure should be done with as little trauma as possible. If excessive postoperative bleeding (slow blood flow and oozing) occurs, one or more of the following measures can be used to control it:

Use a splint constructed before surgery (in cases with multiple extractions)

Pressure using gauze pack

Absorbable gelatin sponge (Gelfoam)

Dental packing blocks:
20 × 20 × 7 mm, can be cut to fit and applied to bleeding site.

Powder: Apply to bleeding site.

Gelfoam with thrombin

Thrombogen: Powder with isotonic saline diluent (5000-unit container with isotonic saline). For bleeding from skin or mucosa, use solution of 100 units/ml. Do not use with Oxycel, Surgicel, or microfibrillar collagen because they inactivate the thrombin.

Oxidized cellulose (Oxycel)

Pad: 3 × 3 inch; pledget: 2 × 1 × 1 inch; strip: 18 × 2, 5 × ½, 36 × ½ inch. Cut to appropriate size and apply dry.

Tranexamic acid (Cyklokapron)

Solution: 100 mg/ml in 10-ml vials; tablets: 500 mg, after surgery 25 mg/kg orally 3 times a day.

Oxidized regenerated cellulose (Surgicel absorbable hemostat)

Surgicel sheets: 2 × 14, 4 × 8, 2 × 3, ½ × 2 inch; Surgicel Nu-Knit sheets: 1 × 1, 3 × 4, 6 × 9 inch. Pick appropriate size and lay over extraction site to control bleeding.

Microfibrillar collagen hemostat (Avitene, CollaTape, Instat MCH)

Avitene sheets: 35 × 35, 70 × 35, 70 × 70 mm; CollaTape: 1 × 3, ¾ × 1½, ⅜ × ¾ inch.

Instat MCH: Coherent fibers packaged in 0.5- and 1.0-g containers. Apply topically, and it adheres firmly to bleeding surfaces.

Collagen hemostat

Pads: 1 × 2, 3 × 4 inch. Apply directly to bleeding surface with pressure. It is more effective when applied dry.

Antiplatelet Therapy

Patients with drug-eluting stents for treatment of coronary artery disease take a combination of aspirin and another antiplatelet drug from the thienopyridine group (clopidogrel, Plavix®; ticlopidine, Ticlid®) for at least 1 yr following placement of the stent. Abrupt discontinuation of this dual antiplatelet therapy in patients prior to routine dental procedures is not recommended. In 2007, the AHA issued an advisory statement that strongly advised against the common practice of discontinuing these agents, which included references to very high mortality rates in at-risk patients who develop thromboemboli.

MANAGEMENT OF ANXIETY IN THE DENTAL PATIENT

Anxiety

The dentist may detect anxiety in a patient on the basis of his or her physical appearance, speech, dress, and presence of certain signs and symptoms. The anxious person looks overalert, displayed in ways such as sitting forward in a chair; moving fingers, arms, or legs; getting up and moving; pacing around the room; checking certain parts of clothing; and straightening ties or scarves.

On the other hand, sloppy dress habits and other signs, just the opposite of a concern with perfection, may also be seen. An anxious person may show signs of being watchful of possessions, always trying to keep them in sight.

The anxious person may speak mechanically and rapidly and at times may seem to block out or not connect thoughts together. The anxious person may respond to questions quickly, often not allowing the dentist to finish a question.

Signs of sweating, tension in muscles, increased breathing, and rapid heart rate may be seen. The patient may complain of an inability to sleep, may wake at an early hour, and may not be able to go back to sleep. Attacks of diarrhea and increased frequency of urination may occur. In general, anxious persons are overalert and tense, feel apprehensive, and have a sense of impending disaster that has no apparent cause. Insomnia, tension, and apprehension lead to fatigue, which makes it even more difficult for the individual to deal with anxiety.

The dentist should talk with the patient and show personal interest. Verbal and nonverbal communication must be consistent. The dentist should confront the patient with the observation that the patient appears anxious, then ask if the individual would like to talk about feelings, which may include the person's attitude toward the dentist. During these discussions, tension-free pauses should be allowed to develop between ideas, as a temporary state of regression will help the patient return to a more anxiety-free state. Some patients may respond well to this approach without ever indicating why they were anxious.

If the patient remains anxious in the dental situation, the dentist can plan to use hypnosis, oral or parenteral sedation agents or nitrous oxide, and oxygen to better manage the dental treatment.

Patients with uncontrolled hyperthyroidism may have associated anxiety. Epinephrine must not be used in these patients, including even the small amounts that are used in local anesthetics. Patients with signs and symptoms of hyperthyroidism should be referred for medical evaluation and treatment.

Dental Management of the Anxious Patient

1. Preoperative
   A. *Behavioral*
      Establish effective communication with the patient; provide instructions
      Be open and honest; let the patient see who you are
      Consistent verbal and nonverbal communication
      Explain procedures and answer any questions
      Explain possible discomfort associated with a procedure
      Explain what you will do to make procedures "pain free"
      Possibly confront patient who appears anxious: "You seem tense today. Would you like to talk about it?"
   B. *Pharmacologic*
      Oral sedation: benzodiazepines

Night before appointment: hypnotic benzodiazepine to aid patient in getting a good night's sleep

Day of appointment: reduce anxiety prior to appointment

Select a drug with an onset of 1 hr or less and at the lowest dosage that will be effective

C. *Informed Consent*

Use a written and verbal informed consent process to ensure that the patient and the patient's perioperative caretaker understand all aspects of the planned sedative and dental procedures

2. Operative

A. *Behavioral*

Allow patient to ask questions

Let patient know if any discomfort will be felt

Reassure patient

B. *Pharmacologic*

Effective local anesthesia

Oral sedation*: benzodiazepines

Inhalation sedation*: nitrous oxide

Intramuscular sedation*

Intravenous sedation*

3. Postoperative

A. *Behavioral*

Explain to patient and patient's caretaker what usually occurs after the procedure

Explain to patient and patient's caretaker what the patient needs to do

Explain to patient and patient's caretaker what the patient needs to avoid

Describe to patient and patient's caretaker what complications can occur and what steps to take to manage them:

Pain

Bleeding

Infection

Allergic reaction to medication

Tell patient and patient's caretaker to inform you if any complications develop

B. *Pharmacologic*

Effective postoperative pain control is essential

Select the most appropriate medication for pain control

Analgesics: nonsteroidal antiinflammatory drugs (NSAIDs) or acetaminophen (in patients who cannot take aspirin/NSAIDs) with codeine, hydrocodone, or oxycodone

Adjunctive medications: antidepressants, muscle relaxants, steroids, anticonvulsants, antibiotics

Specific Drugs and Dosage for Anxiety Control (Dosage for Older Adults and Children Must Be Reduced)

Nitrous oxide, inhalation, titrated to 20%–50%

Diazepam (Valium), oral (2-, 5-, or 10-mg tablets)

Triazolam (Halcion), oral (0.125- or 0.25-mg tablets)

Lorazepam (Ativan), oral (1- or 3-mg tablets)

---

*NOTE: Many states require that dentists have special permits for the use of various sedation modalities; appropriate emergency and monitoring equipment is recommended whenever sedative agents are employed.

Other benzodiazepines or non-benzodiazepines according to practitioner preference and needs of patient (e.g., oxazepam, alprazolam, diphenhydramine, zolpidem)

DEPRESSION IN DENTAL PATIENTS

Signs of low-grade chronic depression include fatigue (even after adequate sleep); difficulty getting up in the morning; restlessness; loss of interest in family, work, and sex; inability to make decisions; anger and resentment; chronic complaining; self-criticism; feelings of inferiority; and excessive daydreaming. Signs of more severe depression include excessive crying, change in sleeping habits, thoughts of food making one sick, weight loss without dieting, strong feelings of guilt, nightmares, thoughts about suicide, feeling unreal or in a "fog," and an inability to concentrate.

Patients with major depression are depressed most of the day, show a marked decrease in interest or pleasure in most activities, have a marked gain or loss in weight, and manifest insomnia or hypersomnia. These symptoms must be present for at least 2 wk before major depression can be diagnosed.

Dental Management
Significant impairment of all personal hygiene may occur during the depth of a depressive episode, including a total lack of oral hygiene. Salivary flow may be reduced, and patients may complain of xerostomia (dry mouth), an increased rate of dental caries, and periodontal disease. The xerostomia may be compounded by the side effects of the medications used to treat depression. Complaints of glossodynia and various facial pain syndromes are common.

The dentist should provide an aggressive preventive dental education program for depressed patients, including the use of artificial salivary products, antiseptic mouthwash, and daily fluoride mouth rinses. Xerostomia provides an excellent environment for overgrowth of *Candida albicans*; as a result, patients are likely to require treatment for candidiasis along with treatment for dry mouth.

Small amounts of epinephrine (0.04 mg or 2 cartridges of a 1 : 100,000 concentration) can be used in patients taking tricyclic or heterocyclic antidepressants, provided the dentist aspirates before injecting and injects the anesthetic slowly. In general, no more than two cartridges should be injected at any appointment. Excessive amounts of epinephrine can result in hypertension. Levonordefrin is contraindicated in patients taking tricyclics or heterocyclics because of the possibility of an exaggerated sympathomimetic response. A lower dosage of sedative medications may be necessary to avoid excessive CNS depression (Table 1).

Patients taking tricyclic or heterocyclic antidepressant drugs may be prone to orthostatic hypotension. Dentists should avoid rapid changes in chair position for these patients and provide support when patients first get out of the dental chair. Atropine should be used with care because increased intraocular pressure can result. Acetaminophen should be used with care because it can decrease the metabolic rate of the heterocyclics, which could lead to toxic levels of the tricyclic antidepressant.

Text continued on p. 47

TABLE 1
Adverse Drug Interactions of Significance to Dentistry

Dental Drug	Interacting Drug	Medical Condition/ Situation	Effect
Antibiotics			
β-Lactams (penicillins, cephalosporins)	Allopurinol (Lopurin, Zyloprim)	Gout	Incidence of minor allergic reactions to ampicillin is increased. Other penicillins have not been implicated. **Recommendation:** Avoid ampicillin.
	β-blockers (Tenormin, Lopressor, Inderal, Corgard)	Hypertension	Serum levels of atenolol are reduced after prolonged use of ampicillin. Anaphylactic reactions to penicillins or other drugs may be more severe in patients taking β-blockers because of increased mediator release from mast cells. **Recommendation:** Use ampicillin cautiously, advise patient of potential reaction.
	Tetracyclines and other bacteriostatic antibiotics	Infection, acne, periodontal disease	Effectiveness of penicillins and cephalosporins may be reduced by bacteriostatic agents. **Recommendation:** Avoid interaction.
Tetracyclines	Antacids	Dyspepsia, gastroesophageal reflux, peptic ulcer	Antacids, dairy products, and other agents containing divalent and trivalent cations will chelate tetracyclines and limit their absorption in the gut. Doxycycline is least influenced by this interaction. **Recommendation:** Avoid interaction.

	Insulin	Diabetes mellitus	
Metronidazole			Doxycycline and oxytetracycline have been documented as enhancing the hypoglycemic effects of exogenously administered insulin. **Recommendation:** Select different antibiotic or increase carbohydrate intake.
	Ethanol	Alcohol use or abuse	Severe disulfiramlike reactions are well documented. **Recommendation:** Avoid interaction.
	Lithium	Manic depression	Inhibits renal excretion of lithium, leading to elevated/toxic levels of lithium. Lithium toxicity produces confusion, ataxia, and kidney damage. **Recommendation:** Avoid interaction.
	Benzodiazepines	Anxiety	Delayed metabolism of benzodiazepine, increasing the pharmacologic effects can result in excessive sedation and irrational behavior. **Recommendation:** Reduce dose of benzodiazepine.
	Carbamazepine (Tegretol)	Seizure disorder	Increased blood levels of carbamazepine leading to toxicity (symptoms include drowsiness, dizziness, nausea, headache, and blurred vision). Hospitalization has been required. **Recommendation:** Avoid interaction.
	Cyclosporine	Organ transplant	Enhanced immunosuppression and nephrotoxicity. **Recommendation:** Avoid interaction, monitor patient.

Continued

TABLE 1
Adverse Drug Interactions of Significance to Dentistry—cont'd

Dental Drug	Interacting Drug	Medical Condition/Situation	Effect
	Lovastatin, pravastatin, simvastatin, other statins	Hyperlipidemia	Muscle (eosinophilia) myalgia and rhabdomyolysis. **Recommendation:** Avoid interaction.
	Prednisone, methylprednisolone	Autoimmune disorders, organ transplant	Increased risk of Cushing's syndrome and immunosuppression. **Recommendation:** Monitor patient, shorten duration of antibiotic administration if possible.
	Theophylline (Theo-Dur)	Asthma	Some macrolide antibiotics (erythromycin, clarithromycin) inhibit metabolism of theophylline, leading to toxic serum levels (symptoms of toxicity: headache, nausea, vomiting, confusion, thirst, cardiac arrhythmias, convulsions). Conversely, theophylline reduces serum levels of erythromycin. **Recommendation:** Avoid prescribing these antibiotics in such patients.
Antibiotics (especially erythromycin and tetracycline)	Digoxin (Lanoxin)	Congestive heart failure	Alters gastrointestinal flora and retards metabolism of digoxin in approximately 10% of patients, resulting in dangerously high digoxin serum levels that may persist for several weeks after discontinuation of antibiotic. Strongest documentation for erythromycin and tetracycline. Patients should be cautioned to report any signs of digitalis toxicity (salivation, visual disturbances, arrhythmias) during antibiotic therapy. **Recommendation:** Avoid interaction by using noninteractive antibiotic.

Antibiotics (cephalosporins, erythromycin, clarithromycin, metronidazole)	Warfarin (Coumadin)	Atrial fibrillation, MI, post major surgery, stroke prevention	Anticoagulant effect of warfarin may be increased by several antibiotic classes. Reduced synthesis of vitamin K by gut flora is a putative mechanism, but several antibiotics have antiplatelet and anticoagulant activity. Most convincing documentation for cephalosporins, macrolide antibiotics, and metronidazole. **Recommendation:** Penicillins, tetracyclines, and clindamycin are preferred choices but must be used cautiously.
Macrolide antibiotics (erythromycin, clarithromycin)	Benzodiazepines with high oral bioavailability (triazolam, midazolam)	Infection	Reduced hepatic first-pass metabolism of benzodiazepine with increased blood level and unpredictably increased levels of CNS depression. **Recommendation:** Avoid interaction with alternative sedative or reduce dose of interacting benzodiazepine.
Azole antifungal agents (e.g., ketoconazole, Nizoral®)	Benzodiazepines	Systemic fungal infection	Reduced hepatic metabolism (CYP 3A4 inhibition) of benzodiazepine results in unpredictably increased CNS depression. **Recommendation:** Avoid interaction with alternative sedative agent or reduce dose of interacting benzodiazepine.
Analgesics			
Acetaminophen	Alcohol	Alcohol use and abuse	Increased risk of liver toxicity, especially during fasting state or over 4 g/day acetaminophen, exacerbated by abrupt discontinuation of alcohol use. **Recommendation:** Use lower dose of acetaminophen, allow patient to continue alcohol use. (NOTE: alcohol-related liver damage may absolutely contraindicate use of acetaminophen.)

Continued

TABLE 1
Adverse Drug Interactions of Significance to Dentistry—cont'd

Dental Drug	Interacting Drug	Medical Condition/Situation	Effect
Aspirin	Oral hypoglycemics (sulfonylureas: glyburide, chlorpropamide, acetohexamide)	Diabetes Type 2	Increased hypoglycemic effects. **Recommendation:** Avoid interaction.
Aspirin, NSAIDs	Anticoagulants (warfarin, Coumadin)	Atrial fibrillation, myocardial infarction, postsurgery	Increased risk of gastrointestinal bleeding. **Recommendation:** Avoid interaction.
Aspirin, NSAIDs	Alcohol	Alcohol use and abuse	Increases risk of GI bleeding. **Recommendation:** Lower dose, encourage discontinuation of alcohol use.
NSAIDs	β-Blocker angiotensin-converting enzyme inhibitor	Hypertension, postmyocardial infarction	Decreased antihypertensive effect. **Recommendation:** Limit duration of NSAID dosage to approximately 4 days.
NSAIDs	Lithium	Manic depression	Produces symptoms of lithium toxicity, including nausea, vomiting, slurred speech, and mental confusion. **Recommendation:** NSAIDs should not be prescribed to patients with manic depression who take lithium. It can result in toxic levels of lithium.

NSAIDs	Methotrexate (MTX)	Connective tissue disease, cancer therapy	Toxic levels of MTX may accumulate. **Recommendation:** Avoid interaction if patient on high-dose MTX for cancer therapy. Low-dose MTX for arthritis is not a concern.
SSRI	Antidepressants	Depressive disease	Increased risk of GI irritation
Anesthetics, local			
All agents	Other local anesthetics		Additive effect of two local anesthetics increases risk. **Recommendation:** Limit dose of each.
	Opioids, sedatives		Sedation with opioids may increase risk of local anesthetic toxicity, especially in children. **Recommendation:** Reduce anesthetic dose.
Sedatives			
Barbiturates	Digoxin, theophylline, corticosteroids, oral anticoagulants	CHF, asthma, autoimmune disease, atrial fibrillation	Barbiturates bind cytochrome P450 system in liver, enhance metabolism of many drugs. **Recommendation:** Limit dose, observe for adverse effects.
	Benzodiazepines, alcohol, antihistamines	Anxiety, alcohol use and abuse, seasonal allergies	Additive effects for sedation and respiratory depression. **Recommendation:** Reduce dose, administer combination of sedatives with extreme caution.

Continued

TABLE 1
Adverse Drug Interactions of Significance to Dentistry—cont'd

Dental Drug	Interacting Drug	Medical Condition/Situation	Effect
Benzodiazepines (BZ; e.g., alprazolam, chlordiazepoxide, diazepam)	Cimetidine, oral contraceptives, fluoxetine, isoniazid (INH), alcohol	Peptic ulcer disease, depression, tuberculosis, alcohol use and abuse	Delayed metabolism of BZDP, increasing pharmacologic effects can result in excessive sedation and irrational behavior. **Recommendation:** Reduce dose of BZDP. Delayed metabolism of BZDP, increasing pharmacologic effects can result in excessive sedation and irrational behavior. **Recommendation:** Reduce dose of BZDP.
	Digoxin (Lanoxin), phenytoin, theophylline (Theo-Dur)	CHF, epilepsy, asthma	Serum concentrations of digoxin, phenytoin may be increased, resulting in toxicity. Antagonize sedative effects of BZDP. **Recommendation:** Avoid interaction.
	Protease inhibitors (Indinavir, Nelfinavir)	HIV, AIDS	Increased bioavailability and effects of BZDP, especially triazolam and oral midazolam. **Recommendation:** Avoid interaction.
Vasoconstrictor			
Epinephrine and levonordefrin (Neo-Cobefrin)	Nonselective β-blockers: propranolol (Inderal), nadolol (Corgard), penbutolol (Levatol), pindolol (Visken), sotalol (Betapace), timolol (Blocadren)	Angina pectoris, hypertension, glaucoma, migraine, headache, hyperthyroidism, panic syndromes	Unopposed effects: increased B/P with secondary bradycardia. **Recommendation:** Limit or avoid epinephrine, aspirate to avoid intravascular injection, inject slowly. Avoid epinephrine-containing retraction cord and higher concentrations of epinephrine in the dental anesthetic.

Cocaine	Illicit use, topical anesthetic for mucous membrane procedures	Blocks reuptake of norepinephrine and intensifies postsynaptic response to epinephrine-like drugs. This potentiates the adrenergic effects on the heart, with potential for a heart attack. **Recommendation:** Recognize signs and symptoms of cocaine abuse. Avoid use of vasoconstrictors in these patients until cocaine has been withheld for at least 24 hr.
Halothane	General anesthetic for surgical procedures	Stimulation of 1 and receptors resulting in arrhythmia at doses greater than 2 g/kg. **Recommendation:** Limit dose to remain below 2 g/kg threshold, aspirate to avoid intravascular injection. Monitor vital signs. Avoid epinephrine-containing retraction cord and concentrations of epinephrine greater than 1:100,000.
Tricyclic antidepressants (amitriptyline [Elavil], doxepin [Sinequan], imipramine [Tofranil])	Depression, severe anxiety, neuropathic pain, attention deficit disorder	Blocks reuptake of norepinephrine resulting in unopposed effects (increased B/P, increased heart rate), potential cardiac arrhythmias; effect is greater with levonordefrin. **Recommendation:** Limit dose or avoid vasoconstrictors, aspirate to avoid intravascular injection. Monitor vital signs. Avoid epinephrine-containing retraction cord and higher concentrations of epinephrine in the dental anesthetic.

Continued

TABLE 1
Adverse Drug Interactions of Significance to Dentistry—cont'd

Dental Drug	Interacting Drug	Medical Condition/Situation	Effect
	Peripheral adrenergic antagonists (reserpine [Serpasil], guanethidine [Ismelin], guanadrel [Hylorell])	Hypertension	Potential for increased sensitivity of adrenergic receptors to epinephrine and levonordefrin. **Recommendation:** Administer cautiously. Monitor vital signs during and following administration of first cartridge. Limit dose or avoid epinephrin. Aspirate to avoid intravascular injection. Avoid epinephrine-containing retraction cord and higher concentrations of epinephrine in the dental anesthetic.
	Catechol-O-methyltransferase inhibitors (tolcapone [Tasmar], entacapone [Comtan])	Parkinson's disease	Potential for increased sensitivity of adrenergic receptors to epinephrine and levonordefrin, resulting in increased heart rate and B/P and arrhythmias. **Recommendation:** Administer cautiously. Monitor vital signs during and after administration of first cartridge. Limit dose or avoid epinephrine. Aspirate to avoid intravascular injection. Avoid epinephrine-containing retraction cord and higher concentrations of epinephrine in the dental anesthetic.

Phenobarbital increases the metabolism of tricyclic antidepressants, which can attenuate their antidepressant effects.

No medical contraindication exists for dental treatment during a depressive episode; however, most depressed patients may be best managed by dealing with their immediate dental needs only during the depression. More complex dental procedures can be performed once the patient has responded to medical treatment.

Patients with signs and symptoms of severe depression must be referred for medical evaluation and treatment. If the patient is not responsive to this recommendation, the problem should be shared with a family member and every attempt made to get the individual to medical attention. During severe depression, suicide is always a possibility; however, medical treatment currently is able to reduce this possibility.

Suicidal Patients

Studies have shown that questions about suicide do not prompt these patients to act. The dentist should ask the very depressed patient if he or she has had any thoughts about suicide. Patients who state they have had these thoughts must be referred for immediate medical care; members of the family need to be involved if possible.

Bisphosphonate-Associated Osteonecrosis of the Jaw (Osteochemonecrosis)

With the increased frequency of bisphosphonate use for the treatment of osteoporosis (e.g., alendronate, Fosamax®), dentists have been alerted to the possibility of osteonecrosis of the jaw related to these drugs. These medications are also used in other resorptive bone diseases, including breast and prostate cancer metastatic to the bones, Paget's disease, and cases of bone fragility related to chronic renal failure. This group of drugs currently includes aminobisphosphonates (alendronate, Fosamax; ibandronate, Boniva; pamidronate, Aredia; risedronate, Actonel; and zoledronate, Zometa) and non-aminobisphosphonates (clodronate, Bonefos; etidronate, Didronel; and tiludronate, Skelid). These agents are used both orally and intravenously, with the intravenous agents appearing to place the patient at a much higher risk for osteonecrosis of the jaw. There are no prospective, randomized scientific studies on which to base dental management algorithms for these patients, but guidelines presently exist, based on retrospective studies and case reports.

Clinically, osteonecrosis of the jaw usually presents as exposed bone in the maxillofacial area, reportedly more frequently in the mandible, spontaneously or following oral surgery, that does not heal within 6 wk (confirmed when other possible causes have been ruled out [e.g., osteoradionecrosis]). Signs and symptoms may include one or more of the following: mucosal ulceration with exposed bone; infection (with or without purulence); pain or swelling in the affected jaw; and/or paresthesia (numbness, tingling) or other sensory alterations (e.g., "heavy jaw"), delayed or incomplete healing, or a sudden deterioration of periodontal health. Additional risk factors include patients in poor health or with a compromised immune system (e.g., long-term corticosteroid therapy) and bony exostoses (e.g., tori). Currently, there are no blood tests that are predictive of the disorder. Endodontically treated teeth in patients with risk factors for bisphosphonate-related osteonecrosis of the jaw must be followed carefully, because low-level, residual infection and inflammation may, over time, result in the condition.

This condition occurs only rarely in patients taking oral bisphosphonates, but a higher risk has been determined for the intravenous agents in this group. The dental management of patients at risk for osteonecrosis includes identification of at-risk patients and the following:

• Patients should have a comprehensive dental exam prior to starting bisphosphonate therapy and should be reevaluated every 6 mo or more frequently, as appropriate
• Oral surgical and other invasive dental procedures should be completed before starting bisphosphonate therapy
• The dental team should emphasize excellent oral hygiene for patients on bisphosphonate therapy
• If dental treatment is necessary after bisphosphonate therapy has been started, the least invasive (nonsurgical) technique is recommended, although routine restorative and dental hygiene procedures may be performed
• The risks and potential benefits of withholding bisphosphonate therapy should be discussed with the patient and the patient's treating physician(s) prior to tooth extraction or other oral surgical procedures. Recently, the American Association of Oral and Maxillofacial Surgeons (AAOMS) has recommended that consideration be given to suspending the use of a bisphosphonate prior to

oral and maxillofacial surgery procedures to reduce the risk of bisphosphonate-related osteonecrosis of the jaw, but this measure is not based on randomized, prospective studies and should not be undertaken without consideration of the potential medical consequences (e.g., fractures) and without the input from the physician prescribing the bisphosphonate
• In patients with oral osteonecrosis, conservative management is recommended and includes the use of antibiotics, antibacterial mouth rinses, limited debridement of the site, and analgesic medications to control pain associated with the osteonecrosis. Steroid drugs may increase the risk for development of osteonecrosis.
• The dental management of patients at risk for bisphosphonate-related osteonecrosis should include appropriate informed consent prior to the performance of actual dental procedures

ADVERSE DRUG INTERACTIONS
Table 1 provides a summary of adverse drug interactions for commonly used dental drugs. Monographs should be referred to for more specific information.

COMPLEMENTARY MEDICINES, NUTRITIONAL/HERBAL SUPPLEMENTS, AND DENTISTRY
The term alternative medicine is used to describe practices that are used instead of mainstream medical practice. Complementary medicine refers to practices that are used as adjuncts to conventional medicine. These systems are divided into five major categories: alternative medical systems (traditional Chinese medicine, Ayurveda medicine of India, and Native American healing

approaches), biologically based therapies (natural products), manipulative and body-based methods (chiropractic and osteopathic manipulation), mind–body interventions (hypnosis, cognitive therapies, and biofeedback), and energy therapies (use of magnets and acupuncture). Both of these systems use treatments that often have no established efficacy. An estimated 42% of Americans use alternative and complementary medicine therapies.

Complementary medicines are defined as herbal medicines, homeopathic remedies, and essential oils. The basic principle of homeopathy is selection of a remedy that if given to a healthy individual, will produce a range of symptoms similar to those observed in the ill patient (like cures like). Only minute amounts are given to avoid toxicity. Only one remedy is used at any one time. Dilute tinctures are used rather than concentrated ones. In homeopathic practice, medication in tablet form is commonly used.

The standard tinctures used in Western tradition herbal medicine are very different from those used in homeopathy. Alcohol is used to dissolve the plant, and the final product is not diluted. Thus, these remedies are concentrated, highly potent preparations and usually are taken as the unmodified liquid tincture. Other preparations used in herbal remedies include lotions and creams for topical application. Tablet form of medication is not used very often (less than 5%).

Efficacy of Herbal Medicines

Many herbal remedies have been used for hundreds of years. However, traditional use is not a good indication of efficacy. The gold standard for testing efficacy is the randomized clinical trial (RCT). This standard should apply as much to herbal medicines as to conventional medicines. A number of RCTs of herbal medical products have been conducted. However, many of these studies differ with regard to how they were conducted and in their findings. Ernst suggests that the best way to evaluate a number of RCTs on the efficacy of a specific herbal medicine is to do a systematic review or meta-analysis of all RCTs for that product.

Herbal medicines with proven efficacy:

Several herbal remedies have been repeatedly tested in placebo-controlled RCTs. Systematic reviews of these studies have shown that some herbal medicines are effective for certain conditions. For example, ginkgo biloba has been shown to be effective for symptomatic treatment of dementia and intermittent claudication. Table 2 lists the more commonly used herbal medicines that have proved to be effective for the condition(s) listed.

Herbal medicines with doubtful or no efficacy:

Asian ginseng, one of the most popular herbal medicines in the United States, showed no convincing evidence for efficacy as a general tonic or in enhancing mental and physical performance. A review of studies regarding the use of valerian as a hypnotic agent was inconclusive because of flaws in the study designs. A systematic review of RCTs found no evidence that evening primrose was effective for treatment of premenstrual syndrome in women. Garlic was not found to be effective as a cholesterol-lowering drug. *For more information on the efficacy of herbal medicines, see on the Companion CD-ROM and*

TABLE 2

Claims for Herbal Actions Supported by Clinical Trials

Herb	Claimed Action	Effectiveness Supported by Clinical Trials
Kava	Used to treat anxiety.	Clinical trials have shown it reduces anxiety significantly more than placebo.
Artichoke	Used to lower the lipid levels in blood.	Only one randomized clinical study shows it moderately lowers elevated total cholesterol levels when given orally for several weeks.
Feverfew	Used for women's ailments and inflammatory diseases. Recently has been suggested for headache and migraine.	Three studies showed greater effect than placebo in alleviating symptoms of headache or migraine.
Garlic	Used to reduce blood pressure and lower blood lipid levels.	Data show a small but statistically significant reduction in systolic and diastolic blood pressures. No data support claims for lipid-lowering properties of garlic.
Ginger	Used to treat nausea and vomiting.	Several studies support the antiemetic use for ginger. Used to treat or prevent nausea or vomiting.
Ginkgo biloba	Used to treat cerebral insufficiency, prevent loss of cognitive function, and tinnitus.	Studies have shown it is effective in the treatment of cerebral insufficiency when given for 4–6 weeks. Data show that regular oral intake of ginkgo biloba slows the loss of cognitive function in patients with dementia.
Hawthorn	Used to treat heart failure.	Various studies show it is effective for the early signs of congestive heart failure.
Horse chestnut	Used to treat venous congestion.	Studies have shown it is effective in reducing signs and symptoms of chronic venous insufficiency.
Saw palmetto	Used in Europe to treat prostate enlargement.	Clinical trials support its use for symptoms of benign prostatic hypertrophy.
St. John's wort	Used to treat depression.	Studies show that it is effective for treating mild to moderate depression. The question of its effectiveness for severe depression remains to be answered.

Evolve site Table 3—Claims for Herbal Actions Unsupported by Clinical Trials.

Side Effects and Adverse Reactions

Recent increased use of herbal remedies seems to come from the public's view that natural products are harmless or at least have fewer side effects than regular drugs. The assumption that phytomedicines (herbal medicines) have only beneficial effects has proved to be incorrect.

Toxicity can be associated with use of herbal remedies. These reactions can be caused by accidental or deliberate contamination of the product. For example, lead, mercury, cadmium, pesticides, microorganisms, and fumigants have been found to contaminate some herbal products. Substitution of animal substances such as enzymes, hormones, or organ extracts and synthetic drugs has accounted for some of the toxic reactions to herbal products. Adulteration by accidental or deliberate substitution of the original plant material by other plant species has been reported to be a source of toxic reactions to herbal products.

Other sources of adverse reactions to herbal products are intrinsic or plant associated. In some cases, the manufacturer ignored the known toxicity of a plant or constituent in the herbal product. In other cases, the product contains plants for which no or insufficient data regarding safety are available. If a highly concentrated or specifically processed extract is used, toxic reactions may occur. If a plant contains constituents known to affect the bioavailability and/or pharmacokinetics of other drugs, serious drug interactions can occur.

Long-term users, consumers of large amounts of phytomedicines, or people who use many different medicinal products may be prone to side effects. Pregnant or nursing women, babies, and the elderly, sick, and undernourished are at higher risk for side effects. Some of the more common side effects associated with herbal remedies include bleeding with ginkgo biloba; upset stomach, fatigue, dizziness, confusion, dry mouth, and photosensitivity with St. John's wort; high blood pressure, arrhythmias, nervousness, headaches, heart attack, or stroke with ephedra; and sleepiness, rash, and motor dysfunction of skeletal muscles with kava kava. *For more information on serious adverse reactions from the use of natural products, see on the Companion CD-ROM and Evolve site Table 4—Selected Herbal Medicines with Potentially Serious Adverse Effects.*

Medical Problems

Certain medical problems can make consumption of herbal medicines unsafe. Individuals with high blood pressure, thyroid disease, psychiatric disorders, Parkinson's disease, enlarged prostate gland, diabetes mellitus, heart disease, epilepsy, glaucoma, blood clotting problems, and a history of stroke should check with their physician before taking any herbal remedies. Patients with a history of aspirin allergy can be at risk if they take an herb containing willow bark.

Drug Interactions

For more information on drug interactions, see on the Companion CD-ROM and Evolve site Table 5—Selected Natural Medicines that Potentiate or Interfere with Approved Prescription and Over-the-Counter Drugs. Important drug interactions can occur between certain herbal products and conventional medications. The most common drug involved with drug–herb interactions is warfarin. The most common herb involved with these interactions is St. John's wort. Long-term administration of St. John's wort may result in diminished clinical effectiveness or increased dosage requirements for all CYP3A4 substrates, which represent approximately 50% of all prescription medications. Garlic extracts alter the disposition of coadministered medications metabolized by the CYP3A4 pathway.

Patients taking aspirin, warfarin, ticlopidine, clopidogrel, or dipyridamole should not take ginkgo biloba because bleeding may occur. Patients taking an antidepressant should not take St. John's wort. Patients taking a decongestant, a stimulant drug, or who drink caffeinated beverages should not take ephedra. Individuals taking a benzodiazepine, a barbiturate, an antipsychotic medication, or any medicine used to treat Parkinson's disease should not take kava kava products. It is important that patients notify their general practitioner if they are taking phytomedicines concurrently with conventional drugs, especially those with cardiac, diuretic, sedative, hypotensive, or other properties. Individuals taking a prescription medicine should check with their physician before taking any herbal health product.

Dental Implications

A limited number of papers describe the use of complementary and alternative medical systems for dental problems. Dentists should accept and encompass science-based advances and reject unproved or disproved methods. Selected unconventional treatments can be incorporated into conventional dentistry in certain patients for specific purposes that will be beneficial to the patient.

Information for Dentists

Herbal remedies have the potential to affect the safety of invasive or prolonged dental procedures. Excessive bleeding can occur with some of these medications. Other herbal medicines may affect the cardiovascular system and render the patient more susceptible to cardiac arrhythmias and other cardiovascular complications. Ginseng may cause hypoglycemia. Chinese cancer patients undergoing chemotherapy who were users of Chinese herbal medicine were found to have higher scores of mucositis. It is important for the dentist to include a section in the patient's medical history on the consumption of herbal medications and over-the-counter drugs. Because most U.S. dental schools teach very little on the use, side effects, toxicity, and drug interactions associated with herbal remedies, the dentist must find a way to become informed regarding these issues.

Important references for dentists are *Mosby's Medical Drug Reference 2007,* by Allan J. Ellsworth, and *Natural Standard Herb and Supplement Reference,* Mosby, 2005. Dentists should use only treatment procedures that have been established to be effective and with minimal risks involved. As clinical trials demonstrate certain alternative and complementary treatments to be effective and safe, they can be incorporated into conventional medicine and dentistry. The dentist may find a medically compromised patient is taking an herbal remedy that is potentially harmful. This should be discussed with the patient and the patient referred to his or her physician for evaluation and management.

MONOCLONAL ANTIBODY THERAPY

Monoclonal antibodies are antibodies that are produced to specifically bind to cells that underlie disease processes (e.g., cancer cells and inflammatory cells involved in autoimmune diseases). They may be produced using viruses, yeasts, or transgenic mice. Monoclonal antibodies that specifically bind to certain substances can also be manufactured and can be used to test for the presence of specific substances within cells, which function as the antigen. Monoclonal antibodies have been produced to treat cancer, cardiovascular disease, inflammatory diseases, macular degeneration, transplant rejection, multiple sclerosis, and viral infections. Dental patients who have received monoclonal antibodies or are in monoclonal antibody therapy have serious systemic medical conditions and should be treated only in consultation with the treating physician(s). Categories of therapeutic monoclonal antibodies include the following specific agents (most named with the suffix—mab to denote their status as a "Monoclonal Antibody"):

• Anti-inflammatory: infliximab, adalimumab, etanercept, basiliximab, daclizumab, omlizumab

• Anti-cancer: alemtuzumab, bevacizumab, cetuximab, gemtuzumab, nimotuzumab, rituximab, trastuzumab

• Other: palivizumab, abciximab

Bibliography

1. ADA: *ADA/PDR Guide to Dental Therapeutics*, ed 5, Chicago, 2006, ADA/Thomson PDR.
2. ADA and AAOS: Antibiotic prophylaxis for dental patients with total joint replacements, *JADA* 134:895, 2003.
3. American Academy of Oral and Maxillofacial Surgeons. Position paper on bisphosphonate-related osteonecrosis of the jaw—2009 update. www.AAOS.org, 2009.
4. American Heart Association Science Advisory: Prevention of premature discontinuation of dual antiplatelet therapy in patients with coronary artery stents, *Circulation* 115(6):813–818, 2007.
5. Baddour LM et al: A summary of the update on cardiovascular implantable electronic device infections and their managment: A scientific statement from the American Heart Association. *JADA* 142(2):159–165, 2011.
6. Jeske AH, Suchko GD: Lack of a scientific basis for routine discontinuation of anticoagulant therapy prior to dental therapy, *JADA* 134:1492–1497, 2003.
7. Little JW: Behavioral and psychiatric disorders. In Little JW, Falace DA, Miller CS, Rhodus NL, editors: *Dental management of the medically compromised patient*, ed 6, St. Louis, 2002, Mosby.
8. Little JW: Anxiety disorders: dental implications, *J Gen Dent* 51:562–570, 2003.
9. Little JW: Dental implication of mood disorders, *J Gen Dent* 52:442, 2004.
10. Little JW: Complementary and alternative medicine: impact on dentistry, *Oral Surg Oral Med Oral Path Oral Radiol Endod* 98:137, 2004.
11. Little JW: Drugs, drugs, and more drugs: their impact on dentistry, *J Northwest Dent* July–August:23, 2005.
12. Little JW, et al: Antithrombotic agents: implications in dentistry, *Oral Surg Oral Med Oral Path Oral Radiol Endod* 93:544, 2002.

54   Medically Compromised Patients

13. Miller CS: Drug interactions of significance to dentistry. In Little JW, Falace DA, Miller CS, Rhodus NL, editors: *Dental management of the medically compromised patient*, ed 6, St. Louis, 2002, Mosby.

14. Miller CS, Little JW, Falace DA: Need of supplemental corticosteroids for dental patients with adrenal insufficiency: reconsideration of the problem, *JADA* 132:1570, 2001.

15. Rhodus NL: Therapeutic management of common oral lesions. In Little JW, Falace DA, Miller CS, Rhodus NL, editors: *Dental management of the medically compromised patient*, ed 6, St. Louis, 2002, Mosby.

16. Ruggiero S, Gralow J, Marx RE, et al: Practice guidelines for the prevention, diagnosis and treatment of osteonecrosis of the jaw in patients with cancer, *J Oncol Prac* 2(1):7–14, 2006.

17. Siegel MA, Silverman S, Sollecato TP, editors: *American Academy of Oral Medicine: clinician's guide to treatment of common oral conditions*, ed 6, Baltimore, 2005, B.C. Decker.

18. Wilson W, Taubert KA, Gewitz M, et al: Prevention of infective endocarditis. Guidelines from the American Heart Association. *JADA* 138:739–760, 2007.

abacavir
ah-**bah'**-cah-veer
(Ziagen)

CATEGORY AND SCHEDULE
Pregnancy Risk Category: C

Drug Class: Antiviral,
nucleoside analog

MECHANISM OF ACTION
An antiretroviral that inhibits the
activity of HIV-1 reverse
transcriptase by competing with the
natural substrate deoxyguanosine-5'-
triphosphate (dGTP) and by its
incorporation into viral DNA.
Therapeutic Effect: Inhibits viral
DNA growth.

USES
Used in combination with other
antiviral drugs for treatment of
HIV-1 infection

PHARMACOKINETICS
Rapidly and extensively absorbed
after PO administration. Protein
binding: 50%. Widely distributed,
including to CSF and erythrocytes.
Metabolized in the liver to inactive
metabolites. Primarily excreted in
urine. Unknown if removed by
hemodialysis. *Half-life:* 1.5 hr.

INDICATIONS AND DOSAGES
▸ **HIV Infection (in combination with
other antiretrovirals)**
PO
Adults. 300 mg twice a day.
Children (3 mo–16 yr). 8 mg/kg
twice a day. Maximum: 300 mg
twice a day.
▸ **Dosage in Hepatic Impairment**
Mild Impairment. 200 mg twice a
day.

Moderate to Severe Impairment. Not
recommended.

SIDE EFFECTS/ADVERSE REACTIONS
Adults
Frequent
Nausea, nausea with vomiting,
diarrhea, decreased appetite
Occasional
Insomnia

Children
Frequent
Nausea with vomiting, fever,
headache, diarrhea, rash
Occasional
Decreased appetite

PRECAUTIONS AND CONTRAINDICATIONS
Hypersensitivity to abacavir or its
components
Caution:
Breast-feeding, bone marrow
depression, renal or hepatic
impairment, use with other antivirals
to avoid emergence of resistant
viruses, avoid alcohol use

DRUG INTERACTIONS OF CONCERN TO DENTISTRY
• None reported

SERIOUS REACTIONS
! A hypersensitivity reaction may
be life threatening. Signs and
symptoms include fever, rash,
fatigue, intractable nausea and
vomiting, severe diarrhea, abdominal
pain, cough, pharyngitis, and
dyspnea.
! Life-threatening hypotension may
occur.
! Lactic acidosis and severe
hepatomegaly may occur.

DENTAL CONSIDERATIONS

General:
• Examine for oral manifestation of opportunistic infection.
• Patient on chronic drug therapy may rarely have symptoms of blood dyscrasias, which include infection, bleeding, and poor healing.
• Avoid dental light in patient's eyes; offer dark glasses for patient comfort.
• Place on frequent recall because of oral side effects.
• Consider semisupine chair position for patient comfort if GI side effects occur.

Consultations:
• In a patient with symptoms of blood dyscrasias, request a medical consultation for blood studies and postpone treatment until normal values are reestablished.
• Medical consultation may be required to assess disease control.

Teach Patient/Family to:
• Encourage effective oral hygiene to prevent soft tissue inflammation.
• Prevent trauma when using oral hygiene aids.
• Be alert for the possibility of secondary oral infection and the need to see dentist immediately if signs of infection occur.

abarelix
ah-**bar**'-eh-lix
(Plenaxis)

CATEGORY AND SCHEDULE
Pregnancy Risk Category: X

Drug Class: Antineoplastic

MECHANISM OF ACTION
A luteinizing hormone-releasing hormone (LHRH) antagonist that inhibits gonadotropin and androgen production by blocking gonadotropin releasing-hormone receptors in the pituitary.
Therapeutic Effect: Suppresses luteinizing hormone, follicle-stimulating hormone secretion, reducing the secretion of testosterone by the testes.

USES
Treatment of cancer of the breasts, endometrium, and prostate

PHARMACOKINETICS
Slowly absorbed following intramuscular administration. Distributed extensively. Protein binding: 96%–99%. *Half-life:* 13.2 days.

INDICATIONS AND DOSAGES
▸ Prostate Cancer
IM
Adults, Elderly. 100 mg on days 1, 15, and 29 and every 4 wk thereafter. Treatment failure can be detected by obtaining serum testosterone concentration prior to abarelix administration, day 19 and every 8 wk thereafter.

SIDE EFFECTS/ADVERSE REACTIONS
Frequent
Hot flashes, sleep disturbances, breast enlargement
Occasional
Breast pain, nipple tenderness, back pain, constipation, peripheral edema, dizziness, upper respiratory tract infection, diarrhea
Rare
Fatigue, nausea, dysuria, micturition frequency, urinary retention, UTI

PRECAUTIONS AND CONTRAINDICATIONS
This drug should not be used in women and children.

DRUG INTERACTIONS OF CONCERN TO DENTISTRY
• Dental drug interactions have not been studied.

SERIOUS REACTIONS
! Immediate-onset systemic allergic reaction characterized by hypotension, urticaria, pruritus, periorbital and/or circumoral edema, shortness of breath, wheezing, and syncope may occur.
! Prolongation of the QT interval may occur. Tightening of throat, tongue swelling, wheezing, shortness of breath, and low blood pressure occur rarely.

DENTAL CONSIDERATIONS
General:
• If additional analgesia is required for dental pain, consider alternative analgesics (NSAIDs) in patients taking narcotics for acute or chronic pain.
• This drug may be used in the hospital or on an outpatient basis. Confirm the patient's disease and treatment status.
Consultations:
• Medical consultation may be required to assess disease control and patient's ability to tolerate stress.
Teach Patient/Family to:
• Encourage effective oral hygiene to prevent soft tissue inflammation.
• Prevent trauma when using oral hygiene aids.
• Update health and medication history if physician makes any changes in evaluation or drug

regimens; include OTC, herbal, and nonherbal remedies in the update.

abatacept
ah-**bat'**-ah-cept
(Orencia)

CATEGORY AND SCHEDULE
Pregnancy Risk Category: C

Drug Class: Antirheumatic, disease modifying

MECHANISM OF ACTION
Selective costimulation modulator; inhibits T-cell activation by binding to CD80 and CD86 on antigen presenting cells, thus blocking the required CD28 interaction and inhibiting autoimmune T-cell activation.

USES
Rheumatoid arthritis (RA), second-line reduction of signs and symptoms of moderate-to-severe active RA, monotherapy or in combination with other disease-modifying antirheumatic drugs (DMARDs) (e.g., methotrexate). Juvenile idiopathic arthritis, moderate-to-severe active

PHARMACOKINETICS
Absorbed completely following parenteral administration. Distribution: 0.02–0.13 L/kg. *Half-life:* 13 days (8–25 days).

INDICATIONS AND DOSAGES
▶ **Rheumatoid Arthritis (moderate to severe) in patients who have had an inadequate response to one or more disease-modifying anti-rheumatic drugs**

IV

Adults. Dose is according to body weight. Administer over a 30-min infusion. Repeat dose at 2 wk and 4 wk after initial dose, and every 4 wk thereafter:

- <60 kg: 500 mg
- 60–100 kg: 750 mg
- >100 kg: 1000 mg

Children. Juvenile idiopathic arthritis (moderate to severe), active, polyarticular

IV Infusion

Children (6 yr and older; weighing less than 75 kg). 10 mg/kg given by IV infusion over 30 min; repeat doses at 2 and 4 wk after first infusion and every 4 wk thereafter.

▶ **Juvenile Idiopathic Arthritis (moderate to severe), active, polyarticular**

IV Infusion

Children (6 yr and older; weighing 75–100 kg). 750 mg given by IV infusion over 30 min; repeat doses at 2 and 4 wk after first infusion and every 4 wk thereafter (MAX dose, 1000 mg).

▶ **Juvenile Idiopathic Arthritis (moderate to severe), active, polyarticular**

IV Infusion

Children (6 yr and older; weighing more than 100 kg). 1000 mg given by IV infusion over 30 min; repeat doses at 2 and 4 wk after first infusion and every 4 wk thereafter (MAX dose, 1000 mg).

Safety and efficacy not established in children less than 6 yr of age. Screen for tuberculosis (TB) and hepatitis before initiating therapy.

SIDE EFFECTS/ADVERSE REACTIONS

Frequent

Infection, antibody formation, headache, dizziness, nasopharyngitis

Occasional

Nausea, hypertension, fever, urinary tract infection, cough, back pain

PRECAUTIONS AND CONTRAINDICATIONS

Hypersensitivity to abatacept or any component of the formulation. Tuberculosis (TB), active or latent; initiate treatment for TB prior to initiating abatacept therapy. Hepatitis B reactivation has been associated with abatacept therapy, screen for viral hepatitis before initiating abatacept therapy. Use with caution in patients with chronic obstructive pulmonary disease (COPD) because of worsening of breathing, COPD exacerbations, cough, and dyspnea.

DRUG INTERACTIONS OF CONCERN TO DENTISTRY

- None reported

SERIOUS REACTIONS

! Infections: should be cautious when considering the use of abatacept in patients with a history of recurrent infection, underlying conditions that may increase risks of infections, or chronic, localized infections. These patients should be monitored closely. If a patient develops a serious infection, the treatment should be discontinued.
! Anaphylaxis/hypersensitivity reaction may occur.

DENTAL CONSIDERATIONS

General:

- Examine for oral manifestation of opportunistic infection.
- Monitor vital signs at every appointment because of cardiovascular side effects.
- Consider semisupine chair position for patients with respiratory disease.

Consultations:
• Consult physician to assess disease control and ability of patient to tolerate dental treatment.
Teach Patient/Family to:
• Encourage effective atraumatic oral hygiene measures to prevent soft-tissue inflammation.
• Use soft tooth brush to reduce risk of bleeding.
• Immediately report any sign of infection to the dentist.

abciximab
ab-**six**′-ih-mab
(c7E3 Fab, ReoPro)

CATEGORY AND SCHEDULE
Pregnancy Risk Category: C

Drug Class: Glycoprotein IIb/IIIa receptor inhibitor

MECHANISM OF ACTION
A glycoprotein IIb/IIIa receptor inhibitor that rapidly inhibits platelet aggregation by preventing the binding of fibrinogen to GP IIb/IIIa receptor sites on platelets.
Therapeutic Effect: Prevents closure of treated coronary arteries. Prevents acute cardiac ischemic complications.

USES
Adjunct to aspirin and heparin therapy to prevent cardiac ischemic complications in patients undergoing percutaneous coronary intervention and those with unstable angina not responding to conventional medical therapy.

PHARMACOKINETICS
Rapidly cleared from plasma. Initial-phase half-life is less than 10 min; second-phase half-life is 30 min. Platelet function generally returns within 48 hr.

INDICATIONS AND DOSAGES
▸ **Percutaneous Coronary Intervention (PCI)**
IV Bolus
Adults. 0.25 mg/kg 10–60 min before angioplasty or atherectomy, then 12-hr IV infusion of 0.125 mcg/kg/min. Maximum: 10 mcg/min.
▸ **PCI (unstable angina)**
IV Bolus
Adults. 0.25 mg/kg, followed by 18- to 24-hr infusion of 10 mcg/min, ending 1 hr after procedure.

SIDE EFFECTS/ADVERSE REACTIONS
Frequent
Nausea, hypotension
Occasional
Vomiting
Rare
Bradycardia, confusion, dizziness, pain, peripheral edema, UTI

PRECAUTIONS AND CONTRAINDICATIONS
Active internal bleeding, arteriovenous malformation or aneurysm, cerebrovascular accident (CVA) with residual neurologic defect, history of CVA (within the past 2 yr) or oral anticoagulant use within the past 7 days unless PT is less than 1.2 times control, history of vasculitis, intracranial neoplasm, prior IV dextran use before or during PTCA, recent surgery or trauma (within the past 6 wk), recent (within the past 6 wk or less) GI or GU bleeding, thrombocytopenia (less than 100,000 cells/mcl), and severe uncontrolled hypertension.

DRUG INTERACTIONS OF CONCERN TO DENTISTRY
• Increased risk of bleeding: drugs that interfere with coagulation or platelet function, such as NSAIDs and aspirin.

SERIOUS REACTIONS
! Major bleeding complications may occur. If complications occur, stop the infusion immediately.
! Hypersensitivity reaction may occur.
! Atrial fibrillation or flutter, pulmonary edema, and complete atrioventricular block occur occasionally.

DENTAL CONSIDERATIONS
General:
• Monitor vital signs at every appointment because of cardiovascular side effects.
• For use in hospitals or emergency rooms.
• Review patient's medical and drug history.
• Provide palliative emergency dental care only during drug use.
• Patients may be at risk of bleeding, check for oral signs.
Consultations:
• Medical consultation may be required to assess disease control and patient's ability to tolerate stress.
• Medical consultation should include routine blood counts including platelet counts and bleeding time.
• Avoid products that affect platelet function, such as aspirin and NSAIDs.
Teach Patient/Family to:
• Encourage effective oral hygiene to prevent soft tissue inflammation.
• Prevent trauma when using oral hygiene aids.

• Report oral lesions, soreness, or bleeding to dentist.
• Update health and medication history if physician makes any changes in evaluation or drug regimens; include OTC, herbal, and nonherbal remedies in the update.
• Use soft tooth brush to reduce risk of bleeding.

absorbable gelatin sponge
(Gelfoam)

CATEGORY AND SCHEDULE
Hemostatic

Drug Class: Hemostatic, purified gelatin sponge

MECHANISM OF ACTION
Absorbs blood, provides area for clot formation

USES
Hemostasis adjunct in dental surgery

PHARMACOKINETICS
IMPLANT: Absorbed in 4–6 wk

INDICATIONS AND DOSAGES
▶ **Dental Use**
Adult. Top can be applied dry or moistened with normal saline solution; blot on sterile gauze to remove excess solution, shape to fit with light finger compression; hold pressure until dry. Apply to bleeding surfaces. Material may be cut to appropriate size or secured in extraction sites with sutures.

SIDE EFFECTS/ADVERSE REACTIONS
None reported

PRECAUTIONS AND CONTRAINDICATIONS

Hypersensitivity, frank infection
Caution:
Avoid use in presence of infection, potential nidus of infection, do not resterilize product.

DENTAL CONSIDERATIONS

Teach Patient/Family to:
• Immediately report any sign of infection to the dentist.

---

acamprosate calcium
(ah-kam′-**proe**-sate)
(Campral)

CATEGORY AND SCHEDULE
Pregnancy Risk Category: C

Drug Class: Alcohol-abuse deterrent

MECHANISM OF ACTIONS

Actual mechanism unknown, may facilitate balance between GABA and glutamate neurotransmitter systems in the CNS to decrease alcohol craving.

USES
Alcohol-abuse deterrent

PHARMACOKINETICS

Partially absorbed from GI tract, steady-state levels reached within 5 days of dosing. Protein binding negligible. *Half-life:* 20–33 hr. Does not undergo metabolism, excreted unchanged in urine.

INDICATIONS AND DOSAGES
▸ **Maintenance of Alcohol Abstinence**
PO
Adult. 666 mg 3 times a day with or without food.

SIDE EFFECTS/ADVERSE REACTIONS

Oral: Dry mouth
CNS: Headache, somnolence, decreased libido, amnesia, abnormal thinking, tremor
CV: Palpitation, syncope, vasodilation, changes in B/P
GI: Vomiting, dyspepsia, constipation, increased appetite
RESP: Rhinitis, cough, dyspnea, pharyngitis, bronchitis
GU: Impotence
EENT: Abnormal vision, taste alterations
INTEG: Rash
MS: Myalgia, arthralgia
SYST: Back pain, infection, flu syndrome, chest pain, chills, attempts at suicide (see Precautions)

PRECAUTIONS AND CONTRAINDICATIONS

Hypersensitivity, severe renal impairment
Caution:
Renal impairment, depression/suicidal tendency

DRUG INTERACTIONS OF CONCERN TO DENTISTRY
• None reported

DENTAL CONSIDERATIONS

General:
• Assess salivary flow as a factor in caries, periodontal disease, and candidiasis.
• After supine positioning, allow patient to sit upright for 2 min to avoid orthostatic hypotension.

• Avoid alcohol-containing products (elixirs, mouth rinses) to assist maintenance of alcohol abstinence.
Consultations:
• Consult physician to assess disease control.
Teach Patient/Family to:
• Encourage effective oral hygiene to prevent caries and periodontal disease.
• Use sugarless gum, frequent sips of water, and saliva substitutes if dry mouth occurs.
• Use home fluoride products for anticaries effect.
• Avoid mouth rinses with high alcohol content because of drying effects.

acarbose
ah-**car**′-bose
(Glucobay[AUS], Prandase[CAN], Precose)
Do not confuse Precose with PreCare.

CATEGORY AND SCHEDULE
Pregnancy Risk Category: B

Drug Class: Oral antidiabetic

MECHANISM OF ACTION
An alpha-glucosidase inhibitor that delays glucose absorption and digestion of carbohydrates, resulting in a smaller rise in blood glucose concentration after meals.
Therapeutic Effect: Lowers postprandial hyperglycemia.

USES
Use as single drug or in combination with insulin or oral hypoglycemics (sulfonylureas, metformin) in type 2 diabetes (non–insulin-dependent diabetes mellitus [NIDDM]) when

diet control is ineffective in controlling blood glucose levels.

PHARMACOKINETICS
PO
Limited oral absorption, absorbed dose excreted in urine, metabolized in the GI tract and major portion of dose excreted in feces.

INDICATIONS AND DOSAGES
▶ Diabetes Mellitus
PO
Adults, Elderly. Initially, 25 mg 3 times a day with first bite of each main meal. Increase at 4- to 8-wk intervals. Maximum: For patients weighing more than 60 kg, 100 mg 3 times a day; for patients weighing 60 kg or less, 50 mg 3 times a day.

SIDE EFFECTS/ADVERSE REACTIONS
Side effects diminish in frequency and intensity over time.
Frequent
Transient GI disturbances: flatulence, diarrhea, abdominal pain

PRECAUTIONS AND CONTRAINDICATIONS
Chronic intestinal diseases associated with marked disorders of digestion or absorption, cirrhosis, colonic ulceration, conditions that may deteriorate as a result of increased gas formation in the intestine, diabetic ketoacidosis, hypersensitivity to acarbose, inflammatory bowel disease, partial intestinal obstruction or predisposition to intestinal obstruction, significant renal dysfunction (serum creatinine level greater than 2 mg/dl)
Caution:
Use glucose for hypoglycemia, monitor blood glucose levels,

pregnancy category B, avoid use in lactation, children.

DRUG INTERACTIONS OF CONCERN TO DENTISTRY
• None reported

SERIOUS REACTIONS
! None known

DENTAL CONSIDERATIONS
General:
• Ensure that patient is following prescribed diet and takes medication regularly.
• Type 2 patients may also be using insulin. If symptomatic hypoglycemia occurs while taking this drug, use dextrose rather than sucrose because of interference with sucrose metabolism.
• Place on frequent recall to evaluate healing response.
• Patients with diabetes may be more susceptible to infection and have delayed wound healing.
• Question the patient about self-monitoring the drug's antidiabetic effect.
• Consider semisupine chair position for patient comfort if GI side effects occur.
Consultations:
• Medical consultation may be required to assess disease control and patient's ability to tolerate stress.
Teach Patient/Family to:
• Encourage effective oral hygiene to prevent soft tissue inflammation.

acebutolol
a-se-**byoo**-toe-lole
(Sectral)

CATEGORY AND SCHEDULE
Pregnancy Risk Category: B (D if used in second or third trimester)

Drug Class: Beta-adrenergic blocker (cardioselective); Antiarrhythmics, class II
Do not confused Sectral with Factrel, Septra, or Seconal.

MECHANISM OF ACTION
A beta$_1$-adrenergic blocker that competitively blocks β_1-adrenergic receptors in cardiac tissue; high doses may competitively block both β_1- and β_2-adrenergic receptors. Reduces the rate of spontaneous firing of the sinus pacemaker and delays AV conduction. Exhibits mild intrinsic sympathomimetic activity (ISA) (partial beta-agonist activity).
Therapeutic Effect: Slows heart rate, decreases cardiac output, decreases B/P, and exhibits antiarrhythmic activity.

USES
Mild to moderate hypertension
Ventricular arrhythmias

PHARMACOKINETICS

Route	Onset	Peak	Duration
PO (hypertension)	1–1.5 hr	2–8 hr	24 hr
PO (antiarrhythmic)	1 hr	4–6 hr	10 hr

Well absorbed from the GI tract. Bioavailability: approximately 40%. Protein binding: 26%. Undergoes extensive first-pass metabolism to active metabolite. Eliminated via bile and excretion into GI tract through intestinal wall, as well as partly excreted in urine. Removed by hemodialysis. *Half-life:* 3–4 hr (parent drug); 8–13 hr (metabolite).

INDICATIONS AND DOSAGES
▶ **Mild to Moderate Hypertension**
PO
Adults. Initially, 400 mg/day in 2 divided doses. Maintenance 400–800 mg/day. Maximum: 1200 mg/day in 2 divided doses.
▶ **Ventricular Arrhythmias**
PO
Adults. Initially, 200 mg twice a day. Increase gradually to 600–1200 mg/day in 2 divided doses.
Elderly. Initially, 200–400 mg/day. Maximum: 800 mg/day.
▶ **Dosage in Renal Impairment**
Dosage is modified based on creatinine clearance.

Creatinine Clearance	% of Usual Dosage
Less than 50 ml/min	50
Less than 25 ml/min	25

SIDE EFFECTS/ADVERSE REACTIONS
Frequent
Hypotension manifested as dizziness, nausea, diaphoresis, headache, cold extremities, fatigue, constipation, or diarrhea
Occasional
Insomnia, urinary frequency, impotence or decreased libido
Rare
Rash, arthralgia, myalgia, confusion (especially in the elderly), altered taste

PRECAUTIONS AND CONTRAINDICATIONS
Hypersensitivity to acebutolol or any component of the formulation
Caution:
Cardiogenic shock
Heart block greater than first degree
Overt heart failure
Severe bradycardia
Caution use in patients with bronchospastic disease, diabetes, hyperthyroidism, impaired renal or hepatic function, inadequate cardiac function, or peripheral vascular disease.

DRUG INTERACTIONS OF CONCERN TO DENTISTRY
• Diuretics, other antihypertensives: May increase hypotensive effect of acebutolol.
• Sympathomimetics, xanthines: May antagonize the effects and reduce bronchodilation.
• Oral hypoglycemics and insulin: May mask symptoms of hypoglycemia and prolong hypoglycemic effect of insulin and oral hypoglycemics.
• Catecholamine-depleting drugs (e.g., reserpine): May have additive effect. Monitor for bradycardia or hypotension.
• NSAIDs: May reduce the antihypertensive effect of acebutolol.
• Digoxin: May cause serious bradycardia.
• Calcium channel blockers (verapamil, diltiazem): May cause hypotension and bradycardia.
• Class I anti-arrhythmic drugs: May increase atrial conduction time and negative inotropic effects.

SERIOUS REACTIONS
! Overdose may produce profound bradycardia and hypotension.

! Abrupt withdrawal may result in diaphoresis, palpitations, headache, rebound hypertension, and tremors.
! Acebutolol administration may precipitate CHF or MI in patients with heart disease; thyroid storm in those with thyrotoxicosis; or peripheral ischemia in those with existing peripheral vascular disease.
! Hypoglycemia may occur in patients with previously controlled diabetes.
! Signs of thrombocytopenia, such as unusual bleeding or bruising, occur rarely.

DENTAL CONSIDERATIONS

General:
• Monitor vital signs at every appointment because of cardiovascular side effects.
• After supine positioning, have patient sit upright for at least 2 min before standing to avoid orthostatic hypotension.
• Assess salivary flow as a factor in caries, periodontal disease, and candidiasis.
• Limit use of sodium-containing products, such as saline IV fluids, for those patients with dietary salt restriction.
• Stress from dental procedures may compromise cardiovascular function; determine patient risk.
Consultations:
• Medical consultation may be required to assess disease control.
Teach Patient/Family to:
Report oral lesions, soreness, or bleeding to dentist.
• When chronic dry mouth occurs, advise patient to:
• Avoid mouth rinses with high alcohol content because of drying effects.
• Use daily home fluoride products for anticaries effect.

• Use sugarless gum, frequent sips of water or saliva substitutes.

acetaminophen
ah-**seet**-ah-min′-oh-fen
(Abenol[CAN], Apo-Acetaminophen[CAN], Atasol[CAN], Dymadon[AUS], Feverall, Panadol[AUS], Panamax[AUS], Paralgin[AUS], Setamol[AUS], Tempra, Tylenol)
Do not confuse with Fiorinal, Hycodan, Indocin, Percodan, or Tuinal.

CATEGORY AND SCHEDULE
Pregnancy Risk Category: B

Drug Class: Nonnarcotic analgesic

MECHANISM OF ACTION
A central analgesic whose exact mechanism is unknown but appears to inhibit prostaglandin synthesis in the CNS and, to a lesser extent, block pain impulses through peripheral action. Acetaminophen acts centrally on hypothalamic heat-regulating center, producing peripheral vasodilation (heat loss, skin erythema, sweating).
Therapeutic Effect: Results in antipyresis. Produces analgesic effect.

USES
Mild-to-moderate pain, fever; also used in combination with other ingredients, including opioids.

PHARMACOKINETICS

Route	Onset	Peak	Duration
PO	15–30 min	1.5 hr	4–6 hr

Rapidly, completely absorbed from GI tract; rectal absorption variable. Protein binding: 20%–50%. Widely distributed to most body tissues. Metabolized in liver; excreted in urine. Removed by hemodialysis. *Half-life:* 1–4 hr (half-life is increased in those with liver disease, elderly, neonates; decreased in children).

INDICATIONS AND DOSAGES
▸ **Analgesia and Antipyresis**
PO
Adults, Elderly. 325–650 mg q4–6h or 1 g 3–4 times a day. Maximum: 4 g/day.
Children. 10–15 mg/kg/dose q4–6h as needed. Maximum: 5 doses/24 hr.
Neonates. 10–15 mg/kg/dose q6–8h as needed.
Rectal
Adults. 650 mg q4–6h. Maximum: 6 doses/24 hr.
Children. 10–20 mg/kg/dose q4–6h as needed.
Neonates. 10–15 mg/kg/dose q6–8h as needed.
▸ **Dosage in Renal Impairment**

Creatinine Clearance	Frequency
10–15 ml/ min	q6h
Less than 10 ml/min	q8h

SIDE EFFECTS/ADVERSE REACTIONS
Rare
Hypersensitivity reaction

PRECAUTIONS AND CONTRAINDICATIONS
Active alcoholism, liver disease, or viral hepatitis, all of which increase the risk of hepatotoxicity
Caution:
Anemia, hepatic disease, renal disease, chronic alcoholism

DRUG INTERACTIONS OF CONCERN TO DENTISTRY
• Decreased effects: barbiturates, oral contraceptives, loop diuretics
• Nephrotoxicity: NSAIDs, salicylates (chronic, high-dose, concurrent use)
• Liver toxicity: chronic use of hydantoins, chronic alcohol use, high-dose carbamazepine
• Possible increased effects of zidovudine
• Possible increased effects of acetaminophen: β-blockers, probenecid
• Increased bleeding: warfarin
• Risk of acetaminophen toxicity when used in combination with OTC products

SERIOUS REACTIONS
! Acetaminophen toxicity is the primary serious reaction.
! Early signs and symptoms of acetaminophen toxicity include anorexia, nausea, diaphoresis, and generalized weakness within the first 12–24 hr.
! Later signs of acetaminophen toxicity include vomiting, right upper quadrant tenderness, and elevated liver function tests within 48–72 hr after ingestion.
! The antidote to acetaminophen toxicity is acetylcysteine (Mucomyst), but it should be administered as soon as possible following toxic dose.

DENTAL CONSIDERATIONS
General:
• Reports regarding the concomitant use of acetaminophen and warfarin seem to suggest a possible increase in anticoagulant effects, especially in patients with other diseases or contributing factors, diarrhea, age, debilitation, etc. Patients taking

warfarin should be questioned about recent use of acetaminophen and current international normalized ratio (INR) values. Acetaminophen has been shown to increase the INR depending on the amount and duration of acetaminophen use. A new PT or INR value may be required if surgical procedures are planned. Data from one study (*JAMA* 279:657–662, 1998) indicated that use of four regular-strength acetaminophen tablets (325 mg) qd for 1 wk can increase the INR values. It is important to closely monitor INR values with use of acetaminophen over a long duration and in higher doses.
• Avoid prolonged use with aspirin-containing products or NSAIDs.
• Determine why the patient is taking the drug.
• Patients on chronic drug therapy may rarely have symptoms of blood dyscrasias, which can include infection, bleeding, and poor healing.
• Question patient about the use of other drug products, including OTC products, that contain acetaminophen because of risk of acetaminophen overdose.
• Severe liver injury can occur when more than 4 g of all products that include acetaminophen are taken in a 24-hr period. Warn patient of detrimental effects.
Consultations:
• For a patient with symptoms of blood dyscrasias, request a medical consult for blood studies and postpone dental treatment until normal values are reestablished.
Teach Patient/Family to:
• Question patient concerning other drugs being taken which include acetaminophen. Caution patient to be aware of products that might include acetaminophen.

• Emphasize the potential risks to liver when consuming alcohol and taking acetaminophen.

acetazolamide
ah-seet-ah-**zole**'-ah-mide
(Apo-Acetazolamide[CAN],
Dazamide, Diamox, Diamox
Sequels)
Do not confuse with
acetohexamide.

CATEGORY AND SCHEDULE
Pregnancy Risk Category: C

Drug Class: Diuretic, carbonic anhydrase inhibitor

MECHANISM OF ACTION
A carbonic anhydrase inhibitor that reduces formation of hydrogen and bicarbonate ions from carbon dioxide and water by inhibiting, in proximal renal tubule, the enzyme carbonic anhydrase, thereby promoting renal excretion of sodium, potassium, bicarbonate, water. Ocular: Reduces rate of aqueous humor formation, lowers intraocular pressure.
Therapeutic Effect: Produces anticonvulsant activity.

USES
Treatment of open-angle glaucoma, narrow-angle glaucoma (preoperatively, if surgery delayed), epilepsy (petit mal, grand mal, mixed), edema in CHF, drug-induced edema, acute mountain sickness in climbers, drug-induced edema

PHARMACOKINETICS
Rapidly absorbed. Protein binding: 95%. Widely distributed throughout

body tissues including erythrocytes, kidneys, and blood-brain barrier. Not metabolized. Excreted unchanged in urine. Removed by hemodialysis. *Half-life:* 2.4–5.8 hr.

INDICATIONS AND DOSAGES
▸ **Glaucoma**
PO
Adults. 250 mg 1–4 times a day. Extended-Release: 500 mg 1–2 times a day usually given in morning and evening.
▸ **Secondary Glaucoma, Preoperative Treatment of Acute Congestive Glaucoma**
PO/IV
Adults. 250 mg q4h, 250 mg q12h; or 500 mg, then 125–250 mg q4h.
PO
Children. 10–15 mg/kg/day in divided doses.
IV
Children. 5–10 mg/kg q6h.
▸ **Edema**
IV
Adults. 25–375 mg once daily.
Children. 5 mg/kg or 150 mg/m² once daily.
▸ **Epilepsy**
PO
Adults, Children. 375–1000 mg/day in 1–4 divided doses.
▸ **Acute Mountain Sickness**
PO
Adults. 500–1000 mg/day in divided doses. If possible, begin 24–48 hr before ascent; continue at least 48 hr at high altitude.
▸ **Usual Elderly Dosage**
PO
Initially, 250 mg 2 times a day; use lowest effective dose.
▸ **Dosage in Renal Impairment**

Creatinine Clearance	Dosage Interval
10–50 ml/min	q12h
Less than 10 ml/min	Avoid use

SIDE EFFECTS/ADVERSE REACTIONS
Frequent
Unusually tired/weak, diarrhea, increased urination/frequency, decreased appetite/weight, altered taste (metallic), nausea, vomiting, numbness in extremities, lips, mouth
Occasional
Depression, drowsiness
Rare
Headache, photosensitivity, confusion, tinnitus, severe muscle weakness, loss of taste

PRECAUTIONS AND CONTRAINDICATIONS
Severe renal disease, adrenal insufficiency, hypochloremic acidosis, hypersensitivity to acetazolamide, to any component of the formulation, or to sulfonamides
Caution:
Hypercalciuria, chronic use of oral sulfonylureas has been associated with increased risk of cardiovascular mortality; risk is controversial.

DRUG INTERACTIONS OF CONCERN TO DENTISTRY
• Toxicity: salicylates (large doses)
• Hypokalemia: corticosteroids (systemic use)
• Crystalluria: ciprofloxacin

SERIOUS REACTIONS
❗ Long-term therapy may result in acidotic state.
❗ Nephrotoxicity/hepatotoxicity occurs occasionally, manifested as dark urine/stools, pain in lower back, jaundice, dysuria, crystalluria, renal colic/calculi.

! Bone marrow depression may be manifested as aplastic anemia, thrombocytopenia, thrombocytopenic purpura, leukopenia, agranulocytosis, hemolytic anemia.

DENTAL CONSIDERATIONS

General:
• Patients on chronic drug therapy may rarely have symptoms of blood dyscrasias, which can include infection, bleeding, and poor healing.
• Assess salivary flow as a factor in caries, periodontal disease, and candidiasis.
• Avoid drugs that may exacerbate glaucoma (e.g., anticholinergics).

Consultations:
• In a patient with symptoms of blood dyscrasias, request a medical consultation for blood studies and postpone dental treatment until normal values are reestablished.
• Consultation may be required to assess disease control.

Teach Patient/Family to:
• Encourage effective oral hygiene to prevent soft tissue inflammation.
• Prevent injury when using oral hygiene aids.
• When chronic dry mouth occurs, advise patient to:
  • Avoid mouth rinses with high alcohol content because of drying effects.
  • Use daily home fluoride products for anticaries effect.
  • Use sugarless gum, frequent sips of water, or saliva substitutes.

acetohexamide
ah-seet-oh-**hex′**-ah-mide
(Dymelor)
Do not confuse with
acetazolamide.

CATEGORY AND SCHEDULE
Pregnancy Risk Category: D

Drug Class: Sulfonylurea (first generation), antidiabetic

MECHANISM OF ACTION
An intermediate-acting sulfonylurea that promotes the release of insulin from beta cells of pancreas, increases insulin sensitivity at peripheral sites.
Therapeutic Effect: Lowers blood glucose concentration.

USES
Treatment of stable adult-onset diabetes mellitus (type 2)

PHARMACOKINETICS
Well absorbed from the GI tract. Protein binding: 65%–90%. Metabolized in liver. Excreted in urine. Not removed by hemodialysis.
Half-life: 1.3 hr.

INDICATIONS AND DOSAGES
▶ **Diabetes Mellitus**
PO
Adults, Elderly. Initially, 250 mg/ day. Adjust dosage in 250- to 500-mg increments at intervals of 5–7 days. Maximum daily dose: 1.5 g. Elderly patients may be more sensitive and should be started at a lower dosage initially.

SIDE EFFECTS/ADVERSE REACTIONS

Frequent
Altered taste sensation, dizziness, drowsiness, weight gain, constipation, diarrhea, heartburn, nausea, vomiting, stomach fullness, headache
Occasional
Increased sensitivity of skin to sunlight, peeling of skin, itching, rash

PRECAUTIONS AND CONTRAINDICATIONS

Diabetic ketoacidosis with or without coma, Type 1 diabetes mellitus, hypersensitivity to acetohexamide or any component of the formulation
Caution:
Elderly, cardiac disease, renal disease, hepatic disease, thyroid disease, severe hypoglycemic reactions

DRUG INTERACTIONS OF CONCERN TO DENTISTRY

• Increased hypoglycemic effects: salicylates (large doses)
• Decreased action: corticosteroids
• Disulfiram-like reaction: alcohol

SERIOUS REACTIONS

! Hypoglycemia may occur because of overdosage or insufficient food intake, especially with increased glucose demands.
! GI hemorrhage, cholestatic hepatic jaundice, leukopenia, thrombocytopenia, pancytopenia, agranulocytosis, aplastic or hemolytic anemia occurs rarely.

DENTAL CONSIDERATIONS

General:
• Monitor vital signs at every appointment because of cardiovascular effects of diabetes.
• Patients on chronic drug therapy may rarely have symptoms of blood dyscrasias, which can include infection, bleeding, and poor healing.
• Place on frequent recall to evaluate healing response.
• Ensure that patient is following prescribed diet and takes medication regularly.
• Question patient about self-monitoring of drug's antidiabetic effect, including self-monitored blood glucose (SMBG) values or finger-stick records.
• Avoid prescribing aspirin-containing products.
• Early-morning appointments and a stress reduction protocol may be required for anxious patients.
• Patients with diabetes may be more susceptible to infection and have delayed wound healing.
Consultations:
• In a patient with symptoms of blood dyscrasias, request a medical consultation for blood studies and postpone dental treatment until normal values are reestablished.
• Medical consultation may include data from patient's blood glucose monitoring, including glycosylated hemoglobin or hemoglobin A1c (HbA1c) testing.
Teach Patient/Family to:
• Encourage effective oral hygiene to prevent soft tissue inflammation.
• Prevent injury when using oral hygiene aids.
• Avoid mouth rinses with high alcohol content.

acetylcholine chloride
ah-seh-teel-**koe'**-leen
(Miochol-E, Miochol-E/
Steri-Tags, Miochol-E System
Pak)

CATEGORY AND SCHEDULE
Pregnancy Risk Category: C

Drug Class: Cholinergic

MECHANISM OF ACTION
A cholinergic agonist that causes
contraction of the sphincter muscles
of the iris.
Therapeutic Effect: Results in
miosis and contraction of ciliary
muscle, leading to accommodation
spasm.

USES
To produce miosis for selected types
of eye surgery

PHARMACOKINETICS
Rapid miosis of short duration

INDICATIONS AND DOSAGES
▶ **Production of Miosis**
Intraocular
Adults, Elderly. 0.5–2 ml instilled
into anterior chamber before or after
securing one or more sutures.

SIDE EFFECTS/ADVERSE REACTIONS
Rare
Corneal clouding, corneal
decompensation

PRECAUTIONS AND CONTRAINDICATIONS
Acute iritis and acute inflammatory
disease of the anterior chamber,
hypersensitivity to acetylcholine

chloride or any component of the
formulation

DRUG INTERACTIONS OF CONCERN TO DENTISTRY
• None reported

SERIOUS REACTIONS
! Systemic effects rarely occur.
These effects include bradycardia,
hypotension, flushing, breathing
difficulties, and sweating.

DENTAL CONSIDERATIONS
General:
• Acute-use drug in selected types
of eye surgery.
• Avoid dental light in patient's eyes;
offer dark glasses for patient
comfort.

acetylcysteine
ah-see-til-**sis'**-tay-een
(Acetadote, Mucomyst,
Parvolex[CAN])
Do not confuse acetylcysteine
with acetylcholine.

CATEGORY AND SCHEDULE
Pregnancy Risk Category: B

Drug Class: Antidotes;
Mucolytics

MECHANISM OF ACTION
An intratracheal respiratory inhalant
that splits the linkage of
mucoproteins, reducing the viscosity
of pulmonary secretions.
Therapeutic Effect: Facilitates the
removal of pulmonary secretions by
coughing, postural drainage,
mechanical means. Protects against
acetaminophen overdose-induced
hepatotoxicity.

USES
Adjuvant therapy for patients with abnormal, viscid, or inspissated mucus secretions

PHARMACOKINETICS
INH/INSTILL: Onset 1 min, duration 5–10 min, metabolized by liver, excreted in urine.
Half-life: 5.6 hr (adult); 11 hr (newborn).

INDICATIONS AND DOSAGES
▶ **Adjunctive Treatment of Viscid Mucus Secretions from Chronic Bronchopulmonary Disease and for Pulmonary Complications of Cystic Fibrosis**
Nebulization
Adults, Elderly, Children. 3–5 ml (20% solution) 3–4 times a day or 6–10 ml (10% solution) 3–4 times a day. Range: 1–10 ml (20% solution) q2–6h or 2–20 ml (10% solution) q2–6h.
Infants. 1–2 ml (20%) or 2–4 ml (10%) 3–4 times a day.
▶ **Treatment of Viscid Mucus Secretions in Patients with a Tracheostomy**
Intratracheal
Adults, Children. 1–2 ml of 10% or 20% solution instilled into tracheostomy q1–4h.
▶ **Acetaminophen Overdose**
PO (Oral Solution 5%)
Adults, Elderly, Children. Loading dose of 140 mg/kg, followed in 4 hr by maintenance dose of 70 mg/kg q4h for 17 additional doses (unless acetaminophen assay reveals nontoxic level).
IV
Adults, Elderly, Children.
150 mg/kg infused over 15 min, then 50 mg/kg infused over 4 hr, then 100 mg/kg infused over 16 hr. See administration and handling. Repeat dose if emesis occurs within

1 hr of administration. Continue until all doses are given, even if acetaminophen plasma level drops below toxic range.
▶ **Prevention of Renal Damage from Dyes Used During Certain Diagnostic Tests**
PO (Oral Solution 5%)
Adults, Elderly. 600 mg twice a day for 4 doses starting the day before the procedure.

SIDE EFFECTS/ADVERSE REACTIONS
Frequent
Inhalation: Stickiness on face, transient unpleasant odor
Occasional
Inhalation: Increased bronchial secretions, throat irritation, nausea, vomiting, rhinorrhea
Rare
Inhalation: Rash

PRECAUTIONS AND CONTRAINDICATIONS
None known

DRUG INTERACTIONS OF CONCERN TO DENTISTRY
• None reported

SERIOUS REACTIONS
! Large doses may produce severe nausea and vomiting.

DENTAL CONSIDERATIONS
General:
• Be aware that aspirin and/or sulfite preservatives in vasoconstrictor-containing products may exacerbate asthma.
• Acute asthmatic episodes may be precipitated in the dental office. A rapid-acting sympathomimetic inhalant (rescue inhaler) should be available for emergency use. Many patients may already have prescribed

rescue inhalers they normally use for acute asthmatic events.
• Consider semisupine chair position for patients with respiratory disease.
• Determine dose and duration of glucocorticoid therapy to assess for risk of stress tolerance and immunosuppression. Patients on chronic glucocorticoid therapy may require supplemental doses for dental treatment.
• Examine for oral manifestation of opportunistic infection.
• Evaluate respiration characteristics and rate.
• Short appointments and a stress reduction protocol may be required for anxious patients.
• Inquire about other drugs patients are using for respiratory disease.
Consultations:
• Consultation with physician may be necessary if sedation or general anesthesia is required.
• Consultation may be required to confirm glucocorticoid dose and duration of use.
• Medical consultation may be required to assess disease control and patient's ability to tolerate stress.
Teach Patient/Family to:
• Encourage effective oral hygiene to prevent soft tissue inflammation.
• Update health and medication history if physician makes any changes in evaluation or drug regimens; include OTC, herbal, and nonherbal remedies in the update.
• Gargle, rinse mouth with water, and expectorate after each aerosol dose.

acitretin
ah-sih-**tre′**-tin
(Soriatane)

CATEGORY AND SCHEDULE
Pregnancy Risk Category: X

Drug Class: Systemic retinoid

MECHANISM OF ACTION
A second-generation retinoid that adjusts factors influencing epidermal proliferation, RNA/DNA synthesis, controls glycoprotein, and governs immune response.
Therapeutic Effect: Regulates keratinocyte growth and differentiation.

USES
Severe psoriasis; unlabeled uses: nonpsoriatic dermatoses, keratinization disorders, palmoplantar keratoses, lichen planus, Darier's disease, Sjögren-Larrson syndrome; should be prescribed only by physicians knowledgeable in the use of systemic retinoids.

PHARMACOKINETICS
Well absorbed from the GI tract. Food increases rate of absorption. Protein binding: greater than 99%. Metabolized in liver. Excreted in bile and urine. Not removed by hemodialysis. *Half-life:* 49 hr.

INDICATIONS AND DOSAGES
▶ **Psoriasis**
PO
Adults, Elderly. 25–50 mg/day as a single dose with main meal. May increase to 75 mg/day if necessary and dose tolerated. Maintenance: 25–50 mg/day after the initial

response is noted. Continue until lesions have resolved.

SIDE EFFECTS/ADVERSE REACTIONS

Frequent
Lip inflammation, alopecia, skin peeling, shakiness, dry eyes, rash, hyperesthesia, paresthesia, sticky skin, dry mouth, epistaxis, dryness/thickening of conjunctiva

Occasional
Eye irritation, brow and lash loss, sweating, chills, sensation of cold, flushing, edema, blurred vision, diarrhea, nausea, thirst

PRECAUTIONS AND CONTRAINDICATIONS

Women who are pregnant or those who intend to become pregnant within 3 yr following discontinuation of therapy; severely impaired liver or kidney function; chronic abnormal elevated lipid levels; concomitant use of methotrexate or tetracyclines; ingestion of alcohol (in females of reproductive potential); hypersensitivity to acitretin, etretinate, or other retinoids; sensitivity to parabenz (used as preservative in gelatin capsule)

Caution:
Women are advised to use effective contraception during use and for 3 yr after use, renal impairment, lactation, hyperlipidemia, cardiovascular disease

DRUG INTERACTIONS OF CONCERN TO DENTISTRY

• Avoid vitamin preparations containing vitamin A.
• Avoid tetracyclines and other drugs that cause photosensitivity.

SERIOUS REACTIONS

! Benign intracranial hypertension (pseudotumor cerebri) occurs rarely.

DENTAL CONSIDERATIONS

General:
• Determine why patient is taking the drug.
• Apply lubricant to dry lips for patient comfort before dental procedures.
• Assess salivary flow as factor in caries, periodontal disease, and candidiasis.
• Palliative medication may be required for management of oral side effects.
• Place on frequent recall because of oral side effects.
• Consider semisupine chair position for patient comfort if GI side effects occur.
• Avoid dental light in patient's eyes; offer dark glasses for patient comfort.

Consultations:
• Medical consultation may be required to assess disease control.

Teach Patient/Family to:
• Encourage effective oral hygiene to prevent soft tissue inflammation.
• Prevent trauma when using oral hygiene aids.
• Report oral lesions, soreness, or bleeding to dentist.
• When chronic dry mouth occurs, advise patient to:
  • Avoid mouth rinses with high alcohol content because of drying effects.
  • Use daily home fluoride products for anticaries effect.
  • Use sugarless gum, frequent sips of water, or saliva substitutes.

acyclovir
ay-**sye′**-kloe-ver
(Aciclovir-BC IV[AUS],
Acihexal[AUS], Acyclo-V[AUS],
Avirax[CAN], Lovir[AUS], Zovirax,
Zyclir[AUS])
Do not confuse with Zostrix,
Zyvox.

CATEGORY AND SCHEDULE
Pregnancy Risk Category: B

Drug Class: Antiviral

MECHANISM OF ACTION
A synthetic nucleoside that converts
to acyclovir triphosphate, becoming
part of the DNA chain.
Therapeutic Effect: Interferes with
DNA synthesis and viral replication.
Virustatic.

USES
Management of initial genital herpes
and in limited non-life-threatening
mucocutaneous herpes simplex
infection in immunocompromised
patients

PHARMACOKINETICS
Poorly absorbed from the GI tract;
minimal absorption following
topical application. Protein binding:
9%–36%. Widely distributed.
Partially metabolized in liver.
Excreted primarily in urine.
Removed by hemodialysis. *Half-life:*
2.5 hr (increased in impaired renal
function).

INDICATIONS AND DOSAGES
▸ **Genital Herpes (initial episode)**
IV
*Adults, Elderly, Children 12 yr and
older.* 5 mg/kg q8h for 5 days.

PO
*Adults, Elderly, Children 12 yr
and older.* 200 mg q4h 5 times a
day.
▸ **Genital Herpes (recurrent) fewer
than 6 episodes per year**
PO
*Adults, Elderly, Children 12 yr and
older.* 200 mg q4h 5 times a day for
5 days.
▸ **Genital Herpes (recurrent) 6
episodes or more per year**
PO
*Adults, Elderly, Children 12 yr and
older.* 400 mg 2 times a day or
200 mg 3–5 times a day for up to
12 mo.
▸ **Herpes Simplex Mucocutaneous**
IV
*Adults, Elderly, Children 12 yr
and older.* 5 mg/kg/dose q8h for 7
days.
Children younger than 12 yr. 10 mg/
kg q8h for 7 days.
▸ **Herpes Simplex Neonatal**
IV
Children younger than 4 mo. 10 mg/
kg q8h for 10 days.
▸ **Herpes Simplex Encephalitis**
IV
*Adults, Elderly, Children 12 yr and
older.* 10 mg/kg q8h for 10 days.
Children younger than 12 yr. 20 mg/
kg q8h for 10 days.
▸ **Herpes Zoster (Caused by
Varicella)**
IV
*Adults, Elderly, Children 12 yr and
older.* 10 mg/kg q8h for 7 days.
Children younger than 12 yr. 20 mg/
kg q8h for 7 days.
▸ **Herpes Zoster (Shingles)**
PO
*Adults, Elderly, Children 12 yr and
older.* 800 mg q4h 5 times a day for
7–10 days.
Topical
Adults, Elderly. Apply to affected
area 3–6 times a day for 7 days.

▸ **Varicella (chickenpox)**
PO
Adults, Elderly, Children older than 12 yr or Children 2–12 yr, weighing 40 kg or more. 800 mg 4 times a day for 5 days.
Children 2–12 yr, weighing less than 40 kg. 20 mg/kg 4 times a day for 5 days. Maximum: 800 mg/dose.
Children younger than 2 yr. 80 mg/kg/day.

▸ **Dosage in Renal Impairment**
Dosage and frequency are modified on the basis of severity of infection and degree of renal impairment.
PO
For creatinine clearance of 10 ml/min or less, dosage is 200 mg q12h.
IV

Creatinine Clearance	Dosage Percent	Dosage Interval
Greater 50 ml/min	100	8 hr
25–50 ml/min	100	12 hr
10–25 ml/min	100	24 hr
Less than 10 ml/min	50	24 hr

SIDE EFFECTS/ADVERSE REACTIONS

Frequent
Parenteral: Phlebitis or inflammation at IV site, nausea, vomiting
Topical: Burning, stinging
Occasional
Parenteral: Pruritus, rash, urticaria
Oral: Malaise, nausea
Topical: Pruritus
Rare
Oral: Vomiting, rash, diarrhea, headache
Parenteral: Confusion, hallucinations, seizures, tremors
Topical: Rash

PRECAUTIONS AND CONTRAINDICATIONS

Use in neonates when acyclovir is reconstituted with bacteriostatic water containing benzyl alcohol.
Caution:
Modify dose with acute or chronic renal impairment, safety of oral doses in pediatric patients less than 2 yr old not established, lactation, hepatic disease, renal disease, electrolyte imbalance, dehydration.

SERIOUS REACTIONS

! Rapid parenteral administration, excessively high doses, or fluid and electrolyte imbalance may produce renal failure exhibited by such signs and symptoms as abdominal pain, decreased urination, decreased appetite, increased thirst, nausea, and vomiting.
! Toxicity has not been reported with oral or topical use.

DENTAL CONSIDERATIONS

General:
• Postpone dental treatment when oral herpetic lesions are present.
Teach Patient/Family to:
• Dispose of tooth brush or other contaminated oral hygiene devices used during period of infection to prevent reinoculation of herpetic infection.
• Apply with a finger cot or latex glove to prevent herpes infection on fingers.
• Avoid mouth rinses with high alcohol content because of irritating effects.

adalimumab
ah-dah-**lim′**-mu-mab
(Humira)

CATEGORY AND SCHEDULE
Pregnancy Risk Category: B

Drug Class: Monoclonal
antibody, antiinflammatory,
immunosuppressant

MECHANISM OF ACTION
A monoclonal antibody that binds
specifically to tumor necrosis factor
(TNF) alpha, blocking its interaction
with cell surface TNF receptors.
Therapeutic Effect: Reduces
inflammation, tenderness, and
swelling of joints; slows or prevents
progressive destruction of joints in
rheumatoid arthritis.

USES
Treatment of signs and symptoms
and inhibition of structural damage
in moderately to severely active
rheumatoid arthritis in adults who
have an inadequate response to one
or more disease-modifying
antirheumatic drugs (DMARDs)

PHARMACOKINETICS
Half-life: 10–20 days.

INDICATIONS AND DOSAGES
▸ **Rheumatoid Arthritis**
Subcutaneous
Adults, Elderly. 40 mg every other
wk. Dose may be increased to
40 mg/wk in those not taking
methotrexate.

SIDE EFFECTS/ADVERSE REACTIONS
Frequent
Injection site, erythema, pruritus,
pain, and swelling

Occasional
Headache, rash, sinusitis, nausea
Rare
Abdominal or back pain,
hypertension

PRECAUTIONS AND CONTRAINDICATIONS
Active infections
Caution:
Appearance of new infection with
use; risk of exacerbation of
demyelinating diseases; risk of
malignancies; risk of TB
reactivation; lactation; elderly; safety
and effectiveness in children not
established.

DRUG INTERACTIONS OF CONCERN TO DENTISTRY
• None known

SERIOUS REACTIONS
❗ Rare reactions include
hypersensitivity reactions,
malignancies, respiratory tract
infections, bronchitis, UTIs, and
more serious infections (such
as pneumonia, tuberculosis,
cellulitis, pyelonephritis, and septic
arthritis).

DENTAL CONSIDERATIONS
General:
• Patient may need assistance in
getting into and out of dental chair.
• Adjust chair position for patient
comfort.
• Determine why patient is taking
the drug.
• Question patient about other drugs
being taken.
• Examine for oral manifestation of
opportunistic infection.
• Report oral infections to patient's
physician; treat infections
aggressively.

• Consider semisupine chair position for patient comfort if GI side effects occur.

Consultations:
• Medical consultation may be required to assess disease control and patient's ability to tolerate stress.

Teach Patient/Family to:
• Encourage effective oral hygiene to prevent soft tissue inflammation.
• Immediately report any signs or symptoms of oral infection.

adapalene
a-**dap**′-ah-leen
(Differin)

CATEGORY AND SCHEDULE
Pregnancy Risk Category: C

Drug Class: Dermatologics, retinoids

MECHANISM OF ACTION
Binds to retinoic acid receptors in cell nuclei modulating cell differentiation, keratinization. Possesses antiinflammatory properties.
Therapeutic Effect: Normalizes differentiation of follicular epithelial cells.

USES
Treatment of acne

PHARMACOKINETICS
Absorption through the skin is low. Trace amount found in plasma following topical application. Excreted primarily by biliary route.

INDICATIONS AND DOSAGES
▶ **Acne Vulgaris**
Topical
Adults, Elderly, Children older than 12 yr. Apply to affected area once daily at bedtime after washing.

SIDE EFFECTS/ADVERSE REACTIONS
Frequent
Erythema, scaling, dryness, pruritus, burning (likely to occur first 2–4 wk, lessens with continued use)
Occasional
Skin irritation, stinging, sunburn, acne flares, erythema, photosensitivity, pruritus, xerosis

PRECAUTIONS AND CONTRAINDICATIONS
Hypersensitivity to adapalene, vitamin A or any one of its components

DRUG INTERACTIONS OF CONCERN TO DENTISTRY
• Avoid use of topical antiinfectives on same skin application site.

SERIOUS REACTIONS
! Concurrent use of other potentially irritating topical products (soaps, cleansers, aftershave, cosmetics) may produce severe topical irritation.

DENTAL CONSIDERATIONS

General:
• Advise patient if dental drugs prescribed have a potential for photosensitivity.
• Apply lubricant to dry lips for patient comfort prior to dental procedures.
• Limit systemic vitamin A doses to no more than the RDA.

Teach Patient/Family to:
• Avoid getting in eyes or mouth, or on other mucous membranes.

adefovir
ah-**deff'**-oh-veer
(Hepsera)

CATEGORY AND SCHEDULE
Pregnancy Risk Category: C

Drug Class: Antiviral

MECHANISM OF ACTION
An antiviral that inhibits the enzyme DNA polymerase, causing DNA chain termination after its incorporation into viral DNA. *Therapeutic Effect:* Prevents cell replication of viral DNA.

USES
Treatment of chronic hepatitis B in adults showing evidence of active viral replication and with persistent elevations of ALT or AST or histologically active disease

PHARMACOKINETICS
Binds to proteins after PO administration. Excreted in urine. *Half-life:* 7 hr (increased in impaired renal function).

INDICATIONS AND DOSAGES
▸ **Chronic Hepatitis B in Patients with Normal Renal Function**
PO
Adults, Elderly. 10 mg once a day.
▸ **Chronic Hepatitis B in Patients with Impaired Renal Function**
PO
Adults, Elderly with creatinine clearance. 20–49 ml/min. 10 mg q48h.
Adults, Elderly with creatinine clearance. 10–19 ml/min. 10 mg q72h.
Adults, Elderly on hemodialysis. 10 mg every 7 days following dialysis.

SIDE EFFECTS/ADVERSE REACTIONS
Frequent
Asthenia
Occasional
Headache, abdominal pain, nausea, flatulence
Rare
Diarrhea, dyspepsia

PRECAUTIONS AND CONTRAINDICATIONS
Hypersensitivity
Caution:
Severe acute exacerbations of hepatitis in patients who have discontinued drug, renal dysfunction with chronic use, HIV resistance, lactic acidosis, severe hepatomegaly with steatosis, monitor renal and hepatic function, safety and effectiveness in children and lactation not established

DRUG INTERACTIONS OF CONCERN TO DENTISTRY
• None reported

SERIOUS REACTIONS
! Nephrotoxicity (characterized by increased serum creatinine and decreased serum phosphorus levels) is a treatment-limiting toxicity of adefovir therapy.
! Lactic acidosis and severe hepatomegaly occur rarely, particularly in female patients.

General:
• Examine for oral manifestation of opportunistic infection.
• Determine why patient is taking the drug.
• Consider semisupine chair position for patient comfort if GI side effects occur.
• Do not provide treatment if clinician does not have seroconversion to protective antibodies to hepatitis B.

Consultations:
• Medical consultation may be required to assess disease control and patient's ability to tolerate stress.
• Patients who report feeling symptoms of lactic acidosis, such as weakness, malaise, with unusual muscle pain, difficulty breathing, stomach pain with nausea, cold feeling in arms or legs, dizziness or light-headedness, and irregular heartbeat, should be immediately referred to their physicians.

Teach Patient/Family to:
• Encourage effective oral hygiene to prevent soft tissue inflammation.
• Prevent trauma when using oral hygiene aids.
• Update health and drug history if physician makes any changes in evaluation or drug regimens.

albendazole
all-**ben′**-dah-zole
(Albenza)

CATEGORY AND SCHEDULE
Pregnancy Risk Category: C

Drug Class: Anthelmintic, systemic

MECHANISM OF ACTION
A benzimidazole carbamate anthelmintic that degrades parasite cytoplasmic microtubules, irreversibly blocks cholinesterase secretion, glucose uptake in helminth and larvae (depletes glycogen, decreases ATP production, depletes energy). Vermicidal.
Therapeutic Effect: Immobilizes and kills worms.

USES
Treatment of infections caused by worms

PHARMACOKINETICS
Poorly and variable absorbed GI tract. Widely distributed, cyst fluid and including CSF. Protein binding: 70%. Extensively metabolized in liver. Primarily excreted in urine and bile. Not removed by hemodialysis.
Half-life: 8–12 hr.

INDICATIONS AND DOSAGES
▸ **Neurocysticercosis**
PO
Adults, Elderly weighing more than 60 kg. 400 mg 2 times a day. Continue for 28 days, rest 14 days, repeat cycle 3 times.
Adults, Elderly weighing less than 60 kg. 15 mg/kg/day. Continue for 28 days, rest 14 days, repeat cycle 3 times.
▸ **Cystic Hydatid**
PO
Adults, Elderly weighing more than 60 kg. 400 mg 2 times a day. Continue for 8–30 days.
Adults, Elderly weighing less than 60 kg. 15 mg/kg/day. Continue for 8–30 days.

SIDE EFFECTS/ADVERSE REACTIONS
Frequent
Neurocysticercosis: Nausea, vomiting, headache
Hydatid: Abnormal liver function tests, abdominal pain, nausea, vomiting
Occasional
Neurocysticercosis: Increased intracranial pressure, meningeal signs
Hydatid: Headache, dizziness, alopecia, fever

PRECAUTIONS AND CONTRAINDICATIONS
Hypersensitivity to albendazole or any component of the formulation, pregnancy

DRUG INTERACTIONS OF CONCERN TO DENTISTRY
• Possible increase in blood levels: glucocorticoids, cimetidine

SERIOUS REACTIONS
! Pancytopenia occurs rarely.
! In presence of cysticercosis, drug may produce retinal damage in presence of retinal lesions.

DENTAL CONSIDERATIONS
General:
• Determine why patient is taking the drug.
• Patient on chronic drug therapy may rarely present with symptoms of blood dyscrasias, which can include infection, bleeding, and poor healing. If dyscrasia is present, caution patient to prevent oral tissue trauma when using oral hygiene aids.
• Question patients about other drugs they may be taking.

Consultations:
• In a patient with symptoms of blood dyscrasias, request a medical consultation for blood studies and postpone treatment until normal values are reestablished.

albuterol
al-**byoo′**-ter-ole
(AccuNeb, Airomir[AUS], Asmol CFC-Free[AUS], Epaq Inhaler[AUS], Novosalmol[CAN], Proventil, Proventil Repetabs, Respax[AUS], Ventolin, Ventolin CFC-Free[AUS], Volmax, Vospire ER)
Do not confuse albuterol with Albutein or atenolol, or Proventil with Prinivil.

CATEGORY AND SCHEDULE
Pregnancy Risk Category: C

Drug Class: Adrenergic β_2-agonist

MECHANISM OF ACTION
A sympathomimetic that stimulates β_2-adrenergic receptors in the lungs, resulting in relaxation of bronchial smooth muscle.
Therapeutic Effect: Relieves bronchospasm and reduces airway resistance.

USES
Prevention and relief of bronchospasm in reversible obstructive airway disease, exercise-induced bronchospasm; unlabeled use acute, serious hyperkalemia in hemodialysis patients

PHARMACOKINETICS

Route	Onset	Peak	Duration
PO	15–30 min	2–3 hr	4–6 hr
PO (extended-release)	30 min	2–4 hr	12 hr
Inhalation	5–15 min	0.5–2 hr	2–5 hr

Rapidly, well absorbed from the GI tract; gradually absorbed from the bronchi after inhalation. Metabolized in the liver. Primarily excreted in urine. *Half-life:* 2.7–5 hr (PO); 3.8 hr (inhalation).

INDICATIONS AND DOSAGES
▸ Bronchospasm
PO
Adults, Children older than 12 yr.
2–4 mg 3–4 times a day.
Maximum: 8 mg 4 times a day.
Elderly. 2 mg 3–4 times a day.
Maximum: 8 mg 4 times a day.
Children 6–12 yr. 2 mg 3–4 times a day. Maximum: 24 mg/day.
PO (Extended-Release)
Adults, Children older than 12 yr.
4–8 mg q12h.
Inhalation
Adults, Elderly, Children older than 12 yr. 1–2 puffs by metered dose inhaler q4–6h as needed.
Children 4–12 yr. 1–2 puffs 4 times a day.
Nebulization
Adults, Elderly, Children older than 12 yr. 2.5 mg 3–4 times a day.
Children 2–12 yr. 0.63–1.25 mg 3–4 times a day.
▸ Exercise-Induced Bronchospasm
Inhalation
Adults, Elderly, Children 4 yr and older. 2 puffs 15–30 min before exercise.

SIDE EFFECTS/ADVERSE REACTIONS
Frequent
Headache; restlessness, nervousness, tremors; nausea; dizziness; throat dryness and irritation, pharyngitis; B/P changes, including hypertension; heartburn, transient wheezing
Occasional
Insomnia, asthenia, altered taste
Inhalation: Dry, irritated mouth or throat; cough; bronchial irritation
Rare
Somnolence, diarrhea, dry mouth, flushing, diaphoresis, anorexia

PRECAUTIONS AND CONTRAINDICATIONS
History of hypersensitivity to sympathomimetics
Caution:
Lactation, cardiac disorders, hyperthyroidism, diabetes mellitus, hypertension, prostatic hypertrophy, narrow-angle glaucoma, seizures, paradoxic bronchospasm

DRUG INTERACTIONS OF CONCERN TO DENTISTRY
• None reported

SERIOUS REACTIONS
! Excessive sympathomimetic stimulation may produce palpitations, extrasystole, tachycardia, chest pain, a slight increase in B/P followed by a substantial decrease, chills, diaphoresis, and blanching of skin.
! Too-frequent or excessive use may lead to decreased bronchodilating effectiveness and severe, paradoxical bronchoconstriction.

General:
• Monitor vital signs at every appointment because of cardiovascular and respiratory side effects.
• Assess salivary flow as a factor in caries, periodontal disease, and candidiasis.
• Consider semisupine chair position for patients with respiratory disease.
• Midday appointments and a stress reduction protocol may be required for anxious patients.
• Be aware that aspirin or sulfite preservatives in vasoconstrictor-containing products can exacerbate asthma.
• Acute asthmatic episodes may be precipitated in the dental office. Sympathomimetic inhalants should be available for emergency use.

Consultations:
• Medical consultation may be required to assess disease control and patient's ability to tolerate stress.

Teach Patient/Family to:
• Rinse mouth with water after each dose to prevent dryness (for inhalation dosage forms).
• When chronic dry mouth occurs, advise patient to:
  • Avoid mouth rinses with high alcohol content because of drying effects.
  • Use daily home fluoride products for anticaries effect.
  • To use sugarless gum, frequent sips of water, or saliva substitutes.

alclometasone
al-kloe-**met**'-ah-sone
(Aclovate)

CATEGORY AND SCHEDULE
Pregnancy Risk Category: C

Drug Class: Antiinflammatory, steroidal

MECHANISM OF ACTION
Topical corticosteroids exhibit antiinflammatory, antipruritic, and vasoconstrictive properties. Clinically, these actions correspond to decreased edema, erythema, pruritus, plaque formation, and scaling of the affected skin.

USES
Provide relief of inflammation/pruritus associated with contact dermatitis, eczema, insect bite reactions.

PHARMACOKINETICS
Approximately 3% is absorbed during an 8-hr period. Metabolized in the liver. Excreted in urine.

INDICATIONS AND DOSAGES
▸ **Atopic Dermatitis, Contact Dermatitis, Dermatitis, Discoid Lupus Erythematosus, Eczema, Exfoliative Dermatitis, Granuloma Annulare, Lichen Planus, Lichen Simplex, Polymorphous Light Eruption, Pruritus, Psoriasis, Rhus Dermatitis, Seborrheic Dermatitis, Xerosis**
Topical
Adults, Adolescents, Children 1 yr and older. Apply a thin film to the affected area 2–3 times a day.

SIDE EFFECTS/ADVERSE REACTIONS
Frequent
Burning, erythema, maculopapular rash, pruritus, skin irritation, xerosis
Occasional
Acneiform rash, contact dermatitis, folliculitis, glycosuria, growth inhibition, headache, hyperglycemia, infection, miliaria, papilledema, skin atrophy, skin hypopigmentation, skin ulcer, striae, telangiectasia
Rare
Adrenalcortical insufficiency, increased intracranial pressure, pseudotumor cerebri, impaired wound healing, Cushing's syndrome, hypothalamic-pituitary-adrenal (HPA) suppression, skin ulcers, tolerance, withdrawal, visual impairment, ocular hypertension, cataracts

PRECAUTIONS AND CONTRAINDICATIONS
Hypersensitivity to alclometasone, other corticosteroids, or any of its components

DRUG INTERACTIONS OF CONCERN TO DENTISTRY
• None reported

SERIOUS REACTIONS
! None listed

DENTAL CONSIDERATIONS

General:
• Determine why patient is taking the drug.
Teach Patient/Family to:
• Avoid use on herpetic lesions.

interleukin-2 (aldesleukin)
in-tur-**lew**′-kin
(IL-2, Proleukin)
Do not confuse interleukin-2 with interferon 2.

CATEGORY AND SCHEDULE
Pregnancy Risk Category: C

Drug Class: Antineoplastic

MECHANISM OF ACTION
A biological response modifier that acts like human recombinant interleukin-2, promoting proliferation, differentiation, and recruitment of T and B cells, lymphokine-activated and natural cells, and thymocytes.
Therapeutic Effect: Enhances cytolytic activity in lymphocytes.

USES
Treatment of metastatic renal cell cancer

PHARMACOKINETICS
Primarily distributed into plasma, lymphocytes, lungs, liver, kidney, and spleen. Metabolized to amino acids in the cell lining the kidneys.
Half-life: 85 min.

INDICATIONS AND DOSAGES
▶ **Metastatic Melanoma, Metastatic Renal Cell Carcinoma**
IV
Adults 18 yr and older. 600,000 units/kg q8h for 14 doses; followed by 9 days of rest, then another 14 doses for a total of 28 doses per course. Course may be repeated after rest period of at least 7 wk from date of hospital discharge.

SIDE EFFECTS/ADVERSE REACTIONS
Side effects are generally self-limiting and reversible within 2–3 days after discontinuing therapy.
Frequent
Fever, chills, nausea, vomiting, hypotension, diarrhea, oliguria or anuria, mental status changes, irritability, confusion, depression, sinus tachycardia, pain (abdominal, chest, back), fatigue, dyspnea, pruritus
Occasional
Edema, erythema, rash, stomatitis, anorexia, weight gain, infection (UTI, injection site, catheter tip), dizziness
Rare
Dry skin, sensory disorders (vision, speech, taste), dermatitis, headache, arthralgia, myalgia, weight loss, hematuria, conjunctivitis, proteinuria

PRECAUTIONS AND CONTRAINDICATIONS
Abnormal pulmonary function or thallium stress test results, bowel ischemia or perforation, coma or toxic psychosis lasting longer than 48 hr, GI bleeding requiring surgery, intubation lasting more than 72 hr, organ allografts, pericardial tamponade, renal dysfunction requiring dialysis for longer than 72 hr, repetitive or difficult-to-control seizures; retreatment in those who experience any of the following toxicities: angina, MI, recurrent chest pain with EKG changes, sustained ventricular tachycardia, uncontrolled or unresponsive cardiac rhythm disturbances

DRUG INTERACTIONS OF CONCERN TO DENTISTRY
• Possible reduction in antitumor efficacy: glucocorticoids

SERIOUS REACTIONS
❗ Anemia, thrombocytopenia, and leukopenia occur commonly.
❗ GI bleeding and pulmonary edema occur occasionally.
❗ Capillary leak syndrome results in hypotension (systolic pressure less than 90 mm Hg or a 20-mm Hg drop from baseline systolic pressure), extravasation of plasma proteins and fluid into extravascular space, and loss of vascular tone. It may result in cardiac arrhythmias, angina, MI, and respiratory insufficiency.
❗ Other rare reactions include fatal malignant hyperthermia, cardiac arrest, CVA, pulmonary emboli, bowel perforation, gangrene, and severe depression leading to suicide.

DENTAL CONSIDERATIONS
General:
• Monitor vital signs at every appointment because of cardiovascular side effects.
• If additional analgesia is required for dental pain, consider alternative analgesics (NSAIDs) in patients taking narcotics for acute or chronic pain.
• Examine for oral manifestation of opportunistic infection.
• Avoid products that affect platelet function, such as aspirin and NSAIDs.
• Chlorhexidine mouth rinse prior to and during chemotherapy may reduce severity of mucositis.
• Patient on chronic drug therapy may rarely present with symptoms of blood dyscrasias, which can include infection, bleeding, and poor healing. If dyscrasia is present, caution patient to prevent oral tissue trauma when using oral hygiene aids.

• Palliative medication may be required for management of oral side effects.
• Short appointments and a stress-reduction protocol may be required for anxious patients.
• Provide emergency dental care only during drug use.
• Patients may be at risk of bleeding; check for oral signs.
• Oral infections should be eliminated and/or treated aggressively.

Consultations:
• Medical consultation should include routine blood counts including platelet counts and bleeding time.
• Consult physician; prophylactic or therapeutic antiinfectives may be indicated if surgery or periodontal treatment is required.
• Medical consultation may be required to assess immunologic status during cancer chemotherapy and determine safety risk, if any, posed by the required dental treatment.
• Medical consultation may be required to assess disease control and patient's ability to tolerate stress.

Teach Patient/Family to:
• See dentist immediately if secondary oral infection occurs.
• Be aware of oral side effects.
• Encourage effective oral hygiene to prevent soft tissue inflammation.
• Report oral lesions, soreness, or bleeding to dentist.
• Prevent trauma when using oral hygiene aids.
• Update health and medication history if physician makes any changes in evaluation or drug regimens; include OTC, herbal, and nonherbal remedies in the update.

alefacept
ale′-fah-sept
(Amevive)

CATEGORY AND SCHEDULE
Pregnancy Risk Category: B

Drug Class: Biologic response modifier, immunosuppressant

MECHANISM OF ACTION
An immunologic agent that interferes with the activation of T lymphocytes by binding to the lymphocyte antigen, thus reducing the number of circulating T lymphocytes.
Therapeutic Effect: Prevents T cells from becoming overactive, which may help reduce symptoms of chronic plaque psoriasis.

USES
Treatment of moderate to severe chronic plaque psoriasis in adults who are candidates for systemic therapy or phototherapy

PHARMACOKINETICS
Half-life: 270 hr.

INDICATIONS AND DOSAGES
▶ Plaque Psoriasis
IV
Adults, Elderly. 7.5 mg once weekly for 12 wk.
IM
Adults, Elderly. 15 mg once weekly for 12 wk.

SIDE EFFECTS/ADVERSE REACTIONS
Frequent
Injection site pain and inflammation (with IM administration)
Occasional
Chills

Rare
Pharyngitis, dizziness, cough, nausea, myalgia

PRECAUTIONS AND CONTRAINDICATIONS
History of systemic malignancy, concurrent use of immunosuppressive agents or phototherapy
Caution:
Live or live-attenuated vaccines require regular monitoring of lymphocyte counts; lactation data not available (caution), elderly, safety and efficacy in pediatric patients not known

DRUG INTERACTIONS OF CONCERN TO DENTISTRY
• None reported

SERIOUS REACTIONS
! Rare reactions include hypersensitivity reactions, lymphopenia, malignancies, and serious infections requiring hospitalization (such as abscess, pneumonia, and postoperative wound infection).
! Coronary artery disease and MI occur in less than 1% of patients.

DENTAL CONSIDERATIONS
• None reported

alemtuzumab
al-em-**two**′-zoo-mab
(Campath)

CATEGORY AND SCHEDULE
Pregnancy Risk Category: C

Drug Class: Antineoplastic

MECHANISM OF ACTION
Binds to CD52, a cell surface glycoprotein, found on the surface of all B and T lymphocytes, most monocytes, macrophages, natural killer cells, and granulocytes.
Therapeutic Effect: Produces cytotoxicity reducing tumor size.

USES
Treatment of B-cell chronic lymphocytic leukemia in patients who have been treated with alkylating agents and who have failed fludarabine therapy

PHARMACOKINETICS
Half-life: About 12 days. Peak and trough levels rise during first few weeks of therapy and approach steady state by about week 6.

INDICATIONS AND DOSAGES
▶ **Chronic Lymphocytic Leukemia**
IV
Adults, Elderly. Initially, 3 mg/day as a 2-hr infusion. When the 3-mg daily dose is tolerated (with only low-grade or no infusion-related toxicities), increase daily dose to 10 mg. When the 10 mg/day dose is tolerated, maintenance dose may be initiated. Maintenance: 30 mg/day 3 times a week on alternate days (such as Monday, Wednesday, and Friday or Tuesday, Thursday, and Saturday) for up to 12 wk. The increase to 30 mg/day is usually achieved in 3–7 days.

SIDE EFFECTS/ADVERSE REACTIONS
Frequent
Rigors, tremors, fever, nausea, vomiting, rash, fatigue, hypotension, urticaria, pruritus, skeletal pain, headache, diarrhea, anorexia

Occasional

Myalgia, dizziness, abdominal pain, throat irritation, vomiting, neutropenia, rhinitis, bronchospasm, urticaria

PRECAUTIONS AND CONTRAINDICATIONS

Active systemic infections, history of hypersensitivity or anaphylactic reaction to the drug, immunosuppression

DRUG INTERACTIONS OF CONCERN TO DENTISTRY

• None reported

SERIOUS REACTIONS

! Neutropenia occurs in 85% of patients, anemia occurs in 80% of patients, and thrombocytopenia occurs in 72% of patients.

! A rash occurs in 40% of patients.

! Respiratory toxicity, manifested as dyspnea, cough, bronchitis, pneumonitis, and pneumonia, occurs in 16%–26% of patients.

DENTAL CONSIDERATIONS

General:

• Monitor vital signs at every appointment because of cardiovascular side effects.

• Examine for oral manifestation of opportunistic infection.

• Avoid products that affect platelet function, such as aspirin and NSAIDs.

• This drug may be used in the hospital or on an outpatient basis. Confirm the patient's disease and treatment status.

• Chlorhexidine mouth rinse prior to and during chemotherapy may reduce severity of mucositis.

• Patient on chronic drug therapy may rarely present with symptoms of blood dyscrasias, which can include infection, bleeding, and poor healing. If dyscrasia is present, caution patient to prevent oral tissue trauma when using oral hygiene aids.

• Palliative medication may be required for management of oral side effects.

• Short appointments and a stress reduction protocol may be required for anxious patients.

• Patients may be taking a prophylactic antiinfective.

• Patients are at risk of bleeding; check for oral signs.

• Place on frequent recall because of oral side effects.

Consultations:

• Medical consultation should include routine blood counts including platelet counts and bleeding time.

• Consult physician; prophylactic or therapeutic antiinfectives may be indicated if surgery or periodontal treatment is required.

• Medical consultation may be required to assess immunologic status during cancer chemotherapy and determine safety risk, if any, posed by the required dental treatment.

• Medical consultation may be required to assess disease control and patient's ability to tolerate stress.

Teach Patient/Family to:

• Inform dentist of unusual bleeding episodes following dental treatment.

• See dentist immediately if secondary oral infection occurs.

• Be aware of oral side effects.

• Encourage effective oral hygiene to prevent soft tissue inflammation.

• Report oral lesions, soreness, or bleeding to dentist.

• Prevent trauma when using oral hygiene aids.

• Update health and medication history if physician makes any changes in evaluation or drug regimens; include OTC, herbal, and nonherbal remedies in the update.

alendronate sodium
ah-**len**´-dro-nate
(Fosamax)
Do not confuse Fosamax with Flomax.

CATEGORY AND SCHEDULE
Pregnancy Risk Category: C

Drug Class: Amino bisphosphonate

MECHANISM OF ACTION
A bisphosphonate that inhibits normal and abnormal bone resorption, without retarding mineralization.
Therapeutic Effect: Leads to significantly increased bone mineral density; reverses the progression of osteoporosis.

USES
Osteoporosis treatment and prevention in men and postmenopausal women, glucocorticoid-induced osteoporosis in men and women receiving glucocorticoids at daily dose of 7.5 mg prednisone, Paget's disease of bone

PHARMACOKINETICS
Poorly absorbed after oral administration. Protein binding: 78%. After oral administration, rapidly taken into bone, with uptake greatest at sites of active bone turnover. Excreted in urine.

Terminal Half-life: Greater than 10 yr (reflects release from skeleton as bone is resorbed).

INDICATIONS AND DOSAGES
▸ **Osteoporosis (in Men)**
PO
Adults, Elderly. 10 mg once a day in the morning.
▸ **Glucocorticoid-Induced Osteoporosis**
PO
Adults, Elderly. 5 mg once a day in the morning.
Postmenopausal women not receiving estrogen. 10 mg once a day in the morning.
▸ **Postmenopausal Osteoporosis**
PO (Treatment)
Adults, Elderly. 10 mg once a day in the morning or 70 mg weekly.
PO (Prevention)
Adults, Elderly. 5 mg once a day in the morning or 35 mg weekly.
▸ **Paget's Disease**
PO
Adults, Elderly. 40 mg once a day in the morning.

SIDE EFFECTS/ADVERSE REACTIONS
Frequent
Back pain, abdominal pain
Occasional
Nausea, abdominal distention, constipation, diarrhea, flatulence
Rare
Rash

PRECAUTIONS AND CONTRAINDICATIONS
GI disease, including dysphagia, frequent heartburn, GI reflux disease, hiatal hernia, and ulcers, inability to stand or sit upright for at least 30 min; renal impairment; sensitivity to alendronate. Carefully evaluate patients when considering the use of dental implants.

Osteonecrosis of the jaw has been reported in patients following oral surgical procedures and who are also taking bisphosphonates.

Caution:
Renal insufficiency, active upper GI disease, may see decrease in serum calcium/phosphate, ensure adequate calcium and vitamin D intake, lactation

DRUG INTERACTIONS OF CONCERN TO DENTISTRY

• Increased risk of GI side effects in doses greater than 10 mg/day: Use NSAIDs, acetylsalicylic acid (ASA) with caution.
• After administration, must wait at least 30 min before taking any other drug.

SERIOUS REACTIONS

! Overdose causes hypocalcemia, hypophosphatemia, and significant GI disturbances.
! Esophageal irritation occurs if alendronate is not given with 6–8 oz of plain water or if the patient lies down within 30 min of drug administration.

DENTAL CONSIDERATIONS

• Bisphosphonate therapy may increase the risk of osteonecrosis of the jaw following dental procedures (see page 38 for management considerations).

General:
• Be aware of oral manifestations of Paget's disease (macrognathia, alveolar pain).
• Consider semisupine chair position for patient comfort because of pain experienced in osteoporosis and GI side effects of drug.
• Consider short appointments for patient comfort.

Consultations:
• Medical consultation may be required to assess disease control and patient's ability to tolerate stress.

Teach Patient/Family to:
• Observe regular recall schedule and use effective oral hygiene measures to minimize risk of osteonecrosis of the jaw.

alfuzosin
ale-few-**zoe**-sin
(Uroxatral, Xatral[CAN])

CATEGORY AND SCHEDULE
Pregnancy Risk Category: B

Drug Class: α_1-adrenergic receptor blocker

MECHANISM OF ACTION
An α_1 antagonist that targets receptors around the bladder base, prostate, prostatic urethra, and prostatic capsule and prostate capsule.
Therapeutic Effect: Relaxes smooth muscle and improves urinary flow and symptoms of prostatic hyperplasia.

USES
Benign prostatic hyperplasia (BPH)

PHARMACOKINETICS
Rapidly absorbed and widely distributed. Food reduces absorption. Protein binding: 90%. Extensively metabolized in the liver via CYP3A4 to inactive metabolites. Primarily excreted in feces (69%) and urine (24%). *Half-life:* 10 hr.

INDICATIONS AND DOSAGES
▶ **BPH**
PO
Adults. 10 mg once a day, immediately after same meal each day.

SIDE EFFECTS/ADVERSE REACTIONS
Frequent
Dizziness, headache, malaise, upper respiratory tract infections (bronchitis, sinusitis, pharyngitis
Occasional
Dry mouth, pain, abdominal pain, constipation, dyspepsia, nausea, impotence, dizziness
Rare
Diarrhea, orthostatic hypotension, tachycardia, drowsiness, priapism, angioedema, chest pain, flushing

PRECAUTIONS AND CONTRAINDICATIONS
Hypersensitivity to alfuzosin or any component of the formulation
Liver disease (moderate or severe)
Concomitant use of cytochrome P450 3A4 inhibitors (e.g., ketoconazole, itraconazole, ritonavir)
Caution:
May increase angina pectoris symptoms
Severe renal impairment, renal failure, renal disease
Known history of QT-interval prolongation
Drugs that prolong QT-interval
Not for use in women and children
Coronary artery disease
Ocular surgery (particularly cataract surgery)

DRUG INTERACTIONS OF CONCERN TO DENTISTRY
• Cimetidine: May increase alfuzosin blood concentration; CYP3A4 inhibitor.

• Cytochrome P450 3A4 inhibitors (e.g., ketoconazole, itraconazole, clarithromycin, ritonavir): May increase alfuzosin blood levels; contraindicated with ketoconazole and itraconazole.
• Antihypertensive agents, other alpha blockers (such as doxazosin, prazosin, tamsulosin, and terazosin): May increase the alpha-blockade effects of both drugs; potential for hypotension.
• Opioids, anticholinergic drugs: May enhance urinary retention in BPH.

SERIOUS REACTIONS
! Priapism has been reported.
! Ischemia-related chest pain may occur rarely.
! Intraoperative floppy iris syndrome (IFIS) has been reported.

DENTAL CONSIDERATIONS

General:
• Monitor vital signs at every appointment because of cardiovascular side effects.
• After supine positioning, have patient sit upright for at least 2 min before standing to avoid orthostatic hypotension.
• Consider semisupine chair position for patient if GI side effects occur.
Consultations:
• Medical consultation may be required to assess disease control.
Teach Patient/Family to:
• Report oral lesions, soreness, or bleeding to dentist.
• When chronic dry mouth occurs, advise patient to:
  • Avoid mouth rinses with high alcohol content because of drying effects.
  • Use daily home fluoride products for anticaries effect.

• Use sugarless gum, frequent sips of water or saliva substitutes.

alglucosidase alfa
al-gloo-ko-**sy**′-dase **al**′-fa
(Myozyme)

CATEGORY AND SCHEDULE
Pregnancy Risk Category: B

Drug Class: Enzyme

MECHANISM OF ACTION
Alglucosidase alfa is a recombinant form of the enzyme acid alpha-glucosidase (GAA), produced in a Chinese hamster ovary cell line. Alglucosidase alfa binds to mannose-6-phosphate receptors on the cell surface and is internalized and transported to lysosomes, resulting in increased enzymatic activity and glycogen cleavage. *Therapeutic Effect:* Provides an exogenous source of GAA, which is the enzyme deficient or absent in Pompe disease.

USES
Used as replacement therapy for Pompe disease (GAA deficiency).

PHARMACOKINETICS
Half-life: 2.3 hr.

INDICATIONS AND DOSAGES
▶ **Replacement Therapy for Pompe Disease**
IV Infusion
Adults. 20 mg/kg over 4 hr, every 2 wk.
Children (1 mo–3.5 yr. at first infusion). 20 mg/kg over 4 hr, every 2 wk.

SIDE EFFECTS/ADVERSE REACTIONS
Frequent
Fever, diarrhea, rash, infusion reaction, vomiting, cough, pneumonia, upper respiratory tract infection, otitis media, oxygen saturation decreased, gastroenteritis, diaper dermatitis, pharyngitis, respiratory distress, oral candidiasis, anemia, respiratory failure, catheter-related infections, pain (postprocedural), gastroesophageal reflux, rhinorrhea, constipation, tachycardia, bronchiolitis, nasopharyngitis, tachypnea, bradycardia, flushing, urticaria. Less frequent adverse effects were not mentioned.

PRECAUTIONS AND CONTRAINDICATIONS
Hypersensitivity to alglucosidase alfa or its components
Caution:
Cardiovascular disease, respiratory impairment, acute underlying illness (increased risk of infusion reactions)

DRUG INTERACTIONS OF CONCERN TO DENTISTRY
• None reported

SERIOUS REACTIONS
! Severe hypersensitivity reactions, including anaphylactic reactions and anaphylactic shock, have been reported during infusion. Infusion-related reactions are common–discontinue immediately for severe hypersensitivity or anaphylactic reaction.
! Cardiac arrhythmia, including ventricular fibrillation, ventricular tachycardia, and bradycardia, resulting in cardiac arrest or death, have been reported.

General:
• Monitor vital signs at every appointment because of cardiovascular side effects.
• Evaluate carefully for drug-related candidiasis and treat in consultation with patient's physician.
• Place patient on frequent recall and use multiple preventive measures to assist with patient's oral hygiene.
• Consult physician to determine disease control and ability of patient to tolerate dental procedures.
Teach Patient/Family to:
• Use atraumatic, effective oral hygiene measures and assist patient with oral care.

aliskiren
(ah-lis-**keer**′-in)
(Tekturna)

CATEGORY AND SCHEDULE
Pregnancy Risk Category: C (first trimester), D (second and third trimesters)

Drug Class: Antihypertensive, direct renin inhibitor

MECHANISM OF ACTION
Directly inhibits renin, decreasing plasma renin activity and inhibiting the conversion of angiotensinogen to angiotensin I.
Therapeutic Effect: Reduces blood pressure by blocking renin-mediated production of angiotensin (vasoconstriction) and aldosterone (salt and water retention).

USES
Hypertension, as monotherapy or in combination with a diuretic

PHARMACOKINETICS
Poorly absorbed after oral administration.
Metabolized primarily in the liver (CYP 3A4); 25% excreted in urine in unmetabolized form, also excreted in feces.

INDICATIONS AND DOSAGES
▸ **Hypertension (Monotherapy)**
Adults. PO 150 mg once daily (antihypertensive effect achieved in 2 wks).
(Daily dose may be increased to 300 mg/day).

SIDE EFFECTS/ADVERSE REACTIONS
Frequent
Diarrhea
Occasional
Dose-related GI disturbances, including abdominal pain, dyspepsia and gastroesophageal reflux; cough
Rare
Rash, elevated uric acid, gout, renal stones

PRECAUTIONS AND CONTRAINDICATIONS
Impaired renal function, hyperkalemia
Hypersensitivity (angioedema), pregnancy
Severe renal dysfunction
Hyperkalemia (especially with an ACE inhibitor in diabetic patients)
Safety during lactation and in pediatric patients not established

DRUG INTERACTIONS OF CONCERN TO DENTISTRY
• CYP3A4 inhibitors: increased blood levels of aliskiren (e.g., azole antifungals, macrolide antibiotics)

SERIOUS REACTIONS
! Head and neck angioedema
! Hypotension

DENTAL CONSIDERATIONS

General:
• Monitor vital signs at every appointment because of underlying disease and cardiovascular side effects of drug.
• Assess salivary flow as a factor in caries, periodontal disease and candidiasis.
• Early-morning appointments and stress-reduction protocol may be needed for anxious patients.
• Use vasoconstrictors with caution, at low doses and with careful aspiration.
• After supine positioning, allow patient to sit upright for 2 min to avoid occurrence of dizziness.

Consultations:
• Consult with physician to determine disease control and ability to tolerate dental procedures.

Teach patient/family to:
• Update medical history when changes in dosage or disease status occur.

alitretinoin

ah-lee-**tret**′-ih-noyn
(Panretin)

CATEGORY AND SCHEDULE
Pregnancy Risk Category: D

Drug Class: Topical retinoid

MECHANISM OF ACTION
Binds to and activates all known retinoid receptors. Once activated, receptors act as transcription factors, regulating genes that control cellular differentiation and proliferation.
Therapeutic Effect: Inhibits growth of Kaposi's sarcoma (KS) cells.

USES
Topical treatment of cutaneous lesions in patients with AIDS-related KS

PHARMACOKINETICS
Minimally absorbed following topical administration.

INDICATIONS AND DOSAGES
▸ **KS Skin Lesions**
Topical
Adults. Initially, apply 2 times a day to lesions. May increase to 3–4 times a day.

SIDE EFFECTS/ADVERSE REACTIONS
Frequent
Rash (erythema, scaling, irritation, redness, dermatitis), itching, exfoliative dermatitis (flaking, peeling, desquamation, exfoliation), stinging, tingling, edema skin disorders (scabbing, crusting, drainage)

PRECAUTIONS AND CONTRAINDICATIONS
When systemic therapy is required (more than 10 new KS lesions in previous month, symptomatic pulmonary KS, symptomatic visceral involvement, symptomatic lymphedema, hypersensitivity to retinoids or alitretinoin ingredients)
Caution:
Avoid pregnancy, discontinue breast-feeding when used, safety in children unknown, patients older than 65 yr, occlusive dressings; do not use products containing DEET

DRUG INTERACTIONS OF CONCERN TO DENTISTRY
• Risk of photosensitivity reaction: tetracyclines, fluoroquinolones, other photosensitizing drugs

SERIOUS REACTIONS

! Severe local skin reaction (intense erythema, edema, vesiculation) may limit treatment.

DENTAL CONSIDERATIONS

General:
• Patients will be taking antiviral drugs; note which drugs are being used because some have potential for significant drug interactions.
• Take a complete medical history, including a current drug history with doses and duration of therapy.

allopurinol

al-oh-**pure**′-ih-nole
(Aloprim, Allohexal[AUS], Allosig[AUS], Apo-Allopurinol[CAN], Capurate[AUS], Progout[AUS] Purinol[CAN], Zyloprim)
Do not confuse Zyloprim with ZORprin.

CATEGORY AND SCHEDULE

Pregnancy Risk Category: C

Drug Class: Antigout drug, antihyperuricemic

MECHANISM OF ACTION

A xanthine oxidase inhibitor that decreases uric acid production by inhibiting xanthine oxidase, an enzyme.
Therapeutic Effect: Reduces uric acid concentrations in both serum and urine.

USES

Chronic gout, hyperuricemia associated with malignancies, recurrent calcium oxalate calculi, uric acid nephropathy

PHARMACOKINETICS

Route	Onset	Peak	Duration
PO/IV	2–3 days	1–3 wk	1–2 wk

Well absorbed from the GI tract. Widely distributed. Metabolized in the liver to active metabolite. Excreted primarily in urine. Removed by hemodialysis. **Half-life:** 1–3 hr; metabolite, 12–30 hr.

INDICATIONS AND DOSAGES
▸ **Chronic Gouty Arthritis**
PO
Adults, Children older than 10 yr. Initially, 100 mg/day; may increase by 100 mg/day at weekly intervals. Maximum: 800 mg/day.
Maintenance: 100–200 mg 2–3 times a day or 300 mg/day.
▸ **To Prevent Uric Acid Nephropathy During Chemotherapy**
PO
Adults. Initially, 600–800 mg/day starting 2–3 days before initiation of chemotherapy or radiation therapy.
Children 6–10 yr. 100 mg 3 times a day or 300 mg once a day.
Children younger than 6 yr. 50 mg 3 times a day.
IV
Adults. 200–400 mg/m^2 day beginning 24–48 hr before initiation of chemotherapy.
Children. 200 mg/m^2 day.
Maximum: 600 mg/day.
▸ **Prevention of Uric Acid Calculi**
PO
Adults. 100–200 mg 1–4 times a day or 300 mg once a day.
▸ **Recurrent Calcium Oxalate Calculi**
PO
Adults. 200–300 mg/day.
Elderly. Initially, 100 mg/day, gradually increased until optimal uric acid level is reached.

▸ **Dosage in Renal Impairment**
Dosage is modified on the basis of creatinine clearance.

Creatinine Clearance	Dosage Adjustment
10–20 ml/min	200 mg/day
3–9 ml/min	100 mg/day
Less than 3 ml/min	100 mg at extended intervals

SIDE EFFECTS/ADVERSE REACTIONS
Occasional
Oral: Somnolence, unusual hair loss
IV: Rash, nausea, vomiting
Rare
Diarrhea, headache

PRECAUTIONS AND CONTRAINDICATIONS
Asymptomatic hyperuricemia
Caution:
Lactation, renal disease, hepatic disease, children

DRUG INTERACTIONS OF CONCERN TO DENTISTRY
• Increased risk of rash: ampicillin, amoxicillin, bacampicillin, hetacillin

SERIOUS REACTIONS
! Pruritic maculopapular rash possibly accompanied by malaise, fever, chills, joint pain, nausea, and vomiting should be considered a toxic reaction.
! Severe hypersensitivity may follow appearance of rash.
! Bone marrow depression, hepatic toxicity, peripheral neuritis, and acute renal failure occur rarely.

DENTAL CONSIDERATIONS
General:
• Patients on chronic drug therapy may rarely have symptoms of blood dyscrasias, which can include infection, bleeding, and poor healing.
Consultations:
• In a patient with symptoms of blood dyscrasias, request a medical consultation for blood studies and postpone dental treatment until normal values are reestablished.
• Medical consultation may be required to assess disease control.
Teach Patient/Family to:
• Encourage effective oral hygiene to prevent soft tissue inflammation.
• Avoid mouth rinses with high alcohol content because of drying effects.

almotriptan malate
al-moe-**trip**′-tan
(Axert)
Do not confuse Axert with Antivert.

CATEGORY AND SCHEDULE
Pregnancy Risk Category: C

Drug Class: Selective serotonin agonist

MECHANISM OF ACTION
A serotonin receptor agonist that binds selectively to vascular receptors, producing a vasoconstrictive effect on cranial blood vessels.
Therapeutic Effect: Produces relief of migraine headache.

USES
Acute treatment of migraine with or without aura in adults

PHARMACOKINETICS
Well absorbed after PO administration. Metabolized by the

liver, excreted in urine. *Half-life:* 3–4 hr.

INDICATIONS AND DOSAGES
▸ **Migraine Headache**
PO
Adults, Elderly. 6.25–12.5 mg. If headache improves but then returns, dose may be repeated after 2 hr. Maximum: 2 doses/24 hr.
▸ **Dosage in Renal Impairment**
For adult and elderly patients, recommended initial dose is 6.25 mg, and maximum daily dose is 12.5 mg.

SIDE EFFECTS/ADVERSE REACTIONS
Frequent
Nausea, dry mouth, paresthesia, flushing
Occasional
Changes in temperature sensation, asthenia, dizziness

PRECAUTIONS AND CONTRAINDICATIONS
Arrhythmias associated with conduction disorders, hemiplegic or basilar migraine, ischemic heart disease (including angina pectoris, history of MI, silent ischemia, and Prinzmetal's angina), uncontrolled hypertension, use within 24 hr of ergotamine-containing preparation or another serotonin receptor antagonist, use within 14 days of MAOIs, Wolff-Parkinson-White syndrome
Caution:
Hypertension, diabetes, hepatitis, renal impairment, elevated cholesterol, obesity, smoking, postmenopause, men older than 40 yr, preexisting heart disease, elderly, lactation, safety/efficacy for pediatric patients not evaluated

DRUG INTERACTIONS OF CONCERN TO DENTISTRY
• Avoid concurrent use of ketoconazole, itraconazole, erythromycin

SERIOUS REACTIONS
! Excessive dosage may produce tremor, red extremities, reduced respirations, cyanosis, seizures, and chest pain.
! Serious arrhythmias occur rarely, particularly in patients with hypertension or diabetes, obese patients, smokers, and those with a strong family history of coronary artery disease.

DENTAL CONSIDERATIONS
General:
• This is an acute-use drug; it is doubtful that patients will undergo dental treatment during acute migraine attacks.
• Be aware of patient's disease, its severity, and frequency.
Consultations:
• If treating chronic orofacial pain, consult with physician of record.
• Medical consultation may be required to assess disease control and patient's ability to tolerate stress.
Teach Patient/Family to:
• Avoid mouth rinses with high alcohol content because of drying effects.
• Update health and drug history if physician makes any changes in evaluation or drug regimens.

alosetron

al-**ohs'**-eh-tron
(Lotronex)
Do not confuse Lotronex with
Lovenox.

CATEGORY AND SCHEDULE
Pregnancy Risk Category: B

Drug Class: Selective serotonin
antagonist, neuroenteric
modulator

MECHANISM OF ACTION
A serotonin (5-HT3) receptor
antagonist that mediates abdominal
pain, bloating, nausea, vomiting,
peristalsis, and secretory reflexes.
Therapeutic Effect: Alleviates
diarrhea, reduces gastric pain.

USES
Treatment of women with diarrhea-
predominant irritable bowel
syndrome (IBS) failing to respond to
conventional therapy

PHARMACOKINETICS
Rapidly absorbed after PO
administration. Extensively
metabolized in liver. Excreted
primarily in urine and, to a lesser
extent, in feces. *Half-life:* 1.5 hr.

INDICATIONS AND DOSAGES
▸ **IBS**
PO
Adults (women older than 18 yr).
1 mg twice a day. Maximum: 2 mg/
day.

SIDE EFFECTS/ADVERSE REACTIONS
Frequent
Constipation

Occasional
Nausea, GI or abdominal discomfort
or pain, dyspepsia, flatulence,
hypertension, clinical depression
Rare
Sedation, abnormal dreams, anxiety

PRECAUTIONS AND CONTRAINDICATIONS
Breast-feeding; constipation;
diverticulitis (active or history of);
GI bleeding, obstruction, or
perforation; history of ischemic
colitis, ulcerative colitis, or Crohn's
disease; thrombophlebitis
Caution:
Food retards absorption, elderly,
reduced hepatic or renal function,
notify physician immediately if
severe constipation or worse occurs,
lactation, children; physicians
prescribing this drug must be
enrolled in the manufacturer's
prescribing program

DRUG INTERACTIONS OF CONCERN TO DENTISTRY
• Does not appear to induce
CYP450 isoenzymes; no interactions
are documented.
• Avoid use of drugs (opioids) that
could lead to increased risk of
constipation.
• Use NSAIDs or acetaminophen for
mild-to-moderate dental pain.

SERIOUS REACTIONS
! Acute ischemic colitis and serious
complications of constipation have
resulted in the need for blood
transfusions and surgery.

DENTAL CONSIDERATIONS

General:
• Short appointments and a
stress-reduction protocol may be
required for anxious patients.

• Consider semisupine chair position for patient comfort because of GI side effects of disease.
• Avoid drugs with anticholinergic activity, such as antihistamines, opioids, benzodiazepines, propantheline, atropine, and scopolamine.
• Question patient about tolerance of NSAIDs or aspirin related to GI disease.
Consultations:
• Consider consulting with physician before prescribing drugs that can cause constipation (opioids).
• Consultation with physician may be necessary if sedation or general anesthesia is required.
• Medical consultation may be required to assess disease control and patient's ability to tolerate stress.
Teach Patient/Family:
• Importance of updating health and drug history if physician makes any changes in evaluation or drug regimens.

alprazolam
al-**praz**'-oe-lam
Schedule IV
(Apo-Alpraz[CAN], Kalma[AUS], Niravam, Novo-Alprazol[CAN], Xanax, Xanax XR)
Do not confuse alprazolam with lorazepam, or Xanax with Tenex or Zantac.

CATEGORY AND SCHEDULE
Pregnancy Risk Category: D
Controlled Substance: Schedule IV

Drug Class: Benzodiazepine

MECHANISM OF ACTION
A benzodiazepine that enhances the action of the inhibitory neurotransmitter gamma-aminobutyric acid in the brain. *Therapeutic Effect:* Produces anxiolytic effect from its CNS depressant action.

USES
Treatment of generalized anxiety disorder, panic disorders, anxiety with depressive symptoms; off-label: agoraphobia

PHARMACOKINETICS
Well absorbed from GI tract. Protein binding: 80%. Metabolized in the liver. Primarily excreted in urine. Minimal removal by hemodialysis. *Half-life:* 11–16 hr.

INDICATIONS AND DOSAGES
▸ **Anxiety Disorders**
PO (Immediate-Release)
Adults. Initially, 0.25–0.5 mg 3 times a day. May titrate q3–4 days. Maximum: 4 mg/day in divided doses.
Elderly, debilitated patients, patients with hepatic disease or low serum albumin. Initially, 0.25 mg 2–3 times a day. Gradually increase to optimum therapeutic response.
PO (Orally Disintegrating)
Adults. 0.25–0.5 mg 3 times a day. Maximum: 4 mg/day in divided doses.
▸ **Anxiety with Depression**
PO
Adults. 2.5–3 mg/day in divided doses.
▸ **Panic Disorder**
PO (Immediate-Release)
Adults. Initially, 0.5 mg 3 times a day. May increase at 3- to 4-day intervals. Range: 5–6 mg/day. Maximum: 10 mg/day.

Elderly. Initially, 0.125–0.25 mg twice a day. May increase in 0.125-mg increments until desired effect attained.
PO (Extended-Release)
▸ **Alert**
To switch from immediate-release to extended-release form, give total daily dose (immediate release) as a single daily dose of extended-release form.
Adults. Initially, 0.5–1 mg once a day. May titrate at 3- to 4-day intervals. Range: 3–6 mg/day. Maximum: 10 mg/day.
Elderly. Initially, 0.5 mg once a day.
PO (Orally Disintegrating)
Adults. Initially, 0.5 mg 3 times a day. May increase at 3- to 4-day intervals. Range: 5–6 mg/day. Maximum: 10 mg/day.
▸ **Premenstrual Syndrome**
PO
Adults. 0.25 mg 3 times a day.

SIDE EFFECTS/ADVERSE REACTIONS

Frequent
Ataxia; lightheadedness; transient, mild somnolence; slurred speech (particularly in elderly or debilitated patients)
Occasional
Confusion, depression, blurred vision, constipation, diarrhea, dry mouth, headache, nausea
Rare
Behavioral problems such as anger, impaired memory, paradoxical reactions such as insomnia, nervousness, or irritability

PRECAUTIONS AND CONTRAINDICATIONS

Acute alcohol intoxication with depressed vital signs, acute angle-closure glaucoma, concurrent use of itraconazole or ketoconazole, myasthenia gravis, severe COPD

Caution:
Elderly, debilitated, hepatic disease, renal disease; dependence, potential for abuse; avoid in lactation, safety and efficacy in patients younger than 18 yr not established

DRUG INTERACTIONS OF CONCERN TO DENTISTRY

• Increased CNS depression: alcohol, other CNS depressants, clarithromycin, erythromycin, fluconazole, miconazole, fluoxetine, isoniazid, fluvoxamine, nefazodone, rifamycin; St. John's wort (herb), kava (herb)
• Contraindicated with ketoconazole, itraconazole, ritonavir, indinavir, saquinavir

SERIOUS REACTIONS

❗ Abrupt or too-rapid withdrawal may result in pronounced restlessness, irritability, insomnia, hand tremors, abdominal and muscle cramps, diaphoresis, vomiting, and seizures.
❗ Overdose results in somnolence, confusion, diminished reflexes, and coma.
❗ Blood dyscrasias have been reported rarely.

DENTAL CONSIDERATIONS

General:
• Monitor vital signs at every appointment because of cardiovascular side effects.
• After supine positioning, have patient sit upright for at least 2 min to avoid orthostatic hypotension.
• Assess salivary flow as a factor in caries, periodontal disease, and candidiasis.
• Psychologic and physical dependence may occur with chronic administration.

Consultations:
• Medical consultation may be required to assess disease control.
Teach Patient/Family:
• When chronic dry mouth occurs, advise patient to:
  • Avoid mouth rinses with high alcohol content because of drying effects.
  • Use daily home fluoride products for anticaries effect.
  • Use sugarless gum, frequent sips of water, or saliva substitutes.

alprostadil (prostaglandin e1, pge1)

al-**pros**′-ta-dil
(Caverject, Edex, Muse, Prostin VR Pediatric)

CATEGORY AND SCHEDULE

Pregnancy Risk Category: C
Naturally occurring prostaglandin (E1, PGE1)

MECHANISM OF ACTION

A prostaglandin that directly affects vascular and ductus arteriosus smooth muscle and relaxes trabecular smooth muscle.
Therapeutic Effect: Causes vasodilation; dilates cavernosal arteries, allowing blood flow to and entrapment in the lacunar spaces of the penis.

USES

Treatment of erectile dysfunction because of neurogenic, vasculogenic, psychogenic, or mixed causes

PHARMACOKINETICS

Rapidly metabolized and cleared from body by urinary excretion

INDICATIONS AND DOSAGES
▶ **Maintain Patency of Ductus Arteriosus**
IV Infusion
Neonates. Initially, 0.05–0.1 mcg/kg/min. Maintenance: 0.01–0.4 mcg/kg/min. Maximum: 0.4 mcg/kg/min.
▶ **Impotence**
Pellet, intracavernosal
Adults. Dosage is individualized.

SIDE EFFECTS/ADVERSE REACTIONS
Frequent
Intracavernosal: Penile pain, prolonged erection, hypertension, localized pain, penile fibrosis, injection site hematoma or ecchymosis, headache, respiratory infection, flu-like symptoms
Intraurethral: Penile pain, urethral pain or burning, testicular pain, urethral bleeding, headache, dizziness, respiratory infection, flu-like symptoms
Systemic: Fever, seizures, flushing, bradycardia, hypotension, tachycardia, apnea, diarrhea, sepsis
Occasional
Intracavernosal: Hypotension, pelvic pain, back pain, dizziness, cough, nasal congestion
Intraurethral: Fainting, sinusitis, back and pelvic pain
Systemic: Anxiety, lethargy, myalgia, arrhythmias, respiratory depression, anemia, bleeding, thrombocytopenia, hematuria

PRECAUTIONS AND CONTRAINDICATIONS

Conditions predisposing to anatomic deformation of penis, hyaline membrane disease, penile implants, priapism, respiratory distress syndrome
Caution:
Patients on anticoagulant therapy, use of sterile technique, care of

syringe, physician instruction in use required, sexually transmitted disease

DRUG INTERACTIONS OF CONCERN TO DENTISTRY

• None reported

SERIOUS REACTIONS

❗ Overdose is manifested as apnea, flushing of the face and arms, and bradycardia.

❗ Cardiac arrest and sepsis occur rarely.

DENTAL CONSIDERATIONS

• None reported

alteplase, recombinant

al-**teep'**-lase

(Activase, Actilyse[AUS], Cathflo Activase)

Do not confuse alteplase or Activase with Altace.

CATEGORY AND SCHEDULE

Pregnancy Risk Category: C

Drug Class: Tissue plasminogen activator

MECHANISM OF ACTION

A tissue plasminogen activator that acts as a thrombolytic by binding to the fibrin in a thrombus and converting entrapped plasminogen to plasmin. This process initiates fibrinolysis.

Therapeutic Effect: Degrades fibrin clots, fibrinogen, and other plasma proteins.

USES

Treatment of acute MI, acute ischemic stroke, acute massive

pulmonary embolism; treatment of occluded central venous catheters

PHARMACOKINETICS

Rapidly metabolized in the liver. Primarily excreted in urine.

Half-life: 35 min.

INDICATIONS AND DOSAGES

▸ **Acute MI**

IV Infusion

Adults weighing greater than 67 kg. 100 mg over 90 min, starting with 15-mg bolus over 1–2 min, then 50 mg over 30 min, then 35 mg over 60 min. Or a 3-hr infusion, giving 60 mg over first hr (6–10 mg as bolus over 1–2 min), 20 mg over second hr, and 20 mg over third hr.

Adults weighing 67 kg or less. 100 mg over 90 min, starting with 15-mg bolus, then 0.75 mg/kg over 30 min (maximum: 50 mg), then 0.5 mg/kg over 60 min (maximum: 35 mg). Or 3-hr infusion of 1.25 mg/kg giving 60% of dose over first hr (6%–10% as 1- to 2-min bolus), 20% over second hr, and 20% over third hr.

▸ **Acute Pulmonary Emboli**

IV Infusion

Adults. 100 mg over 2 hr. Institute or reinstitute heparin near end or immediately after infusion when aPTT or TT returns to twice normal or less.

▸ **Acute Ischemic Stroke**

IV Infusion

Adults. 0.9 mg/kg over 60 min (10% total dose as initial IV bolus over 1 min).

▸ **Central Venous Catheter Clearance**

IV

Adults, Elderly. 2 mg; may repeat after 2 hr.

SIDE EFFECTS/ADVERSE REACTIONS
Frequent
Superficial bleeding at puncture sites, decreased B/P
Occasional
Allergic reaction, such as rash or wheezing; bruising

PRECAUTIONS AND CONTRAINDICATIONS
Active internal bleeding, AV malformation or aneurysm, bleeding diathesis, intracranial neoplasm, intracranial or intraspinal surgery or trauma, recent (within past 2 mo) cerebrovascular accident, severe uncontrolled hypertension

DRUG INTERACTIONS OF CONCERN TO DENTISTRY
• Increased risk of bleeding: drugs that interfere with coagulation or platelet function, such as NSAIDs and aspirin

SERIOUS REACTIONS
! Severe internal hemorrhage may occur.
! Lysis of coronary thrombi may produce atrial or ventricular arrhythmias or stroke.

DENTAL CONSIDERATIONS
General:
• An acute use drug for use in hospitals or emergency rooms.
• Patients are at risk of bleeding; check for oral signs.
• Avoid products that affect platelet function, such as aspirin and NSAIDs.
• Monitor vital signs every appointment because of cardiovascular side effects.
• Patients who have been treated with drug may present with

cardiovascular disease or stroke; review medical and drug history.
Consultations:
• Consultation should include data on bleeding time.
• Medical consultation should include routine blood counts including platelet counts and bleeding time.
• In a patient with symptoms of blood dyscrasias, request a medical consultation for blood studies and postpone treatment until normal values are reestablished.
• Medical consultation may be required to assess disease control and patient's ability to tolerate stress.
Teach Patient/Family to:
• Use soft tooth brush to reduce risk of bleeding.
• Encourage effective oral hygiene to prevent soft tissue inflammation.
• Report oral lesions, soreness, or bleeding to dentist.
• Prevent trauma when using oral hygiene aids.
• Update health and medication history if physician makes any changes in evaluation/drug regimens; include OTC, herbal, and nonherbal remedies in the update.

alvimopan
(al-**vim'**-oh-pan)
(Entereg)

CATEGORY AND SCHEDULE
Pregnancy Risk Category: B

Drug Class: Opioid antagonist

MECHANISM OF ACTION
Peripherally acting mu opioid receptor antagonist (PAM-OR).

Therapeutic Effect: Blocks the adverse side effects of opioid analgesics in the GI tract without interfering with their beneficial CNS effect (analgesia), accelerates time to upper and lower GI recovery following bowel surgery.

USES
Short-term, inpatient control of post-operative ileus (to accelerate recovery following bowel surgery) as an adjunct to opioid pain control (for hospital use only)

PHARMACOKINETICS
Poorly absorbed (absolute bioavailability approximately 6%). Protein binding: 80%. No significant hepatic metabolism, excreted primarily in bile, also in urine (35%). *Half-life:* 10–17 hr.

INDICATIONS AND DOSAGES
▸ **Postoperative Control of Ileus**
Adult. PO 12 mg capsule administered 30 min to 5 hr prior to surgery, followed by 12 mg twice daily beginning the day after surgery for a maximum of 7 days or until discharge. Maximum number of doses: 15.

SIDE EFFECTS/ADVERSE REACTIONS
Frequent
Constipation, flatulence, dyspepsia
Occasional
Anemia, back pain, urinary retention, hypokalemia

PRECAUTIONS AND CONTRAINDICATIONS
May be administered only under the Entereg Access Support and Education program.
Myocardial infarction
Recent use of opioids (increased GI adverse effects)

DRUG INTERACTIONS OF CONCERN TO DENTISTRY
• None reported

SERIOUS REACTIONS
! Hypersensitivity, severe diarrhea, bowel cramping

DENTAL CONSIDERATIONS

General:
• Know status of patient GI disease and surgical recovery.
Consultations:
• Consult with physician to determine disease status of patient and ability to tolerate dental procedures.
Teach patient/family to:
• Update medical history as surgical recovery and GI disease status occur.

amantadine hydrochloride
ah-**man**′-ta-deen hi-droh-**klor**′-ide (Endantadine[CAN], PMS-Amantadine[CAN], Symmetrel)

CATEGORY AND SCHEDULE
Pregnancy Risk Category: C

Drug Class: Antiviral, antiparkinsonian agent

MECHANISM OF ACTION
A dopaminergic agonist that blocks the uncoating of influenza A virus, preventing penetration into the host and inhibiting M2 protein in the assembly of progeny virions. Amantadine also blocks the reuptake of dopamine into presynaptic neurons and causes direct stimulation of postsynaptic receptors.

Therapeutic Effect: Antiviral and antiparkinsonian activity.

USES

Prophylaxis or treatment of respiratory tract illness caused by influenza type A; drug-induced extrapyramidal reactions; parkinsonism

PHARMACOKINETICS

Rapidly and completely absorbed from the GI tract. Protein binding: 67%. Widely distributed. Primarily excreted in urine. Minimally removed by hemodialysis. *Half-life:* 11–15 hr (increased in the elderly, decreased in impaired renal function).

INDICATIONS AND DOSAGES

▸ **Prevention and Symptomatic Treatment of Respiratory Illness Caused by Influenza A Virus**
PO
Adults older than 64 yr. 100 mg/day.
Adults 13–64 yr. 200 mg/day.
Children 10–12 yr. 5 mg/kg/day up to 200 mg/day.
Children 1–9 yr. 5 mg/kg/day (up to 150 mg/day).
▸ **Parkinson's Disease, Extrapyramidal Symptoms**
PO
Adults, Elderly. 100 mg twice a day. May increase up to 300 mg/day in divided doses.
▸ **Dosage in Renal Impairment**
Dose and frequency are modified on the basis of creatinine clearance.

Creatinine Clearance	Dosage
30–50 ml/min	200 mg first day; 100 mg/day thereafter
15–29 ml/min	200 mg

SIDE EFFECTS/ADVERSE REACTIONS

Frequent
Nausea, dizziness, poor concentration, insomnia, nervousness
Occasional
Orthostatic hypotension, anorexia, headache, livedo reticularis (reddish blue, netlike blotching of skin), blurred vision, urine retention, dry mouth or nose
Rare
Vomiting, depression, irritation or swelling of eyes, rash

PRECAUTIONS AND CONTRAINDICATIONS

Hypersensitivity, lactation, child younger than 1 yr
Caution:
Epilepsy, CHF, orthostatic hypotension, psychiatric disorders, hepatic disease, renal disease (necessitates dose adjustment)

DRUG INTERACTIONS OF CONCERN TO DENTISTRY

• Increased anticholinergic response: anticholinergic drugs
• Increased CNS depression: alcohol, other CNS depressants

SERIOUS REACTIONS

! CHF, leukopenia, and neutropenia occur rarely.
! Hyperexcitability, seizures, and ventricular arrhythmias may occur.

DENTAL CONSIDERATIONS

General:
• Monitor vital signs at every appointment because of cardiovascular side effects.
• Assess salivary flow as a factor in caries, periodontal disease, and candidiasis.

• After supine positioning, have patient sit upright for at least 2 min to avoid orthostatic hypotension.
• Avoid dental light in patient's eyes; offer dark glasses for patient comfort.
• Short appointments and stress-reduction protocol may be required for anxious patients.
• Consider semisupine chair position for patients with respiratory distress.

Teach Patient/Family to:
• Avoid mouth rinses with high alcohol content because of drying effects.
• Use powered tooth brush if patient has difficulty holding conventional device.

ambenonium
am-be-**noe′**-nee-um
(Mytelase)

CATEGORY AND SCHEDULE
Pregnancy Risk Category: C

Drug Class: Cholinesterase inhibitor

MECHANISM OF ACTION
A cholinesterase inhibitor that enhances and prolongs cholinergic function by increasing the concentration of acetylcholine through inhibition of the hydrolysis of acetylcholine.
Therapeutic Effect: Increases muscle strength in myasthenia gravis.

USES
Treatment of myasthenia gravis, when other drugs cannot be used

PHARMACOKINETICS
Poorly absorbed after PO administration.

INDICATIONS AND DOSAGES
▶ Myasthenia Gravis
PO
Adults. 5–25 mg 3 or 4 times a day. If well tolerated, after 1 or 2 days, may increase to 50–75 mg 3 times a day. Range: 5–200 mg/day in divided doses.

SIDE EFFECTS/ADVERSE REACTIONS
Frequent
Abdominal pain, diarrhea, increased salivation, miosis, sweating, and vomiting
Occasional
Anxiety, blurred vision, and urinary urgency
Rare
Trembling, difficulty moving or controlling movement of the tongue, neck, or arms

PRECAUTIONS AND CONTRAINDICATIONS
Not recommended in patients receiving routine administration of atropine or other belladonna derivatives. Not recommended in patients receiving mecamylamine
Caution:
Seizure disorders, bronchial asthma, coronary occlusion, hyperthyroidism, dysrhythmias, peptic ulcer, megacolon, poor GI motility, bradycardia, hypotension, lactation, children

DRUG INTERACTIONS OF CONCERN TO DENTISTRY
• Avoid drugs with anticholinergic activity and neuromuscular blocking agents.

• Avoid systemic use of ester-type local anesthetics because of reduced plasma cholinesterase activity.
• Use glucocorticoids with caution.

SERIOUS REACTIONS

! Overdosage may result in cholinergic crisis, characterized by severe nausea, vomiting, diarrhea, increased salivation, diaphoresis, bradycardia, hypotension, flushed skin, stomach pain, respiratory depression, seizures, and paralysis of muscles.
! Increasing muscle weakness of myasthenia gravis may occur. Antidote: 0.5–1 mg IV atropine sulfate with other supportive treatment.

DENTAL CONSIDERATIONS

General:
• Control excessive salivary flow with rubber dam and suction.
• Avoid drugs that reduce salivary flow because they will antagonize this drug.
• Patient may be unable to keep mouth open for long periods because of disease; short appointments may be necessary.
• Monitor vital signs at every appointment because of cardiovascular side effects.
• Evaluate respiration characteristics and rate.
• Consider semisupine chair position for patient comfort if GI side effects occur.
• After supine positioning, have patient sit upright for at least 2 min to avoid orthostatic hypotension.
Consultations:
• Consultation with physician may be necessary if sedation or general anesthesia is required.
• Medical consultation may be required to assess disease control and patient's ability to tolerate stress.
Teach Patient/Family to:
• Use powered tooth brush if patient has difficulty holding conventional devices.
• Update health and drug history, reporting changes in health status, drug regimen changes, or disease/treatment status.

ambrisentan
am-bri-**sin**′-tan
(Letairis [U.S.], Volibris [E.U.])

CATEGORY AND SCHEDULE
Pregnancy Risk Category: X

Drug Class: Endothelin receptor antagonist

MECHANISM OF ACTION
Blocks type A endothelin receptor. *Therapeutic Effect:* Blocks effects of endothelin on vascular smooth muscle, produces vasodilation.

USES
Treatment of pulmonary arterial hypertension to improve exercise capacity and delay clinical worsening

PHARMACOKINETICS
Well absorbed after oral administration. Protein binding: 99%.
Metabolized primarily in the liver (CYP 3A4, 2C19, UGTs); metabolites excreted primarily by non-renal pathways.

INDICATIONS AND DOSAGES
▶ Pulmonary Arterial Hypertension
Adult. PO 5 mg once daily, with or without food, may be increased to 10 mg.

A

SIDE EFFECTS/ADVERSE REACTIONS
Frequent
Reduced red blood cell count, peripheral edema, nasal congestion, sinusitis, flushing, palpitations, pharyngitis, constipation, dyspnea, headache
Occasional
Hepatic injury

PRECAUTIONS AND CONTRAINDICATIONS
May be administered only under the Letairis Education and Access Program.
Women of childbearing potential (Pregnancy Category X)
Pre-existing hepatic disease (see "SERIOUS REACTIONS")

DRUG INTERACTIONS OF CONCERN TO DENTISTRY
• Increased blood levels: CYP3A4 inhibitors, e.g., azole antifungals and macrolide antibiotics (erythromycin, clarithromycin)

SERIOUS REACTIONS
! Potential liver injury (manifested as elevations of aminotransferases)

DENTAL CONSIDERATIONS
General:
• Monitor vital signs at every appointment because of underlying disease and cardiovascular side effects of drug.
• Position patient for comfort because of underlying respiratory disease.
Consultations:
• Consult with physician to determine disease control and ability to tolerate dental procedures.
Teach patient/family to:
• Update medical history as disease and medication status change.

amcinonide
am-**sin**′-oh-nide
(Cylocort)

CATEGORY AND SCHEDULE
Pregnancy Risk Category: C

Drug Class: Antiinflammatory steroidal, topical

MECHANISM OF ACTION
Topical corticosteroids have antiinflammatory, antipruritic, and vasoconstrictive properties. The exact mechanism of the antiinflammatory process is unclear.
Therapeutic Effect: Reduces or prevents tissue response to inflammatory process.

USES
Relief of redness, swelling, itching, and discomfort of many skin problems

PHARMACOKINETICS
Well absorbed systemically. Large variation in absorption among sites: forearm 1%; scalp 4%, forehead 7%, scrotum 36%. Greatest penetration occurs at groin, axillae, and face. Protein binding in varying degrees. Metabolized in liver. Primarily excreted in urine.

INDICATIONS AND DOSAGES
▸ **Dermatoses**
Topical
Adults, Elderly. Apply sparingly 2–3 times a day.

SIDE EFFECTS/ADVERSE REACTIONS
Frequent
Itching, redness, irritation, burning

Occasional
Dryness, folliculitis, hypertrichosis, acneiform eruptions, hypopigmentation, perioral dermatitis
Rare
Allergic contact dermatitis, maceration of the skin, secondary infection, skin atrophy
Systemic: Absorption more likely with occlusive dressings or extensive application in young children.

PRECAUTIONS AND CONTRAINDICATIONS
History of hypersensitivity to amcinonide or other corticosteroids

DRUG INTERACTIONS OF CONCERN TO DENTISTRY
• None reported

SERIOUS REACTIONS
! The serious reactions of long-term therapy and the addition of occlusive dressings are reversible hypothalamic-pituitary-adrenal (HPA) axis suppression, manifestations of Cushing's syndrome, hyperglycemia and glucosuria.
! Abruptly withdrawing the drug after long-term therapy may require supplemental systemic corticosteroids.

DENTAL CONSIDERATIONS

General:
• Determine why patient is taking the drug.
• Side effects include a variety of skin lesions.
Teach Patient/Family to:
• Avoid use on oral herpetic ulcerations.

amifostine
am-ih-**fos**´-teen
(Ethyol)
Do not confuse Ethyol with ethanol.

CATEGORY AND SCHEDULE
Pregnancy Risk Category: C

Drug Class: Cytoprotective, radioprotective

MECHANISM OF ACTION
An antineoplastic adjunct and cytoprotective agent that is converted to an active metabolite by alkaline phosphatase in tissues. The active metabolite binds to and detoxifies metabolites of cisplatin. These actions occur more readily in normal tissues than in tumor tissue.
Therapeutic Effect: Reduces the toxic effect of the chemotherapeutic agent cisplatin.

USES
(1) Incidence reduction in moderate to severe xerostomia in patients undergoing postoperative head and neck radiation for cancer where the radiation port includes a substantial part of the parotid gland; (2) reduction in cumulative renal toxicity associated with repeated cisplatin use in patients with advanced ovarian or non-small cell lung cancers

PHARMACOKINETICS
Rapidly cleared from plasma. Converted in tissue to active free thiol metabolite. Tissue uptake highest in bone marrow, skin, GI mucosa, salivary glands. *Half-life:* less than 1 min. Less than 10% remains in plasma 6 min after drug administration.

INDICATIONS AND DOSAGES

▶ **To Reduce Cumulative Renal Toxicity from Repeated Administration of Cisplatin in Patients with Advanced Ovarian Cancer**
IV
Adults. 910 mg/m² once a day as 15-min infusion, beginning 30 min before chemotherapy. A 15-min infusion is better tolerated than extended infusions. If the full dose cannot be administered, dose for subsequent cycles should be 740 mg/m².

▶ **Treatment of Postoperative Radiation-Induced Xerostomia in Patients with Head and Neck Cancer**
IV
Adults. 200 mg/m² once a day as 3-min infusion, starting 15–30 min before radiation therapy.
Subcutaneous
Adults. 500 mg/day during radiation therapy.

SIDE EFFECTS/ADVERSE REACTIONS

Frequent
Transient reduction in B/P (usually starts 14 min into infusion, lasts about 6 min and returns to normal in 5–15 min); severe nausea, vomiting
Occasional
Flushing or feeling of warmth or chills or feeling of coldness; dizziness, hiccups, sneezing, somnolence
Rare
Clinically relevant hypocalcemia, mild rash

PRECAUTIONS AND CONTRAINDICATIONS

Sensitivity to aminothiol compounds or mannitol

Caution:
Patients should be well hydrated, monitor blood pressure, safety not established in CV disease; elderly, cerebrovascular disease, lactation, children

DRUG INTERACTIONS OF CONCERN TO DENTISTRY

• None reported

SERIOUS REACTIONS

❗ A pronounced drop in B/P may require temporary cessation of amifostine and fluid resuscitation.

DENTAL CONSIDERATIONS

General:
• This is an in-hospital or outpatient chemotherapy drug. Confirm the patient's disease and treatment status.
• Dental treatment may be provided if necessary during treatment.
• Monitor vital signs at every appointment because of cardiovascular side effects.
• Consider semisupine chair position for patient comfort if GI side effects occur.
• Patients taking opioids for acute or chronic pain should be given alternative analgesics for dental pain.
• Short appointments and a stress-reduction protocol may be required for anxious patients.
• Palliative medication may be required for management of oral side effects caused by chemotherapeutic drugs.
• Assess salivary flow as a factor in caries, periodontal disease, and candidiasis.

• Chlorhexidine mouth rinse before and during chemotherapy may reduce severity of mucositis.
• Apply lubricant to dry lips for patient comfort before dental procedures.
• Examine for oral manifestation of opportunistic infection.
Consultations:
• Medical consultation may be required to assess immunologic status during cancer therapy and determine safety risks posed by dental treatment.
• Consultation with physician may be necessary if sedation or general anesthesia is required.
Teach Patient/Family to:
• Prevent trauma when using oral hygiene aids.
• Encourage effective oral hygiene to prevent soft tissue inflammation, infection.
• Report oral lesions, soreness, or bleeding to dentist.
• When chronic dry mouth occurs, advise patient to:
  • Avoid mouth rinses with high alcohol content because of drying effects.
  • Use daily home fluoride products for anticaries effect.
  • Use sugarless gum, frequent sips of water, or saliva substitutes.
  • Update health and drug history, reporting changes in health status, drug regimen changes, or disease/treatment status.

amiloride hydrochloride

a-**mill′**-oh-ride hi-droh-**klor′**-ide
(Kaluril[AUS], Midamor)
Do not confuse amiloride with amiodarone or amlodipine.

CATEGORY AND SCHEDULE
Pregnancy Risk Category: B (D if used in pregnancy-induced hypertension)

Drug Class: Potassium-sparing diuretic

MECHANISM OF ACTION
A guanidine derivative that acts as a potassium-sparing diuretic, antihypertensive, and antihypokalemic by directly interfering with sodium reabsorption in the distal tubule.
Therapeutic Effect: Increases sodium and water excretion and decreases potassium excretion.

USES
Edema in CHF in combination with other diuretics, for hypertension as an adjunct with other diuretics to maintain potassium

PHARMACOKINETICS

Route	Onset	Peak	Duration
PO	2 hr	6–10 hr	24 hr

Incompletely absorbed from the GI tract. Protein binding: Minimal. Primarily excreted in urine; partially eliminated in feces. *Half-life:* 6–9 hr.

INDICATIONS AND DOSAGES
▸ To Counteract Potassium Loss Induced by Other Diuretics
PO
Adults, Children weighing more than 20 kg. 5–10 mg/day up to 20 mg.
Elderly. Initially, 5 mg/day or every other day.
Children weighing 6–20 kg.
0.625 mg/kg/day. Maximum: 10 mg/day.
▸ Dosage in Renal Impairment

Creatinine Clearance	Dosage
10–50 ml/min	Less than 10 ml/min
50% of normal	Avoid

SIDE EFFECTS/ADVERSE REACTIONS
Frequent
Headache, nausea, diarrhea, vomiting, decreased appetite
Occasional
Dizziness, constipation, abdominal pain, weakness, fatigue, cough, impotence
Rare
Tremors, vertigo, confusion, nervousness, insomnia, thirst, dry mouth, heartburn, shortness of breath, increased urination, hypotension, rash

PRECAUTIONS AND CONTRAINDICATIONS
Acute or chronic renal insufficiency, anuria, diabetic nephropathy, patients on other potassium-sparing diuretics, serum potassium greater than 5.5 mEq/L
Caution:
Dehydration, diabetes, acidosis, lactation

DRUG INTERACTIONS OF CONCERN TO DENTISTRY
• Decreased effects: corticosteroids, NSAIDs, indomethacin

SERIOUS REACTIONS
! Severe hyperkalemia may produce irritability; anxiety; a feeling of heaviness in the legs; paresthesia of hands, face, and lips; hypotension; bradycardia; tented T waves; widening of QRS, and ST depression.

DENTAL CONSIDERATIONS
General:
• Monitor vital signs at every appointment because of cardiovascular side effects.
• Assess salivary flow as a factor in caries, periodontal disease, and candidiasis.
• After supine positioning, have patient sit upright for at least 2 min to avoid orthostatic hypotension.
• Patients on chronic drug therapy may rarely have symptoms of blood dyscrasias, which can include infection, bleeding, and poor healing.
• Limit use of sodium-containing products, such as saline IV fluids, for those patients with a dietary salt restriction.
Consultations:
• Medical consultation may be required to assess patient's ability to tolerate stress.
• Medical consultation may be required to assess disease control.
• In a patient with symptoms of blood dyscrasias, request a medical consultation for blood studies and postpone dental treatment until normal values are reestablished.
Teach Patient/Family to:
• Encourage effective oral hygiene to prevent soft tissue inflammation.

• Prevent injury when using oral hygiene aids.
• When chronic dry mouth occurs, advise patient to:
  • Avoid mouth rinses with high alcohol content because of drying effects.
  • Use daily home fluoride products for anticaries effect.
  • Use sugarless gum, frequent sips of water, or saliva substitutes.

aminoglutethimide
ah-mee-noe-gloo-**teth′**-ih-mide
(Cytadren)

CATEGORY AND SCHEDULE
Pregnancy Risk Category: D

Drug Class: Antineoplastic, antiadrenal

MECHANISM OF ACTION
An antiadrenal agent that partially inhibits the conversion of cholesterol to pregnenolone in the adrenal glands and blocks the conversion of androstenedione to estrone and estradiol in peripheral tissues.
Therapeutic Effect: Suppresses adrenal function.

USES
Treatment of some kinds of tumors that affect the adrenal cortex

PHARMACOKINETICS
Rapidly and completely absorbed from the GI tract. Protein binding: Low (20%–25%). Metabolized in the liver by acetylation. Primarily excreted in urine. *Half-life:* 12.5 hr.

INDICATIONS AND DOSAGES
▶ **Cushing's Syndrome**
PO
Adults. Initially, 250 mg q6h. May increase by 250 mg daily every 1–2 wk. Maximum: 2 g/day.

SIDE EFFECTS/ADVERSE REACTIONS
Frequent
Drowsiness, rash, loss of appetite, nausea
Occasional
Dizziness, headache, fever, myalgia, hypotension, tachycardia, pruritus, depression
Rare
Neck tenderness, swelling, increased hair growth in females

PRECAUTIONS AND CONTRAINDICATIONS
Hypersensitivity to glutethimide or aminoglutethimide

DRUG INTERACTIONS OF CONCERN TO DENTISTRY
• None reported

SERIOUS REACTIONS
! Adrenal insufficiency, agranulocytosis, leukopenia, neutropenia, and pancytopenia may occur.

DENTAL CONSIDERATIONS
General:
• Determine why patient is taking the drug.
• Monitor vital signs at every appointment because of cardiovascular side effects.
• Determine dose and duration of glucocorticoid therapy to assess for risk of stress tolerance and immunosuppression. Patients on chronic glucocorticoid therapy may

require supplemental doses for dental treatment.

• Precaution if dental surgery is anticipated or general anesthesia is required.

• Patient on chronic drug therapy may rarely present with symptoms of blood dyscrasias, which can include infection, bleeding, and poor healing. If dyscrasia is present, caution patient to prevent oral tissue trauma when using oral hygiene aids.

• After supine positioning, have patient sit upright for at least 2 min before standing to avoid orthostatic hypotension.

• Patient may need assistance in getting into and out of dental chair. Adjust chair position for patient comfort.

• Examine for oral manifestation of opportunistic infection.

• Caution: use of additional CNS depressants.

• If cancer is present, evaluate surgical, radiation, and chemotherapy history.

Consultations:

• Consultation may be required to confirm glucocorticoid dose and duration of use.

• Medical consultation may be required to assess disease control and patient's ability to tolerate stress.

• In a patient with symptoms of blood dyscrasias, request a medical consultation for blood studies and postpone treatment until normal values are reestablished.

Teach Patient/Family to:

• Update health and medication history if physician makes any changes in evaluation or drug regimens; include OTC, herbal, and nonherbal remedies in the update.

• Report oral lesions, soreness, or bleeding to dentist.

• Avoid driving or performing other tasks requiring mental alertness while taking aminoglutethimide.

• Encourage effective oral hygiene to prevent soft tissue inflammation.

• Prevent trauma when using oral hygiene aids.

aminophylline/ theophylline

am-in-**off**'-ih-lin

(aminophylline) Phyllocontin, (theophylline) Elixophyllin, Quibron-T, Quibron-T/SR, Nuelin[AUS], Nuelin SR[AUS], Slo-Bid Gyrocaps, Theo-24, Thoechron, Theodur, Theolair, T-Phyl, Uniphyl

Do not confuse aminophylline with amitriptyline or ampicillin, or Slo-Bid with Dolobid.

CATEGORY AND SCHEDULE
Pregnancy Risk Category: C

Drug Class: Xanthine

MECHANISM OF ACTION
A xanthine derivative that acts as a bronchodilator by directly relaxing smooth muscle of the bronchial airways and pulmonary blood vessels.

Therapeutic Effect: Relieves bronchospasm and increases vital capacity.

USES
Treatment of bronchial asthma, bronchospasm, Cheyne-Stokes respirations

PHARMACOKINETICS
PO: Peak 1 hr; metabolized in liver; excreted in urine, breast milk; crosses placenta.

INDICATIONS AND DOSAGES
▸ **Chronic Bronchospasm**
PO
Adults, Elderly, Children. 16 mg/kg or 400 mg/day (whichever is less) in 3–4 divided doses (8-hr intervals); may increase by 25% every 2–3 days. Maximum: 13 mg/kg/day (children 13–16 yr); 18 mg/kg/day (children 9–12 yr); 20 mg/kg/day (children 1–8 yr). Maximum dosages are based on serum theophylline concentrations, clinical condition, and presence of toxicity.

▸ **Acute Bronchospasm in Patients Not Currently Taking Theophylline**
PO
Adults, Children older than 1 yr. Initially, loading dose of 5 mg/kg (theophylline); then maintenance dosage of theophylline based on patient group (shown below).

Patient Group	Maintenance Theophylline Dosage
Healthy, nonsmoking adults	3 mg/kg q8h
Elderly patients, patients with cor pulmonale	2 mg/kg q8h
Patients with CHF or hepatic disease	1–2 mg/kg q12h
Children 9–16 yr, young adult smokers	3 mg/kg q6h
Children 1–8 yr	4 mg/kg q6h

IV
Adults, Children older than 1 yr. Initially, loading dose of 6 mg/kg (aminophylline); maintenance dosage of aminophylline based on patient group (shown below).

Patient Group	Maintenance Aminophylline Dosage
Healthy, nonsmoking adults	0.7 mg/kg/hr
Elderly patients, patients with cor pulmonale, CHF, or hepatic impairment	0.25 mg/kg/hr
Children 13–16 yr	0.7 mg/kg/hr
Children 9–12 yr, young adult smokers	0.9 mg/kg/hr
Children 1–8 yr	1–1.2 mg/kg/hr
Children 6 mo–1 yr	0.6–0.7 mg/kg/hr
Children 6 wk–6 mo	0.5 mg/kg/hr
Neonates	5 mg/kg q12h

▸ **Acute Bronchospasm In Patients Currently Taking Theophylline**
PO, IV
Adults, Children older than 1 yr. Obtain serum theophylline level. If not possible and patient is in respiratory distress and not experiencing toxic effects, may give 2.5 mg/kg dose. Maintenance: Dosage based on peak serum theophylline concentration, clinical condition, and presence of toxicity.

SIDE EFFECTS/ADVERSE REACTIONS
Frequent
Altered smell (during IV administration), restlessness, tachycardia, tremor
Occasional
Heartburn, vomiting, headache, mild diuresis, insomnia, nausea

PRECAUTIONS AND CONTRAINDICATIONS
History of hypersensitivity to caffeine or xanthine
Caution:
Elderly, CHF, cor pulmonale, hepatic disease, active peptic ulcer disease, diabetes mellitus, hyperthyroidism,

hypertension, children, glaucoma, prostatic hypertrophy

DRUG INTERACTIONS OF CONCERN TO DENTISTRY
• Increased action: erythromycin (macrolides), ciprofloxacin
• Cardiac dysrhythmia: CNS stimulants, hydrocarbon inhalation anesthetics
• Decreased effects: barbiturates, carbamazepine
• Decreased effects of benzodiazepines

SERIOUS REACTIONS
! Too-rapid IV administration may produce marked hypotension with accompanying faintness, light-headedness, palpitations, tachycardia, hyperventilation, nausea, vomiting, angina-like pain, seizures, ventricular fibrillation, and cardiac standstill.

DENTAL CONSIDERATIONS

General:
• Monitor vital signs at every appointment because of cardiovascular and respiratory side effects.
• Consider semisupine chair position for patient comfort because of respiratory disease and GI side effects of drug.
• Midday appointments and a stress reduction protocol may be required for anxious patients.
• Be aware that aspirin or sulfite preservatives in vasoconstrictor-containing products can exacerbate asthma.
• Acute asthmatic episodes may be precipitated in the dental office. Sympathomimetic inhalants should be available for emergency use.

Consultations:
• Medical consultation may be required to assess disease control.

aminosalicylic acid
ah-**mee′**-noe-sal-ih-sil-ik as-id
(Nemasol[CAN], Paser)

CATEGORY AND SCHEDULE
Pregnancy Risk Category: C

Drug Class: Antitubercular antiinfective

MECHANISM OF ACTION
An antitubercular agent active against *M. tuberculosis*. Thought to exhibit competitive antagonism of folic acid synthesis.
Therapeutic Effect: Bacteriostatic activity in susceptible microorganisms.

USES
Tuberculosis, in combination with other *M. tuberculosis* antiinfectives

PHARMACOKINETICS
Readily absorbed from the GI tract. Protein binding: 50%–60%. Widely distributed (including CSF). Metabolized in liver. Primarily excreted in urine. Removed by hemodialysis. *Half-life:* 1.1–1.62 hr.

INDICATIONS AND DOSAGES
▸ **Tuberculosis**
PO
Adults, Elderly. 4 g in divided doses 3 times a day.
Children. 150 mg/kg/day in divided doses 3 times a day. Maximum: 12 g/day.

SIDE EFFECTS/ADVERSE REACTIONS
Occasional
Abdominal pain, diarrhea, nausea, vomiting
Rare
Hypersensitivity reactions, hepatotoxicity, thrombocytopenia

PRECAUTIONS AND CONTRAINDICATIONS
End-stage renal disease, hypersensitivity to aminosalicylic acid products
Caution:
Hepatic dysfunction, refrigeration required for storage, malabsorption of vitamin B_{12}, no data on safe use in children or lactation

DRUG INTERACTIONS OF CONCERN TO DENTISTRY
• None reported

SERIOUS REACTIONS
! Liver toxicity and hepatitis, blood dyscrasias occur rarely.
! Agranulocytosis, methemoglobinemia, thrombocytopenia have been reported.

DENTAL CONSIDERATIONS
General:
• Determine that noninfectious status exists by ensuring that:
  • **Anti-tuberculosis (TB) drugs have been taken for more than 3 wk.**
  • Culture confirmed TB susceptibility to antiinfectives.
  • Patient has had three consecutive negative sputum smears.
  • Patient is not in the coughing stage.

• Determine why patient is taking drug (i.e., for prophylaxis or active therapy).
• Explain importance of taking medication for full length of regimen to ensure effectiveness of treatment and to prevent the emergence of resistant strains.
• Patients on chronic drug therapy may rarely have symptoms of blood dyscrasias, which can include infection, bleeding, and poor healing.
• Consider semisupine chair position for patient comfort if GI side effects occur.
Consultations:
• Medical consultation may be required to assess disease control and patient's ability to tolerate stress.
• In a patient with symptoms of blood dyscrasias, request a medical consultation for blood studies and postpone treatment until normal values are reestablished.
Teach Patient/Family to:
• Update health and drug history if physician makes any changes in evaluation or drug regimens.
• Prevent trauma when using oral hygiene aids.

amiodarone hydrochloride
ay′-mee-oh-da-rone hi-droh-**klor′**-ide
(Aratac[AUS], Cordarone, Cordarone X[AUS], Pacerone)
Do not confuse amiodarone with amiloride or Cordarone with Cardura.

CATEGORY AND SCHEDULE
Pregnancy Risk Category: D

Drug Class: Antidysrhythmic (class III)

MECHANISM OF ACTION

A cardiac agent that prolongs duration of myocardial cell action potential and refractory period by acting directly on all cardiac tissue. Decreases AV and SN function. *Therapeutic Effect:* Suppresses arrhythmias.

USES

Documented life-threatening ventricular tachycardia; unapproved: ventricular fibrillation not controlled by first-line agents

PHARMACOKINETICS

Route	Onset	Peak	Duration
PO	3 days– 1 wk	1 wk– 5 mo	7–50 days after discontinuation

Slowly, variably absorbed from GI tract. Protein binding: 96%. Extensively metabolized in the liver to active metabolite. Excreted via bile; not removed by hemodialysis. *Half-life:* 26–107 days; metabolite, 61 days.

INDICATIONS AND DOSAGES
▸ **Life-Threatening Recurrent Ventricular Fibrillation or Hemodynamically Unstable Ventricular Tachycardia**
PO
Adults, Elderly. Initially, 800–1600 mg/day in 2–4 divided doses for 1–3 wk. After arrhythmia is controlled or side effects occur, reduce to 600–800 mg/day for about 4 wk. Maintenance: 200–600 mg/day.
Children. Initially, 10–15 mg/kg/day for 4–14 days, then 5 mg/kg/day for several wk. Maintenance: 2.5 mg/kg or lowest effective maintenance dose for 5 of 7 days/wk.

IV Infusion
Adults. Initially, 1050 mg over 24 hr; 150 mg over 10 min, then 360 mg over 6 hr; then 540 mg over 18 hr. May continue at 0.5 mg/min for up to 2–3 wk regardless of age or renal or left ventricular function.

SIDE EFFECTS/ADVERSE REACTIONS
Expected
Corneal microdeposits are noted in almost all patients treated for more than 6 mo (can lead to blurry vision).
Frequent
Parenteral: Hypotension, nausea, fever, bradycardia
Oral: Constipation, headache, decreased appetite, nausea, vomiting, paresthesias, photosensitivity, muscular incoordination
Occasional
Oral: Bitter or metallic taste; decreased libido; dizziness; facial flushing; blue-gray coloring of skin (face, arms, and neck); blurred vision; bradycardia; asymptomatic corneal deposits
Rare
Oral: Rash, vision loss, blindness

PRECAUTIONS AND CONTRAINDICATIONS
Bradycardia-induced syncope (except in the presence of a pacemaker), second- and third-degree AV block, severe hepatic disease, severe SN dysfunction
Caution:
Goiter, Hashimoto's thyroiditis, SN dysfunction, second- or third-degree AV block, electrolyte imbalances, bradycardia; lactation, not recommended for children

DRUG INTERACTIONS OF CONCERN TO DENTISTRY

• Bradycardia, hypotension: inhalation anesthetics, lidocaine, anticholinergics, vasoconstrictors
• Increased photosensitization: tetracyclines
• Do not use with grapefruit juice, gatifloxacin, moxifloxacin, or sparfloxacin.
• Amiodarone is both a substrate and an inhibitor of CYP3A4; potential interactions with strong inhibitors of CYP3A4 isoenzymes.

SERIOUS REACTIONS

! Serious, potentially fatal pulmonary toxicity (alveolitis, pulmonary fibrosis, pneumonitis, acute respiratory distress syndrome) may begin with progressive dyspnea and cough with crackles, decreased breath sounds, pleurisy, CHF, or hepatotoxicity.
! Amiodarone may worsen existing arrhythmias or produce new arrhythmias (called proarrhythmias).

DENTAL CONSIDERATIONS

General:
• Monitor vital signs at every appointment because of cardiovascular and respiratory side effects.
• Assess salivary flow as a factor in caries, periodontal disease, and candidiasis.
• Avoid dental light in patient's eyes; offer dark glasses for patient comfort.
• After supine positioning, have patient sit upright for at least 2 min before standing to avoid orthostatic hypotension.
• Use vasoconstrictors with caution, in low doses, and with careful aspiration. Avoid gingival retraction cord with epinephrine.

• Stress from dental procedures may compromise cardiovascular function; determine patient risk.
• Delay or avoid dental treatment if patient shows signs of cardiac symptoms or respiratory distress.
Consultations:
• Medical consultation may be required to assess patient's ability to tolerate stress.
• Medical consultation may be required to assess disease control.
Teach Patient/Family to:
• Update health and drug history, reporting changes in health status, drug regimen changes, or disease/treatment status.
• When chronic dry mouth occurs, advise patient to:
  • Avoid mouth rinses with high alcohol content because of drying effects.
  • Use daily home fluoride products for anticaries effect.
  • Use sugarless gum, frequent sips of water, or saliva substitutes.

amitriptyline hydrochloride

ah-mee-**trip**′-ti-leen hi-droh-**klor**′-ide
(Apo-Amitriptyline[CAN], Elavil, Endep[AUS], Levate[CAN], Novo-Triptyn[CAN], Tryptanol[AUS])
Do not confuse amitriptyline with aminophylline or nortriptyline, or Elavil with Equanil or Mellaril.

CATEGORY AND SCHEDULE
Pregnancy Risk Category: C

Drug Class:
Antidepressant-tricyclic

MECHANISM OF ACTION

A tricyclic antidepressant that blocks the reuptake of neurotransmitters, including norepinephrine and serotonin, at presynaptic membranes, thus increasing their availability at postsynaptic receptor sites. Also has strong anticholinergic activity.
Therapeutic Effect: Relieves depression.

USES

Treatment of major depression; unapproved: treatment of enuresis and neurogenic pain

PHARMACOKINETICS

Rapidly and well absorbed from the GI tract. Protein binding: 90%. Undergoes first-pass metabolism in the liver. Primarily excreted in urine. Minimal removal by hemodialysis.
Half-life: 10–26 hr.

INDICATIONS AND DOSAGES

▸ **Depression**
PO
Adults. 30–100 mg/day as a single dose at bedtime or in divided doses. May gradually increase up to 300 mg/day. Titrate to lowest effective dosage.
Elderly. Initially, 10–25 mg at bedtime. May increase by 10–25 mg at weekly intervals. Range: 25–150 mg/day.
Children 6–12 yr. 1–5 mg/kg/day in 2 divided doses.
IM
Adults. 20–30 mg 4 times a day.
▸ **Pain Management**
PO
Adults, Elderly. 25–100 mg at bedtime.

SIDE EFFECTS/ADVERSE REACTIONS

Frequent
Dizziness, somnolence, dry mouth, orthostatic hypotension, headache, increased appetite, weight gain, nausea, unusual fatigue, unpleasant taste
Occasional
Blurred vision, confusion, constipation, hallucinations, delayed micturition, eye pain, arrhythmias, fine muscle tremors, parkinsonian syndrome, anxiety, diarrhea, diaphoresis, heartburn, insomnia
Rare
Hypersensitivity, alopecia, tinnitus, breast enlargement, photosensitivity

PRECAUTIONS AND CONTRAINDICATIONS

Acute recovery period after MI, use within 14 days of MAOIs.
Caution:
Suicidal patients, convulsive disorders, prostatic hypertrophy, asthma, schizophrenia, psychotic disorders, severe depression, increased intraocular pressure, narrow-angle glaucoma, urinary retention, cardiac disease, hepatic disease, renal disease, hyperthyroidism, electroshock therapy, elective surgery, children younger than 12 yr, elderly, MAOIs, St. John's wort

DRUG INTERACTIONS OF CONCERN TO DENTISTRY

• Increased anticholinergic effects: muscarinic blockers, antihistamines, phenothiazines
• Increased effects of direct-acting sympathomimetics (epinephrine, levonordefrin)
• Possible risk of increased CNS depression: alcohol, barbiturates, benzodiazepines, CNS depressants, antidepressants

• Possible increase in serum levels: fluconazole, ketoconazole, bupropion, fluvoxamine, paroxetine, sertraline
• Decreased antihypertensive effect: clonidine, guanadrel, guanethidine
• Possible decrease in serum levels: barbiturates, St. John's wort (herb)

SERIOUS REACTIONS

! Overdose may produce confusion, seizures, severe somnolence, arrhythmias, fever, hallucinations, agitation, dyspnea, vomiting, and unusual fatigue or weakness.
! Abrupt discontinuation after prolonged therapy may produce headache, malaise, nausea, vomiting, and vivid dreams.
! Blood dyscrasias and cholestatic jaundice occur rarely.

DENTAL CONSIDERATIONS

General:
• Take vital signs every appointment because of cardiovascular side effects.
• Assess salivary flow as a factor in caries, periodontal disease, and candidiasis.
• Patients on chronic drug therapy may rarely have symptoms of blood dyscrasias, which can include infection, bleeding, and poor healing.
• After supine positioning, have patient sit upright for at least 2 min to avoid orthostatic hypotension.
• Use vasoconstrictors with caution, in low doses, and with careful aspiration. Avoid use of gingival retraction cord with epinephrine.
• Place on frequent recall because of oral side effects.
Consultations:
• In a patient with symptoms of blood dyscrasias, request a medical consultation for blood studies and

postpone dental treatment until normal values are reestablished.
• Medical consultation may be required to assess disease control.
• Physician should be informed if significant xerostomic side effects occur (e.g., increased caries, sore tongue, problems eating or swallowing, difficulty wearing prosthesis) so that a medication change can be considered.
Teach Patient/Family to:
• Encourage effective oral hygiene to prevent soft tissue inflammation.
• Prevent injury when using oral hygiene aids.
• When chronic dry mouth occurs, advise patient to:
  • **Avoid mouth rinses with high alcohol content because of drying effects.**
  • Use daily home fluoride products for anticaries effect.
  • Use sugarless gum, frequent sips of water, or saliva substitutes.

---

amlexanox
am-**lecks**′-ah-knocks
(Apthasol)
Do not confuse with Ambesol.

CATEGORY AND SCHEDULE
Pregnancy Risk Category: B

Drug Class: Topical antiinflammatory

MECHANISM OF ACTION
A mouth agent that has antiallergic and antiinflammatory properties. Appears to inhibit formation and/or release of inflammatory mediators (e.g., histamine) from mast cells, neutrophils, mononuclear cells.

Therapeutic Effect: Alleviates signs and symptoms of aphthous ulcers.

USES
Treatment of aphthous ulcers in patients with normal immune systems

PHARMACOKINETICS
After topical application, most systemic absorption occurs from the GI tract. Metabolized to inactive metabolite. Excreted in urine. *Half-life:* 3.5 hr.

INDICATIONS AND DOSAGES
▶ Aphthous Ulcers
Topical
Adults, Elderly. Administer ¼ inch directly to ulcers 4 times a day (after meals and at bedtime) following oral hygiene.

SIDE EFFECTS/ADVERSE REACTIONS
Rare
Stinging, burning at administration site, transient pain, rash

PRECAUTIONS AND CONTRAINDICATIONS
Hypersensitivity
Caution:
Wash hands immediately before and after each use; discontinue if mucositis appears, lactation, children

DRUG INTERACTIONS OF CONCERN TO DENTISTRY
• None reported

SERIOUS REACTIONS
! Ingestion of a full tube would result in nausea, vomiting, and diarrhea.

DENTAL CONSIDERATIONS
General:
• Recurrent aphthous ulcers may be associated with systemic conditions; evaluate as needed if healing has not occurred after 10 days.
Teach Patient/Family to:
• Apply paste as directed and wash hands immediately before and after each use.
• Report oral lesions or soreness to dentist.

amlodipine
am-**loh′**-dip-een
(Norvasc)

CATEGORY AND SCHEDULE
Pregnancy Risk Category: C

Drug Class: Calcium channel antagonist, dihydropyridine class

MECHANISM OF ACTION
Antianginal and antihypertensive agent that inhibits calcium ion movement across cell members, depressing contraction of cardiac and vascular smooth muscle.
Therapeutic Effect: Decreases myocardial oxygen demand, decreases systemic vascular resistance and blood pressure.

USES
Essential hypertension, chronic stable angina, vasospastic angina (Prinzmetal's or variant angina)

PHARMACOKINETICS
64%–90% bioavailable after oral administration. Protein binding 93%. Primarily metabolized in the liver (90%), primarily excreted in urine. *Half-life:* 30–50 hr.

INDICATIONS AND DOSAGES
▸ **Essential Hypertension, Stable Angina and Vasospastic Angina**
Adult. PO 5 mg once daily, titrated over 7–14 days up to 10 mg daily maximum.
Child (6–17 yr). PO 2.5 to 5 mg once daily.

SIDE EFFECTS/ADVERSE REACTIONS
Frequent
Peripheral edema, headache, flushing, dizziness, palpitation
Occasional
Headache, fatigue, nausea, abdominal pain, somnolence
Rare
Arrhythmias (ventricular tachycardia, atrial fibrillation), bradycardia, chest pain, hypotension, peripheral ischemia, syncope, tachycardia, postural hypotension, vasculitis
Hypoesthesia, peripheral neuropathy, paresthesia, tremor, vertigo
Anorexia, constipation, dyspepsia, dysgeusia, diarrhea, flatulence, pancreatitis, vomiting, gingival enlargement, dry mouth, hyperglycemia, thirst
Allergy, back pain, arthralgia, myalgia, pruritus, rash
Angioedema, erythema multiforme, leukopenia, thrombocytopenia

PRECAUTIONS AND CONTRAINDICATIONS
Advanced aortic stenosis, severe hypotension
CHF, hypotension, hepatic disease, lactation, children under the age of 6, hepatic disease, beta-blocker withdrawal

DRUG INTERACTIONS OF CONCERN TO DENTISTRY
• Decreased effect: NSAIDs (antagonize antihypertensive effect)

• Increased hypotension: sedatives, opioids with hypotensive actions

SERIOUS REACTIONS
❗ Amlodipine may precipitate CHF and MI in patients with chronic cardiac disease and peripheral ischemia.
❗ Overdose produces nausea, somnolence, confusion, and slurred speech.

DENTAL CONSIDERATIONS
General:
• Monitor vital signs at every appointment because of underlying disease and possible cardiovascular side effects.
• After supine positioning, have patient sit upright for at least 2 min before standing to avoid orthostatic hypotension.
• Use stress-reduction protocol.
• Use vasoconstrictors with caution, in low doses and with careful aspiration.
• Place on frequent recall to monitor gingival condition for possible gingival enlargement.
Consultations:
• Consult with physician to determine disease control and ability of patient to tolerate dental treatment.
• Consult with physician if gingival enlargement occurs, to discuss use of alternative medical drug or to emphasize need for frequent monitoring of gingival condition.
Teach Patient/Family to:
• Encourage effective oral hygiene to minimize gingivitis and gingival enlargement.
• Schedule frequent oral hygiene recall visits to control gingivitis and gingival enlargement.
• When chronic dry mouth occurs, advise patient to

• Avoid mouth rinses with high alcohol content because of drying effects.
• Use daily home fluoride products for anticaries effect.
• Use sugarless gum, frequent sips of water, or saliva substitutes.

amoxapine
ah-**moks'**-ah-peen
(Ascendin)
Do not confuse amoxapine with atomoxetine or atropine.

CATEGORY AND SCHEDULE
Pregnancy Risk Category: C

Drug Class: Antidepressant, tricyclic

MECHANISM OF ACTION
A tricyclic antidepressant that blocks the reuptake of neurotransmitters, such as norepinephrine and serotonin, at CNS presynaptic membranes, increasing their availability at postsynaptic receptor sites. The metabolite 7-OH-amoxapine has significant dopamine receptor blocking activity similar to haloperidol.
Therapeutic Effect: Produces antidepressant effects.

USES
Treatment of depression

PHARMACOKINETICS
Rapidly, well absorbed from the GI tract. Protein binding: 90%. Metabolized in liver. Excreted in urine and feces. *Half-life:* 8 hr.

INDICATIONS AND DOSAGES
▸ **Depression**
PO
Adults. 25 mg 2–3 times a day. May increase to 100 mg 2–3 times a day.
Adolescents. Initially, 25–50 mg/day as single or divided doses. May increase to 100 mg/day.
Elderly. Initially, 25 mg at bedtime. May increase by 25 mg/day q3–7 days. Maximum: 400 mg/day (outpatient), 600 mg/day (inpatient).

SIDE EFFECTS/ADVERSE REACTIONS
Frequent
Drowsiness, fatigue, xerostomia, constipation, weight gain
Occasional
Nausea, dizziness, headache, confusion, nervousness, restlessness, insomnia, edema, tremor, blurred vision, aggressiveness, muscle weakness
Rare
Paradoxical reactions (agitation, restlessness, nightmares, insomnia, extrapyramidal symptoms, particularly fine hand tremor), laryngitis, seizures

PRECAUTIONS AND CONTRAINDICATIONS
Acute recovery period following MI, within 14 days of MAOI ingestion, hypersensitivity to dibenzoxazepine compounds
Caution:
Suicidal patients, severe depression, increased intraocular pressure, narrow-angle glaucoma, urinary retention, cardiac disease, hepatic disease, hyperthyroidism, electroshock therapy, elective surgery, elderly, MAOIs

DRUG INTERACTIONS OF CONCERN TO DENTISTRY
• Increased anticholinergic effects: muscarinic blockers, antihistamines, phenothiazines
• Increased effects of direct-acting sympathomimetics (epinephrine, levonordefrin)
• Potential risk of increased CNS depression: alcohol, barbiturates, benzodiazepines, CNS depressants
• Decreased antihypertensive effect: clonidine, guanadrel, guanethidine

SERIOUS REACTIONS
! High dosage may produce cardiovascular effects, including severe postural hypotension, dizziness, tachycardia, palpitations, arrhythmias, and seizures. High dosage may also result in altered temperature regulation, such as hyperpyrexia or hypothermia.
! Abrupt withdrawal from prolonged therapy may produce headache, malaise, nausea, vomiting, and vivid dreams.

DENTAL CONSIDERATIONS

General:
• Take vital signs every appointment because of cardiovascular side effects.
• Assess salivary flow as a factor in caries, periodontal disease, and candidiasis.
• Patients on chronic drug therapy may rarely have symptoms of blood dyscrasias, which can include infection, bleeding, and poor healing.
• After supine positioning, have patient sit upright for at least 2 min to avoid orthostatic hypotension.
• Use vasoconstrictors with caution, in low doses, and with careful aspiration. Avoid use of gingival retraction cord with epinephrine.

• Place on frequent recall because of oral side effects.
Consultations:
• In a patient with symptoms of blood dyscrasias, request a medical consultation for blood studies and postpone dental treatment until normal values are reestablished.
• Medical consultation may be required to assess disease control.
• Physician should be informed if significant xerostomic side effects occur (e.g., increased caries, sore tongue, problems eating or swallowing, difficulty wearing prosthesis) so that a medication change can be considered.
Teach Patient/Family to:
• Encourage effective oral hygiene to prevent soft tissue inflammation.
• Prevent injury when using oral hygiene aids.
• When chronic dry mouth occurs, advise patient to:
  • Avoid mouth rinses with high alcohol content because of drying effects.
  • Use daily home fluoride products for anticaries effect.
  • Use sugarless gum, frequent sips of water, or saliva substitutes.

amoxicillin
ah-mox-eh-**sill**'-in
(Amoxil, Moxage, others)

CATEGORY AND SCHEDULE
Pregnancy Risk Category: B

Drug Class: Antibacterial aminopenicillin, extended spectrum

MECHANISM OF ACTION

Inhibits bacterial cell wall synthesis, resulting in death of susceptible bacteria (bactericidal).
Therapeutic Effect: Bactericidal effect on susceptible microorganisms, reduces severity of or eliminates infection.

USES

For treatment of infections caused by susceptible bacterial species in the orofacial region, upper and lower respiratory tract (including pneumonia), sinuses, pharyngeal/tonsillar region, middle ear, genitourinary tract, skin structures, and in otitis media and sinusitis. Used as a single dose for prophylaxis in patients at high risk of infective endocarditis and to prevent infections of artificial joints in susceptible patients (see section on "Medically Compromised Patients"). Also used in combination therapy of *H. pylori*–related GI disease.

PHARMACOKINETICS

Well absorbed after oral administration. Protein binding 20%. Widely distributed, does not cross blood-brain barrier except in the presence of inflamed meninges. Partially metabolized in the liver, primarily excreted unchanged in urine. *Half-life:* 1–1.5 hr.

INDICATIONS AND DOSAGES
▶ **Ear, Nose, and Throat Infections**
Adult. PO 250 mg q8h or 500 mg q12h (mild to moderate).
PO 500 mg q8h or 875 mg q12h (severe).
Child. PO 20 mg/kg/day in divided doses q8h or 25 mg/kg/day in divided doses q12h (mild to moderate).

PO 40 mg/kg/day in divided doses q8h or 45 mg/kg/day in divided doses q12h (severe).
▶ **Lower Respiratory Tract**
Adult. PO 500 mg q8h or 875 mg q12h (mild, moderate or severe).
Child. PO 40 mg/kg/day in divided doses q8h or 45 mg/kg/day in divided doses q12h (mild, moderate or severe).
▶ **Skin/Skin Structure**
Adult. PO 250 mg q8h or 500 mg q12h (mild to moderate).
PO 500 mg q8h or 875 mg q12h (severe).
Child. PO 20 mg/kg/day in divided doses q8h or 25 mg/kg/day in divided doses q12h (mild to moderate).
PO 40 mg/kg/day in divided doses q8h or 45 mg/kg/day in divided doses q12h (severe).
▶ **Genitourinary Tract**
Adult. PO 250 mg q8h or 500 mg q12h (mild to moderate).
PO 500 mg q8h or 875 mg q1h (severe).
Child. 20 mg/kg/day in divided doses q8h or 25 mg/kg/day in divided doses q12h (mild to moderate).
40 mg/kg/day in divided doses q8h or 45 mg/kg/day in divided doses q12h (severe).

SIDE EFFECTS/ADVERSE REACTIONS
Frequent
Mild GI disturbances (nausea, vomiting, mild diarrhea), headache, oral or vaginal candidiasis
Occasional
Generalized rash, urticaria
Rare
Severe allergic reactions, fatal anaphylaxis

PRECAUTIONS AND CONTRAINDICATIONS

Hypersensitivity to penicillins and cross-sensitivity to cephalosporins, including fatal anaphylaxis
Superinfections
Phenylketonuria (chewable tablets contain phenylalanine)
False-positive urinary glucose tests (if amoxicillin reaches high concentration in urine)

DRUG INTERACTIONS OF CONCERN TO DENTISTRY

• Decreased antimicrobial effectiveness: tetracyclines, macrolide antibiotics, lincosamide antibiotic

SERIOUS REACTIONS

! Antibiotic-associated colitis and other superinfections may result from altered bacterial flora.
! Severe hypersensitivity reactions, including anaphylaxis and acute interstitial nephritis

DENTAL CONSIDERATIONS

General:
• Take precautions regarding allergy to medications.
• If medically prescribed, determine why patient is taking drug.
• If used for prophylaxis, determine that patient has taken drug prior to dental procedure.
• Amoxicillin may be considered among first-choice antibiotics for odontogenic infections, and may be taken with food and liquid if needed.
• May be associated with brown, yellow, or gray tooth staining in pediatric patients (can be removed with brushing or prophylaxis paste).

Consultations:
• Consult with physician to determine disease control and ability of patient to tolerate dental procedures.
Teach Patient/Family to:
• When used for dental infection, advise patient to take at prescribed intervals and complete dosage regimen.
• Discontinue taking drug and immediately notify dentist if signs/symptoms of allergy or diarrhea occur.
• Immediately notify dentist if signs/symptoms of infection are not relieved or increase.

amoxicillin/clavulanate potassium

ah-**mox**′-ih-sill-in /clav-u-**lan**′-ate poh-**tass**′-ee-um
(Augmentin, Augmentin ES 600, Augmentin XR, Ausclay[AUS], Ausclay Duo Forte[AUS], Ausclay Duo 400[AUS], Clamoxyl[AUS], Clamoxyl Duo 400[AUS], Clamoxyl Duo Forte[AUS], Clavulin[CAN], Clavulin Duo Forte[AUS])
Do not confuse amoxicillin with amoxapine.

CATEGORY AND SCHEDULE
Pregnancy Risk Category: B

Drug Class: Aminopenicillin with a β-lactamase inhibitor

MECHANISM OF ACTION
Amoxicillin inhibits bacterial cell wall synthesis, while clavulanate inhibits bacterial β-lactamase.

Therapeutic Effect: Amoxicillin is bactericidal in susceptible microorganisms. Clavulanate protects amoxicillin from enzymatic degradation.

USES

For treatment of infections caused by susceptible ß-lactamase-producing strains of microorganisms as listed: lower respiratory tract infections, otitis media, and sinusitis caused by *H. influenzae, M. catarrhalis;* skin and skin structure infections caused by *S. aureus, E. coli, Klebsiella* species; UTIs caused by *E. coli, Klebsiella, Enterobacter* species; Augmentin ES-600: treatment of recurrent or persistent otitis media, *S. pneumoniae,* and β-lactamase-producing strains of *H. influenzae* or *M. catarrhalis*

PHARMACOKINETICS

Well absorbed from the GI tract. Protein binding: 20%. Partially metabolized in the liver. Primarily excreted in urine. Removed by hemodialysis. *Half-life:* 1–1.3 hr (increased in impaired renal function).

INDICATIONS AND DOSAGES

▸ **Mild-to-Moderate Infections**
PO
Adults, Elderly. 500 mg q12h or 250 mg q8h.
▸ **Severe Infections, Respiratory Tract Infections**
PO
Adults, Elderly. 875 mg q12h or 500 mg q8h.
▸ **Community-Acquired Pneumonia, Sinusitis**
PO
Adults, Elderly. 2 g (extended-release tablets) q12h for 7–10 days.

▸ **Usual Pediatric Dosage**
PO
Children weighing 40 kg and less. 25–45 mg/kg/day (200 or 400 mg/5 ml powder or 200 or 400 mg chewable tablets) in 2 divided doses or 20–40 mg/kg/day (125 or 250 mg/5 ml powder or 125 or 250 mg chewable tablets) in 3 divided doses.
▸ **Otitis Media**
PO
Children. 90 mg/kg/day (600 mg/5 ml suspension) in divided doses q12h for 10 days.
▸ **Usual Neonate Dosage**
PO
Neonates, Children younger than 3 mo. 30 mg/kg/day (125 mg/5 ml suspension) in divided doses q12h.
▸ **Dosage in Renal Impairment**
Dosage and frequency are modified on the basis of creatinine clearance.
Creatinine clearance 10–30 ml/min. 250–500 mg q12h. Creatinine clearance less than 10 ml/min. 250–500 mg q24h.

SIDE EFFECTS/ADVERSE REACTIONS

Frequent
GI disturbances (mild diarrhea, nausea, vomiting), headache, oral or vaginal candidiasis
Occasional
Generalized rash, urticaria

PRECAUTIONS AND CONTRAINDICATIONS

Hypersensitivity to any penicillins, infectious mononucleosis
Caution:
Hypersensitivity to cephalosporins, hepatic function impairment

DRUG INTERACTIONS OF CONCERN TO DENTISTRY
• Decreased antimicrobial effectiveness: tetracyclines, erythromycins, lincomycins
• Increased amoxicillin concentrations: probenecid
• Increased risk of skin rashes: allopurinol

SERIOUS REACTIONS
! Antibiotic-associated colitis and other superinfections may result from altered bacterial balance.
! Severe hypersensitivity reactions including anaphylaxis and acute interstitial nephritis occur rarely.

DENTAL CONSIDERATIONS
General:
• Take precautions regarding allergy to medication.
• Determine why the patient is taking the drug.
Consultations:
• Medical consultation may be required to assess disease control.
Teach Patient/Family:
• Importance of good oral hygiene to prevent soft tissue inflammation.
• Caution to prevent injury when using oral hygiene aids.
• When used for dental infection, advise patient:
  • To report sore throat, oral burning sensation, fever, and fatigue, any of which could indicate superinfection.
  • To take at prescribed intervals and complete dosage regimen.
  • To immediately notify the dentist if signs or symptoms of infection increase.

amphetamine
am-**fet′**-ah-meen

CATEGORY AND SCHEDULE
Pregnancy Risk Category: C
Controlled substance: Schedule II

Drug Class: Amphetamine

MECHANISM OF ACTION
A sympathomimetic amine that produces CNS and respiratory stimulation, mydriasis, bronchodilation, a pressor response, and contraction of the urinary sphincter. Directly affects α and β receptor sites in peripheral system. Enhances release of norepinephrine by blocking reuptake, inhibiting monoamine oxidase.
Therapeutic Effect: Increases motor activity, mental alertness; decreases drowsiness, fatigue.

USES
Narcolepsy, attention-deficit/hyperactivity disorder (ADHD)

PHARMACOKINETICS
Well absorbed from the GI tract. Protein binding: 20%. Widely distributed (including CSF). Metabolized in liver. Excreted in urine. Unknown if removed by hemodialysis. *Half-life:* 7–31 hr.

INDICATIONS AND DOSAGES
▸ ADHD
PO
Adults. 5–20 mg 1–3 times a day.
Adults, Children older than 12 yr. Initially, 5 mg twice a day. Increase by 10 mg at weekly intervals until therapeutic response achieved.
Children 6–12 yr. Initially, 2.5 mg twice a day. Increase by 5 mg/day at

weekly intervals until therapeutic response achieved.
Children 3–6 yr. Initially, 2.5 mg twice a day. Increase by 2.5 mg/day at weekly intervals until therapeutic response achieved.
▸ **Narcolepsy**
PO
Adults. 5–20 mg 1–3 times a day.
Adults, Children older than 12 yr. Initially, 5 mg twice a day. Increase by 10 mg at weekly intervals until therapeutic response achieved.
Children 6–12 yr. Initially, 2.5 mg twice a day. Increase by 5 mg/day at weekly intervals until therapeutic response achieved.

SIDE EFFECTS/ADVERSE REACTIONS

Frequent
Irregular pulse, increased motor activity, talkativeness, nervousness, mild euphoria, insomnia
Occasional
Headache, chills, dry mouth, GI distress, worsening depression in patients who are clinically depressed, tachycardia, palpitations, chest pain

PRECAUTIONS AND CONTRAINDICATIONS

Advanced arteriosclerosis, agitated states, glaucoma, history of drug abuse, history of hypersensitivity to sympathomimetic amines, hyperthyroidism, moderate to severe hypertension, symptomatic cardiovascular disease, within 14 days following discontinuation of a MAOI
Caution:
Gilles de la Tourette's syndrome, lactation, children younger than 3 yr

DRUG INTERACTIONS OF CONCERN TO DENTISTRY

• Increased sensitivity to effects of sympathomimetics; increased risk of serotonin syndrome with selective serotonin reuptake inhibitors (SSRIs)
• Increased pressor response: tricyclic antidepressants

SERIOUS REACTIONS

! Overdose may produce skin pallor or flushing, arrhythmias, and psychosis.
! Abrupt withdrawal following prolonged administration of high dosage may produce lethargy (may last for weeks).
! Prolonged administration to children with ADHD may produce a temporary suppression of normal weight and height patterns.

DENTAL CONSIDERATIONS

General:
• Monitor vital signs at every appointment because of cardiovascular side effects.
• Assess salivary flow as a factor in caries, periodontal disease, and candidiasis.
• Psychologic and physical dependence may occur with chronic use.
• Consider short appointments, frequent recall if patient becomes restless during a dental appointment.
Consultations:
• Medical consultation may be required to assess disease control and patient's ability to tolerate stress.
Teach Patient/Family to:
• Update health and drug history, reporting changes in health status, drug regimen changes, or disease/treatment status.

- Encourage effective oral hygiene to prevent soft tissue inflammation, infection.
- Prevent trauma when using oral hygiene aids.
- When chronic dry mouth occurs, advise patient to:
  - Avoid mouth rinses with high alcohol content because of drying effects.
  - Use daily home fluoride products for anticaries effect.
  - Use sugarless gum, frequent sips of water, or saliva substitutes.

amphotericin b
am-foe-ter′-ih-sin bee
(Abelcet, AmBisome, Amphocin, Amphotec, Fungizone)

CATEGORY AND SCHEDULE
Pregnancy Risk Category: B

Drug Class: Polyene antifungal

MECHANISM OF ACTION
An antifungal and antiprotozoal that is generally fungistatic but may become fungicidal with high dosages or very susceptible microorganisms. This drug binds to sterols in the fungal cell membrane.
Therapeutic Effect: Increases fungal cell-membrane permeability, allowing loss of potassium and other cellular components.

USES
Oral mucocutaneous infections caused by *Candida* species

PHARMACOKINETICS
Protein binding: 90%. Widely distributed. Metabolic fate unknown.
Cleared by nonrenal pathways. Minimal removal by hemodialysis. Amphotec and Abelcet are not dialyzable. *Half-life:* Fungizone, 24 hr (increased in neonates and children); Amphotec, 26–28 hr; Abelcet, 7.2 days; AmBisome, 100–153 hr.

INDICATIONS AND DOSAGES
▸ **Cryptococcosis; Blastomycosis; Systemic Candidiasis; Disseminated Forms of Moniliasis, Coccidioidomycosis, and Histoplasmosis; Zygomycosis; Sporotrichosis; Aspergillosis**
IV Infusion (Fungizone)
Adults, Elderly. Dosage based on patient tolerance and severity of infection. Initially, 1-mg test dose is given over 20–30 min. If test dose is tolerated, 5-mg dose may be given the same day. Subsequently, dosage is increased by 5 mg q12–24h until desired daily dose is reached. Alternatively, if test dose is tolerated, 0.25/kg is given on same day and 0.5 mg on second day; then dosage is increased until desired daily dose reached. Total daily dose: 1 mg/kg/day up to 1.5 mg/kg every other day. Maximum: 1.5 mg/kg/day.
Children. Test dose of 0.1 mg/kg/dose (maximum 1 mg) is infused over 20–60 min. If test dose is tolerated, initial dose of 0.4 mg/kg may be given on same day; dosage is then increased in 0.25-mg/kg increments as needed. Maintenance dose: 0.25–1 mg/kg/day.
▸ **Invasive Fungal Infections Unresponsive to or Intolerant of Fungizone**
IV Infusion (Abelcet)
Adults, Children. 5 mg/kg at rate of 2.5 mg/kg/hr.

▶ Empiric Treatment of Fungal
Infections in Patients with Febrile
Neutropenia; Aspergillosis,
Candidiasis, or Cryptococcosis in
Patients with Renal Impairment and
Those Who Have Experienced
Toxicity or Treatment Failure with
Fungizone
IV Infusion (Ambisome)
Adults, Children. 3–5 mg/kg over
1 hr.
▶ Invasive Aspergillosis in Patients
with Renal Impairment and Those
Who Have Experienced Toxicity or
Treatment Failure with Fungizone
IV Infusion (Amphotec)
Adults, Children. 3–4 mg/kg over
2–4 hr.
▶ Cutaneous and Mucocutaneous
Infections Caused by *Candida
albicans,* such as Paronychia, Oral
Thrush, Perléche, Diaper Rash, and
Intertriginous Candidiasis
Topical
Adults, Elderly, Children. Apply
liberally to affected area and rub in
2–4 times a day.

SIDE EFFECTS/ADVERSE
REACTIONS
Frequent
Abelcet: Chills, fever, increased
serum creatinine level, multiple
organ failure
AmBisome: Hypokalemia,
hypomagnesemia, hyperglycemia,
hypocalcemia, edema, abdominal
pain, back pain, chills, chest pain,
hypotension, diarrhea, nausea,
vomiting, headache, fever, rigors,
insomnia, dyspnea, epistaxis,
increased hepatic or renal function
test results
Amphotec: Chills, fever,
hypotension, tachycardia, increased
serum creatinine level, hypokalemia,
bilirubinemia
Fungizone: Fever, chills, headache,
anemia, hypokalemia,

hypomagnesemia, anorexia, malaise,
generalized pain, nephrotoxicity
Topical: Local irritation, dry skin
Rare
Topical: Rash

PRECAUTIONS AND
CONTRAINDICATIONS
Hypersensitivity to amphotericin B
or sulfites
Caution:
Lactation; not for systemic fungal
infections

DRUG INTERACTIONS OF
CONCERN TO DENTISTRY
• None reported

SERIOUS REACTIONS
! Cardiovascular toxicity (as
evidenced by hypotension,
ventricular fibrillation, and
anaphylaxis) occurs rarely.
! Altered vision and hearing,
seizures, hepatic failure, coagulation
defects, multiple organ failure, and
sepsis may be noted.

DENTAL CONSIDERATIONS

General:
• Determine why the patient is
taking the drug.
• Broad-spectrum antibiotics may
contribute to oral *Candida*
infections.
Teach Patient/Family to:
• Complete entire course of
medication.
• Not use commercial mouthwashes
for mouth infection unless
prescribed by dentist.
• Soak removable appliance in
antifungal agent overnight.
• Prevent reinoculation of *Candida*
infection by disposing of tooth brush
or other contaminated oral hygiene
devices used during period of
infection.

amphotericin b, lipid-based
am-foe-**ter'**-ih-sin bee
(Abelcet, Amphotec, AmBisome)

CATEGORY AND SCHEDULE
Pregnancy Risk Category: B

Drug Class: Antifungal

MECHANISM OF ACTION
An antifungal and antiprotozoal that is generally fungistatic but may become fungicidal with high dosages or very susceptible microorganisms. This drug binds to sterols in the fungal cell membrane. *Therapeutic Effect:* Increases fungal cell-membrane permeability, allowing loss of potassium and loss of other cellular components.

USES
Treatment of infections caused by fungus

PHARMACOKINETICS
Protein binding: 90%. Widely distributed. Metabolic fate unknown. Cleared by nonrenal pathways. Minimal removal by hemodialysis. Not dialyzable. *Half-life:* 7.2 days.

INDICATIONS AND DOSAGES
▸ **Invasive Fungal Infections Unresponsive to, or Intolerant of, Fungizone.**
IV Infusion
Adults, Children. 5 mg/kg at rate of 2.5 mg/kg/hr.

SIDE EFFECTS/ADVERSE REACTIONS
Frequent
Chills, fever, increased serum creatinine, multiple organ failure

Occasional
Nausea, hypotension, vomiting, dyspnea, diarrhea, headache, hypokalemia, abdominal pain, rash

PRECAUTIONS AND CONTRAINDICATIONS
Hypersensitivity to amphotericin B or sulfites

DRUG INTERACTIONS OF CONCERN TO DENTISTRY
• Risk of hypokalemia: glucocorticoids and mineralocorticoids

SERIOUS REACTIONS
! Cardiovascular toxicity (as evidenced by hypotension, ventricular fibrillation, and anaphylaxis) occurs rarely.
! Altered vision and hearing, seizures, hepatic failure, coagulation defects, multiple organ failure, and sepsis may be noted.

DENTAL CONSIDERATIONS
General:
• Intended for serious systemic fungal infections; palliative emergency dental care only.
• Determine why patient is taking the drug.
• Patient on chronic drug therapy may rarely present with symptoms of blood dyscrasias, which can include infection, bleeding, and poor healing. If dyscrasia is present, caution patient to prevent oral tissue trauma when using oral hygiene aids.
• Monitor vital signs at every appointment because of cardiovascular side effects.
• Avoid prescribing aspirin-containing products.

Consultations:
• In a patient with symptoms of blood dyscrasias, request a medical consultation for blood studies and postpone treatment until normal values are reestablished.
• Medical consultation may be required to assess disease control and patient's ability to tolerate stress.

Teach Patient/Family to:
• Encourage effective oral hygiene to prevent soft tissue inflammation.
• Report oral lesions, soreness, or bleeding to dentist.
• Prevent trauma when using oral hygiene aids.

ampicillin
am´-pi-sill-in
(Alpovex[AUS], Amficot, Apo-Ampi[CAN], Novo-Ampicillin[CAN], Nu-Ampi[CAN], Omnipen, Omnipen-N, Polycillin, Polycillin-N, Principen, Totacillin, Totacillin-N)
Do not confuse with aminophylline, Imipenem, or Unipen.

CATEGORY AND SCHEDULE
Pregnancy Risk Category: B

Drug Class: Aminopenicillin

MECHANISM OF ACTION
A penicillin that inhibits cell wall synthesis in susceptible microorganisms.
Therapeutic Effect: Produces bactericidal effect.

USES
Treatment of sinus infections, pneumonia, otitis media, skin infections, UTIs; effective for susceptible strains of β-lactamase negative *E. coli, P. mirabilis, H. influenzae, S. faecalis, S. pneumoniae, S. typhosa, N. gonorrhoeae, N. meningitidis, L. monocytogenes,* shigella, enterococci

PHARMACOKINETICS
Moderately absorbed from the GI tract. Protein binding: 28%. Widely distributed. Partially metabolized in liver. Primarily excreted in urine. Removed by hemodialysis. **Half-life:** 1–1.9 hr (half-life increased in impaired renal function).

INDICATIONS AND DOSAGES
▸ **Respiratory Tract, Skin/Skin-Structure Infections**
PO
Adults, Elderly, Children weighing more than 20 kg. 250–500 mg q6h.
Children weighing less than 20 kg. 50 mg/kg/day in divided doses q6h.
IM/IV
Adults, Elderly, Children weighing more than 40 kg. 250–500 mg q6h.
Children weighing less than 40 kg. 25–50 mg/kg/day in divided doses q6–8h.
▸ **Bacterial Meningitis, Septicemia**
IM/IV
Adults, Elderly. 2 g q4h or 3 g q6h.
Children. 100–200 mg/kg/day in divided doses q4h.
▸ **Gonococcal Infections**
PO
Adults. 3.5 g one time with 1 g probenecid.
▸ **Perioperative Prophylaxis**
IM/IV
Adults, Elderly. 2 g 30 min before procedure. May repeat in 8 hr.

Children. 50 mg/kg using same dosage regimen.
▸ **Usual Neonate Dosage**
IM/IV
Neonates 7–28 days old. 75 mg/kg/day in divided doses q8h up to 200 mg/kg/day in divided doses q6h.
Neonates 0–7 days old. 50 mg/kg/day in divided doses q12h up to 150 mg/kg/day in divided doses q8h.

SIDE EFFECTS/ADVERSE REACTIONS
Frequent
Pain at IM injection site, GI disturbances, including mild diarrhea, nausea, or vomiting, oral or vaginal candidiasis
Occasional
Generalized rash, urticaria, phlebitis, thrombophlebitis with IV administration, headache
Rare
Dizziness, seizures, especially with IV therapy

PRECAUTIONS AND CONTRAINDICATIONS
Hypersensitivity to any penicillin, infectious mononucleosis

DRUG INTERACTIONS OF CONCERN TO DENTISTRY
• Decreased antimicrobial effectiveness: tetracyclines, erythromycins, lincomycins
• Increased ampicillin concentrations: probenecid
• Increased skin rash: allopurinol
• Decreased effects of atenolol
• Suspected increased risk of methotrexate toxicity

SERIOUS REACTIONS
! Altered bacterial balance may result in potentially fatal superinfections and antibiotic-associated colitis as evidenced by abdominal cramps, watery or severe diarrhea, and fever.
! Severe hypersensitivity reactions including anaphylaxis and acute interstitial nephritis occur rarely.

DENTAL CONSIDERATIONS
General:
• Take precautions regarding allergy to medication.
• Determine why the patient is taking the drug.
Consultations:
• Medical consultation may be required to assess disease control.
Teach Patient/Family to:
• Encourage effective oral hygiene to prevent soft tissue inflammation.
• Prevent injury when using oral hygiene aids.
• When used for dental infection, advise patient to:
  • Report sore throat, oral burning sensation, fever, and fatigue, any of which could indicate superinfection.
  • Take at prescribed intervals and complete dosage regimen.
  • Immediately notify the dentist if signs or symptoms of infection increase.

ampicillin sodium

am-pi-**sill'**-in **soe'**-dee-um
(Alphacin[AUS], Apo-Ampi[CAN],
Novo-Ampicillin[CAN],
Nu-Ampi[CAN], Polycillin,
Principen)
Do not confuse ampicillin with
aminophylline, Imipenem, or
Unipen.

CATEGORY AND SCHEDULE
Pregnancy Risk Category: B

Drug Class: Aminopenicillin

MECHANISM OF ACTION
A penicillin that inhibits cell wall
synthesis in susceptible
microorganisms.
Therapeutic Effect: Bactericidal.

USES
Sinus infections, pneumonia, otitis
media, skin infections, UTIs;
effective for susceptible strains of
β-lactamase negative) E. coli,
P. mirabilis, H. influenzae,
S. faecalis, S. pneumoniae,
S. typhosa, N. gonorrhoeae,
N. meningitidis, L. monocytogenes,
shigella, enterococci

PHARMACOKINETICS
Moderately absorbed from the GI
tract. Protein binding: 28%. Widely
distributed. Partially metabolized in
the liver. Primarily excreted in urine.
Removed by hemodialysis. *Half-life:*
1–1.5 hr (increased in impaired
renal function).

INDICATIONS AND DOSAGES
▸ **Respiratory Tract, Skin and**
Skin-Structure Infections
PO
Adults, Elderly. 250–500 mg q6h.

Children. 50–100 mg/kg/day in
divided doses q6h. Maximum: 3 g/
day.
IV, IM
Adults, Elderly. 500 mg to 3 g q6h.
Maximum: 14 g/day.
Children. 100–200 mg/kg/day in
divided doses q6h.
Neonates. 50–100 mg/kg/day in
divided doses q6–12h.
▸ **Meningitis**
IV
Children. 200–400 mg/kg/day in
divided doses q6h. Maximum: 12 g/
day.
Neonates. 100–200 mg/kg/day in
divided doses q6–12h.
▸ **Gonococcal Infections**
PO
Adults. 3.5 g one time with 1 g
probenecid.
▸ **Perioperative Prophylaxis**
IV, IM
Adults, Elderly. 2 g 30 min before
procedure. May repeat in 8 hr.
Children. 50 mg/kg 30 min before
procedure. May repeat in 8 hr.
▸ **Dosage in Renal Impairment**

Creatinine Clearance	% of Normal Dosage
10–30 ml/min	Give q6–12h
Less than 10 ml/min	Give q12h

SIDE EFFECTS/ADVERSE REACTIONS
Frequent
Pain at IM injection site, GI
disturbances (mild diarrhea, nausea,
vomiting), oral or vaginal
candidiasis
Occasional
Generalized rash, urticaria, phlebitis
or thrombophlebitis (with IV
administration), headache

Rare
Dizziness, seizures (especially with
IV therapy)

PRECAUTIONS AND CONTRAINDICATIONS
Hypersensitivity to any penicillin,
infectious mononucleosis

DRUG INTERACTIONS OF CONCERN TO DENTISTRY
• Decreased antimicrobial
effectiveness: tetracyclines,
erythromycins, lincomycins
• Increased ampicillin
concentrations: probenecid
• Increased skin rash: allopurinol
• Decreased effects of atenolol
• Suspected increased risk of
methotrexate toxicity

SERIOUS REACTIONS
! Antibiotic-associated colitis and
other superinfections may result
from altered bacterial balance.
! Severe hypersensitivity reactions,
including anaphylaxis and acute
interstitial nephritis, occur rarely.

DENTAL CONSIDERATIONS

General:
• Take precautions regarding allergy
to medication.
• Determine why the patient is
taking the drug.
Consultations:
• Medical consultation may be
required to assess disease control.
Teach Patient/Family to:
• Encourage effective oral hygiene
to prevent soft tissue inflammation.
• Prevent injury when using oral
hygiene aids.
• When used for dental infection,
advise patient to:
 • Report sore throat, oral
 burning sensation, fever, and

fatigue, any of which could
indicate superinfection.
• Take at prescribed intervals
and complete dosage regimen.
• Immediately notify the dentist
if signs or symptoms of infection
increase.

ampicillin/sulbactam sodium
am′-pi-sill-in/sul-**bac′**-tam
so′-dee-um
(Unasyn)

CATEGORY AND SCHEDULE
Pregnancy Risk Category: B

Drug Class: Aminopenicillin

MECHANISM OF ACTION
Ampicillin inhibits bacterial cell
wall synthesis, while sulbactam
inhibits bacterial β-lactamase.
Therapeutic Effect: Ampicillin is
bactericidal in susceptible
microorganisms. Sulbactam protects
ampicillin from enzymatic
degradation.

USES
Elimination of bacteria

PHARMACOKINETICS
Protein binding: 28%–38%. Widely
distributed. Partially metabolized in
the liver. Primarily excreted in urine.
Removed by hemodialysis. *Half-life:*
1 hr (increased in impaired renal
function).

INDICATIONS AND DOSAGES
▸ **Skin and Skin-Structure, Intraabdominal, and Gynecologic Infections**
IV, IM
Adults, Elderly. 1.5 g (1 g ampicillin/500 mg sulbactam) to 3 g (2 g ampicillin/1 g sulbactam) q6h.
▸ **Dosage in Renal Impairment**
Dosage and frequency are modified based on creatinine clearance and the severity of the infection.

Creatinine Clearance	Dosage
Greater than 30 ml/min	0.5–3 g q6–8h
15–29 ml/min	1.5–3 g q12h
5–14 ml/min	1.5–3 g q24h
Less than 5 ml/min	Not recommended

SIDE EFFECTS/ADVERSE REACTIONS
Frequent
Diarrhea and rash (most common), urticaria, pain at IM injection site, thrombophlebitis with IV administration, oral or vaginal candidiasis
Occasional
Nausea, vomiting, headache, malaise, urine retention

PRECAUTIONS AND CONTRAINDICATIONS
Hypersensitivity to any penicillin, infectious mononucleosis

DRUG INTERACTIONS OF CONCERN TO DENTISTRY
• Decreased antimicrobial effectiveness: tetracyclines, erythromycins, lincomycins
• Increased ampicillin concentration: probenecid
• Increased skin rash: allopurinol
• Decreased effects of atenolol
• Suspected increased risk of methotrexate toxicity

• Increased risk of bleeding with anticoagulants: large IV doses of penicillins
• When used for dental infection:
  • **Oral contraceptives: advise patient of a low potential risk for decreased contraceptive action, to maintain compliance with oral contraceptive use while using antibiotics, and to consider the use of additional nonhormonal contraception**

SERIOUS REACTIONS
❗ Severe hypersensitivity reactions including anaphylaxis, acute interstitial nephritis, and blood dyscrasias may occur.
❗ Antibiotic-associated colitis and other superinfections may result from altered bacterial balance.
❗ Overdose may produce seizures.

DENTAL CONSIDERATIONS
General:
• For selected infections in the hospital setting, provide emergency dental treatment only.
• Caution regarding allergy to medication.
• Examine for oral manifestation of opportunistic infection.
• Determine why patient is taking the drug.
Consultations:
• Medical consultation may be required to assess disease control.
• Consult patient's physician if an acute dental infection occurs and another antiinfective is required.
Teach Patient/Family to:
• Encourage effective oral hygiene to prevent soft tissue inflammation.
• Report oral lesions, soreness, or bleeding to dentist.
• Prevent trauma when using oral hygiene aids.

- See dentist immediately if secondary oral infection occurs.
- When used for dental infection, advise patient to:
  - Report sore throat, oral burning sensation, fever, or fatigue, any of which could indicate superinfection.
  - Take at prescribed intervals and complete dosage regimen.
  - Immediately notify the dentist if signs or symptoms of infection increase.

amprenavir
am-**pren**′-eh-veer
(Agenerase)
Do not confuse Agenerase with asparaginase.

CATEGORY AND SCHEDULE
Pregnancy Risk Category: C

Drug Class: Antiviral

MECHANISM OF ACTION
An antiretroviral that inhibits HIV-1 protease by binding to the enzyme's active site, thus preventing processing of viral precursors and resulting in the formation of immature, noninfectious viral particles.
Therapeutic Effect: Impairs HIV replication and proliferation.

USES
HIV-1 infection, in combination with other antiretroviral agents

PHARMACOKINETICS
Rapidly absorbed after PO administration. Protein binding: 90%. Metabolized in the liver. Primarily excreted in feces.
Half-life: 7.1–10.6 hr.

INDICATIONS AND DOSAGES
▸ **HIV-1 Infection (in combination with other antiretrovirals)**
PO
Adults, Children 13–16 yr. 1200 mg capsules twice a day.
Children 4–12 yr, and children 13–16 yr weighing less than 50 kg. 20 mg/kg twice a day or 15 mg/kg 3 times a day. Maximum: 2400 mg/day.
Oral Solution
Adults. 1400 mg 2 times/day.
Children 4–12 yr, and children 13–16 yr weighing less than 50 kg. 22.5 mg/kg/day (1.5 ml/kg) oral solution twice a day or 17 mg/kg/day (1.1 ml/kg) 3 times a day. Maximum: 2800 mg/day.
▸ **Dosage in Hepatic Impairment**
Dosage and frequency are modified on the basis of the Child-Pugh score.

Child-Pugh Scores	Capsules	Oral Solution
5–8	450 mg bid	513 mg bid
9–12	300 mg bid	342 mg bid

SIDE EFFECTS/ADVERSE REACTIONS
Frequent
Diarrhea or loose stools, nausea, oral paresthesia, rash, vomiting
Occasional
Peripheral paresthesia, depression

PRECAUTIONS AND CONTRAINDICATIONS
Concurrent use with midazolam, triazolam, bepridil, disulfiram, metronidazole, pimozide, and ergot-like drugs; hypersensitivity; serious reactions could occur with lidocaine (systemic) or other antiarrhythmics and tricyclic antidepressants; avoid use of drugs

metabolized by CYP3A4 enzymes; lactation

Caution:
Exacerbation of diabetes, hyperglycemia, use of additional vitamin E, hemophilia, viral resistance, risk of cross allergy with sulfonamides, fat redistribution, hepatic disease, patients on oral contraceptives, sildenafil; oral solution contains propylene glycol with risk of toxicity to children younger than 4 yr

DRUG INTERACTIONS OF CONCERN TO DENTISTRY

• Contraindicated with midazolam, triazolam, tricyclic antidepressants
• Increased plasma levels of erythromycin, clarithromycin, itraconazole, alprazolam, clorazepate, diazepam, carbamazepine, loratadine, flurazepam, ketoconazole, itraconazole; lidocaine (systemic use for cardiac arrhythmias)
• Decreased effectiveness: dexamethasone, St. John's wort (herb)
• Use with caution: sildenafil, vardenafil, todalafil

SERIOUS REACTIONS

! Severe hypersensitivity reactions or Stevens-Johnson syndrome as evidenced by blisters, peeling of the skin, loosening of skin and mucous membranes, and fever may occur.

DENTAL CONSIDERATIONS

General:
• Palliative medication may be required for management of oral side effects.
• Examine for oral manifestation of opportunistic infection.

• Patients on chronic drug therapy may rarely have symptoms of blood dyscrasias, which can include infection, bleeding, and poor healing.
• Consider semisupine chair position for patient comfort if GI side effects occur.

Consultations:
• In a patient with symptoms of blood dyscrasias, request a medical consultation for blood studies and postpone treatment until normal values are reestablished.
• Medical consultation may be required to assess disease control and patient's ability to tolerate stress.

Teach Patient/Family to:
• Encourage effective oral hygiene to prevent soft tissue inflammation.
• Prevent trauma when using oral hygiene aids.
• Update health and drug history if physician makes any changes in evaluation or drug regimens.
• See dentist immediately if secondary oral infection occurs.

amyl nitrite
am′-il nye′-trite
(Amyl Nitrite)
Do not confuse with Nicobid, Nicoderm, Nilstat, nitroprusside, Nizoral, or Nystatin.

CATEGORY AND SCHEDULE
Pregnancy Risk Category: C

Drug Class: Antianginal

MECHANISM OF ACTION
A nitrite vasodilator that relaxes smooth muscles. Reduces afterload

and improves vascular supply to the myocardium.
Therapeutic Effect: Dilates coronary arteries, improves blood flow to ischemic areas within myocardium. Following inhalation, systemic vasodilation occurs.

USES
Pain relief of anginal attacks

PHARMACOKINETICS
The vapors are absorbed rapidly through the pulmonary alveoli and metabolized rapidly. Partially excreted in the urine.

INDICATIONS AND DOSAGES
▸ **Acute Relief of Angina Pectoris**
Nasal Inhalation
Adults, Elderly. Place crushed capsule to nostrils for 0.18–0.3 ml inhalation of vapors. Repeat at 5–10 min intervals. No more than 3 doses in a 15–30 min period.

SIDE EFFECTS/ADVERSE REACTIONS
Frequent
Headache (may be severe) occurs mostly in early therapy, diminishes rapidly in intensity, usually disappears during continued treatment; transient flushing of face and neck; dizziness (especially if patient is standing immobile or is in a warm environment); weakness; postural hypotension
Occasional
Nausea, rash, vomiting
Rare
Involuntary passage of urine and feces, restlessness, weakness

PRECAUTIONS AND CONTRAINDICATIONS
Closed-angle glaucoma, severe anemia, head injury, postural hypotension, pregnancy, hypersensitivity to nitrates

DRUG INTERACTIONS OF CONCERN TO DENTISTRY
• None reported

SERIOUS REACTIONS
❗ Large doses may produce hemolytic anemia or methemoglobinemia.
❗ Severe postural hypotension manifested by fainting, pulselessness, cold or clammy skin, and profuse sweating may occur.
❗ Tolerance may occur with repeated, prolonged therapy.
❗ High dose tends to produce severe headache.

DENTAL CONSIDERATIONS
General:
• For emergency relief of acute angina; if angina is not relieved, call 911 for transfer of patient to a medical emergency facility.
• Prior to treatment, inquire about disease control and frequency of angina episodes.
• Ensure that patient's rescue antianginal drug is available for use.
• Monitor vital signs at every appointment because of cardiovascular side effects.
• Postpone elective dental treatment if patient shows signs of cardiac symptoms or respiratory distress.
• After supine positioning, have patient sit upright for at least 2 min before standing to avoid orthostatic hypotension.
Consultations:
• Medical consultation may be required to assess disease control and patient's ability to tolerate stress.

Teach Patient/Family to:
• Report angina symptoms to physician.
• Update health and medication history if physician makes any changes in evaluation or drug regimens; include OTC, herbal, and nonherbal remedies in the update.
• Encourage effective oral hygiene to prevent soft tissue inflammation.

anagrelide
ah-**na**′-greh-lide
(Agrylin)

CATEGORY AND SCHEDULE
Pregnancy Risk Category: C

Drug Class: Platelet count-reducing agent

MECHANISM OF ACTION
A hematologic agent that reduces platelet production and prevents platelet shape changes caused by platelet aggregating agents.
Therapeutic Effect: Inhibits platelet aggregation.

USES
Decreases the risk of blood clots in patients who have too many platelet cells

PHARMACOKINETICS
After oral administration, plasma concentration peak within 1 hr. Extensively metabolized. Primarily excreted in urine. *Half-life:* About 3 days.

INDICATIONS AND DOSAGES
▸ Thrombocythemia
PO
Adults, Elderly. Initially, 0.5 mg 4 times a day or 1 mg twice a day. Adjust to lowest effective dosage, increasing by up to 0.5 mg/day or less in any 1 wk. Maximum: 10 mg/day or 2.5 mg/dose.

SIDE EFFECTS/ADVERSE REACTIONS
Frequent
Headache, palpitations, diarrhea, abdominal pain, nausea, flatulence, bloating, asthenia, pain, dizziness
Occasional
Tachycardia, chest pain, vomiting, paresthesia, peripheral edema, anorexia, dyspepsia, rash
Rare
Confusion, insomnia

PRECAUTIONS AND CONTRAINDICATIONS
Caution:
Cardiac disease, renal impairment, hepatic impairment, monitor reduction in platelets, risk of thrombocytopenia especially while correct dose is being found, sudden discontinuance of use, lactation, children younger than 16 yr

DRUG INTERACTIONS OF CONCERN TO DENTISTRY
• Possible risk of hemorrhage: NSAIDs, aspirin

SERIOUS REACTIONS
! Angina, heart failure, and arrhythmias occur rarely.

DENTAL CONSIDERATIONS

General:
• Laboratory studies should include routine complete blood counts (CBCs).

• Patients have risk of thrombohemorrhagic complications; prolonged bleeding time, anemia, or splenomegaly may occur in some patients with this disease. However, thrombosis may also occur in some patients.
• Mucosal bleeding can be a symptom of disease.
• Patients with severe symptoms may be taking chemotherapy.
• Monitor vital signs at every appointment because of cardiovascular side effects.
• Consider semisupine chair position for patient comfort if GI side effects occur.

Consultations:
• Medical consultation with hematologist or physician directing therapy is essential before dental treatment.

Teach Patient/Family to:
• Inform dentist of unusual bleeding episodes following dental treatment.
• Update health and drug history if physician makes any changes in evaluation or drug regimens.

anakinra
an-ah-**kin**′-ra
(Kineret)

CATEGORY AND SCHEDULE
Pregnancy Risk Category: B

Drug Class: Antirheumatic

MECHANISM OF ACTION
An interleukin-1 (IL-1) receptor antagonist that blocks the binding of IL-1, a protein that is a major mediator of joint disease and is present in excess amounts in patients with rheumatoid arthritis.

Therapeutic Effect: Inhibits the inflammatory response.

USES
Treatment of moderate to severe symptoms of rheumatoid arthritis

PHARMACOKINETICS
No accumulation of anakinra in tissues or organs was observed after daily subcutaneous doses. Excreted in urine. *Half-life:* 4–6 hr.

INDICATIONS AND DOSAGES
▸ **Rheumatoid Arthritis**
Subcutaneous
Adults, Children older than 18 yr, Elderly. 100 mg/day, given at same time each day.

SIDE EFFECTS/ADVERSE REACTIONS
Occasional
Injection site ecchymosis, erythema, and inflammation
Rare
Headache, nausea, diarrhea, abdominal pain

PRECAUTIONS AND CONTRAINDICATIONS
Known hypersensitivity to *Escherichia coli*-derived proteins, serious infection

DRUG INTERACTIONS OF CONCERN TO DENTISTRY
• None reported

SERIOUS REACTIONS
! Infections, including upper respiratory tract infection, sinusitis, flu-like symptoms, and cellulitis, have been noted.
! Neutropenia may occur, particularly when anakinra is used in combination with tumor necrosis factor-blocking agents.

DENTAL CONSIDERATIONS

General:
• Question patient about other drugs or products he or she may be taking for arthritis.
• Patient may be at risk for infection.
• Oral infections should be eliminated and/or treated aggressively.
• Evaluate efficacy of oral hygiene home care; preventive instruction appointment may be necessary.
• Patient on chronic drug therapy may rarely present with symptoms of blood dyscrasias, which can include infection, bleeding, and poor healing. If dyscrasia is present, caution patient to prevent oral tissue trauma when using oral hygiene aids.
• Patient may need assistance in getting into and out of dental chair. Adjust chair position for patient comfort.

Consultations:
• Medical consultation may be required to assess disease control.
• In a patient with symptoms of blood dyscrasias, request a medical consultation for blood studies and postpone treatment until normal values are reestablished.

Teach Patient/Family to:
• Use powered tooth brush if patient has difficulty holding conventional devices.
• Prevent trauma when using oral hygiene aids.
• Encourage effective oral hygiene to prevent soft tissue inflammation.
• Update health and medication history if physician makes any changes in evaluation or drug regimens; include OTC, herbal, and nonherbal remedies in the update.

anastrozole
ah-**nas'**-trow-zole
(Arimidex)
Do not confuse Arimidex with Imitrex.

CATEGORY AND SCHEDULE
Pregnancy Risk Category: D

Drug Class: Antineoplastic

MECHANISM OF ACTION
Decreases the circulating estrogen level by inhibiting aromatase, the enzyme that catalyzes the final step in estrogen production.
Therapeutic Effect: Inhibits the growth of breast cancers that are stimulated by estrogens.

USES
Treatment of breast cancer

PHARMACOKINETICS
Well absorbed into systemic circulation (absorption not affected by food). Protein binding: 40%. Extensively metabolized in the liver. Eliminated by biliary system and, to a lesser extent, kidneys. *Mean Half-life:* 50 hr in postmenopausal women. Steady-state plasma levels reached in about 7 days.

INDICATIONS AND DOSAGES
▶ **Breast Cancer**
PO
Adults, Elderly. 1 mg once a day.

SIDE EFFECTS/ADVERSE REACTIONS
Frequent
Asthenia, nausea, headache, hot flashes, back pain, vomiting, cough, diarrhea

Occasional

Constipation, abdominal pain, anorexia, bone pain, pharyngitis, dizziness, rash, dry mouth, peripheral edema, pelvic pain, depression, chest pain, paresthesia

Rare

Weight gain, diaphoresis

PRECAUTIONS AND CONTRAINDICATIONS

None known

DRUG INTERACTIONS OF CONCERN TO DENTISTRY

• None reported

SERIOUS REACTIONS

! Thrombophlebitis, anemia, leukopenia, and vaginal hemorrhage occur rarely.

! Vaginal hemorrhage occurs rarely (2%).

DENTAL CONSIDERATIONS

General:

• Monitor vital signs at every appointment because of cardiovascular side effects.

• If additional analgesia is required for dental pain, consider alternative analgesics (NSAIDs) in patients taking narcotics for acute or chronic pain.

• Avoid products that affect platelet function, such as aspirin and NSAIDs.

• Consider semisupine chair position for patient comfort if GI side effects occur.

• Examine for oral manifestation of opportunistic infection.

• Patient on chronic drug therapy may rarely present with symptoms of blood dyscrasias, which can include infection, bleeding, and poor healing. If dyscrasia is present, caution patient to prevent oral tissue

trauma when using oral hygiene aids.

• Assess salivary flow as a factor in caries, periodontal disease, and candidiasis.

Consultations:

• Consider consulting with physician before prescribing drugs that may cause constipation (narcotics).

• Consultation with physician may be necessary if sedation or general anesthesia is required.

• In a patient with symptoms of blood dyscrasias, request a medical consultation for blood studies and postpone treatment until normal values are reestablished.

• Medical consultation may be required to assess disease control and patient's ability to tolerate stress.

Teach Patient/Family to:

• Encourage effective oral hygiene to prevent soft tissue inflammation.

• Prevent trauma when using oral hygiene aids.

• Update health and medication history if physician makes any changes in evaluation or drug regimens; include OTC, herbal, and nonherbal remedies in the update.

• When chronic dry mouth occurs, advise patient to:

• Avoid mouth rinses with high alcohol content because of drying effects.

• Use daily home fluoride products for anticaries effect.

• Use sugarless gum, frequent sips of water, or saliva substitutes.

anidulafungin
ann-id-yoo-la-**fun**´-jin
(Eraxis)

CATEGORY AND SCHEDULE
Pregnancy Risk Category: C

Drug Class: Antifungal

MECHANISM OF ACTION
An antifungal that inhibits the synthesis of 1,3-β-D-glucan, an essential component of the fungal cell wall.
Therapeutic Effect: Fungistatic.

USES
Treatment of fungal infections including candidemia and esophageal candidiasis.

PHARMACOKINETICS
Protein binding: 84%. Metabolism in the liver has not been observed. Approximately 30% eliminated in feces; less than 1% excreted in the urine. *Half-life:* 26.5 hr.

INDICATIONS AND DOSAGES
▸ Candidemia
IV
Adults. 200 mg loading dose on day 1, followed by 100 mg daily thereafter. Continue for at least 14 days after the last positive culture.
▸ Esophageal Candidiasis
IV
Adult. 100 mg loading dose on day 1, followed by 50 mg daily for a minimum of 14 days and for at least 7 days following resolution of symptoms.
Children. Safety and efficacy have not been established.

SIDE EFFECTS/ADVERSE REACTIONS
Rare
Diarrhea, hypokalemia, abnormal liver function, rash, urticaria, flushing, pruritus, dyspnea, hypotension, deep vein thrombosis

PRECAUTIONS AND CONTRAINDICATIONS
Hypersensitivity to anidulafungin or its components
Caution:
Do not breast-feed, hepatic impairment

DRUG INTERACTIONS OF CONCERN TO DENTISTRY
• None reported

SERIOUS REACTIONS
! Histamine-mediated symptoms including rash, urticaria, flushing, pruritus, dyspnea, and hypotension have been reported.

DENTAL CONSIDERATIONS

General:
• Determine why the patient is taking the drug.
• Examine oral mucous membranes for signs of residual fungal infection.
• Monitor vital signs at each appointment because of cardiovascular side effects.
• Consult physician to determine control of disease.
• Consider removable prostheses as source of residual source of candidal organisms.
Teach Patient/Family to:
• Soak full or partial dentures in an antifungal solution at night until lesions are absent; prolonged infections may require fabrication of new prosthesis.

• Dispose of tooth brush used during oral infection after oral lesions are absent to prevent reinoculation.
• Comply with antifungal therapy completely to eliminate infection and complete entire course of medication.

anthralin
anth-**rah**′-lin
(A-Fil, Anthra-Derm, Anthraforte[CAN], Anthranol[CAN], Anthrascalp[CAN], Dithrocream[AUS], Drithocreme, Dritho-Scalp, Micanol, Psoriatec) (capsules, tablets, chewable tablets, syrup, elixir, cream, spray) Do not confuse with Antagon, Antabuse, or Andriol.

CATEGORY AND SCHEDULE
Pregnancy Risk Category: C

Drug Class: Antipsoriatic

MECHANISM OF ACTION
A topical agent that binds DNA, inhibiting synthesis of nucleic protein, and reduces mitotic activity.
Therapeutic Effect: Results in damage to DNA sugar and enhances membrane lipid peroxidation, which may play a critical role in the antipsoriatic action.

USES
Treatment of psoriasis

PHARMACOKINETICS
Poorly absorbed systemically, but excellent epidermal absorption. Auto-oxidized to inactive metabolites-danthrone and dianthrone. Rapid urinary excretion,

so significant levels do not accumulate in the blood or other tissues. *Half-life:* 6 hr.

INDICATIONS AND DOSAGES
▶ **Psoriasis**
Topical
Adults, Elderly. Apply in a thin layer to affected areas q12h or q24h.

SIDE EFFECTS/ADVERSE REACTIONS
Frequent
Irritation
Rare
Neutrophilia, proteinuria, staining of the skin

PRECAUTIONS AND CONTRAINDICATIONS
Acute psoriasis where inflammation is present, erythroderma, hypersensitivity to anthralin

DRUG INTERACTIONS OF CONCERN TO DENTISTRY
• None reported

SERIOUS REACTIONS
! Patients with renal disease should have routine urine tests for albuminuria.
! Hypersensitivity reaction, such as burning, erythema, and dermatitis, may occur.

DENTAL CONSIDERATIONS
General:
• Determine why patient is taking the drug.
• Arthritic symptoms may occur in some patients; inquire about use of other medications.

apomorphine
ah-poe-**more**'-feen
(Apokyn)

CATEGORY AND SCHEDULE
Pregnancy Risk Category: C

Drug Class: Anti-Parkinson's
agent

MECHANISM OF ACTION
Stimulation of postsynaptic
dopamine receptors in the brain,
counteracting the excess cholinergic
activity responsible for striatal
excitation and involuntary
movements.

USES
Control of acute loss of control of
body movements in advanced
Parkinson's disease

PHARMACOKINETICS
Rapidly absorbed after subcutaneous
injection. Protein binding: 99.9%.
Widely distributed. ***Half-life:***
45 min; rapidly metabolized, not
detectable in urine or bodily
secretions in unchanged form.

INDICATIONS AND DOSAGES
▶ **Acute, Intermittent Treatment of**
Hypomobility ("Off Episodes")
Associated with Advanced
Parkinson's Disease
Injection Pen for Subcutaneous
Administration
Adult, Elderly. Subcutaneous, 0.2 ml
(2 mg) initially; may be increased in
0.1-ml (1-mg) increments every few
days, up to a maximum of 0.6 ml
(6 mg).

SIDE EFFECTS/ADVERSE
REACTIONS
ORAL: Stomatitis, taste alterations

CNS: Somnolence, dizziness,
headache, depression, hallucinations
(rare)
CV: Chest pain, tachycardia,
shortness of breath
GI: Nausea, vomiting
RESP: Respiratory depression,
tachypnea
INTEG: Injection site discomfort
MS: May exacerbate preexisting
dyskinesias

PRECAUTIONS AND
CONTRAINDICATIONS
Hypersensitivity, irritable bowel or
antiemetic therapy with 5-HT3
antagonists (e.g., ondansetron).
Do not administer with antiemetics
other than 5-HT3 antagonists. Use
with caution in patients with cardiac
decompensation or impaired hepatic
or renal function. Do not use if
solution is cloudy, contains
particulates, or is discolored.

DRUG INTERACTIONS OF
CONCERN TO DENTISTRY
• CNS depressants may intensify
adverse effects of therapy (e.g.,
dizziness).
• Phenothiazines may reduce
effectiveness of apomorphine.

DENTAL CONSIDERATIONS

General:
• Monitor vital signs because of
possible cardiovascular and
respiratory effects.
• Understand limitations of
Parkinson's disease on dental
treatment.
• After supine positioning, have
patient sit upright for 2 min before
standing to avoid orthostatic
hypotension.
• Assist patient with ambulation if
dizziness or loss of coordination
occurs.

• Differentiate taste alterations because of drug from those associated with restorative materials.
Consultations:
• Consult physician to determine degree of disease control and patient's ability to tolerate dental treatment.
Teach Patient/Family to:
• Encourage effective oral hygiene measures to prevent soft-tissue inflammation.
• Help patient with effective dental home care to minimize oral diseases if patient lacks adequate motor coordination.

apraclonidine hydrochloride

ap-ra-**kloe'**-ni-deen
hi-droh-**klor'**-ide
(Iopidine)
Do not confuse with Cetapred, clomiphene, Klonopin, or quinidine.

CATEGORY AND SCHEDULE
Pregnancy Risk Category: C

Drug Class: Selective α_2-adrenergic agonist

MECHANISM OF ACTION
An ocular α-adrenergic agent that is relatively selective for α_2 receptor agonist.
Therapeutic Effect: Reduces intraocular pressure.

USES
Control or prevention of increases in intraocular pressure related to laser surgery of eye; short-term control of increased intraocular pressure as an adjunctive drug

PHARMACOKINETICS
Onset of action occurs within 1 hr. The duration of a single dose is about 12 hr. *Half-life:* 8 hr.

INDICATIONS AND DOSAGES
▸ **Glaucoma**
Ophthalmic
Adults, Elderly. Instill 1 drop of 0.5% solution to affected eye(s) 3 times a day.
▸ **Intraocular Hypertension, Post Laser Surgery**
Ophthalmic
Adults, Elderly. Instill 1 drop of 1% solution in operative eye(s) 1 hr before surgery and 1 drop postoperatively.

SIDE EFFECTS/ADVERSE REACTIONS
Frequent
Eye discomfort, dry mouth
Occasional
Headache, constipation, redness around eye, conjunctivitis, changes in visual acuity, mydriasis, ocular inflammation
Rare
Nasal decongestion

PRECAUTIONS AND CONTRAINDICATIONS
Hypersensitivity to apraclonidine or clonidine or any component of the formulation
Caution:
Tachyphylaxis, impaired renal or liver function, depression, lactation, children, cardiovascular disease, cardiovascular drugs

DRUG INTERACTIONS OF CONCERN TO DENTISTRY
• No drug interactions have been reported; this is a new drug and data are lacking.

• Avoid using drugs that can exacerbate glaucoma: anticholinergic drugs.

SERIOUS REACTIONS

! Allergic reaction occurs rarely.
! Peripheral edema and arrhythmias have been reported.

DENTAL CONSIDERATIONS

General:
• Protect patient's eyes from accidental spatter during dental treatment.
• Avoid dental light in patient's eyes; offer dark glasses for patient comfort.
• Determine why the patient is taking the drug.
• Assess salivary flow as a factor in caries, periodontal disease, and candidiasis.
Consultations:
• Medical consultation may be required to assess disease control.
Teach Patient/Family to:
• When chronic dry mouth occurs, advise patient to:
  • Avoid mouth rinses with high alcohol content because of drying effects.
  • Use daily home fluoride to prevent caries.
  • Use sugarless gum, frequent sips of water, or saliva substitutes.

aprepitant
ah-**prep**´-ih-tant
(Emend)

CATEGORY AND SCHEDULE
Pregnancy Risk Category: B

Drug Class: Antiemetic

MECHANISM OF ACTION
A selective human substance P and neurokinin-1 (NK1) receptor antagonist that inhibits chemotherapy-induced nausea and vomiting centrally in the chemoreceptor trigger zone.
Therapeutic Effect: Prevents the acute and delayed phases of chemotherapy-induced emesis, including vomiting caused by high-dose cisplatin.

USES
Prevention of acute and delayed nausea/vomiting associated with cancer chemotherapy, including high-dose cisplatin; for acute use only

PHARMACOKINETICS
Crosses the blood-brain barrier. Extensively metabolized in the liver. Eliminated primarily by liver metabolism (not excreted renally). *Half-life:* 9–13 hr.

INDICATIONS AND DOSAGES
▸ **Prevention of Chemotherapy-Induced Nausea and Vomiting**
PO
Adults, Elderly. 125 mg 1 hr before chemotherapy on day 1 and 80 mg once a day in the morning on days 2 and 3.

SIDE EFFECTS/ADVERSE REACTIONS
Frequent
Fatigue, nausea, hiccups, diarrhea, constipation, anorexia
Occasional
Headache, vomiting, dizziness, dehydration, heartburn
Rare
Abdominal pain, epigastric discomfort, gastritis, tinnitus, insomnia

PRECAUTIONS AND CONTRAINDICATIONS

Breast-feeding, concurrent use of pimozide (Orap)

Caution:
Patients taking drugs metabolized by CYP3A4 enzymes; not for chronic use; acts as a moderate inhibitor of CYP3A4 and an inducer of CYP3A4 and CYP2C9; use with caution in lactation, safety and efficacy in pediatric patients not established

DRUG INTERACTIONS OF CONCERN TO DENTISTRY

• Increased plasma concentrations of midazolam and other benzodiazepines metabolized by CYP3A4
• Increased plasma levels: concurrent use of drugs that inhibit CYP3A4 enzymes (fluconazole, itraconazole, ketoconazole, erythromycin, and clarithromycin)
• Decreased plasma levels: concurrent use of drugs that induce CYP3A4 enzymes (carbamazepine)

SERIOUS REACTIONS

! Neutropenia and mucous membrane disorders occur rarely.

DENTAL CONSIDERATIONS

General:
• Patients using this drug are also undergoing or have recently undergone cancer chemotherapy; take a complete health history.
• Chemotherapy patients may show stomatitis and ulceration; palliative therapy may be required.
• Consider semisupine chair position for patient comfort if GI side effects occur.
• Examine for oral manifestation of opportunistic infection.

• Short appointments and a stress-reduction protocol may be required for anxious patients.
• Patients taking opioids for acute or chronic pain should be given alternative analgesics for dental pain.
• Patients on chronic drug therapy may rarely have symptoms of blood dyscrasias, which can include infection, bleeding, and poor healing.
• Consult physician; prophylactic or therapeutic antibiotics may be indicated to prevent or treat infection if surgery or periodontal debridement is required for patients undergoing chemotherapy.

Consultations:
• Medical consultation may be required to assess immunologic status during cancer therapy and determine safety risks posed by dental treatment.
• Consultation with physician may be necessary if sedation or general anesthesia is required.
• Medical consultation may be required to assess disease control and patient's ability to tolerate stress.

Teach Patient/Family to:
• Encourage effective oral hygiene to prevent soft tissue inflammation.
• Prevent trauma when using oral hygiene aids.
• Importance of updating health and drug history if physician makes any changes in evaluation or drug regimens.

arformoterol tartrate
ar-for-**moe′**-ter-ole **tar′**-trate
(Brovana)

CATEGORY AND SCHEDULE
Pregnancy Risk Category: C

Drug Class: β_2 agonist

MECHANISM OF ACTION
A long-acting β_2 agonist that stimulates adrenergic receptors in bronchial smooth muscle causing relaxation of smooth muscle.
Therapeutic Effect: Produces bronchodilation.

USES
Used for chronic obstructive pulmonary disease (COPD).

PHARMACOKINETICS
Primarily absorbed by the pulmonary system following inhalation. Protein binding: 52%–65%. Primarily metabolized by glucuronidation. Primarily excreted in urine; partial elimination in feces.
Half-life: 26 hr.

INDICATIONS AND DOSAGES
▶ COPD
Oral Inhalation
Adults. 15 mcg (2 ml) twice a day by nebulization.
Children. Safety and efficacy have not been established in children.

SIDE EFFECTS/ADVERSE REACTIONS
Occasional
Pain, chest pain, back pain, sinusitis, rash, leg cramps, dyspnea, peripheral edema
Rare
Oral candidiasis, pulmonary congestion

PRECAUTIONS AND CONTRAINDICATIONS
Hypersensitivity to arformoterol or its components
Caution:
Acutely deteriorating COPD, cardiovascular disorders, convulsive disorders, diabetes mellitus, thyrotoxicosis, coadministration with other long-acting β_2 agonists

DRUG INTERACTIONS OF CONCERN TO DENTISTRY
• Methylxanthines (e.g., aminophylline, theophylline), steroids, diuretics: may potentiate hypokalemic effects.
• Tricyclic antidepressants, drugs that prolong QT interval: may potentiate cardiovascular effects.

SERIOUS REACTIONS
! May increase the risk of asthma-related death.
! May exacerbate cardiovascular conditions including arrhythmias and hypertension.
! Hypersensitivity reactions including urticaria, angioedema, rash, bronchospasm, and anaphylaxis may occur.

DENTAL CONSIDERATIONS

General:
• Monitor vital signs at every appointment because of cardiovascular and respiratory side effects.
• Evaluate oral mucous membranes for signs of candidiasis.
• Consider semisupine chair position for patients with respiratory disease.
• Midday appointments and stress-reduction protocol may be required for anxious patients.
• Aspirin, NSAIDs, and bisulfites in local anesthetics may exacerbate asthma.

• Acute asthmatic episodes may be precipitated in the dental office. Sympathomimetic/bronchodilator inhalants should be available for emergency use.

Consultations:
• Consult physician to determine control of disease and ability of patient to tolerate dental procedures.

Teach Patient/Family to:
• Rinse mouth with water after each dose of drug to prevent dryness.

argatroban
ar-**gat′**-tro-ban
(Acova)
Do not confuse argatroban with Aggrestat or Orgaran.

CATEGORY AND SCHEDULE
Pregnancy Risk Category: B

Drug Class: Anticoagulants

MECHANISM OF ACTION
A direct thrombin inhibitor that reversibly binds to thrombin-active sites. Inhibits thrombin-catalyzed or thrombin-induced reactions, including fibrin formation, activation of coagulant factors V, VIII, and XIII; also inhibits protein C formation; and platelet aggregation. *Therapeutic Effect:* Produces anticoagulation.

USES
An anticoagulant for prophylaxis or treatment of thrombosis in patients with heparin-induced thrombocytopenia

PHARMACOKINETICS
Following IV administration, distributed primarily in extracellular fluid. Protein binding: 54%. Metabolized in the liver. Primarily excreted in the feces, presumably through biliary secretion. *Half-life:* 39–51 min.

INDICATIONS AND DOSAGES
▸ **To Prevent and Treat Heparin-Induced Thrombocytopenia**
IV Infusion
Adults, Elderly. Initially, 2 mcg/kg/min administered as a continuous infusion. After initial infusion, dose may be adjusted until steady state aPTT is 1.5–3 times initial baseline value, not to exceed 100 sec.
▸ **Percutaneous Coronary Intervention**
IV Infusion
Adults, Elderly. Initially, 25 mcg/kg/min and administer bolus of 350 mcg/kg over 3–5 min. ACT (activated clotting time) checked in 5–10 min following bolus. If ACT is less than 300 sec, give additional bolus 150 mcg/kg, increase infusion to 30 mcg/kg/min. If ACT is greater than 450 sec, decrease infusion to 15 mcg/kg/min. Once ACT of 300–450 sec achieved, proceed with procedure.
▸ **Dosage in Hepatic Impairment**
Adults, Elderly. Initially, 0.5 mcg/kg/min.

SIDE EFFECTS/ADVERSE REACTIONS
Frequent
Dyspnea, hypotension, fever, diarrhea, nausea, pain, vomiting, infection, cough

PRECAUTIONS AND CONTRAINDICATIONS
Overt major bleeding

DRUG INTERACTIONS OF CONCERN TO DENTISTRY
• Increased risk of bleeding: drugs that interfere with coagulation or

platelet function, such as NSAIDs and aspirin

SERIOUS REACTIONS
! Ventricular tachycardia and atrial fibrillation occur occasionally.
! Major bleeding and sepsis occur rarely.

DENTAL CONSIDERATIONS
General:
• Patients are at risk of bleeding, check for oral signs.
• Delay elective dental treatment until patient completes parenteral anticoagulant therapy.
• Determine why patient is taking the drug.
• Avoid products that affect platelet function, such as aspirin and NSAIDs.
• Consider local hemostasis measures to prevent excessive bleeding.
Consultations:
• Medical consultation should include partial prothrombin time, prothrombin time, or INR.
• Medical consultation should include routine blood counts including platelet counts and bleeding time.
Teach Patient/Family to:
• Use soft tooth brush to reduce risk of bleeding.
• Encourage effective oral hygiene to prevent soft tissue inflammation.
• Report oral lesions, soreness, or bleeding to dentist.
• Prevent trauma when using oral hygiene aids.
• Update health and medication history if physician makes any changes in evaluation or drug regimens; include OTC, herbal, and nonherbal remedies in the update.
• Inform dentist of unusual bleeding episodes following dental treatment.

aripiprazole
ar-ah-**pip**′-rah-zole
(Abilify)

CATEGORY AND SCHEDULE
Pregnancy Risk Category: C

Drug Class: Antipsychotic

MECHANISM OF ACTION
An antipsychotic agent that provides partial agonist activity at dopamine and serotonin (5-HT1A) receptors and antagonist activity at serotonin (5-HT2A) receptors.
Therapeutic Effect: Diminishes schizophrenic behavior.

USES
Treatment of schizophrenia

PHARMACOKINETICS
Well absorbed through the GI tract. Protein binding: 99% (primarily albumin). Reaches steady levels in 2 wk. Metabolized in the liver. Eliminated primarily in feces and, to a lesser extent, in urine. Not removed by hemodialysis. *Half-life:* 75 hr.

INDICATIONS AND DOSAGES
▸ Schizophrenia, Bipolar Disorder
PO
Adults, Elderly. Initially, 10–15 mg once a day. May increase up to 30 mg/day.

SIDE EFFECTS/ADVERSE REACTIONS
Frequent
Weight gain, headache, insomnia, vomiting
Occasional
Light-headedness, nausea, akathisia, somnolence

Rare
Blurred vision, constipation, asthenia or loss of energy and strength, anxiety, fever, rash, cough, rhinitis, orthostatic hypotension

PRECAUTIONS AND CONTRAINDICATIONS
Hypersensitivity
Caution:
Known cardiovascular diseases, cerebrovascular disease, or other conditions predisposing the patient to hypotension; seizures, may impair judgment or motor skills, elevated body temperature, suicide, dysphagia, dehydration, severe renal or hepatic impairment, avoid breast-feeding and use in children

DRUG INTERACTIONS OF CONCERN TO DENTISTRY
• Possible lowering of blood levels: carbamazepine and other inducers of CYP3A4 isoenzymes
• Increased blood levels: ketoconazole and other inhibitors of CYP3A4 or CYP2D6 isoenzymes
• Caution with CNS depressants and alcohol

SERIOUS REACTIONS
! Extrapyramidal symptoms and neuroleptic malignant syndrome occur rarely.

DENTAL CONSIDERATIONS
General:
• Assess for presence of extrapyramidal motor symptoms, such as tardive dyskinesia and akathisia. Extrapyramidal motor activity may complicate dental treatment.
• Consider semisupine chair position for patient comfort if GI side effects occur.

Consultations:
• Consultation with physician may be necessary if sedation or general anesthesia is required.
• Medical consultation may be required to assess disease control and patient's ability to tolerate stress.
Teach Patient/Family to:
• Consult physician if signs of tardive dyskinesia or akathisia are present.
• Encourage effective oral hygiene to prevent soft tissue inflammation.
• Use powered tooth brush if patient has difficulty holding conventional devices.
• Update health and drug history if physician makes any changes in evaluation or drug regimens.

armodafinil
ar-moe-**daf**′-i-nil
(Nuvigil)

CATEGORY AND SCHEDULE
Pregnancy Risk Category: C
Controlled Substance: Schedule IV

Drug Class: CNS stimulant

MECHANISM OF ACTION
Alpha-1 agonist and the R-enantiomer of modafinil. The exact mechanism of action is unknown. Binds to dopamine transporter and inhibits dopamine reuptake.

USES
Narcolepsy; obstructive sleep apnea/hypopnea syndrome (OSAHS); shift-work sleep disorder (SWSD)

PHARMACOKINETICS

Readily absorbed after oral administration. Food may delay absorption. Protein binding: 60%. Widely distributed. Metabolized in liver to R-modafinil acid and modafinil sulfone. Excreted primarily in urine (80%, and <10% unchanged drug). *Half-life*: 15 hr.

INDICATIONS AND DOSAGES

▶ **Narcolepsy, Improve Wakefulness in Patients with Excessive Sleepiness; Obstructive Sleep Apnea**
PO
Adults. 150 mg or 250 mg as a single dose in the morning.
▶ **Shift-Work Sleep Disorder**
PO
Adults. 150 mg daily approximately 1 hr before to the start of work shift.
Pediatric. Not approved for use in children.
Dose Adjustments. Severe hepatic impairment: dose should be reduced by half.
Renal impairment: Inadequate data to determine safety and efficacy.

SIDE EFFECTS/ADVERSE REACTIONS

Frequent
Neurologic: dizziness, headache (dose-related), insomnia
Gastrointestinal: diarrhea, nausea, xerostomia
Occasional
Rash, indigestion, increase heart rate, anxiety
Rare
Stevens-Johnson syndrome, anaphylaxis, angioedema, dyspnea

PRECAUTIONS AND CONTRAINDICATIONS

Contraindications: hypersensitivity to modafinil, armodafinil, or any component of the formulation.

Serious and life-threatening rashes, including Stevens-Johnson syndrome, and rare cases of multi-organ hypersensitivity reactions have occurred with armodafinil use.
Use with caution in patients with cardiovascular diseases (increased risk of cardiac adverse events), hepatic impairment, psychiatric disorder (increased risk of psychiatric adverse effects), renal impairment (drug clearance may be reduced); and excessive sleepiness. Avoid or limit alcohol.

DRUG INTERACTIONS OF CONCERN TO DENTISTRY

• CYP3A4 substrates: Armodafinil may decrease the levels and effects of CYP3A4 substrates (e.g., lidocaine).
• CYP3A4 inhibitors: May increase the concentrations of armodafinil.

SERIOUS REACTIONS

! Serious and life-threatening rashes, including Stevens-Johnson syndrome. Patients should be advised to discontinue drug at first sign of rash.
! Rare cases of angioedema reactions have been reported with the use of armodafinil.

DENTAL CONSIDERATIONS

General:
• Xerostomia may complicate dental treatment and oral hygiene.
• Monitor vital signs at every appointment because of cardiovascular effects.
• Consider semisupine chair position for patient comfort if GI side effects occur.
• Use vasoconstrictors with caution, at low doses and with careful aspiration.

Teach Patient/Family to:
• Encourage effective oral hygiene to prevent soft tissue inflammation.
• Prevent injury when using oral hygiene aids.
• When chronic dry mouth (xerostomia) occurs, advise patient to:
  • Avoid mouth rinses with high alcohol content because of drying effects.
  • Use daily home fluoride products for anticaries effect.
  • Use sugarless gum, frequent sips of water, or saliva substitutes.

artemether/ lumefantrine

ar-**tem**-e-ther / **loo**-me-**fan**-tree
(Coartem)

CATEGORY AND SCHEDULE

Pregnancy Risk Category: C

Drug Class: Antimalarial

MECHANISM OF ACTION

A semisynthetic derivative of artemisinin that destroys the malarial pathogen, *Plasmodium falciparum*. Artemether is rapidly metabolized into an active metabolite dihydroartemisinin (DHA). The antimalarial activity of artemether and DHA has been attributed to endoperoxide moiety. Both artemether and lumefantrine were shown to inhibit nucleic acid and protein synthesis.
Therapeutic Effect: Inhibits parasite growth.

USES

Malaria due to *Plasmodium falciparum*

PHARMACOKINETICS

Well absorbed after PO administration. Protein binding: 95.4% (artemether); 99.7% (lumefantrine). Binds to α_1-acid glycoprotein and erythrocytes. Rapidly and extensively metabolized in liver. Food enhances absorption.
Half-life: 1–7 hr (artemether); 130 hr (lumefantrine).

INDICATIONS AND DOSAGES
▸ **Malaria due to *Plasmodium falciparum***
PO
Adults, 16 yr and older (who weigh 35 kg or greater). Four tablets of oral combination of artemether (20 mg) and lumefantrine (120 mg) as an initial dose; 4 more tablets 8 hr later; 4 tablets in the morning and 4 tablets in the evening for the next 2 days (total course of 24 tablets).
Children younger than 16 yr old who weigh 25 to less than 35 kg. Three tablets as an initial dose; take 3 more tablets 8 hr later; 3 tablets in the morning and 3 tablets in the evening for the next 2 days.
Children younger than 16 yr old who weigh 15 to less than 25 kg. Two tablets as an initial dose; 2 more tablets 8 hr later; 2 tablets in the morning and 2 tablets in the evening for the next 2 days.
Children younger than 16 yr old who weigh 5 to less than 15 kg. One tablet as an initial dose; second tablet 8 hr later. One tablet in the morning and 1 tablet in the evening for the next 2 days.

SIDE EFFECTS/ADVERSE REACTIONS
Frequent
Adults: Headache, anorexia, dizziness, asthenia, arthralgia, myalgia, nausea, vomiting,

abdominal pain, sleep disorder, palpitations, fatigue, fever, shivering
Children: Pyrexia, cough, vomiting, anorexia, headache
Occasional
Adults: diarrhea, insomnia, hepatomegaly, splenomegaly, headache
Children: abdominal pain, diarrhea, splenomegaly, anemia, hepatomegaly
Rare
Adults: Anemia, cough, pruritus, rash, vertigo, nasopharyngitis
Children: Chills, asthenia, fatigue, nausea, rhinitis, dizziness, aspartate aminotransferase increased, arthralgia, myalgia, rash

PRECAUTIONS AND CONTRAINDICATIONS
Hypersensitivity to artemether, lumefantrine, or its components
Caution:
Hypokalemia
Hypomagnesemia
Drugs that prolong the QT interval (e.g. quinine, quinidine)
Cardiovascular disease
Hepatic impairment
Renal insufficiency
Halofantrine (within one month of Coartem therapy)
CYP450 3A4 substrates, inhibitors, inducers
Food aversion: increased risk of recrudescence due to reduce drug absorption

DRUG INTERACTIONS OF CONCERN TO DENTISTRY
• Antiretroviral agents: May increase the risk of QT prolongation, loss of antiviral efficacy, or loss of Coartem efficacy.
• Aurothioglucose: May increase risk of blood dyscrasias.
• CYP 450 3A4 inhibitors (ketoconazole, itraconazole): May increase Coartem levels; increase risk of QT prolongation.
• CYP450 2D6: May increase the risk of adverse effects and QT prolongation.
• Clarithromycin, telithromycin: May increase Coartem concentrations; increase risk of QT prolongation.
• Drugs that prolong the QT interval: May increase the risk of QT prolongation.
• Halofantrine: May cause additive effects and increase the risk of QT prolongation.
• Hormonal contraceptives: May reduce hormone contraceptive concentrations.
• Mefloquine: May decrease efficacy of Coartem.
• Grapefruit juice: This can increase concentrations of artemether/ lumefantrine and increase risk of QT interval prolongation; avoid.

SERIOUS REACTIONS
! QTc prolongation may occur.
! Ototoxicity has been reported.
! Angioedema may occur.
! Hepatomegaly and splenomegaly have been reported.

DENTAL CONSIDERATIONS
General:
• QTc prolongation has been reported.
• Use caution with coadministration of CYP3A4 substrates, inducers or inhibitors.
• Examine for oral manifestation of opportunistic infection.
• Patient on chronic drug therapy may rarely have symptoms of blood dyscrasias, which include infection, bleeding, and poor healing.
• Avoid dental light in patient's eyes; offer dark glasses for patient comfort.

• Place on frequent recall because of oral side effects.
• Consider semisupine chair position for patient comfort if GI side effects occur.
Consultations:
• In a patient with symptoms of blood dyscrasias, request a medical consultation for blood studies and postpone treatment until normal values are reestablished.
• Medical consultation may be required to assess disease control.
Teach Patient/Family to:
• Encourage effective oral hygiene to prevent soft tissue inflammation.
• Prevent trauma when using oral hygiene aids.
• Be alert for the possibility of secondary oral infection and the need to see dentist immediately if signs of infection occur.
• Recommend using an additional non-hormonal method of birth control.
• Instruct patient to take drug with food.
• Advise patient to avoid drinking grapefruit juice while taking this drug.

articaine hydrochloride
ar-ti-kane hi-droh-**klor'**-ide
(Astracaine[CAN], Astracaine Forte[CAN], Septocaine, Zorcaine)

CATEGORY AND SCHEDULE
Pregnancy Risk Category: C

Drug Class: Amide local anesthetic with vasoconstrictor (epinephrine)

MECHANISM OF ACTION
An amide anesthetic that inhibits conduction of nerve impulses. ***Therapeutic Effect:*** Causes temporary loss of feeling and sensation.

USES
Local, infiltrative, or conductive anesthesia in both simple and complex dental and periodontal procedures

PHARMACOKINETICS
Onset of action occurs within 1–6 min depending on route of administration. Complete anesthesia lasts approximately 1 hr. Well absorbed. Protein binding: 60%–80%. Rapidly metabolized by plasma carboxyesterase to its primary metabolite, articainic acid, which is inactive. Excreted in urine. ***Half-life:*** 20–120 min.

INDICATIONS AND DOSAGES
These recommended doses serve only as a guide to the amount of anesthetic required for most routine procedures. The actual volumes to be used depend on a number of factors, such as type and extent of surgical procedure, depth of anesthesia, degree of muscular relaxation, and condition of the patient.
▶ **Local, Infiltrative, or Conductive Anesthesia in Both Simple and Complex Dental or Periodontal Procedures**
Infiltration
Adults, Elderly, Children older than 4 yr. 0.5–2.5 ml of a 4% solution, which corresponds to 20–100 mg. Maximum dose administered should not exceed 7 mg/kg (0.175 ml/kg) or 3.2 mg/lb (0.0795 ml/lb) of body weight (up to 500 mg).

SIDE EFFECTS/ADVERSE REACTIONS

Rare
Drowsiness, dizziness, disorientation, light-headedness, tremors, blurred or double vision, nausea, sensation of heat, cold, numbness

PRECAUTIONS AND CONTRAINDICATIONS

History of hypersensitivity to local anesthetics of the amide type or sodium metabisulfite
Caution:
Accidental intravascular injections may be associated with convulsions, CNS depression, or cardiorespiratory depression; reduce dose for elderly, debilitated, or pediatric patients; exaggerated response to intravascular epinephrine, severe hepatic impairment, lactation

DRUG INTERACTIONS OF CONCERN TO DENTISTRY

• CNS depressants: increased risk of CNS depression with all CNS depressants, especially in children and when larger doses are used.
• Avoid placing dental cartridges in disinfectant solutions with heavy metals or surface-active agents; may see release of metal ions into local anesthetic solutions with tissue irritation following injection.
• Risk of cardiovascular side effects; rapid intravascular administration of local anesthetic containing vasoconstrictor, either alone or in patients taking tricyclic antidepressants, MAOIs, digitalis drugs, cocaine, phenothiazines, β-blockers, and in presence of halogenated hydrocarbon general anesthetics; use smallest effective vasoconstrictor dose and careful aspiration technique.

• Avoid use of vasoconstrictors in patients with uncontrolled hyperthyroidism, diabetes, angina, or hypertension; refer these patients for medical treatment before elective dental procedures.

SERIOUS REACTIONS

! Tachycardia or bradycardia, B/P changes, syncope, cardiac arrest, and seizures have been observed in some patients during dental procedures.

DENTAL CONSIDERATIONS

General:
• Monitor vital signs at every appointment because of cardiovascular side effects.
• Apply lubricant to dry lips for patient comfort before dental procedures.
• Use vasoconstrictor with caution, in low doses, and with careful aspiration.
Teach Patient/Family to:
• Use care to prevent injury while numbness exists and to not chew gum or eat following dental anesthesia.
• Report any signs of infection, muscle pain, or fever to dentist when feeling returns.
• Report any unusual soft tissue reactions.

ascorbic acid (vitamin c)

ah-**skor**′-bic **as**′-id
(Apo-C[CAN], Cecon, Cenolate, Pro-C[AUS], Redoxon[CAN])

CATEGORY AND SCHEDULE
Pregnancy Risk Category: C
OTC

Drug Class: Vitamin C, water-soluble vitamin

MECHANISM OF ACTION
Assists in collagen formation and tissue repair and is involved in oxidation reduction reactions and other metabolic reactions.
Therapeutic Effect: Involved in carbohydrate use and metabolism, as well as synthesis of carnitine, lipids, and proteins. Preserves blood vessel integrity.

USES
Vitamin C deficiency, scurvy, urine acidification, and supplemental use in a variety of debilitated patients with poor vitamin C intake

PHARMACOKINETICS
Readily absorbed from the GI tract. Protein binding: 25%. Metabolized in the liver. Excreted in urine. Removed by hemodialysis.

INDICATIONS AND DOSAGES
▸ **Dietary Supplement**
PO
Adults, Elderly. 50–200 mg/day.
Children. 35–100 mg/day.
▸ **Acidification of Urine**
PO
Adults, Elderly. 4–12 g/day in 3–4 divided doses.
Children. 500 mg q6–8h.

▸ **Scurvy**
PO
Adults, Elderly. 100–250 mg 1–2 times a day.
Children. 100–300 mg/day in divided doses.
▸ **Prevention and Reduction of Severity of Colds**
PO
Adults, Elderly. 1–3 g/day in divided doses.

SIDE EFFECTS/ADVERSE REACTIONS
Rare
Abdominal cramps, nausea, vomiting, diarrhea, increased urination with doses exceeding 1 g
Parenteral: Flushing, headache, dizziness, sleepiness or insomnia, soreness at injection site

PRECAUTIONS AND CONTRAINDICATIONS
Caution:
Gout

DRUG INTERACTIONS OF CONCERN TO DENTISTRY
• Increased urinary excretion: salicylates, barbiturates

SERIOUS REACTIONS
! Ascorbic acid may acidify urine, leading to crystalluria.
! Large doses of IV ascorbic acid may lead to deep vein thrombosis.
! Abrupt discontinuation after prolonged use of large doses may produce rebound ascorbic acid deficiency.

DENTAL CONSIDERATIONS
General:
• An increased incidence of caries and soft tissue injury has been

reported with excessive use of chewable ascorbic acid tablets.

aspirin/ acetylsalicylic acid

as′-pir-in/ah-**seet′**-il-sill-ic **as′**-id (Ascriptin, Aspro[AUS], Bayer, Bex[AUS], Bufferin, Disprin[AUS], Ecotrin, Entrophen[CAN], Halfprin, Novasen[CAN], Solprin[AUS], Spren[AUS])
Do not confuse aspirin or Ascriptin with Aricept, Afrin, or Asendin, or Ecotrin with Edecrin.

CATEGORY AND SCHEDULE
Pregnancy Risk Category: D
OTC

Drug Class: Nonnarcotic analgesic salicylate

MECHANISM OF ACTION
A nonsteroidal salicylate that inhibits prostaglandin synthesis, acts on the hypothalamus heat-regulating center, and interferes with the production of thromboxane A_2, a substance that stimulates platelet aggregation.
Therapeutic Effect: Reduces inflammatory response and intensity of pain; decreases fever; inhibits platelet aggregation.

USES
Treatment of mild-to-moderate pain or fever, including arthritis, thromboembolic disorders, transient ischemic attacks in men, rheumatic fever, post-MI

PHARMACOKINETICS

Route	Onset	Peak	Duration
PO	1 hr	2–4 hr	24 hr

Rapidly and completely absorbed from GI tract; enteric-coated absorption delayed; rectal absorption delayed and incomplete. Protein binding: High. Widely distributed. Rapidly hydrolyzed to salicylate. **Half-life:** 15–20 min (aspirin); 2–3 hr (salicylate at low dose); more than 20 hr (salicylate at high dose).

INDICATIONS AND DOSAGES
▸ **Analgesia, Fever**
PO, Rectal
Adults, Elderly. 325–1000 mg q4–6h.
Children. 10–15 mg/kg/dose q4–6h. Maximum: 4 g/day.
▸ **Antiinflammatory**
PO
Adults, Elderly. Initially, 2.4–3.6 g/ day in divided doses; then 3.6–5.4 g/ day.
Children. Initially, 60–90 mg/kg/day in divided doses; then 80–100 mg/ kg/day.
▸ **Suspected MI**
PO
Adults, Elderly. 162 mg as soon as the MI is suspected, then daily for 30 days after the MI.
▸ **Prevention of MI**
PO
Adults, Elderly. 75–325 mg/day.
▸ **Prevention of Stroke after Transient Ischemic Attack**
PO
Adults, Elderly. 50–325 mg/day.
▸ **Kawasaki Disease**
PO
Children. 80–100 mg/kg/day in divided doses.

SIDE EFFECTS/ADVERSE REACTIONS
Occasional
GI distress (including abdominal distention, cramping, heartburn, and mild nausea); allergic reaction

(including bronchospasm, pruritus, and urticaria)

PRECAUTIONS AND CONTRAINDICATIONS

Allergy to tartrazine dye, bleeding disorders, chickenpox or flu in children and teenagers, GI bleeding or ulceration, hepatic impairment, history of hypersensitivity to aspirin or NSAIDs

Caution:
Anemia, hepatic disease, renal disease, Hodgkin's disease, preoperative, postoperative

DRUG INTERACTIONS OF CONCERN TO DENTISTRY

- Increased risk of GI complaints and occult blood loss: alcohol, NSAIDs, corticosteroids
- Buffered aspirin: Decreased absorption of tetracycline
- Recent report indicated ibuprofen may block clot-preventing effects of aspirin
- Interactions when used as a dental drug:
  - Increased risk of bleeding: oral anticoagulants, valproic acid, dipyridamole
  - Increased risk of hypoglycemia: sulfonylureas
  - Increased risk of toxicity: methotrexate, lithium, zidovudine
  - Decreased effects of probenecid, sulfinpyrazone
- Avoid prolonged or concurrent use with NSAIDs, corticosteroids, acetaminophen
- Suspected reduction in antihypertensives and vasodilator effects of angiotensin-converting enzyme (ACE) inhibitors; monitor blood pressure if used concurrently

SERIOUS REACTIONS

! High doses of aspirin may produce GI bleeding and gastric mucosal lesions.
! Dehydrated, febrile children may experience aspirin toxicity quickly. Reye's syndrome may occur in children with the chickenpox or the flu.
! Low-grade toxicity is characterized by tinnitus, generalized pruritus (possibly severe), headache, dizziness, flushing, tachycardia, hyperventilation, diaphoresis, and thirst.
! Marked toxicity is characterized by hyperthermia, restlessness, seizures, abnormal breathing patterns, respiratory failure, and coma.

DENTAL CONSIDERATIONS

General:
- Patients on chronic drug therapy may rarely have symptoms of blood dyscrasias, which can include infection, bleeding, and poor healing.
- Avoid prescribing buffered aspirin-containing products if patient is on a sodium-restricted diet.
- Chewable forms of aspirin should not be used for 7 days following oral surgery because of possible soft tissue injury.
- Evaluate allergic reactions: rash, urticaria; patients with allergy to salicylates may not be able to take NSAIDs; drug may need to be discontinued.
- Severe stomach bleeding may occur in patients who regularly use NSAIDs in recommended doses, when the patient is also taking another NSAID, a blood thinning or steroid drug, if the patient has GI or peptic ulcer disease, if they are 60 yr or older, or when NSAIDs are taken longer than directed. Warn

patients of the potential for severe stomach bleeding.

Consultations:

• In a patient with symptoms of blood dyscrasias, request a medical consultation for blood studies and postpone dental treatment until normal values are reestablished.

• Take precautions if dental surgery is anticipated because of risk of increased bleeding; avoid prescribing aspirin before dental surgery.

• Tinnitus, ringing, roaring in ears after high-dose and long-term therapy necessitates referral for salicylism.

Teach Patient/Family to:

• Not place aspirin or buffered aspirin tablets directly on a tooth or mucosal surface because of the risk of chemical burn.

• Read label on other OTC drugs; may contain aspirin.

• Avoid alcohol ingestion; GI bleeding may occur.

• Warn patient of potential risks of NSAIDs.

atazanavir sulfate
ah-tah-**zan**′-ah-veer **sul**′-fate
(Reyataz)
Do not confuse Reyataz with Retavase.

CATEGORY AND SCHEDULE
Pregnancy Risk Category: B

Drug Class: Antiviral, HIV-1 protease inhibitor

MECHANISM OF ACTION
An antiviral that acts as an HIV-1 protease inhibitor, selectively preventing the processing of viral precursors found in cells infected with HIV-1.

Therapeutic Effect: Prevents the formation of mature HIV cells.

USES
HIV-1 infection in combination with other antiretroviral medications

PHARMACOKINETICS
Rapidly absorbed after PO administration. Protein binding: 86%. Extensively metabolized in the liver. Excreted primarily in urine and, to a lesser extent, in feces. ***Half-life:*** 5–8 hr.

INDICATIONS AND DOSAGES
▸ **HIV-1 Infection**
PO
Adults, Elderly (antiretroviral-naive). 400 mg (2 capsules) once a day with food.
Adults, Elderly (antiretroviral-experienced). 300 mg and ritonavir (Norvir) 100 mg once a day.
▸ **HIV-1 Infection (concurrent therapy with efavirenz)**
PO
Adults, Elderly. 300 mg atazanavir, 100 mg ritonavir, and 600 mg efavirenz as a single daily dose with food.
▸ **HIV-1 Infection (concurrent therapy with didanosine)**
PO
Adults, Elderly. Give atazanavir with food 2 hr before or 1 hr after didanosine.
▸ **HIV-1 Infection (concurrent therapy with tenofovir)**
PO
Adults, Elderly. 300 mg atazanavir and 100 mg ritonavir and 300 mg tenofovir given as a single daily dose with food.
▸ **HIV-1 Infection in Patients with Mild-to-Moderate Hepatic Impairment**

PO
Adults, Elderly. 300 mg once a day
with food.

SIDE EFFECTS/ADVERSE REACTIONS

Frequent
Nausea, headache
Occasional
Rash, vomiting, depression,
diarrhea, abdominal pain, fever
Rare
Dizziness, insomnia, cough, fatigue,
back pain

PRECAUTIONS AND CONTRAINDICATIONS

Concurrent use with ergot
derivatives, midazolam, pimozide, or
triazolam; severe hepatic
insufficiency
Caution:
Prolongs PR interval, use with
caution in preexisting conduction
disorders; diabetes mellitus,
hyperglycemia, hepatic impairment;
monitor liver function, HBV
infection, redistribution of body fat,
do not breast-feed infants, safety
and efficacy in children not
established

DRUG INTERACTIONS OF CONCERN TO DENTISTRY

• Avoid drugs metabolized by
CYP3A4 isoenzymes; however, the
package insert notes that significant
drug interactions are not expected
with azithromycin, erythromycin,
itraconazole, or ketoconazole; use
with caution and monitor.

SERIOUS REACTIONS

! A severe hypersensitivity reaction
(marked by angioedema and chest
pain) and jaundice may occur.

DENTAL CONSIDERATIONS

General:
• Short appointments and a
stress-reduction protocol may be
required for anxious patients.
• Use precaution if sedation or
general anesthesia is required; risk
of hypotensive episode.
• Consider semisupine chair position
for patient comfort if GI side effects
occur.
• Patient history should include all
medications and herbal or nonherbal
remedies taken by the patient.
• Assess salivary flow as a factor in
caries, periodontal disease, and
candidiasis.
• Examine for oral manifestation of
opportunistic infection.
• Palliative medication may be
required for management of oral
side effects.
• Advise patient if dental drugs
prescribed have a potential for
photosensitivity.
• Take precautions if dental surgery
is anticipated and general anesthesia
required.
• Patients on chronic drug therapy
may rarely have symptoms of blood
dyscrasias, which can include
infection, bleeding, and poor
healing.
Consultations:
• Consultation with physician may
be necessary if sedation or general
anesthesia is required.
• Medical consultation may be
required to assess disease control
and patient's ability to tolerate
stress.
Teach Patient/Family to:
• Be aware of oral side effects and
potential sequelae.
• Update health and drug history,
reporting changes in health status,
drug regimen changes, or disease/
treatment status.

• Encourage effective oral hygiene to prevent soft tissue inflammation, infection.
• Prevent trauma when using oral hygiene aids.

atenolol
ah-ten′-oh-lol
(Apo-Atenol[CAN],
AteHexal[AUS], Noten[AUS],
Tenolin[CAN], Tenormin,
Tensig[AUS])
Do not confuse atenolol with albuterol or timolol.

CATEGORY AND SCHEDULE
Pregnancy Risk Category: D

Drug Class: Antihypertensive, selective β₁-blocker

MECHANISM OF ACTION
A β₁-adrenergic blocker that acts as an antianginal, antiarrhythmic, and antihypertensive agent by blocking β1-adrenergic receptors in cardiac tissue.
Therapeutic Effect: Slows SN heart rate, decreasing cardiac output and BP. Decreases myocardial oxygen demand.

USES
Treatment of mild-to-moderate hypertension, treatment and prophylaxis of angina pectoris, arrhythmia, adjunct therapy in hypertrophic cardiomyopathy, MI therapy and prophylaxis, adjunct therapy in pheochromocytoma, prophylaxis for vascular headache, adjunct therapy in thyrotoxicosis, mitral valve prolapse syndrome, mild to moderate heart failure

PHARMACOKINETICS

Route	Onset	Peak	Duration
PO	1 hr	2–4 hr	24 hr

Incompletely absorbed from the GI tract. Protein binding: 6%–16%. Minimal liver metabolism. Primarily excreted unchanged in urine. Removed by hemodialysis. *Half-life:* 6–7 hr (increased in impaired renal function).

INDICATIONS AND DOSAGES
▸ **Hypertension**
PO
Adults. Initially, 25–50 mg once a day. May increase dose up to 100 mg once a day.
Elderly. Usual initial dose, 25 mg a day.
Children. Initially, 0.8–1 mg/kg/dose given once a day. Range: 0.8–1.5 mg/kg/day. Maximum: 2 mg/kg/day or 100 mg/day.
▸ **Angina Pectoris**
PO
Adults. Initially, 50 mg once a day. May increase dose up to 200 mg once a day.
Elderly. Usual initial dose, 25 mg a day.
▸ **Acute MI**
IV
Adults. Give 5 mg over 5 min; may repeat in 10 min. In those who tolerate full 10-mg IV dose, begin 50-mg tablets 10 min after last IV dose followed by another 50-mg oral dose 12 hr later. Thereafter, give 100 mg once a day or 50 mg twice a day for 6–9 days. Or, for those who do not tolerate full IV dose, give 50 mg orally twice a day or 100 mg once a day for at least 7 days.
▸ **Dosage in Renal Impairment**
Dosage interval is modified on the basis of creatinine clearance.

Creatinine Clearance	Dosage Interval
15–35 ml/min	50 mg a day
Less than 15 ml/min	50 mg every other day

SIDE EFFECTS/ADVERSE REACTIONS

Atenolol is generally well tolerated, with mild and transient side effects.

Frequent

Hypotension manifested as cold extremities, constipation or diarrhea, diaphoresis, dizziness, fatigue, headache, and nausea

Occasional

Insomnia, flatulence, urinary frequency, impotence or decreased libido, depression

Rare

Rash, arthralgia, myalgia, confusion (especially in the elderly), altered taste

PRECAUTIONS AND CONTRAINDICATIONS

Cardiogenic shock, overt heart failure, second- or third-degree heart block, severe bradycardia

Caution:

Major surgery, lactation, diabetes mellitus, severe renal disease, thyroid disease, COPD, asthma, well-compensated heart failure

DRUG INTERACTIONS OF CONCERN TO DENTISTRY

• Decreased antihypertensive effects: NSAIDs, indomethacin, salicylates
• May slow metabolism of lidocaine
• Decreased β-blocking effects (or decreased β-adrenergic effects) of epinephrine, levonordefrin, isoproterenol, and other sympathomimetics
• Reduced bioavailability suspected with ampicillin

SERIOUS REACTIONS

❗ Overdose may produce profound bradycardia and hypotension.
❗ Abrupt atenolol withdrawal may result in diaphoresis, palpitations, headache, and tremors.
❗ Atenolol administration may precipitate CHF or MI in patients with cardiac disease; thyroid storm in those with thyrotoxicosis; and peripheral ischemia in those with existing peripheral vascular disease.
❗ Hypoglycemia may occur in patients with previously controlled diabetes.
❗ Thrombocytopenia, manifested as unusual bruising or bleeding, occurs rarely.

DENTAL CONSIDERATIONS

General:

• Monitor vital signs at every appointment because of cardiovascular and respiratory side effects.
• After supine positioning, have patient sit upright for at least 2 min before standing to avoid orthostatic hypotension.
• Patients on chronic drug therapy may rarely have symptoms of blood dyscrasias, which can include infection, bleeding, and poor healing.
• Assess salivary flow as a factor in caries, periodontal disease, and candidiasis.
• Stress from dental procedures may compromise cardiovascular function; determine patient risk.
• Short appointments and a stress-reduction protocol may be required for anxious patients.
• Use vasoconstrictors with caution, in low doses, and with careful aspiration. Avoid use of gingival retraction cord with epinephrine.

• Patient should never abruptly discontinue.

Consultations:

• In a patient with symptoms of blood dyscrasias, request a medical consultation for blood studies and postpone dental treatment until normal values are reestablished.

• Medical consultation may be required to assess disease control and stress tolerance of patient.

• Use precautions if general anesthesia is required for dental surgery.

Teach Patient/Family to:

• Encourage effective oral hygiene to prevent soft tissue inflammation.

• Use caution to prevent injury when using oral hygiene aids.

• When chronic dry mouth occurs, advise patient to:

  • Avoid mouth rinses with high alcohol content because of drying effects.

  • Use daily home fluoride products for anticaries effect.

  • Use sugarless gum, frequent sips of water, or saliva substitutes.

atomoxetine
ah-toh-**mox**′-eh-teen
(Strattera)

CATEGORY AND SCHEDULE
Pregnancy Risk Category: C

Drug Class: Selective norepinephrine reuptake inhibitor

MECHANISM OF ACTION
A norepinephrine reuptake inhibitor that enhances noradrenergic function by selective inhibition of the presynaptic norepinephrine transporter.

Therapeutic Effect: Improves symptoms of attention-deficit hyperactivity disorder (ADHD).

USES
Treatment of ADHD

PHARMACOKINETICS
Rapidly absorbed after PO administration. Protein binding: 98% (primarily to albumin). Eliminated primarily in urine and, to a lesser extent, in feces. Not removed by hemodialysis. *Half-life:* 4–5 hr in general population, 22 hr in 7% of Caucasians and 2% of African-Americans (increased in moderate to severe hepatic insufficiency).

INDICATIONS AND DOSAGES
▸ **ADHD**
PO
Adults, Children weighing 70 kg and more. 40 mg once a day. May increase after at least 3 days to 80 mg as a single daily dose or in divided doses. Maximum: 100 mg.
Children weighing less than 70 kg. Initially, 0.5 mg/kg/day. May increase after at least 3 days to 1.2 mg/kg/day. Maximum: 1.4 mg/kg/day or 100 mg.
▸ **Dosage in Hepatic Impairment**
Expect to administer 50% of normal atomoxetine dosage to patients with moderate hepatic impairment and 25% of normal dosage to those with severe hepatic impairment.

SIDE EFFECTS/ADVERSE REACTIONS
Frequent
Headache, dyspepsia, nausea, vomiting, fatigue, decreased appetite, dizziness, altered mood
Occasional
Tachycardia, hypertension, weight loss, delayed growth in children, irritability

Rare
Insomnia, sexual dysfunction in adults, fever

PRECAUTIONS AND CONTRAINDICATIONS
Angle-closure glaucoma, use within 14 days of MAOIs
Caution:
Hypertension, tachycardia, CV disease, urinary retention, nursing, use of herbs, poor metabolizers of CYP2D6 drugs, hepatic impairment, monitor weight and growth changes, use in geriatric patients not established

DRUG INTERACTIONS OF CONCERN TO DENTISTRY
• No dental drug interactions reported; however, drugs that inhibit CYP2D6 enzymes (paroxetine, fluoxetine) can increase plasma levels.
• Albuterol and other β_2-agonists should be used with caution because of potential effects on the cardiovascular system.

SERIOUS REACTIONS
! Urine retention or urinary hesitance may occur.
! In overdose, gastric emptying and repeated use of activated charcoal may prevent systemic absorption.

DENTAL CONSIDERATIONS
General:
• Assess salivary flow as a factor in caries, periodontal disease, and candidiasis.
• Monitor vital signs at every appointment because of cardiovascular side effects.
• Consider semisupine chair position for patient comfort if GI side effects occur.

• Use vasoconstrictor with caution, in low doses, and with careful aspiration.
Consultations:
• Medical consultation may be required to assess disease control and patient's ability to tolerate stress.
Teach Patient/Family to:
• Encourage effective oral hygiene to prevent soft tissue inflammation, infection.
• When chronic dry mouth occurs, advise patient to:
  • **Avoid mouth rinses with high alcohol content because of drying effects.**
  • Use daily home fluoride products for anticaries effect.
  • Use sugarless gum, frequent sips of water, or saliva substitutes.

atorvastatin
ah-tore-**vah'**-stah-tin
(Lipitor)
Do not confuse Lipitor with Levatol.

CATEGORY AND SCHEDULE
Pregnancy Risk Category: X

Drug Class: Cholesterol-lowering agent

MECHANISM OF ACTION
An antihyperlipidemic that inhibits HMG-CoA reductase, the enzyme that catalyzes the early step in cholesterol synthesis.
Therapeutic Effect: Decreases LDL and VLDL cholesterol, and plasma triglyceride levels; increases HDL cholesterol concentration.

USES
An adjunct in homozygous familial hypercholesterolemia, mixed lipidemia, elevated serum triglyceride levels, and type IV hyperproteinemia, also reduces total cholesterol, LDL-C, apo B, and triglyceride levels; patient should first be placed on cholesterol-lowering diet; familial hypercholesterolemia age 10–17 yr

PHARMACOKINETICS
Poorly absorbed from the GI tract. Protein binding: greater than 98%. Metabolized in the liver. Minimally eliminated in urine. Plasma levels are markedly increased in chronic alcoholic hepatic disease but are unaffected by renal disease.
Half-life: 14 hr.

INDICATIONS AND DOSAGES
▶ **Hyperlipidemia, Reduction of Risk of MI, Angina Revascularization Procedures**
PO
Adults, Elderly. Initially, 10–40 mg a day given as a single dose. Dose range: Increase at 2- to 4-wk intervals to maximum of 80 mg/day.
Children 10–17 yr. Initially, 10 mg/day, may increase to 20 mg/day.
▶ **Familial Hypercholesterolemia**
PO
Children 10–17 yr. Initially, 10 mg/day. May increase to 20 mg/day.

SIDE EFFECTS/ADVERSE REACTIONS
Atorvastatin is generally well tolerated. Side effects are usually mild and transient.
Frequent
Headache
Occasional
Myalgia, rash or pruritus, allergy
Rare
Flatulence, dyspepsia

PRECAUTIONS AND CONTRAINDICATIONS
Active hepatic disease, lactation, pregnancy, unexplained elevated hepatic function test results
Caution:
Chronic alcohol liver disease, pregnancy risk category X, monitor liver function and lipid levels

DRUG INTERACTIONS OF CONCERN TO DENTISTRY
• Severe myopathy or rhabdomyolysis: erythromycin, niacin, itraconazole, ketoconazole
• Increase in plasma levels: erythromycin, itraconazole, alcohol, ketoconazole
• Suspected increase in midazolam effects when used in general anesthesia (*Anesthesia* 58:899–904, 2003)

SERIOUS REACTIONS
! Cataracts may develop, and photosensitivity may occur.

DENTAL CONSIDERATIONS
General:
• Consider semisupine chair position for patient comfort if GI side effects occur.

atropine sulfate
a′-troe-peen
(Atropine Sulfate, Atropt[AUS])
Do not confuse atropine sulfate with Akarpine or Aplisol.

CATEGORY AND SCHEDULE
Pregnancy Risk Category: C

Drug Class: Anticholinergic

MECHANISM OF ACTION
An acetylcholine antagonist that inhibits the action of acetylcholine by competing with acetylcholine for common binding sites on muscarinic receptors, which are located on exocrine glands, cardiac and smooth-muscle ganglia, and intramural neurons. This action blocks all muscarinic effects. *Therapeutic Effect:* Decreases GI motility and secretory activity, and GU muscle tone (ureter, bladder); produces ophthalmic cycloplegia and mydriasis.

USES
Reduction of salivary and bronchial secretions

PHARMACOKINETICS
Onset 0.5–1 hr, moderate protein binding, duration of action 4–6 hr, renal excretion

INDICATIONS AND DOSAGES
▶ **Asystole, Slow, Pulseless Electrical Activity**
IV
Adults, Elderly. 1 mg; may repeat q3–5 min up to total dose of 0.04 mg/kg.
▶ **Preanesthetic**
IV/IM/Subcutaneous
Adults, Elderly. 0.4–0.6 mg 30–60 min preoperatively.
Children weighing 5 kg and more. 0.01–0.02 mg/kg/dose to maximum of 0.4 mg/dose.
Children weighing less than 5 kg. 0.02 mg/kg/dose 30–60 min pre-op.
▶ **Bradycardia**
IV
Adults, Elderly. 0.5–1 mg q5min not to exceed 2 mg or 0.04 mg/kg.
Children. 0.02 mg/kg with a minimum of 0.1 mg to a maximum of 0.5 mg in children and 1 mg in adolescents. May repeat in 5 min.

Maximum total dose: 1 mg in children, 2 mg in adolescents.

SIDE EFFECTS/ADVERSE REACTIONS
Frequent
Dry mouth, nose, and throat that may be severe; decreased sweating, constipation, irritation at subcutaneous or IM injection site
Occasional
Swallowing difficulty, blurred vision, bloated feeling, impotence, urinary hesitancy
Rare
Allergic reaction, including rash and urticaria; mental confusion or excitement, particularly in children, fatigue

PRECAUTIONS AND CONTRAINDICATIONS
Bladder neck obstruction because of prostatic hypertrophy, cardiospasm, intestinal atony, myasthenia gravis in those not treated with neostigmine, narrow-angle glaucoma, obstructive disease of the GI tract, paralytic ileus, severe ulcerative colitis, tachycardia secondary to cardiac insufficiency or thyrotoxicosis, toxic megacolon, unstable cardiovascular status in acute hemorrhage

DRUG INTERACTIONS OF CONCERN TO DENTISTRY
• Increased anticholinergic effects: tricyclic antidepressants, antihistamines, opioid analgesics, antipsychotic medications, or other drugs with anticholinergic activity
• Decreased absorption of ketoconazole

SERIOUS REACTIONS
! Overdosage may produce tachycardia, palpitations, hot, dry or flushed skin, absence of bowel sounds, increased respiratory rate,

nausea, vomiting, confusion, somnolence, slurred speech, dizziness, and CNS stimulation.
! Overdosage may also produce psychosis as evidenced by agitation, restlessness, rambling speech, visual hallucinations, paranoid behavior, and delusions, followed by depression.

DENTAL CONSIDERATIONS

General:
• Give PO dose 30–60 min before drying effects are required for dental procedures.
• Request that patient remove contact lenses before using drug because of possible drying effects in the eyes.
• Caution patients that they may feel a dry, burning sensation in the throat and experience blurred vision.
• This drug is intended for acute use, usually in single doses only; therefore, chronic dry mouth should not be a concern.
• Avoid dental light in patient's eyes; offer dark glasses for patient comfort.
Consultations:
• Medical consultation is advisable before using this drug in patients with a history of GI disease, cardiac disease, or glaucoma.

aurothioglucose/ gold sodium thiomalate

ŏr-o-thī-o-**glu′**-kos
(Gold-50[AUS], Solganal);
(Myochrysine, Myocrisin[AUS])

CATEGORY AND SCHEDULE
Pregnancy Risk Category: C

Drug Class: Antiinflammatory gold compound

MECHANISM OF ACTION
Aurothioglucose: A gold compound that alters cellular mechanisms, collagen biosynthesis, enzyme systems, and immune responses.
Therapeutic Effect: Suppresses synovitis of the active stage of rheumatoid arthritis.
Gold sodium thiomalate: A gold compound whose mechanism of action is unknown. May decrease prostaglandin synthesis or alter cellular mechanisms by inhibiting sulfhydryl systems.
Therapeutic Effect: Decreases synovial inflammation, retards cartilage and bone destruction, suppresses or prevents but does not cure, arthritis, synovitis.

USES
Treatment of rheumatoid arthritis; juvenile arthritis; unapproved: psoriatic arthritis, Felty's syndrome

PHARMACOKINETICS
Aurothioglucose (50% gold): Slow, erratic absorption after IM administration. Protein binding: 95%–99%. Primarily excreted in urine. **Half-life:** 3–27 days (half-life increased with increased number of doses).
Gold sodium thiomalate: Well absorbed. Protein binding: 95%. Widely distributed. Metabolized in liver. Excreted in urine and feces. Not removed by hemodialysis. **Half-life:** 5 days.

INDICATIONS AND DOSAGES
▸ **Rheumatoid Arthritis (Aurothioglucose)**
IM
Adults, Elderly. Initially, 10 mg, then 25 mg for 2 doses, then 50 mg weekly thereafter until total dose of 0.8–1 g given. If patient is improved

and there are no signs of toxicity, may give 50 mg at 3- to 4-wk intervals for many months.
Children. 0.25 mg/kg, may increase by 0.25 mg/kg each week.
Maintenance: 0.75–1 mg/kg/dose.
Maximum: 25-mg dose for total of 20 doses, then q2–4wk.
▸ **Rheumatoid Arthritis (Gold Sodium Thiomalate)**
IM
Adults, Elderly. Initially, 10 mg, then 25 mg for second dose. Follow with 25–50 mg/wk until improvement noted or total of 1 g administered. Maintenance: 25–50 mg q2wk for 2–20 wk; if stable, may increase to q3–4wk intervals.
Children. Initially, 10 mg, then 1 mg/kg/wk. Maximum single dose: 50 mg. Maintenance: 1 mg/kg/dose at 2- to 4-wk intervals.
▸ **Dosage in Renal Impairment**

Creatinine Clearance	Dosage
50–80 ml/min	50% of usual dosage
Less than 50 ml/min	Not recommended

SIDE EFFECTS/ADVERSE REACTIONS
Frequent
Aurothioglucose: Rash, stomatitis, diarrhea
Gold sodium thiomalate: Pruritic dermatitis, stomatitis, marked by erythema, redness, shallow ulcers of oral mucous membranes, sore throat, and difficulty swallowing, diarrhea or loose stools, abdominal pain, nausea
Occasional
Aurothioglucose: Nausea, vomiting, anorexia, abdominal cramps
Gold sodium thiomalate: Vomiting, anorexia, flatulence, dyspepsia, conjunctivitis, photosensitivity

Rare
Gold sodium thiomalate:
Constipation, urticaria, rash

PRECAUTIONS AND CONTRAINDICATIONS
Aurothioglucose: Bone marrow aplasia, history of gold-induced pathologies, including blood dyscrasias, exfoliative dermatitis, necrotizing enterocolitis, and pulmonary fibrosis, serious adverse effects with previous gold therapy, severe blood dyscrasias
Gold sodium thiomalate: Colitis, concurrent use of antimalarials, immunosuppressive agents, penicillamine, or phenylbutazone, CHF, exfoliative dermatitis, history of blood dyscrasias, severe liver or renal impairment, systemic lupus erythematosus

DRUG INTERACTIONS OF CONCERN TO DENTISTRY
• None reported

SERIOUS REACTIONS
! Gold toxicity is the primary serious reaction. Signs and symptoms of gold toxicity include decreased hemoglobin, leukopenia (WBC count less than 4000/mm^3), reduced granulocyte counts (less than 150,000/mm^3), proteinuria, hematuria, stomatitis (sores, ulcers, and white spots in the mouth and throat), blood dyscrasias (anemia, leukopenia, thrombocytopenia, and eosinophilia), glomerulonephritis, nephritic syndrome, and cholestatic jaundice.

DENTAL CONSIDERATIONS
General:
• Patients on chronic drug therapy may rarely have symptoms of blood dyscrasias, which can include

infection, bleeding, and poor healing.

• Palliative medication may be required for management of oral side effects.

• Consider semisupine chair position for patient comfort because of arthritic disease.

Consultations:

• Medical consultation may be required to assess disease control and patient's ability to tolerate stress.

• In a patient with symptoms of blood dyscrasias, request a medical consultation for blood studies and postpone dental treatment until normal values are reestablished.

Teach Patient/Family to:

• Encourage effective oral hygiene to prevent soft tissue inflammation.

• Be aware of the possibility of secondary oral infection and the need to see dentist immediately if infection occurs.

• Report oral lesions, soreness, or bleeding to dentist.

• Avoid mouth rinses with high alcohol content because of drying effects.

azatadine maleate
ah-**za**′-ta-deen **mal**′-ee-ate
(Optimine)
Do not confuse with azelastine or azacitidine.

CATEGORY AND SCHEDULE
Pregnancy Risk Category: B

Drug Class: Antihistamine, H1-receptor antagonist

MECHANISM OF ACTION
A piperazine-derivative antihistamine that has both anticholinergic and antiserotonin activity. Inhibits mediator release from mast cells and prevents calcium entry into mast cells through voltage-dependent calcium channels.

Therapeutic Effect: Relieves allergic conditions, including urticaria and pruritus. Anticholinergic effects cause drying of nasal mucosa.

USES
Allergy symptoms, rhinitis, chronic urticaria, pruritus

PHARMACOKINETICS
Rapidly and extensively absorbed from the GI tract. Protein binding: minimal. Metabolized in liver. Excreted in urine. **Half-life:** 8.7 hr.

INDICATIONS AND DOSAGES
▶ Allergic Rhinitis
PO
Adults, Elderly, Children 12 yr or older. 1–2 mg 2 times a day.

SIDE EFFECTS/ADVERSE REACTIONS
Frequent
Slight to moderate drowsiness, thickening of bronchial secretions
Rare
Headache, fatigue, nervousness, dizziness, appetite increase, weight gain, nausea, diarrhea, abdominal pain, dry mouth, arthralgia, pharyngitis

PRECAUTIONS AND CONTRAINDICATIONS
History of hypersensitivity to azatadine, antihistamines, or any other component of the formulation or to other related antihistamines including cyproheptadine, concomitant use of MAOIs

DRUG INTERACTIONS OF CONCERN TO DENTISTRY
• Increased CNS depression: all CNS depressants, alcohol
• Increased anticholinergic effect: anticholinergics

SERIOUS REACTIONS
! Hepatitis, bronchospasm, and epistaxis have been reported.

General:
• Assess salivary flow as a factor in caries, periodontal disease, and candidiasis.
• Patients on chronic drug therapy may rarely have symptoms of blood dyscrasias, which can include infection, bleeding, and poor healing.
• Consider semisupine chair position for patient comfort because of respiratory disease.
• Monitor vital signs at every appointment because of cardiovascular side effects.
Consultations:
• In a patient with symptoms of blood dyscrasia, request a medical consultation for blood studies and postpone dental treatment until normal values are reestablished.
Teach Patient/Family to:
• Encourage effective oral hygiene to prevent soft tissue inflammation.
• Prevent injury when using oral hygiene aids.
• When chronic dry mouth occurs, advise patient to:
  • **Avoid mouth rinses with high alcohol content because of drying effects.**
  • Use daily home fluoride products for anticaries effect.
  • Use sugarless gum, frequent sips of water, or saliva substitutes.

azathioprine
ay-za-**thye′**-oh-preen
(Alti-Azathioprine[CAN], Azasan, Imuran, Thioprine[AUS])
Do not confuse azathioprine with Azulfidine or azatadine, or Imuran with Elmiron or Imferon.

CATEGORY AND SCHEDULE
Pregnancy Risk Category: D

Drug Class: Immunosuppressant

MECHANISM OF ACTION
An immunologic agent that antagonizes purine metabolism and inhibits DNA, protein, and RNA synthesis.
Therapeutic Effect: Suppresses cell-mediated hypersensitivities; alters antibody production and immune response in transplant recipients; reduces the severity of arthritis symptoms.

USES
Renal transplants to prevent graft rejection, refractory rheumatoid arthritis; unapproved use in refractory ITP, glomerulonephritis, nephrotic syndrome, bone marrow transplant; unapproved: pemphigoid and pemphigus, chronic ulcerative colitis, Behçet's syndrome, Crohn's disease

PHARMACOKINETICS
Metabolized in liver; excreted in urine (active metabolite); crosses placenta.

INDICATIONS AND DOSAGES
▸ **Adjunct in Prevention of Renal Allograft Rejection**

PO, IV
Adults, Elderly, Children. 2–5 mg/kg/day on day of transplant, then 1–3 mg/kg/day as maintenance dose.

▸ **Rheumatoid Arthritis**
PO
Adults. Initially, 1 mg/kg/day as a single dose or in 2 divided doses. May increase by 0.5 mg/kg/day after 6–8 wk at 4-wk intervals up to maximum of 2.5 mg/kg/day. Maintenance: Lowest effective dosage. May decrease dose by 0.5 mg/kg or 25 mg/day q4wk (while other therapies, such as rest, physiotherapy, and salicylates, are maintained).
Elderly. Initially, 1 mg/kg/day (50–100 mg); may increase by 25 mg/day until response or toxicity.

▸ **Dosage in Renal Impairment**
Dosage is modified on the basis of creatinine clearance.

Creatinine Clearance	Dose
10–50 ml/min	75% of usual dose
Less than 10 ml/min	50% of usual dose

SIDE EFFECTS/ADVERSE REACTIONS

Frequent
Nausea, vomiting, anorexia (particularly during early treatment and with large doses)
Occasional
Rash
Rare
Severe nausea and vomiting with diarrhea, abdominal pain, hypersensitivity reaction

PRECAUTIONS AND CONTRAINDICATIONS

Pregnant patients with rheumatoid arthritis

DRUG INTERACTIONS OF CONCERN TO DENTISTRY

• Increased blood dyscrasias: NSAIDs, especially phenylbutazone, dapsone, phenothiazines
• Increased immunosuppression, risk of infection: corticosteroids

SERIOUS REACTIONS

! Azathioprine use increases the risk of developing neoplasia (new abnormal-growth tumors).
! Significant leukopenia and thrombocytopenia may occur, particularly in those undergoing kidney transplant rejection.
! Hepatotoxicity occurs rarely.

DENTAL CONSIDERATIONS

General:
• Patients on chronic drug therapy may rarely have symptoms of blood dyscrasias, which can include infection, bleeding, and poor healing.
• To prevent infection if surgery or deep scaling is planned, prophylactic antibiotics may be indicated in patients who develop neutropenia.
• Determine why the patient is taking the drug.
• Alert the patient to the possibility of secondary oral infection; must see dentist immediately if infection occurs.
Consultations:
• In a patient with symptoms of blood dyscrasias, request a medical consultation for blood studies and postpone dental treatment until normal values are reestablished.
• Medical consultation may be required to assess disease control and patient's ability to tolerate stress.
Teach Patient/Family to:
• Encourage effective oral hygiene to prevent soft tissue inflammation.

• Use caution to prevent injury when using oral hygiene aids.
• Avoid mouth rinses with high alcohol content because of drying effects and irritation of mucous membranes.

azelaic acid
aye-zeh-**lay′**-ick **as′**-id
(Azelex, Finacea, Finevin)

CATEGORY AND SCHEDULE
Pregnancy Risk Category: B

Drug Class: Topical antimicrobial, antiacne

MECHANISM OF ACTION
The exact mechanism of action of azelaic acid is not known. Possesses antimicrobial activity against *Propionibacterium acnes* and *Staphylococcus epidermidis.*
Therapeutic Effect: Inhibits microbial cellular protein synthesis.

USES
Topical therapy of mild-to-moderate inflammatory acne vulgaris; unapproved: melasma

PHARMACOKINETICS
Minimal absorption after topical administration. Metabolized in liver. Excreted in urine as unchanged drug. *Half-life:* 12 hr.

INDICATIONS AND DOSAGES
▶ **Mild-to-Moderate Acne**
Topical
Adults, Adolescents. Apply cream or gel to affected area twice daily (morning and evening).

SIDE EFFECTS/ADVERSE REACTIONS
Occasional
Pruritus, stinging, burning, tingling, erythema, dryness, rash, peeling, irritation, contact dermatitis
Rare
Worsening of asthma, vitiligo depigmentation, small depigmented spots, hypertrichosis, reddening (signs of keratosis pilaris), exacerbation of recurrent cold sore, fever blister, or oral herpes simplex

PRECAUTIONS AND CONTRAINDICATIONS
Hypersensitivity to azelaic acid or any component of the formulation

DRUG INTERACTIONS OF CONCERN TO DENTISTRY
• None reported

SERIOUS REACTIONS
! None reported

DENTAL CONSIDERATIONS

General:
• Topical use rarely causes exacerbation of recurrent herpes labialis.
• Keep away from mouth and other mucous membranes; wash eyes if cream comes in contact; irritation can occur.

azelastine
ah-zel-ah-steen
(Astelin, Optivar)
Do not confuse Optivar with Optiray.

CATEGORY AND SCHEDULE
Pregnancy Risk Category: C

Drug Class: Antihistamine

MECHANISM OF ACTION
An antihistamine that competes with histamine for histamine receptor sites on cells in the blood vessels, GI tract, and respiratory tract. *Therapeutic Effect:* Relieves symptoms associated with seasonal allergic rhinitis such as increased mucus production and sneezing and symptoms associated with allergic conjunctivitis, such as redness, itching, and excessive tearing.

USES
Temporary relief of signs and symptoms of allergic conjunctivitis. Control of symptoms associated with seasonal allergic rhinitis, nonallergic vasomotor rhinitis, nasal pruritus.

PHARMACOKINETICS

Route	Onset	Peak	Duration
Nasal spray	0.5–1 hr	2–3 hr	12 hr
Ophthalmic	N/A	3 min	8 hr

Well absorbed through nasal mucosa. Primarily excreted in feces. *Half-life:* 22 hr.

INDICATIONS AND DOSAGES
▶ **Allergic Rhinitis**
Nasal
Adults, Elderly, Children 12 yr and older. 2 sprays in each nostril twice a day.
Children 5–11 yr. 1 spray in each nostril twice a day.
▶ **Allergic Conjunctivitis**
Ophthalmic
Adults, Elderly, Children 3 yr or older. 1 drop into affected eye twice a day.

SIDE EFFECTS/ADVERSE REACTIONS
Frequent
Headache, bitter taste
Rare
Nasal burning, paroxysmal sneezing
Ophthalmic: Transient eye burning or stinging, bitter taste, headache

PRECAUTIONS AND CONTRAINDICATIONS
Breast-feeding women, history of hypersensitivity to antihistamines, neonates or premature infants, third trimester of pregnancy

DRUG INTERACTIONS OF CONCERN TO DENTISTRY
• Increased risk of anticholinergic effects: anticholinergics
• Possible additive sedation: alcohol, anxiolytics, opioid analgesics

SERIOUS REACTIONS
❗ Epistaxis occurs rarely.

DENTAL CONSIDERATIONS
General:
• Protect patient's eyes from accidental spatter during dental treatment.
• Assess salivary flow as factor in caries, periodontal disease, and candidiasis.
Teach Patient/Family:
• When chronic dry mouth occurs, advise patient to:
  • Avoid mouth rinses with high alcohol content because of drying effects.
  • Use daily home fluoride products for anticaries effect.
  • Use sugarless gum, frequent sips of water, or saliva substitutes.

azithromycin

ah-zi-thro-**mye**´-sin
(Zithromax, Zithromax TRI-PAK,
Zithromax Z-PAK)
Do not confuse azithromycin with
erythromycin.

CATEGORY AND SCHEDULE

Pregnancy Risk Category: B

Drug Class: Macrolide antibiotic

MECHANISM OF ACTION

A macrolide antibiotic that binds to
ribosomal receptor sites of
susceptible organisms, inhibiting
RNA-dependent protein synthesis.
Therapeutic Effect: Bacteriostatic or
bactericidal, depending on the drug
dosage.

USES

Treatment of mild-to-moderate
infections of the upper or lower
respiratory tract; COPD
exacerbations caused by *H.
influenzae, M. catarrhalis,* or *S.
pneumoniae;* gonorrhea, chancroid,
uncomplicated skin and skin
structure infections caused by *M.
catarrhalis, S. pneumoniae, S.
pyogenes, S. aureus, S. agalactiae,
H. influenzae, Clostridium,* or *L.
pneumophila;* nongonococcal
urethritis; cervicitis caused by *C.
trachomatis;* otitis media caused by
H. influenzae, S. pneumoniae, or *M.
catarrhalis;* chlamydia;
Mycobacterium avium complex
(MAC) in HIV infection

PHARMACOKINETICS

Rapidly absorbed from the GI tract.
Protein binding: 7%–50%. Widely
distributed. Eliminated primarily
unchanged by biliary excretion.
Half-life: 68 hr.

INDICATIONS AND DOSAGES

▶ **Respiratory Tract, Skin, and
Skin-Structure Infections**
PO
Adults, Elderly. 500 mg once, then
250 mg/day for 4 days.
Children 6 mo and older. 10 mg/kg
once (maximum 500 mg) then 5 mg/
kg/day for 4 days (maximum
250 mg).
▶ **Acute Bacterial Exacerbations of
COPD**
PO
Adults. 500 mg/day for 3 days.
▶ **Otitis Media**
PO
Children 6 mo and older. 10 mg/kg
once (maximum 500 mg) then 5 mg/
kg/day for 4 days (maximum
250 mg). Single dose: 30 mg/kg.
Maximum: 1500 mg. Three-day
regimen: 10 mg/kg/day as single
daily dose. Maximum: 500 mg/day.
▶ **Pharyngitis, Tonsillitis**
PO
Children older than 2 yr. 12 mg/kg/
day (maximum 500 mg) for 5 days.
▶ **Chancroid**
PO
Adults, Elderly. 1 g as single dose.
Children. 20 mg/kg as single dose.
Maximum: 1 g.
▶ **Treatment of MAC**
PO
Adults, Elderly. 500 mg/day in
combination.
Children. 5 mg/kg/day (maximum
250 mg) in combination.
▶ **Prevention of MAC**
PO
Adults, Elderly. 1200 mg/wk alone
or with rifabutin.
Children. 5 mg/kg/day (maximum
250 mg) or 20 mg/kg/wk (maximum
1200 mg) alone or with rifabutin.
▶ **Nongonococcal Urethritis and
Cervicitis Caused by *Chlamydia
trachomatis***

PO
Adults. 1 g as a single dose.
▶ **Usual Pediatric Dosage**
PO
Children older than 6 mo. 10 mg/kg
once (maximum: 500 mg) then
5 mg/kg/day for 4 days (maximum
250 mg).
▶ **Usual Parenteral Dosage
(Community-Acquired Pneumonia,
PID)**
IV
Adults. 500 mg/day, followed by oral
therapy.

SIDE EFFECTS/ADVERSE REACTIONS

Occasional
Nausea, vomiting, diarrhea,
abdominal pain
Rare
Headache, dizziness, allergic
reaction

PRECAUTIONS AND CONTRAINDICATIONS

Hypersensitivity to azithromycin or
other macrolide antibiotics

DRUG INTERACTIONS OF CONCERN TO DENTISTRY

• Increased serum levels:
carbamazepine, cyclosporine,
pimozide
• Risk of severe myopathy,
rhabdomyolysis:
hydroxymethylglutaryl coenzyme A
(HMG-CoA) reductase inhibitors
(statins)
• Decreased action of clindamycin,
penicillin, lincomycin
• Possible increase in anticoagulant
effect: warfarin
• Increased serum levels of
theophylline

SERIOUS REACTIONS

❗ Antibiotic-associated colitis and
other superinfections may result
from altered bacterial balance.
❗ Acute interstitial nephritis and
hepatotoxicity occur rarely.

DENTAL CONSIDERATIONS

General:
• An alternative drug of choice for
mild infection caused by susceptible
organisms in patients allergic to
penicillin.
• Determine why the patient is
taking the drug.
• Consider semisupine chair position
for patient comfort if GI side effects
occur.
Teach Patient/Family:
• When used for dental infection,
advise patient to:
• Report sore throat, oral
burning sensation, fever, and
fatigue, any of which could
indicate superinfection.
• Take at prescribed intervals
and complete dosage regimen.
• Immediately notify the dentist
if signs or symptoms of infection
increase.

---

aztreonam
az-**tree**′-oo-nam
(Azactam)

CATEGORY AND SCHEDULE
Pregnancy Risk Category: B

Drug Class: Antibacterial

MECHANISM OF ACTION
A monobactam antibiotic that inhibits bacterial cell wall synthesis. *Therapeutic Effect:* Bactericidal.

USES
Treatment of infections caused by bacteria

PHARMACOKINETICS
Completely absorbed after IM administration. Protein binding: 56%–60%. Partially metabolized by hydrolysis. Primarily excreted unchanged in urine. Removed by hemodialysis. *Half-life:* 1.4–2.2 hr (increased in impaired renal or hepatic function).

INDICATIONS AND DOSAGES
▸**UTIs**
IV, IM
Adults, Elderly. 500 mg–1 g q8–12h.
▸**Moderate to Severe Systemic Infections**
IV, IM
Adults, Elderly. 1–2 g q8–12h.
▸**Severe or Life-Threatening Infections**
IV
Adults, Elderly. 2 g q6–8h.
▸**Cystic Fibrosis**
IV
Children. 50 mg/kg/dose q6–8h up to 200 mg/kg/day. Maximum: 8 g/d.
▸**Mild to Severe Infections in Children**
IV
Children. 30 mg/kg q6–8h. Maximum: 120 mg/kg/day.
Neonates. 60–120 mg/kg/day q6–12h.
▸**Dosage in Renal Impairment**
Dosage and frequency are modified on the basis of creatinine clearance and the severity of the infection.

Creatinine Clearance	Dosage
10–30 ml/min	1–2 g initially, then usual dose at usual intervals
Less than 10 ml/min	1–2 g initially; then usual dose at usual intervals

SIDE EFFECTS/ADVERSE REACTIONS
Occasional
Discomfort and swelling at IM injection site, nausea, vomiting, diarrhea, rash
Rare
Phlebitis or thrombophlebitis at IV injection site, abdominal cramps, headache, hypotension

PRECAUTIONS AND CONTRAINDICATIONS
None known

DRUG INTERACTIONS OF CONCERN TO DENTISTRY
• None reported

SERIOUS REACTIONS
❗Antibiotic-associated colitis and other superinfections may result from altered bacterial balance.
❗Severe hypersensitivity reactions, including anaphylaxis, occur rarely.

DENTAL CONSIDERATIONS
General:
• For selected infections in the hospital setting.
• Provide palliative dental care for dental emergencies only.
• Caution regarding allergy to medication.
• Examine for oral manifestation of opportunistic infection.
• Determine why patient is taking the drug.

Consultations:
• Medical consultation may be required to assess disease control.
• Consult patient's physician if an acute dental infection occurs and another antiinfective is required.

Teach Patient/Family to:
• Encourage effective oral hygiene to prevent soft tissue inflammation.
• Report oral lesions, soreness, or bleeding to dentist.
• Prevent trauma when using oral hygiene aids.

bacitracin

bass-ih-**tray**′-sin
(Baciguent, Baci-IM, Bacitracin)
Do not confuse bacitracin with
Bactrim or Bactroban.

CATEGORY AND SCHEDULE
Pregnancy Risk Category: C
OTC

Drug Class: Antiinfective;
antibiotic

MECHANISM OF ACTION
An antibiotic that interferes with
plasma membrane permeability and
inhibits bacterial cell wall synthesis
in susceptible bacteria.
Therapeutic Effect: Bacteriostatic.

USES
Treatment of superficial ocular
infections (conjunctivitis, keratitis,
corneal ulcers, blepharitis). Minor
skin abrasions, superficial infections.
Treatment, prophylaxis of surgical
procedures.

INDICATIONS AND DOSAGES
▶ **Superficial Ocular Infections**
Ophthalmic
Adults. $\frac{1}{2}$-inch ribbon in
conjunctival sac q3–4h.
▶ **Skin Abrasions, Superficial Skin
Infections**
Topical
Adults, Children. Apply to affected
area 1–5 times a day.
▶ **Surgical Treatment and
Prophylaxis**
Irrigation
Adults, Elderly. 50,000–150,000
units, as needed.

SIDE EFFECTS/ADVERSE REACTIONS
Rare
Ophthalmic: Burning, itching,
redness, swelling, pain
Topical: Hypersensitivity reaction
(allergic contact dermatitis, burning,
inflammation, pruritus)

PRECAUTIONS AND CONTRAINDICATIONS
None known

DRUG INTERACTIONS OF CONCERN TO DENTISTRY
• None reported

SERIOUS REACTIONS
! Severe hypersensitivity reactions,
including apnea and hypotension,
occur rarely.

DENTAL CONSIDERATIONS
General:
• Use protective glove or finger cot
to apply.
• Determine why patient is taking
the drug.
Teach Patient/Family to:
• Report burning, itching, or rash.

baclofen

bak′-loe-fen
(Apo-Baclofen[CAN], Baclo[AUS],
Clofen[AUS], Lioresal,
Liotec[CAN], Novo-
Baclofen[CAN],
Nu-Baclofen[CAN], Stelax[AUS])
Do not confuse baclofen with
Bactroban or Beclovent.

CATEGORY AND SCHEDULE
Pregnancy Risk Category: C

Drug Class: Skeletal muscle
relaxant, central acting

B

MECHANISM OF ACTION

A direct-acting skeletal muscle relaxant that inhibits transmission of reflexes at the spinal cord level. *Therapeutic Effect:* Relieves muscle spasticity.

USES

Treatment of skeletal muscle spasticity in multiple sclerosis, spinal cord injury, children with cerebral palsy; intrathecal dose form for severe spasticity in spinal cord injury or those not responsive to oral dose form; unapproved: trigeminal neuralgia

PHARMACOKINETICS

Well absorbed from the GI tract. Protein binding: 30%. Partially metabolized in the liver. Primarily excreted in urine. *Half-life:* 2.5–4 hr; intrathecal: 1.5 hr.

INDICATIONS AND DOSAGES
▸ **Spasticity**
PO
Adults. Initially, 5 mg 3 times a day. May increase by 15 mg/day at 3-day intervals. Range: 40–80 mg/day. Maximum: 80 mg/day.
Elderly. Initially, 5 mg 2–3 times a day. May gradually increase dosage.
Children. Initially, 10–15 mg/day in divided doses q8h. May increase by 5–15 mg/day at 3-day intervals. Maximum: 40 mg/day (children 2–7 yr); 60 mg/day (children 8 yr and older).
Usual intrathecal dosage
Adults, Elderly, Children older than 12 yr. 300–800 mcg/day.
Children 12 yr and younger. 100–300 mcg/day.

SIDE EFFECTS/ADVERSE REACTIONS

Frequent
Transient somnolence, asthenia, dizziness, light-headedness, nausea, vomiting
Occasional
Headache, paresthesia, constipation, anorexia, hypotension, confusion, nasal congestion
Rare
Paradoxical CNS excitement or restlessness, slurred speech, tremor, dry mouth, diarrhea, nocturia, impotence

PRECAUTIONS AND CONTRAINDICATIONS

Skeletal muscle spasm due to cerebral palsy, Parkinson's disease, rheumatic disorders, CVA, cough, intractable hiccups, neuropathic pain

DRUG INTERACTIONS OF CONCERN TO DENTISTRY

• Increased CNS depression: alcohol, all CNS depressants
• Muscle hypertonia: tricyclic antidepressants
• Warn patient of sedative effects while taking medication

SERIOUS REACTIONS

❗ Abrupt discontinuation of baclofen may produce hallucinations and seizures.
❗ Overdose results in blurred vision, seizures, myosis, mydriasis, severe muscle weakness, strabismus, respiratory depression, and vomiting.

DENTAL CONSIDERATIONS

General:
• Monitor vital signs at every appointment because of cardiovascular side effects.

• Assess salivary flow as a factor in caries, periodontal disease, and candidiasis.
• After supine positioning, have patient sit upright for at least 2 min to avoid orthostatic hypotension.

Teach Patient/Family:
• When chronic dry mouth occurs, advise patient to:
  • Avoid mouth rinses with high alcohol content because of drying effects.
  • Use daily home fluoride products for anticaries effect.
  • Use sugarless gum, frequent sips of water, or saliva substitutes.

balsalazide
ball-**sal'**-ah-zide
(Colazal)

CATEGORY AND SCHEDULE
Pregnancy Risk Category: B

Drug Class: Antiinflammatory

MECHANISM OF ACTION
A 5-aminosalicylic acid derivative that changes intestinal microflora, altering prostaglandin production and inhibiting function of natural killer cells, mast cells, neutrophils, and macrophages.
Therapeutic Effect: Diminishes inflammatory effect in colon.

USES
Treatment of mild to moderately active ulcerative colitis

PHARMACOKINETICS
PO: Drug reaches colon intact; bacterial azoreductases release 5-aminobenzyl-B-analine and mesalamine (active metabolite); low, variable systemic absorption; peak concentration 1–2 hr, protein binding ≈99%; less than 1% renal excretion; most excreted in feces (65%).

INDICATIONS AND DOSAGES
▸ **Ulcerative Colitis**
PO
Adults, Elderly. Three 750-mg capsules 3 times a day for 8 wk.

SIDE EFFECTS/ADVERSE REACTIONS
Frequent
Headache, abdominal pain, nausea, diarrhea
Occasional
Vomiting, arthralgia, rhinitis, insomnia, fatigue, flatulence, coughing, dyspepsia

PRECAUTIONS AND CONTRAINDICATIONS
Hypersensitivity, including hypersensitivity to mesalamine or salicylates

DRUG INTERACTIONS OF CONCERN TO DENTISTRY
• None reported

SERIOUS REACTIONS
! Liver toxicity occurs rarely.

DENTAL CONSIDERATIONS
General:
• Consider semisupine chair position for patient comfort because of GI side effects of disease.
Consultations:
• To reduce any potential risk of antibiotic-associated pseudomembranous colitis, a consultation is recommended before selecting an antibiotic for a dental infection.

B

becaplermin
beh-**kap'**-lear-min
(Regranex)

CATEGORY AND SCHEDULE
Pregnancy Risk Category: C

Drug Class: Topical wound repair

MECHANISM OF ACTION
A platelet-derived growth factor that heals open wounds.
Therapeutic Effect: Stimulates body to grow new tissue.

USES
An adjunct to good ulcer care practices in lower extremity diabetic, neuropathic ulcers that extend into subcutaneous tissues or beyond and have adequate blood supply

PHARMACOKINETICS
None reported

INDICATIONS AND DOSAGES
▸ **Ulcers**
Topical
Adults, Elderly. Apply once daily (spread evenly; cover with saline-moistened gauze dressing). After 12 hr, rinse ulcer, re-cover with saline gauze.

SIDE EFFECTS/ADVERSE REACTIONS
Occasional
Local rash near ulcer
Precautions and Contraindications
Hypersensitivity, neoplasms at the site of application, ulcers caused by vascular insufficiency
Caution:
Nonsterile, low-bioburden product that is not for use in ulcers that heal by primary intention, lactation,

children younger than 16 yr, external use only, do not apply with fingers

DRUG INTERACTIONS OF CONCERN TO DENTISTRY
• Unknown

SERIOUS REACTIONS
! None reported

DENTAL CONSIDERATIONS
General:
• Patients requiring use of this medication probably will be limited in activities or bedridden.
• Determine why patient is taking the drug.
• Diabetes: question patient about self-monitoring of blood glucose values or finger-stick records.
• Diabetics may be more susceptible to infection and have delayed wound healing.
• Examine for oral manifestation of opportunistic infection.
• Patients with advanced diabetes should be questioned about any limitations in activities or stress tolerance. Some will also be receiving dialysis treatment if renal function is compromised. Dental treatment usually can be performed the day after dialysis.
Consultations:
• Medical consultation may be required to assess disease control and patient's ability to tolerate stress.
• Medical consultation may include data from patient's blood glucose monitoring, including glycosylated hemoglobin or HbA1c testing.
• Patients in dialysis may require antibiotic prophylaxis; determine need.
Teach Patient/Family to:
• Encourage effective oral hygiene to prevent soft tissue inflammation.

- Prevent trauma when using oral hygiene aids.
- Update health and drug history if physician makes any changes in evaluation or drug regimens.

beclomethasone dipropionate/ beclomethasone dipropionate hfa

be-kloe-**meth′**-ah-sone
di-**pro′**-pi-o-nate
Oral inhalation: Qvar
Nasal inhalation: Beconase, Beconase AQ Nasal, Vancenase AQ 84 mcg, Vancenase Pockethaler

CATEGORY AND SCHEDULE

Pregnancy Risk Category: C

Drug Class: Corticosteroid, synthetic

MECHANISM OF ACTION

Glucocorticoids have multiple actions that include antiinflammatory and immunosuppressant effects. They inhibit phospholipase A_2, interfering with or reducing the synthesis of prostaglandins and leukotrienes. They also bind to cytoplasmic glucocorticoid receptors (GRs) and enter the cell nucleus to bind with DNA. This results in the synthesis of various enzymes such as collagenase, elastase, and cytokines that play important roles in inflammation control and immunosuppression. They also suppress the production of lymphocytes, monocytes, and eosinophils.

USES

Treatment of chronic asthma, prevention of recurrent nasal polyps, allergic and nonallergic rhinitis

PHARMACOKINETICS

Inhalation: Onset 10 min, half-life 3–15 hr; crosses placenta; metabolized in lungs, liver, GI system; excreted in feces (metabolites).

INDICATIONS AND DOSAGES

Oral Inhalation (QVAR only)
Adults, Adolescents. 40–160 mcg bid; limit to 320 mcg bid.
Children 5–11 yr. 40 mcg bid; limit 80 mcg bid.
Nasal Inhalation
Adults, Children older than 12 yr. 1–2 sprays in each nostril bid-qid; 84 mcg double strength: use once daily.
Children 6–12 yr. 1 spray in each nostril once daily.
Pockethaler
Adults, Children older than 12 yr. 1 spray in each nostril bid–qid.

SIDE EFFECTS/ADVERSE REACTIONS

Occasional
Dry mouth, candidiasis
Rare
Bronchospasm, hoarseness, sore throat

PRECAUTIONS AND CONTRAINDICATIONS

Hypersensitivity; status asthmaticus (primary treatment); nonasthmatic bronchial disease; bacterial, fungal, or viral infections of mouth, throat, or lungs; children younger than 3 yr
Caution:
Nasal disease/surgery

DRUG INTERACTIONS OF CONCERN TO DENTISTRY

- None reported

B

SERIOUS REACTIONS
❗ Potential acute adrenal insufficiency if used to replace systemic corticosteroid use
❗ Signs and symptoms of hypercorticism

DENTAL CONSIDERATIONS
General:
• Evaluate respiration characteristics and rate.
• Assess salivary flow as a factor in caries, periodontal disease, and candidiasis.
• Place on frequent recall because of oral side effects.
• Be aware that aspirin or sulfite preservatives in vasoconstrictor-containing products can exacerbate asthma.
• Acute asthmatic episodes may be precipitated in the dental office. Sympathomimetic inhalants should be available for emergency use.
• Midday appointments and a stress-reduction protocol may be required for anxious patients.
Consultations:
• Medical consultation may be required to assess patient's ability to tolerate stress.
Teach Patient/Family:
• Gargling and rinsing with water after each dose helps prevent candidiasis.
• When chronic dry mouth occurs, advise patient to:
  • Avoid mouth rinses with high alcohol content because of drying effects.
  • Use daily home fluoride products for anticaries effect.
  • Use sugarless gum, frequent sips of water, or saliva substitutes.

benazepril
be-**naze'**-ah-pril
(Lotensin)
Do not confuse benazepril with Benadryl, or Lotensin with Loniten or lovastatin.

CATEGORY AND SCHEDULE
Pregnancy Risk Category: C (D if used in second or third trimester)

Drug Class: Angiotensin-converting enzyme (ACE) inhibitor

MECHANISM OF ACTION
An ACE inhibitor that decreases the rate of conversion of angiotensin I to angiotensin II, a potent vasoconstrictor. Reduces peripheral arterial resistance.
Therapeutic Effect: Lowers B/P.

USES
Treatment of hypertension, alone or in combination with thiazide diuretics

PHARMACOKINETICS

Route	Onset	Peak	Duration
PO	1 hr	2–4 hr	24 hr

Partially absorbed from the GI tract. Protein binding: 97%. Metabolized in the liver to active metabolite. Primarily excreted in urine. Minimal removal by hemodialysis. *Half-life:* 35 min; metabolite 10–11 hr.

INDICATIONS AND DOSAGES
▶ Hypertension (monotherapy)
PO
Adults. Initially, 10 mg/day.
Maintenance: 20–40 mg/day as

single or in 2 divided doses.
Maximum: 80 mg/day.
Elderly. Initially, 5–10 mg/day.
Range: 20–40 mg/day.
▶ **Hypertension (combination therapy)**
PO
Adults. Discontinue diuretic 2–3 days prior to initiating benazepril, then dose as noted above. If unable to discontinue diuretic, begin benazepril at 5 mg/day.
▶ **Dosage in Renal Impairment**
For adult patients with creatinine clearance less than 30 ml/min, initially, 5 mg/day titrated up to maximum of 40 mg/day.

SIDE EFFECTS/ADVERSE REACTIONS
Frequent
Cough, headache, dizziness
Occasional
Fatigue, somnolence or drowsiness, nausea
Rare
Rash, fever, myalgia, diarrhea, loss of taste

PRECAUTIONS AND CONTRAINDICATIONS
History of angioedema from previous treatment with ACE inhibitors
Caution:
Impaired renal or liver function, dialysis patients, hypovolemia, blood dyscrasias, CHF, chronic obstructive pulmonary disease (COPD), asthma, elderly

DRUG INTERACTIONS OF CONCERN TO DENTISTRY
• Increased hypotension: alcohol, phenothiazines
• Decreased hypotensive effects: indomethacin and possibly other NSAIDs, sympathomimetics
• Suspected reduction in the antihypertensive and vasodilator effects by salicylates; monitor blood pressure if used concurrently

SERIOUS REACTIONS
❗ Excessive hypotension ("first-dose syncope") may occur in patients with CHF and in those who are severely salt or volume depleted.
❗ Angioedema (swelling of the face and lips) and hyperkalemia occur rarely.
❗ Agranulocytosis and neutropenia may be noted in those with collagen vascular disease, including scleroderma and systemic lupus erythematosus, and impaired renal function.
❗ Nephrotic syndrome may be noted in patients with history of renal disease.

DENTAL CONSIDERATIONS

General:
• Monitor vital signs at every appointment because of cardiovascular and respiratory side effects.
• After supine positioning, have patient sit upright for at least 2 min to avoid orthostatic hypotension.
• Patients on chronic drug therapy may rarely have symptoms of blood dyscrasias, which can include infection, bleeding, and poor healing.
• Assess salivary flow as a factor in caries, periodontal disease, and candidiasis.
• Limit use of sodium-containing products, such as saline IV fluids, for those patients with a dietary salt restriction.
• Use vasoconstrictors with caution, in low doses, and with careful aspiration.

B

• Stress from dental procedures may compromise cardiovascular function; determine patient risk.

• Short appointments and a stress-reduction protocol may be required for anxious patients.

Consultations:

• Medical consultation may be required to assess disease control and patient's ability to tolerate stress.

• In a patient with symptoms of blood dyscrasias, request a medical consultation for blood studies and postpone dental treatment until normal values are reestablished.

• Take precautions if dental surgery is anticipated and sedation or general anesthesia is required; risk of hypotensive episode.

Teach Patient/Family to:

• Use effective oral hygiene to prevent soft tissue inflammation.

• Use caution to prevent injury when using oral hygiene aids.

• When chronic dry mouth occurs, advise patient to:

• Avoid mouth rinses with high alcohol content because of drying effects.

• Use daily home fluoride products for anticaries effect.

• Use sugarless gum, frequent sips of water, or saliva substitutes.

bendamustine
ben-da-**mus'**-teen
(Treanda)

CATEGORY AND SCHEDULE
Pregnancy Risk Category: D

Drug Class: Antineoplastic agent, alkylating agent

MECHANISM OF ACTION
The exact mechanism of action of bendamustine is unknown. Bendamustine is an alkylating drug and (PARP) modulator. Dissociates into electrophilic alkyl groups, forms covalent bonds with electron-rich nucleophilic moieties, which results in tumor cell death through different pathways.

USES
Chronic lymphocytic leukemia (CLL)

PHARMACOKINETICS
Protein binding: 94%–96%. Metabolism occurs in liver primarily by hydrolysis; active minor metabolites formed primarily by CYP 1A2. Excreted primarily in the feces (90%). **Half-life**: 40 min.

INDICATIONS AND DOSAGES
IV
Adult. CLL: 100 mg/m^2 on days 1 and 2 of a 28-day treatment cycle (maximum: 6 cycles).
Allopurinol may be given to prevent tumor lysis syndrome. Prophylactic antibiotics may be considered.
Pediatric Dosing. Safety and efficacy has not been established.
Dose Adjustments. Renal impairment: Creatinine clearance less than 40 ml/min: DO NOT USE.
Hematologic toxicity, grade 3 or higher: reduce dose to 50 mg/m^2 on days 1 and 2 of each 28-day cycle. For recurrent hematologic toxicity, grade 3 or higher: reduce dose to 25 mg/m^2 on days 1 and 2 of each 28-day cycle.
Delay treatment for hematologic toxicity of grade 4 or high until ANC = 1000/mm^3, platelets = 75,000/mm^3.

For nonhematologic toxicity, grade 2 or higher: delay treatment until resolves to grade 1 or higher.
Hepatic impairment: Moderate (AST or ALT 2.5–10 times ULN and total bilirubin 1.5–3 times ULN) or severe (total bilirubin >3 times ULN): DO NOT USE.

SIDE EFFECTS/ADVERSE REACTIONS
Frequent
Fever, nausea and vomiting, anemia, bilirubin increased, myelosuppression, neutropenia, pyrexia, thrombocytopenia, and leukopenia
Occasional
Hypertension, fatigue, chills, rash, diarrhea, weight loss, cough

PRECAUTIONS AND CONTRAINDICATIONS
Hypersensitivity to bendamustine, mannitol, or any component of the formulation.
May cause fetal harm if administered to a woman during pregnancy.
Use appropriate precautions for handling and disposal.
Do not administer to children.
Hepatic impairment, moderate to severe: not recommended.
Smoking tobacco may decrease the levels and effects of bendamustine.
May increase the levels and effects of the active metabolites of bendamustine.

DRUG INTERACTIONS OF CONCERN TO DENTISTRY
• CYP1A2 inhibitors (e.g., ciprofloxacin): May increase the levels and effects of bendamustine. May decrease the levels and effects of the active metabolites of bendamustine.

SERIOUS REACTIONS
! Bone marrow suppression has occurred.
! Dermatologic toxicity including hypersensitivity/infusion reaction (chills, fever, pruritus, and rash) may occur.
! Infection such as pneumonia and sepsis have been reported.
! Tumor lysis syndrome occurring in the first treatment cycle. May lead to life-threatening acute renal failure.

DENTAL CONSIDERATIONS
General:
• Monitor vital signs at every appointment because of cardiovascular side effects.
• Patients on chronic drug therapy may have symptoms of blood dyscrasias, which can include infection, bleeding and poor healing.
• Examine for oral manifestation of opportunistic infection.
• Consider semisupine chair position for patient comfort if GI side effects occur.
• Evaluate allergic reactions: rash, urticaria.
• Stomatitis and xerostomia may complicate dental treatment and oral hygiene.
Consultations:
• Medical consultation may be required to assess disease control and ability of patient to tolerate dental treatment.
Teach Patient/Family to:
• Use effective atraumatic oral hygiene measures to prevent soft tissue inflammation.
• Report oral lesions, soreness, or bleeding to dentist.
• Be alert for the possibility of stomatitis and xerostomia and the need to see dentist immediately if signs of inflammation.

B

* If dry mouth occurs:
  * Avoid mouth rinse with high alcohol content because of dryness effects.
  * Use sugarless gum, frequent sips of water, or saliva substitutes.

bendroflumethiazide

ben-droe-floo-meth-**eye′**-ah-zide
(Naturetin-5)

CATEGORY AND SCHEDULE
Pregnancy Risk Category: C

Drug Class: Antidiuretic, central and nephrogenic diabetes insipidus; Antihypertensive; Antiurolithic, calcium calculi; Diuretic

MECHANISM OF ACTION
A benzothiadiazine derivative that acts as a thiazide diuretic and antihypertensive. As a diuretic blocks reabsorption of water, sodium, and potassium at cortical diluting segment of distal tubule. As an antihypertensive reduces plasma, extracellular fluid volume, peripheral vascular resistance by direct effect on blood vessels.
Therapeutic Effect: Promotes diuresis, reduces B/P.

USES
Commonly used to treat high B/P. May also be used to help reduce the amount of water in the body by increasing the flow of urine.

PHARMACOKINETICS

Route	Onset	Peak	Duration
PO	2 hr	4 hr	6–12 hr

Variably absorbed from the GI tract. Primarily excreted unchanged in urine. Not removed by hemodialysis.
Half-life: 5.6–14.8 hr.

INDICATIONS AND DOSAGES
▶ **Edema**
PO
Adults. 5 mg/day, preferably given in the morning. To initiate therapy, doses up to 20 mg may be given once a day or divided into 2 doses.
▶ **Hypertension**
PO
Adults. 5–20 mg/day, preferably given in the morning. Maintenance: 2.5–15 mg/day.

SIDE EFFECTS/ADVERSE REACTIONS
Expected
Increase in urine frequency and volume
Frequent
Potassium depletion
Occasional
Postural hypotension, headache, GI disturbances, photosensitivity reaction

PRECAUTIONS AND CONTRAINDICATIONS
Anuria, history of hypersensitivity to sulfonamides or thiazide diuretics

DRUG INTERACTIONS OF CONCERN TO DENTISTRY
* Decreased hypotensive response: NSAIDs, especially indomethacin

SERIOUS REACTIONS
! Vigorous diuresis may lead to profound water and electrolyte depletion, resulting in hypokalemia, hyponatremia, and dehydration.
! Acute hypotensive episodes may occur.

! Hyperglycemia may be noted during prolonged therapy.

! Pancreatitis, blood dyscrasias, pulmonary edema, allergic pneumonitis, and dermatologic reactions occur rarely.

! Overdose can lead to lethargy and coma without changes in electrolytes or hydration.

DENTAL CONSIDERATIONS

General:

* Monitor vital signs at every appointment due to cardiovascular side effects.
* Patient on chronic drug therapy may rarely present with symptoms of blood dyscrasias, which can include infection, bleeding, and poor healing. If dyscrasia is present, caution patient to prevent oral tissue trauma when using oral hygiene aids.
* After supine positioning, have patient sit upright for at least 2 min before standing to avoid orthostatic hypotension.
* Limit use of sodium-containing products, such as saline IV fluids, for patients with a dietary salt restriction.
* Stress from dental procedures may compromise cardiovascular function; determine patient risk.
* Short appointments and a stress-reduction protocol may be required for anxious patients.
* Advise patient if dental drugs prescribed have a potential for photosensitivity.
* Patients taking diuretics should be monitored for serum K levels.

Consultations:

* In a patient with symptoms of blood dyscrasias, request a medical consultation for blood studies and postpone treatment until normal values are reestablished.

* Medical consultation may be required to assess disease control and patient's ability to tolerate stress.

Teach Patient/Family to:

* Use effective oral hygiene to prevent soft tissue inflammation.
* Prevent trauma when using oral hygiene aids.
* Update health and medication history if physician makes any changes in evaluation or drug regimens; include OTC, herbal, and nonherbal remedies in the update.

benzocaine

ben'-zoe-kane

(Americaine Anesthetic Lubricant, Americaine Otic, Anbesol, Anbesol Baby Gel, Anbesol Maximum Strength, Babee Teething, Benzodent, Cepacol, Cetacaine, Chiggerex, Chigger-Tox, Cylex, Dermoplast, Detaine, Foille, Foille Medicated First Aid, Foille Plus, HDA Toothache, Hurricaine, Lanacaine, Mycinettes, Omedia, Orabase-B, Orajel, Orajel Baby, Orajel Baby Nighttime, Orajel Maximum Strength, Orasol, Otricaine, Otocain, Retre-Gel, Solarcaine, Topicaine[AUS], Trocaine, Zilactin, Zilactin Baby) Topicale

CATEGORY AND SCHEDULE

Pregnancy Risk Category: C

Drug Class: Topical ester, local anesthetic. Action: Inhibits conduction of nerve impulses from sensory nerves

B

MECHANISM OF ACTION

A local anesthetic that blocks nerve conduction in the autonomic, sensory, and motor nerve fibers. Reduces permeability of resting nerves to potassium and sodium ions.
Therapeutic Effect: Produces local analgesic effect.

USES

Treatment of oral irritation, toothache, cold sore, canker sore, pain, teething pain, pain caused by dental prostheses or orthodontic appliances

PHARMACOKINETICS

Poorly absorbed by topical administration. Well absorbed from mucous membranes and traumatized skin. Metabolized in liver and by hydrolysis with cholinesterase. Minimal excretion in urine.

INDICATIONS AND DOSAGES

▸ **Canker Sores**
Topical
Adults, Elderly, Children older than 2 yr. Apply gel, liquid, or ointment to affected area. Maximum: 4 times a day.
▸ **Denture Irritation**
Topical
Adults, Elderly. Apply thin layer of gel to affected area up to 4 times a day or until pain is relieved.
▸ **General Lubrication**
Topical
Adults, Elderly, Children older than 2 yr. Apply gel to exterior of tube or instrument prior to use.
▸ **Otitis Externa, Otitis Media**

Otic
Adults, Elderly, Children older than 1 yr. Instill 4–5 drops into external ear canal of affected ears. Repeat q1–2h as needed.
▸ **Pain and Itching Associated with Sunburn, Insect Bites, Minor Cuts, Scrapes, Minor Burns, Minor Skin Irritations**
Topical
Adults, Elderly, Children older than 2 yr. Apply to affected area 3–4 times a day.
▸ **Pharyngitis**
PO
Adults, Elderly. 1 lozenge q2h. Maximum 8 lozenges a day.
▸ **Toothache/Teething Pain**
Topical
Adults, Elderly, Children older than 2 yr. Apply gel, liquid, or ointment to affected areas. Maximum: 4 times a day.
▸ **Anesthesia**
Topical
Adults, Elderly. Apply aerosol, gel, ointment, liquid q4–12h as needed.

SIDE EFFECTS/ADVERSE REACTIONS

Occasional
Burning, stinging, angioedema, contact dermatitis, taste disorders
Rare
Allergic ulceration of oral mucosa

PRECAUTIONS AND CONTRAINDICATIONS

Hypersensitivity to benzocaine or ester-type local anesthetics, perforated tympanic membrane or ear discharge (otic preparations)

DRUG INTERACTIONS OF CONCERN TO DENTISTRY

• None reported

SERIOUS REACTIONS
! Methemoglobinemia occurs rarely in infants and young children.

DENTAL CONSIDERATIONS
General:
• Do not use for topical anesthesia if medical history reveals allergy to procaine, PABA, parabens, or other ester-type local anesthetics.
• Use smallest effective amount in infants and children.
• Avoid applying to large denuded areas of mucosa to prevent excessive systemic absorption and potential toxicity.

benzonatate
ben-**zoe'**-na-tate
(Tessalon Perles)

CATEGORY AND SCHEDULE
Pregnancy Risk Category: C

Drug Class: Antitussive, non-narcotic

MECHANISM OF ACTION
A non-narcotic antitussive that anesthetizes stretch receptors in respiratory passages, lungs, and pleura.
Therapeutic Effect: Reduces cough.

USES
Relief of nonproductive cough

PHARMACOKINETICS
PO: Onset 15–20 min, duration 3–8 hr; metabolized by liver; excreted in urine.

INDICATIONS AND DOSAGES
▶ **Antitussive**
PO
Adults, Elderly, Children older than 10 yr. 100 mg 3 times a day or every 4 hr up to 600 mg/day.

SIDE EFFECTS/ADVERSE REACTIONS
Occasional
Mild somnolence, mild dizziness, constipation, GI upset, skin eruptions, nasal congestion

PRECAUTIONS AND CONTRAINDICATIONS
Hypersensitivity
Caution:
Lactation

DRUG INTERACTIONS OF CONCERN TO DENTISTRY
• Increased CNS depression: slight risk of increased sedation with other CNS depressants

SERIOUS REACTIONS
! A paradoxical reaction, including restlessness, insomnia, euphoria, nervousness, and tremor, has been noted.

DENTAL CONSIDERATIONS
General:
• Elective dental treatment may not be possible with significant coughing episodes.

B

benzoyl peroxide

ben′-zoe-ill per-ox′-ide
(Acetoxyl[CAN], Benoxyl[CAN],
Benzac, Benzac AC, Benzac AC
Wash, Benzac W, Benzac W
Wash, Benzagel, Benzagel Wash,
Benzashave, Brevoxyl, Brevoxyl
Cleansing, Brevoxyl Wash,
Clearplex, Clinac BPO, Del Aqua,
Desquam-E, Desquam-X, Exact
Acne Medication, Fostex 10%
BPO, Loroxide, Neutrogena Acne
Mask, Neutrogena On the Spot
Acne Treatment, Oxy[AUS], Oxy
10 Balanced Medicated Face
Wash, Oxy 10 Balance Spot
Treatment, Palmer's Skin Success
Acne, Oxyderm[CAN], PanOxyl,
PanOxyl-AQ, PanOxyl Aqua Gel,
PanOxyl Bar, Seba-Gel,
Solugel[CAN], Triaz, Triaz
Cleanser, Zapzyt)

CATEGORY AND SCHEDULE

Pregnancy Risk Category: C
OTC

Drug Class: Antiacne agent,
topical; keratolytic, topical

MECHANISM OF ACTION

A keratolytic agent that releases
free-radical oxygen, which oxidizes
bacterial proteins in the sebaceous
follicles, decreasing the number of
anaerobic bacteria and decreasing
irritating-type free fatty acids.
Therapeutic Effect: Bactericidal
action against *Propionibacterium
acnes* and *Staphylococcus
epidermidis.*

USES

Treatment of acne

PHARMACOKINETICS

Minimal absorption through skin.
Gel is more penetrating than cream.
Metabolized to benzoic acid in skin.
Excreted in urine as benzoate.

INDICATIONS AND DOSAGES

▶ Acne
Topical
Adults. Apply 2.5%–10%
concentration 1–2 times a day.

SIDE EFFECTS/ADVERSE REACTIONS

Occasional

Irritation, dryness, burning, peeling,
stinging, contact dermatitis,
bleaching of hair

PRECAUTIONS AND CONTRAINDICATIONS

Hypersensitivity to benzoyl
peroxide or any component of the
formulation

DRUG INTERACTIONS OF CONCERN TO DENTISTRY

• None reported

SERIOUS REACTIONS

! Hypersensitivity reactions have
been reported with benzoyl peroxide
use.

DENTAL CONSIDERATIONS

General:
• Determine why patient is taking
the drug.
• Advise patient if dental drugs
prescribed have a potential for
photosensitivity.
• Inquire about other drugs the
patient may be using for acne.
Teach Patient/Family to:
• Avoid application to eyes, nose,
mouth and mucous membranes.
• Update health and medication
history if physician makes any

changes in evaluation or drug regimens; include OTC, herbal, and nonherbal remedies in the update.

benzthiazide
benz-**thigh′**-ah-zide
(Exna)

CATEGORY AND SCHEDULE
Pregnancy Risk Category: C

Drug Class: Diuretic, Thiazide

MECHANISM OF ACTION
Thiazide diuretic and antihypertensive. As a diuretic, blocks reabsorption of water, sodium, and potassium at cortical diluting segment of distal tubule. As an antihypertensive, reduces plasma and extracellular fluid volume and reduces peripheral vascular resistance by direct effect on blood vessels.
Therapeutic Effect: Promotes diuresis, reduces B/P.

USES
Treatment of high B/P

PHARMACOKINETICS

Route	Onset	Peak	Duration
PO	2 hr	4 hr	6–12 hr

Variably absorbed from the GI tract. Primarily excreted unchanged in urine. Not removed by hemodialysis.
Half-life: Unknown.

INDICATIONS AND DOSAGES
▸ **Edema**
PO
Adults. Initially, 50–200 mg/day. Maintenance: 50–150 mg/day.

▸ **Hypertension**
PO
Adults. Initially, 50–100 mg/day. Dosage should be adjusted according to the patient response, either upward to as much as 50 mg 4 times a day or downward to the minimal effective dosage level.

SIDE EFFECTS/ADVERSE REACTIONS
Expected

Increase in urine frequency and volume
Frequent

Potassium depletion
Occasional

Postural hypotension, headache, GI disturbances, photosensitivity reaction

PRECAUTIONS AND CONTRAINDICATIONS
Anuria, history of hypersensitivity to sulfonamide-derived drugs or thiazide diuretics

DRUG INTERACTIONS OF CONCERN TO DENTISTRY
• Decreased hypotensive response: NSAIDs

SERIOUS REACTIONS
❗ Vigorous diuresis may lead to profound water and electrolyte depletion, resulting in hypokalemia, hyponatremia, and dehydration.
❗ Acute hypotensive episodes may occur.
❗ Hyperglycemia may be noted during prolonged therapy.
❗ Pancreatitis, blood dyscrasias, pulmonary edema, allergic pneumonitis, and dermatologic reactions occur rarely.
❗ Overdose can lead to lethargy and coma without changes in electrolytes or hydration.

B

DENTAL CONSIDERATIONS
General:
• Monitor vital signs at every appointment due to cardiovascular side effects.
• Patient on chronic drug therapy may rarely present with symptoms of blood dyscrasias, which can include infection, bleeding and poor healing. If dyscrasia is present, caution patient to prevent oral tissue trauma when using oral hygiene aids.
• Observe appropriate limitations of vasoconstrictor doses.
• After supine positioning, have patient sit upright for at least 2 min before standing to avoid orthostatic hypotension.
• Limit use of sodium-containing products, such as saline IV fluids, for patients with a dietary salt restriction.
• Stress from dental procedures may compromise cardiovascular function; determine patient risk.
• Short appointments and a stress-reduction protocol may be required for anxious patients.
• Advise patient if dental drugs prescribed have a potential for photosensitivity.
• Patients taking diuretics should be monitored for serum K levels.
Consultations:
• In a patient with symptoms of blood dyscrasias, request a medical consultation for blood studies and postpone treatment until normal values are reestablished.
• Medical consultation may be required to assess disease control and patient's ability to tolerate stress.
Teach Patient/Family to:
• Use effective oral hygiene to prevent soft tissue inflammation.

• Prevent trauma when using oral hygiene aids.
• Update health and medication history if physician makes any changes in evaluation or drug regimens; include OTC, herbal, and nonherbal remedies in the update.

benztropine mesylate
benz′-troe-peen mess′-ah-late
(Apo-Benztropine[CAN], Bentrop[AUS], Cogentin)
Do not confuse benztropine with bromocriptine.

CATEGORY AND SCHEDULE
Pregnancy Risk Category: C

Drug Class: Anticholinergic, antidyskinetic

MECHANISM OF ACTION
An antiparkinson agent that selectively blocks central cholinergic receptors, helping to balance cholinergic and dopaminergic activity.
Therapeutic Effect: Reduces the incidence and severity of akinesia, rigidity, and tremor.

USES
Treatment of Parkinson symptoms, extrapyramidal symptoms associated with neuroleptic drugs

PHARMACOKINETICS
IM/IV: Onset 15 min, duration 6–10 hr. **PO:** Onset 1 hr, duration 6–10 hr.

INDICATIONS AND DOSAGES
▸ **Parkinsonism**
PO
Adults. 0.5–6 mg/day as a single dose or in 2 divided doses. Titrate by 0.5 mg at 5–6 day intervals.
Elderly. Initially, 0.5 mg once or twice a day. Titrate by 0.5 mg at 5–6 day intervals. Maximum: 4 mg/day.
▸ **Drug-Induced Extrapyramidal Symptoms**
PO, IM
Adults. 1–4 mg once or twice a day.
Children older than 3 yr. 0.02–0.05 mg/kg/dose once or twice a day.
▸ **Acute Dystonic Reactions**
IV, IM
Adults. Initially, 1–2 mg; then 1–2 mg PO twice a day to prevent recurrence.

SIDE EFFECTS/ADVERSE REACTIONS
Frequent
Somnolence, dry mouth, blurred vision, constipation, decreased sweating or urination, GI upset, photosensitivity
Occasional
Headache, memory loss, muscle cramps, anxiety, peripheral paresthesia, orthostatic hypotension, abdominal cramps
Rare
Rash, confusion, eye pain

PRECAUTIONS AND CONTRAINDICATIONS
Angle-closure glaucoma, benign prostatic hyperplasia, children younger than 3 yr, GI obstruction, intestinal atony, megacolon, myasthenia gravis, paralytic ileus, severe ulcerative colitis
Caution:
Elderly, lactation, tachycardia, prostatic hypertrophy, liver or kidney disease, drug abuse history,

dysrhythmias, hypotension, hypertension, psychiatric patients

DRUG INTERACTIONS OF CONCERN TO DENTISTRY
• Increased anticholinergic effect: antihistamines, anticholinergics, and meperidine
• Decreased effects of phenothiazines

SERIOUS REACTIONS
❗ Overdose may produce severe anticholinergic effects, such as unsteadiness, somnolence, tachycardia, dyspnea, skin flushing, and severe dryness of the mouth, nose, or throat.
❗ Severe paradoxical reactions, marked by hallucinations, tremor, seizures, and toxic psychosis, may occur.

DENTAL CONSIDERATIONS

General:
• Monitor vital signs at every appointment because of cardiovascular side effects.
• Assess salivary flow as a factor in caries, periodontal disease, and candidiasis.
• After supine positioning, have patient sit upright for at least 2 min to avoid orthostatic hypotension.
• Avoid dental light in patient's eyes; offer dark glasses for patient comfort.
• Do not use ingestible sodium bicarbonate products, such as the Prophy-Jet air polishing system, within 1 hr of taking benztropine.
• Place on frequent recall because of oral side effects.
Consultations:
• Medical consultation may be required to assess disease control and patient's ability to tolerate stress.

B

Teach Patient/Family to:
• Use effective oral hygiene to prevent soft tissue inflammation.
• Use a powered tooth brush if patient has difficulty holding conventional devices.
• When chronic dry mouth occurs, advise patient to:
  • Avoid mouth rinses with high alcohol content because of drying effects.
  • Use daily home fluoride products for anticaries effect.
  • Use sugarless gum, frequent sips of water, or saliva substitutes.

bepridil
beh′-prih-dill
(Bapadin, Vascor)

CATEGORY AND SCHEDULE
Pregnancy Risk Category: C

Drug Class: Calcium channel blocker

MECHANISM OF ACTION
A calcium channel blocker that inhibits calcium ion entry across cell membranes of cardiac and vascular smooth muscle; decreases heart rate, myocardial contractility, slows SA and AV conduction.
Therapeutic Effect: Dilates coronary arteries, peripheral arteries/arterioles.

USES
Treatment of stable angina, used alone or in combination with propranolol

PHARMACOKINETICS
Rapidly, completely absorbed from GI tract. Undergoes first-pass metabolism in liver to active metabolite. Primarily excreted in urine. Not removed by hemodialysis.
Half-life: less than 24 hr.

INDICATIONS AND DOSAGES
▶ **Chronic Stable Angina**
PO
Adults, Elderly. Initially, 200 mg/day; after 10 days, dosage may be adjusted. Maintenance: 200–400 mg/day.

SIDE EFFECTS/ADVERSE REACTIONS
Frequent
Dizziness, lightheadedness, nervousness, headache, asthenia (loss of strength), hand tremor, nausea, diarrhea
Occasional
Drowsiness, insomnia, tinnitus, abdominal discomfort, palpitations, dry mouth, shortness of breath, wheezing, anorexia, constipation
Rare
Peripheral edema, anxiety, flatulence, nasal congestion, paresthesia

PRECAUTIONS AND CONTRAINDICATIONS
Sick sinus syndrome/second- or third-degree AV block (except in presence of pacemaker), severe hypotension (90 mm Hg, systolic), history of serious ventricular arrhythmias, uncompensated cardiac insufficiency, congenital QT interval prolongation, use with other drugs prolonging QT interval
Caution:
CHF, hypotension, hepatic injury, lactation, children, renal disease, may induce new arrhythmias, prolongs QT interval with risk of torsades de pointes

DRUG INTERACTIONS OF CONCERN TO DENTISTRY
* Decreased effect: NSAIDs, phenobarbital
* Increased effect: parenteral and inhalational general anesthetics or other drugs with hypotensive actions
* Increased effects of carbamazepine

SERIOUS REACTIONS
! CHF, second-and third-degree AV block occur rarely.
! Serious arrhythmias can be induced.
! Overdosage produces nausea, drowsiness, confusion, slurred speech, profound bradycardia.

DENTAL CONSIDERATIONS

General:
* Monitor cardiac status; take vital signs at every appointment because of cardiovascular side effects.
* Consider a stress-reduction protocol to prevent stress-induced angina during the dental appointment.
* Observe appropriate limitations of vasoconstrictor doses.
* After supine positioning, have patient sit upright for at least 2 min to avoid orthostatic hypotension.
* Limit use of sodium-containing products, such as saline IV fluids, for those patients with a dietary salt restriction.
* Assess salivary flow as a factor in caries, periodontal disease, and candidiasis.
Consultations:
* Medical consultation may be required to assess disease control and stress tolerance of patient.
Teach Patient/Family to:
* Schedule frequent oral prophylaxis if gingival overgrowth occurs.

* When chronic dry mouth occurs, advise patient to:
  * Avoid mouth rinses with high alcohol content because of drying effects.
* Use daily home fluoride products for anticaries effect.
* Use sugarless gum, frequent sips of water, or saliva substitutes.

B

---

besifloxacin
(bess-ih-**flox**-ah-sin)
(Besivance)

CATEGORY AND SCHEDULE
Pregnancy Risk Category: C

Drug class: Antibacterial, ophthalmic

MECHANISM OF ACTION
A bactericidal, broad-spectrum fluoroquinolone that inhibits bacterial DNA gyrase and topoisomerase.

USES
Bacterial conjunctivitis

PHARMACOKINETICS
Following single topical application to the eye, tear concentration averages 610 mcg/ml. Peak plasma concentrations less than 1.3 ng/ml. Distribution not reported. Protein binding: 39%–44%. Does not undergo hepatic metabolism.
Half-life: 7 hr. Primarily excreted unchanged in feces (73%) and urine (23%).

B

INDICATIONS AND DOSAGES
▸ **Conjunctivitis**
Adult, children over 1 yr. Shake
bottle, instill 1 drop in the affected
eye every 8 hr for 7 days.

SIDE EFFECTS/ADVERSE REACTIONS
Frequent
Conjunctival redness
Occasional
Blurred vision, eye pain, eye
irritation, itching eyes, headache

PRECAUTIONS AND CONTRAINDICATIONS
Hypersensitivity to besifloxacin or
any of its ingredients

DRUG INTERACTIONS OF CONCERN TO DENTISTRY
• None reported

SERIOUS REACTIONS
! Increased risk of congestive
circulatory failure in patients at-risk
for peripheral edema

DENTAL CONSIDERATIONS

General:
Protect patient's eyes from irritants
(splatter, excessive gas flow from
nitrous oxide nasal hood).

betamethasone
bay-ta-**meth′**-ah-sone
(Alphatrex, Betaderm[CAN],
Betatrex, Beta-Val,
Betnesol[CAN], Celestone,
Diprolene, Luxiq, Maxivate)

CATEGORY AND SCHEDULE
Pregnancy Risk Category: C (D if
used in first trimester)

Drug Class: Antiinflammatory

MECHANISM OF ACTION
An adrenocortical steroid that
controls the rate of protein synthesis,
depresses the migration of
polymorphonuclear leukocytes and
fibroblasts, reduces capillary
permeability, and prevents or
controls inflammation.
Therapeutic Effect: Decreases
tissue response to inflammatory
process.

USES
Treatment of psoriasis, eczema,
contact dermatitis, pruritus, oral
ulcerative inflammatory lesions,
mild-to-moderate ulcerative colitis.
Also used to relieve swelling,
itching, and discomfort of some
other rectal problems, including
hemorrhoids and inflammation of
the rectum caused by radiation
therapy.

PHARMACOKINETICS:
PO: Onset 1–2 hr, peak 1 hr,
duration 3 days.
IM/IV: Onset 10 min, peak 4–8 hr,
duration 1–1.5 days.
Metabolized in liver, excreted in
urine as steroids, crosses placenta.

INDICATIONS AND DOSAGES
▸ **Antiinflammation, Immunosuppression, Corticosteroid Replacement Therapy**
PO
Adults, Elderly. 0.6–7.2 mg/day.
Children. 0.063–0.25 mg/kg/day in
3–4 divided doses.
▸ **Relief of Inflamed and Pruritic Dermatoses**
Topical
Adults, Elderly. 1–3 times a day.
Foam: Apply twice a day.

SIDE EFFECTS/ADVERSE REACTIONS
Frequent
Systemic: Increased appetite, abdominal distention, nervousness, insomnia, false sense of well-being
Topical: Burning, stinging, pruritus
Occasional
Systemic: Dizziness, facial flushing, diaphoresis, decreased or blurred vision, mood swings
Topical: Allergic contact dermatitis, purpura or blood-containing blisters, thinning of skin with easy bruising, telangiectases, or raised dark red spots on skin

PRECAUTIONS AND CONTRAINDICATIONS
Hypersensitivity to betamethasone, systemic fungal infections

DRUG INTERACTIONS OF CONCERN TO DENTISTRY
• Decreased action: barbiturates
• Increased GI side effects: alcohol, salicylates, and other NSAIDs
• Increased action: ketoconazole, macrolide antibiotics

SERIOUS REACTIONS
! Overdose may cause systemic hypercorticism and adrenal suppression.

DENTAL CONSIDERATIONS
General:
• Monitor vital signs at every appointment because of cardiovascular side effects.
• Patients on chronic drug therapy may rarely have symptoms of blood dyscrasias, which can include infection, bleeding, and poor healing.
• Symptoms of oral infections may be masked.

• Determine dose and duration of steroid therapy for each patient to assess risk for stress tolerance and immunosuppression.
• Avoid prescribing aspirin-containing products.
• Place on frequent recall to evaluate healing response.
• Prophylactic antibiotics may be indicated to prevent infection if surgery or deep scaling is planned.
• Patients who have been or are currently on chronic steroid therapy (longer than 2 wk) may require supplemental steroids for dental treatment.
Consultations:
• In a patient with symptoms of blood dyscrasias, request a medical consultation for blood studies and postpone dental treatment until normal values are reestablished.
• Medical consultation may be required to assess disease control.
• Consultation may be required to confirm steroid dose and duration of use.
Teach Patient/Family to:
• Use effective oral hygiene to prevent soft tissue inflammation.
• Use caution to prevent injury when using oral hygiene aids.

betaxolol
bee-**tax**′-oh-lol
(Betoptic[AUS], Betoptic-S, Betoquin[AUS], Kerlone)
Do not confuse betaxolol with bethanechol.

CATEGORY AND SCHEDULE
Pregnancy Risk Category: C (D if used in second or third trimester)

Drug Class: Antihypertensive, selective β₁-blocker

B

MECHANISM OF ACTION

An antihypertensive and antiglaucoma agent that blocks β_1-adrenergic receptors in cardiac tissue. Reduces aqueous humor production.
Therapeutic Effect: Slows sinus heart rate, decreases B/P, and reduces intraocular pressure (IOP).

USES

Treatment of hypertension, alone or in combination with other antihypertensive drugs, especially thiazide diuretics

PHARMACOKINETICS

PO: Peak 3–4 hr. *Half-life:* 14–22 hr; protein binding 50%; some hepatic metabolism; excreted in urine mostly unchanged.

INDICATIONS AND DOSAGES
▸ **Hypertension**
PO
Adults. Initially, 5–10 mg/day. May increase to 20 mg/day after 7–14 days.
Elderly. Initially, 5 mg/day.
▸ **Chronic Open-Angle Glaucoma and Ocular Hypertension**
Ophthalmic (Eye Drops)
Adults, Elderly. 1 drop twice a day.
▸ **Dosage in Renal Impairment**
For adult and elderly patients who are on dialysis, initially give 5 mg/day; increase by 5 mg/day q2wk. Maximum: 20 mg/day.

SIDE EFFECTS/ADVERSE REACTIONS

Betaxolol is generally well tolerated, with mild and transient side effects.
Frequent
Systemic: Hypotension manifested as dizziness, nausea, diaphoresis, headache, fatigue, constipation or diarrhea, dyspnea

Ophthalmic: Eye irritation, visual disturbances
Occasional
Systemic: Insomnia, flatulence, urinary frequency, impotence or decreased libido
Ophthalmic: Increased light sensitivity, watering of eye
Rare
Systemic: Rash, arrhythmias, arthralgia, myalgia, confusion, altered taste, increased urination
Ophthalmic: Dry eye, conjunctivitis, eye pain

PRECAUTIONS AND CONTRAINDICATIONS

Cardiogenic shock, overt cardiac failure, second- or third-degree heart block, sinus bradycardia
Caution:
Major surgery, lactation, diabetes mellitus, renal disease, thyroid disease, COPD, asthma, well-compensated heart failure, aortic or mitral valve disease

DRUG INTERACTIONS OF CONCERN TO DENTISTRY
• Decreased antihypertensive effects: NSAIDs, indomethacin
• May slow metabolism of lidocaine
• Decreased β-blocking effects (or decreased β-adrenergic effects) of epinephrine, levonordefrin, isoproterenol, and other sympathomimetics

SERIOUS REACTIONS
! Overdose may produce profound bradycardia, hypotension, and bronchospasm.
! Abrupt withdrawal may result in diaphoresis, palpitations, headache, and tremors.
! Betaxolol administration may precipitate CHF or MI in patients with cardiac disease; thyroid storm

in those with thyrotoxicosis; and peripheral ischemia in those with existing peripheral vascular disease.
! Hypoglycemia may occur in patients with previously controlled diabetes.
! Ophthalmic overdose may produce bradycardia, hypotension, bronchospasm, and acute cardiac failure.

DENTAL CONSIDERATIONS

General:
• Monitor vital signs at every appointment because of cardiovascular and respiratory side effects.
• After supine positioning, have patient sit upright for at least 2 min to avoid orthostatic hypotension.
• Assess salivary flow as a factor in caries, periodontal disease, and candidiasis.
• Stress from dental procedures may compromise cardiovascular function; determine patient risk.
• Short appointments and a stress-reduction protocol may be required for anxious patients.
• Use vasoconstrictors with caution, in low doses, and with careful aspiration. Avoid use of gingival retraction cord with epinephrine.
Consultations:
• Medical consultation may be required to assess disease control and stress tolerance of patient.
• Use precautions if general anesthesia is required for dental surgery.
Teach Patient/Family to:
• Use effective oral hygiene to prevent soft tissue inflammation.
• Use caution to prevent injury when using oral hygiene aids.
• When chronic dry mouth occurs, advise patient to:

• Avoid mouth rinses with high alcohol content because of drying effects.
• Use daily home fluoride products for anticaries effect.
• Use sugarless gum, frequent sips of water, or saliva substitutes.

bethanechol chloride
beh-**than'**-eh-kole
(Duvoid[CAN], Myotonachol[CAN], Urecholine, Urocarb[AUS])
Do not confuse bethanechol with betaxolol.

CATEGORY AND SCHEDULE
Pregnancy Risk Category: C

Drug Class: Cholinergic stimulant

MECHANISM OF ACTION
A cholinergic that acts directly at cholinergic receptors in the smooth muscle of the urinary bladder and GI tract. Increases detrusor muscle tone.
Therapeutic Effect: May initiate micturition and bladder emptying. Improves gastric and intestinal motility.

USES
Treatment of urinary retention (postoperative, postpartum), neurogenic atony of bladder with retention; unapproved: gastric atony

PHARMACOKINETICS
PO: Onset 30–90 min, duration 6 hr. SC: Onset 5–15 min, duration 2 hr; excreted by kidneys.

B

INDICATIONS AND DOSAGES
▸ **Postoperative and Postpartum Urine Retention, Atony of Bladder**
PO
Adults, Elderly. 10–50 mg 3–4 times a day. Minimum effective dose determined by giving 5–10 mg initially, then repeating same amount at 1-hr intervals until desired response is achieved, or maximum of 50 mg is reached.
Children. 0.6 mg/kg/day in 3–4 divided doses.

SIDE EFFECTS/ADVERSE REACTIONS
Occasional
Belching, blurred or changed vision, diarrhea, urinary urgency

PRECAUTIONS AND CONTRAINDICATIONS
Active or latent bronchial asthma, acute inflammatory GI tract conditions, anastomosis, bladder wall instability, cardiac or coronary artery disease, epilepsy, hypertension, hyperthyroidism, hypotension, GI or urinary tract obstruction, parkinsonism, peptic ulcer, pronounced bradycardia, recent GI resection, vasomotor instability
Caution:
Hypertension, lactation, children younger than 8 yr, urinary retention

DRUG INTERACTIONS OF CONCERN TO DENTISTRY
• Decreased effects: anticholinergics

SERIOUS REACTIONS
! Overdosage produces CNS stimulation (including insomnia, anxiety, and orthostatic hypotension), and cholinergic stimulation (such as headache, increased salivation diaphoresis,

nausea, vomiting, flushed skin, abdominal pain, and seizures).

DENTAL CONSIDERATIONS

General:
• Monitor vital signs at every appointment because of cardiovascular and respiratory side effects.
• After supine positioning, have patient sit upright for at least 2 min to avoid orthostatic hypotension.
Consultations:
• For excessive, troublesome salivation, reassure patient that treatment duration usually is limited to a few days; otherwise consult to lower bethanechol dose.

bevacizumab
beh-vah-**siz**'-you-mab
(Avastin)

CATEGORY AND SCHEDULE
Pregnancy Risk Category: C

Drug Class: Antineoplastic monoclonal antibody; vascular endothelial growth factor (VEGF) inhibitor

MECHANISM OF ACTION
An antineoplastic that binds to and inhibits VEGF, a protein that plays a major role in the formation of new blood vessels to tumors.
Therapeutic Effect: Inhibits metastatic disease progression.

USES
Prevents the growth of certain types of blood vessels to cancer cells by starving the cells of nutrients needed to grow

PHARMACOKINETICS

Clearance varies by body weight, gender, and tumor burden. *Half-life:* 20 days (range, 11–50 days).

INDICATIONS AND DOSAGES

▶ **First-Line Treatment of Metastatic Carcinoma of the Colon or Rectum in Combination with 5-Fluorouracil (5-FU)**
IV
Adults, Elderly. 5 mg/kg once every 14 days.

SIDE EFFECTS/ADVERSE REACTIONS

Frequent
Asthenia, vomiting, anorexia, hypertension, epistaxis, stomatitis, constipation, headache, dyspnea
Occasional
Altered taste, dry skin, exfoliative dermatitis, dizziness, flatulence, excessive lacrimation, skin discoloration, weight loss, myalgia
Rare
Nail disorder, skin ulcer, alopecia, confusion, abnormal gait, dry mouth

PRECAUTIONS AND CONTRAINDICATIONS

GI perforation, hypertensive crisis, nephrotic syndrome, recent hemoptysis, serious bleeding, wound dehiscence requiring medical intervention

DRUG INTERACTIONS OF CONCERN TO DENTISTRY

• None reported

SERIOUS REACTIONS

! UTIs, manifested as urinary frequency or urgency and proteinuria, occur frequently.
! CHF, deep vein thrombosis, GI perforation, hypertensive crisis, nephrotic syndrome, and severe hemorrhage are the most serious reactions that occur.
! Anemia, neutropenia, and thrombocytopenia occur occasionally.
! Hypersensitivity reactions occur rarely.

DENTAL CONSIDERATIONS

General:
• Assess salivary flow as a factor in caries, periodontal disease, and candidiasis.
• If additional analgesia is required for dental pain, consider alternative analgesics (NSAIDs) in patients taking opioids for acute or chronic pain.
• Avoid products that affect platelet function, such as aspirin and NSAIDs.
• This drug may be used in the hospital or on an outpatient basis. Confirm the patient's disease and treatment status.
• Consider semisupine chair position for patient comfort if GI side effects occur.
• Chlorhexidine mouth rinse prior to and during chemotherapy may reduce severity of mucositis.
• Patient on chronic drug therapy may rarely present with symptoms of blood dyscrasias, which can include infection, bleeding, and poor healing. If dyscrasia is present, caution patient to prevent oral tissue trauma when using oral hygiene aids.
• Palliative medication may be required for management of oral side effects.
• Short appointments and a stress-reduction protocol may be required for anxious patients.
• Monitor vital signs at every appointment for cardiovascular side effects.

B

• Patients may have received other chemotherapy or radiation; confirm medical and drug history.

• Patients may be taking a prophylactic antiinfective.

• Patients may be at risk of bleeding, check for oral signs.

• Oral infections should be eliminated and/or treated aggressively.

• Place on frequent recall due to oral side effects.

Consultations:

• Medical consultation should include routine blood counts including platelet counts and bleeding time.

• Consult physician; prophylactic or therapeutic antiinfectives may be indicated if surgery or periodontal treatment is required.

• Medical consultation may be required to assess immunologic status during cancer chemotherapy and determine safety risk, if any, posed by the required dental treatment.

• Medical consultation may be required to assess disease control and patient's ability to tolerate stress.

Teach Patient/Family to:

• Inform dentist of unusual bleeding episodes following dental treatment.

• Be aware of oral side effects.

• Use effective oral hygiene to prevent soft tissue inflammation.

• Report oral lesions, soreness, or bleeding to dentist.

• Prevent trauma when using oral hygiene aids.

• Update health and medication history if physician makes any changes in evaluation or drug regimens; include OTC, herbal, and nonherbal remedies in the update.

• If abdominal pain associated with constipation and/or vomiting occur,

advise patient to consult physician immediately.

• When chronic dry mouth occurs advise patient to:

• Avoid mouth rinses with high alcohol content due to drying effects.

• Use daily home fluoride products for anticaries effect.

• Use sugarless gum, frequent sips of water, or saliva substitutes.

---

bexarotene
becks-**aye′**-row-teen
(Targretin)

CATEGORY AND SCHEDULE
Pregnancy Risk Category: X

Drug Class: Antineoplastic

MECHANISM OF ACTION
Retinoid antineoplastic agent that binds to and activates retinoid X receptor subtypes, which regulate the genes that control cellular differentiation and proliferation.
Therapeutic Effect: Inhibits growth of tumor cell lines of hematopoietic and squamous cell origin and induces tumor regression.

USES
Treatment of a form a cancer called cutaneous T-cell lymphoma (CTCL)

PHARMACOKINETICS
Moderately absorbed from the GI tract. Protein binding: greater than 99%. Metabolized in the liver. Primarily eliminated through the hepatobiliary system. *Half-life:* 7 hr.

INDICATIONS AND DOSAGES
▶ **Cutaneous T-Cell Lymphoma Refractory to at Least One Prior Systemic Therapy**
PO
Adults. 300 mg/m²/day. If no response and initial dose is well tolerated, may be increased to 400 mg/m²/day. If not tolerated, may decrease to 200 mg/m²/day, then to 100 mg/m²/day.
Topical
Adults. Initially, apply once every other day. May increase at weekly intervals up to 4 times a day.

SIDE EFFECTS/ADVERSE REACTIONS
Frequent
Hyperlipidemia, headache, hypothyroidism, asthenia
Occasional
Rash, nausea, peripheral edema, dry skin, abdominal pain, chills, exfoliative dermatitis, diarrhea

PRECAUTIONS AND CONTRAINDICATIONS
Hypersensitivity to bexarotene or any component of the formulation

DRUG INTERACTIONS OF CONCERN TO DENTISTRY
• Erythromycin, itraconazole

SERIOUS REACTIONS
❗ Pancreatitis, hepatic failure, and pneumonia occur rarely.

DENTAL CONSIDERATIONS
• Consult patient for ability to tolerate dental procedure and to determine why patient is taking drug.

bicalutamide
by-kal-**yew**′-tah-myd
(Casodex, Cosudex[AUS])

CATEGORY AND SCHEDULE
Pregnancy Risk Category: X

Drug Class: Nonsteroidal antiandrogen, antineoplastic

MECHANISM OF ACTION
An antiandrogen antineoplastic agent that competitively inhibits androgen action by binding to androgen receptors in target tissue.
Therapeutic Effect: Decreases growth of prostatic carcinoma.

USES
Combination therapy with a luteinizing hormone-releasing hormone (LHRH) analog for advanced prostate cancer

PHARMACOKINETICS
Well absorbed from the GI tract. Protein binding: 96%. Metabolized in the liver to inactive metabolite. Excreted in urine and feces. Not removed by hemodialysis. *Half-life:* 5.8 days.

INDICATIONS AND DOSAGES
▶ **Prostatic Carcinoma**
PO
Adults, Elderly. 50–100 mg once a day in morning or evening, given concurrently with a LHRH analog or after surgical castration.

SIDE EFFECTS/ADVERSE REACTIONS
Frequent
Hot flashes, breast pain, muscle pain, constipation, asthenia, nausea, diarrhea

Occasional
Nocturia, abdominal pain, peripheral edema
Rare
Vomiting, weight loss, dizziness, insomnia, rash, impotence, gynecomastia

PRECAUTIONS AND CONTRAINDICATIONS

Hypersensitivity, women who may become pregnant, pregnancy category X
Caution:
Hepatic impairment, lactation, children

DRUG INTERACTIONS OF CONCERN TO DENTISTRY

• Avoid drugs that could exacerbate urinary retention, such as anticholinergics.

SERIOUS REACTIONS

! Sepsis, CHF, hypertension, and iron deficiency anemia may occur.

DENTAL CONSIDERATIONS

General:
• Patients taking opioids for acute or chronic pain should be given alternative analgesics for dental pain.
• Palliative medication may be required for management of oral side effects.
• Assess salivary flow as a factor in caries, periodontal disease, and candidiasis.
• Monitor vital signs at every appointment because of cardiovascular and respiratory side effects.
• Short appointments may be required for patient comfort.
• Consider semisupine chair position for patient comfort because of disease and drug side effects.

• Place on frequent recall because of oral side effects.
Consultations:
• Medical consultation may be required to assess disease control and patient's ability to tolerate stress.
Teach Patient/Family to:
• Update medical/drug record if physician makes any changes in evaluation or drug regimens.
• When chronic dry mouth occurs, advise patient to:
  • Avoid mouth rinses with high alcohol content because of drying effects.
  • Use daily home fluoride products for anticaries effect.
  • Use sugarless gum, frequent sips of water, or saliva substitutes.

---

bimatoprost
bye-**mat'**-oh-prost
(Lumigan)

CATEGORY AND SCHEDULE
Pregnancy Risk Category: C

Drug Class: A prostamide (synthetic structural analog of prostaglandin)

MECHANISM OF ACTION
A synthetic analog of prostaglandin with ocular hypotensive activity.
Therapeutic Effect: Reduces intraocular pressure (IOP) by increasing the outflow of aqueous humor.

USES
Reduction of elevated IOP in patients with open-angle glaucoma or ocular hypertension who are intolerant of, or insufficiently

responsive to, other IOP-lowering drugs

PHARMACOKINETICS
Absorbed through the cornea and hydrolyzed to the active free acid form. Protein binding: 88%. Moderately distributed into body tissues. Metabolized in liver. Primarily excreted in urine; some elimination in feces. *Half-life:* 45 min.

INDICATIONS AND DOSAGES
▸ **Glaucoma, Ocular Hypertension**
Ophthalmic
Adults, Elderly. 1 drop in affected eye(s) once daily, in the evening.

SIDE EFFECTS/ADVERSE REACTIONS
Frequent
Conjunctival hyperemia, growth of eyelashes, and ocular pruritus
Occasional
Ocular dryness, visual disturbance, ocular burning, foreign body sensation, eye pain, pigmentation of the periocular skin, blepharitis, cataract, superficial punctate keratitis, eyelid erythema, ocular irritation, and eyelash darkening
Rare
Intraocular inflammation (iritis)

PRECAUTIONS AND CONTRAINDICATIONS
Hypersensitivity to bimatoprost or any other component of the formulation
Caution:
Increased pigmentation in iris and eyelid, change in eye color, changes in eyelashes (color, length, shape); uveitis, macular edema; renal or hepatic impairment, lactation, pediatric use, remove contact lenses to apply

DRUG INTERACTIONS OF CONCERN TO DENTISTRY
• None reported

SERIOUS REACTIONS
! Systemic adverse events, including infections (colds and upper respiratory tract infections), headaches, asthenia, and hirsutism, have been reported.

DENTAL CONSIDERATIONS
General:
• Avoid drugs with anticholinergic activity, such as antihistamines, opioids, benzodiazepines, propantheline, atropine, and scopolamine.
• Protect patient's eyes from accidental spatter during dental treatment.
• Avoid dental light in patient's eyes; offer dark glasses for patient comfort.
Consultations:
• Medical consultation may be required to assess disease control.
Teach Patient/Family to:
• Update health and drug history if physician makes any changes in evaluation or drug regimens.

biperiden
bye-per'-ih-den
(Akineton HCl)

CATEGORY AND SCHEDULE
Pregnancy Risk Category: C

Drug Class: Anticholinergic

MECHANISM OF ACTION
A weak anticholinergic that exhibits competitive antagonism of acetylcholine at cholinergic

B

receptors in the corpus striatum, which restores balance.
Therapeutic Effect: Antiparkinson activity.

USES
Treatment of Parkinson symptoms, extrapyramidal symptoms secondary to neuroleptic drug therapy

PHARMACOKINETICS
Well absorbed from GI tract. Protein binding: 23%–33%. Widely distributed. *Half-life:* 18–24 hr.

INDICATIONS AND DOSAGES
▶ Extrapyramidal Symptoms
PO
Adults, Elderly. 2 mg 3–4 times a day. Dosage in renal impairment.
▶ Parkinsonism
PO
Adults, Elderly. 2 mg 1–3 times a day.

SIDE EFFECTS/ADVERSE REACTIONS
Frequent
Orthostatic hypotension, anorexia, headache, blurred vision, urinary retention, dry mouth or nose
Occasional
Insomnia, agitation, euphoria
Rare
Vomiting, depression, irritation or swelling of eyes, rash

PRECAUTIONS AND CONTRAINDICATIONS
Hypersensitivity, narrow-angle glaucoma, myasthenia gravis, GI/GU obstruction, megacolon, stenosing peptic ulcers
Caution:
Elderly, lactation, tachycardia, prostatic hypertrophy, dysrhythmias, liver or kidney disease, drug abuse, hypotension, hypertension, psychiatric patients, children

DRUG INTERACTIONS OF CONCERN TO DENTISTRY
• Increased anticholinergic effect: antihistamines, anticholinergic-acting drugs, meperidine
• Increased CNS depression: alcohol, CNS depressants
• Decreased effects of phenothiazines

SERIOUS REACTIONS
❗ Overdosage may vary from severe anticholinergic effects, such as unsteadiness, severe drowsiness, dryness of mouth, nose, or throat, tachycardia, shortness of breath, and skin flushing.
❗ Also produces severe paradoxical reaction, marked by hallucinations, tremor, seizures, and toxic psychosis.

DENTAL CONSIDERATIONS
General:
• Monitor vital signs at every appointment because of cardiovascular side effects.
• After supine positioning, have patient sit upright for at least 2 min to avoid orthostatic hypotension.
• Assess salivary flow as a factor in caries, periodontal disease, and candidiasis.
• Avoid dental light in patient's eyes; offer dark glasses for patient comfort.
Consultations:
• Medical consultation may be required to assess disease control and patient's ability to tolerate stress.
Teach Patient/Family to:
• Use powered tooth brush if patient has difficulty holding conventional devices.
• Use effective hygiene to prevent soft tissue inflammation.

• When chronic dry mouth occurs, advise patient to:
  • Avoid mouth rinses with high alcohol content because of drying effects.
  • Use daily home fluoride products for anticaries effect.
  • Use sugarless gum, frequent sips of water, or saliva substitutes.

bisacodyl
bis-ah-**koe**′-dill
(Alophen, Apo-Bisacodyl[CAN], Bisa-Lax[AUS], Dulcolax, Femilax, Gentlax, Modane, Veracolate)
Do not confuse Veracolate with Accolate or Modane with Mudrane.

CATEGORY AND SCHEDULE
Pregnancy Risk Category: C
OTC

Drug Class: Laxative, carbon dioxide-releasing; hyperosmotic; laxative, hyperosmotic, saline; laxative, lubricant; laxative, stimulant (contact); laxative, stool softener (emollient)

MECHANISM OF ACTION
A GI stimulant that has a direct effect on colonic smooth musculature by stimulating the intramural nerve plexus.
Therapeutic Effect: Promotes fluid and ion accumulation in the colon, increasing peristalsis and producing a laxative effect.

USES
As enemas or suppositories to produce bowel movements in a short time

PHARMACOKINETICS

Route	Onset	Peak	Duration
PO	6–12 hr	N/A	N/A
Rectal	15–30 min	N/A	N/A

Minimal absorption following oral and rectal administration. Absorbed drug is excreted in urine; remainder is eliminated in feces.

INDICATIONS AND DOSAGES
▸Treatment of Constipation
PO
Adults, Children older than 12 yr. 5–15 mg as needed. Maximum: 30 mg.
Children 3–12 yr. 5–10 mg or 0.3 mg/kg at bedtime or after breakfast.
Elderly. Initially, 5 mg/day.
Rectal
Adults, Children 12 yr and older. 10 mg to induce bowel movement.
Children 2–11 yr. 5–10 mg as a single dose.
Children younger than 2 yr. 5 mg.
Elderly. 5–10 mg/day.

SIDE EFFECTS/ADVERSE REACTIONS
Frequent
Some degree of abdominal discomfort, nausea, mild cramps, faintness
Occasional
Rectal administration: burning of rectal mucosa, mild proctitis

PRECAUTIONS AND CONTRAINDICATIONS
Abdominal pain, appendicitis, intestinal obstruction, nausea, undiagnosed rectal bleeding, vomiting

DRUG INTERACTIONS OF CONCERN TO DENTISTRY
• None reported; however, a delayed absorption time may be expected for orally administered drugs.

SERIOUS REACTIONS
! Long-term use may result in laxative dependence, chronic constipation, and loss of normal bowel function.
! Prolonged use or overdose may result in electrolyte or metabolic disturbances (such as hypokalemia, hypocalcemia, and metabolic acidosis or alkalosis), as well as persistent diarrhea, vomiting, muscle weakness, malabsorption, and weight loss.

DENTAL CONSIDERATIONS

General:
• Determine why patient is taking the drug.
• Consider semisupine chair position for patient comfort if GI side effects occur.
• Avoid the use of drugs that may exacerbate constipation, e.g., opioids.

bismuth subsalicylate
bis′-muth sub-sal-ih′-sah-late
(Bismed[CAN], Colo-Fresh, Devrom, Kaopectate, Pepto-Bismol)

CATEGORY AND SCHEDULE
Pregnancy Risk Category: C
OTC

Drug Class: Antidiarrheal

MECHANISM OF ACTION
An antinauseant and antiulcer agent that absorbs water and toxins in the large intestine and forms a protective coating in the intestinal mucosa. Also possesses antisecretory and antimicrobial effects.
Therapeutic Effect: Prevents diarrhea. Helps treat *Helicobacter pylori*-associated peptic ulcer disease.

USES
Treatment of diarrhea (cause undetermined), prevention of diarrhea when traveling

PHARMACOKINETICS
PO: Onset 1 hr, peak 2 hr, duration 4 hr.

INDICATIONS AND DOSAGES
▶ **Diarrhea, Gastric Distress**
PO
Adults, Elderly. 2 tablets (30 ml) q30–60 min. Maximum: 8 doses in 24 hr.
Children 9–12 yr. 1 tablet or 15 ml q30–60 min. Maximum: 8 doses in 24 hr.
Children 6–8 yr. Two-thirds of a tablet or 10 ml q30–60 min. Maximum: 8 doses in 24 hr.
Children 3–5 yr. One-third of a tablet or 5 ml q30–60 min. Maximum: 8 doses in 24 hr.
▶ **H. pylori-Associated Duodenal Ulcer, Gastritis**
PO
Adults, Elderly. 525 mg 4 times a day, with 500 mg amoxicillin and 500 mg metronidazole, 3 times a day after meals, for 7–14 days.

▸ **Chronic Infant Diarrhea**
PO
Children 2–24 mo. 2.5 ml q4h.

SIDE EFFECTS/ADVERSE REACTIONS
Frequent
Grayish-black stools
Rare
Constipation

PRECAUTIONS AND CONTRAINDICATIONS
Bleeding ulcers, gout, hemophilia, hemorrhagic states, renal impairment
Caution:
Anticoagulant therapy

DRUG INTERACTIONS OF CONCERN TO DENTISTRY
• Salicylate toxicity: other salicylates
• Decreased absorption of tetracyclines
• Suspected reduction in antihypertensives and vasodilator effects of ACE inhibitors; monitor blood pressure if used concurrently

SERIOUS REACTIONS
! Debilitated patients and infants may develop impaction.

DENTAL CONSIDERATIONS
General:
• Avoid prescribing aspirin-containing products for analgesia.

bisoprolol fumarate   B
bis-**ope**′-pro-lal
(Bicor[AUS], Zebeta)
Do not confuse Zebeta with DiaBeta.

CATEGORY AND SCHEDULE
Pregnancy Risk Category: C (D if used in second or third trimester)

Drug Class: Antihypertensive, selective β₁-blocker

MECHANISM OF ACTION
An antihypertensive that blocks β_1-adrenergic receptors in cardiac tissue.
Therapeutic Effect: Slows sinus heart rate and decreases B/P.

USES
Treatment of hypertension as a single agent or in combination with other antihypertensives, mild to moderate heart failure

PHARMACOKINETICS
Well absorbed from the GI tract. Protein binding: 26%–33%. Metabolized in the liver. Primarily excreted in urine. Not removed by hemodialysis. *Half-life:* 9–12 hr (increased in impaired renal function).

INDICATIONS AND DOSAGES
▸ **Hypertension**
PO
Adults. Initially, 5 mg/day. May increase up to 20 mg/day.
Elderly. Initially, 2.5–5 mg/day. May increase by 2.5–5 mg/day. Maximum: 20 mg/day.
▸ **Dosage in Hepatic Impairment**
For adults and elderly patients with cirrhosis or hepatitis whose

creatinine clearance is less than 40 ml/min, initially give 2.5 mg.

SIDE EFFECTS/ADVERSE REACTIONS

Frequent
Hypotension manifested as dizziness, nausea, diaphoresis, headache, cold extremities, fatigue, constipation, or diarrhea
Occasional
Insomnia, flatulence, urinary frequency, impotence, or decreased libido
Rare
Rash, arthralgia, myalgia, confusion (especially in the elderly), altered taste

PRECAUTIONS AND CONTRAINDICATIONS

Cardiogenic shock, overt cardiac failure, second-or third-degree heart block
Caution:
Major surgery, lactation, diabetes mellitus, renal disease, thyroid disease, COPD, heart failure, CAD, nonallergic bronchospasm, hepatic disease

DRUG INTERACTIONS OF CONCERN TO DENTISTRY

• Decreased antihypertensive effects: NSAIDs, indomethacin, sympathomimetics
• May slow metabolism of lidocaine
• Decreased β-blocking effects (or decreased β-adrenergic effects) of epinephrine, levonordefrin, isoproterenol, and other sympathomimetics

SERIOUS REACTIONS

! Overdose may produce profound bradycardia and hypotension.
! Abrupt withdrawal may result in diaphoresis, palpitations, headache, and tremulousness.

! Bisoprolol administration may precipitate CHF and MI in patients with heart disease, thyroid storm in those with thyrotoxicosis, and peripheral ischemia in those with existing peripheral vascular disease.
! Hypoglycemia may occur in patients with previously controlled diabetes.
! Thrombocytopenia, including unusual bruising and bleeding, occurs rarely.

DENTAL CONSIDERATIONS

General:
• Monitor vital signs at every appointment because of cardiovascular side effects.
• After supine positioning, have patient sit upright for at least 2 min to avoid orthostatic hypotension.
• Patients on chronic drug therapy may rarely have symptoms of blood dyscrasias, which can include infection, bleeding, and poor healing.
• Patient should never abruptly discontinue.
• Assess salivary flow as a factor in caries, periodontal disease, and candidiasis.
• Stress from dental procedures may compromise cardiovascular function; determine patient risk.
• Short appointments and a stress-reduction protocol may be required for anxious patients.
• Use vasoconstrictors with caution, in low doses, and with careful aspiration. Avoid use of gingival retraction cord with epinephrine.
Consultations:
• In a patient with symptoms of blood dyscrasias, request a medical consultation for blood studies and postpone dental treatment until normal values are reestablished.

• Medical consultation may be required to assess disease control and patient's ability to tolerate stress.

• Take precautions if general anesthesia is required for dental surgery.

Teach Patient/Family:
• When chronic dry mouth occurs, advise patient to:
  • Avoid mouth rinses with high alcohol content because of drying effects.
  • Use daily home fluoride products for anticaries effect.
  • Use sugarless gum, frequent sips of water, or saliva substitutes.

bivalirudin
bye-va-**leer'**-uh-din
(Angiomax)

CATEGORY AND SCHEDULE
Pregnancy Risk Category: B

Drug Class: Anticoagulants, thrombin inhibitors

MECHANISM OF ACTION
An anticoagulant that specifically and reversibly inhibits thrombin by binding to its receptor sites. *Therapeutic Effect:* Decreases acute ischemic complications in patients with unstable angina pectoris.

USES
Treatment of unstable angina in patients undergoing percutaneous transluminal coronary angioplasty

PHARMACOKINETICS

Route	Onset	Peak	Duration
IV	Immediate	N/A	1 hr

Primarily eliminated by kidneys. Twenty-five percent removed by hemodialysis. *Half-life:* 25 min (increased in moderate to severe renal impairment).

INDICATIONS AND DOSAGES
▸ **Anticoagulant in Patients with Unstable Angina Who Are Undergoing Percutaneous Transluminal Coronary Angioplasty (PTCA) in Conjunction with Aspirin**
IV
Adults, Elderly. 1 mg/kg as IV bolus followed by 4-hr IV infusion at rate of 2.5 mg/kg/hr. After initial 4-hr infusion is completed, give additional IV infusion at rate of 0.2 mg/kg/hr for 20 hr or less, if necessary.
Dosage in renal impairment

GFR	Dosage Reduced By
30–59 ml/min	20%
10–29 ml/min	60%
Dialysis	90%

SIDE EFFECTS/ADVERSE REACTIONS
Frequent
Back pain
Occasional
Nausea, headache, hypotension, generalized pain
Rare
Injection site pain, insomnia, hypertension, anxiety, vomiting, pelvic or abdominal pain, bradycardia, nervousness, dyspepsia, fever, urine retention

B

PRECAUTIONS AND CONTRAINDICATIONS
Active major bleeding

DRUG INTERACTIONS OF CONCERN TO DENTISTRY
• Increased risk of bleeding: anticoagulants, antiplatelet agents, thrombolytics, ginkgo biloba (herb)

SERIOUS REACTIONS
❗ A hemorrhagic event occurs rarely and is characterized by a fall in B/P or HCT.

DENTAL CONSIDERATIONS
General:
• Intended for use in hospitals or emergency rooms.
• Patients are at risk of bleeding; check for oral signs.
• Provide palliative dental care for dental emergencies only.
Consultations:
• Medical consultation should include routine blood counts including platelet counts and bleeding time.
• In a patient with symptoms of blood dyscrasias, request a medical consultation for blood studies and postpone treatment until normal values are reestablished.
Teach Patient/Family to:
• Use soft tooth brush to reduce risk of bleeding.
• Use effective oral hygiene to prevent soft tissue inflammation.
• Report oral lesions, soreness, or bleeding to dentist.
• Prevent trauma when using oral hygiene aids.
• Update health and medication history if physician makes any changes in evaluation or drug regimens; include OTC, herbal,

and nonherbal remedies in the update.

bleomycin sulfate
blee-oh-**my′**-sin **sull′**-fate
(Blenamax[AUS], Blenoxane)

CATEGORY AND SCHEDULE
Pregnancy Risk Category: D

Drug Class: Antineoplastic

MECHANISM OF ACTION
A glycopeptide antibiotic whose mechanism of action is unknown. Is most effective in the G2 phase of cell division.
Therapeutic Effect: Appears to inhibit DNA synthesis and, to a lesser extent, RNA and protein synthesis.

USES
Treatment of cancer of head, neck, penis, cervix, vulva of squamous cell origin, Hodgkin's and non-Hodgkin's disease, lymphosarcoma, reticulum cell sarcoma, testicular carcinoma, as a sclerosing agent for malignant pleural effusion

PHARMACOKINETICS
Half-life: 2 hr; when creatinine clearance is greater than 35 ml/min, half-life is increased in lower clearance; metabolized in liver, 50% excreted in urine (unchanged).

INDICATIONS AND DOSAGES
▸ **As Monotherapy to Treat Testicular Carcinoma; Lymphomas (Including Hodgkin's Disease, Choriocarcinoma, Reticulum Cell Sarcoma, and Lymphosarcoma); and Squamous Cell Carcinomas of the**

Head and Neck (Including Mouth, Tongue, Tonsil, Nasopharynx, Oropharynx, Sinus, Palate, Lip, Buccal Mucosa, Gingiva, Epiglottis, and Larynx)
IV, IM, Subcutaneous
Adults, Elderly. 10–20 units/m^2 (0.25–0.5 units/kg) 1–2 times/wk.
IV (Continuous)
Adults, Elderly. 15 units/m^2 over 24 hr for 4 days.
▶ **In Combination Therapy to Treat Testicular Carcinoma; Lymphomas (Including Hodgkin's Disease, Choriocarcinoma, Reticulum Cell Sarcoma, and Lymphosarcoma); and Squamous Cell Carcinomas of the Head and Neck (Including Mouth, Tongue, Tonsil, Nasopharynx, Oropharynx, Sinus, Palate, Lip, Buccal Mucosa, Gingiva, Epiglottis, and Larynx)**
IV, IM
Adults, Elderly. 3–4 units/m^2.
▶ **As a Sclerosing Agent to Treat Malignant Pleural Effusions and Prevent Recurrent Pleural Effusions**
Intrapleural
Adults, Elderly. 60–240 units as a single injection.

SIDE EFFECTS/ADVERSE REACTIONS
Frequent
Anorexia, weight loss, erythematous skin swelling, urticaria, rash, striae, vesiculation, hyperpigmentation (particularly at areas of pressure, skin folds, cuticles, IM injection sites, and scars); stomatitis (usually evident 1–3 wk after initial therapy); may also be accompanied by decreased skin sensitivity followed by skin hypersensitivity, nausea, vomiting, alopecia, and—with parenteral form—fever or chills (typically occurring a few hours after large single dose and lasting 4–12 hr)

PRECAUTIONS AND CONTRAINDICATIONS
Previous allergic reaction

DRUG INTERACTIONS OF CONCERN TO DENTISTRY
• None reported

SERIOUS REACTIONS
❗ Interstitial pneumonitis occurs in 10% of patients and occasionally progresses to pulmonary fibrosis. This condition appears to be dose or age related, occurring more often in patients receiving a total dose greater than 400 units and those older than 70 yr.
❗ Nephrotoxicity and hepatotoxicity occur infrequently.

DENTAL CONSIDERATIONS
General:
• Monitor vital signs at every appointment due to cardiovascular side effects.
• Examine for oral manifestation of opportunistic infection.
• This drug may be used in the hospital or on an outpatient basis. Confirm the patient's disease and treatment status.
• Chlorhexidine mouth rinse prior to and during chemotherapy may reduce severity of mucositis.
• Patient on chronic drug therapy may rarely present with symptoms of blood dyscrasias, which can include infection, bleeding, and poor healing. If dyscrasia is present, caution patient to prevent oral tissue trauma when using oral hygiene aids.
• Palliative medication may be required for management of oral side effects.
• Patients may have received other chemotherapy or radiation; confirm medical and drug history.

B

• Patients may be taking a prophylactic antiinfective.
• Place on frequent recall due to oral side effects.

Consultations:

• Consult physician; prophylactic or therapeutic antiinfectives may be indicated if surgery or periodontal treatment is required.
• Medical consultation may be required to assess immunologic status during cancer chemotherapy and determine safety risk, if any, posed by the required dental treatment.
• Medical consultation may be required to assess disease control and patient's ability to tolerate stress.

Teach Patient/Family to:

• Be aware of oral side effects.
• Use effective oral hygiene to prevent soft tissue inflammation.
• Report oral lesions, soreness, or bleeding to dentist.
• Prevent trauma when using oral hygiene aids.
• Update health and medication history if physician makes any changes in evaluation or drug regimens; include OTC, herbal, and nonherbal remedies in the update.

bosentan

bo′-sen-tan
(Tracleer)
Do not confuse with TriCor.

CATEGORY AND SCHEDULE

Pregnancy Risk Category: X

Drug Class: Antihypertensive

MECHANISM OF ACTION

An endothelin receptor antagonist that blocks endothelin-1, the neurohormone that constricts pulmonary arteries.
Therapeutic Effect: Improves exercise ability and slows clinical worsening of pulmonary arterial hypertension (PAH).

USES

Treatment of pulmonary arterial hypertension in patients with World Health Organization (WHO) class III and IV symptoms

PHARMACOKINETICS

Highly bound to plasma proteins, mainly albumin. Metabolized in the liver. Eliminated by biliary excretion. *Half-life:* Approximately 5 hr.

INDICATIONS AND DOSAGES

▶ **PAH in Those With WHO Class III or IV Symptoms**
PO
Adults, Elderly. 62.5 mg twice a day for 4 wk; then increase to maintenance dosage of 125 mg twice a day.
Children weighing less than 40 kg. 62.5 mg twice a day.

SIDE EFFECTS/ADVERSE REACTIONS

Occasional
Headache, nasopharyngitis, flushing
Rare
Dyspepsia (heartburn, epigastric distress), fatigue, pruritus, hypotension

PRECAUTIONS AND CONTRAINDICATIONS

Administration with cyclosporine or glyburide, pregnancy

Caution:
Hepatic impairment, pregnancy category X, use during lactation or in children has not been determined, necessitates monthly tests for pregnancy during use

DRUG INTERACTIONS OF CONCERN TO DENTISTRY
• Increased plasma concentrations: ketoconazole and possibly other drugs that inhibit or induce CYP450 enzymes involved with metabolism
• See contraindications for other drugs

SERIOUS REACTIONS
! Abnormal hepatic function, lower extremity edema, and palpitations occur rarely.

DENTAL CONSIDERATIONS
General:
• Acute PAH rarely occurs and is a major medical problem. Patients are at high risk.
• Chronic PAH also occurs. Patients may be taking a variety of antihypertensive medications. It is advisable to consult with the physician of record to determine quality of disease control, patient's ability to tolerate stress, and, with this particular drug, liver function.
Teach Patient/Family to:
• Use effective oral hygiene to prevent tissue inflammation and dental caries.
• Update health and drug history if physician makes any changes in evaluation or drug regimens; include OTC, herbal, and nonherbal drugs in the update.

brimonidine B
bry-**mo′**-nih-deen
(Alphagan P)
Do not confuse with bromocriptine.

CATEGORY AND SCHEDULE
Pregnancy Risk Category: B

Drug Class: α-adrenergic receptor agonist

MECHANISM OF ACTION
An ophthalmic agent that is a selective α_2-adrenergic agonist. ***Therapeutic Effect:*** Reduces intraocular pressure (IOP).

USES
Lowering of intraocular pressure in open-angle glaucoma or ocular hypertension; prevention of postoperative intraocular pressure elevation after argon laser trabeculoplasty

PHARMACOKINETICS
Plasma concentrations peak within 0.5–2.5 hr after ocular administration. Distributed into aqueous humor. Metabolized in liver. Primarily excreted in urine. ***Half-life:*** 3 hr.

INDICATIONS AND DOSAGES
▶ **Glaucoma, Ocular Hypertension**
Ophthalmic
Adults, Elderly, Children 2 yr and older. 1 drop in affected eye(s) 3 times a day.

SIDE EFFECTS/ADVERSE REACTIONS
Occasional
Allergic conjunctivitis, conjunctival hyperemia, eye pruritus, burning

B

sensation, conjunctival folliculosis, oral dryness, visual disturbances

PRECAUTIONS AND CONTRAINDICATIONS

Concurrent use of MAOI therapy, hypersensitivity to brimonidine tartrate or any other component of the formulation

Caution:

Wait 15 min after using before inserting contact lens; tricyclic antidepressants, β-blockers, CNS depressants; severe CV disease, hepatic or renal impairment, depression, cerebral or coronary insufficiency, Raynaud's phenomenon, orthostatic hypotension, thromboangiitis obliterans, lactation, children younger than 2 yr

DRUG INTERACTIONS OF CONCERN TO DENTISTRY

• Drug interactions have not been studied; however, the following possibilities exist:
  • Increased CNS depression: opioids, sedatives, alcohol, and general anesthetics
  • Possible risk of interference with lowering intraocular pressure: anticholinergic drugs or drugs with anticholinergic actions; tricyclic antidepressants; benzodiazepines

SERIOUS REACTIONS

! Bradycardia, hypotension, iritis, miosis, skin reactions, including erythema, eyelid, pruritus, rash, vasodilation, and tachycardia have been reported.

DENTAL CONSIDERATIONS

General:

• Assess salivary flow as factor in caries, periodontal disease, and candidiasis.
• Avoid dental light in patient's eyes; offer dark glasses for patient comfort.
• Question patient about compliance with prescribed drug regimen for glaucoma.
• Avoid drugs with anticholinergic activity, such as antihistamines, opioids, benzodiazepines, propantheline, atropine, and scopolamine.
• Monitor vital signs at every appointment because of cardiovascular side effects.

Consultations:

• Consultation with physician may be necessary if sedation or general anesthesia is required.

Teach Patient/Family to:

• Update health and drug history if physician makes any changes in evaluation or drug regimens.
• When chronic dry mouth occurs, advise patient to:
  • Avoid mouth rinses with high alcohol content because of drying effects.
  • Use daily home fluoride products for anticaries effect.
  • Use sugarless gum, frequent sips of water, or saliva substitutes.

brinzolamide

brin-**zol**'-ah-mide
(Azopt)

CATEGORY AND SCHEDULE

Pregnancy Risk Category: C

Drug Class: Carbonic anhydrase inhibitor

MECHANISM OF ACTION

An ophthalmic agent that inhibits carbonic anhydrase. Decreases aqueous humor secretion. *Therapeutic Effect:* Reduces intraocular pressure (IOP).

USES

Treatment of ocular hypertension, open-angle glaucoma

PHARMACOKINETICS

Systemically absorbed to some degree. Protein binding: 60%. Distributed extensively in red blood cells. Site of metabolism has not been established. Metabolized to active and inactive metabolites. Primarily excreted unchanged in urine.

INDICATIONS AND DOSAGES

▸ **Glaucoma, Ocular Hypertension**
Ophthalmic
Adults, Elderly. Instill 1 drop in affected eye(s) 3 times a day.

SIDE EFFECTS/ADVERSE REACTIONS

Occasional
Blurred vision, bitter taste, dry eye, ocular discharge, ocular discomfort and pain, ocular pruritus, headache, rhinitis
Rare
Allergic reactions, alopecia, chest pain, conjunctivitis, diarrhea, diplopia, dizziness, dry mouth, dyspnea, dyspepsia, eye fatigue, hypertonia, keratoconjunctivitis, keratopathy, kidney pain, lid margin crusting or sticky sensation, nausea, pharyngitis, tearing, urticaria

PRECAUTIONS AND CONTRAINDICATIONS

Hypersensitivity to brinzolamide or any other component of the formulation

Caution:
Lactation, no data for pediatric use

DRUG INTERACTIONS OF CONCERN TO DENTISTRY

• Avoid drugs that can exacerbate glaucoma (e.g., anticholinergics).

SERIOUS REACTIONS

! Electrolyte imbalance, development of an acidotic state, and possible CNS effects may occur.

DENTAL CONSIDERATIONS

General:
• Avoid dental light in patient's eyes; offer dark glasses for patient comfort.
• Question patient about compliance with prescribed drug regimen for glaucoma.
Consultations:
• Medical consult may be required to assess disease control.

bromocriptine mesylate

broe-moe-**krip'**-teen **mess'**-ah-late
(Apo-Bromocriptine[CAN], Bromohexal[AUS], Kripton[AUS], Parlodel)
Do not confuse bromocriptine with benztropine, or Parlodel with pindolol.

CATEGORY AND SCHEDULE

Pregnancy Risk Category: C

Drug Class: Dopamine receptor agonist, ovulation stimulant

MECHANISM OF ACTION

A dopamine agonist that directly stimulates dopamine receptors in the corpus striatum and inhibits prolactin secretion. Also suppresses secretion of growth hormone. *Therapeutic Effect:* Improves symptoms of parkinsonism, suppresses galactorrhea, and reduces serum growth hormone concentrations in acromegaly.

USES

Treatment of female infertility, Parkinson's disease, prevention of postpartum lactation, amenorrhea caused by hyperprolactinemia, acromegaly

PHARMACOKINETICS

Indication	Onset	Peak	Duration
Prolactin lowering	2 hr	8 hr	24 hr
Antiparkinson	0.5–1.5 hr	2 hr	N/A
Growth hormone suppressant	1–2 hr	4–8 wk	4–8 hr

Minimally absorbed from the GI tract. Protein binding: 90%–96%. Metabolized in the liver. Excreted in feces by biliary secretion. *Half-life:* 15 hr.

INDICATIONS AND DOSAGES
▶ **Hyperprolactinemia**
PO
Adults, Elderly. Initially, 1.25–2.5 mg/day. May increase by 2.5 mg/day at 3- to 7-day intervals. Range: 2.5 mg 2–3 times a day.
▶ **Parkinson's Disease**
PO
Adults, Elderly. Initially, 1.25 mg twice a day. May increase by 2.5 mg/day every 14–28 days. Range: 30–90 mg/day.

▶ **Acromegaly**
PO
Adults, Elderly. Initially, 1.25–2.5 mg. May increase at 3- to 7-day intervals. Usual dose 20–30 mg/day.

SIDE EFFECTS/ADVERSE REACTIONS
Frequent
Nausea, headache, dizziness
Occasional
Fatigue, lightheadedness, vomiting, abdominal cramps, diarrhea, constipation, nasal congestion, somnolence, dry mouth
Rare
Muscle cramps, urinary hesitancy

PRECAUTIONS AND CONTRAINDICATIONS
Hypersensitivity to ergot alkaloids, peripheral vascular disease, pregnancy, severe ischemic heart disease, uncontrolled hypertension
Caution:
Lactation, hepatic disease, renal disease, children

DRUG INTERACTIONS OF CONCERN TO DENTISTRY
• None reported

SERIOUS REACTIONS
! Visual or auditory hallucinations have been noted in patients with Parkinson's disease.
! Long-term, high-dose therapy may produce continuing rhinorrhea, syncope, GI hemorrhage, peptic ulcer, and severe abdominal pain.

DENTAL CONSIDERATIONS

General:
• Monitor vital signs at every appointment because of cardiovascular side effects.

* After supine positioning, have patient sit upright for at least 2 min to avoid orthostatic hypotension.
* Assess salivary flow as a factor in caries, periodontal disease, and candidiasis.
* Short appointments may be required because of disease effects on musculature.

Consultations:
* Medical consultation may be required to assess disease control.

Teach Patient/Family to:
* Avoid mouth rinses with high alcohol content because of drying effects.

brompheniramine
brome-fen-**ir**'-ah-meen
(BroveX, BroveX CT, Codimal A, Colhist, Dimetane, Dimetane Extentabs, Dimetapp, Lodrane 12 Hour, Nasahist B, ND Stat)

CATEGORY AND SCHEDULE
Pregnancy Risk Category: B
OTC (tablets, elixir)

Drug Class: Antihistamine, H1-receptor antagonist

MECHANISM OF ACTION
An alkylamine that competes with histamine at histaminic receptor (H_1) sites. Inhibits central acetylcholine.
Therapeutic Effect: Results in anticholinergic, antipruritic, antitussive, antiemetic effects. Produces antidyskinetic, sedative effect.

USES
Allergy symptoms, rhinitis, hay fever

PHARMACOKINETICS
Rapidly absorbed after PO administration. Widely distributed. Metabolized in liver. Primarily excreted in urine. *Half-life:* 25 hr.

INDICATIONS AND DOSAGES
▶ **Allergic Rhinitis, Anaphylaxis, Urticarial Transfusion Reactions, Urticaria**
PO
Adults, Elderly, Children 12 yr and older. 4 mg q4–6h or 8–12 mg extended/timed-release q12h.
Children younger than 12 yr. 1–2 mg q4–6h.
▶ **Amelioration of Allergic Reactions to Blood or Plasma, Anaphylaxis as an Adjunct to Epinephrine and Other Standard Measures After the Acute Symptoms Have Been Controlled, Other Uncomplicated Allergic Conditions of the Immediate Type When Oral Therapy Is Impossible or Contraindicated**
IM/IV/SC
Adults, Elderly, Children 12 yr and older. 5–20 mg/day in 2 divided doses. Maximum: 40 mg/day.
Children younger than 12 yr. 0.125 mg/kg/day or 3.75 mg/m^2 in 3–4 divided doses.

SIDE EFFECTS/ADVERSE REACTIONS
Frequent
Drowsiness; dizziness; dry mouth, nose, or throat; urinary retention; thickening of bronchial secretions
Elderly. Sedation, dizziness, hypotension
Occasional
Epigastric distress, flushing, blurred vision, tinnitus, paresthesia, sweating, chills

B

PRECAUTIONS AND CONTRAINDICATIONS

Concurrent MAOI therapy, focal CNS lesions, newborn or premature infants, hypersensitivity to brompheniramine or related drugs
Caution:
Increased intraocular pressure, renal disease, cardiac disease, hypertension, bronchial asthma, seizure disorder, stenosed peptic ulcers, hyperthyroidism, prostatic hypertrophy, bladder neck obstruction

DRUG INTERACTIONS OF CONCERN TO DENTISTRY

• Increased CNS depression: alcohol, all CNS depressants
• Additive photosensitization: tetracyclines
• Increased drying effect: anticholinergics
• Hypotension: general anesthetics

SERIOUS REACTIONS

! Children may experience dominant paradoxical reactions, including restlessness, insomnia, euphoria, nervousness, and tremors.
! Overdosage in children may result in hallucinations, seizures, and death.
! Hypersensitivity reaction, such as eczema, pruritus, rash, cardiac disturbances, and photosensitivity, may occur.

DENTAL CONSIDERATIONS

General:
• Assess salivary flow as a factor in caries, periodontal disease, and candidiasis.
• Consider semisupine chair position for patients with respiratory disease.
• Determine why the patient is taking the drug.

Teach Patient/Family to:
• Use effective oral hygiene to prevent soft tissue inflammation.
• Avoid mouth rinses with high alcohol content because of drying effects.

bucindolol

byoo-sin-doe-lole
(Gencaro)—currently unavailable in the U.S.

CATEGORY AND SCHEDULE

Drug Class: β-adrenergic blocker, nonselective

MECHANISM OF ACTION

Nonselective β-blocking activity. Mild vasodilatory activity.
Therapeutic Effect: Decreases B/P, increases left ventricular ejection fraction, reduces plasma rennin activity.

USES

Hypertension
Congestive heart failure

PHARMACOKINETICS

Route	Onset	Peak	Duration
PO (hypertension)	1 hr	2–3 hr	6–12 hr
PO (CHF)	4 hr	3 months	< 24 hr

Well absorbed from the GI tract. Bioavailability: approximately 30%. Undergoes extensive first-pass metabolism to active metabolite.
Half-life: 3.6 hr.

INDICATIONS AND DOSAGES
▸ **Hypertension**
PO
Adults. Initially, 50 mg three times/day, followed by weekly increases until target blood pressure is achieved.
▸ **Congestive Heart Failure**
PO
Adults. Initially, 12.5mg every 12 hr. If tolerated, may increase. Maximum dose: 100 mg twice/day.

SIDE EFFECTS/ADVERSE REACTIONS
Frequent
Drowsiness, nausea, vomiting, abdominal cramps, dyspepsia, hypotension manifested as dizziness, faintness, lightheadedness
Occasional
Facial flushing, hypo-/hyperglycemia, arthralgias, myalgias, bronchospasms
Rare
Elevated liver enzymes

PRECAUTIONS AND CONTRAINDICATIONS
Hypersensitivity to bucindolol or any component of the formulation
Cardiogenic shock
Overt cardiac failure
Second- or third-degree AV block
Severe sinus bradycardia or hypotension
Caution:
Anesthesia/surgery
Abrupt withdrawal
Bronchial asthma or related bronchospastic conditions
Cerebrovascular insufficiency
Diabetes mellitus
Hyperthyroidism/thyrotoxicosis
Myasthenic conditions
Peripheral vascular disease
Renal disease

DRUG INTERACTIONS OF CONCERN TO DENTISTRY
• Amiodarone: Increased risk of hypotension, bradycardia, or cardiac arrest
• β_2-agonists: Decreased effectiveness
• Calcium channel blockers: Increase risk of conduction disturbances
• Digoxin: Increases concentrations of digoxin
• Diuretics, other antihypertensives: May increase hypotensive effect
• Insulin, oral hypoglycemics: May mask symptoms of hypoglycemia and prolong hypoglycemic effect of these drugs
• NSAIDs: Decreased antihypertensive effect
• Epinephrine: May cause reflex tachycardia, hypertension, resistance to epinephrine

SERIOUS REACTIONS
! Overdose may produce profound bradycardia and hypotension.
! Abrupt withdrawal may result in rebound hypertension.
! Bucindolol administration may precipitate CHF or MI in patients with heart disease; thyroid storm in those with thyrotoxicosis; or peripheral ischemia in those with existing peripheral vascular disease.
! Hypoglycemia may occur in patients with previously controlled diabetes.

DENTAL CONSIDERATIONS
General:
• Monitor vital signs at every appointment because of cardiovascular side effects.
• After supine positioning, have patient sit upright for at least 2 min before standing to avoid orthostatic hypotension.

B

• Assess salivary flow as a factor in caries, periodontal disease, and candidiasis.
• Limit use of sodium-containing products, such as saline IV fluids, for those patients with dietary salt restriction.
• Stress from dental procedures may compromise cardiovascular function; determine patient risk.
• Limit or avoid vasoconstrictors.
Consultations:
• Medical consultation may be required to assess disease control.
Teach Patient/Family to:
• Report oral lesions, soreness, or bleeding to dentist.
• When chronic dry mouth occurs, advise patient to:
  • Avoid mouth rinses with high alcohol content because of drying effects.
  • Use daily home fluoride products for anticaries effect.
  • Use sugarless gum, frequent sips of water, or saliva substitutes.

buclizine hydrochloride
bew'-klih-zeen hi-droh-**klor**'-ide
(Bucladin-S)

CATEGORY AND SCHEDULE
Pregnancy Risk Category: C

Drug Class: Antiemetic

MECHANISM OF ACTION
A centrally acting agent that suppresses nausea and vomiting. Buclizine is an anticholinergic that reduces labyrinth excitability and diminishes vestibular stimulation of labyrinth, affecting chemoreceptor trigger zone (CTZ). Possesses anticholinergic activity.

Therapeutic Effect: Reduces nausea, vomiting, vertigo.

USES
Prophylaxis of nausea, vomiting, and dizziness associated with motion sickness

PHARMACOKINETICS
None reported

INDICATIONS AND DOSAGES
▶ Motion Sickness
PO
Adults, Elderly, Children 12 yr and older. 50 mg 30 min before travel. Dose may be repeated every 4–6 hr as needed. Maximum: 150 mg/day.

SIDE EFFECTS/ADVERSE REACTIONS
Frequent
Drowsiness
Occasional
Dryness of mouth, headache, jitteriness

PRECAUTIONS AND CONTRAINDICATIONS
Early pregnancy, hypersensitivity to buclizine or other components of the formulation, including tartrazine

DRUG INTERACTIONS OF CONCERN TO DENTISTRY
• None reported

SERIOUS REACTIONS
! Children may experience dominant paradoxical reaction, including restlessness, insomnia, euphoria, nervousness, and tremors.
! Overdosage in children may result in hallucinations, convulsions, and death.
! Hypersensitivity reaction, marked by eczema, pruritus, rash, cardiac disturbances, and photosensitivity, may occur.

! Overdosage may vary from CNS depression, such as sedation, apnea, cardiovascular collapse, or death, to severe paradoxical reaction, including hallucinations, tremors, or seizures.

DENTAL CONSIDERATIONS

General:
* Symptoms may preclude elective dental treatment.
* Assess salivary flow as a factor in caries, periodontal disease, and candidiasis.
* Consider semisupine chair position for patient comfort because of GI effects of disease.

Teach Patient/Family to:
* Use effective oral hygiene to prevent soft tissue inflammation.
* When chronic dry mouth occurs, advise patient to:
  * Avoid mouth rinses with high alcohol content because of drying effects.
  * Use daily home fluoride products for anticaries effect.
  * Use sugarless gum, frequent sips of water, or saliva substitutes.

budesonide
bu-**dess'**-ah-nide
(Burinex[AUS], Entocort EC, Pulmicort Respules, Pulmicort Turbuhaler, Rhinocort Aqua, Rhinocort Aqueous[AUS], Rhinocort Hayfever[AUS])

CATEGORY AND SCHEDULE
Pregnancy Risk Category: B

Drug Class: Glucocorticoid, long-acting

MECHANISM OF ACTION
A glucocorticoid that inhibits the accumulation of inflammatory cells and decreases and prevents tissues from responding to the inflammatory process.
Therapeutic Effect: Relieves symptoms of allergic rhinitis or Crohn's disease.

USES
Treatment of mild-to-moderate active Crohn's disease of the ileum or ascending colon

PHARMACOKINETICS
Minimally absorbed from nasal tissue; moderately absorbed from inhalation. Protein binding: 88%. Primarily metabolized in the liver.
Half-life: 2–3 hr.

INDICATIONS AND DOSAGES
▸ **Rhinitis**
Intranasal (Rhinocort Aqua)
Adults, Elderly, Children 6 yr and older. 1 spray in each nostril once a day. Maximum: 8 sprays a day for adults and children 12 yr and older; 4 sprays a day for children younger than 12 yr.
▸ **Bronchial Asthma**
Nebulization
Children 6 mo–8 yr. 0.25–1 mg/day titrated to lowest effective dosage.
Inhalation
Adults, Elderly, Children 6 yr and older. Initially, 200–400 mcg twice a day. Maximum: Adults: 800 mcg twice a day. Children: 400 mcg twice a day.
▸ **Crohn's Disease**
PO
Adults, Elderly. 9 mg once a day for up to 8 wk.

SIDE EFFECTS/ADVERSE REACTIONS

Frequent

Nasal: Mild nasopharyngeal irritation, burning, stinging, or dryness; headache; cough

Inhalation: Flu-like symptoms, headache, pharyngitis

Occasional

Nasal: Dry mouth, dyspepsia, rebound congestion, rhinorrhea, loss of taste

Inhalation: Back pain, vomiting, altered taste, voice changes, abdominal pain, nausea, dyspepsia

PRECAUTIONS AND CONTRAINDICATIONS

Hypersensitivity to any corticosteroid or its components, persistently positive sputum cultures for *Candida albicans,* primary treatment of status asthmaticus, systemic fungal infections, untreated localized infection involving nasal mucosa

Caution:

Tuberculosis, hypertension, diabetes mellitus, osteoporosis, peptic ulcer, glaucoma, cataracts, suppression of the hypothalamic-pituitary-adrenal (HPA) axis, discontinue use during nursing or discontinue drug, safety in children has not been established, geriatric patients

SERIOUS REACTIONS

! An acute hypersensitivity reaction marked by urticaria, angioedema, and severe bronchospasm; occurs rarely.

DENTAL CONSIDERATIONS

General:

• Evaluate respiration characteristics and rate.

• Assess salivary flow as a factor in caries, periodontal disease, and candidiasis.

• Midday appointments are suggested with stress-reduction protocol for anxious patients.

• Place on frequent recall because of oral side effects.

• Acute asthmatic episodes may be precipitated in the dental office. Rapid-acting sympathomimetic inhalants should be available for emergency use. Budesonide is not a rapid-acting drug and is not intended for use in acute asthmatic attacks.

Consultations:

• Medical consultation may be required to assess disease control.

Teach Patient/Family to:

• Use effective oral hygiene to prevent soft tissue inflammation.

• Gargle and rinse with water after each dose.

• When chronic dry mouth occurs, advise patient to:

   • Avoid mouth rinses with high alcohol content because of drying effects.

   • Use daily home fluoride products for anticaries effect.

   • Use sugarless gum, frequent sips of water, or artificial saliva substitutes.

bumetanide
byoo-**met'**-ah-nide
(Bumex, Burinex[CAN])

CATEGORY AND SCHEDULE
Pregnancy Risk Category: C (D if used in pregnancy-induced hypertension)

Drug Class: Loop diuretic

MECHANISM OF ACTION
A loop diuretic that enhances excretion of sodium, chloride, and, to lesser degree, potassium, by direct action at the ascending limb of the loop of Henle and in the proximal tubule.
Therapeutic Effect: Produces diuresis.

USES
Treatment of edema in CHF, liver disease, renal disease (nephrotic syndrome), pulmonary edema, ascites (nephrotic syndrome), hypertension

PHARMACOKINETICS

Route	Onset	Peak	Duration
PO	30–60 min	60–120 min	60–120 min
IV	Rapid	15–30 min	2–3 hr
IM	40 min	4–6 hr	4–6 hr

Completely absorbed from the GI tract (absorption decreased in CHF and nephrotic syndrome). Protein binding: 94%–96%. Partially metabolized in the liver. Primarily excreted in urine. Not removed by hemodialysis. *Half-life:* 1–1.5 hr.

INDICATIONS AND DOSAGES
▸ **Edema**
PO
Adults, Children older than 18 yr. 0.5–2 mg as a single dose in the morning. May repeat at q4–5 hr.
Elderly. 0.5 mg/day, increased as needed.
IV, IM
Adults, Elderly. 0.5–2 mg/dose; may repeat in 2–3 hr. Or 0.5–1 mg/hr by continuous IV infusion.
▸ **Hypertension**
PO
Adults, Elderly. Initially, 0.5 mg/day. Range: 1–4 mg/day. Maximum:

5 mg/day. Larger doses may be given 2–3 doses a day.
▸ **Usual Pediatric Dosage**
PO, IV, IM
Children. 0.015–0.1 mg/kg/dose q6–24h.

SIDE EFFECTS/ADVERSE REACTIONS
Expected
Increased urinary frequency and urine volume
Frequent
Orthostatic hypotension, dizziness
Occasional
Blurred vision, diarrhea, headache, anorexia, premature ejaculation, impotence, dyspepsia
Rare
Rash, urticaria, pruritus, asthenia, muscle cramps, nipple tenderness

PRECAUTIONS AND CONTRAINDICATIONS
Anuria, hepatic coma, severe electrolyte depletion
Caution:
Dehydration, ascites, severe renal disease

DRUG INTERACTIONS OF CONCERN TO DENTISTRY
• Decreased diuretic effect: NSAIDs, indomethacin
• Masked ototoxicity: phenothiazines
• Increased electrolyte imbalance: nondepolarizing skeletal muscle relaxants, corticosteroids

SERIOUS REACTIONS
! Vigorous diuresis may lead to profound water and electrolyte depletion, resulting in hypokalemia, hyponatremia, dehydration, coma, and circulatory collapse.
! Ototoxicity—manifested as deafness, vertigo, or tinnitus—may occur, especially in patients with

severe renal impairment and those taking other ototoxic drugs.
! Blood dyscrasias and acute hypotensive episodes have been reported.

DENTAL CONSIDERATIONS

General:
• Monitor vital signs at every appointment because of cardiovascular side effects.
• Patients on chronic drug therapy may rarely have symptoms of blood dyscrasias, which can include infection, bleeding, and poor healing.
• After supine positioning, have patient sit upright for at least 2 min to avoid orthostatic hypotension.
• Assess salivary flow as a factor in caries, periodontal disease, and candidiasis.
• Limit or avoid vasoconstrictors.
• Limit use of sodium-containing products, such as saline IV fluids, for patients with a dietary salt restriction.
• Patients on high-potency diuretics should be monitored for serum K^+ levels.
Consultations:
• In a patient with symptoms of blood dyscrasias, request a medical consultation for blood studies and postpone dental treatment until normal values are reestablished.
• Medical consultation may be required to assess disease control.
Teach Patient/Family to:
• Use effective oral hygiene to prevent soft tissue inflammation.
• Use caution to prevent injury when using oral hygiene aids.
• When chronic dry mouth occurs, advise patient to:

• Avoid mouth rinses with high alcohol content because of drying effects.
• Use daily home fluoride products for anticaries effect.
• Use sugarless gum, frequent sips of water, or saliva substitutes.

bupivacaine
byoo-**piv**′-ah-caine
(Marcaine, Marcaine Spinal, Sensorcaine, Sensorcaine-MPF)

CATEGORY AND SCHEDULE
Pregnancy Risk Category: C

Drug Class: Amide local anesthetic

MECHANISM OF ACTION
An amide-type anesthetic that stabilizes neuronal membranes and prevents initiation and transmission of nerve impulses, thereby effecting local anesthetic actions.
Therapeutic Effect: Produces local analgesia.

USES
Local dental anesthesia, epidural anesthesia, peripheral nerve block, caudal anesthesia

PHARMACOKINETICS
Onset of action occurs within 4–10 min depending on route of administration. Duration is 1.5–8.5 hr, depending on site of administration. Well absorbed. Protein binding: 95%. Metabolized in liver. Excreted in urine. **Half-life:** 1.5–5.5 hr (adults), 8.1 hr (neonates).

INDICATIONS AND DOSAGES

Dose varies with procedure, depth of anesthesia, vascularity of tissues, duration of anesthesia and condition of patient.

▶ **Analgesic, Epidural (partial to moderate motor blockade)**
IV

Adults, Elderly. 10–20 ml (25–50 mg) of a 0.25% solution. Repeat once q3h as needed.

Children weighing more than 10 kg. 1–2.5 mg/kg single dose as a 0.125% or 0.25% solution or 0.2–0.4 mg/kg/hr continuous infusion as a 0.1%, 0.125%, or 0.25% solution. Maximum: 0.4 mg/kg/hr.

Children weighing less than 10 kg. 1–1.25 mg/kg single dose as a 0.125% or 0.25% solution or 0.1–0.2 mg/kg/hr continuous infusion as a 0.1%, 0.125%, or 0.25% solution. Maximum: 0.2 mg/kg/hr.

▶ **Analgesic, Epidural (moderate to complete motor blockade)**
IV

Adults, Elderly. 10–20 ml (50–100 mg) as a 0.5% solution. Repeat once q3h as needed.

Children weighing more than 10 kg. 1–2.5 mg/kg single dose as a 0.125% or 0.25% solution or 0.2–0.4 mg/kg/hr continuous infusion as a 0.1%, 0.125%, or 0.25% solution. Maximum: 0.4 mg/kg/hr.

Children weighing less than 10 kg. 1–1.25 mg/kg single dose as a 0.125% or 0.25% solution or 0.1–0.2 mg/kg/hr continuous infusion as a 0.1%, 0.125%, or 0.25% solution. Maximum: 0.2 mg/kg/hr.

▶ **Analgesic, Epidural (complete motor blockade)**
IV

Adults. 10–20 ml (75–150 mg) as a 0.75% solution. Repeat once q3h as needed.

Children weighing more than 10 kg. 1–2.5 mg/kg single dose as a 0.125% or 0.25% solution or 0.2–0.4 mg/kg/hr continuous infusion as a 0.1%, 0.125%, or 0.25% solution. Maximum: 0.4 mg/kg/hr.

Children weighing less than 10 kg. 1–1.25 mg/kg single dose as a 0.125% or 0.25% solution or 0.1–0.2 mg/kg/hr continuous infusion as a 0.1%, 0.125%, or 0.25% solution. Maximum: 0.2 mg/kg/hr.

▶ **Analgesic, Intrapleural**
IV

Adults, Elderly. 10–30 ml bolus of 0.25%, 0.375%, or 0.5% q4–8h or 0.375% solution with epinephrine continuous infusion at 6 ml/hr after 20-ml loading dose.

▶ **Analgesic, Caudal (moderate to complete blockade)**
IV

Adults, Elderly. 15–30 ml of 0.5% solution (75–150 mg) or 0.25% solution (37.5–75 mg), repeated once every 3 hr as needed.

Children weighing more than 10 kg. 1–2.5 mg/kg single dose as a 0.125% or 0.25% solution or 0.2–0.4 mg/kg/hr continuous infusion as a 0.1%, 0.125%, or 0.25% solution. Maximum: 0.4 mg/kg/hr.

Children weighing less than 10 kg. 1–1.25 mg/kg single dose as a 0.125% or 0.25% solution or 0.1–0.2 mg/kg/hr continuous infusion as a 0.1%, 0.125%, or 0.25% solution. Maximum: 0.2 mg/kg/hr.

▸ **Analgesic, Dental**
IV
Adults, Elderly. 1.8–3.6 ml of 0.5% solution (9–18 mg) with epinephrine. A second dose of 9 mg may be administered. Maximum: 90 mg total dose.

▸ **Analgesic, Peripheral Nerve Block (moderate to complete motor blockade)**
IV
Adults, Elderly. 5–37.5 ml (25–175 mg) of 0.5% solution or 5–70 ml (12.5–175 mg) of 0.25% solution. Repeat q3h as needed. Maximum: up to 400 mg/day.
Children 12 yr and older. 0.3–2.5 mg/kg as a 0.25% or 0.5% solution. Maximum: 1 ml/kg of 0.25% solution or 0.5 ml/kg of 0.5% solution.

▸ **Analgesic, Retrobulbar (complete motor blockade)**
IV
Adults, Elderly. 2–4 ml (15–30 mg) of 0.75% solution.

▸ **Analgesic, Sympathetic Blockade**
IV
Adults, Elderly. 20–50 ml (50–125 mg) of 0.25% (no epinephrine) solution. Repeat once q3h as needed.

▸ **Analgesic, Hyperbaric Spinal (obstetrical, normal vaginal delivery)**
IV
Adults, Elderly. 0.8 ml (6 mg) bupivacaine in dextrose as 0.75% solution.

▸ **Analgesic, Hyperbaric Spinal (obstetrical, cesarean section)**
IV
Adults, Elderly. 1–1.4 ml (7.5–10.5 mg) bupivacaine in dextrose as 0.75% solution.

▸ **Anesthesia, Hyperbaric Spinal (surgical, lower extremity, and perineal procedures)**
IV
Adults, Elderly. 1 ml (7.5 mg) bupivacaine in dextrose as 0.75% solution.
Children 12 yr and older. 0.3–0.6 mg/kg bupivacaine in dextrose as a 0.75% solution.

▸ **Anesthesia, Spinal (surgical, lower abdominal procedures)**
IV
Adults, Elderly. 1.6 ml (12 mg) bupivacaine in dextrose as 0.75% solution.
Children 12 yr and older. 0.3–0.6 mg/kg bupivacaine in dextrose as a 0.75% solution.

▸ **Anesthesia, Spinal (surgical, hyperbaric, upper abdominal procedures)**
IV
Adults, Elderly. 2 ml (15 mg) bupivacaine in dextrose administered in horizontal position.
Children 12 yr and older. 0.3–0.6 mg/kg bupivacaine in dextrose as a 0.75% solution.

▸ **Analgesic, Local Infiltration**
IV
Adults, Elderly. 0.25% solution. Maximum: 225 mg with epinephrine or 175 mg without epinephrine.
Children 12 yr and older. 0.5–2.5 mg/kg as a 0.25% or 0.5% solution. Maximum: 1 ml/kg of 0.25% solution or 0.5 ml/kg of 0.5% solution.

SIDE EFFECTS/ADVERSE REACTIONS

Occasional

Hypotension, bradycardia, palpitations, respiratory depression, dizziness, headache, vomiting, nausea, restlessness, weakness, blurred vision, tinnitus, apnea

PRECAUTIONS AND CONTRAINDICATIONS

Local infection at the site of proposed lumbar puncture (spinal anesthesia), obstetrical paracervical block anesthesia, septicemia (spinal anesthesia), severe hemorrhage, severe hypotension or shock, arrhythmias such as complete heart block, which severely restricts cardiac output (spinal anesthesia), sulfite allergy (epinephrine containing solutions only), hypersensitivity to bupivacaine products or to other amide-type anesthetics

Caution:

Elderly, severe drug allergies, use in children (risk of local injury because of long duration of anesthesia)

DRUG INTERACTIONS OF CONCERN TO DENTISTRY

• CNS depressants: may see increased risk of CNS depression with all CNS depressants, especially in children and when larger doses are used.

• Avoid placing dental cartridges in disinfectant solutions with heavy metals or surface-active agents; may see release of metal ions into local anesthetic solutions, with tissue irritation following injection.

• Avoid excessive exposure of dental cartridges to light or heat; it hastens deterioration of vasoconstrictors; color change in local anesthetic solution indicates breakdown of vasoconstrictor.

• Risk of cardiovascular side effects: rapid intravascular administration of local anesthetic containing vasoconstrictors, either alone or in patients taking tricyclic antidepressants, MAOIs, digitalis drugs, cocaine, phenothiazines, ß-blockers, and in the presence of halogenated hydrocarbon general anesthetics; always use the smallest effective vasoconstrictor dose and careful aspiration technique.

• Avoid use of vasoconstrictors in patients with uncontrolled hyperthyroidism, diabetes, angina, or hypertension; refer these patients for medical treatment before elective dental procedures.

SERIOUS REACTIONS

! Arterial hypotension, bradycardia, ventricular arrhythmias, central nervous system (CNS) depression and excitation, convulsions, respiratory arrest, tinnitus have been reported.

! Solutions with epinephrine contain metabisulfite, a sulfite that may cause allergic-type reactions, including anaphylaxis.

DENTAL CONSIDERATIONS

General:

• Monitor vital signs at every appointment because of cardiovascular and respiratory side effects.

• Lubricate dry lips before injection or dental treatment as required.

Teach Patient/Family to:

• Use care to prevent injury while numbness exists; do not chew gum or eat following dental anesthesia.

• Remember that numbness with this drug is expected to last for a considerable period.

• Report any signs of infection, muscle pain, or fever to dentist when oral sensations return.

• Report any unusual soft tissue reactions.

B

buprenorphine hydrochloride

byoo-pre-**nor'**-feen
hi-droh-**klor'**-ide
Schedule V
(Buprenex, Subutex,
Temgesic[CAN])

CATEGORY AND SCHEDULE

Pregnancy Risk Category: C
Controlled Substance: Schedule V
(opioid agonist), III (tablet)

Drug Class: Opioid
agonist-antagonist

MECHANISM OF ACTION

An opioid agonist-antagonist that
binds with opioid receptors in the
CNS.
Therapeutic Effect: Alters the
perception of and emotional
response to pain; blocks the effects
of heroin and produces minimal
opioid withdrawal symptoms.

USES

Relief of moderate to severe pain
(injection) and for treatment of
opioid dependence (tablets)

PHARMACOKINETICS:

IM: Onset 15–30 min, duration
4–6 hr; absorption 90%–100%;
hepatic metabolism; excreted in
feces (68%–71%); also renal
excretion.

INDICATIONS AND DOSAGES

▸ **Analgesia**
IV, IM
Adults, Children older than 12 yr.
0.3 mg q6–8h as needed. May repeat
once in 30–60 min. Range:
0.15–0.6 mg q4–8h as needed.
Children 2–12 yr. 2–6 mcg/kg q4–6h
as needed.

Elderly. 0.15 mg q6h as needed.
▸ **Opioid Dependence**
Sublingual
*Adults, Elderly, Children older than
16 yr.* Initially, 12–16 mg/day,
beginning at least 4 hr after last use
of heroin or short-acting opioid.
Maintenance: 16 mg/day. Range:
4–24 mg/day. Patients should be
switched to buprenorphine and
naloxone combination, preferred for
maintenance treatment.

SIDE EFFECTS/ADVERSE REACTIONS

Frequent
Tablet: Headache, pain, insomnia,
anxiety, depression, nausea,
abdominal pain, constipation, back
pain, weakness, rhinitis, withdrawal
syndrome, infection, diaphoresis
Injection (more than 10%): Sedation
Occasional
Injection: Hypotension, respiratory
depression, dizziness, headache,
vomiting, nausea, vertigo

PRECAUTIONS AND CONTRAINDICATIONS

Hypersensitivity to buprenorphine;
hypersensitivity to naloxone for
those receiving the fixed
combination product containing
naloxone (Suboxone)
Caution:
Hepatic impairment, hepatitis, risk
of allergic reaction, bile tract
disease, impaired respiration
(COPD, cor pulmonale, decreased
respiratory reserve, hypoxia,
hypercapnia, preexisting respiratory
depression); naloxone may not be
effective as a narcotic reversal agent,
head injury, impairment of reaction
time, low abuse potential, opioid-
dependent patients, debilitated
patients, elderly, children younger
than 2 yr, use not advised during
lactation

DRUG INTERACTIONS OF CONCERN TO DENTISTRY

• Increased risk of respiratory and cardiovascular collapse: benzodiazepines
• Increased CNS depression: all CNS depressants, concomitant use of other opioids

SERIOUS REACTIONS

! Overdose results in cold and clammy skin, weakness, confusion, severe respiratory depression, cyanosis, pinpoint pupils, and extreme somnolence progressing to seizures, stupor, and coma.

DENTAL CONSIDERATIONS

General:
• Patients taking this drug for opioid dependence; avoid the use of any drug with abuse potential.
• Consider aspirin, acetaminophen, or NSAIDs for the management of dental-related pain.
• Monitor vital signs at every appointment because of cardiovascular side effects.
• After supine positioning, have patient sit upright for at least 2 min to avoid orthostatic hypotension.
• Assess salivary flow as a factor in caries, periodontal disease, and candidiasis.
• Consider semisupine chair position for patient comfort if GI or respiratory side effects occur.
• Take precautions if dental surgery is anticipated and general anesthesia is required.
• If opioid or sedative drugs are required for patient management and comfort, advise current drug abuse care facility or aftercare program as appropriate.
Consultations:
• Consultations may be difficult to obtain where treatment

confidentiality of drug dependence is followed.
• Medical consultation may be required to assess disease control.
Teach Patient/Family to:
• Use effective oral hygiene to prevent soft tissue inflammation.
• When chronic dry mouth occurs, advise patient to:
   • Avoid mouth rinses with high alcohol content because of drying effects.
   • Use daily home fluoride products for anticaries effect.
   • Use sugarless gum, frequent sips of water, or saliva substitutes.

bupropion

byoo-**proe**′-pee-on
(Wellbutrin, Wellbutrin SR, Wellbutrin XL, Zyban, Zyban sustained release[AUS])
Do not confuse bupropion with buspirone, Wellbutrin with Wellcovorin or Wellferon, or Zyban with Zagam.

CATEGORY AND SCHEDULE

Pregnancy Risk Category: B

Drug Class: Antidepressant

MECHANISM OF ACTION

An aminoketone that blocks the reuptake of neurotransmitters, including serotonin and norepinephrine at CNS presynaptic membranes, increasing their availability at postsynaptic receptor sites. Also reduces the firing rate of noradrenergic neurons.
Therapeutic Effect: Relieves depression and nicotine withdrawal symptoms.

USES
Treatment of depression; smoking cessation treatment (Zyban)

PHARMACOKINETICS
Rapidly absorbed from the GI tract. Protein binding: 84%. Crosses the blood-brain barrier. Undergoes extensive first-pass metabolism in the liver to active metabolite. Primarily excreted in urine.
Half-life: 14 hr.

INDICATIONS AND DOSAGES
▸ **Depression**
PO (Immediate-Release)
Adults. Initially, 100 mg twice a day. May increase to 100 mg 3 times a day no sooner than 3 days after beginning therapy. Maximum: 450 mg/day.
Elderly. 37.5 mg twice a day. May increase by 37.5 mg q3–4 days. Maintenance: Lowest effective dosage.
PO (Sustained-Release)
Adults. Initially, 150 mg/day as a single dose in the morning. May increase to 150 mg twice a day as early as day 4 after beginning therapy. Maximum: 400 mg/day.
Elderly. 50–100 mg/day. May increase by 50–100 mg/day q3–4 days. Maintenance: Lowest effective dosage.
PO (Extended-Release)
Adults. 150 mg once a day. May increase to 300 mg once a day. Maximum: 450 mg a day.
▸ **Smoking Cessation**
PO
Adults. Initially, 150 mg a day for 3 days; then 150 mg twice a day for 7–12 wk.

SIDE EFFECTS/ADVERSE REACTIONS
Frequent
Constipation, weight gain or loss, nausea, vomiting, anorexia, dry mouth, headache, diaphoresis, tremors, sedation, insomnia, dizziness, agitation
Occasional
Diarrhea, akinesia, blurred vision, tachycardia, confusion, hostility, fatigue

PRECAUTIONS AND CONTRAINDICATIONS
Current or prior diagnosis of anorexia nervosa or bulimia, seizure disorder, use within 14 days of MAOIs
Caution:
Renal and hepatic disease, recent MI, cranial trauma, lactation, children, low abuse potential; increased CNS or psychiatric symptoms may occur with use

DRUG INTERACTIONS OF CONCERN TO DENTISTRY
• Increased adverse reactions (seizures): tricyclic antidepressants, phenothiazines, benzodiazepines, alcohol, haloperidol, and trazodone
• Decreased serum levels with carbamazepine
• Inhibits CYP2D6 isoenzymes; use with caution; other drugs metabolized by this enzyme

SERIOUS REACTIONS
❗ The risk of seizures increases in patients taking more than 150 mg/dose of bupropion, in patients with a history of bulimia or seizure disorders, and in patients

discontinuing drugs that may lower the seizure threshold.

DENTAL CONSIDERATIONS

General:
• Assess salivary flow as a factor in caries, periodontal disease, and candidiasis.
• Short appointments and a stress-reduction protocol may be required for anxious patients.
• See nicotine dose forms for additional smoking cessation considerations.

Consultations:
• Medical consultation may be required to assess disease control and patient's ability to tolerate stress.
• Physician should be informed if significant xerostomic side effects occur (e.g., increased caries, sore tongue, problems eating or swallowing, difficulty wearing prosthesis) so that a medication change can be considered.

Teach Patient/Family:
• When chronic dry mouth occurs, advise patient to:
  • Avoid mouth rinses with high alcohol content because of drying effects.
  • Use daily home fluoride products for anticaries effect.
  • Use sugarless gum, frequent sips of water, or saliva substitutes.

buspirone hydrochloride

byoo-**spir′**-own hi-droh-**klor′**-ide
(BuSpar, Buspirex[CAN], Bustab[CAN])
Do not confuse buspirone with bupropion.

CATEGORY AND SCHEDULE
Pregnancy Risk Category: B

Drug Class: Antianxiety agent

MECHANISM OF ACTION
Although its exact mechanism of action is unknown, this nonbarbiturate is thought to bind to serotonin and dopamine receptors in the CNS. The drug may also increase norepinephrine metabolism in the locus ceruleus.
Therapeutic Effect: Produces anxiolytic effect.

USES
Management and short-term relief of anxiety disorders; unapproved: PMS

PHARMACOKINETICS
Rapidly and completely absorbed from the GI tract. Protein binding: 95%. Undergoes extensive first-pass metabolism. Metabolized in the liver to active metabolite. Primarily excreted in urine. Not removed by hemodialysis. *Half-life:* 2–3 hr.

INDICATIONS AND DOSAGES
▶ **Short-Term Management (up to 4 wk) of Anxiety Disorders**
PO
Adults. 5 mg 2–3 times a day or 7.5 mg twice a day. May increase by 5 mg/day every 2–4 days.
Maintenance: 15–30 mg/day in 2–3

divided doses. Maximum: 60 mg/day.
Elderly. Initially, 5 mg twice a day. May increase by 5 mg/day every 2–3 days. Maximum: 60 mg/day.
Children. Initially, 5 mg/day. May increase by 5 mg/day at weekly intervals. Maximum: 60 mg/day.

SIDE EFFECTS/ADVERSE REACTIONS

Frequent
Dizziness, somnolence, nausea, headache

Occasional
Nervousness, fatigue, insomnia, dry mouth, lightheadedness, mood swings, blurred vision, poor concentration, diarrhea, paraesthesia

Rare
Muscle pain and stiffness, nightmares, chest pain, involuntary movements

PRECAUTIONS AND CONTRAINDICATIONS

Concurrent use of MAOIs, severe hepatic or renal impairment

Caution:
Lactation, elderly, impaired hepatic/renal function

DRUG INTERACTIONS OF CONCERN TO DENTISTRY

• Increased sedation: alcohol, all CNS depressants
• Increased plasma levels: fluconazole, ketoconazole, itraconazole, miconazole, erythromycin, clarithromycin, troleandomycin

SERIOUS REACTIONS

❗ Buspirone does not appear to cause drug tolerance, psychological or physical dependence, or withdrawal syndrome.
❗ Overdose may produce severe nausea, vomiting, dizziness, drowsiness, abdominal distention, and excessive pupil contraction.

DENTAL CONSIDERATIONS

General:
• Monitor vital signs at every appointment because of cardiovascular side effects.
• Assess salivary flow as a factor in caries, periodontal disease, and candidiasis.
• Short appointments and a stress-reduction protocol may be required for anxious patients.
• Determine why the patient is taking the drug.

Consultations:
• Medical consultation may be required to assess disease control.

Teach Patient/Family:
• When chronic dry mouth occurs, advise patient to:
   • Avoid mouth rinses with high alcohol content because of drying effects.
   • Use daily home fluoride products for anticaries effect.
   • Use sugarless gum, frequent sips of water, or saliva substitutes.

busulfan
byoo-**sull'**-fan
(Busulfex, Myleran)
Do not confuse Myleran with Alkeran, Leukeran, or Mylicon.

CATEGORY AND SCHEDULE
Pregnancy Risk Category: D

Drug Class: Antineoplastic

MECHANISM OF ACTION
An alkylating agent that interferes with DNA replication and RNA

synthesis. Cell cycle-phase nonspecific.
Therapeutic Effect: Disrupts nucleic acid function and causes myelosuppression.

USES
Treatment of chronic myelogenous leukemia, orphan drug in preparative therapy for malignancies treated with bone marrow transplant

PHARMACOKINETICS
Completely absorbed from the GI tract. Protein binding: 33%. Metabolized in the liver. Primarily excreted in urine. Minimally removed by hemodialysis. *Half-life:* 2.5 hr.

INDICATIONS AND DOSAGES
▸ **Remission Induction in Chronic Myelogenous Leukemia (CML)**
PO
Adults, Elderly. 4–8 mg/day up to 12 mg/day. Maintenance: 1–4 mg/day to 2 mg/wk. Continue until WBC count is 10,000–20,000/mm³, resume when WBC count reaches 50,000/mm³.
Children. 0.06–0.12 mg/kg/day. Maintenance: Titrate to maintain leukocyte count above 40,000/mm³, reduce dose by 50% if count is 30,000–40,000/mm³, and discontinue if the count is 20,000/mm³ or less.
▸ **Marrow Ablative Conditioning for Bone Marrow Transplantation**
IV
Adults, Elderly, Children weighing more than 12 kg. 0.8 mg/kg/dose q6h for total of 16 doses. (Use IBW or ABW, whichever is lower.)
Children weighing 12 kg or less. 1.1 mg/kg/dose (IBW) q6h for 16 doses.
PO
Adults, Elderly, Children. 1 mg/kg/dose (IBW) q6h for 16 doses.

SIDE EFFECTS/ADVERSE REACTIONS
Expected
Nausea, stomatitis, vomiting, anorexia, insomnia, diarrhea, fever, abdominal pain, anxiety
Frequent
Headache, rash, asthenia, infection, chills, tachycardia, dyspepsia
Occasional
Constipation, dizziness, edema, pruritus, cough, dry mouth, depression, abdominal enlargement, pharyngitis, hiccups, back pain, alopecia, myalgia
Rare
Injection site pain, arthralgia, confusion, hypotension, lethargy

PRECAUTIONS AND CONTRAINDICATIONS
Disease resistance to previous therapy with this drug
Caution:
Women of childbearing age, leukopenia, thrombocytopenia, anemia, hepatotoxicity, renal toxicity

DRUG INTERACTIONS OF CONCERN TO DENTISTRY
• Acetaminophen may reduce clearance if given within 72 hr before busulfan administration.

SERIOUS REACTIONS
! Busulfan's major adverse effect is myelosuppression, resulting in hematologic toxicity, as evidenced by anemia, severe leukopenia, and severe thrombocytopenia.
! Very high busulfan dosages may produce blurred vision, muscle twitching, and tonic-clonic seizures.
! Long-term therapy (more than 4 yr) may produce pulmonary syndrome ("busulfan lung"), characterized by persistent cough, congestion, crackles, and dyspnea.

B

! Hyperuricemia may produce uric acid nephropathy, renal calculi, and acute renal failure.

DENTAL CONSIDERATIONS

General:
• Patients taking opioids for acute or chronic pain should be given alternative analgesics for dental pain.
• Consider semisupine chair position for patient comfort if GI side effects occur.
• Chlorhexidine mouth rinse (nonalcoholic) before and during chemotherapy may reduce severity of mucositis.
• Patients on chronic drug therapy may rarely have symptoms of blood dyscrasias, which can include infection, bleeding, and poor healing.
• Palliative medication may be required for management of oral side effects.
• Apply lubricant to dry lips for patient comfort before dental procedures.
• Assess salivary flow as factor in caries, periodontal disease, and candidiasis.
• Patients in active chemotherapy treatment should have adequate WBC count before completing dental procedures that may produce a wound. Consultation with the oncologist may be required to determine WBC counts before treatment.

Consultations:
• Medical consultation may be required to assess disease control and patient's ability to tolerate stress.
• In a patient with symptoms of blood dyscrasias, request a medical consultation for blood studies and postpone dental treatment until normal values are reestablished.
• Consult oncologist; prophylactic or therapeutic antibiotics may be indicated to prevent or treat infection if surgery or deep scaling is planned.

Teach Patient/Family to:
• Use effective oral hygiene to prevent soft tissue inflammation.
• Prevent trauma when using oral hygiene aids.
• Report oral lesions, soreness, or bleeding to dentist.
• See dentist immediately if secondary oral infection occurs.
• Update medical/drug record if physician makes any changes in evaluation or drug regimen.
• When chronic dry mouth occurs, advise patient to:
  • Avoid mouth rinses with high alcohol content because of drying effects.
  • Use daily home fluoride products for anticaries effect.
  • Use sugarless gum, frequent sips of water, or artificial saliva substitutes.

butabarbital sodium
byoo-tah-**bar**′-bi-tal
(Butisol)

CATEGORY AND SCHEDULE
Pregnancy Risk Category: D
Controlled Substance: Schedule III

Drug Class: Anticonvulsant; antihyperbilirubinemic; sedative-hypnotic

MECHANISM OF ACTION
A barbiturate and nonselective CNS depressant that binds at GABA receptor complex, enhancing GABA activity.
Therapeutic Effect: Produces hypnotic effect caused by CNS depression.

USES
May be used before surgery to relieve anxiety or tension. In addition, some are used as anticonvulsants to help control seizures in certain disorders or diseases, such as epilepsy.

PHARMACOKINETICS
Widely distributed. Metabolized in liver. Minimally excreted unchanged in urine. *Half-life:* 34–100 hr.

INDICATIONS AND DOSAGES
▶ **Insomnia, Short-Term**
PO
Adults. 50–100 mg at bedtime.
▶ **Preoperative Sedation**
PO
Adults. 50–100 mg, 60–90 min before surgery.
Children. 2–6 mg/kg. Maximum: 100 mg.
▶ **Sedation, Daytime**
PO
Adults. 15–30 mg 3–4 times a day.

SIDE EFFECTS/ADVERSE REACTIONS
Occasional
Somnolence
Rare
Confusion, dizziness, agitation, nausea, vomiting, constipation, headache, hypotension, acne

PRECAUTIONS AND CONTRAINDICATIONS
Porphyria, barbiturate sensitivity

DRUG INTERACTIONS OF CONCERN TO DENTISTRY
• Nephrotoxicity and/or hepatotoxicity: halogenated hydrocarbon anesthetics
• Increased CNS depression: alcohol and all other CNS depressants
• Increased metabolism of oral anticoagulants, glucocorticoids, carbamazepine, tricyclic antidepressants

SERIOUS REACTIONS
! Skin eruptions appear as hypersensitivity reaction.
! Blood dyscrasias, liver disease, and hypocalcemia occur rarely.

DENTAL CONSIDERATIONS
General:
• Determine why patient is taking the drug.
• Monitor vital signs at every appointment due to cardiovascular side effects.
• Patient on chronic drug therapy may rarely present with symptoms of blood dyscrasias, which can include infection, bleeding and poor healing. If dyscrasia is present, caution patient to prevent oral tissue trauma when using oral hygiene aids.
• When used for sedation in dentistry:
   • Have responsible person drive patient to and from dental office when drug used for conscious sedation.
   • After supine positioning, have patient sit upright for at least 2 min before standing to avoid orthostatic hypotension.
   • Geriatric patients are more susceptible to drug effects; use lower dose.
   • Barbiturates induce certain liver enzymes that can alter the

metabolism of other drugs (see drug interactions).

Consultations:

• In a patient with symptoms of blood dyscrasias, request a medical consultation for blood studies and postpone treatment until normal values are reestablished.

Teach Patient/Family to:

• Avoid driving or other activities requiring mental alertness.

• Avoid alcohol ingestion or CNS depressants; serious CNS depression may result.

• Avoid OTC preparations that contain CNS depressants (antihistamine, cold remedies).

• Update health and medication history if physician makes any changes in evaluation or drug regimens; include OTC, herbal, and nonherbal remedies in the update.

butenafine
byoo-**ten′**-ah-feen
(Mentax)

CATEGORY AND SCHEDULE
Pregnancy Risk Category: B

Drug Class: Antifungal

MECHANISM OF ACTION
An antifungal agent that locks biosynthesis of ergosterol, essential for fungal cell membrane. Fungicidal.
Therapeutic Effect: Relieves athlete's foot.

USES
Treatment of tinea pedis caused by *E. floccosum, T. mentagrophytes* or *T. rubrum;* and tinea versicolor caused by *Malassezia furfur*

PHARMACOKINETICS
Total amount absorbed into systemic circulation has not been determined. Metabolized in liver. Excreted in urine. *Half-life:* 35 hr.

INDICATIONS AND DOSAGES
▶ **Tinea Pedis, Tinea Corporis, Tinea Cruris, Tinea Versicolor**
Topical
Adults, Elderly, Children 12 yr and older. Apply to affected area and immediate surrounding skin daily for 4 wk.

SIDE EFFECTS/ADVERSE REACTIONS
Occasional
Contact dermatitis, burning/stinging, worsening of the condition
Rare
Erythema, irritation, pruritus

PRECAUTIONS AND CONTRAINDICATIONS
Hypersensitivity to butenafine or any component of the formulation
Caution:
External use only, lactation, children younger than 12 yr, not for oral use

DRUG INTERACTIONS OF CONCERN TO DENTISTRY
• None reported

SERIOUS REACTIONS
! None known

butoconazole
byoo-toe-**ko′**-na-zole
(Gynazole-1, Femstat One[CAN])
Mycelex-32%

CATEGORY AND SCHEDULE
Pregnancy Risk Category: C

Drug Class: Antifungal

MECHANISM OF ACTION
An antifungal similar to imidazole derivatives that inhibits the steroid synthesis, a vital component of fungal cell formation, thereby damaging the fungal cell membrane. *Therapeutic Effect:* Fungistatic.

USES
Treatment of vulvovaginal infections caused by *Candida* spp.

PHARMACOKINETICS
Not known

INDICATIONS AND DOSAGES
▸ **Treatment of Candidiasis**
Topical
Adults, Elderly. Insert 1 full applicator intravaginally at bedtime for up to 6 days.

SIDE EFFECTS/ADVERSE REACTIONS
Occasional
Vaginal itching, burning, irritation

PRECAUTIONS AND CONTRAINDICATIONS
Hypersensitivity to butoconazole or any of its components
Caution:
Lactation

SERIOUS REACTIONS
! Soreness, swelling, pelvic pain, or cramping rarely occurs.

DENTAL CONSIDERATIONS

General:
• Examine oral mucous membranes for signs of yeast infection.
• Broad-spectrum antibiotics for dental infections may cause vaginal yeast infection.

butorphanol tartrate
byoo-**tor**'-fa-nole
Schedule IV
(Stadol, Stadol NS)
Do not confuse butorphanol with butabarbital or Stadol with Haldol.

CATEGORY AND SCHEDULE
Pregnancy Risk Category: C, D if used for prolonged time, high dose at term
Controlled Substance: Schedule IV

Drug Class: Analgesic; anesthesia adjunct; anesthesia adjunct, opioid analgesic; antidiarrheal; antitussive; pulmonary edema therapy adjunct; suppressant, narcotic abstinence syndrome

MECHANISM OF ACTION
An opioid that binds to opiate receptor sites in the CNS. Reduces intensity of pain stimuli incoming from sensory nerve endings. *Therapeutic Effect:* Alters pain perception and emotional response to pain.

USES
Pain relief

PHARMACOKINETICS

Route	Onset	Peak	Duration
IM	10–30 min	30–60 min	3–4 hr
IV	Less than 1 min	30 min	2–4 hr
Nasal	15 min	1–2 hr	4–5 hr

Rapidly absorbed after IM injection. Protein binding: 80%. Extensively metabolized in the liver. Primarily

B

excreted in urine. *Half-life:*
2.5–4 hr.

INDICATIONS AND DOSAGES
▸ **Analgesia**
IV
Adults. 0.5–2 mg q3–4h as needed.
Elderly. 1 mg q4–6h as needed.
IM
Adults. 1–4 mg q3–4h as needed.
Elderly. 1 mg q4–6h as needed.
▸ **Migraine**
Nasal
Adults. 1 mg or 1 spray in one
nostril. May repeat in 60–90 min.
May repeat 2-dose sequence q3–4h
as needed. Alternatively, 2 mg or 1
spray each nostril if patient remains
recumbent, may repeat in 3–4 hr.

SIDE EFFECTS/ADVERSE
REACTIONS
Frequent
Parenteral: Somnolence, dizziness
Nasal: Nasal congestion, insomnia
Occasional
Parenteral: Confusion, diaphoresis,
clammy skin, lethargy, headache,
nausea, vomiting, dry mouth
Nasal: Vasodilation, constipation,
unpleasant taste, dyspnea, epistaxis,
nasal irritation, upper respiratory
tract infection, tinnitus
Rare
Parenteral: Hypotension, pruritus,
blurred vision, sensation of heat,
CNS stimulation, insomnia
Nasal: Hypertension, tremor, ear
pain, paresthesia, depression,
sinusitis

PRECAUTIONS AND
CONTRAINDICATIONS
CNS disease that affects
respirations, physical dependence on
other opioid analgesics, preexisting
respiratory depression, pulmonary
disease

DRUG INTERACTIONS OF
CONCERN TO DENTISTRY
• Increased CNS depression: alcohol
and all CNS depressants
• Decreased effects of:
buprenorphine
• Use caution or avoid use in
patients taking MAOIs
• Avoid use in narcotic-dependent
persons
• Possible decrease in effects: drugs
that induce CYP3A4 isoenzymes
(phenobarbital, carbamazepine)
• Possible increase in effects: drugs
that inhibit CYP3A4 isoenzymes
(ketoconazole, itraconazole,
erythromycin, protease inhibitors)

SERIOUS REACTIONS
! Abrupt withdrawal after prolonged
use may produce symptoms of
narcotic withdrawal, such as
abdominal cramping, rhinorrhea,
lacrimation, anxiety, increased
temperature, and piloerection or
goose bumps.
! Overdose results in severe
respiratory depression, skeletal
muscle flaccidity, cyanosis, and
extreme somnolence progressing to
seizures, stupor, and coma.
! Tolerance to analgesic effect and
physical dependence may occur with
chronic use.

DENTAL CONSIDERATIONS
General:
• Monitor vital signs at every
appointment due to cardiovascular
side effects.
• This is an acute-use drug; it is
doubtful that patients will undergo
dental treatment during severe
migraine attacks.
• After supine positioning, have
patient sit upright for at least 2 min
before standing to avoid orthostatic
hypotension.

• Psychologic and physical dependence may occur with chronic administration.
• Determine why patient is taking the drug.
• If additional analgesia is required for dental pain, consider alternative analgesics (NSAIDs) in patients taking narcotics for acute or chronic pain.

Teach Patient/Family to:
• Avoid driving or other activities requiring mental alertness.

• Avoid alcohol ingestion or CNS depressants; serious CNS depression may result.
• Avoid OTC preparations that contain CNS depressants (antihistamine, cold remedies).
• Update health and medication history if physician makes any changes in evaluation or drug regimens; include OTC, herbal, and nonherbal remedies in the update.

C

cabergoline
kab-err-**go**′-leen
(Dostinex)

CATEGORY AND SCHEDULE
Pregnancy Risk Category: B

Drug Class: Dopamine agonist;
antihyperprolactinemic

MECHANISM OF ACTION
Agonist at dopamine D_2 receptors,
suppressing prolactin secretion.
Therapeutic Effects: Shrinks
prolactinomas, restores gonadal
function.

USES
Treatment of different types of
medical problems that occur when
too much of the hormone prolactin
is produced. It can be used to treat
certain menstrual problems, fertility
problems in men and women, and
pituitary prolactinomas (tumors of
the pituitary gland).

PHARMACOKINETICS
Cabergoline is administered orally
and undergoes significant first-pass
metabolism following systemic
absorption. Extensively metabolized
in the liver. Elimination is
primarily in the feces. *Half-life:*
80 hr.

INDICATIONS AND DOSAGES
▸ **Hyperprolactinemia (Idiopathic or
Primary Pituitary Adenomas)**
PO
Adults, Elderly. 0.25 mg 2 times a
week, titrate by 0.25 mg/dose no
more than every 4 wk up to 1 mg 2
times a week.
PV
Adults. 0.5 mg 2 to 5 times a
week.

▸ **Parkinson's Disease**
PO
Adults. 0.5 mg/day and titrate to
response. Mean effective dose is
3 mg/day and ranges from 0.5 to
6 mg/day.
▸ **Restless Legs Syndrome (RLS)**
PO
Adults. 0.5 mg once daily at
bedtime, slowly titrate until
symptoms resolve or drug-
intolerance limits further
adjustment. Mean effective dose is
2 mg/day and ranges from 1 to
4 mg/day.

SIDE EFFECTS/ADVERSE REACTIONS
Frequent
Nausea, orthostatic hypotension,
confusion, dyskinesia,
hallucinations, peripheral edema
Occasional
Headache, vertigo, dizziness,
dyspepsia, postural hypotension,
constipation, asthenia, fatigue,
abdominal pain, drowsiness
Rare
Vomiting, dry mouth, diarrhea,
flatulence, anxiety, depression,
dysmenorrhea, dyspepsia,
mastalgia, paresthesias,
vertigo, visual impairment,
pleuropulmonary changes, pleural
effusion, pulmonary fibrosis, heart
failure, peptic ulcer

PRECAUTIONS AND CONTRAINDICATIONS
Hypersensitivity to cabergoline,
ergot alkaloids or any one of its
components. Uncontrolled
hypertension.

DRUG INTERACTIONS OF CONCERN TO DENTISTRY
• None reported

SERIOUS REACTIONS

! Overdosage may produce nasal congestion, syncope, or hallucinations.

DENTAL CONSIDERATIONS

General:
• Determine why patient is taking the drug.
• Monitor vital signs at every appointment for cardiovascular side effects.
• After supine positioning, have patient sit upright for at least 2 min before standing to avoid orthostatic hypotension.
• Use precaution if sedation or general anesthesia is required; risk of hypotensive episode.
• Assess salivary flow as a factor in caries, periodontal disease, and candidiasis.
• Consider semisupine chair position for patient comfort if GI side effects occur.
Consultations:
• Medical consultation may be required to assess disease control.
Teach Patient/Family:
• When chronic dry mouth occurs, advise patient to:
  • Avoid mouth rinses with high alcohol content because of drying effects.
  • Use daily home fluoride products for anticaries effect.
  • Use sugarless gum, frequent sips of water, or saliva substitutes.
• Update health and medication history if physician makes any changes in evaluation or drug regimens; include OTC, herbal, and nonherbal remedies in the update.

calcitonin

kal-si-**toe**'-nin
(Calcimar, Caltine[CAN], Cibacalcin, Miacalcin)
Do not confuse calcitonin with calcitriol.

CATEGORY AND SCHEDULE

Pregnancy Risk Category: C

Drug Class: Synthetic polypeptide calcitonins

MECHANISM OF ACTION

A synthetic hormone that decreases osteoclast activity in bones, decreases tubular reabsorption of sodium and calcium in the kidneys, and increases absorption of calcium in the GI tract.
Therapeutic Effect: Regulates serum calcium concentrations.

USES

Treatment of Paget's disease, postmenopausal osteoporosis, hypercalcemia

PHARMACOKINETICS

Injection form rapidly metabolized (primarily in kidneys); primarily excreted in urine. Nasal form rapidly absorbed. *Half-life:* 70–90 min (injection); 43 min (nasal).

INDICATIONS AND DOSAGES
▸ Skin Testing Before Treatment in Patients with Suspected Sensitivity to Calcitonin-Salmon
Intracutaneous
Adults, Elderly. Prepare a 10-international units/ml dilution; withdraw 0.05 ml from a 200-international units/ml vial in a tuberculin syringe; fill up to 1 ml with 0.9% NaCl. Take 0.1 ml and inject intracutaneously on inner

C

aspect of forearm. Observe after 15 min; a positive response is the appearance of more than mild erythema or wheal.

▸ **Paget's Disease**
IM, Subcutaneous
Adults, Elderly. Initially, 100 international units/day.
Maintenance: 50 international units/day or 50–100 international units every 1–3 days.
Intranasal
Adults, Elderly. 200–400 international units/day.

▸ **Osteoporosis Imperfecta**
IM, Subcutaneous
Adults. 2 international units/kg 3 times a wk.

▸ **Postmenopausal Osteoporosis**
IM, Subcutaneous
Adults, Elderly. 100 international units/day with adequate calcium and vitamin D intake.
Intranasal
Adults, Elderly. 200 international units/day as a single spray, alternating nostrils daily.

▸ **Hypercalcemia**
IM, Subcutaneous
Adults, Elderly. Initially, 4 international units/kg q12h; may increase to 8 international units/kg q12h if no response in 2 days; may further increase to 8 international units/kg q6h if no response in another 2 days.

SIDE EFFECTS/ADVERSE REACTIONS
Frequent
IM, Subcutaneous: Nausea (may occur 30 min after injection, usually diminishes with continued therapy), inflammation at injection site
Nasal: Rhinitis, nasal irritation, redness, sores
Occasional
IM, Subcutaneous: Flushing of face or hands

Nasal: Back pain, arthralgia, epistaxis, headache
Rare
IM, Subcutaneous: Epigastric discomfort, dry mouth, diarrhea, flatulence
Nasal: Itching of earlobes, edema of feet, rash, diaphoresis

PRECAUTIONS AND CONTRAINDICATIONS
Hypersensitivity to gelatin desserts or salmon protein
Caution:
Allergy, hypocalcemic tetany, routine monitoring of urine sediment, osteogenic sarcoma in Paget's disease, lactation, children

DRUG INTERACTIONS OF CONCERN TO DENTISTRY
• Supplemental calcium and vitamin D may already be used; do not use additional amounts.

SERIOUS REACTIONS
! Patients with a protein allergy may develop a hypersensitivity reaction.

DENTAL CONSIDERATIONS
General:
• Consider semisupine chair position for patient comfort because of effects of disease or if GI side effects occur.
• Assess salivary flow as factor in caries, periodontal disease, and candidiasis.
Teach Patient/Family to:
• Encourage effective oral hygiene to prevent soft tissue inflammation.
• When chronic dry mouth occurs, advise patient to:
  • Avoid mouth rinses with high alcohol content because of drying effects.
• Use daily home fluoride products for anticaries effect.

• Use sugarless gum, frequent sips of water, or saliva substitutes.

calcitriol
kal-si-**trye**-ole
(Calcijex, Rocaltrol, Vectical)

CATEGORY AND SCHEDULE
Pregnancy Risk Category: C

Drug Class: Fat-soluble vitamin, vitamin D analog

MECHANISM OF ACTION
A fat-soluble vitamin that is essential for absorption, utilization of calcium and phosphate, and normal calcification of bone. *Therapeutic Effect:* Stimulates calcium and phosphate absorption from small intestine, promotes secretion of calcium from bone to blood, promotes renal tubule phosphate resorption, acts on bone cells to stimulate skeletal growth and on parathyroid gland to suppress hormone synthesis and secretion.

USES
Renal failure
Hypoparathyroidism/
pseudohypoparathyroidism
Mild-to-moderate plaque psoriasis
Vitamin D-dependent rickets
Vitamin D-resistant rickets

PHARMACOKINETICS
Rapidly absorbed from small intestine. Extensive metabolism in kidneys. Primarily excreted in feces; minimal excretion in urine. Topical: some systemic absorption. *Half-life:* 5–8 hr. Topical: 3–6 hr.

INDICATIONS AND DOSAGES
▸ **Renal Failure**
PO
Adults, Elderly. 0.25 mcg/day or 0.5–1 mcg every other day. Increases can be made every 4–8 wk, if necessary.
Children. 0.25–2 mcg/day with hemodialysis; 0.014–0.41 mcg/kg/day without hemodialysis.
IV
Adults, Elderly. Initially, 1–2 mcg (0.02 mcg/kg) 3 times/wk. Dose range: 0.5–4 mcg (0.01–0.05 mcg/kg) 3 times/wk. Adjust dose at 2- to 4-wk intervals.
Children. 0.01–0.05 mcg/kg 3 times/wk with hemodialysis.
▸ **Hypoparathyroidism/Pseudohypoparathyroidism**
PO
Adults, Elderly. Initially, 0.25 mcg/day. Range: 0.5–2 mcg/day.
Children 6 yr and older. Initially, 0.25 mcg/day. Range: 0.5–2 mcg/day.
Children 1–5 yr. 0.25–0.75 mcg once daily.
Children less than 1 yr. 0.04–0.08 mcg/kg once daily.
▸ **Psoriasis, Mild-Moderate Plaque**
Topical
Adults. Apply twice/day. Max: 200 g/wk.
▸ **Vitamin D-Dependent Rickets**
PO
Adults, Elderly, Children. 1 mcg once daily.
▸ **Vitamin D-Resistant Rickets**
PO
Adults, Elderly, Children. 0.015–0.02 mcg/kg once daily. Maintenance: 0.03–0.06 mcg/kg once daily. Maximum: 2 mcg once daily.

C

C

SIDE EFFECTS/ADVERSE REACTIONS

Occasional

Oral: Hypercalcemia, headache, irritability, constipation, metallic taste, nausea, polyuria, photophobia, dry mouth, hypercalciuria, nephrolithiasis

Topical: skin discomfort, pruritus, psoriasis (worsening)

PRECAUTIONS AND CONTRAINDICATIONS

Hypersensitivity to calcitriol or other vitamin D products or analogs

Hypercalcemia

Malabsorption syndrome

Vitamin D toxicity

Caution:

Concurrent use with digitalis

Surgery or prolonged immobilization

Ocular exposure

Cardiac disease

Breast-feeding

DRUG INTERACTIONS OF CONCERN TO DENTISTRY

• Aluminum-containing antacid (long-term use): May increase aluminum concentration and aluminum bone toxicity.

• Calcium-containing preparations, thiazide diuretics: May increase the risk of hypercalcemia.

• Didanosine: May alter intestinal PO4 absorption; increased risk of hypermagnesemia.

• Digoxin: May increase risk of arrhythmia.

• Magnesium-containing antacids: May increase magnesium concentration.

• Mineral oil: May cause fat-soluble vitamin malabsorption.

• Vitamin D analogs: Increased risk of hypervitaminosis D, hypercalcemia.

SERIOUS REACTIONS

! Early signs of overdosage are manifested as weakness, headache, somnolence, nausea, vomiting, dry mouth, constipation, muscle and bone pain, and metallic taste sensation.

! Later signs of overdosage are evidenced by polyuria, polydipsia, anorexia, weight loss, nocturia, photophobia, rhinorrhea, pruritus, disorientation, hallucinations, hyperthermia, hypertension, and cardiac arrhythmias.

DENTAL CONSIDERATIONS

General:

• Monitor the patient's BUN, serum alkaline phosphatase, serum calcium, serum creatinine, serum magnesium, serum phosphate, and urinary calcium levels. Know that the therapeutic serum calcium level is 9 to 10 mg/dl.

• Estimate the patient's daily dietary calcium intake.

• Encourage the patient to maintain adequate fluid intake.

• Avoid bright light in the patient's eyes; offer dark glasses for patient comfort.

• Consider semisupine position if the patient experiences GI discomfort.

Consultations:

• Medical consultation may be required to assess disease control.

Teach Patient/Family to:

• Encourage the patient to consume foods rich in vitamin D including eggs, leafy vegetables, margarine, meats, milk, vegetable oils, and vegetable shortening.

• Warn the patient not to take mineral oil during calcitriol therapy.

• Advise the patient receiving chronic renal dialysis not to take

magnesium-containing antacids during calcitriol therapy.
• Encourage the patient to drink plenty of liquids.

candesartan cilexetil
kan-de-**sar′**-tan sill-**ex′**-eh-till
(Atacand)

CATEGORY AND SCHEDULE
Pregnancy Risk Category: C (D if used in second or third trimester)

Drug Class: Angiotensin II (AT1) receptor antagonist, antihypertensive

MECHANISM OF ACTION
An angiotensin II receptor, type AT_1, antagonist that blocks the vasoconstrictor and aldosterone-secreting effects of angiotensin II, inhibiting the binding of angiotensin II to the AT_1 receptors.
Therapeutic Effect: Causes vasodilation, decreases peripheral resistance, and decreases B/P.

USES
Treatment of hypertension, as a single drug or in combination with other antihypertensives

PHARMACOKINETICS
Rapidly, completely absorbed. Protein binding: greater than 99%. Undergoes minor hepatic metabolism to inactive metabolite. Excreted unchanged in urine and in the feces through the biliary system. Not removed by hemodialysis.
Half-life: 9 hr.

INDICATIONS AND DOSAGES
▶ **Hypertension Alone or in Combination with Other Antihypertensives**
PO
Adults, Elderly, Patients with mildly impaired liver or renal function.
Initially, 16 mg once a day in those who are not volume depleted. Can be given once or twice a day with total daily doses of 8–32 mg. Give lower dosage in those treated with diuretics or with severely impaired renal function.

SIDE EFFECTS/ADVERSE REACTIONS
Occasional
Upper respiratory tract infection, dizziness, back and leg pain
Rare
Pharyngitis, rhinitis, headache, fatigue, diarrhea, nausea, dry cough, peripheral edema

PRECAUTIONS AND CONTRAINDICATIONS
Hypersensitivity to candesartan
Caution:
Discontinue drug if pregnancy occurs, risk of fetal and neonatal injury, correct volume depletion if present, renal impairment, pregnancy category C (first trimester) and D (second and third trimesters), lactation

DRUG INTERACTIONS OF CONCERN TO DENTISTRY
• Potential for increased hypotensive effects with other hypotensive and sedative drugs

SERIOUS REACTIONS
❗ Overdosage may manifest as hypotension and tachycardia. Bradycardia occurs less often.
❗ Institute supportive measures.

C

DENTAL CONSIDERATIONS

General:
• Monitor vital signs at every appointment in patients with history of hypertension.
• Evaluate respiration characteristics and rate.
• Consider semisupine chair position for patient comfort if GI side effects occur.
• Observe appropriate limitations of vasoconstrictor doses.
• Limit use of sodium-containing products, such as saline IV fluids, for those patients with a dietary salt restriction.
• Stress from dental procedures may compromise cardiovascular function; determine patient risk.
• Short appointments and a stress-reduction protocol may be required for anxious patients.
• Use precaution if sedation or general anesthesia is required; risk of hypotensive episode.
Consultations:
• Medical consultation may be required to assess disease control and patient's ability to tolerate stress.
Teach Patient/Family to:
• Update health and drug history if physician makes any changes in evaluation or drug regimens.

capecitabine
cap-eh-**site'**-ah-bean
(Xeloda)
Do not confuse Xeloda with Xenical.

CATEGORY AND SCHEDULE
Pregnancy Risk Category: D

Drug Class: Antineoplastic

MECHANISM OF ACTION
An antimetabolite that is enzymatically converted to 5-fluorouracil. Inhibits enzymes necessary for synthesis of essential cellular components.
Therapeutic Effect: Interferes with DNA synthesis, RNA processing, and protein synthesis.

USES
First-line treatment of patients with metastatic colorectal cancer and metastatic breast cancer resistant to both paclitaxel and anthracycline-containing chemotherapy regimens; colorectal cancer when treatment with a fluoropyrimidine alone is preferred

PHARMACOKINETICS
Readily absorbed from the GI tract. Protein binding: less than 60%. Metabolized in the liver. Primarily excreted in urine. **Half-life:** 45 min.

INDICATIONS AND DOSAGES
▸ **Metastatic Breast Cancer, Colon Cancer**
PO
Adults, Elderly. Initially, 2500 mg/m^2/day in 2 equally divided doses approximately q12h for 2 wk. Follow with a 1-wk rest period; given in 3-wk cycles.

SIDE EFFECTS/ADVERSE REACTIONS
Frequent
Diarrhea (sometimes severe), nausea, vomiting, stomatitis, hand-and-foot syndrome (painful palmar-plantar swelling with paresthesia, erythema, and blistering), fatigue, anorexia, dermatitis

Occasional
Constipation, dyspepsia, nail
disorder, headache, dizziness,
insomnia, edema, myalgia

PRECAUTIONS AND CONTRAINDICATIONS
Severe renal impairment
Caution:
Food reduces absorption, renal
insufficiency, altered coagulation
when taken with Coumadin, patients
older than 80 yr, pregnancy category
D, hepatic dysfunction because of
liver metastases, lactation, children
younger than 18 yr, avoid use of
folic acid

DRUG INTERACTIONS OF CONCERN TO DENTISTRY
• Dental drug interactions not
reported; however, patients taking
this drug with coumarin oral
anticoagulants have altered
coagulation parameters, bleeding, or
both; INR or PT should be
physician-monitored.

SERIOUS REACTIONS
! Serious reactions may include
myelosuppression (evidenced by
neutropenia, thrombocytopenia, and
anemia), cardiovascular toxicity
(marked by angina, cardiomyopathy,
and deep vein thrombosis),
respiratory toxicity (marked by
dyspnea, epistaxis, and pneumonia),
and lymphedema.

DENTAL CONSIDERATIONS

General:
• Monitor vital signs at every
appointment because of
cardiovascular side effects.
• Patients on chronic drug therapy
may have symptoms of blood
dyscrasias, which can include

infection, bleeding, and poor
healing.
• Patients taking opioids for acute or
chronic pain should be given
alternative analgesics for dental
pain.
• Short appointments and a stress
reduction protocol may be required
for anxious patients.
• Consider semisupine chair position
for patient comfort if GI side effects
occur.
• Question patient about tolerance of
NSAIDs or aspirin related to GI side
effects of drug.
• Consider local hemostasis
measures to control and prevent
excessive bleeding.
• Examine for oral manifestation of
opportunistic infection.
• Be aware of oral side effects and
potential sequelae.
• Palliative medication may be
required for management of oral
side effects.
• Avoid dental light in patient's eyes;
offer dark glasses for patient
comfort.
• Prophylactic or therapeutic
antibiotics may be indicated to
prevent or treat infection if surgery
or periodontal debridement is
required.
Consultations:
• In a patient with symptoms
of blood dyscrasias, request a
medical consultation for blood
studies and postpone treatment
until normal values are
reestablished.
• Medical consultation may be
required to assess disease control
and patient's ability to receive dental
treatment.
• Consultation with physician may
be necessary if sedation or general
anesthesia is required.

C

Teach Patient/Family to:
• Prevent trauma when using oral hygiene aids.
• See dentist immediately if secondary oral infection occurs.
• Encourage effective oral hygiene to prevent soft tissue inflammation.
• Report oral lesions, soreness, or bleeding to dentist.
• Update health and drug history if physician makes any changes in evaluation or drug regimens.

capsaicin
kap-**say**′-sin
(Zostrix)
Do not confuse with Zovirax.

CATEGORY AND SCHEDULE
Pregnancy Risk Category: C
OTC

Drug Class: Topical analgesic

MECHANISM OF ACTION
A topical analgesic that depletes and prevents reaccumulation of the chemomediator of pain impulses (substance P) from peripheral sensory neurons to CNS.
Therapeutic Effect: Relieves pain.

USES
Treatment of neuralgia associated with herpes zoster or diabetic neuropathy; pain of osteoarthritis and rheumatoid arthritis

PHARMACOKINETICS
None reported

INDICATIONS AND DOSAGES
▸ **Treatment of Neuralgia, Osteoarthritis, Rheumatoid Arthritis**
Topical
Adults, Elderly, Children older than 2 yr. Apply directly to affected area 3–4 times a day. Continue for 14–28 days for optimal clinical response.

SIDE EFFECTS/ADVERSE REACTIONS
Frequent
Burning, stinging, erythema at site of application

PRECAUTIONS AND CONTRAINDICATIONS
Hypersensitivity to capsaicin or any component of the formulation
Caution:
Lactation, avoid use on broken skin

DRUG INTERACTIONS OF CONCERN TO DENTISTRY
• None reported

SERIOUS REACTIONS
! None known

DENTAL CONSIDERATIONS
General:
• Determine why the patient is taking the drug.
• Consider location of lesions and alter dental procedures accordingly.
Teach Patient/Family to:
• Wash hands thoroughly after use and avoid contact with mouth or eyes.

captopril

kap′-toe-pril

(Acenorm[AUS], Capoten, Captohexal[AUS], Novo-Captoril[CAN], Topace[AUS])

Do not confuse captopril with Capitrol.

CATEGORY AND SCHEDULE

Pregnancy Risk Category: C (D if used in second or third trimester)

Drug Class: Angiotensin-converting enzyme (ACE) inhibitor

MECHANISM OF ACTION

An ACE inhibitor that suppresses the renin-angiotensin-aldosterone system and prevents conversion of angiotensin I to angiotensin II, a potent vasoconstrictor; may also inhibit angiotensin II at local vascular and renal sites. Decreases plasma angiotensin II, increases plasma renin activity, and decreases aldosterone secretion.

Therapeutic Effect: Reduces peripheral arterial resistance, pulmonary capillary wedge pressure; improves cardiac output and exercise tolerance.

USES

Treatment of hypertension, heart failure not responsive to conventional therapy, left ventricular dysfunction (LVD) after MI, diabetic nephropathy

PHARMACOKINETICS

Rapidly, well absorbed from the GI tract (absorption is decreased in the presence of food). Protein binding: 25%–30%. Metabolized in the liver. Primarily excreted in urine. Removed by hemodialysis.

Half-life: less than 3 hr (increased in those with impaired renal function).

INDICATIONS AND DOSAGES

▸ **Hypertension**

PO

Adults, Elderly. Initially, 12.5–25 mg 2–3 times a day. After 1–2 wk, may increase to 50 mg 2–3 times a day. Diuretic may be added if no response in additional 1–2 wk. If taken in combination with diuretic, may increase to 100–150 mg 2–3 times a day after 1–2 wk. Maintenance: 25–150 mg 2–3 times a day. Maximum: 450 mg/day.

▸ **CHF**

PO

Adults, Elderly. Initially, 6.25–25 mg 3 times a day. Increase to 50 mg 3 times a day. After at least 2 wk, may increase to 50–100 mg 3 times a day. Maximum: 450 mg/day.

▸ **Post-Myocardial Infarction, Impaired Liver Function**

PO

Adults, Elderly. 6.25 mg a day, then 12.5 mg 3 times a day. Increase to 25 mg 3 times a day over several days up to 50 mg 3 times a day over several week.

▸ **Diabetic Nephropathy Prevention of Kidney Failure**

PO

Adults, Elderly. 25 mg 3 times a day.

Children. Initially 0.3–0.5 mg/kg/dose titrated up to a maximum of 6 mg/kg/day in 2–4 divided doses.

Neonates. Initially, 0.05–0.1 mg/kg/dose q8–24h titrated up to 0.5 mg/kg/dose given q6–24 hr.

Dosage in Renal Impairment.
Creatinine clearance 10–50 ml/min. 75% of normal dosage. Creatinine clearance less than 10 ml/min. 50% of normal dosage.

C

SIDE EFFECTS/ADVERSE REACTIONS
Frequent
Rash
Occasional
Pruritus, dysgeusia (altered taste)
Rare
Headache, cough, insomnia, dizziness, fatigue, paraesthesia, malaise, nausea, diarrhea or constipation, dry mouth, tachycardia

PRECAUTIONS AND CONTRAINDICATIONS
History of angioedema from previous treatment with ACE inhibitors
Caution:
Dialysis patients, hypovolemia, leukemia, scleroderma, lupus erythematosus, blood dyscrasias, CHF, diabetes mellitus, renal disease, thyroid disease, COPD, asthma, discontinue drug if pregnancy is detected

DRUG INTERACTIONS OF CONCERN TO DENTISTRY
• Increased hypotension: alcohol, phenothiazines
• Decreased hypotensive effects: indomethacin and possibly other NSAIDs, sympathomimetics
• Suspected reduction in the antihypertensive and vasodilator effects by salicylates; monitor blood pressure if used concurrently

SERIOUS REACTIONS
❗ Excessive hypotension ("first-dose syncope") may occur in patients with CHF and in those who are severely salt and volume depleted.
❗ Angioedema (swelling of face and lips) and hyperkalemia occur rarely.
❗ Agranulocytosis and neutropenia may be noted in those with collagen vascular disease, including

scleroderma and systemic lupus erythematosus, and impaired renal function.
❗ Nephrotic syndrome may be noted in those with history of renal disease.

DENTAL CONSIDERATIONS

General:
• Monitor vital signs at every appointment because of cardiovascular side effects.
• Observe appropriate limitations of vasoconstrictor doses.
• After supine positioning, have patient sit upright for at least 2 min before standing to avoid orthostatic hypotension.
• Patients on chronic drug therapy may rarely have symptoms of blood dyscrasias, which can include infection, bleeding, and poor healing.
• Assess salivary flow as a factor in caries, periodontal disease, and candidiasis.
• Limit use of sodium-containing products, such as saline IV fluids, for patients with a dietary salt restriction.
• Stress from dental procedures may compromise cardiovascular function; determine patient risk.
• Short appointments and a stress-reduction protocol may be required for anxious patients.
Consultations:
• Medical consultation may be required to assess patient's ability to tolerate stress.
• In a patient with symptoms of blood dyscrasias, request a medical consultation for blood studies and postpone dental treatment until normal values are reestablished.
• Take precautions if dental surgery is anticipated and sedation or

general anesthesia is required; risk of hypotensive episode.

Teach Patient/Family to:
• Encourage effective oral hygiene to prevent soft tissue inflammation.
• Use caution to prevent injury when using oral hygiene aids.
• When chronic dry mouth occurs, advise patient to:
  • Avoid mouth rinses with high alcohol content because of drying effects.
  • Use daily home fluoride products for anticaries effect.
  • Use sugarless gum, frequent sips of water, or saliva substitutes.

carbachol
kar′-ba-kole
(Caroptic, Isopto Carbachol, Miostat)

CATEGORY AND SCHEDULE
Pregnancy Risk Category: C

Drug Class: Antiglaucoma agent, ophthalmic; Antihypertensive agent, ocular, postsurgical; Miotic

MECHANISM OF ACTION
A direct-acting parasympathomimetic agent that stimulates cholinergic receptors resulting in muscarinic and nicotinic effects. Indirectly promotes release of acetylcholine.
Therapeutic Effect: Produces contraction of the iris sphincter muscle, resulting in miosis, and reduction in intraocular pressure associated with decreased resistance to aqueous humor outflow.

USES
Used in the eye to treat glaucoma

PHARMACOKINETICS
None reported

INDICATIONS AND DOSAGES
▸ **Glaucoma**
Ophthalmic
Adults, Elderly. Instill 1–2 drops of 0.75%–3% solution in affected eye(s) up to 3 times a day.
▸ **Miosis, Ophthalmic Surgery**
Ophthalmic
Adults, Elderly. Instill 0.5 ml of 0.01% solution into anterior chamber before or after securing sutures.

SIDE EFFECTS/ADVERSE REACTIONS
Occasional
Blurred vision, burning/irritation of eye, decreased night vision, headache

PRECAUTIONS AND CONTRAINDICATIONS
Acute iritis, hypersensitivity to carbachol or any component of the formulation

DRUG INTERACTIONS OF CONCERN TO DENTISTRY
• None reported

SERIOUS REACTIONS
! None reported

DENTAL CONSIDERATIONS
General:
• Determine why patient is taking the drug.
• Avoid drugs with anticholinergic activity, such as antihistamines, opioids, benzodiazepines, propantheline, atropine, and scopolamine.

C

• Avoid dental light in patient's eyes; offer dark glasses for patient comfort.
• Protect patient's eyes from accidental spatter during dental treatment.
• Question glaucoma patient about compliance with prescribed drug regimen.
Consultations:
• Medical consultation may be required to assess disease control.
Teach Patient/Family to:
• Update health and medication history if physician makes any changes in evaluation or drug regimens; include OTC, herbal, and nonherbal remedies in the update.

carbamazepine

kar-ba-**maz**′-eh-peen
(Apo-Carbamazepine[CAN], Carbatrol, Epitol, Equetro, Tegretol, Tegretol CR[AUS], Tegretol XR, Teril[AUS])
Do not confuse Tegretol with Cartrol, Toradol, or Trental.

CATEGORY AND SCHEDULE
Pregnancy Risk Category: D

Drug Class: Anticonvulsant

MECHANISM OF ACTION
An iminostilbenes derivative that decreases sodium and calcium ion influx into neuronal membranes, reducing post-tetanic potentiation at synapses.
Therapeutic Effect: Reduces seizure activity.

USES
Treatment of tonic-clonic, complex-partial, and mixed seizures; trigeminal neuralgia; unapproved: neurogenic pain, some psychotic disorders, diabetes insipidus, alcohol withdrawal

PHARMACOKINETICS
Slowly and completely absorbed from the GI tract. Protein binding: 75%. Metabolized in the liver to active metabolite. Primarily excreted in urine. Not removed by hemodialysis. *Half-life:* 25–65 hr (decreased with chronic use).

INDICATIONS AND DOSAGES
▶ Seizure Control
PO
Adults, Children older than 12 yr. Initially, 200 mg twice a day. May increase dosage by 200 mg/day at weekly intervals. Range: 400–1200 mg/day in 2–4 divided doses. Maximum: 1.6–2.4 g/day.
Children 6–12 yr. Initially, 100 mg twice a day. May increase by 100 mg/day at weekly intervals. Range: 20–30 mg/kg/day. Maximum: 1000 mg/day.
Children younger than 6 yr. Initially 5 mg/kg/day. May increase at weekly intervals to 10 mg/kg/day up to 20 mg/kg/day.
Elderly. Initially 100 mg 1–2 times a day. May increase by 100 mg/day at weekly intervals. Usual dose 400–1000 mg/day.
▶ Trigeminal Neuralgia, Diabetic Neuropathy
PO
Adults. Initially, 100 mg twice a day. May increase by 100 mg twice a day up to 400–800 mg/day. Maximum: 1200 mg/day.
Elderly. Initially 100 mg 1–2 times a day. May increase by 100 mg/day at weekly intervals. Usual dose 400–1000 mg/day.

SIDE EFFECTS/ADVERSE REACTIONS
Frequent

Drowsiness, dizziness, nausea, vomiting
Occasional

Visual abnormalities (spots before eyes, difficulty focusing, blurred vision), dry mouth or pharynx, tongue irritation, headache, fluid retention, diaphoresis, constipation or diarrhea, behavioral changes in children

PRECAUTIONS AND CONTRAINDICATIONS
Concomitant use of MAOIs, history of myelosuppression, hypersensitivity to tricyclic antidepressants.
Caution:

Glaucoma, hepatic disease, renal disease, cardiac disease, psychosis, lactation, children younger than 6 yr

DRUG INTERACTIONS OF CONCERN TO DENTISTRY
• Decreased metabolism: erythromycin, clarithromycin, propoxyphene, troleandomycin, metronidazole, ketoconazole, fluconazole, itraconazole, or any drug that inhibits CYP450 3A4 enzymes
• Increased serum levels: tricyclic antidepressants, fluoxetine, fluvoxamine, nefazodone, ketoconazole, itraconazole
• Increased CNS depression: haloperidol, phenothiazines
• Decreased half-life: doxycycline
• Potential hepatotoxicity: chronic high doses of carbamazepine with acetaminophen
• Decreased effects of phenobarbital, corticosteroids, benzodiazepines, doxycycline, sertraline

SERIOUS REACTIONS
! Toxic reactions may include blood dyscrasias (such as aplastic anemia, agranulocytosis, thrombocytopenia, leukopenia, leukocytosis, and eosinophilia), cardiovascular disturbances (such as CHF, hypotension or hypertension, thrombophlebitis, and arrhythmias), and dermatologic effects (such as rash, urticaria, pruritus, and photosensitivity).
! Abrupt withdrawal may precipitate status epilepticus.

DENTAL CONSIDERATIONS
General:

• Monitor vital signs at every appointment because of cardiovascular side effects.
• Patients on chronic drug therapy may rarely have symptoms of blood dyscrasias, which can include infection, bleeding, and poor healing.
• Assess salivary flow as a factor in caries, periodontal disease, and candidiasis.
• Short appointments and a stress-reduction protocol may be required for anxious patients.
• Talk with patient about type of epilepsy, seizure frequency, and quality of seizure control.
• Recommend sealants and home fluoride therapy if patient is using the chewable dose form.
Consultations:

• In a patient with symptoms of blood dyscrasias, request a medical consultation for blood studies and postpone dental treatment until normal values are reestablished.
• Medical consultation may be required to assess disease control and patient's ability to tolerate stress.

C

Teach Patient/Family to:
• Encourage effective oral hygiene to prevent soft tissue inflammation.
• Use caution to prevent injury when using oral hygiene aids.
• Use caution when driving or performing other tasks requiring alertness.
• When chronic dry mouth occurs, advise patient to:
  • Avoid mouth rinses with high alcohol content because of drying effects.
  • Use daily home fluoride products for anticaries effect.
  • Use sugarless gum, frequent sips of water, or saliva substitutes.

carbamide peroxide
kahr′-buh-mahyd
(Auro Ear Drops, Debrox, E • R • O Ear, Gly-Oxide, Mollifene Ear Wax Removing, Murine Ear Drops, Orajel Perioseptic, Proxigel) (gel, solution)

CATEGORY AND SCHEDULE
Pregnancy Risk Category: C

Drug Class: Ceruminolytic; topical oral antiinflammatory

MECHANISM OF ACTION
A ceruminolytic that releases oxygen on contact with moist mouth tissues to provide cleansing effects, reduce inflammation, relieve pain, and inhibit odor-forming bacteria. In the ear, oxygen is released and hydrogen peroxide is reduced to water, which enables the chemical reaction.
Therapeutic Effect: Relieves inflammation of gums and lips. Emulsifies and disperses ear wax.

USES
Dental whitener

PHARMACOKINETICS
Not known

INDICATIONS AND DOSAGES
▶ **Earwax Removal**
Topical, Solution
Adults, Elderly, Children 12 yr or older. Tilt head and administer 5–10 drops twice a day for up to 4 days.
Children 12 yr or younger. Tilt head and administer 1–5 drops twice a day for up to 4 days.
▶ **Oral Lesions**
Topical, gel
Adults, Elderly, Children. Apply to affected area 4 times a day.
Topical, solution
Adults, Elderly, Children. Apply several drops undiluted on affected area 4 times a day after meals and at bedtime.

SIDE EFFECTS/ADVERSE REACTIONS
Occasional
Oral: Gingival sensitivity

PRECAUTIONS AND CONTRAINDICATIONS
Dizziness, ear discharge or drainage, ear injury, ear pain, irritation, or rash, hypersensitivity to carbamide peroxide or any one of its components

DRUG INTERACTIONS OF CONCERN TO DENTISTRY
• None reported

SERIOUS REACTIONS
❗ Opportunistic infections caused by organisms like *Candida albicans* are possible with prolonged use.

General:
• For oral ulcers, perform an oral exam to rule out possible local contributing factors such as broken tooth or filling or ill-fitting dentures.
• Question patient about symptom history; onset, duration, and frequency.
• This drug is the principal ingredient in tooth bleaching or whitening agents; avoid excessive use.

Teach Patient/Family:
• To see the dentist if symptoms worsen or do not abate within 7 days.

carbinoxamine maleate

kar-bi-**nox**'-ah-meen **mal**'-ee-ate
(Carboxine, Histex CT, Histex I/E, Histex PD, Histex Pd 12, Palgic, Pediatex, Pediox)

CATEGORY AND SCHEDULE
Pregnancy Risk Category: C

Drug Class: Antihistaminic (H₁-receptor)-decongestant

MECHANISM OF ACTION
An antihistamine that exhibits H1 receptor blocking action.
Therapeutic Effect: Prevents allergic responses mediated by histamine, such as rhinitis.

USES
Treatment of the nasal congestion (stuffy nose), sneezing, and runny nose caused by colds and hay fever

PHARMACOKINETICS
Virtually no intact drug is excreted in urine. ***Half-life:*** 1–20 hr.

INDICATIONS AND DOSAGES
▸ **Allergic Rhinitis**
PO
Adults, Children 6 yr and older. 1 tsp 4 times a day.
Children 18 mo–6 yr. ½ tsp 4 times a day.
Children 9–18 mo. ¼–½ tsp 4 times a day.

SIDE EFFECTS/ADVERSE REACTIONS
Frequent
Somnolence, dizziness, muscle weakness, hypotension, urine retention, thickening of bronchial secretions, dry mouth, nose, throat, or lips; in elderly, sedation, dizziness, hypotension
Occasional
Epigastric distress, vomiting, headache
Rare
Excitability in children

PRECAUTIONS AND CONTRAINDICATIONS
Hypersensitivity or idiosyncrasy to any ingredients, patients taking MAOIs

DRUG INTERACTIONS OF CONCERN TO DENTISTRY
• Increased sedation: alcohol and all CNS depressants
• Prolonged sedative and anticholinergic effects: MAOIs

SERIOUS REACTIONS
! Overdose symptoms may vary from CNS depression, including sedation, apnea, hypotension, cardiovascular collapse, and death, to severe paradoxical reactions, such

as hallucinations, tremor, and seizures.

DENTAL CONSIDERATIONS

General:
• Assess salivary flow as a factor in caries, periodontal disease, and candidiasis.
• Determine why patient is taking the drug.
Teach Patient/Family to:
• Encourage effective oral hygiene to prevent soft tissue inflammation.
• Prevent trauma when using oral hygiene aids.
• When chronic dry mouth occurs, advise patient to:
  • Avoid mouth rinses with high alcohol content because of drying effects.
  • Use daily home fluoride products for anticaries effect.
  • Use sugarless gum, frequent sips of water, or saliva substitutes.

---

carboplatin
kar-bow-**play**'-tin
(Paraplatin)
Do not confuse carboplatin with Cisplatin or Platinol.

CATEGORY AND SCHEDULE
Pregnancy Risk Category: D

Drug Class: Antineoplastic

MECHANISM OF ACTION
A platinum coordination complex that inhibits DNA synthesis by cross-linking with DNA strands, preventing cell division. Cell cycle-phase nonspecific.
Therapeutic Effect: Interferes with DNA function.

USES
Treatment of cancer of the ovaries

PHARMACOKINETICS
Protein binding: Low. Hydrolyzed in solution to active form. Primarily excreted in urine. *Half-life:* 2.6–5.9 hr.

INDICATIONS AND DOSAGES
▶ **Ovarian Carcinoma (Monotherapy)**
IV
Adults. 360 mg/m^2 on day 1, every 4 wk. Do not repeat dose until neutrophil and platelet counts are within acceptable levels. Adjust drug dosage in previously treated patients based on lowest post-treatment platelet or neutrophil count. Increase dosage only once to no more than 125% of starting dose.
▶ **Ovarian Carcinoma (Combination Therapy)**
IV
Adults. 300 mg/m^2 (with cyclophosphamide) on day 1, every 4 wk. Don't repeat dose until neutrophil and platelet counts are within acceptable levels.
Children. 300–600 mg/m^2 every 4 wk for solid tumor, or 175 mg/m^2 every 4 wk for brain tumor.
▶ **Dosage in Renal Impairment**
Initial dosage is based on creatinine clearance; subsequent dosages are based on the patient's tolerance and degree of myelosuppression.

Creatinine Clearance	Dosage Day 1
60 ml/min or greater	360 mg/m^2
41–59 ml/min	250 mg/m^2
16–40 ml/min	200 mg/m^2

SIDE EFFECTS/ADVERSE REACTIONS
Frequent
Nausea, vomiting

C

Occasional

Generalized pain, diarrhea or
constipation, peripheral neuropathy

Rare

Alopecia, asthenia, hypersensitivity
reaction (erythema, pruritus, rash,
urticaria)

PRECAUTIONS AND CONTRAINDICATIONS

History of severe allergic reaction to
cisplatin, platinum compounds, or
mannitol; severe bleeding, severe
myelosuppression

DRUG INTERACTIONS OF CONCERN TO DENTISTRY

• None reported

SERIOUS REACTIONS

! Myelosuppression may be severe,
resulting in anemia, infection,
(sepsis, pneumonia), and bleeding.

! Prolonged treatment may result in
peripheral neurotoxicity.

DENTAL CONSIDERATIONS

General:

• Determine why patient is taking
the drug.

• If additional analgesia is required
for dental pain, consider alternative
analgesics (NSAIDs) in patients
taking narcotics for acute or chronic
pain.

• Examine for oral manifestation of
opportunistic infection.

• Avoid prescribing aspirin-
containing products.

• This drug may be used in the
hospital or on an outpatient basis.
Confirm the patient's disease and
treatment status.

• Patient on chronic drug therapy
may rarely present with symptoms
of blood dyscrasias, which can
include infection, bleeding, and poor
healing. If dyscrasia is present,
caution patient to prevent oral tissue
trauma when using oral hygiene
aids.

• Short appointments and a
stress-reduction protocol may be
required for anxious patients.

• Patients may have received other
chemotherapy or radiation; confirm
medical and drug history.

• Patients may be at risk of
bleeding; check for oral signs.

• Patients may be at risk of
infection.

• Patients may be taking
prophylactic antiinfectives.

• Oral infections should be
eliminated and/or treated
aggressively.

Consultations:

• Medical consultation should
include routine blood counts
including platelet counts and
bleeding time.

• Consult physician; prophylactic or
therapeutic antiinfectives may be
indicated if surgery or periodontal
treatment is required.

• Medical consultation may be
required to assess immunologic
status during cancer chemotherapy
and determine safety risk, if any,
posed by the required dental
treatment.

• Medical consultation may be
required to assess disease control
and patient's ability to tolerate
stress.

Teach Patient/Family to:

• See dentist immediately if
secondary oral infection occurs.

• Encourage effective oral
hygiene to prevent soft tissue
inflammation.

• Report oral lesions, soreness, or
bleeding to dentist.

• Prevent trauma when using oral
hygiene aids.

• Updating health and medication
history if physician makes any

C

changes in evaluation or drug regimens; include OTC, herbal, and nonherbal remedies in the update.

carglumic acid
kar-**gloo**-mik **as**-id
(Carbaglu)

CATEGORY AND SCHEDULE
Pregnancy Risk Category: C

Drug Class: Antidote, metabolic acidosis agent, urea cycle disorder (UCD) treatment agent

MECHANISM OF ACTION
A synthetic analogue of N-acetylglutamate (NAG) that activates carbamoyl phosphate synthetase 1 (CPS 1) in liver mitochondria, which is responsible for converting ammonia to urea during the first step of the urea cycle.
Therapeutic Effect: Allows conversion of ammonia, and thus the excretion of ammonia.

USES
Adjunctive therapy for the treatment of acute hyperammonemia due to the deficiency of the hepatic enzyme N-acetylglutamate synthase (NAGS)
Maintenance therapy for the treatment of chronic hyperammonemia due to the deficiency of the hepatic enzyme NAGS

PHARMACOKINETICS
Metabolized slightly by intestinal bacteria. Primarily excreted in feces. Minimal excretion in urine.
Half-life: 4.3–9.5 hr.

INDICATIONS AND DOSAGES
▸ **Adjunctive Therapy for the Treatment of Acute Hyperammonemia due to the Deficiency of the Hepatic Enzyme N-Acetylglutamate Synthase**
PO or Via Nasogastric Tube
Adults, Adolescents, Children, Infants, Neonates. 100–250 mg/kg/day; divide total daily dose into 2 to 4 doses and give immediately before meals or feeding. Disperse each tablet (200 mg) in a minimum of 2.5 mL of water and take immediately. Titrate dose based on plasma ammonia levels and clinical symptoms.
▸ **Maintenance Therapy for the Treatment of Chronic Hyperammonemia due to the Deficiency of the Hepatic Enzyme N-Acetylglutamate Synthase**
PO
Adults, Adolescents, Children, Infants, Neonates. 100 mg/kg/day; divide total daily dose into 2–4 doses before meals. Disperse each tablet (200 mg) in a minimum of 2.5 mL of water and take immediately. Titrate dose based on plasma ammonia levels and clinical symptoms.

SIDE EFFECTS/ADVERSE REACTIONS
Adults/Children
Frequent
Infections, vomiting, abdominal pain, pyrexia, tonsillitis, anemia, ear infection, diarrhea, nasopharyngitis, headache
Occasional
Diaphoresis, rash, weight reduction, loss of appetite, altered taste, asthenia, somnolence, pneumonia, influenza

PRECAUTIONS AND CONTRAINDICATIONS

Hypersensitivity to carglumic acid or its components
Caution:
Breast-feeding
Elderly

DRUG INTERACTIONS OF CONCERN TO DENTISTRY

• None reported

SERIOUS REACTIONS

! Prolonged exposure to elevated ammonia levels can result in brain injury or death.
! Anemia has been reported.

DENTAL CONSIDERATIONS

General:
• Avoid dental light in patient's eyes; offer dark glasses for patient comfort.
• Place on frequent recall because of oral side effects.
• Consider semisupine chair position for patient comfort if GI side effects occur.
• Monitor for any neurological changes.
Consultations:
• Plasma ammonia levels must be monitored throughout therapy.
• Medical consultation may be required to assess disease control.
Teach Patient/Family to:
• Encourage effective oral hygiene to prevent soft tissue inflammation.
• Prevent trauma when using oral hygiene aids.
• Be alert for the possibility of secondary oral infection and the need to see dentist immediately if signs of infection occur.
• Adhere to dietary recommendations from doctor, such as a low-protein diet.

carisoprodol

kar-ih-so-**pro'**-dol
(Soma)

C

CATEGORY AND SCHEDULE

Pregnancy Risk Category: C

Drug Class: Skeletal muscle relaxant, central acting

MECHANISM OF ACTION

A centrally acting skeletal muscle relaxant whose exact mechanism is unknown. Effects may be because of its CNS depressant actions.
Therapeutic Effect: Relieves muscle spasms and pain.

USES

Adjunct for relief of acute, painful musculoskeletal conditions

PHARMACOKINETICS

Onset 2 hr, duration 4–6 hr.
Half-life: 2.5 hr. Metabolized in liver to meprobamate by the CYP 2C19 isoenzyme; excreted by kidneys.

INDICATIONS AND DOSAGES

▸ **Adjunct to Rest, Physical Therapy, Analgesics, and Other Measures for Relief of Discomfort from Acute, Painful Musculoskeletal Conditions**
PO
Adults, Elderly. 350 mg 4 times a day.

SIDE EFFECTS/ADVERSE REACTIONS

Frequent
Somnolence
Occasional
Tachycardia, facial flushing, dizziness, headache, lightheadedness, dermatitis, nausea,

C

vomiting, abdominal cramps, dyspnea

PRECAUTIONS AND CONTRAINDICATIONS
Acute intermittent porphyria, sensitivity to meprobamate
Caution:
Renal disease, hepatic disease, addictive personalities, elderly, children younger than 12 yr

DRUG INTERACTIONS OF CONCERN TO DENTISTRY
• Increased CNS depression: alcohol, all CNS depressants

SERIOUS REACTIONS
! Overdose may cause CNS and respiratory depression, shock, and coma.

DENTAL CONSIDERATIONS
General:
• When used in dentistry, may be more effective when used in combination with aspirin or NSAIDs.
Teach Patient/Family to:
• Use powered tooth brush if patient has difficulty holding conventional devices.

carmustine
kar-**muss**'-teen
(BiCNU, Gliadel)

CATEGORY AND SCHEDULE
Pregnancy Risk Category: D

Drug Class: Antineoplastic

MECHANISM OF ACTION
An alkylating agent and nitrosourea that inhibits DNA and RNA synthesis by cross-linking with DNA and RNA strands, preventing cell division. Cell cycle-phase nonspecific.
Therapeutic Effect: Interferes with DNA and RNA function.

USES
Treatment of certain types of brain cancer

PHARMACOKINETICS
Degraded within 15 min; crosses blood-brain barrier; 70% excreted in urine within 96 hr; 10% excreted as CO_2; fate of 20% is unknown.

INDICATIONS AND DOSAGES
▶ **Disseminated Hodgkin's Disease, Non-Hodgkin's Lymphoma, Multiple Myeloma, and Primary and Metastatic Brain Tumors in Previously Untreated Patients (Monotherapy)**
IV (BiCNU)
Adults, Elderly. 150–200 mg/m^2 as a single dose or 75–100 mg/m^2 on 2 successive days.
Children. 200–250 mg/m^2 every 4–6 wk as a single dose.
▶ **Implantation (Gliadel)**
Adults, Elderly, Children. Up to 8 wafers may be placed in resection cavity.

SIDE EFFECTS/ADVERSE REACTIONS
Frequent
Nausea and vomiting within min to 2 hr after administration (may last up to 6 hr)
Occasional
Diarrhea, esophagitis, anorexia, dysphagia
Rare
Thrombophlebitis

PRECAUTIONS AND CONTRAINDICATIONS
None known

DRUG INTERACTIONS OF CONCERN TO DENTISTRY
• None reported

SERIOUS REACTIONS
❗ Hematologic toxicity because of myelosuppression occurs frequently. Thrombocytopenia occurs about 4 wk after carmustine treatment begins and lasts 1–2 wk.

❗ Leukopenia is evident 5–6 wk after treatment begins and lasts 1–2 wk. Anemia occurs less frequently and is less severe.

❗ Mild, reversible hepatotoxicity also occurs frequently.

❗ Prolonged high-dose carmustine therapy may produce impaired renal function and pulmonary toxicity (pulmonary infiltrate or fibrosis).

DENTAL CONSIDERATIONS

General:
• Determine why patient is taking the drug.
• If additional analgesia is required for dental pain, consider alternative analgesics in patients taking narcotics for acute or chronic pain.
• Avoid products that affect platelet function, such as aspirin and NSAIDs.
• This drug may be used in the hospital or on an outpatient basis. Confirm the patient's disease and treatment status.
• Consider semisupine chair position for patient comfort if GI side effects occur.
• Patient on chronic drug therapy may rarely present with symptoms of blood dyscrasias, which can include infection, bleeding, and poor

healing. If dyscrasia is present, caution patient to prevent oral tissue trauma when using oral hygiene aids.
• Examine for oral manifestation of opportunistic infection.
• Consider local hemostasis measures to prevent excessive bleeding.
• Monitor vital signs at every appointment because of cardiovascular side effects.
• Use caution with use of potentially hepatotoxic drugs.

Consultations:
• Medical consultation should include routine blood counts including platelet counts and bleeding time.
• Consult physician; prophylactic or therapeutic antiinfectives may be indicated if surgery or periodontal treatment is required.
• In a patient with symptoms of blood dyscrasias, request a medical consultation for blood studies and postpone treatment until normal values are reestablished.
• Medical consultation may be required to assess disease control and patient's ability to tolerate stress.

Teach Patient/Family to:
• Encourage effective oral hygiene to prevent soft tissue inflammation.
• Prevent trauma when using oral hygiene aids.
• Update health and medication history if physician makes any changes in evaluation or drug regimens; include OTC, herbal, and nonherbal remedies in the update.
• Report oral lesions, soreness, or bleeding to dentist.

C

carteolol
kar-**tee**'-oh-lole
(Cartrol, Ocupress)
Do not confuse carteolol with
carvedilol.

CATEGORY AND SCHEDULE
Pregnancy Risk Category: C (D if
after first trimester)

Drug Class: β-adrenergic
blocker

MECHANISM OF ACTION
An antihypertensive that blocks
β_1-adrenergic receptor at normal
doses and β_2-adrenergic receptors at
large doses. Predominantly blocks
β_1-adrenergic receptors in cardiac
tissue. Reduces aqueous humor
production.
Therapeutic Effect: Slows sinus
heart rate, decreases cardiac output,
decreases B/P, increases airway
resistance, decreases intraocular
pressure.

USES
Treatment of chronic open-angle
glaucoma, ocular hypertension

PHARMACOKINETICS
Well absorbed from the GI tract.
Protein binding: unknown.
Minimally metabolized in liver.
Primarily excreted unchanged in
urine. Not removed by hemodialysis.
Half-life: 6 hr (increased in
decreased renal function).

INDICATIONS AND DOSAGES
▸ Ocular Hypertension
PO
Adults, Elderly. Initially, 2.5 mg/day
as single dose either alone or in
combination with diuretic. May

increase gradually to 5–10 mg/day
as a single dose. Maintenance:
2.5–5 mg/day.
▸ **Dosage in Renal Impairment**

Creatinine Clearance	Dosage Interval
Greater than 60 ml/min	24 hr
20–60 ml/min	48 hr
Less than 20 ml/min	72 hr

▸ **Open-Angle Glaucoma, Ocular Hypertension**
Ophthalmic
Adults, Elderly. 1 drop 2 times
a day.

SIDE EFFECTS/ADVERSE REACTIONS
Frequent
Oral: Hypotension manifested as
dizziness, nausea, diaphoresis,
headache, cold extremities, fatigue,
constipation/diarrhea
Ophthalmic: Redness of eye or
inside of eyelids, decreased night
vision
Occasional
Oral: Insomnia, flatulence, urinary
frequency, impotence or decreased
libido
Ophthalmic: Blepharoconjunctivitis,
edema, droopy eyelid, staining of
cornea, blurred vision, brow ache,
increased light sensitivity, burning,
stinging
Rare
Rash, arthralgia, myalgia, confusion
(especially elderly), taste
disturbances

PRECAUTIONS AND CONTRAINDICATIONS
Bronchial asthma, COPD,
bronchospasm, overt cardiac failure,
cardiogenic shock, heart block
greater than first degree, persistently
severe bradycardia.

C

Caution:
Major surgery, lactation, diabetes mellitus, renal disease, thyroid disease, COPD, well-compensated heart failure, coronary artery disease (CAD), nonallergic bronchospasm

DRUG INTERACTIONS OF CONCERN TO DENTISTRY
• Decreased hypotensive effect: indomethacin, NSAIDs
• Increased hypotension, myocardial depression: hydrocarbon inhalation anesthetics
• Hypertension, bradycardia: sympathomimetics (epinephrine, ephedrine)
• Bradycardia: fluoxetine, paroxetine

SERIOUS REACTIONS
! Abrupt withdrawal (particularly in those with CAD) may produce angina or precipitate MI.
! May precipitate thyroid crisis in those with thyrotoxicosis.
! β-blockers may mask signs and symptoms of acute hypoglycemia (tachycardia, B/P changes) in diabetic patients.

DENTAL CONSIDERATIONS
General:
• Monitor vital signs at every appointment because of cardiovascular side effects.
• After supine positioning, have patient sit upright for at least 2 min before standing to avoid orthostatic hypotension.
• Assess salivary flow as a factor in caries, periodontal disease, and candidiasis.
• Patients on chronic drug therapy may rarely have symptoms of blood dyscrasias, which can include infection, bleeding, and poor healing.

• Limit use of sodium-containing products, such as saline IV fluids, for those patients with a dietary salt restriction.
• Stress from dental procedures may compromise cardiovascular function; determine patient risk.
• Short appointments and a stress-reduction protocol may be required for anxious patients.
Consultations:
• In a patient with symptoms of blood dyscrasias, request a medical consultation for blood studies and postpone dental treatment until normal values are reestablished.
• Medical consultation may be required to assess disease control and patient's ability to tolerate stress.
Teach Patient/Family to:
• Report oral lesions, soreness, or bleeding to dentist.
• When chronic dry mouth occurs, advise patient to:
  • Avoid mouth rinses with high alcohol content because of drying effects.
  • Use daily home fluoride products for anticaries effect.
  • Use sugarless gum, frequent sips of water, or saliva substitutes.

carvedilol
kar-vea-die-lole
(Coreg, Coreg CR)

CATEGORY AND SCHEDULE
Pregnancy Risk Category: C (D if used in second or third trimester)

Drug Class: β-Adrenergic Blocker with α-Blocking Activity
Do not confuse carvedilol with carteolol or captopril.

C

MECHANISM OF ACTION
A cardiovascular agent that possesses nonselective β-blocking and α-adrenergic blocking activity. Causes vasodilation.
Therapeutic Effect: Reduces cardiac output, exercise-induced tachycardia, and reflex orthostatic tachycardia; reduces peripheral vascular resistance; inhibits renin release.

USES
Hypertension
Left ventricular dysfunction following myocardial infarction
Heart failure

PHARMACOKINETICS
Rapidly and extensively absorbed from the GI tract following oral administration. Bioavailability: 25%–35% (immediate release formulation); 85% (extended-release). Protein binding: 98%, primarily to albumin. Metabolized in the liver primarily through CYP450 3A4, 2C19, and 2D6 pathway to active metabolites. Excreted primarily via bile into feces. Minimally removed by hemodialysis. *Half-life:* 7–10 hr. Food delays rate of absorption.

INDICATIONS AND DOSAGES
▶ **Hypertension**
PO (Immediate Release)
Adults, Elderly. Initially, 6.25 mg twice a day. May double at 7- to 14-day intervals to highest tolerated dosage. Maximum: 50 mg/day. (25 mg twice a day); if pulse drops below 55 bpm, reduce dose.
PO (Extended Release)
Adults, Elderly. Initially, 20 mg once a day, in the morning with food. May double the dose at 7- to 14-day intervals. Maximum: 80 mg/day.

Note: 6.25 mg of immediate release is equivalent to 20 mg of extended release.
▶ **Myocardial Infarction Prophylaxis in Stable Patients with Left Ventricular Dysfunction**
PO (Immediate Release)
Adults, Elderly. Initially, 3.125–6.25 mg twice a day with food. May increase at intervals of 3–10 days up to target dose of 25 mg twice a day. Maximum: 50 mg/day.
PO (Extended Release)
Adults, Elderly. Initially, 20 mg once a day, in the morning with food. Increase at 3- to 10-day intervals to a target dose of 80 mg a day.

SIDE EFFECTS/ADVERSE REACTIONS
Carvedilol is generally well tolerated, with mild and transient side effects.

Adults
Frequent
Fatigue, dizziness, hyperglycemia, diarrhea, weight gain, hypotension, weakness
Occasional
Bradycardia, rhinitis, back pain, syncope, headache, blurred vision, impotence, nausea, vomiting, angina
Rare
Orthostatic hypotension, somnolence, UTI, viral infection, rash, hypercholesterolemia, gout, weight loss

PRECAUTIONS AND CONTRAINDICATIONS
Hypersensitivity to carvedilol or any component of the formulation
Caution:
Bronchial asthma or related bronchospastic conditions
Cardiogenic shock
Pulmonary edema
Second- or third-degree AV block

Severe bradycardia
Hepatic disease
Heart rate below 55 bpm
Caution use in patients undergoing anesthesia and in those with CHF controlled with ACE inhibitor, digoxin or diuretics; diabetes mellitus; hypoglycemia; impaired hepatic function; peripheral vascular disease; and thyrotoxicosis
Avoid abrupt withdrawal

DRUG INTERACTIONS OF CONCERN TO DENTISTRY

• Calcium blockers: Increase risk of conduction disturbances, hypotension, and/or bradycardia.
• Cimetidine: May increase carvedilol blood concentration.
• Digoxin: Increases concentrations of digoxin.
• Diuretics, other antihypertensives: May increase hypotensive effect.
• Insulin, oral hypoglycemics: May mask symptoms of hypoglycemia and prolong hypoglycemic effect of these drugs.
• Rifampin: Decreases carvedilol blood concentration.
• CYP450 2D6 inhibitors: May decrease the metabolism of CYP2D6 substrates.
• Cyclosporine: Increases concentrations of cyclosporine.

SERIOUS REACTIONS

! Overdose may produce profound bradycardia and hypotension.
! Abrupt withdrawal may result in diaphoresis, palpitations, headache, and tremors.
! Carvedilol administration may precipitate CHF or MI in patients with heart disease; thyroid storm in those with thyrotoxicosis; or peripheral ischemia in those with existing peripheral vascular disease.

! Hypoglycemia may occur in patients with previously controlled diabetes.
! Signs of thrombocytopenia, such as unusual bleeding or bruising, occur rarely.

DENTAL CONSIDERATIONS

General:
• Monitor vital signs at every appointment because of cardiovascular side effects.
• After supine positioning, have patient sit upright for at least 2 min before standing to avoid orthostatic hypotension.
• Assess salivary flow as a factor in caries, periodontal disease, and candidiasis.
• Limit use of sodium-containing products, such as saline IV fluids, for those patients with dietary salt restriction.
• Stress from dental procedures may compromise cardiovascular function; determine patient risk.
Consultations:
• Medical consultation may be required to assess disease control.
Teach Patient/Family to:
Report oral lesions, soreness, or bleeding to dentist.
• When chronic dry mouth occurs, advise patient to:
  • Avoid mouth rinses with high alcohol content because of drying effects.
  • Use daily home fluoride products for anticaries effect.
  • Use sugarless gum, frequent sips of water, or saliva substitutes.

C

caspofungin acetate
kas-poe-**fun**′-gin **ass**′-eh-tayte
(Cancidas)

CATEGORY AND SCHEDULE
Pregnancy Risk Category: C

Drug Class: Antifungal,
systemic

MECHANISM OF ACTION
An antifungal that inhibits the
synthesis of glucan, a vital
component of fungal cell formation,
thereby damaging the fungal cell
membrane.
Therapeutic Effect: Fungistatic.

USES
Help the body overcome serious
fungus infections

PHARMACOKINETICS
Distributed in tissue. Extensively
bound to albumin. Protein binding:
97%. Slowly metabolized in liver to
active metabolite. Excreted primarily
in urine and to a lesser extent in
feces. Not removed by hemodialysis.
Half-life: 40–50 hr.

INDICATIONS AND DOSAGES
▸ **Aspergillosis**
IV
*Adults, Elderly, Children older than
12 yr.* Give single 70-mg loading
dose on day 1, followed by 50 mg/
day thereafter. For patients with
moderate hepatic insufficiency, daily
dose reduced to 35 mg.
▸ **Invasive Candidiasis**
IV
Adults, Elderly. Initially, 70 mg
followed by 50 mg daily.
▸ **Esophageal Candidiasis**
IV
Adult, Elderly. 50 mg a day.

SIDE EFFECTS/ADVERSE REACTIONS
Frequent
Fever
Occasional
Headache, nausea, phlebitis
Rare
Paresthesia, vomiting, diarrhea,
abdominal pain, myalgia, chills,
tremor, insomnia

PRECAUTIONS AND CONTRAINDICATIONS
None known

DRUG INTERACTIONS OF CONCERN TO DENTISTRY
• Reduction in concentration:
dexamethasone, carbamazepine

SERIOUS REACTIONS
! Hypersensitivity reactions
(characterized by rash, facial
swelling, pruritus, and a sensation of
warmth) may occur.

DENTAL CONSIDERATIONS

General:
• For selected infections in the
hospital setting.
• Provide palliative dental care for
dental emergencies only.
• Patient on chronic drug therapy
may rarely present with symptoms
of blood dyscrasias, which can
include infection, bleeding, and poor
healing. If dyscrasia is present,
caution patient to prevent oral tissue
trauma when using oral hygiene
aids.
Consultations:
• In a patient with symptoms of
blood dyscrasias, request a medical
consultation for blood studies and
postpone treatment until normal
values are reestablished.
• Medical consultation may be
required to assess disease control

and patient's ability to tolerate stress.

• Medical consultation should include PPT, PT, or INR.

Teach Patient/Family to:

• Encourage effective oral hygiene to prevent soft tissue inflammation.

• Report oral lesions, soreness, or bleeding to dentist.

• Prevent trauma when using oral hygiene aids.

cefaclor

sef'-ah-klor

(Apo-Cefaclor[CAN], Ceclor, Ceclor CD, Cefkor[AUS], Cefkor CD[AUS], Keflor[AUS])

CATEGORY AND SCHEDULE

Pregnancy Risk Category: B

Drug Class: Antibiotic, cephalosporin (second generation)

MECHANISM OF ACTION

A second-generation cephalosporin that binds to bacterial cell membranes and inhibits cell wall synthesis.

Therapeutic Effect: Bactericidal.

USES

For use in the treatment of the following infections when caused by susceptible strains of named microorganisms: otitis media caused by S. pneumoniae, H. influenzae, staphylococci, and S. pyogenes; lower respiratory tract infections caused by S. pneumoniae, H. influenzae, and S. pyogenes; pharyngitis and tonsillitis caused by S. pyogenes; UTIs caused by E. coli, P. mirabilis, Klebsiella species, and coagulase-negative staphylococci;

skin and skin structure infections caused by S. aureus and S. pyogenes; and in vitro activity against Peptococcus, Peptostreptococcus, and Propionibacterium (clinical significance unknown)

PHARMACOKINETICS

Well absorbed from the GI tract. Protein binding: 25%. Widely distributed. Primarily excreted unchanged in urine. Moderately removed by hemodialysis. *Half-life:* 0.6–0.9 hr (increased in impaired renal function).

INDICATIONS AND DOSAGES

▶ **Bronchitis**

PO (Extended-Release)

Adults, Elderly. 500 mg q12h for 7 days.

▶ **Lower Respiratory Tract Infections**

PO

Adults, Elderly. 250–500 mg q8h.

▶ **Otitis Media**

PO

Children. 20–40 mg/kg/day in 2–3 divided doses. Maximum: 1 g/day.

▶ **Pharyngitis, Skin/Skin Structure Infections, Tonsillitis**

PO (Extended-Release)

Adults, Elderly. 375 mg q12h.

PO (Regular-Release)

Adults, Elderly. 250–500 mg q8h.

Children. 20–40 mg/kg/day in 2–3 divided doses. Maximum: 1 g/day.

▶ **UTIs**

PO

Adults, Elderly. 250–500 mg q8h.

Children. 20–40 mg/kg/day in 2–3 divided doses q8h. Maximum: 1 g/day.

PO (Extended-Release)

Adults, Children older than 16 yr. 375–500 mg q12h.

C

▸ **Otitis Media**
PO
Children older than 1 mo. 40 mg/kg/ day in divided doses q8h.
Maximum: 1 g/day.
▸ **Dosage in Renal Impairment**
Decreased dosage may be necessary in patients with creatinine clearance less than 40 ml/min.

SIDE EFFECTS/ADVERSE REACTIONS
Frequent
Oral candidiasis, mild diarrhea, mild abdominal cramping, vaginal candidiasis
Occasional
Nausea, serum sickness-like reaction (marked by fever and joint pain; usually occurs after the second course of therapy and resolves after the drug is discontinued)
Rare
Allergic reaction (pruritus, rash, and urticaria)

PRECAUTIONS AND CONTRAINDICATIONS
History of anaphylactic reaction to penicillins or hypersensitivity to cephalosporins
Caution:
Hypersensitivity to penicillins, lactation, renal disease

DRUG INTERACTIONS OF CONCERN TO DENTISTRY
• Decreased bactericidal effects: tetracyclines, erythromycins
• Increased and prolonged serum levels: probenecid

SERIOUS REACTIONS
! Antibiotic-associated colitis and other superinfections may result from altered bacterial balance.

! Nephrotoxicity may occur, especially in patients with preexisting renal disease.
! Patients with a history of allergies, especially to penicillin, are at increased risk for developing a severe hypersensitivity reaction, marked by severe pruritus, angioedema, bronchospasm, and anaphylaxis.

DENTAL CONSIDERATIONS
General:
• Take precautions regarding allergy to medication.
• Determine why the patient is taking the drug.
Consultations:
• Medical consultation may be required to assess disease control.
Teach Patient/Family to:
• Encourage effective oral hygiene to prevent soft tissue inflammation.
• Avoid mouth rinses with high alcohol content because of drying effects and possible drug-drug reaction.
• When used for dental infection, advise patient to:
    • Report sore throat, oral burning sensation, fever, and fatigue, any of which could indicate superinfection.
    • Take at prescribed intervals and complete dosage regimen.
    • Immediately notify the dentist if signs or symptoms of infection increase.

cefadroxil
sef-ah-**drox'**-ill
(Duricef)

CATEGORY AND SCHEDULE
Pregnancy Risk Category: B

Drug Class: Cephalosporin (first
generation)

MECHANISM OF ACTION
A first-generation cephalosporin
that binds to bacterial cell
membranes and inhibits cell wall
synthesis.
Therapeutic Effect: Bactericidal.

USES
Treatment of gram-negative bacilli:
E. coli, P. mirabilis, Klebsiella
(UTI only); gram-positive
organisms: *S. pneumoniae,
S. pyogenes, S. aureus*; upper/lower
respiratory tract, urinary tract, skin
infections; otitis media; tonsillitis;
particularly for UTI

PHARMACOKINETICS
Well absorbed from the GI tract.
Protein binding: 15%–20%. Widely
distributed. Primarily excreted
unchanged in urine. Removed by
hemodialysis. **Half-life:** 1.2–1.5 hr
(increased in impaired renal
function).

INDICATIONS AND DOSAGES
▸ **UTIs**
PO
Adults, Elderly. 1–2 g/day as a
single dose or in 2 divided
doses.
Children. 30 mg/kg/day in 2 divided
doses. Maximum: 2 g/day.

▸ **Skin and Skin-Structure Infections,
Group A β-Hemolytic Streptococcal
Pharyngitis, Tonsillitis**
PO
Adults, Elderly. 1–2 g in 2 divided
doses.
Children. 30 mg/kg/day in 2 divided
doses. Maximum: 2 g/day.
▸ **Impetigo**
PO
Children. 30 mg/kg/day as a single
or in 2 divided doses. Maximum:
2 g/day.
▸ **Dosage in Renal Impairment**
After an initial 1-g dose, dosage and
frequency are modified on the basis
of creatinine clearance and the
severity of the infection.

Creatinine Clearance	Dosage Interval
25–50 ml/min	500 mg q12h
10–25 ml/min	500 mg q24h
0–10 ml/min	500 mg q36h

SIDE EFFECTS/ADVERSE REACTIONS
Frequent
Oral candidiasis, mild diarrhea, mild
abdominal cramping, vaginal
candidiasis
Occasional
Nausea, unusual bruising or
bleeding, serum sickness-like
reaction (marked by fever and joint
pain; usually occurs after the second
course of therapy and resolves after
the drug is discontinued)
Rare
Allergic reaction (rash, pruritus,
urticaria), thrombophlebitis
(pain, redness, swelling at
injection site)

PRECAUTIONS AND CONTRAINDICATIONS

History of anaphylactic reaction to penicillins or hypersensitivity to cephalosporins

Caution:

Hypersensitivity to penicillins, lactation, renal disease

DRUG INTERACTIONS OF CONCERN TO DENTISTRY

• Decreased bactericidal effects: tetracyclines, erythromycins
• Increased and prolonged serum levels: probenecid

SERIOUS REACTIONS

! Antibiotic-associated colitis and other superinfections may result from altered bacterial balance.
! Nephrotoxicity may occur, especially in patients with preexisting renal disease.
! Patients with a history of allergies, especially to penicillin, are at increased risk for developing a severe hypersensitivity reaction, marked by severe pruritus, angioedema, bronchospasm, and anaphylaxis.

DENTAL CONSIDERATIONS

General:

• Take precautions regarding allergy to medication.
• Determine why the patient is taking the drug.

Consultations:

• Medical consultation may be required to assess disease control.

Teach Patient/Family to:

• Encourage effective oral hygiene to prevent soft tissue inflammation.

• Avoid mouth rinses with high alcohol content because of drying effects and possible drug-drug reaction.
• When used for dental infection, advise patient to:
  • Report sore throat, oral burning sensation, fever, and fatigue, any of which could indicate superinfection.
  • Take at prescribed intervals and complete dosage regimen.
  • Immediately notify the dentist if signs or symptoms of infection increase.

cefazolin sodium

sef-**a**′-zoe-lin **so**′-dee-um
(Ancef, Kefzol)
Do not confuse cefazolin with cefprozil or Cefzil.

CATEGORY AND SCHEDULE

Pregnancy Risk Category: B

Drug Class: Cephalosporin (first generation)

MECHANISM OF ACTION

A first-generation cephalosporin that binds to bacterial cell membranes and inhibits cell wall synthesis.
Therapeutic Effect: Bactericidal.

USES

Indicated for use when infection is caused by susceptible microorganisms: respiratory tract infections caused by *S. pneumoniae, Klebsiella* species, *H. influenzae, S. aureus,* and group A β-hemolytic streptococci; UTI infections caused by *E. coli, P. mirabilis, Klebsiella* species, and some Enterobacter and enterococci; skin and skin structure infections caused by *S. aureus,* group A β-hemolytic streptococci; biliary tract infections caused by *E. coli, P. mirabilis, S. aureus, Klebsiella* species, and various strains of streptococci; bone and joint infections caused by *S. aureus*; genital infections caused by *E. coli, P. mirabilis, Klebsiella* species, and some enterococci; septicemia caused by *S. aureus, S. viridans, P. mirabilis, E. coli,* and *Klebsiella* species, group A β-hemolytic streptococci

PHARMACOKINETICS
Widely distributed. Protein binding: 85%. Primarily excreted unchanged in urine. Moderately removed by hemodialysis. *Half-life:* 1.4–1.8 hr (increased in impaired renal function).

INDICATIONS AND DOSAGES
▸ **Uncomplicated UTIs**
IV, IM
Adults, Elderly. 1 g q12h.
▸ **Mild to Moderate Infections**
IV, IM
Adults, Elderly. 250–500 mg q8–12h.
▸ **Severe Infections**
IV, IM
Adults, Elderly. 0.5–1 g q6–8h.
▸ **Life-Threatening Infections**
IV, IM
Adults, Elderly. 1–1.5 g q6h. Maximum: 12 g/day.
▸ **Perioperative Prophylaxis**
IV, IM
Adults, Elderly. 1 g 30–60 min before surgery, 0.5–1 g during surgery, and q6–8h for up to 24 hr postoperatively.

▸ **Usual Pediatric Dosage**
Children. 50–100 mg/kg/day in divided doses q8h. Maximum: 6 g/day.
Neonates older than 7 days. 40–60 mg/kg/day in divided doses q8–12h.
Neonates 7 days and younger. 40 mg/kg/day in divided doses q12h.
▸ **Dosage in Renal Impairment**
Dosing frequency is modified on the basis of creatinine clearance.

Creatinine Clearance	Dosage Interval
10–30 ml/min	Usual dose q12h
Less than 10 ml/min	Usual dose q24h

SIDE EFFECTS/ADVERSE REACTIONS
Frequent
Discomfort with IM administration, oral candidiasis, mild diarrhea, mild abdominal cramping, vaginal candidiasis
Occasional
Nausea, serum sickness-like reaction (marked by fever and joint pain; usually occurs after the second course of therapy and resolves after the drug is discontinued)
Rare
Allergic reaction (rash, pruritus, urticaria), thrombophlebitis (pain, redness, swelling at injection site)

PRECAUTIONS AND CONTRAINDICATIONS
History of anaphylactic reaction to penicillins or hypersensitivity to cephalosporins
Caution:
Hypersensitivity to penicillins, lactation, renal disease

C

DRUG INTERACTIONS OF CONCERN TO DENTISTRY
• Decreased bactericidal effects: tetracyclines, erythromycins
• Increased and prolonged serum levels: probenecid

SERIOUS REACTIONS
! Antibiotic-associated colitis and other superinfections may result from altered bacterial balance.
! Nephrotoxicity may occur, especially in patients with preexisting renal disease.
! Patients with a history of allergies, especially to penicillin, are at increased risk for developing a severe hypersensitivity reaction, marked by severe pruritus, angioedema, bronchospasm, and anaphylaxis.

DENTAL CONSIDERATIONS

General:
• Take precautions regarding allergy to medication.
• Determine why the patient is taking the drug.
Consultations:
• Medical consultation may be required to assess disease control.
Teach Patient/Family to:
• Encourage effective oral hygiene to prevent soft tissue inflammation.
• Avoid mouth rinses with high alcohol content because of drying effects and possible drug-drug reaction.
• When used for dental infection, advise patient to:
  • Report sore throat, oral burning sensation, fever, and fatigue, any of which could indicate superinfection.

• Take at prescribed intervals and complete dosage regimen.
• Immediately notify the dentist if signs or symptoms of infection increase.

cefdinir
sef´-di-neer
(Omnicef)

CATEGORY AND SCHEDULE
Pregnancy Risk Category: B

Drug Class: Cephalosporin (third generation)

MECHANISM OF ACTION
A third-generation cephalosporin that binds to bacterial cell membranes and inhibits cell wall synthesis.
Therapeutic Effect: Bactericidal.

USES
Community-acquired pneumonia, acute exacerbations of chronic bronchitis, acute maxillary sinusitis, pharyngitis/tonsillitis

PHARMACOKINETICS
Moderately absorbed from the GI tract. Protein binding: 60%–70%. Widely distributed. Not appreciably metabolized. Primarily excreted unchanged in urine. Minimally removed by hemodialysis. *Half-life:* 1–2 hr (increased in impaired renal function).

INDICATIONS AND DOSAGES
▸ **Community-Acquired Pneumonia**
PO

Adults, Elderly, Children 13 yr and older. 300 mg q12h for 10 days.
▸ **Acute Exacerbation of Chronic Bronchitis**
PO

Adults, Elderly. 300 mg q12h for 5–10 days.
▸ **Acute Maxillary Sinusitis**
PO

Adults, Elderly, Children 13 yr and older. 300 mg q12h or 600 mg q24h for 10 days.

Children 6 mo–12 yr. 7 mg/kg q12h or 14 mg/kg q24h for 10 days.
▸ **Pharyngitis or Tonsillitis**
PO

Adults, Elderly, Children 13 yr and older. 300 mg q12h for 5–10 days or 600 mg q24h for 10 days.

Children 6 mo–12 yr. 7 mg/kg q12h for 5–10 days or 14 mg/kg q24h for 10 days.
▸ **Uncomplicated Skin or Skin-Structure Infections**
PO

Adults, Elderly, Children 13 yr and older. 300 mg q12h for 10 days.

Children 6 mo–12 yr. 7 mg/kg q12h for 10 days.
▸ **Acute Bacterial Otitis Media**
PO (Capsules)

Children 6 mo–12 yr. 7 mg/kg q12h or 14 mg/kg q24h for 10 days.
▸ **Usual Pediatric Dosage for Oral Suspension**

Children weighing 81–95 lb (37–43 kg). 12.5 ml (2.5 tsp) q12h or 25 ml (5 tsp) q24h.

Children weighing 61–80 lb (28–36 kg). 10 ml (2 tsp) q12h or 20 ml (4 tsp) q24h.

Children weighing 41–60 lb (19–27 kg). 7.5 ml (1 tsp) q12h or 15 ml (3 tsp) q24h.

Children weighing 20–40 lb (9–18 kg). 5 ml (1 tsp) q12h or 10 ml (2 tsp) q24h.

Infants weighing less than 20 lb (9 kg). 2.5 ml (1/2 tsp) q12h or 5 ml (1 tsp) q24h.
▸ **Dosage in Renal Impairment**
For patients with creatinine clearance less than 30 ml/min, dosage is 300 mg/day as single daily dose. For hemodialysis patients, dosage is 300 mg or 7 mg/kg/dose every other day.

SIDE EFFECTS/ADVERSE REACTIONS
Frequent
Oral candidiasis, mild diarrhea, mild abdominal cramping, vaginal candidiasis
Occasional
Nausea, serum sickness-like reaction (marked by fever and joint pain; usually occurs after the second course of therapy and resolves after the drug is discontinued)
Rare
Allergic reaction (rash, pruritus, urticaria)

PRECAUTIONS AND CONTRAINDICATIONS
History of anaphylactic reaction to penicillins or hypersensitivity to cephalosporins
Caution:
Hypersensitivity to other cephalosporins, penicillins, or penicillamine; renal impairment (need dose reduction); ulcerative colitis, pseudomembranous colitis, bleeding disorders, renal impairment, hemodialysis, β-lactamase-resistant organisms, not detected in breast milk, children younger than 6 mo

C

DRUG INTERACTIONS OF CONCERN TO DENTISTRY
• Absorption retarded by iron salts, magnesium, or aluminum antacids: take antiinfective dose at least 2 hr before antacids or iron preparations
• Increased plasma levels: probenecid

SERIOUS REACTIONS
! Antibiotic-associated colitis and other superinfections may result from altered bacterial balance.
! Nephrotoxicity may occur, especially in patients with preexisting renal disease.
! Patients with a history of allergies, especially to penicillin, are at increased risk for developing a severe hypersensitivity reaction, marked by severe pruritus, angioedema, bronchospasm, and anaphylaxis.

DENTAL CONSIDERATIONS
General:
• Use precaution regarding allergy to medication.
• Determine why patient is taking the drug.
• Examine for oral manifestation of opportunistic infection.
Consultations:
• Medical consultation may be required to assess disease control.
Teach Patient/Family to:
• Encourage effective oral hygiene to prevent soft tissue inflammation.

cefditoren pivoxil
seff-di-**tore**'-en
(Spectracef)

CATEGORY AND SCHEDULE
Pregnancy Risk Category: B

Drug Class: Cephalosporin, third generation

MECHANISM OF ACTION
A third-generation cephalosporin that binds to bacterial cell membranes and inhibits cell wall synthesis.
Therapeutic Effect: Bactericidal.

USES
Treatment of mild-to-moderate infections in adults and children older than 12 yr; for susceptible microorganisms causing (1) acute bacterial exacerbation of chronic bronchitis (*H. influenzae, H. parainfluenzae, S. pneumoniae* (penicillin susceptible only), or *M. catarrhalis*); (2) pharyngitis/tonsillitis (*S. pyogenes*); (3) uncomplicated skin and skin-structure infections (*S. aureus* and *S. pyogenes*)

PHARMACOKINETICS
Moderately absorbed from the GI tract. Protein binding: 88%. Not metabolized. Excreted in the urine. Minimally removed by hemodialysis.
Half-life: 1.6 hr (half-life increased with impaired renal function).

INDICATIONS AND DOSAGES
▶ **Pharyngitis, Tonsillitis, Skin Infections**
PO
Adults, Elderly, Children older than 12 yr. 200 mg twice a day for 10 days.

▶ **Acute Exacerbation of Chronic Bronchitis**
PO
Adults, Elderly, Children older than 12 yr. 400 mg twice a day for 10 days.
▶ **Community-Acquired Pneumonia**
PO
Adults, Elderly, Children older than 12 yr. 400 mg 2 twice a day for 14 days.
▶ **Dosage in Renal Impairment**
Dosage and frequency are modified on the basis of creatinine clearance.

Creatinine Clearance	Dosage Interval
50–80 ml/min	No adjustment necessary
30–49 ml/min	200 mg twice a day
Less than 30 ml/min	200 mg twice a day

SIDE EFFECTS/ADVERSE REACTIONS
Occasional
Diarrhea
Rare
Nausea, headache, abdominal pain, vaginal candidiasis, dyspepsia, vomiting

PRECAUTIONS AND CONTRAINDICATIONS
Carnitine deficiency, inborn errors of metabolism, known allergy to cephalosporins, hypersensitivity to milk protein
Caution:
Penicillin-allergic patients, diarrhea, not for prolonged treatment, risk of resistance emergence, alteration of normal GI flora, decrease in prothrombin activity (long-term use, renal or hepatic impairment, taking anticoagulants), take with meals, lactation, safety and efficiency has not been established in children younger than 12 yr, elderly patients

with impaired renal function, reduce dose in severe renal impairment

DRUG INTERACTIONS OF CONCERN TO DENTISTRY
• Reduced absorption: concurrent use with antacids, H2-receptor antagonist
• Increased and prolonged serum levels: probenecid

SERIOUS REACTIONS
❗ Antibiotic-associated colitis and other superinfections may occur.
❗ Patients with a history of allergies, especially to penicillin, are at increased risk for developing a severe hypersensitivity reaction, marked by severe pruritus, angioedema, bronchospasm, and anaphylaxis.

DENTAL CONSIDERATIONS
General:
• Caution regarding allergy to medication.
• Assess salivary flow as a factor in caries, periodontal disease, and candidiasis.
• Determine why patient is taking the drug.
• Consider semisupine chair position for patient comfort if GI side effects occur.
• Consult with patient's physician if an acute dental infection occurs and another antiinfective is required.
• Examine for oral manifestation of opportunistic infection.
• Patients on chronic drug therapy may rarely have symptoms of blood dyscrasias, which can include infection, bleeding, and poor healing.

C

Consultations:
• Medical consultation may be required to assess disease control.
• In a patient with symptoms of blood dyscrasias, request a medical consultation for blood studies and postpone treatment until normal values are reestablished.

Teach Patient/Family to:
• Encourage effective oral hygiene to prevent soft tissue inflammation and infection.
• When chronic dry mouth occurs, advise patient to:
  • Avoid mouth rinses with high alcohol content because of drying effects.
  • Use daily home fluoride products for anticaries effect.
  • Use sugarless gum, frequent sips of water, or saliva substitutes.

cefepime

sef´-eh-peem
(Maxipime)
Do not confuse cefepime with ceftidine.

CATEGORY AND SCHEDULE

Pregnancy Risk Category: B

Drug Class: Cephalosporin (fourth generation)

MECHANISM OF ACTION

A fourth-generation cephalosporin that binds to bacterial cell membranes and inhibits cell wall synthesis.
Therapeutic Effect: Bactericidal.

USES

Treatment of UTIs (uncomplicated and complicated), uncomplicated skin and soft tissue infections, complicated intraabdominal infections (in combination with metronidazole), and pneumonia caused by susceptible strains of microorganisms, including *S. pneumoniae*; febrile neutropenia

PHARMACOKINETICS

Well absorbed after IM administration. Protein binding: 20%. Widely distributed. Primarily excreted unchanged in urine. Removed by hemodialysis.
Half-life: 2–2.3 hr (increased in impaired renal function, and in the elderly).

INDICATIONS AND DOSAGES

▸ **Pneumonia**
IV
Adults, Elderly. 1–2 g q12h for 7–10 days.
Children 2 mo and older. 50 mg/kg q12h. Maximum: 2 g/dose.

▸ **Intraabdominal Infections**
IV
Adults, Elderly. 2 g q12h for 10 days.

▸ **Skin and Skin-Structure Infections**
IV
Adults, Elderly. 2 g q12h for 10 days.
Children 2 mo and older.
50 mg/kg q12h. Maximum: 2 g/dose.

▸ **UTIs**
IV
Adults, Elderly. 0.5–2 g q12h for 7–10 days.
Children 2 mo and older.
50 mg/kg q12h. Maximum: 2 g/dose.

▸ **Febrile Neutropenia**
IV
Adults, Elderly. 2 g q8h.
Children 2 mo and older. 50 mg/kg q8h. Maximum: 2 g/dose.

C

▶ Dosage in Renal Impairment

Dosage and frequency are modified on the basis of creatinine clearance and the severity of the infection.

Creatinine Clearance	Dosage
30–60 ml/min	0.5–2 g q24h
11–29 ml/min	0.5–1 g q24h
10 ml/min or less	0.25–0.5 g q24h

SIDE EFFECTS/ADVERSE REACTIONS

Frequent

Discomfort with IM administration, oral candidiasis, mild diarrhea, mild abdominal cramping, vaginal candidiasis

Occasional

Nausea, serum sickness-like reaction (marked by fever and joint pain; usually occurs after the second course of therapy and resolves after the drug is discontinued)

Rare

Allergic reaction (rash, pruritus, urticaria), thrombophlebitis (pain, redness, swelling at injection site)

PRECAUTIONS AND CONTRAINDICATIONS

History of anaphylactic reaction to penicillins or hypersensitivity to cephalosporins

Caution:

Renal impairment, overgrowth of resistant organisms, colitis, monitor prothrombin, lactation, children younger than 12 yr; renal insufficiency patient at risk for encephalopathy, myoclonus, seizures, renal failure

DRUG INTERACTIONS OF CONCERN TO DENTISTRY

• Increased risk of nephrotoxicity, ototoxicity: aminoglycosides in high doses, furosemide

SERIOUS REACTIONS

! Antibiotic-associated colitis manifested and other superinfections may result from altered bacterial balance.

! Nephrotoxicity may occur, especially in patients with preexisting renal disease.

! Patients with a history of allergies, especially penicillin, are at increased risk for developing a severe hypersensitivity reaction, marked by severe pruritus, angioedema, bronchospasm, and anaphylaxis.

DENTAL CONSIDERATIONS

General:

• Precaution regarding allergy to medication.

• Determine why patient is taking the drug.

Consultation:

• Medical consultation may be required to assess disease control.

Teach Patient/Family to:

• Encourage effective oral hygiene to prevent soft tissue inflammation.

• Report sore throat, oral burning sensation, fever, and fatigue, any of which could indicate presence of a superinfection.

cefixime

sef-**ix**′-zeem

(Suprax)

Do not confuse Suprax with Sporanox, Surbex, or Surfak.

CATEGORY AND SCHEDULE

Pregnancy Risk Category: B

Drug Class: Cephalosporin (third generation)

MECHANISM OF ACTION
A third-generation cephalosporin that binds to bacterial cell membranes and inhibits cell wall synthesis.
Therapeutic Effect: Bactericidal.

USES
Treatment of uncomplicated UTI (*E. coli, P. mirabilis*), pharyngitis and tonsillitis (*S. pyogenes*), otitis media (*H. influenzae, M. catarrhalis*), acute bronchitis, and acute exacerbations of chronic bronchitis (*S. pneumoniae, H. influenzae*)

PHARMACOKINETICS
Moderately absorbed from the GI tract. Protein binding: 65%–70%. Widely distributed. Primarily excreted unchanged in urine. Minimally removed by hemodialysis.
Half-life: 3–4 hr (increased in renal impairment).

INDICATIONS AND DOSAGES
▸ **Otitis Media, Acute Bronchitis, Acute Exacerbations of Chronic Bronchitis, Pharyngitis, Tonsillitis, and Uncomplicated UTIs**
PO
Adults, Elderly, Children weighing more than 50 kg. 400 mg/day as a single dose or in 2 divided doses.
Children 6 mo–12 yr weighing less than 50 kg. 8 mg/kg/day as a single dose or in 2 divided doses.
Maximum: 400 mg.
▸ **Uncomplicated Gonorrhea**
PO
Adults. 400 mg as a single dose.
▸ **Dosage in Renal Impairment**
Dosage is modified on the basis of creatinine clearance.

Creatinine Clearance	% of Usual Dose
21–60 ml/min	75%
20 ml/min or less	50%

SIDE EFFECTS/ADVERSE REACTIONS
Frequent
Oral candidiasis, mild diarrhea, mild abdominal cramping, vaginal candidiasis
Occasional
Nausea, serum sickness-like reaction (marked by arthralgia and fever; usually occurs after second course of therapy and resolves after drug is discontinued)
Rare
Allergic reaction (rash, pruritus, urticaria)

PRECAUTIONS AND CONTRAINDICATIONS
History of anaphylactic reaction to penicillins, hypersensitivity to cephalosporins.
Caution:
Hypersensitivity to penicillins, lactation, renal disease

DRUG INTERACTIONS OF CONCERN TO DENTISTRY
• Decreased bactericidal effects: tetracyclines, erythromycins
• Increased and prolonged serum levels: probenecid

SERIOUS REACTIONS
! Antibiotic-associated colitis and other superinfections may result from altered bacterial balance.
! Nephrotoxicity may occur, especially in patients with preexisting renal disease.

! Patients with a history of allergies, especially to penicillin, are at increased risk for developing a severe hypersensitivity reaction, marked by severe pruritus, angioedema, bronchospasm, and anaphylaxis.

DENTAL CONSIDERATIONS

General:
• Take precautions regarding allergy to medication.
• Determine why the patient is taking the drug.

Consultations:
• Medical consultation may be required to assess disease control.

Teach Patient/Family to:
• Encourage effective oral hygiene to prevent soft tissue inflammation.
• Avoid mouth rinses with high alcohol content because of drying effects and possible drug-drug reaction.
• When used for dental infection, advise patient to:
  • Report sore throat, oral burning sensation, fever, and fatigue, any of which could indicate superinfection.
  • Take at prescribed intervals and complete dosage regimen.
  • Immediately notify the dentist if signs or symptoms of infection increase.

cefonicid sodium
sef-on-**ih′**-sid
(Monocid)
Do not confuse with cefoxitin.

C

CATEGORY AND SCHEDULE
Pregnancy Risk Category: B

Drug Class: Antibacterial, systemic

MECHANISM OF ACTION
A second-generation cephalosporin that binds to bacterial cell membranes and inhibits cell wall synthesis.
Therapeutic Effect: Bactericidal.

USES
Treatment of infections caused by bacteria

PHARMACOKINETICS
Protein binding: greater than 90%. Widely distributed. Not metabolized. Primarily excreted unchanged in urine. Not removed by hemodialysis.
Half-life: 4.5 hr.

INDICATIONS AND DOSAGES
▸ **UTIs**
IV, IM
Adults, Elderly. 0.5 g q24h.
▸ **Mild to Moderate Infections**
IV, IM
Adults, Elderly. 1 g q24h.
▸ **Severe or Life-Threatening Infections**
IV, IM
Adults, Elderly. 2 g q24h.

C

▶ **Surgical Prophylaxis**
IV
Adults, Elderly. 1 g 60 min before
surgery.
▶ **Dosage in Renal Impairment**
Dosage and frequency are modified
on the basis of creatinine clearance
and the severity of infection.

Creatinine Clearance	Dosage (mild to moderate infections)
60–79 ml/min	10 mg/kg q24h
59–40 ml/min	8 mg/kg q24h
39–20 ml/min	4 mg/kg q24h
19–10 ml/min	4 mg/kg q48h
9–5 ml/min	4 mg/kg q3–5days
Less than 5 ml/min	3 mg/kg q3–5days

SIDE EFFECTS/ADVERSE REACTIONS

Frequent
Discomfort with IM administration,
oral candidiasis, mild diarrhea, mild
abdominal cramping, vaginal
candidiasis
Occasional
Nausea, unusual bleeding or
bruising, serum sickness-like
reaction (marked by fever and joint
pain)
Rare
Allergic reaction (rash, pruritus,
urticaria), thrombophlebitis
(pain, redness, swelling at injection
site)

PRECAUTIONS AND CONTRAINDICATIONS

History of anaphylactic reaction to
penicillins or hypersensitivity to
cephalosporins

DRUG INTERACTIONS OF CONCERN TO DENTISTRY

• Increased or prolonged plasma
levels: probenecid

SERIOUS REACTIONS

! Antibiotic-associated colitis and
other superinfections may result
from altered bacterial balance.
! Nephrotoxicity may occur,
especially in patients with
preexisting renal disease.
! Patients with a history of allergies,
especially to penicillin, are at an
increased risk for developing a
severe hypersensitivity reaction,
marked by severe pruritus,
angioedema, bronchospasm, and
anaphylaxis.

DENTAL CONSIDERATIONS

General:
• For selected infections in
the hospital setting; provide
palliative emergency dental care
only.
• Use with caution in patients with a
history of antibiotic-associated
colitis.
• Determine why patient is taking
the drug.
• Examine for oral manifestation of
opportunistic infection.
• Caution regarding allergy to
medication.
Consultations:
• Medical consultation may be
required to assess disease control
and patient's ability to tolerate
stress.
Teach Patient/Family to:
• Encourage effective oral
hygiene to prevent soft tissue
inflammation.
• Report sore throat, oral burning
sensation, fever, or fatigue, any of
which could indicate presence of a
superinfection.

cefoperazone
sef-oh-**per'**-ah-zone
(Cefobid)
Do not confuse with Ceftin,
cefotetan, and cefamandole.

CATEGORY AND SCHEDULE
Pregnancy Risk Category: B

Drug Class: Antibacterial,
systemic

MECHANISM OF ACTION
A third-generation cephalosporin
that binds to bacterial cell
membranes.
Therapeutic Effect: Inhibits
synthesis of bacterial cell wall.
Bactericidal.

USES
Treatment of infections caused by
bacteria

PHARMACOKINETICS
Widely distributed, including CSF.
Protein binding: 82%–93%.
Metabolized and excreted in kidney
and urine. Removed by
hemodialysis. *Half-life:* 1.6–2.4 hr
(half-life is increased with impaired
renal function).

INDICATIONS AND DOSAGES
▸ **Mild to Moderate Infections**
IM/IV
Adults, Elderly. 2–4 g/day in 2
divided doses q12h.
▸ **Severe or Life-Threatening
Infections**
IM/IV
Adults, Elderly. Total daily dose and/
or frequency may be increased to
6–12 g/day divided into 2, 3, or 4
equal doses of 1.5–4 g per dose.

▸ **Dosage in Renal and/or Hepatic
Impairment**
Do not exceed 4 g/day in those with
liver disease and/or biliary
obstruction. Modification of dose
usually not necessary in those with
renal impairment. Dose should not
exceed 1–2 g/day in those with both
hepatic and substantial renal
impairment.

SIDE EFFECTS/ADVERSE REACTIONS
Frequent
Discomfort with IM administration,
oral candidiasis, mild diarrhea, mild
abdominal cramping, vaginal
candidiasis
Occasional
Nausea, unusual bruising/bleeding,
serum sickness reaction
Rare
Allergic reaction, rash, pruritus,
urticaria, thrombophlebitis
(pain, redness, swelling at
injection site)

PRECAUTIONS AND CONTRAINDICATIONS
Anaphylactic reaction to penicillins,
history of hypersensitivity to
cephalosporins or any one of its
components

DRUG INTERACTIONS OF CONCERN TO DENTISTRY
• Avoid alcohol, risk of disulfiram-
like reaction.
• Increased risk of bleeding:
drugs that interfere with platelet
action.

SERIOUS REACTIONS
❗ Antibiotic-associated colitis
manifested as severe abdominal pain
and tenderness, fever, and watery
and severe diarrhea, and other
superinfections may result from
altered bacterial balance.

C

! Nephrotoxicity may occur, especially in patients with preexisting renal disease. Severe hypersensitivity reaction including severe pruritus, angioedema, bronchospasm, and anaphylaxis, particularly in patients with a history of allergies, especially to penicillins, may occur.

General:
• For selected infections in the hospital setting; provide palliative emergency dental treatment only.
• Use with caution in patients with a history of antibiotic-associated colitis.
• May interfere with prothrombin levels.
• Examine for oral manifestation of opportunistic infection.
• Determine why patient is taking the drug.
• Caution regarding allergy to medication.

Consultations:
• Medical consultation may be required to assess disease control and patient's ability to tolerate stress.
• Medical consultation should include partial prothrombin time, prothrombin time, or INR.

Teach Patient/Family to:
• Encourage effective oral hygiene to prevent soft tissue inflammation.
• Report sore throat, oral burning sensation, fever, or fatigue, any of which could indicate presence of a superinfection.

cefotaxime sodium
sef-oh-**taks**′-eem **so**′-dee-um
(Claforan)
Do not confuse cefotaxime with cefoxitin, ceftizoxime, or cefuroxime, or Claforan with Claritin.

CATEGORY AND SCHEDULE
Pregnancy Risk Category: B

Drug Class: Antibacterial, systemic

MECHANISM OF ACTION
A third-generation cephalosporin that binds to bacterial cell membranes and inhibits cell wall synthesis.
Therapeutic Effect: Bactericidal.

USES
Treatment of infections caused by bacteria

PHARMACOKINETICS
Widely distributed, including to CSF. Protein binding: 30%–50%. Partially metabolized in the liver to active metabolite. Primarily excreted in urine. Moderately removed by hemodialysis. *Half-life:* 1 hr (increased in impaired renal function).

INDICATIONS AND DOSAGES
▶ **Uncomplicated Infections**
IV, IM
Adults, Elderly. 1 g q12h.
▶ **Mild to Moderate Infections**
IV, IM
Adults, Elderly. 1–2 g q8h.
▶ **Severe Infections**
IV, IM
Adults, Elderly. 2 g q6–8h.

▸ **Life-Threatening Infections**
IV, IM
Adults, Elderly. 2 g q4h.
Children. 2 g q4h. Maximum: 12 g/day.
▸ **Gonorrhea**
IM
Adults (Male). 1 g as a single dose.
Adults (Female). 0.5 g as a single dose.
▸ **Perioperative Prophylaxis**
IV, IM
Adults, Elderly. 1 g 30–90 min before surgery.
▸ **Cesarean Section**
IV
Adults. 1 g as soon as umbilical cord is clamped, then 1 g 6 and 12 hr after first dose.
▸ **Usual Pediatric Dosage**
Children weighing 50 kg or more. 1–2 g q6–8h.
Children 1 mo–12 yr weighing less than 50 kg. 100–200 mg/kg/day in divided doses q6–8h.
▸ **Dosage in Renal Impairment**
For patients with creatinine clearance less than 20 ml/min give half of dose at usual dosing intervals.

SIDE EFFECTS/ADVERSE REACTIONS
Frequent
Discomfort with IM administration, oral candidiasis, mild diarrhea, mild abdominal cramping, vaginal candidiasis
Occasional
Nausea, serum sickness-like reaction (marked by fever and joint pain; usually occurs after the second course of therapy and resolves after the drug is discontinued)
Rare
Allergic reaction (rash, pruritus, urticaria), thrombophlebitis (pain, redness, swelling at injection site)

PRECAUTIONS AND CONTRAINDICATIONS
History of anaphylactic reaction to penicillins or hypersensitivity to cephalosporins

DRUG INTERACTIONS OF CONCERN TO DENTISTRY
• Increased or prolonged plasma levels: probenecid

SERIOUS REACTIONS
❗ Antibiotic-associated colitis and other superinfections may result from altered bacterial balance.
❗ Nephrotoxicity may occur, especially in patients with preexisting renal disease.
❗ Patients with a history of allergies, especially to penicillin, are at increased risk for developing a severe hypersensitivity reaction, marked by severe pruritus, angioedema, bronchospasm, and anaphylaxis.

DENTAL CONSIDERATIONS
General:
• For selected infections in the hospital setting; provide palliative emergency dental treatment only.
• Use caution in patients with a history of antibiotic-associated colitis.
• Examine for oral manifestation of opportunistic infection.
• Determine why patient is taking the drug.
• Caution regarding allergy to medication.
Consultations:
• Medical consultation may be required to assess disease control and patient's ability to tolerate stress.

C

Teach Patient/Family to:
• Encourage effective oral hygiene to prevent soft tissue inflammation.
• Report sore throat, oral burning sensation, fever, or fatigue, any of which could indicate presence of a superinfection.

cefotetan disodium
sef´-oh-tee-tan die-**so**´-dee-um
(Apatef[AUS], Cefotan)
Do not confuse cefotetan with cefoxitin or Ceftin.

CATEGORY AND SCHEDULE
Pregnancy Risk Category: B

Drug Class: Antibacterial, systemic

MECHANISM OF ACTION
A second-generation cephalosporin that binds to bacterial cell membranes and inhibits cell wall synthesis.
Therapeutic Effect: Bactericidal.

USES
Treatment of infections caused by bacteria

PHARMACOKINETICS
Protein binding: 78%–91%. Primarily excreted unchanged in urine. Minimally removed by hemodialysis. ***Half-life:*** 3–4.6 hr (increased in impaired renal function).

INDICATIONS AND DOSAGES
▶ **UTIs**
IV, IM
Adults, Elderly. 1–2 g in divided doses q12–24h.

▶ **Mild to Moderate Infections**
IV, IM
Adults, Elderly. 1–2 g q12h.
▶ **Severe Infections**
IV, IM
Adults, Elderly. 2 g q12h.
▶ **Life-Threatening Infections**
IV, IM
Adults, Elderly. 3 g q12h.
▶ **Perioperative Prophylaxis**
IV
Adults, Elderly. 1–2 g 30–60 min before surgery.
▶ **Cesarean Section**
IV
Adults. 1–2 g as soon as umbilical cord is clamped.
▶ **Usual Pediatric Dosage**
Children. 40–80 mg/kg/day in divided doses q12h. Maximum: 6 g/day.
▶ **Dosage in Renal Impairment**
Dosing frequency is modified on the basis of creatinine clearance and the severity of the infection.

Creatinine Clearance	Dosage Interval
10–30 ml/min	Usual dose q24h
Less than 10 ml/min	Usual dose q48h

SIDE EFFECTS/ADVERSE REACTIONS
Frequent
Discomfort with IM administration, oral candidiasis, mild diarrhea, mild abdominal cramping, vaginal candidiasis
Occasional
Nausea, unusual bleeding or bruising, serum sickness-like reaction (marked by fever and joint pain; usually occurs after the second course of therapy and resolves after the drug is discontinued)

Rare

Allergic reaction (rash, pruritus, urticaria), thrombophlebitis (pain, redness, swelling at injection site)

PRECAUTIONS AND CONTRAINDICATIONS

History of anaphylactic reaction to penicillins or hypersensitivity to cephalosporins

DRUG INTERACTIONS OF CONCERN TO DENTISTRY

• Avoid alcohol, risk of disulfiram-like reaction
• Increased or prolonged plasma levels: probenecid
• Increased risk of bleeding: drugs that interfere with platelet action

SERIOUS REACTIONS

! Antibiotic-associated colitis and other superinfections may result from altered bacterial balance.
! Nephrotoxicity may occur, especially in patients with preexisting renal disease.
! Patients with a history of allergies, especially to penicillin, are at increased risk for developing a severe hypersensitivity reaction, marked by severe pruritus, angioedema, bronchospasm, and anaphylaxis.

DENTAL CONSIDERATIONS

General:

• For selected infections in the hospital setting; provide palliative emergency dental treatment only.
• Use with caution in patients with a history of antibiotic-associated colitis.
• May interfere with prothrombin levels.
• Examine for oral manifestation of opportunistic infection.

• Determine why patient is taking the drug.
• Caution regarding allergy to medication.

Consultations:

• Medical consultation may be required to assess disease control and patient's ability to tolerate stress.
• Medical consultation should include partial prothrombin time, prothrombin time or INR.

Teach Patient/Family to:

• Encourage effective oral hygiene to prevent soft tissue inflammation.
• Report sore throat, oral burning sensation, fever, or fatigue, any of which could indicate presence of a superinfection.

cefoxitin sodium

se-**fox'**-ih-tin so'-dee-um
(Mefoxin)
Do not confuse cefoxitin with cefotaxime, cefotetan, or Cytoxan.

CATEGORY AND SCHEDULE

Pregnancy Risk Category: B

Drug Class: Antibacterial, systemic

MECHANISM OF ACTION

A second-generation cephalosporin that binds to bacterial cell membranes and inhibits cell wall synthesis.
Therapeutic Effect: Bactericidal.

USES

Treatment of infections caused by bacteria

PHARMACOKINETICS

Peak levels reached within 5 min following IV infusion. *Half-life:* 45 m–1 hr; 85% excreted unchanged in urine.

INDICATIONS AND DOSAGES

▶ **Mild to Moderate Infections**

IV, IM

Adults, Elderly. 1–2 g q6–8h.

▶ **Severe Infections**

IV, IM

Adults, Elderly. 1 g q4h or 2 g q6–8h up to 2 g q4h.

▶ **Uncomplicated Gonorrhea**

IM

Adults. 2 g one time with 1 g probenecid.

▶ **Perioperative Prophylaxis**

IV, IM

Adults, Elderly. 2 g 30–60 min before surgery, then q6h for up to 24 hr after surgery.

Children older than 3 mo. 30–40 mg/kg 30–60 min before surgery, then q6h for up to 24 hr after surgery.

▶ **Cesarean Section**

IV

Adults. 2 g as soon as umbilical cord is clamped, then 2 g 4 and 8 hr after first dose, then q6h for up to 24 hr.

▶ **Usual Pediatric Dosage**

Children older than 3 mo. 80–160 mg/kg/day in 4–6 divided doses. Maximum: 12 g/day.

Neonates. 90–100 mg/kg/day in divided doses q6–8h.

▶ **Dosage in Renal Impairment**

After a loading dose of 1–2 g, dosage and frequency are modified on the basis of creatinine clearance and the severity of the infection.

Creatinine Clearance	Dosage
30–50 ml/min	1–2 g q8–12h
10–29 ml/min	1–2 g q12–24h
5–9 ml/min	500 mg–1 g q12–24h
Less than 5 ml/min	500 mg–1 g q24–48h

SIDE EFFECTS/ADVERSE REACTIONS

Frequent

Discomfort with IM administration, oral candidiasis, mild diarrhea, mild abdominal cramping, vaginal candidiasis

Occasional

Nausea, serum sickness-like reaction (marked by fever and joint pain; usually occurs after the second course of therapy and resolves after the drug is discontinued)

Rare

Allergic reaction (pruritus, rash, urticaria), thrombophlebitis (pain, redness, swelling at injection site)

PRECAUTIONS AND CONTRAINDICATIONS

History of anaphylactic reaction to penicillins or hypersensitivity to cephalosporins

DRUG INTERACTIONS OF CONCERN TO DENTISTRY

• Increased or prolonged plasma levels: probenecid

SERIOUS REACTIONS

‼ Antibiotic-associated colitis and other superinfections may result from altered bacterial balance.

‼ Nephrotoxicity may occur, especially in patients with preexisting renal disease.

‼ Patients with a history of allergies, especially to penicillin, are at increased risk for developing a severe hypersensitivity reaction, marked by severe pruritus, angioedema, bronchospasm, and anaphylaxis.

DENTAL CONSIDERATIONS
General:
• For selected infections in the hospital setting; provide palliative emergency dental treatment only.
• Use with caution in patients with a history of antibiotic-associated colitis.
• Examine for oral manifestation of opportunistic infection.
• Determine why patient is taking the drug.
• Caution regarding allergy to medication.
Consultations:
• Consult patient's physician if an acute dental infection occurs and another antiinfective is required.
• Medical consultation may be required to assess disease control and patient's ability to tolerate stress.
Teach Patient/Family to:
• Encourage effective oral hygiene to prevent soft tissue inflammation.
• Report sore throat, oral burning sensation, fever, or fatigue, any of which could indicate presence of a superinfection.

cefpodoxime proxetil
sef-poe-**dox**'-ime **prox**'-eh-til (Vantin)
Do not confuse Vantin with Ventolin.

CATEGORY AND SCHEDULE
Pregnancy Risk Category: B

Drug Class: Cephalosporin (third generation)

MECHANISM OF ACTION
A third-generation cephalosporin that binds to bacterial cell membranes and inhibits cell wall synthesis.
Therapeutic Effect: Bactericidal.

USES
Treatment of upper and lower respiratory tract infections, pharyngitis (tonsillitis), gonorrhea, UTI, uncomplicated skin and skin structure infections caused by susceptible organisms, acute otitis media, community-acquired pneumonia, acute bacterial exacerbation of chronic bronchitis, anorectal infections in women

PHARMACOKINETICS
Well absorbed from the GI tract (food increases absorption). Protein binding: 21%–40%. Widely distributed. Primarily excreted unchanged in urine. Partially removed by hemodialysis. *Half-life:* 2.3 hr (increased in impaired renal function and elderly patients).

INDICATIONS AND DOSAGES
▶ **Chronic Bronchitis, Pneumonia**
PO
Adults, Elderly, Children older than 13 yr. 200 mg q12h for 10–14 days.
▶ **Gonorrhea, Rectal Gonococcal Infection (Female Patients Only)**
PO
Adults, Children older than 13 yr. 200 mg as a single dose.
▶ **Skin and Skin-Structure Infections**
PO
Adults, Elderly, Children older than 13 yr. 400 mg q12h for 7–14 days.
▶ **Pharyngitis, Tonsillitis**
PO
Adults, Elderly, Children older than 13 yr. 100 mg q12h for 5–10 days.

C

Children 6 mo–13 yr. 5 mg/kg q12h for 5–10 days. Maximum: 100 mg/dose.

▸**Acute Maxillary Sinusitis**
PO
Adults, Children older than 13 yr. 200 mg twice a day for 10 days.
Children 2 mo–13 yr. 5 mg/kg q12h for 10 days. Maximum: 400 mg/day.

▸**UTIs**
PO
Adults, Elderly, Children older than 13 yr. 100 mg q12h for 7 days.

▸**Acute Otitis Media**
PO
Children 6 mo–13 yr. 5 mg/kg q12h for 5 days. Maximum: 400 mg/dose.

▸**Dosage in Renal Impairment**
For patients with creatinine clearance less than 30 ml/min, usual dose is given q24h. For patients on hemodialysis, usual dose is given 3 times a wk after dialysis.

SIDE EFFECTS/ADVERSE REACTIONS
Frequent
Oral candidiasis, mild diarrhea, mild abdominal cramping, vaginal candidiasis
Occasional
Nausea, serum sickness-like reaction (marked by fever and joint pain; usually occurs after the second course of therapy and resolves after the drug is discontinued)
Rare
Allergic reaction (pruritus, rash, urticaria)

PRECAUTIONS AND CONTRAINDICATIONS
History of anaphylactic reaction to penicillins or hypersensitivity to cephalosporins
Caution:
Hypersensitivity to penicillins, lactation, renal disease, safety and

efficacy in infants younger than 5 mo not established

DRUG INTERACTIONS OF CONCERN TO DENTISTRY
• Decreased bactericidal effects: tetracyclines, erythromycins
• Increased and prolonged serum levels: probenecid
• Oral contraceptives: advise patient of a potential risk for decreased contraceptive action, to maintain compliance with oral contraceptive use while using antibiotics, and to consider the use of additional nonhormonal contraception

SERIOUS REACTIONS
❗ Antibiotic-associated colitis and other superinfections may result from altered bacterial balance.
❗ Nephrotoxicity may occur, especially in patients with preexisting renal disease.
❗ Patients with a history of allergies, especially to penicillin, are at increased risk for developing a severe hypersensitivity reaction, marked by severe pruritus, angioedema, bronchospasm, and anaphylaxis.

DENTAL CONSIDERATIONS

General:
• Take precautions regarding allergy to medication.
• Determine why the patient is taking the drug.
Consultations:
• Medical consultation may be required to assess disease control.
Teach Patient/Family to:
• Encourage effective oral hygiene to prevent soft tissue inflammation.
• Avoid mouth rinses with high alcohol content because of drying effects and possible drug-drug reaction.

- When used for dental infection, advise patient to:
  - Report sore throat, oral burning sensation, fever, and fatigue, any of which could indicate superinfection.
  - Take at prescribed intervals and complete dosage regimen.
  - Immediately notify the dentist if signs or symptoms of infection increase.

cefprozil
sef-**pro**′-zil
(Cefzil)
Do not confuse cefprozil with Cefazolin or Cefzil with Cefol, Ceftin or Kefzol.

CATEGORY AND SCHEDULE
Pregnancy Risk Category: B

Drug Class: Cephalosporin (second generation)

MECHANISM OF ACTION
A second-generation cephalosporin that binds to bacterial cell membranes and inhibits cell wall synthesis.
Therapeutic Effect: Bactericidal.

USES
Treatment of pharyngitis/tonsillitis, otitis media, secondary bacterial infection of acute bronchitis, sinusitis; acute bacterial sinusitis; acute bacterial exacerbation of chronic bronchitis and uncomplicated skin and skin structure infections

PHARMACOKINETICS
Well absorbed from the GI tract. Protein binding: 36%–45%. Widely distributed. Primarily excreted unchanged in urine. Moderately removed by hemodialysis. **Half-life:** 1.3 hr (increased in impaired renal function).

INDICATIONS AND DOSAGES
▶ **Pharyngitis, Tonsillitis**
PO
Adults, Elderly. 500 mg q24h for 10 days.
Children 2–12 yr. 7.5 mg/kg q12h for 10 days.
▶ **Acute Bacterial Exacerbation of Chronic Bronchitis, Secondary Bacterial Infection of Acute Bronchitis**
PO
Adults, Elderly. 500 mg q12h for 10 days.
▶ **Skin and Skin-Structure Infections**
PO
Adults, Elderly. 250–500 mg q12h for 10 days.
Children. 20 mg/kg q24h for 10 days.
▶ **Acute Sinusitis**
PO
Adults, Elderly. 250–500 mg q12h for 10 days.
Children 6 mo–12 yr. 7.5–15 mg/kg q12h for 10 days.
▶ **Otitis Media**
PO
Children 6 mo–12 yr. 15 mg/kg q12h for 10 days. Maximum: 1 g/day.
▶ **Dosage in Renal Impairment**
Patients with creatinine clearance less than 30 ml/min receive 50% of usual dose at usual interval.

SIDE EFFECTS/ADVERSE REACTIONS
Frequent
Oral candidiasis, mild diarrhea, mild abdominal cramping, vaginal candidiasis

C

Occasional
Nausea, serum sickness reaction (marked by fever and joint pain; usually occurs after the second course of therapy and resolves after the drug is discontinued)
Rare
Allergic reaction (pruritus, rash, urticaria)

PRECAUTIONS AND CONTRAINDICATIONS

History of anaphylactic reaction to penicillins or hypersensitivity to cephalosporins
Caution:
Lactation, elderly, hypersensitivity to penicillins, renal disease

DRUG INTERACTIONS OF CONCERN TO DENTISTRY

• Decreased bactericidal effects: tetracyclines, erythromycins
• Increased and prolonged serum levels: probenecid

SERIOUS REACTIONS

! Antibiotic-associated colitis and other superinfections may result from altered bacterial balance.
! Nephrotoxicity may occur, especially in patients with preexisting renal disease.
! Patients with a history of allergies, especially to penicillin, are at increased risk for developing a severe hypersensitivity reaction, marked by severe pruritus, angioedema, bronchospasm, and anaphylaxis.

DENTAL CONSIDERATIONS

General:
• Take precautions regarding allergy to medication.

• Determine why the patient is taking the drug.
• Examine for evidence of oral manifestations of blood dyscrasia (infection, bleeding, poor healing) and superinfection.
Consultations:
• Medical consultation may be required to assess disease control.
Teach Patient/Family to:
• Encourage effective oral hygiene to prevent soft tissue inflammation.
• Avoid mouth rinses with high alcohol content because of drying effects and possible drug-drug reaction.
• When used for dental infection, advise patient to:
    • Report sore throat, oral burning sensation, fever, and fatigue, any of which could indicate superinfection.
    • Take at prescribed intervals and complete dosage regimen.
    • Immediately notify the dentist if signs or symptoms of infection increase.

ceftazidime

sef-**taz**'-ih-deem
(Ceptaz, Fortaz, Fortum[AUS], Tazicef, Tazidime)
Do not confuse ceftazidime with ceftizoxime.

CATEGORY AND SCHEDULE
Pregnancy Risk Category: B

Drug Class: Third-generation cephalosporin; antibiotic

MECHANISM OF ACTION

A third-generation cephalosporin that binds to bacterial cell membranes and inhibits cell wall synthesis.
Therapeutic Effect: Bactericidal.

USES

Treatment of intraabdominal, biliary tract, respiratory tract, GU tract, skin, bone infections; meningitis; septicemia

PHARMACOKINETICS

Widely distributed (including to CSF). Protein binding: 5%–17%. Primarily excreted unchanged in urine. Removed by hemodialysis.
Half-life: 2 hr (increased in impaired renal function).

INDICATIONS AND DOSAGES
▸ **UTIs**
IV, IM
Adults. 250–500 mg q8–12h.
▸ **Mild-to-Moderate Infections**
IV, IM
Adults. 1 g q8–12h.
▸ **Uncomplicated Pneumonia, Skin and Skin-Structure Infections**
IV, IM
Adults. 0.5–1 g q8h.
▸ **Bone and Joint Infections**
IV, IM
Adults. 2 g q12h.
▸ **Meningitis, Serious Gynecologic and Intraabdominal Infections**
IV, IM
Adults. 2 g q8h.
▸ **Pseudomonal Pulmonary Infections in Patients with Cystic Fibrosis**
IV
Adults. 30–50 mg/kg q8h.
Maximum: 6 g/day.
▸ **Usual Elderly Dosage**
Elderly (normal renal function).
500 mg–1 g q12h.

▸ **Usual Pediatric Dosage**
Children 1 mo–12 yr. 100–150 mg/ kg/day in divided doses q8h.
Maximum: 6 g/day.
Neonates 0–4 wk. 100–150 mg/kg/ day in divided doses q8–12h.
▸ **Dosage in Renal Impairment**
After an initial 1-g dose, dosage and frequency are modified on the basis of creatinine clearance and the severity of the infection.

Creatinine Clearance	Dosage
31–50 ml/min	1 g q12h
16–30 ml/min	1 g q24h
6–15 ml/min	500 mg q24h
Less than 5 ml/min	500 mg q48h

SIDE EFFECTS/ADVERSE REACTIONS

Frequent
Discomfort with IM administration, oral candidiasis, mild diarrhea, mild abdominal cramping, vaginal candidiasis
Occasional
Nausea, serum sickness-like reaction (marked by fever and joint pain; usually occurs after the second course of therapy and resolves after the drug is discontinued)
Rare
Allergic reaction (pruritus, rash, urticaria), thrombophlebitis (pain, redness, swelling at injection site)

PRECAUTIONS AND CONTRAINDICATIONS

History of anaphylactic reaction to penicillins or hypersensitivity to cephalosporins

DRUG INTERACTIONS OF CONCERN TO DENTISTRY

• None reported

C

SERIOUS REACTIONS

! Antibiotic-associated colitis and other superinfections may result from altered bacterial balance.
! Nephrotoxicity may occur, especially in patients with preexisting renal disease.
! Patients with a history of allergies, especially to penicillin, are at increased risk for developing a severe hypersensitivity reaction, marked by severe pruritus, angioedema, bronchospasm, and anaphylaxis.

DENTAL CONSIDERATIONS

General:
• For selected infections in the hospital setting; provide palliative emergency dental treatment only.
• Use with caution in patients with a history of antibiotic-associated colitis.
• Examine for oral manifestation of opportunistic infection.
• Determine why patient is taking the drug.
• Caution regarding allergy to medication.
Consultations:
• Medical consultation may be required to assess disease control and patient's ability to tolerate stress.
Teach Patient/Family to:
• Encourage effective oral hygiene to prevent soft tissue inflammation.
• Report sore throat, oral burning sensation, fever, or fatigue, any of which could indicate presence of a superinfection.

ceftibuten
cef'-te-bute-in
(Cedax)

CATEGORY AND SCHEDULE
Pregnancy Risk Category: B

Drug Class: Cephalosporin (third generation)

MECHANISM OF ACTION
A third-generation cephalosporin that binds to bacterial cell membranes and inhibits cell wall synthesis.
Therapeutic Effect: Bactericidal.

USES
Treatment of acute exacerbations of chronic bronchitis caused by susceptible strains of *H. influenzae, M. catarrhalis,* or *S. pneumoniae*; acute otitis media caused by susceptible strains of *H. influenzae, M. catarrhalis,* or *S. pyogenes*; pharyngitis and tonsillitis caused by *S. pyogenes*

PHARMACOKINETICS
Rapidly absorbed from the GI tract. Excreted primarily in urine.
Half-life: 2–3 hr.

INDICATIONS AND DOSAGES
▸ Chronic Bronchitis
PO
Adults, Elderly. 400 mg/day once a day for 10 days.
▸ Pharyngitis, Tonsillitis
PO
Adults, Elderly. 400 mg once a day for 10 days.
Children older than 6 mo. 9 mg/kg once a day for 10 days. Maximum: 400 mg/day.

▶ **Otitis Media**
PO
Children older than 6 mo. 9 mg/kg
once a day for 10 days. Maximum:
400 mg/day.
▶ **Dosage in Renal Impairment**
Dosage is modified on the basis of
creatinine clearance.

Creatinine Clearance	Dosage
50 ml/min and higher	400 mg or 9 mg/kg q24h
30–49 ml/min	200 mg or 4.5 mg/kg q24h
Less than 30 ml/min	100 mg or 2.25 mg/kg q24h

SIDE EFFECTS/ADVERSE REACTIONS
Frequent
Oral candidiasis, mild diarrhea
(discharge, itching)
Occasional
Nausea, serum sickness-like reaction
(marked by fever and joint pain;
usually occurs after the second
course of therapy and resolves after
the drug is discontinued)
Rare
Allergic reaction (rash, pruritus,
urticaria)

PRECAUTIONS AND CONTRAINDICATIONS
History of anaphylactic reaction to
penicillins or hypersensitivity to
cephalosporins
Caution:
Hypersensitivity to penicillins, renal
impairment, lactation, infants
younger than 6 mo,
pseudomembranous colitis, oral
suspension contains 1 g
sucrose/5 ml

DRUG INTERACTIONS OF CONCERN TO DENTISTRY
• Decreased bactericidal effects:
tetracyclines, erythromycins

• Increased and prolonged serum
levels: probenecid
• Aminoglycosides increase
nephrotoxic potential

SERIOUS REACTIONS
! Antibiotic-associated colitis and
other superinfections may result
from altered bacterial balance.
! Nephrotoxicity may occur,
especially in patients with
preexisting renal disease.
! Patients with a history of allergies,
especially to penicillin, are at
increased risk for developing a
severe hypersensitivity reaction,
marked by severe pruritus,
angioedema, bronchospasm, and
anaphylaxis.

DENTAL CONSIDERATIONS
General:
• Take precautions regarding allergy
to medication.
• Assess salivary flow as factor in
caries, periodontal disease, and
candidiasis.
• Oral suspension contains
sucrose; patient should rinse mouth
after use.
• Determine why the patient is
taking the drug.
Consultations:
• Medical consultation may be
required to assess disease control.
Teach Patient/Family to:
• Encourage effective oral
hygiene to prevent soft tissue
inflammation.
• When used for dental infection,
advise patient to:
  • Report sore throat, oral
  burning sensation, fever, and
  fatigue, any of which could
  indicate superinfection.
  • Take at prescribed intervals
  and complete dosage regimen.

C

• Immediately notify the dentist if signs or symptoms of infection increase.

ceftizoxime sodium
sef-ti-zox'-eem so'-dee-um
(Cefizox)
Do not confuse ceftizoxime with cefotaxime or ceftazidime.

CATEGORY AND SCHEDULE
Pregnancy Risk Category: B

Drug Class: Third-generation cephalosporin; antibiotic

MECHANISM OF ACTION
A third-generation cephalosporin that binds to bacterial cell membranes and inhibits cell wall synthesis.
Therapeutic Effect: Bactericidal.

USES
Treatment of intraabdominal, biliary tract, respiratory tract, GU tract, skin, bone infections; gonorrhea; meningitis; septicemia; pelvic inflammatory disease (PID)

PHARMACOKINETICS
Widely distributed (including to CSF). Protein binding: 30%. Primarily excreted unchanged in urine. Moderately removed by hemodialysis. *Half-life:* 1.7 hr (increased in impaired renal function).

INDICATIONS AND DOSAGES
▸ **Uncomplicated UTIs**
IV, IM
Adults, Elderly. 500 mg q12h.

▸ **Mild, Moderate, or Severe Infections of the Biliary, Respiratory, and GU Tracts; Skin, Bone, and Intraabdominal Infections; Meningitis; and Septicemia**
IV, IM
Adults, Elderly. 1–2 g q8–12h.
▸ **Life-Threatening Infections of the Biliary, Respiratory, and GU Tracts; Skin, Bone and Intraabdominal Infections; Meningitis; and Septicemia**
IV
Adults, Elderly. 3–4 g q8h, up to 2 g q4h.
▸ **PID**
IV
Adults. 2 g q4–8h.
▸ **Uncomplicated Gonorrhea**
IM
Adults. 1 g 1 time.
▸ **Usual Pediatric Dosage**
Children older than 6 mo. 50 mg/kg q6–8h. Maximum: 12 g/day.
▸ **Dosage in Renal Impairment**
After a loading dose of 0.5–1 g, dosage and frequency are modified on the basis of creatinine clearance and the severity of the infection.

Creatinine Clearance	Dosage
50–79 ml/min	0.5 g–1.5 g q8h
5–49 ml/min	0.25 g–1 g q12h
Less than 5 ml/min	0.25–0.5 g q24h or 0.5 g–1 g q48h

SIDE EFFECTS/ADVERSE REACTIONS
Frequent
Discomfort with IM administration, oral candidiasis, mild diarrhea, mild abdominal cramping, vaginal candidiasis

Occasional
Nausea, serum sickness-like reaction (fever, joint pain; usually occurs after the second course of therapy and resolves after the drug is discontinued)
Rare
Allergic reaction (rash, pruritus, urticaria), thrombophlebitis (pain, redness, swelling at injection site)

PRECAUTIONS AND CONTRAINDICATIONS
History of anaphylactic reaction to penicillins or hypersensitivity to cephalosporins

DRUG INTERACTIONS OF CONCERN TO DENTISTRY
• Increased or prolonged plasma levels: probenecid

SERIOUS REACTIONS
! Antibiotic-associated colitis manifested and other superinfections may result from altered bacterial balance.
! Nephrotoxicity may occur, especially in patients with preexisting renal disease.
! Patients with a history of allergies, especially to penicillin, are at increased risk for developing a severe hypersensitivity reaction, marked by severe pruritus, angioedema, bronchospasm, and anaphylaxis.

DENTAL CONSIDERATIONS
General:
• For selected infections in the hospital setting; provide palliative emergency dental treatment only.
• Use with caution in patients with a history of antibiotic-associated colitis.
• Examine for oral manifestation of opportunistic infection.
• Determine why patient is taking the drug.
• Caution regarding allergy to medication.
Consultations:
• Medical consultation may be required to assess disease control and patient's ability to tolerate stress.
Teach Patient/Family to:
• Encourage effective oral hygiene to prevent soft tissue inflammation.
• Report sore throat, oral burning sensation, fever, or fatigue, any of which could indicate presence of a superinfection.

ceftriaxone sodium
sef-try-**ax**'-one **so**'-dee-um
(Rocephin)

CATEGORY AND SCHEDULE
Pregnancy Risk Category: B

Drug Class: Third-generation cephalosporin; antibiotic

MECHANISM OF ACTION
A third-generation cephalosporin that binds to bacterial cell membranes and inhibits cell wall synthesis.
Therapeutic Effect: Bactericidal.

USES
Treatment of respiratory tract, GU tract, skin, bone, intraabdominal, biliary tract infections; septicemia; meningitis; gonorrhea; Lyme disease; acute bacterial otitis media

PHARMACOKINETICS
Widely distributed (including to CSF). Protein binding: 83%–96%. Primarily excreted unchanged in

C

urine. Not removed by hemodialysis.
Half-life: 4.3–4.6 hr IV; 5.8–8.7 hr
IM (increased in impaired renal
function).

INDICATIONS AND DOSAGES
▸ **Mild to Moderate Infections**
IV, IM
Adults, Elderly. 1–2 g as a single
dose or in 2 divided doses.
▸ **Serious Infections**
IV, IM
Adults, Elderly. Up to 4 g/day in 2
divided doses.
Children. 50–75 mg/kg/day in
divided doses q12h. Maximum: 2 g/
day.
▸ **Skin and Skin-Structure Infections**
IV, IM
Children. 50–75 mg/kg/day as a
single dose or in 2 divided doses.
Maximum: 2 g/day.
▸ **Meningitis**
IV
Children. Initially, 75 mg/kg, then
100 mg/kg/day as a single dose or in
divided doses q12h. Maximum: 4 g/
day.
▸ **Lyme Disease**
IV
Adults, Elderly. 2–4 g a day for
10–14 days.
▸ **Acute Bacterial Otitis Media**
IM
Children. 50 mg/kg once a day for 3
days. Maximum: 1 g/day.
▸ **Perioperative Prophylaxis**
IV, IM
Adults, Elderly. 1 g 0.5–2 hr before
surgery.
▸ **Uncomplicated Gonorrhea**
IM
Adults. 250 mg plus doxycycline
one time.
▸ **Dosage in Renal Impairment**
Dosage modification is usually
unnecessary, but liver and renal
function test results should be
monitored in those with both renal

and liver impairment or severe renal
impairment.

SIDE EFFECTS/ADVERSE
REACTIONS
Frequent
Discomfort with IM administration,
oral candidiasis, mild diarrhea, mild
abdominal cramping, vaginal
candidiasis
Occasional
Nausea, serum sickness-like reaction
(marked by fever and joint pain;
usually occurs after the second
course of therapy and resolves after
the drug is discontinued)
Rare
Allergic reaction (rash, pruritus,
urticaria), thrombophlebitis (pain,
redness, swelling at injection site)

PRECAUTIONS AND
CONTRAINDICATIONS
History of anaphylactic reaction to
penicillins or hypersensitivity to
cephalosporins
Caution:
Hypersensitivity to penicillins,
lactation, renal disease

DRUG INTERACTIONS OF
CONCERN TO DENTISTRY
• None reported

SERIOUS REACTIONS
! Antibiotic-associated colitis and
other superinfections may result
from altered bacterial balance.
! Nephrotoxicity may occur,
especially in patients with
preexisting renal disease.
! Patients with a history of allergies,
especially to penicillin, are at
increased risk for developing a
severe hypersensitivity reaction,
marked by severe pruritus,
angioedema, bronchospasm, and
anaphylaxis.

DENTAL CONSIDERATIONS

General:
• For selected infections in the hospital setting; provide palliative emergency dental treatment only.
• Use with caution in patients with a history of antibiotic-associated colitis.
• May interfere with prothrombin levels.
• Examine for oral manifestation of opportunistic infection.
• Determine why patient is taking the drug.
• Caution regarding allergy to medication.

Consultations:
• Medical consultation may be required to assess disease control and patient's ability to tolerate stress.
• Medical consultation should include partial prothrombin time, prothrombin time, or INR.

Teach Patient/Family to:
• Encourage effective oral hygiene to prevent soft tissue inflammation.
• Report sore throat, oral burning sensation, fever, or fatigue, any of which could indicate presence of a superinfection.

cefuroxime axetil/ cefuroxime sodium

sef-yur-**ox**'-ime
(cefuroxime axetil) Ceftin, Zinnat[AUS] (cefuroxime sodium), Kefurox, Zinacef
Do not confuse cefuroxime with cefotaxime or deferoxamine or Ceftin with Cefzil.

CATEGORY AND SCHEDULE

Pregnancy Risk Category: B

Drug Class: Cephalosporin (second generation)

MECHANISM OF ACTION

A second-generation cephalosporin that binds to bacterial cell membranes and inhibits cell wall synthesis.
Therapeutic Effect: Bactericidal.

USES

Gram-negative bacilli (*H. influenzae, E. coli, Neisseria, P. mirabilis, Klebsiella*); gram-positive organisms (*S. pneumoniae, S. pyogenes, S. aureus*); serious lower respiratory tract, urinary tract, skin, gonococcal infections; septicemia; meningitis; early Lyme disease; acute bronchitis, acute bacterial maxillary sinusitis, pharyngitis, tonsillitis, impetigo, bone and joint infections

PHARMACOKINETICS

Rapidly absorbed from the GI tract. Protein binding: 33%–50%. Widely distributed (including to CSF). Primarily excreted unchanged in urine. Moderately removed by hemodialysis. *Half-life:* 1.3 hr (increased in impaired renal function).

INDICATIONS AND DOSAGES

▶ **Ampicillin-Resistant Influenza; Bacterial Meningitis; Early Lyme Disease; GU Tract, Gynecologic, Skin and Bone Infections; Septicemia; Gonorrhea and Other Gonococcal Infections**

IV, IM
Adults, Elderly. 750 mg–1.5 g q8h.
Children. 75–100 mg/kg/day divided q8h. Maximum: 8 g/day.
Neonates. 50–100 mg/kg/day divided q12h.
PO
Adults, Elderly. 125–500 mg twice a day, depending on the infection.

▶ **Pharyngitis, Tonsillitis**
PO
Children 3 mo–12 yr. 125 mg
(tablets) q12h or 20 mg/kg/day
(suspension) in 2 divided doses.
▶ **Acute Otitis Media, Acute
Bacterial Maxillary Sinusitis,
Impetigo**
PO
Children 3 mo–12 yr. 250 mg
(tablets) q12h or 30 mg/kg/day
(suspension) in 2 divided doses.
▶ **Bacterial Meningitis**
IV
Children 3 mo–12 yr. 200–240 mg/
kg/day in divided doses q6–8h.
▶ **Perioperative Prophylaxis**
IV
Adults, Elderly. 1.5 g 30–60 min
before surgery and 750 mg q8h after
surgery.
▶ **Usual Neonatal Dosage**
IV, IM
Neonates. 20–100 mg/kg/day in
divided doses q12h.
▶ **Dosage in Renal Impairment**
Adult dosage and frequency are
modified based on creatinine
clearance and the severity of the
infection.

SIDE EFFECTS/ADVERSE
REACTIONS
Frequent
Discomfort with IM administration,
oral candidiasis, mild diarrhea, mild
abdominal cramping, vaginal
candidiasis
Occasional
Nausea, serum sickness-like reaction
(marked by fever and joint pain;
usually occurs after the second
course of therapy and resolves after
the drug is discontinued)
Rare
Allergic reaction (rash, pruritus,
urticaria), thrombophlebitis
(pain, redness, swelling at injection
site)

PRECAUTIONS AND
CONTRAINDICATIONS
History of anaphylactic reaction to
penicillins or hypersensitivity to
cephalosporins

DRUG INTERACTIONS OF
CONCERN TO DENTISTRY
• Decreased bactericidal effects:
tetracyclines, erythromycins
• Increased and prolonged serum
levels: probenecid

SERIOUS REACTIONS
! Antibiotic-associated colitis and
other superinfections may result
from altered bacterial balance.
! Nephrotoxicity may occur,
especially in patients with
preexisting renal disease.
! Patients with a history of allergies,
especially to penicillin, are at
increased risk for developing a
severe hypersensitivity reaction,
marked by severe pruritus,
angioedema, bronchospasm, and
anaphylaxis.

DENTAL CONSIDERATIONS
General:
• Take precautions regarding allergy
to medication.
• Determine why the patient is
taking the drug.
Consultations:
• Medical consultation may be
required to assess disease
control.
Teach Patient/Family to:
• Encourage effective oral hygiene
to prevent soft tissue inflammation.
• Avoid mouth rinses with high
alcohol content because of drying
effects and possible drug-drug
reaction.

- When used for dental infection, advise patient to:
  - Report sore throat, oral burning sensation, fever, and fatigue, any of which could indicate superinfection.
  - Take at prescribed intervals and complete dosage regimen.
  - Immediately notify the dentist if signs or symptoms of infection increase.

celecoxib
sel-eh-**kox**′-ib
(Celebrex, DisperDose, Panixine)
Do not confuse Celebrex with Cerebyx or Celexa.

CATEGORY AND SCHEDULE
Pregnancy Risk Category: C (D if used in third trimester or near delivery)

Drug Class: Nonsteroidal antiinflammatory, analgesic

MECHANISM OF ACTION
An NSAID that inhibits cyclo-oxygenase-2, the enzyme responsible for prostaglandin synthesis. Mechanism of action in treating familial adenomatous polyposis is unknown.
Therapeutic Effect: Reduces inflammation and relieves pain.

USES
Relief of signs and symptoms of osteoarthritis and relief of signs and symptoms of rheumatoid arthritis in adults; also approved for reducing the number of intestinal polyps in patients with familial adenomatous polyposis; acute pain and primary dysmenorrhea

PHARMACOKINETICS
Widely distributed. Protein binding: 97%. Metabolized in the liver. Primarily eliminated in feces.
Half-life: 11.2 hr.

INDICATIONS AND DOSAGES
▸ **Osteoarthritis**
PO
Adults, Elderly. 200 mg/day as a single dose or 100 mg twice a day.
▸ **Rheumatoid Arthritis**
PO
Adults, Elderly. 100–200 mg twice a day.
▸ **Acute Pain**
PO
Adults, Elderly. Initially, 400 mg with additional 200 mg on day 1, if needed. Maintenance: 200 mg twice a day as needed.
▸ **Familial Adenomatous Polyposis**
PO
Adults, Elderly. 400 mg twice daily (with food).

SIDE EFFECTS/ADVERSE REACTIONS
Frequent
Diarrhea, dyspepsia, headache, upper respiratory tract infection
Occasional
Abdominal pain, flatulence, nausea, back pain, peripheral edema, dizziness, rash

PRECAUTIONS AND CONTRAINDICATIONS
NSAIDs may cause an increased risk of serious cardiovascular thrombotic events, including myocardial infarction and stroke, which may be fatal. Patients with cardiovascular disease may be at greater risk.

Hypersensitivity to aspirin, NSAIDs, or sulfonamides

Caution:
Geriatric patients weighing less than 50 kg use lowest dose, children younger than 18 yr, severe hepatic or renal impairment, upper active GI disease, GI bleeding, avoid in late pregnancy (category D after 34 wk), lactation, dehydrated patients, heart failure, hypertension, asthma, patients suspected or known to be poor CYP2C9 isoenzyme metabolizers

DRUG INTERACTIONS OF CONCERN TO DENTISTRY

• Increased plasma levels: fluconazole
• Increased risk of thromboembolism
• Increased risk of GI bleeding: long-duration NSAIDs, aspirin (except low doses), oral glucocorticoids, alcoholism, smoking, older age, generally poor health
• Increased plasma levels of lithium
• Possible risk of increased INR in elderly patients taking warfarin
• Possible reduction in blood pressure control: ACE inhibitors
• Users of SSRIs also taking NSAIDs may have a higher risk of GI side effects; until more data are available, it may be advisable to avoid use of NSAIDs in these patients (*Br J Clin Pharmacol* 55:591–595, 2003)

SERIOUS REACTIONS

! None known

DENTAL CONSIDERATIONS

General:
• Patients on chronic drug therapy may rarely have symptoms of blood dyscrasias, which can include infection, bleeding, and poor healing.
• Assess salivary flow as a factor in caries, periodontal disease, and candidiasis.
• Consider semisupine chair position for patient comfort because of effects of disease and GI side effects of drug.
• Severe stomach bleeding may occur in patients who regularly use NSAIDs in recommended doses, when the patient is also taking another NSAID, a blood thinning, or steroid drug, if the patient has GI or peptic ulcer disease, if they are 60 yr or older, or when NSAIDs are taken longer than directed. Warn patients of the potential for severe stomach bleeding.

Teach Patient/Family to:
• Encourage effective oral hygiene to prevent soft tissue inflammation.
• Update health and drug history if physician makes any changes in evaluation or drug regimens.
• Use powered tooth brush if patient has difficulty holding conventional devices.
• When chronic dry mouth occurs, advise patient to:
  • Avoid mouth rinses with high alcohol content because of drying effects.
  • Use daily home fluoride products for anticaries effect.
  • Use sugarless gum, frequent sips of water, or saliva substitutes.
• Warn patient of potential risks of NSAIDs.

cephalexin
sef-ah-**lex**′-in
(Apo-Cephalex[CAN], Biocef,
Ceporex[AUS], Ibilex[AUS],
Keflex, Keftab, Novolexin[CAN])

CATEGORY AND SCHEDULE
Pregnancy Risk Category: B

Drug Class: Cephalosporin (first
generation)

MECHANISM OF ACTION
A first-generation cephalosporin that
binds to bacterial cell membranes
and inhibits cell wall synthesis.
Therapeutic Effect: Bactericidal.

USES
Treatment of the following
infections when caused by
susceptible microorganisms:
respiratory tract infections caused by
S. pneumoniae and group A
β-hemolytic streptococci; otitis
media caused by *S. pneumoniae,
H. influenzae, M. catarrhalis,*
staphylococci, and streptococci; skin
and skin structure infections caused
by staphylococci and streptococci;
bone infections caused by
staphylococci and *P. mirabilis;* and
GU tract infections caused by
E. coli, P. mirabilis, and
K. pneumoniae

PHARMACOKINETICS
Rapidly absorbed from the GI tract.
Protein binding: 10%–15%. Widely
distributed. Primarily excreted
unchanged in urine. Moderately
removed by hemodialysis. *Half-life:*
0.9–1.2 hr (increased in impaired
renal function).

INDICATIONS AND DOSAGES
▶ Bone Infections, Prophylaxis of
Rheumatic Fever, Follow-up to
Parenteral Therapy
PO
Adults, Elderly. 250–500 mg q6h up
to 4 g/day.
▶ Streptococcal Pharyngitis, Skin
and Skin-Structure Infections,
Uncomplicated Cystitis
PO
Adults, Elderly. 500 mg q12h.
▶ Usual Pediatric Dosage
Children. 25–100 mg/kg/day in 2–4
divided doses.
▶ Otitis Media
PO
Children. 75–100 mg/kg/day in 4
divided doses.
▶ Dosage in Renal Impairment
After usual initial dose, dosing
frequency is modified on the basis
of creatinine clearance and the
severity of the infection.

Creatinine Clearance	Dosage Interval
10–50 ml/min	250 mg q6h
0–10 ml/min	125 mg q6h

SIDE EFFECTS/ADVERSE REACTIONS
Frequent
Oral candidiasis, mild diarrhea, mild
abdominal cramping, vaginal
candidiasis
Occasional
Nausea, serum sickness-like reaction
(marked by fever and joint pain;
usually occurs after the second
course of therapy and resolves after
the drug is discontinued)
Rare
Allergic reaction (rash, pruritus,
urticaria)

PRECAUTIONS AND CONTRAINDICATIONS

History of anaphylactic reaction to penicillins or hypersensitivity to cephalosporins
Caution:
Hypersensitivity to penicillins, lactation, renal disease

DRUG INTERACTIONS OF CONCERN TO DENTISTRY

• Decreased bactericidal effects: tetracyclines, erythromycins
• Increased and prolonged serum levels: probenecid

SERIOUS REACTIONS

! Antibiotic-associated colitis and other superinfections may result from altered bacterial balance.
! Nephrotoxicity may occur, especially in patients with preexisting renal disease.
! Patients with a history of allergies, especially to penicillin, are at increased risk for developing a severe hypersensitivity reaction, marked by severe pruritus, angioedema, bronchospasm, and anaphylaxis.

DENTAL CONSIDERATIONS

General:
• Take precautions regarding allergy to medication.
• Determine why the patient is taking the drug.
Consultations:
• Medical consultation may be required to assess disease control.
Teach Patient/Family to:
• Encourage effective oral hygiene to prevent soft tissue inflammation.
• Avoid mouth rinses with high alcohol content because of drying effects and possible drug-drug reaction.

• When used for dental infection, advise patient to:
  • Report sore throat, oral burning sensation, fever, and fatigue, any of which could indicate superinfection.
  • Take at prescribed intervals and complete dosage regimen.
  • Immediately notify the dentist if signs or symptoms of infection increase.

cephradine

sef´-ra-deen
(Velosef)

CATEGORY AND SCHEDULE

Pregnancy Risk Category: B

Drug Class: Cephalosporin (first generation)

MECHANISM OF ACTION

A first-generation cephalosporin that binds to bacterial cell membranes. Inhibits synthesis of bacterial cell wall.
Therapeutic Effect: Bactericidal.

USES

Treatment of gram-negative bacilli: *H. influenzae, E. coli, P. mirabilis, Klebsiella*; gram-positive organisms: *S. pneumoniae, S. pyogenes, S. aureus*; serious respiratory tract, urinary tract, skin, and skin structure infections; otitis media

PHARMACOKINETICS

Well absorbed from the GI tract. Protein binding: 18%–20%. Widely distributed. Primarily excreted unchanged in urine. Removed by hemodialysis. **Half-life:** 1–2 hr (half-life is increased with impaired renal function).

C

INDICATIONS AND DOSAGES

▶ **Mild, Moderate or Severe Infections of the Respiratory and GU Tracts; Bone, Joint and Skin Infections; Prostatitis; Otitis Media**
PO

Adults, Elderly. 250–500 mg q6h.
Maximum: 8 g/day.
Children older than 9 mo.
25–50 mg/kg/day in divided doses
q6–12h. Maximum: 4 g/day.

▶ **Dosage in Renal Impairment**
Dosage and frequency are based on the degree of renal impairment and the severity of infection. In patients with renal impairment, starting doses of 250 mg are recommended, with longer dosing intervals of up to 12 hr. Consult physician for use in patients on dialysis.

SIDE EFFECTS/ADVERSE REACTIONS

Frequent
Diarrhea, mild abdominal cramping, vaginal candidiasis (discharge, itching)
Occasional
Nausea, headache, unusual bruising or bleeding, serum sickness-like reaction (fever, joint pain)
Rare
Allergic reaction (rash, pruritus, urticaria)

PRECAUTIONS AND CONTRAINDICATIONS

History of hypersensitivity to penicillins and cephalosporins
Caution:
Hypersensitivity to penicillins, lactation, renal disease

DRUG INTERACTIONS OF CONCERN TO DENTISTRY

• Decreased bactericidal effects: tetracyclines, erythromycins
• Increased and prolonged serum levels: probenecid

SERIOUS REACTIONS

! Antibiotic-associated colitis as evidenced by severe abdominal pain and tenderness, fever, and watery and severe diarrhea, and other superinfections may result from altered bacterial balance.
! Nephrotoxicity may occur, especially in patients with preexisting renal disease.
! Severe hypersensitivity reaction including severe pruritus, angioedema, bronchospasm, and anaphylaxis, particularly in patients with history of allergies, especially penicillin, may occur.

DENTAL CONSIDERATIONS

General:
• Take precautions regarding allergy to medication.
• Determine why the patient is taking the drug.
Consultations:
• Medical consultation may be required to assess disease control.
Teach Patient/Family to:
• Encourage effective oral hygiene to prevent soft tissue inflammation.
• Avoid mouth rinses with high alcohol content because of drying effects and possible drug-drug reaction.
• When used for dental infection, advise patient to:
  • Report sore throat, oral burning sensation, fever, and fatigue, any of which could indicate superinfection.
  • Take at prescribed intervals and complete dosage regimen.
  • Immediately notify the dentist if signs or symptoms of infection increase.

C

certolizumab

cer-to-**liz**′-u-mab
(Cimzia)

CATEGORY AND SCHEDULE
Pregnancy Risk Category: B

Drug Class: Antiinflammatory, monoclonal antibody

MECHANISM OF ACTION
Humanized, pegylated tumor necrosis factor alpha (TNF-α) inhibitor. Reduces infiltration of inflammatory cells. Higher binding affinity for TNF-α than adalimumab or infliximab.

USES
Crohn's disease, moderately to severely active disease in patients who have inadequate response to conventional therapy

PHARMACOKINETICS
Approximately 80% bioavailability following SC administration.
Half-life: 14 days.

INDICATIONS AND DOSAGES
Adult. Subcutaneous (sc)
Crohn's disease: Initially, 400 mg (as 2 SC injections of 200 mg) once and then repeat at weeks 2 and 4.
Maintenance: 400 mg (as 2 SC injections of 200 mg) once every 4 wk.
Note: Evaluate patients for tuberculosis (TB) risk factors and test for latent TB infection before starting therapy.
Do not start therapy with certolizumab in patients with an active infection.

Evaluate patients at risk for hepatitis B virus infection for signs of prior HBV infection.
Pediatric. Safety and efficacy have not been established.

SIDE EFFECTS/ADVERSE REACTIONS
Frequent
Upper respiratory infection, urinary tract infectious disease, headache, nausea, infection
Occasional
Dizziness, vomiting, abdominal pain, arthralgia, injection site reactions (bleeding, burning, inflammation, pain, rash), cough
Rare
Congestive heart failure, myocardial infarction, bowel obstruction, opportunistic infection, sepsis

PRECAUTIONS AND CONTRAINDICATIONS
There are no contraindications listed within the manufacturer's labeling.
Caution:
Tuberculosis, children and young adults, cytopenias (e.g., leucopenia), heart failure, hepatitis B virus, infection

DRUG INTERACTIONS OF CONCERN TO DENTISTRY
• None reported

SERIOUS REACTIONS
❗ Sepsis and occasionally serious infections have occurred.
❗ Heart failure, hypersensitivity reactions, and opportunistic infections have been reported.
❗ Lupus-like syndrome may occur; discontinue if symptoms occur.

! Immunogenicity: Patients develop antibodies to certolizumab during therapy.

General:
• Patients on chronic drug therapy may rarely have symptoms of blood dyscrasias, which can include infection, bleeding, and poor healing.
• Aphthous ulcers may require postponement of dental treatment.
• Examine for oral manifestations of opportunistic infection.
• Monitor vital signs at every appointment because of cardiovascular side effects.
Consultations:
• In a patient with symptoms of blood dyscrasias, request a medical consultation for blood studies and postpone treatment until normal values are reestablished.
Teach Patient/Family to:
• Encourage effective oral hygiene to prevent soft tissue inflammation, infection.
• Report oral lesions, soreness, or bleeding to dentist.
• Prevent trauma when using oral hygiene aids.

cetirizine
si-**tear′**-ah-zeen
(Reactine[CAN], Zyrtec)
Do not confuse Zyrtec with Zantac or Zyprexa.

CATEGORY AND SCHEDULE
Pregnancy Risk Category: B

Drug Class: Antihistamine

MECHANISM OF ACTION
A second-generation piperazine that competes with histamine for H_1-receptor sites on effector cells in the GI tract, blood vessels, and respiratory tract.
Therapeutic Effect: Prevents allergic response, produces mild bronchodilation, blocks histamine-induced bronchitis.

USES
Treatment of symptoms of seasonal allergic rhinitis, perennial allergic rhinitis, chronic urticaria

PHARMACOKINETICS
Rapidly and almost completely absorbed from the GI tract (absorption not affected by food). Protein binding: 93%. Undergoes low first-pass metabolism; not extensively metabolized. Primarily excreted in urine (more than 80% as unchanged drug). *Half-life:* 6.5–10 hr.

INDICATIONS AND DOSAGES
▸ **Allergic Rhinitis, Urticaria**
PO
Adults, Elderly, Children older than 5 yr. Initially, 5–10 mg/day as a single or in 2 divided doses.
Children 2–5 yr. 2.5 mg/day. May increase up to 5 mg/day as a single or in 2 divided doses.
Children 12–23 mo. Initially, 2.5 mg/day. May increase up to 5 mg/day in 2 divided doses.
Children 6–11 mo. 2.5 mg once a day.
▸ **Dosage in Renal or Hepatic Impairment**
For adult and elderly patients with renal impairment (creatinine clearance of 11–31 ml/min), those receiving hemodialysis (creatinine clearance of 7 ml/min), and those

C

with hepatic impairment, dosage is decreased to 5 mg once a day.

SIDE EFFECTS/ADVERSE REACTIONS

Occasional

Pharyngitis; dry mucous membranes, nose, or throat; nausea and vomiting; abdominal pain; headache; dizziness; fatigue; thickening of mucus; somnolence; photosensitivity; urine retention

PRECAUTIONS AND CONTRAINDICATIONS

Hypersensitivity to cetirizine or hydroxyzine

Caution:

Renal impairment (requires dose reduction), elderly, glaucoma, urinary obstruction, lactation

DRUG INTERACTIONS OF CONCERN TO DENTISTRY

• No drug interactions reported, but should be similar to other antihistamines; anticipate increased sedation with other CNS depressants and increased anticholinergic effects with anticholinergic drugs.

SERIOUS REACTIONS

! Children may experience paradoxical reactions, including restlessness, insomnia, euphoria, nervousness, and tremor.

! Dizziness, sedation, and confusion are more likely to occur in elderly patients.

DENTAL CONSIDERATIONS

General:

• Assess salivary flow as factor in caries, periodontal disease, and candidiasis.

Teach Patient/Family:
• When chronic dry mouth occurs, advise patient to:
  • Avoid mouth rinses with high alcohol content because of drying effects.
  • Use daily home fluoride products for anticaries effect.
  • Use sugarless gum, frequent sips of water, or saliva substitutes.

cetuximab

ceh-**tux′**-ih-mab
(Erbitux)

CATEGORY AND SCHEDULE

Pregnancy Risk Category: C

Drug Class: Monoclonal antibody; antineoplastic

MECHANISM OF ACTION

A monoclonal antibody that binds to the epidermal growth factor receptor (EGFR), a glycoprotein on normal and tumor cells, thus inhibiting cell growth and inducing apoptosis.
Therapeutic Effect: Inhibits the growth and survival of tumor cells that overexpress EGFR.

USES

As a single agent or in combination with irinotecan for treatment of EGFR-expressing, metastatic colorectal carcinoma in patients who are refractory or intolerant to irinotecan-based chemotherapy

PHARMACOKINETICS

Reaches steady state levels by the third weekly infusion. Clearance decreases as dose increases.
Half-life: 114 hr (range, 75–188 hr).

INDICATIONS AND DOSAGES
▶ **Metastatic Colorectal Carcinoma**
IV
Adults, Elderly. Initially, 400 mg/m² as a loading dose. Maintenance: 250 mg/m² infused over 60 min weekly.

SIDE EFFECTS/ADVERSE REACTIONS
Frequent
Acneiform rash, malaise, fever, nausea, diarrhea, constipation, headache, abdominal pain, anorexia, vomiting
Occasional
Nail disorder, back pain, stomatitis, peripheral edema, pruritus, cough, insomnia
Rare
Weight loss, depression, dyspepsia, conjunctivitis, alopecia

PRECAUTIONS AND CONTRAINDICATIONS
None known

DRUG INTERACTIONS OF CONCERN TO DENTISTRY
• None reported

SERIOUS REACTIONS
! Anemia occurs in 10% of patients.
! A severe infusion reaction, characterized by rapid onset of airway obstruction, a precipitous drop in B/P, and severe urticaria, occurs rarely.
! Dermatologic toxicity, pulmonary embolus, leukopenia, and renal failure occur rarely.

DENTAL CONSIDERATIONS

General:
• Monitor vital signs at every appointment because of cardiovascular side effects.

• If additional analgesia is required for dental pain, consider alternative analgesics (NSAIDs) in patients taking narcotics for acute or chronic pain.
• Examine for oral manifestation of opportunistic infection.
• Consider semisupine chair position for patient comfort because of GI effects of disease.
• Patient on chronic drug therapy may rarely present with symptoms of blood dyscrasias, which can include infection, bleeding, and poor healing. If dyscrasia is present, caution patient to prevent oral tissue trauma when using oral hygiene aids.
• Advise patient if dental drugs prescribed have a potential for photosensitivity.
• Patients may be taking a prophylactic antiinfective.
• Use caution in the use of drugs that may cause diarrhea or constipation.
• Patients may have received other chemotherapy or radiation; confirm medical and drug history.
Consultations:
• Consult physician; prophylactic or therapeutic antiinfectives may be indicated if surgery or periodontal treatment is required.
• Medical consultation may be required to assess immunologic status during cancer chemotherapy and determine safety risk, if any, posed by the required dental treatment.
• Medical consultation may be required to assess disease control and patient's ability to tolerate stress.
• Medical consultation should include routine blood counts including platelet counts and bleeding time.

Teach Patient/Family to:
• Encourage effective oral hygiene to prevent soft tissue inflammation.
• Report oral lesions, soreness, or bleeding to dentist.
• Prevent trauma when using oral hygiene aids.
• Update health and medication history if physician makes any changes in evaluation or drug regimens; include OTC, herbal, and nonherbal remedies in the update.

cevimeline
sev-**im**′-el-ine
(Evoxac)
Do not confuse Evoxac with Eurax.

CATEGORY AND SCHEDULE
Pregnancy Risk Category: C

Drug Class: Cholinergic (muscarinic) agonist

MECHANISM OF ACTION
A cholinergic agonist that binds to muscarinic receptors of effector cells, thereby increasing secretion of exocrine glands, such as salivary glands.
Therapeutic Effect: Relieves dry mouth.

USES
Treatment of symptoms of dry mouth associated with Sjögren's syndrome

PHARMACOKINETICS
Rapid absorption after oral administration, peak levels 1.5–2 hr. Protein binding: 20%. Metabolized in liver by CYP 2D6 and CYP 3A4

isoenzymes. ***Half-life:*** 5 hr. 84% excreted in urine within 24 hr.

INDICATIONS AND DOSAGES
▶ **Dry Mouth**
PO
Adults. 30 mg 3 times a day.

SIDE EFFECTS/ADVERSE REACTIONS
Frequent
Diaphoresis, headache, nausea, sinusitis, rhinitis, upper respiratory tract infection, diarrhea
Occasional
Dyspepsia, abdominal pain, cough, UTI, vomiting, back pain, rash, dizziness, fatigue
Rare
Skeletal pain, insomnia, hot flashes, excessive salivation, rigors, anxiety

PRECAUTIONS AND CONTRAINDICATIONS
Acute iritis, angle-closure glaucoma, uncontrolled asthma
Caution:
Has the potential to alter heart rate or cardiac conduction; use with care in cardiovascular disease, asthma, bronchitis, COPD, seizure disorders, Parkinson's disease, urinary tract/ bladder obstruction, cholecystitis, cholangitis, biliary obstruction, GI ulcers, lactation, children (no data), history of adverse effects to other cholinergic agonists

DRUG INTERACTIONS OF CONCERN TO DENTISTRY
• Use with caution in patients taking β-adrenergic blockers: possible conduction disturbances.
• There are no specific data on dental drug interactions; however, use caution with other cholinergic agonists.

• Possibility that a cholinergic antagonist could interfere with this drug's action.
• Although there are no supporting data, use with caution in patients taking drugs that inhibit cytochrome P-450 (CYP3A3/4 and CYP2D6 isoenzymes).

SERIOUS REACTIONS

! Cevimeline use may result in decreased visual acuity, especially at night, and impaired depth perception.

DENTAL CONSIDERATIONS

General:
• Assess salivary flow as a factor in caries, periodontal disease, and candidiasis.
• Place on frequent recall to assess effectiveness.
• Consider semisupine chair position for patient comfort if GI side effects occur.
Consultations:
• Medical consultation may be required to assess disease control.
• Medical consultation may be necessary before prescribing for those patients with cardiovascular or respiratory disease.
Teach Patient/Family to:
• Be aware that this drug may cause visual disturbances, especially with night driving, which may impair driving safety.
• Drink extra fluids (water) to compensate for excessive sweating.
• When chronic dry mouth occurs, advise patient to:
  • Avoid mouth rinses with high alcohol content because of drying effects.
  • Use daily home fluoride to prevent caries.

• Use sugarless gum, frequent sips of water, or saliva substitutes.

chloral hydrate
klor′-al hye′-drate
(Aquachloral Supprettes, PMS-Chloral Hydrate[CAN], Somnote)

CATEGORY AND SCHEDULE
Pregnancy Risk Category: C
Controlled Substance Schedule IV

Drug Class: Sedative hypnotic, chloral derivative

MECHANISM OF ACTION
A nonbarbiturate chloral derivative that produces CNS depression. *Therapeutic Effect:* Induces quiet, deep sleep, with only a slight decrease in respiratory rate and B/P.

USES
Sedation, insomnia

PHARMACOKINETICS
Rapid absorption after oral administration, peak levels 30–45 min. Duration: 2–5 hr. Metabolized to trichloroethanol in liver and other tissues and, to a lesser extent, trichloroacetic acid, in liver. *Half-life:* 7–9.5 hr. Glucuronide conjugate excreted in urine.

INDICATIONS AND DOSAGES
▸ **Premedication for Dental or Medical Procedures**
PO, Rectal
Adults. 0.5–1 g.
Children. 75 mg/kg up to 1 g total. (Dosage reduced when combined with other sedatives.)

c

▸ **Premedication for EEG**
PO, Rectal
Adults. 0.5–1.5 g.
Children. 25–50 mg/kg/dose
30–60 min prior to EEG. May repeat
in 30 min. Maximum: 1 g for
infants, 2 g for children.

SIDE EFFECTS/ADVERSE REACTIONS
Occasional
Gastric irritation (nausea, vomiting,
flatulence, diarrhea), rash,
sleepwalking
Rare
Headache, paradoxical CNS
hyperactivity or nervousness in
children, excitement or restlessness
in the elderly (particularly in
patients with pain)

PRECAUTIONS AND CONTRAINDICATIONS
Gastritis, marked hepatic or
renal impairment, severe cardiac
disease
Caution:
Severe cardiac disease, depression,
suicidal individuals, asthma,
intermittent porphyria, lactation,
elderly; no specific reversal agent
available, use extreme caution in
dose calculation when used in
pediatric patients for sedation

DRUG INTERACTIONS OF CONCERN TO DENTISTRY
• Increased action of both drugs:
alcohol, all CNS depressants,
including nitrous oxide
• Sensitization of myocardium to
vasoconstrictors

SERIOUS REACTIONS
! Overdose may produce
somnolence, confusion, slurred
speech, severe incoordination,
respiratory depression, and coma.

DENTAL CONSIDERATIONS
General:
• Consider semisupine chair position
for patient comfort because of GI
side effects of drug.
• Administer syrup in juice or
beverage to mask taste and reduce
GI upset.
• Contraindicated for use in patients
with GI ulcerative disease.
• Have someone drive patient to and
from dental office when drug used
for conscious sedation.
• Geriatric patients are more
susceptible to drug effects; use lower
dose.
• Psychologic and physical
dependence may occur with chronic
administration.

chlordiazepoxide
klor-dye-az-eh-**pox**′-ide
(Apo-Chlordiazepoxide[CAN],
Librium, Novopoxide[CAN])
Do not confuse Librium with
Librax.

CATEGORY AND SCHEDULE
Pregnancy Risk Category: D
Controlled Substance Schedule IV

Drug Class: Benzodiazepine
antianxiety

MECHANISM OF ACTION
A benzodiazepine that enhances the
action of the inhibitory
neurotransmitter gamma-
aminobutyric acid in the CNS.
Therapeutic Effect: Produces
anxiolytic effect.

USES
Short-term management of anxiety,
acute alcohol withdrawal,
preoperatively for relaxation

PHARMACOKINETICS

Slow onset after oral administration, peak levels 2 hr. Metabolized in liver (active metabolites). *Half-life:* 24–48 hr. Metabolites excreted in urine.

INDICATIONS AND DOSAGES

▶ **Alcohol Withdrawal Symptoms**
PO
Adults, Elderly. 50–100 mg. May repeat q2–4h. Maximum: 300 mg/24 hr.

▶ **Anxiety**
PO
Adults. 15–100 mg/day in 3–4 divided doses.
Elderly. 5 mg 2–4 times a day.
IV, IM
Adults. Initially, 50–100 mg, then 25–50 mg 3–4 times a day as needed.

SIDE EFFECTS/ADVERSE REACTIONS

Frequent
Pain at IM injection site; somnolence, ataxia, dizziness, confusion with oral dose (particularly in elderly or debilitated patients)

Occasional
Rash, peripheral edema, GI disturbances

Rare
Paradoxical CNS reactions, such as hyperactivity or nervousness in children and excitement or restlessness in the elderly (generally noted during first 2 wk of therapy, particularly in presence of uncontrolled pain)

PRECAUTIONS AND CONTRAINDICATIONS

Acute alcohol intoxication, acute angle-closure glaucoma

Caution:
Elderly, debilitated, hepatic disease, renal disease

DRUG INTERACTIONS OF CONCERN TO DENTISTRY

• Delayed elimination: erythromycin
• Increased CNS depression: CNS depressants, alcohol, disulfiram, nefazodone
• Increased serum levels and prolonged effects of benzodiazepines: ketoconazole, itraconazole, fluconazole, miconazole (systemic), cimetidine, fluvoxamine, omeprazole, rifabutin, rifampin
• Contraindicated with ritonavir, indinavir, saquinavir
• Possible increase in CNS side effects: kava kava (herb)
• Decreased plasma levels: St. John's wort (herb)

SERIOUS REACTIONS

! IV administration may produce pain, swelling, thrombophlebitis, and carpal tunnel syndrome.
! Abrupt or too-rapid withdrawal may result in pronounced restlessness, irritability, insomnia, hand tremors, abdominal or muscle cramps, diaphoresis, vomiting, and seizures.
! Overdose results in somnolence, confusion, diminished reflexes, and coma.

DENTAL CONSIDERATIONS

General:
• After supine positioning, have patient sit upright for at least 2 min to avoid orthostatic hypotension.
• Assess salivary flow as a factor in caries, periodontal disease, and candidiasis.

C

• Psychologic and physical dependence may occur with chronic administration.
• Geriatric patients are more susceptible to drug effects; use lower dose.
• Have someone drive patient to and from dental office if used for conscious sedation.
Consultations:
• Medical consultation may be required to assess disease control.
Teach Patient/Family to:
• Encourage effective oral hygiene to prevent soft tissue inflammation.
• Avoid mouth rinses with high alcohol content because of drying effects.

chlorhexidine gluconate

klor-**hex**′-ih-deen **gloo**′-ko-nate
(Chlorhexidine Mouthwash[AUS], Chlorhexidine Obstetric Lotion[AUS], Chlorhex Gel[AUS], Chlorhex Gel Forte[AUS], Chlorhex Mouth Rinse[AUS], Peridex, PerioChip, PerioGard, Perisol)

CATEGORY AND SCHEDULE
Pregnancy Risk Category: C

Drug Class: Antiinfective-oral rinse

MECHANISM OF ACTION
An antiseptic and antimicrobial agent that is active against a broad spectrum of microbes. The chlorhexidine molecule, because of its positive charge, reacts with the microbial cell surface, destroys the integrity of the cell membrane, penetrates into the cell, precipitates the cytoplasm, and the cell dies.

Therapeutic Effect: Causes cell death.

USES
Treatment of gingivitis; unlabeled use: acute aphthous ulcers and denture stomatitis

PHARMACOKINETICS
Initially, the chlorhexidine gluconate dental chip releases approximately 40% of the drug within the first 24 hr, then releases the remainder in an almost linear fashion for 7–10 days.
Approximately 30% of the active ingredient, chlorhexidine gluconate, is retained in the oral cavity following oral rinsing. This retained drug is slowly released into the oral fluids. Poorly absorbed from the GI track. Primarily excreted in feces.
Half-life: Unknown.

INDICATIONS AND DOSAGES
▶ **Gingivitis**
Oral Rinse
Adults, Elderly. Swish and spit for 30 sec twice daily.
▶ **Periodontitis**
Oral Insert
Adults, Elderly. One chip is inserted into a periodontal pocket; insert a new chip q3mo; maximum of 8 chips per dental visit.

SIDE EFFECTS/ADVERSE REACTIONS
Occasional
Altered taste, staining of tooth, toothache

PRECAUTIONS AND CONTRAINDICATIONS
Hypersensitivity to chlorhexidine gluconate or any component of the formulation

Caution:
Lactation, efficacy not established for children younger than 18 yr, not intended for periodontitis

DRUG INTERACTIONS OF CONCERN TO DENTISTRY
• Disulfiram-like effects resulting from alcohol content: Antabuse, metronidazole

SERIOUS REACTIONS
! Anaphylaxis has been reported.

DENTAL CONSIDERATIONS
General:
• Perform dental examination and prophylaxis/scaling/root planing before starting rinse.
• Place on frequent recall because of oral side effects.
• Use discretion when prescribing to patients with anterior facial restorations with rough surfaces or margins.
Teach Patient/Family to:
• Eat, brush, and floss before using rinse.
• Not rinse with water after using chlorhexidine.
• Not dilute solution; not swallow solution.
• Beware of oral side effects.
• Not brush or use dental floss at site of chip placement.

chlorhexidine gluconate chip
klor-**hex**′-ih-deen **gloo**′-ko-nate
(Perio Chip)

C

CATEGORY AND SCHEDULE
Pregnancy Risk Category: C

Drug Class: Antiinfective

MECHANISM OF ACTION
Interferes with the integrity of the bacterial cell membrane, causing leakage of the intracellular components; penetrates into the cell, precipitates the cytoplasm, and the cell dies; effective against numerous supragingival and subgingival bacteria.

USES
Adjunct to scaling and root planing for reduction of the subgingival bacterial flora

PHARMACOKINETICS
40% of chlorhexidine released in first 24 hr, remainder released over 7–10 days; no detectable plasma levels.

INDICATIONS AND DOSAGES
Adults. Insert chip into a periodontal pocket with probing depth 5 mm or greater; up to 8 chips may be inserted per single visit; treatment 5 mm in depth; if chip dislodges within 48 hr of placement, replace with new chip; do not replace chips lost after 48 hr, but reevaluate in 3 mo and insert a new chip if pocket depth has not been reduced to less than 5mm; if chip is dislodged 7 days or more after placement, consider this a full course of treatment.

SIDE EFFECTS/ADVERSE REACTIONS

Oral: Localized pain, tenderness, aching, throbbing, toothache
Note: All other side effects reported did not differ from placebo chip

PRECAUTIONS AND CONTRAINDICATIONS

Hypersensitivity
Caution:
Not recommended for acutely abscessed periodontal pocket, use in children not established

DRUG INTERACTIONS OF CONCERN TO DENTISTRY

• None reported

DENTAL CONSIDERATIONS

General:
• Do not brush or use dental floss at site of chip placement.
Teach Patient/Family to:
• Notify dentist immediately if chip is dislodged or if pain, swelling, or other symptoms occur.

chloroquine/ chloroquine phosphate

klor'-oh-kwin/**klor'**-oh-kwin **foss'**-fate
(Aralen hydrochloride, Aralen[CAN]) (Aralen phosphate)

CATEGORY AND SCHEDULE

Pregnancy Risk Category: C

Drug Class: Antimalarial

MECHANISM OF ACTION

An amebacide that concentrates in parasite acid vesicles and may interfere with parasite protein synthesis.
Therapeutic Effect: Increases pH and inhibits parasite growth.

USES

Treatment of malaria caused by *P. vivax, P. malariae, P. ovale, P. falciparum* (some strains); rheumatoid arthritis; amebiasis

PHARMACOKINETICS

Rate of absorption is variable. Chloroquine is almost completely absorbed from the GI tract. Protein binding: 50%–65%. Widely distributed into body tissues such as eyes, heart, kidneys, liver, and lungs. Partially metabolized to active de-ethylated metabolites (principal metabolite is desethylchloroquine). Excreted in urine. Removed by hemodialysis. *Half-life:* 1–2 mo.

INDICATIONS AND DOSAGES

Chloroquine Phosphate
▸ **Treatment of Malaria (Acute Attack): Dose (mg Base)**

Dose	Time	Adults	Children
Initial	1 hr	600 mg	10 mg/kg
Second	6 hr later	300 mg	5 mg/kg
Third	Day 2	300 mg	5 mg/kg
Fourth	Day 3	300 mg	5 mg/kg

▸ **Suppression of Malaria**
PO
Adults. 300 mg (base)/wk on same day each week beginning 2 wk before exposure; continue for 6–8 wk after leaving endemic area.
Children. 5 mg (base)/kg/wk.
▸ **Malaria Prophylaxis**
PO
Adults. 600 mg base initially given in 2 divided doses 6 hr apart.
Children. 10 mg base/kg.

▸ **Amebiasis**
PO
Adults. 1 g (600 mg base) daily for 2 days; then, 500 mg (300 mg base)/ day for at least 2–3 wk.
Chloroquine HCL
▸ **Treatment of Malaria**
IM
Adults. Initially, 160–200 mg base (4–5 ml), repeat in 6 hr. Maximum: 800 mg base in first 24 hr. Begin oral therapy as soon as possible and continue for 3 days until approximately 1.5 g base given.
Children. Initially, 5 mg base/kg, repeat in 6 hr. Do not exceed 10 mg base/kg/24 hr.
▸ **Amebiasis**
IM
Adults. 160–200 mg base (4–5 ml) daily for 10–12 days. Change to oral therapy as soon as possible.

SIDE EFFECTS/ADVERSE REACTIONS

Frequent
Discomfort with IM administration, mild transient headache, anorexia, nausea, vomiting
Occasional
Visual disturbances (blurring, difficulty focusing); nervousness, fatigue, pruritus especially of palms, soles, scalp; bleaching of hair, irritability, personality changes, diarrhea, skin eruptions
Rare
Phlebitis or thrombophlebitis at IV injection site, abdominal cramps, headache, hypotension

PRECAUTIONS AND CONTRAINDICATIONS

Hypersensitivity to 4-aminoquinoline compounds, retinal or visual field changes

DRUG INTERACTIONS OF CONCERN TO DENTISTRY

• Hepatotoxicity: alcohol, hepatotoxic drugs

SERIOUS REACTIONS

❗ Ocular toxicity and ototoxicity have been reported.
❗ Prolonged therapy: peripheral neuritis and neuromyopathy, hypotension, ECG changes, agranulocytosis, aplastic anemia, thrombocytopenia, convulsions, psychosis.
❗ Overdosage includes symptoms of headache, vomiting, visual disturbance, drowsiness, convulsions, hypokalemia followed by cardiovascular collapse, and death.

DENTAL CONSIDERATIONS

General:
• Patients on chronic drug therapy may rarely have symptoms of blood dyscrasias, which can include infection, bleeding, and poor healing.
• Avoid dental light in patient's eyes; offer dark glasses for patient comfort.
• Determine why the patient is taking the drug.
Consultations:
• In a patient with symptoms of blood dyscrasias, request a medical consultation for blood studies and postpone dental treatment until normal values are reestablished.
Teach Patient/Family to:
• Encourage effective oral hygiene to prevent soft tissue inflammation.
• Avoid mouth rinses with high alcohol content because of drying effects.

C

chlorothiazide
klor-oh-**thye′**-ah-zide
(Diuril, Diuril Sodium)

CATEGORY AND SCHEDULE
Pregnancy Risk Category: C

Drug Class: Thiazide diuretic

MECHANISM OF ACTION
A sulfonamide derivative that acts as
a thiazide diuretic and
antihypertensive. As a diuretic
blocks reabsorption of water, the
electrolytes sodium and potassium at
cortical diluting segment of distal
tubule. As an antihypertensive
reduces plasma, extracellular fluid
volume, decreases peripheral
vascular resistance (PVR) by direct
effect on blood vessels.
Therapeutic Effect: Promotes
diuresis, reduces B/P.

USES
Treatment of edema, hypertension,
diuresis

PHARMACOKINETICS
Poorly absorbed from the GI tract.
Not metabolized. Primarily excreted
unchanged in urine. Not removed by
hemodialysis. *Half-life:*
45–120 min.

INDICATIONS AND DOSAGES
▸ **Edema, Hypertension**
PO
Adults. 0.5–1 g 1–2 times a day.
May give every other day or 3–5
days a wk.
Children 12 yr and older. 10–20 mg/
kg/dose in divided doses q8–12h.
Maximum: 2g/day.
Children 2–12 yr. 1 g/day.

Children 6 mo–2 yr. 10–20 mg/kg/
day in divided doses q12–24h.
Maximum: 375 mg/day.
Children younger than 6 mo.
20–30 mg/kg/day in divided
doses q12h. Maximum:
375 mg/day.
▸ **Hypertension**
IV
Adults. 0.5–1 g in divided doses
q12–24h.

SIDE EFFECTS/ADVERSE REACTIONS
Expected
Increase in urine frequency and
volume
Frequent
Potassium depletion
Occasional
Postural hypotension, headache, GI
disturbances, photosensitivity
reaction, muscle spasms, alopecia,
rash, urticaria

PRECAUTIONS AND CONTRAINDICATIONS
Anuria, history of hypersensitivity to
sulfonamides or thiazide diuretics,
renal decompensation
Caution:
Hypokalemia, renal disease, hepatic
disease, gout, COPD, lupus
erythematosus, diabetes mellitus,
elderly

DRUG INTERACTIONS OF CONCERN TO DENTISTRY
• Increased photosensitization:
tetracyclines
• Decreased hypotensive response,
nephrotoxicity: NSAIDs

SERIOUS REACTIONS
! Vigorous diuresis may lead to
profound water loss and electrolyte

depletion, resulting in hypokalemia, hyponatremia, and dehydration.

! Acute hypotensive episodes may occur.

! Hyperglycemia may be noted during prolonged therapy.

! GI upset, pancreatitis, dizziness, paresthesias, headache, blood dyscrasias, pulmonary edema, allergic pneumonitis, and dermatologic reactions occur rarely.

! Overdosage can lead to lethargy and coma without changes in electrolytes or hydration.

DENTAL CONSIDERATIONS

General:

• Monitor vital signs at every appointment because of cardiovascular side effects.

• After supine positioning, have patient sit upright for at least 2 min before standing to avoid orthostatic hypotension.

• Patients on chronic drug therapy may rarely have symptoms of blood dyscrasias, which can include infection, bleeding, and poor healing.

• Observe appropriate limitations of vasoconstrictor doses.

• Assess salivary flow as a factor in caries, periodontal disease, and candidiasis.

• Limit use of sodium-containing products, such as saline IV fluids, for patients with a dietary salt restriction.

• Stress from dental procedures may compromise cardiovascular function; determine patient risk.

• Short appointments and a stress-reduction protocol may be required for anxious patients.

• Patients taking diuretics should be monitored for serum K levels.

Consultations:

• In a patient with symptoms of blood dyscrasias, request a medical consultation for blood studies and postpone dental treatment until normal values are reestablished.

• Medical consultation may be required to assess disease control and patient's ability to tolerate stress.

• Physician should be informed if significant xerostomic side effects occur (increased caries, sore tongue, problems eating or swallowing, difficulty wearing prosthesis) so that a medication change can be considered.

Teach Patient/Family to:

• Encourage effective oral hygiene to prevent soft tissue inflammation.

• Use caution to prevent injury when using oral hygiene aids.

• When chronic dry mouth occurs, advise patient to:

  • Avoid mouth rinses with high alcohol content because of drying effects.

  • Use daily home fluoride products for anticaries effect.

  • Use sugarless gum, frequent sips of water, or saliva substitutes.

C

chlorpheniramine

klor-fen-**ir**′-ah-meen
(Aller-Chlor, Chlor-Trimeton,
Chlor-Trimeton Allergy,
Chlor-Trimeton Allergy 12
Hour, Chlor-Trimeton Allergy 8
Hour, Chlor-Tripolon[CAN],
Chlorate, Chlorphen, Diabetic
Tussin Allergy Relief)
Do not confuse with
chlorpromazine or
chlorpropamide.

CATEGORY AND SCHEDULE

Pregnancy Risk Category: C
OTC (tablets, syrup)

Drug Class: Antihistamine,
H₁-receptor antagonist

MECHANISM OF ACTION

A propylamine derivative
antihistamine that competes with
histamine for H₁ histamine receptor
sites on cells in the blood vessels,
GI tract, and respiratory tract.
Therapeutic Effect: Inhibits
symptoms associated with
seasonal allergic rhinitis such as
increased mucus production and
sneezing.

USES

Allergy symptoms, rhinitis

PHARMACOKINETICS

Well absorbed after PO and
parenteral administration. Food
delays absorption. Widely
distributed. Metabolized in liver.
Primarily excreted in urine. Not
removed by dialysis. *Half-life:*
20 hr.

INDICATIONS AND DOSAGES
▸ **Allergic Rhinitis, Common Cold**
PO
Adults, Elderly. 4 mg q6–8h or
8–12 mg (sustained-release) q8–12h.
Maximum: 24 mg/day.
Children 12 yr and older. 4 mg
q6–8h or 8 mg (sustained-release)
q12h. Maximum: 24 mg/day.
Children 6–11 yr. 2 mg q4–6h.
Maximum: 12 mg/day.
IM/IV/SC
Adults, Elderly. 5–40 mg as a single
dose. Maximum: 40 mg/day.
SC
Children 6 yr and older.
87.5 mcg/kg or 2.5 mg/m² 4 times
a day.

SIDE EFFECTS/ADVERSE REACTIONS
Frequent
Drowsiness, dizziness, muscular
weakness, hypotension, dry mouth,
nose, throat, and lips, urinary
retention, thickening of bronchial
secretions
Elderly: Sedation, dizziness,
hypotension
Occasional
Epigastric distress, flushing, visual
or hearing disturbances, paresthesia,
diaphoresis, chills

PRECAUTIONS AND CONTRAINDICATIONS
Hypersensitivity to chlorpheniramine
or its components

DRUG INTERACTIONS OF CONCERN TO DENTISTRY
• Increased CNS depression:
alcohol, all CNS depressants
• Increased anticholinergic effect:
other anticholinergics,
phenothiazines, tricyclic
antidepressants

SERIOUS REACTIONS

! Children may experience dominant paradoxical reactions, including restlessness, insomnia, euphoria, nervousness, and tremors.
! Overdosage in children may result in hallucinations, seizures, and death.
! Hypersensitivity reaction, such as eczema, pruritus, rash, cardiac disturbances, and photosensitivity, may occur.
! Overdosage may vary from CNS depression, including sedation, apnea, hypotension, cardiovascular collapse, or death to severe paradoxical reaction, such as hallucinations, tremors, and seizures.

DENTAL CONSIDERATIONS

General:
• Assess salivary flow as a factor in caries, periodontal disease, and candidiasis.
• Consider semisupine chair position for patients with respiratory disease.
• Determine why the patient is taking the drug.
Teach Patient/Family to:
• Encourage effective oral hygiene to prevent soft tissue inflammation.
• Use caution to prevent injury when using oral hygiene aids.
• When chronic dry mouth occurs, advise patient to:
  • Avoid mouth rinses with high alcohol content because of drying effects.
  • Use daily home fluoride products for anticaries effect.
  • Use sugarless gum, frequent sips of water, or saliva substitutes.

chlorpromazine
klor-**proe**′-ma-zeen
(Chlorpromanyl[CAN], Largactil[CAN], Thorazine)
Do not confuse chlorpromazine with chlorpropamide, clomipramine, or prochlorperazine, or Thorazine with thiamide or thioridazine.

CATEGORY AND SCHEDULE
Pregnancy Risk Category: C

Drug Class: Phenothiazine antipsychotic

MECHANISM OF ACTION
A phenothiazine that blocks dopamine neurotransmission at postsynaptic dopamine receptor sites. Possesses strong anticholinergic, sedative, and antiemetic effects; moderate extrapyramidal effects; and slight antihistamine action.
Therapeutic Effect: Relieves nausea and vomiting; improves psychotic conditions; controls intractable hiccups and porphyria.

USES
Psychotic disorders, mania, schizophrenia, anxiety, intractable hiccups, nausea, vomiting, preoperatively for relaxation, acute intermittent porphyria, behavioral problems in children

PHARMACOKINETICS
Rapidly absorbed after oral or IM administration. Protein binding: 92%–97%. Metabolized in the liver. Excreted in urine. *Half-life:* 6 hr.

INDICATIONS AND DOSAGES

▶ **Severe Nausea or Vomiting**

PO
Adults, Elderly. 10–25 mg q4–6h.
Children. 0.5–1 mg/kg q4–6h.
IV, IM
Adults, Elderly. 25–50 mg q4–6h.
Children. 0.5–1 mg/kg q6–8h.
Rectal
Adults, Elderly. 50–100 mg q6–8h.
Children. 1 mg/kg q6–8h.

▶ **Psychotic Disorders**

PO
Adults, Elderly. 30–800 mg/day in
1–4 divided doses.
Children older than 6 mo. 0.5–1 mg/
kg q4–6h.
IV, IM
Adults, Elderly. Initially, 25 mg; may
repeat in 1–4 hr. May gradually
increase to 400 mg q4–6h.
Maximum: 300–800 mg/day.
Children older than 6 mo. 0.5–1 mg/
kg q6–8h. Maximum: 75 mg/day for
children 5–12 yr; 40 mg/day for
children younger than 5 yr.

▶ **Intractable Hiccups**

PO, IV, IM
Adults. 25–50 mg 3 times a day.

▶ **Porphyria**

PO
Adults. 25–50 mg 3–4 times a day.
IM
Adults, Elderly. 25 mg 3–4 times a
day.

SIDE EFFECTS/ADVERSE REACTIONS

Frequent

Somnolence, blurred vision,
hypotension, color vision or night
vision disturbances, dizziness,
decreased sweating, constipation,
dry mouth, nasal congestion

Occasional

Urinary retention, photosensitivity,
rash, decreased sexual function,
swelling or pain in breasts, weight
gain, nausea, vomiting, abdominal
pain, tremors

PRECAUTIONS AND CONTRAINDICATIONS

Comatose states, myelosuppression,
severe cardiovascular disease, severe
CNS depression, subcortical brain
damage
Caution:
Lactation, seizure disorders,
hypertension, hepatic disease,
cardiac disease, elderly

DRUG INTERACTIONS OF CONCERN TO DENTISTRY

• Increased sedation: other CNS
depressants, alcohol, barbiturate
anesthetics, opioid analgesics
• Hypotension, tachycardia:
epinephrine (systemic)
• Increased extrapyramidal
effects: related drugs, such as
haloperidol, droperidol, and
metoclopramide
• Additive photosensitization:
tetracyclines
• Increased anticholinergic effects:
anticholinergics

SERIOUS REACTIONS

! Extrapyramidal symptoms appear
to be dose related and are divided
into three categories: akathisia
(including inability to sit still,
tapping of feet), parkinsonian
symptoms (such as masklike face,
tremors, shuffling gait,
hypersalivation), and acute dystonias
(including torticollis, opisthotonos,
and oculogyric crisis). A dystonic
reaction may also produce
diaphoresis and pallor.
! Tardive dyskinesia, including
tongue protrusion, puffing of the
cheeks, and puckering of the mouth
is a rare reaction that may be
irreversible.

! Abrupt discontinuation after long-term therapy may precipitate nausea, vomiting, gastritis, dizziness, and tremors.

! Blood dyscrasias, particularly agranulocytosis and mild leukopenia, may occur.

! Chlorpromazine may lower the seizure threshold.

DENTAL CONSIDERATIONS

General:
• Monitor vital signs at every appointment because of cardiovascular side effects.
• Patients on chronic drug therapy may rarely have symptoms of blood dyscrasias, which can include infection, bleeding, and poor healing.
• After supine positioning, have patient sit upright for at least 2 min before standing to avoid orthostatic hypotension.
• Assess salivary flow as a factor in caries, periodontal disease, and candidiasis.
• Avoid dental light in patient's eyes; offer dark glasses for patient comfort.
• Assess for presence of extrapyramidal motor symptoms, such as tardive dyskinesia and akathisia. Extrapyramidal motor activity may complicate dental treatment.
• Geriatric patients are more susceptible to drug effects; use a lower dose.

Consultations:
• In a patient with symptoms of blood dyscrasias, request a medical consultation for blood studies and postpone dental treatment until normal values are reestablished.
• Take precautions if dental surgery is anticipated and anesthesia is required.

• If signs of tardive dyskinesia or akathisia are present, refer to physician.
• Physician should be informed if significant xerostomic side effects occur (increased caries, sore tongue, problems eating or swallowing, difficulty wearing prosthesis) so that a medication change can be considered.

Teach Patient/Family to:
• Encourage effective oral hygiene to prevent soft tissue inflammation.
• Use caution to prevent injury when using oral hygiene aids.
• Use powered tooth brush if patient has difficulty holding conventional devices.
• When chronic dry mouth occurs, advise patient to:
  • Avoid mouth rinses with high alcohol content because of drying effects.
  • Use daily home fluoride products for anticaries effect.
  • Use sugarless gum, frequent sips of water, or saliva substitutes.

chlorpropamide
klor-**pro**′-pa-mide
(Apo-Chlorpropamide[CAN], Diabinese)
Do not confuse with chlorpromazine.

CATEGORY AND SCHEDULE
Pregnancy Risk Category: C

Drug Class: Antidiabetic, sulfonylurea (first generation)

MECHANISM OF ACTION
A first-generation sulfonylurea that promotes release of insulin from beta cells of pancreas.

Therapeutic Effect: Lowers blood glucose concentration.

USES
Treatment of stable adult-onset diabetes mellitus (Type 2)

PHARMACOKINETICS
Rapidly absorbed from the GI tract. Protein binding: 60%–90%. Extensively metabolized in liver. Excreted primarily in urine. Removed by hemodialysis. *Half-life:* 30–42 hr.

INDICATIONS AND DOSAGES
▶ **Diabetes Mellitus, Combination Therapy**
PO
Adults. Initially, 250 mg once a day. Maintenance: 250–500 mg once a day. Maximum: 750 mg/day.
Elderly. Initially, 100–125 mg once a day. Maintenance: 100–250 mg once a day. Increase or decrease by 50–125 mg a day for 3- to 5-day intervals.
▶ **Renal Function Impairment**
Not recommended.

SIDE EFFECTS/ADVERSE REACTIONS
Frequent
Headache, upper respiratory tract infection
Occasional
Sinusitis, myalgia (muscle aches), pharyngitis, aggravated diabetes mellitus

PRECAUTIONS AND CONTRAINDICATIONS
Diabetic complications, such as ketosis, acidosis, and diabetic coma, severe liver or renal impairment, sole therapy for type 1 diabetes mellitus, or hypersensitivity to sulfonylureas

Caution:
Elderly, cardiac disease, thyroid disease, renal disease, hepatic disease, severe hypoglycemic reactions, avoid use in lactation, use in children not established

DRUG INTERACTIONS OF CONCERN TO DENTISTRY
• Increased hypoglycemic effects: salicylates, NSAIDs, ketoconazole, miconazole
• Decreased action: corticosteroids, sympathomimetics
• Disulfiram-like reaction: alcohol

SERIOUS REACTIONS
❗ Possible increased risk of cardiovascular mortality with this class of drugs.
❗ Overdosage can cause severe hypoglycemia prolonged by extended half-life.

DENTAL CONSIDERATIONS
General:
• Patients on chronic drug therapy may rarely have symptoms of blood dyscrasias, which can include infection, bleeding, and poor healing.
• Short appointments and a stress-reduction protocol may be required for anxious patients.
• Question patient about self-monitoring of drug's antidiabetic effect, including blood glucose values or finger-stick records.
• Ensure that patient is following prescribed diet and regularly takes medication.
• Determine if medication controls disease. Patients with diabetes may be more susceptible to infection and have delayed wound healing.
• Avoid prescribing aspirin-containing products.

Consultations:
• In a patient with symptoms of blood dyscrasias, request a medical consultation for blood studies and postpone dental treatment until normal values are reestablished.
• Medical consultation may be required to assess disease control.
• Medical consultation may include data from patient's blood glucose monitoring, including glycosylated hemoglobin or HbA1c testing.

Teach Patient/Family to:
• Encourage effective oral hygiene to prevent soft tissue inflammation.
• Use caution to prevent injury when using oral hygiene aids.
• Avoid mouth rinses with high alcohol content because of drying effects.

chlorthalidone

klor-**thal′**-ih-doan
(Apo-Chlorthalidone[CAN],
Hygroton[AUS], Thalitone)

CATEGORY AND SCHEDULE
Pregnancy Risk Category: B (D if used in pregnancy-induced hypertension)

Drug Class: Diuretic with thiazide-like effects

MECHANISM OF ACTION
A thiazide diuretic that blocks reabsorption of sodium, potassium, and water at the distal convoluted tubule; also decreases plasma and extracellular fluid volume and peripheral vascular resistance.
Therapeutic Effect: Produces diuresis; lowers B/P.

USES
Treatment of edema, hypertension, diuresis, CHF

PHARMACOKINETICS
Rapidly absorbed from the GI tract. Excreted unchanged in urine.
Half-life: 35–50 hr. Onset of antihypertensive effect: 3–4 days; optimal therapeutic effect: 3–4 wk.

INDICATIONS AND DOSAGES
▸ **Hypertension, Edema**
PO
Adults. 25–100 mg/day or 100 mg 3 times a week.
Elderly. Initially, 12.5–25 mg/day or every other day.

SIDE EFFECTS/ADVERSE REACTIONS
Expected
Increase in urinary frequency and urine volume
Frequent
Potassium depletion (rarely produces symptoms)
Occasional
Anorexia, impotence, diarrhea, orthostatic hypotension, GI disturbances, photosensitivity
Rare
Rash

PRECAUTIONS AND CONTRAINDICATIONS
Anuria, history of hypersensitivity to sulfonamides or thiazide diuretics, renal decompensation
Caution:
Hypokalemia, renal disease, hepatic disease, gout, diabetes mellitus, elderly, lactation

DRUG INTERACTIONS OF CONCERN TO DENTISTRY
• Increased photosensitization: tetracyclines

C

• Decreased hypotensive response, nephrotoxicity: NSAIDs, indomethacin

SERIOUS REACTIONS

! Vigorous diuresis may lead to profound water and electrolyte depletion, resulting in hypokalemia, hyponatremia, and dehydration.

! Acute hypotensive episodes may occur.

! Hyperglycemia may occur during prolonged therapy.

! Overdose can lead to lethargy and coma without changes in electrolytes or hydration.

DENTAL CONSIDERATIONS

General:

• Monitor vital signs at every appointment because of cardiovascular side effects.

• After supine positioning, have patient sit upright for at least 2 min before standing to avoid orthostatic hypotension.

• Patients on chronic drug therapy may rarely have symptoms of blood dyscrasias, which can include infection, bleeding, and poor healing.

• Assess salivary flow as a factor in caries, periodontal disease, and candidiasis.

• Limit use of sodium-containing products, such as saline IV fluids, for those patients with a dietary salt restriction.

• Short appointments and a stress-reduction protocol may be required for anxious patients.

• Observe appropriate limitations of vasoconstrictor doses.

• Stress from dental procedures may compromise cardiovascular function; determine patient risk.

Consultations:

• In a patient with symptoms of blood dyscrasias, request a medical consultation for blood studies and postpone dental treatment until normal values are reestablished.

• Medical consultation may be required to assess disease control and patient's ability to tolerate stress.

Teach Patient/Family to:

• Encourage effective oral hygiene to prevent soft tissue inflammation.

• Use caution to prevent injury when using oral hygiene aids.

• When chronic dry mouth occurs, advise patient to:

  • Avoid mouth rinses with high alcohol content because of drying effects.

  • Use daily home fluoride products for anticaries effect.

  • Use sugarless gum, frequent sips of water, or saliva substitutes.

chlorzoxazone

klor-zox´-ah-zone

(Parafon Forte DSC, Remular, Remular-S)

Do not confuse with chlorthalidone.

CATEGORY AND SCHEDULE

Pregnancy Risk Category: C

Drug Class: Skeletal muscle relaxant, centrally acting

MECHANISM OF ACTION

A skeletal muscle relaxant that inhibits transmission of reflexes at the spinal cord level.

Therapeutic Effect: Relieves muscle spasticity.

USES
Adjunct for relief of muscle spasm in musculoskeletal conditions

PHARMACOKINETICS
Readily absorbed from the GI tract. Metabolized in liver. Primarily excreted in urine. *Half-life:* 1.1 hr.

INDICATIONS AND DOSAGES
▶ **Musculoskeletal Pain**
PO
Adults, Elderly. 250–500 mg 3–4 times a day. Maximum: 750 mg 3–4 day.
Children. 20 mg/kg/day in 3–4 divided doses.

SIDE EFFECTS/ADVERSE REACTIONS
Frequent
Drowsiness, fever, headache
Occasional
Nausea, vomiting, stomach cramps, rash

PRECAUTIONS AND CONTRAINDICATIONS
Hypersensitivity to chlorzoxazone or any one of its components
Caution:
Lactation, hepatic disease, elderly

DRUG INTERACTIONS OF CONCERN TO DENTISTRY
• Increased CNS depression: alcohol, narcotics, barbiturates, sedatives, hypnotics

SERIOUS REACTIONS
❗ Overdosage results in nausea, vomiting, diarrhea, and hypotension.

DENTAL CONSIDERATIONS
General:
• Determine why the patient is taking the drug.

• Consider semisupine chair position if back is involved.
• When used for dental-related problems, consider aspirin or NSAIDs to improve response.

cholestyramine resin
koe-less-**tir**′-ah-meen
(Novo-Cholamine[CAN], Prevalite, Questran[CAN], Questran Lite[AUS])
Do not confuse Questran with Quarzan.

CATEGORY AND SCHEDULE
Pregnancy Risk Category: B

Drug Class: Antihyperlipidemic

MECHANISM OF ACTION
An antihyperlipoproteinemic that binds with bile acids in the intestine, forming an insoluble complex. Binding results in partial removal of bile acid from enterohepatic circulation.
Therapeutic Effect: Blocks absorption of cholesterol from GI tract.

USES
Treatment of primary hypercholesterolemia, pruritus associated with biliary obstruction, diarrhea caused by excess bile acid, digitalis toxicity, xanthomas

PHARMACOKINETICS
Not absorbed from the GI tract. Decreases in serum LDL apparent in 5–7 days and in serum cholesterol in 1 mo. Serum cholesterol returns to baseline levels about 1 mo after drug is discontinued.

INDICATIONS AND DOSAGES
▶ **Primary Hypercholesterolemia**
PO
Adults, Elderly. 3–4 g 3–4 times a day. Maximum: 16–32 g/day in 2–4 divided doses.
Children older than 10 yr. 2 g/day. Maximum: 8 g/day in 2 or more divided doses.
Children 10 yr and younger. Initially, 2 g/day. Range: 1–4 g/day.
▶ **Pruritus**
PO
Adults, Elderly. 4 g 1–2 times a day. Maintenance: Up to 24 g/day in divided doses.

SIDE EFFECTS/ADVERSE REACTIONS
Frequent
Constipation (may lead to fecal impaction), nausea, vomiting, abdominal pain, indigestion
Occasional
Diarrhea, belching, bloating, headache, dizziness
Rare
Gallstones, peptic ulcer disease, malabsorption syndrome

PRECAUTIONS AND CONTRAINDICATIONS
Complete biliary obstruction, hypersensitivity to cholestyramine or tartrazine (frequently seen in aspirin hypersensitivity)
Caution:
Lactation, children

DRUG INTERACTIONS OF CONCERN TO DENTISTRY
• Decreased absorption of tetracyclines, cephalexin, phenobarbital, corticosteroids, clindamycin, penicillins; administer doses several hours apart

SERIOUS REACTIONS
❗ GI tract obstruction, hyperchloremic acidosis, and osteoporosis secondary to calcium excretion may occur.
❗ High dosage may interfere with fat absorption, resulting in steatorrhea.

DENTAL CONSIDERATIONS
General:
• Consider semisupine chair position for patient comfort because of GI side effects of disease.

ciclesonide
sye-**kles′**-oh-nide
(Alvesco, Omnaris)

CATEGORY AND SCHEDULE
Pregnancy Risk Category: C

Drug Class: Glucocorticoid

MECHANISM OF ACTION
The exact mechanism of action of corticosteroids in asthma is unknown. Ciclesonide a is non-halogenated glucocorticoid prodrug, hydrolyzed to a pharmacologically-active metabolite, C21-desisobutyryl-ciclesonide (des-ciclesonide or RM1) following oral inhalation. Has antiinflammatory and inhibitory activities against various mediators (e.g., histamine) and cell types (e.g., mast cells).

PHARMACOKINETICS
Absorption: minimal systemic absorption (intranasal); about 52% following oral inhalation. Protein binding: 99% or higher. Metabolized in the liver by CYP 3A4 and 2D6. It is hydrolyzed into active metabolites, des-ciclesonide by

esterases enzymes in nasal mucosa and lungs. Excreted primarily in feces (66% [intranasal]); partially in urine (20% [intranasal]); Oral inhalation: feces (78%). *Half-life*: Oral inhalation: 5–7 hr (metabolites); less than 1 hr (parent compound).

INDICATIONS AND DOSAGES
▸ **Asthma**
Oral Inhalation (Alvesco)
Adults, Children 12 yr and older.
Prior therapy with bronchodilators alone: 80 mcg twice daily (max: 160 mcg twice day). Prior therapy with inhaled corticosteroids: 80 mcg twice daily (max: 320 mcg twice daily). Prior therapy with oral corticosteroids: 320 mcg twice daily (max: 320 mcg twice daily).
▸ **Allergic Rhinitis**
Nasal (Omnaris)
Adults, Children 6 yr and older.
200 mcg daily (2 sprays [50 mcg/ spray]) in each nostril once daily. Do not exceed a total daily dose of 2 sprays in each nostril.

SIDE EFFECTS/ADVERSE REACTIONS
Frequent
Nasal: Mild nasopharyngeal irritation, burning, stinging, or dryness; headache, cough
Oral inhalation: Flu-like symptoms, headache, pharyngitis
Occasional
Nasal: Dry mouth, dyspepsia, rebound congestion, rhinorrhea, loss of taste
Inhalation: Back pain, vomiting, altered taste, voice changes, abdominal pain, nausea, dyspepsia
Rare
Facial edema, oral candidiasis, arthralgia, back pain, weight gain, cough, rash, rhinorrhea

PRECAUTIONS AND CONTRAINDICATIONS
Hypersensitivity to ciclesonide, corticosteroids, or any component of the formulations
Acute asthma and status asthmaticus (oral inhalation)
Untreated fungal, bacterial, or tuberculosis infections of the respiratory tract
Hypertension, diabetes mellitus, osteoporosis, peptic ulcer, glaucoma, cataracts, suppression of the hypothalamic-pituitary-adrenal (HPA) axis

DRUG INTERACTIONS OF CONCERN TO DENTISTRY
• Antifungals (azole): May increase levels of ciclesonide.
• CYP3A4 inhibitors (e.g., azole antifungals): May increase the levels and effects of ciclesonide.
• Quinolone antibiotics: May enhance the adverse effects of corticosteroids.

SERIOUS REACTIONS
! May cause adrenocortical suppression, which can lead to adrenal crisis, especially in younger children or in patients receiving high doses for prolonged periods.

DENTAL CONSIDERATIONS
General:
• Determine frequency and severity of asthmatic attacks.
• Assess salivary flow as a factor in caries, periodontal disease, and candidiasis.
• Mid-day appointments are suggested with stress-reduction protocol for anxious patients.
• Place on frequent recall because of oral side effects, including oropharyngeal candidiasis.

C

• Acute asthmatic episodes may be precipitated in dental office. Rapid-acting sympathomimetic inhalants should be available for emergency use.

Consultations:
• Medical consultation may be required to assess disease control and ability of patient to tolerate dental treatment.

Teach Patient/Family to:
• Encourage effective oral hygiene to prevent soft tissue inflammation.
• When chronic dry mouth occurs, advise patient to:
  • Avoid mouth rinses with high alcohol content because of drying effects.
  • Use daily home fluoride products for anticaries effect.
  • Use sugarless gum, frequent sips of water or artificial saliva substitutes.

ciclopirox

sye-kloe-**peer**′-ox
(Loprox, Penlac)
Do not confuse with ciprofloxacin.

CATEGORY AND SCHEDULE

Pregnancy Risk Category: B

Drug Class: Topical antifungal

MECHANISM OF ACTION

An antifungal that inhibits the transport of essential elements in the fungal cell, thereby interfering with biosynthesis in fungi.
Therapeutic Effect: Results in fungal cell death.

USES

Treatment of tinea cruris, tinea corporis, tinea pedis, tinea versicolor, cutaneous candidiasis, nail solution for immunocompetent patients with mild to moderate onychomycosis of nails without lunula involvement; caused by *T. rubrum*

PHARMACOKINETICS

Absorbed through intact skin. Distributed to epidermis, dermis, including hair, hair follicles, and sebaceous glands. Protein binding: 98%. Primarily excreted in urine and to a lesser extent in feces. *Half-life:* 1.7 hr.

INDICATIONS AND DOSAGES

▶ **Tinea Pedis**
Topical
Adults, Elderly, Children 10 yr and older. Apply 2 times a day until signs and symptoms significantly improve.

▶ **Tinea Cruris, Tinea Corporis**
Topical
Adults, Elderly, Children 10 yr and older. Apply 2 times a day until signs and symptoms significantly improve.

▶ **Onychomycosis**
Topical (Solution)
Adults, Elderly, Children 10 yr and older. Apply to the affected area (nails) daily. Remove with alcohol every 7 days.

▶ **Seborrheic Dermatitis**
Shampoo
Adults, Elderly, Children 10 yr and older. Apply to affected scalp areas 2 times a day, in the morning and evening for 4 wk.

SIDE EFFECTS/ADVERSE REACTIONS

Rare
Topical: Irritation, burning, redness, pain at the site of application

PRECAUTIONS AND CONTRAINDICATIONS

Hypersensitivity to ciclopirox or any one of its components
Caution:
Lactation, children younger than 10 yr

DRUG INTERACTIONS OF CONCERN TO DENTISTRY

• None reported

SERIOUS REACTIONS

! None known

DENTAL CONSIDERATIONS

General:
• There are neither dental drug interactions nor relevant considerations to dentistry for this drug.

cimetidine

sye-**met**′-ih-deen
(Apo-Cimetidine[CAN], Cimehexal[AUS], Magicul[AUS], Novocimetine[CAN], Peptol[CAN], Sigmetadine[AUS], Tagamet, Tagamet HB)
Do not confuse cimetidine with simethicone.

CATEGORY AND SCHEDULE

Pregnancy Risk Category: B

Drug Class: H_2 histamine receptor antagonist
OTC (100 mg tablets)

MECHANISM OF ACTION

An antiulcer agent and gastric acid secretion inhibitor that inhibits histamine action at H_2 receptor sites of parietal cells.
Therapeutic Effect: Inhibits gastric acid secretion during fasting, at night, or when stimulated by food, caffeine, or insulin.

USES

Short-term treatment of duodenal and benign gastric ulcers and maintenance; gastroesophageal reflux disease (GERD), upper GI bleeding, pathologic hypersecretory diseases and heartburn with acid indigestion

PHARMACOKINETICS

Well absorbed from the GI tract. Protein binding: 15%–20%. Widely distributed. Metabolized in the liver. Primarily excreted in urine. Not removed by hemodialysis. *Half-life:* 2 hr; increased with impaired renal function.

INDICATIONS AND DOSAGES
▸ **Active Ulcer**
PO
Adults, Elderly. 300 mg 4 times a day or 400 mg twice a day or 800 mg at bedtime.
IV, IM
Adults, Elderly. 300 mg q6h or 150 mg as single dose followed by 37.5 mg/hr continuous infusion.
▸ **Prevention of Duodenal Ulcer**
PO
Adults, Elderly. 400–800 mg at bedtime.
▸ **Gastric Hypersecretory Secretions**
PO, IV, IM
Adults, Elderly. 300–600 mg q6h. Maximum: 2400 mg/day.
Children. 20–40 mg/kg/day in divided doses q6h.
Infants. 10–20 mg/kg/day in divided doses q6–12h.
Neonates. 5–10 mg/kg/day in divided doses q8–12h.

> **GERD**

PO

Adults, Elderly. 800 mg twice a day or 400 mg 4 times a day for 12 wk.

> **OTC Use**

PO

Adults, Elderly. 100 mg up to 30 min before meals. Maximum: 2 doses a day.

> **Prevention of Upper GI Bleeding**

IV Infusion

Adults, Elderly. 50 mg/hr.

> **Dosage in Renal Impairment**

Dosage is based on a 300-mg dose in adults. Dosage interval is modified on the basis of creatinine clearance.

Creatinine Clearance	Dosage Interval
Greater than 40 ml/min	q6h
20–40 ml/min	q8h or decrease dose by 25%
Less than 20 ml/min	q12h or decrease dose by 50%

Give after hemodialysis and q12h between dialysis sessions.

SIDE EFFECTS/ADVERSE REACTIONS

Occasional

Headache

Elderly and severely ill patients, patients with impaired renal function: Confusion, agitation, psychosis, depression, anxiety, disorientation, hallucinations. Effects reverse 3–4 days after discontinuance

Rare

Diarrhea, dizziness, somnolence, nausea, vomiting, gynecomastia, rash, impotence

PRECAUTIONS AND CONTRAINDICATIONS

Hypersensitivity to other H_2-antagonists

Caution:

Lactation, children younger than 12 yr, organic brain syndrome, hepatic disease, renal disease, smoking

DRUG INTERACTIONS OF CONCERN TO DENTISTRY

• GI ulceration, bleeding: aspirin, NSAIDs

• Decreased absorption: sodium bicarbonate, anticholinergics

• Decreased absorption of fluconazole, ketoconazole, tetracycline (take doses 2 hr apart), ferrous salts

• Increased blood levels of metronidazole, alcohol, lidocaine, narcotic analgesics, benzodiazepines, carbamazepine

SERIOUS REACTIONS

! Rapid IV administration may produce cardiac arrhythmias and hypotension.

DENTAL CONSIDERATIONS

General:

• Monitor vital signs at every appointment because of cardiovascular side effects.

• Consider semisupine chair position for patient comfort because of GI side effects of disease.

• Avoid prescribing aspirin- or NSAID-containing products in patients with active upper GI disease; risk of irritation and ulceration exists.

• Sodium bicarbonate products can be used 1 hr before or 1 hr after cimetidine dose.

Teach Patient/Family to:

• Encourage effective oral hygiene to prevent soft tissue inflammation.

• Use caution to prevent injury when using oral hygiene aids.

ciprofloxacin hydrochloride

sip-ro-**floks'**-ah-sin
hi-droe-**klor'**-ide
(C-Flox[AUS], Ciloquin[AUS], Ciloxan, Cipro, Ciproxin[AUS])
Do not confuse ciprofloxacin or Ciproxin with Ciloxan, cinoxacin, or Cytoxan.

CATEGORY AND SCHEDULE
Pregnancy Risk Category: C

Drug Class: Topical fluoroquinolone antiinfective

MECHANISM OF ACTION
A fluoroquinolone that inhibits the enzyme DNA gyrase in susceptible bacteria, interfering with bacterial cell replication.
Therapeutic Effect: Bactericidal.

USES
Infections caused by susceptible strains of microorganisms in conjunctivitis or corneal ulcers

PHARMACOKINETICS
Well absorbed from the GI tract (food delays absorption). Protein binding: 20%–40%. Widely distributed (including to CSF). Metabolized in the liver to active metabolite. Primarily excreted in urine. Minimal removal by hemodialysis. ***Half-life:*** 4–6 hr (increased in impaired renal function and the elderly).

INDICATIONS AND DOSAGES
▶ **Mild to Moderate UTIs**
PO
Adults, Elderly. 250 mg q12h.
IV
Adults, Elderly. 200 mg q12h.

▶ **Complicated UTIs; Mild to Moderate Respiratory Tract, Bone, Joint, Skin, and Skin-Structure Infections; Infectious Diarrhea**
PO
Adults, Elderly. 500 mg q12h.
IV
Adults, Elderly. 400 mg q12h.

▶ **Severe, Complicated Infections**
PO
Adults, Elderly. 750 mg q12h.
IV
Adults, Elderly. 400 mg q12h.

▶ **Prostatitis**
PO
Adults, Elderly. 500 mg q12h for 28 days.

▶ **Uncomplicated Bladder Infection**
PO
Adults. 100 mg twice a day for 3 days.

▶ **Acute Sinusitis**
PO
Adults. 500 mg q12h.

▶ **Uncomplicated Gonorrhea**
PO
Adults. 250 mg as a single dose.

▶ **Cystic Fibrosis**
IV
Children. 30 mg/kg/day in 2–3 divided doses. Maximum: 1.2 g/day.
PO
Children. 40 mg/kg/day. Maximum: 2 g/day.

▶ **Corneal Ulcer**
Ophthalmic
Adults, Elderly. 2 drops q15min for 6 hr, then 2 drops q30min for the remainder of first day, 2 drops q1h on second day, and 2 drops q4h on days 3–14.

▶ **Conjunctivitis**
Ophthalmic
Adults, Elderly. 1–2 drops q2h for 2 days, then 2 drops q4h for next 5 days.

C

▸ **Dosage in Renal Impairment**
Dosage and frequency are modified on the basis of creatinine clearance and the severity of the infection.

Creatinine Clearance	Dosage Interval
Less than 30 ml/min	Usual dose q18–24h

▸ **Hemodialysis**
Adults, Elderly. 250–500 mg q24h (after dialysis).
▸ **Peritoneal Dialysis**
Adults, Elderly. 250–500 mg q24h (after dialysis).

SIDE EFFECTS/ADVERSE REACTIONS
Frequent
Nausea, diarrhea, dyspepsia, vomiting, constipation, flatulence, confusion, crystalluria
Ophthalmic: Burning, crusting in corner of eye
Occasional
Abdominal pain or discomfort, headache, rash
Ophthalmic: Bad taste, sensation of something in eye, eyelid redness or itching
Rare
Dizziness, confusion, tremors, hallucinations, hypersensitivity reaction, insomnia, dry mouth, paresthesia

PRECAUTIONS AND CONTRAINDICATIONS
Hypersensitivity to ciprofloxacin or other quinolones; for ophthalmic administration: vaccinia, varicella, epithelial herpes simplex, keratitis, mycobacterial infection, fungal disease of ocular structure, use after uncomplicated removal of a foreign body

Caution:
Lactation, children, renal disease, tendon ruptures of shoulder, hand, and Achilles tendons, epilepsy, severe cerebral arteriosclerosis; monitor blood glucose levels, extended release tablets can be taken with meals, defects in glucose-6-phosphate dehydrogenase activity, myasthenia gravis

DRUG INTERACTIONS OF CONCERN TO DENTISTRY
• Decreased absorption: divalent, trivalent antacids, iron and zinc salts, calcium fortified juices.
• Increased serum levels: probenecid.
• Increased risk of bleeding with warfarin (monitor).
• Serious adverse effects with theophylline, caffeine.
• Specific studies have not been conducted with topical ciprofloxacin. See systemic drug for interactions.

SERIOUS REACTIONS
! Superinfection (especially enterococcal or fungal), nephropathy, cardiopulmonary arrest, chest pain, and cerebral thrombosis may occur.
! Hypersensitivity reactions, including photosensitivity (as evidenced by rash, pruritus, blisters, edema, and burning skin), have occurred in patients receiving fluoroquinolones.
! Arthropathy may occur if the drug is given to children younger than 18 yr.
! Sensitization to the ophthalmic form of the drug may contraindicate later systemic use of ciprofloxacin.

DENTAL CONSIDERATIONS

General:
• Determine why the patient is taking the drug.
• Avoid dental light in patient's eyes; offer dark glasses for patient comfort.
• Minimize exposure to sunlight and wear sunscreen if sun exposure is planned.
• Ruptures of the shoulder, hand, and Achilles tendon requiring surgical repair or resulting in prolonged disability have been reported with this drug.
• Protect patient's eyes from accidental spatter during dental treatment.
• Avoid dental light in patient's eyes; offer dark glasses for patient comfort.

Consultations:
• Consult with patient's physician if an acute dental infection occurs and another antiinfective is required.

Teach Patient/Family to:
• Discontinue treatment and inform dentist immediately if patient experiences pain or inflammation of a tendon, and to rest and refrain from exercise.

cisplatin
sis-**plah'**-tin
(Platinol-AQ)
Do not confuse cisplatin with carboplatin, or Platinol with Paraplatin or Patanol.

CATEGORY AND SCHEDULE
Pregnancy Risk Category: D

Drug Class: Platinum coordination complex; antineoplastic

MECHANISM OF ACTION
A platinum coordination complex that inhibits DNA and to a lesser extent, RNA, protein synthesis by cross-linking with DNA strands, preventing cell division. Cell cycle-phase nonspecific.
Therapeutic Effect: Interferes with DNA function.

USES
Treatment of metastatic testicular tumors, metastatic ovarian tumors, advanced bladder carcinoma

PHARMACOKINETICS
Widely distributed. Protein binding: greater than 90%. Undergoes rapid nonenzymatic conversion to inactive metabolite. Excreted in urine. Removed by hemodialysis. *Half-life:* 58–73 hr (increased with impaired renal function).

INDICATIONS AND DOSAGES
▶ **Advanced Bladder Carcinoma, Metastatic Ovarian Tumors, Metastatic Testicular Tumors**
IV
Adults, Elderly, Children. For intermittent dosage schedule, 37–75 mg/m² once every 2–3 wk or 50–100 mg/m² over 4–8 hr once every 21–28 days. For daily dosage schedule, 15–20 mg/m²/day for 5 days every 3–4 wk.
▶ **Dosage in Renal Impairment**
Dosage is modified on the basis of creatinine clearance.

Creatinine Clearance	Dosage Interval
10–50 ml/min	75%
Less than 10 ml/min	50%

C

SIDE EFFECTS/ADVERSE REACTIONS

Frequent

Nausea, vomiting (generally beginning 1–4 hr after administration and lasting up to 24 hr); myelosuppression (affecting 25%–30% of patients with recovery generally occurring in 18–23 days)

Occasional

Peripheral neuropathy (with prolonged therapy [4–7 mo]). Pain or redness at injection site, loss of taste or appetite

Rare

Hemolytic anemia, blurred vision, stomatitis

PRECAUTIONS AND CONTRAINDICATIONS

Hearing impairment, myelosuppression, pregnancy

DRUG INTERACTIONS OF CONCERN TO DENTISTRY

• Risk of masking ototoxicity: antihistamines

SERIOUS REACTIONS

! An anaphylactic reaction manifested as angioedema, wheezing, tachycardia, and hypotension, may occur in the first few minutes of IV administration in patients previously exposed to cisplatin.

! Nephrotoxicity occurs in 28%–36% of patients treated with a single dose of cisplatin, usually during the second week of therapy.

! Ototoxicity, including tinnitus and hearing loss, occurs in 31% of patients treated with a single dose of cisplatin. It may be more severe in children and may become more frequent or severe with repeated doses.

DENTAL CONSIDERATIONS

General:

• Determine why patient is taking the drug.

• If additional analgesia is required for dental pain, consider alternative analgesics (NSAIDs) in patients taking narcotics for acute or chronic pain.

• Examine for oral manifestation of opportunistic infection.

• Avoid prescribing aspirin-containing products.

• This drug may be used in the hospital or on an outpatient basis. Confirm the patient's disease and treatment status.

• Chlorhexidine mouth rinse prior to and during chemotherapy may reduce severity of mucositis.

• Patient on chronic drug therapy may rarely present with symptoms of blood dyscrasias, which can include infection, bleeding, and poor healing. If dyscrasia is present, caution patient to prevent oral tissue trauma when using oral hygiene aids.

• Palliative medication may be required for management of oral side effects.

• Short appointments and a stress-reduction protocol may be required for anxious patients.

• Patients may have received other chemotherapy or radiation; confirm medical and drug history.

• Patients may be at risk of bleeding; check for oral signs.

• Oral infections should be eliminated and/or treated aggressively.

• Patients may be at risk of infection.

Consultations:

• Medical consultation should include routine blood counts

including platelet counts and
bleeding time.

• Consult physician; prophylactic or
therapeutic antiinfectives may be
indicated if surgery or periodontal
treatment is required.

• Medical consultation may be
required to assess immunologic
status during cancer chemotherapy
and determine safety risk, if any,
posed by the required dental
treatment.

• Medical consultation may be
required to assess disease control
and patient's ability to tolerate
stress.

Teach Patient/Family to:

• See dentist immediately if
secondary oral infection occurs.

• Be aware of oral side effects.

• Encourage effective oral
hygiene to prevent soft tissue
inflammation.

• Report oral lesions, soreness, or
bleeding to dentist.

• Prevent trauma when using oral
hygiene aids.

• Update health and medication
history if physician makes any
changes in evaluation or drug
regimens; include OTC, herbal, and
nonherbal remedies in the update.

clarithromycin
clare-ih-thro-**mye**´-sin
(Biaxin, Biaxin XL, Klacid[AUS])

CATEGORY AND SCHEDULE
Pregnancy Risk Category: C

Drug Class: Macrolide antibiotic

MECHANISM OF ACTION
A macrolide that binds to ribosomal
receptor sites of susceptible
organisms, inhibiting protein
synthesis of the bacterial cell wall.
Therapeutic Effect: Bacteriostatic;
may be bactericidal with high
dosages or very susceptible
microorganisms.

USES
Treatment of mild-to-moderate
infections of the upper and lower
respiratory tract; community-
acquired pneumonia caused by
H. influenzae; uncomplicated skin
and skin structure infections caused
by *S. pneumoniae, M. pneumoniae,*
C. diphtheriae, B. pertussis,
L. monocytogenes, H. influenzae,
S. pyogenes, and *S. aureus;* otitis
media; maxillary sinusitis, bronchitis
(XL dose form); middle ear
infection; disseminated
Mycobacterium avium complex
(MAC); in combination with
other drugs for *H. pylori* duodenal
ulcer

PHARMACOKINETICS
Well absorbed from the GI tract.
Protein binding: 65%–75%.
Widely distributed. Metabolized in
the liver to active metabolite.
Primarily excreted in urine. Not
removed by hemodialysis.
Half-life: 3–7 hr; metabolite 5–7 hr
(increased in impaired renal
function).

INDICATIONS AND DOSAGES
▶ **Bronchitis**
PO
Adults, Elderly. 500 mg q12h for
7–14 days.
▶ **Skin, Soft Tissue Infections**
PO
Adults, Elderly. 250 mg q12h for
7–14 days.
Children. 7.5 mg/kg q12h for 10
days.

C

▶ **MAC Prophylaxis**
PO
Adults, Elderly. 500 mg 2 times a day.
Children. 7.5 mg/kg q12h.
Maximum: 500 mg 2 times a day.

▶ **MAC Treatment**
PO
Adults, Elderly. 500 mg 2 times a day in combination.
Children. 7.5 mg/kg q12h in combination. Maximum: 500 mg 2 times a day.

▶ **Pharyngitis, Tonsillitis**
PO
Adults, Elderly. 250 mg q12h for 10 days.
Children. 7.5 mg/kg q12h for 10 days.

▶ **Pneumonia**
PO
Adults, Elderly. 250 mg q12h for 7–14 days.
Children. 7.5 mg/kg q12h.

▶ **Maxillary Sinusitis**
PO
Adults, Elderly. 500 mg q12h for 14 days.
Children. 7.5 mg/kg q12h.
Maximum: 500 mg 2 times a day.

▶ *H. pylori*
PO
Adults, Elderly. 500 mg q12h for 10–14 days in combination.

▶ **Acute Otitis Media**
PO
Children. 7.5 mg/kg q12h for 10 days.

▶ **Dosage in Renal Impairment**
For patients with creatinine clearance less than 30 ml/min, reduce dose by 50% and administer once or twice a day.

SIDE EFFECTS/ADVERSE REACTIONS
Occasional
Diarrhea, nausea, altered taste, abdominal pain

Rare
Headache, dyspepsia

PRECAUTIONS AND CONTRAINDICATIONS
Hypersensitivity to clarithromycin or other macrolide antibiotics
Caution:
Lactation, hepatic and renal disease

DRUG INTERACTIONS OF CONCERN TO DENTISTRY
• Decreased effect: anticholinergic drugs
• Use with caution, possible reduced metabolism: drugs metabolized by CYP450 3A4 isoenzymes
• Increased effects of cyclosporine, warfarin, cilostazol, tacrolimus, pimozide, methylprednisolone, fluconazole, buspirone
• Decreased action of clindamycin, penicillins, lincomycin, rifabutin, rifampin, zidovudine
• Increased serum levels of carbamazepine, theophylline, digoxin
• Contraindicated with indinavir
• Increased CNS depression with alprazolam, diazepam, midazolam, triazolam
• Suspected increase in plasma levels of repaglinide
• Risk of severe myopathy or rhabdomyolysis: atorvastatin, fluvastatin, lovastatin, pravastatin

SERIOUS REACTIONS
❗ Antibiotic-associated colitis and other superinfections may result from altered bacterial balance.
❗ Hepatotoxicity and thrombocytopenia occur rarely.

DENTAL CONSIDERATIONS

General:

• Determine why the patient is taking the drug.

• May prove to be an alternative drug of choice for mild infections caused by a susceptible organism in patients who are allergic to penicillin.

Teach Patient/Family to:

• Encourage effective oral hygiene to prevent soft tissue inflammation.

• When used for dental infection, advise patient to:

• Report sore throat, oral burning sensation, fever, and fatigue, any of which could indicate superinfection.

• Take at prescribed intervals and complete dosage regimen.

• Immediately notify the dentist if signs or symptoms of infection increase.

---

clemastine fumarate
klem′-as-teen fyoo′-mer-ate
(Dayhistol Allergy, Tavist Allergy)

CATEGORY AND SCHEDULE
Pregnancy Risk Category: B

Drug Class: Antihistamine, H₁-receptor antagonist

MECHANISM OF ACTION
An ethanolamine that competes with histamine on effector cells in the GI tract, blood vessels, and respiratory tract.

Therapeutic Effect: Relieves allergy symptoms, including urticaria, rhinitis, and pruritus.

USES
Treatment of allergy symptoms, rhinitis, angioedema, urticaria, common cold

PHARMACOKINETICS

Route	Onset	Peak	Duration
PO	15–60 min	5–7 hr	10–12 hr

Well absorbed from the GI tract. Metabolized in the liver. Excreted primarily in urine.

INDICATIONS AND DOSAGES
▸ **Allergic Rhinitis, Urticaria**
PO
Adults, Children older than 11 yr.
1.34 mg twice a day up to 2.68 mg 3 times a day. Maximum: 8.04 mg/day.
Children 6–11 yr. 0.67–1.34 mg twice a day. Maximum: 4.02 mg/day.
Children younger than 6 yr.
0.05 mg/kg/day divided into 2–3 doses per day. Maximum: 1.34 mg/day.
Elderly. 1.34 mg 1–2 times a day.

SIDE EFFECTS/ADVERSE REACTIONS
Frequent
Somnolence, dizziness, urine retention, thickening of bronchial secretions, dry mouth, nose, or throat; in elderly, sedation, dizziness, hypotension
Occasional
Epigastric distress, flushing, blurred vision, tinnitus, paresthesia, diaphoresis, chills

PRECAUTIONS AND CONTRAINDICATIONS
Angle-closure glaucoma, hypersensitivity to clemastine, use within 14 days of MAOIs

Caution:
Increased intraocular pressure, renal disease, cardiac disease, hypertension, bronchial asthma, seizure disorder, stenosed peptic ulcers, hyperthyroidism, prostatic hypertrophy, bladder neck obstruction, elderly

DRUG INTERACTIONS OF CONCERN TO DENTISTRY
• Increased CNS depression: all CNS depressants, alcohol
• Increased anticholinergic effect of anticholinergics, phenothiazines, tricyclic antidepressants

SERIOUS REACTIONS
❗ A hypersensitivity reaction, marked by eczema, pruritus, rash, cardiac disturbances, angioedema, and photosensitivity, may occur.
❗ Overdose symptoms may vary from CNS depression, including sedation, apnea, cardiovascular collapse, and death to severe paradoxical reaction, such as hallucinations, tremors, and seizures.
❗ Children may experience paradoxical reactions, such as restlessness, insomnia, euphoria, nervousness, and tremors.
❗ Overdose in children may result in hallucinations, seizures, and death.

DENTAL CONSIDERATIONS
General:
• Assess salivary flow as a factor in caries, periodontal disease, and candidiasis.
• Determine why the patient is taking the drug.
Teach Patient/Family to:
• Encourage effective oral hygiene to prevent soft tissue inflammation.
• Use caution to prevent injury when using oral hygiene aids.

• When chronic dry mouth occurs, advise patient to:
   • Avoid mouth rinses with high alcohol content because of drying effects.
   • Use daily home fluoride products for anticaries effect.
   • Use sugarless gum, frequent sips of water, or saliva substitutes.

clevidipine
klev-**id**-i-peen
(Cleviprex)

CATEGORY AND SCHEDULE
Pregnancy Risk Category: C

Drug Class: Antihypertensive; Calcium Channel Blocker, third-generation dihydropyridine

MECHANISM OF ACTION
A short-acting dihydropyridine calcium channel antagonist that selectively relaxes smooth muscle cells that line the small arteries. Decreases systemic vascular resistance; does not reduce preload. It is associated with greater inotropic versus chronotropic selectivity; increase in stroke volume.
Therapeutic Effect: Reduces blood pressure.

USES
Hypertension when oral therapy is not feasible or desired, perioperative hypertension, hypertensive urgency, and hypertensive emergency

PHARMACOKINETICS
IV administration results in complete bioavailability. Protein

binding: 99.5%. Rapidly metabolized by hydrolysis, primarily esterases in plasma and tissue to inactive metabolites; metabolites are excreted in urine (63%–74%) and feces (7%–22%). *Half-life:* 1 min (initial phase); 15 min (terminal phase).

INDICATIONS AND DOSAGES
▸ **Hypertension when Oral Therapy Is Not Feasible or Desired, Perioperative Hypertension, Hypertensive Urgency, and Hypertensive Emergency**
IV
Adults. Initial dose: 1–2 mg/hr; Dose titration: Double dose every 90 sec initially; as blood pressure approaches goal, increase dose by less than double and lengthen the time between dose adjustments to every 5–10 min. Usual dose required is 4–6 mg/hr. Severe hypertensive patients may require higher doses with a maximum of 16 mg/hr or less. Doses up to 32 mg/hr have been used, but generally should not exceed 21 mg/hr in a 24-hr period due to lipid load.

SIDE EFFECTS/ADVERSE REACTIONS
Frequent
Atrial fibrillation, nausea, fever, insomnia
Occasional
Headache, CHF, hypotension, rebound hypertension, reflex tachycardia, vomiting, arthralgia, acute renal failure

PRECAUTIONS AND CONTRAINDICATIONS
Hypersensitivity to clevidipine or any component of the formulation
Allergy to soybeans or eggs/egg products

Defective lipid metabolism including pathologic hyperlipidemia, lipoid nephrosis or acute pancreatitis
Severe aortic stenosis
Caution:
Elderly
Heart failure
Concurrent β-blocker use; gradually reduce dose

DRUG INTERACTIONS OF CONCERN TO DENTISTRY
• Other antihypertensives: May increase risk of hypotension.
• Anesthetics: General anesthetics may be potentiated by calcium-channel blockers' additive hypotension, depression of cardiac contractility, conductivity, and automaticity. Local anesthetics may cause additive hypotension as well.
• NSAIDS: Inhibits vasodilatory prostaglandins and may affect the response to antihypertensive agents.

SERIOUS REACTIONS
! Hypotension and reflex tachycardia may occur with rapid upward titration.

DENTAL CONSIDERATIONS
General:
• Monitor vital signs at every appointment because of cardiovascular side effects.
• After supine positioning, have patient sit upright for at least 2 min before standing to avoid orthostatic hypotension.
• Assess salivary flow as a factor in caries, periodontal disease, and candidiasis.
• Stress from dental procedures may compromise cardiovascular function; determine patient risk.

Consultations:
• Medical consultation may be required to assess disease control.
Teach Patient/Family to:
• Report oral lesions, soreness, or bleeding to dentist.
• When chronic dry mouth occurs, advise patient to:
  • Avoid mouth rinses with high alcohol content because of drying effects.
  • Use daily home fluoride products for anticaries effect.
  • Use sugarless gum, frequent sips of water, or saliva substitutes.

clindamycin
klin-da-**mye'**-sin
(Cleocin, Cleocin HCl[AUS], Clindesse, Dalacin[CAN], Dalacin C[AUS])

CATEGORY AND SCHEDULE
Pregnancy Risk Category: B

Drug Class: Lincomycin derivative antiinfective

MECHANISM OF ACTION
A lincosamide antibiotic that inhibits protein synthesis of the bacterial cell wall by binding to bacterial ribosomal receptor sites. Topically, it decreases fatty acid concentration on the skin.
Therapeutic Effect: Bacteriostatic. Prevents outbreaks of acne vulgaris.

USES
Indications for use include serious infections caused by susceptible anaerobic bacteria and the treatment of serious infections caused by susceptible strains of pneumococci and streptococci; includes infections of the respiratory tract, serious skin and soft tissue infections, intraabdominal abscess, and infections of the female GU tract.

PHARMACOKINETICS
Rapidly absorbed from the GI tract. Protein binding: 92%–94%. Widely distributed. Metabolized in the liver to some active metabolites. Primarily excreted in urine. Not removed by hemodialysis. *Half-life:* 2.4–3 hr (increased in impaired renal function and premature infants).

INDICATIONS AND DOSAGES
▶ **Chronic Bone and Joint, Respiratory Tract, Skin and Soft Tissue, Intraabdominal, and Female GU Infections; Endocarditis; Septicemia**
PO
Adults, Elderly. 150–450 mg/dose q6–8h.
Children. 10–30 mg/kg/day in 3–4 divided doses. Maximum: 1.8 g/day.
IV, IM
Adults, Elderly. 1.2–1.8 g/day in 2–4 divided doses.
Children. 25–40 mg/kg/day in 3–4 divided doses. Maximum: 4.8 g/day.
▶ **Bacterial Vaginosis**
PO
Adults, Elderly. 300 mg twice a day for 7 days.
▶ **Intravaginal**
Adults. One full applicator at bedtime for 3–7 days or 1 suppository at bedtime for 3 days.
▶ **Acne Vulgaris**
Topical
Adults. Apply thin layer to affected area twice a day.

SIDE EFFECTS/ADVERSE REACTIONS

Frequent
Systemic: Abdominal pain, nausea, vomiting, diarrhea
Topical: Dry scaly skin
Vaginal: Vaginitis, pruritus
Occasional
Systemic: Phlebitis or thrombophlebitis with IV administration, pain and induration at IM injection site, allergic reaction, urticaria, pruritus
Topical: Contact dermatitis, abdominal pain, mild diarrhea, burning, or stinging
Vaginal: Headache, dizziness, nausea, vomiting, abdominal pain
Rare
Vaginal: Hypersensitivity reaction

PRECAUTIONS AND CONTRAINDICATIONS

History of antibiotic-associated colitis, regional enteritis, or ulcerative colitis; hypersensitivity to clindamycin or lincomycin
Caution:
Renal disease, liver disease, GI disease, elderly, lactation, tartrazine sensitivity

DRUG INTERACTIONS OF CONCERN TO DENTISTRY

• Decreased action: erythromycin, absorbent antidiarrheals (e.g., aluminum salts)
• Increased effects of nondepolarizing muscle relaxants, hydrocarbon inhalation anesthetics
• Avoid antiperistaltic drugs if diarrhea occurs
• Possible reduced blood levels of cyclosporine
• Oral contraceptives: advise patient of a potential low risk for decreased contraceptive action, to maintain compliance with oral contraceptive use while using antibiotics, and to consider the use of additional nonhormonal contraception

SERIOUS REACTIONS

! Antibiotic-associated colitis and other superinfections may occur during and several weeks after clindamycin therapy (including topical form).
! Blood dyscrasias (leukopenia, thrombocytopenia) and nephrotoxicity (proteinuria, azotemia, oliguria) occur rarely.

DENTAL CONSIDERATIONS

General:
• Determine why the patient is taking the drug.
Consultations:
• Medical consultation may be required to assess disease control.
Teach Patient/Family to:
• Encourage effective oral hygiene to prevent soft tissue inflammation.
• Use caution to prevent injury when using oral hygiene aids.
• When used for dental infection, advise patient to:
    • Report sore throat, oral burning sensation, fever, and fatigue, any of which could indicate superinfection.
    • Take at prescribed intervals and complete dosage regimen.
    • Immediately notify the dentist if signs or symptoms of infection increase.

C

clobetasol

klo-**bet**′-ah-sol
(Alti-Clobetasol[CAN], Cormax,
Dermovate[CAN], Gen-
Clobetasol[CAN], Olux, Novo-
Clobetasol[CAN], Temovate)

CATEGORY AND SCHEDULE
Pregnancy Risk Category: C

Drug Class: Topical
corticosteroid, very high potency

MECHANISM OF ACTION
A corticosteroid that inhibits
accumulation of inflammatory cells
at inflammation sites, phagocytosis,
lysosomal enzyme release, and
synthesis or release of mediators of
inflammation.
Therapeutic Effect: Decreases or
prevents tissue response to
inflammatory process.

USES
Treatment of inflammatory and
pruritic manifestations of moderate
to severe corticosteroid-responsive
dermatitis of the scalp; other uses
include psoriasis.

PHARMACOKINETICS
May be absorbed from intact skin.
Metabolized in liver. Excreted in the
urine.

INDICATIONS AND DOSAGES
▶ **Antiinflammatory, Corticosteroid
Replacement Therapy**
Topical
*Adults, Elderly, Children 12 yr
and older.* Apply 2 times a day for
2 wk.
Foam
*Adults, Elderly, Children 12 yr
and older.* Apply 2 times a day for
2 wk.

SIDE EFFECTS/ADVERSE REACTIONS
Frequent
Local irritation, dry skin, itching,
redness
Occasional
Allergic contact dermatitis
Rare
Cushing's syndrome, numbness of
fingers, skin atrophy

PRECAUTIONS AND CONTRAINDICATIONS
Hypersensitivity to clobetasol or
other corticosteroids
Caution:
Lactation, bacterial infections

DRUG INTERACTIONS OF CONCERN TO DENTISTRY
• None reported

SERIOUS REACTIONS
! Overdosage can occur from
topically applied clobetasol
propionate absorbed in sufficient
amounts to produce systemic effects
producing reversible adrenal
suppression, manifestations of
Cushing's syndrome, hyperglycemia,
and glucosuria in some patients.

DENTAL CONSIDERATIONS
**Clobetasol Propionate (Topical
Foam)**
General:
• Determine why patient is taking
the drug.
• Avoid use of systemic
corticosteroids unless a consultation
is made.
Clobetasol Propionate
General:
• Place on frequent recall to evaluate
healing response.
• Topical adrenocorticosteroids are
not indicated for treating plaque-
related gingivitis, which should be

treated by removal of local irritants and improved oral hygiene.

Teach Patient/Family to:
• Encourage effective oral hygiene to prevent soft tissue inflammation.
• Use on oral herpetic ulcerations is contraindicated.
• Apply at bedtime or after meals for maximum effect.
• Apply with cotton-tipped applicator by pressing, not rubbing, paste on lesion.
• Return for oral evaluation if response of oral tissues has not occurred in 7–14 days.

clocortolone
klo-**kort**'-oh-lone
(Cloderm, Cloderm[CAN])

CATEGORY AND SCHEDULE
Pregnancy Risk Category: C

Drug Class: Topical corticosteroid, group III medium potency

MECHANISM OF ACTION
A topical corticosteroid that inhibits accumulation of inflammatory cells at inflammation sites, suppresses mitotic activity, and causes vasoconstriction.
Therapeutic Effect: Decreases or prevents tissue response to inflammatory process.

USES
Psoriasis, eczema, contact dermatitis, pruritus

PHARMACOKINETICS
Absorption is variable and dependent upon many factors including integrity of skin, dose, vehicle used, and use of occlusive dressings. Small amounts may be absorbed from the skin. Metabolized in liver. Excreted in the urine and feces.

INDICATIONS AND DOSAGES
▸ **Dermatoses**
Topical
Adults, Elderly, Children 12 yr and older. Apply 1–4 times a day.

SIDE EFFECTS/ADVERSE REACTIONS
Occasional
Local irritation, burning, itching, redness
Allergic contact dermatitis
Rare
Hypertrichosis, hypopigmentation, maceration of skin, miliaria, perioral dermatitis, skin atrophy, striae

PRECAUTIONS AND CONTRAINDICATIONS
Hypersensitivity to clocortolone pivalate or other corticosteroids; viral, fungal, or tubercular skin lesions
Caution:
Lactation, viral infections, bacterial infections

DRUG INTERACTIONS OF CONCERN TO DENTISTRY
• None reported

SERIOUS REACTIONS
! Overdosage can occur from topically applied clocortolone pivalate absorbed in sufficient amounts to produce systemic effects in some patients.

DENTAL CONSIDERATIONS
General:
• Determine why the patient is taking the drug.

C

• Place on frequent recall to evaluate healing response if used on a chronic basis.
• Apply lubricant to dry lips for patient comfort before dental procedures.

clofarabine
kloe-**far′**-ah-been
(Clolar)

CATEGORY AND SCHEDULE
Pregnancy Risk Category: D

Drug Class: Antineoplastic

MECHANISM OF ACTION
An antineoplastic agent that inhibits DNA synthesis by decreasing deoxynucleotide triphosphate pools. It inhibits ribonucleoside reductase, terminates elongation of the DNA chain, and inhibits repair through incorporation into the DNA chain by competitive inhibition of DNA polymerases.
Therapeutic Effect: Inhibits synthesis of DNA.

USES
Treatment of acute lymphoid leukemia (ALL) in patients who have failed prior regimens

PHARMACOKENETICS
Protein binding: 47%. Negligible liver metabolism. Primarily excreted in urine. ***Half-life:*** 5.2 hr.

INDICATIONS AND DOSAGES
▶ ALL
IV
Adults. 52 mg/m^2 over 2 hr daily for 5 consecutive days. Repeat every 2–6 wk following recovery or return to baseline organ function.

Children. 52 mg/m^2 over 2 hr daily for 5 consecutive days. Repeat every 2–6 wk following recovery or return to baseline organ function.

SIDE EFFECTS/ADVERSE REACTIONS:
Frequent
Infection, vomiting, nausea, febrile neutropenia, diarrhea, pruritus, headache, ALT increased, dermatitis, pyrexia, AST increased, rigors, abdominal pain, fatigue, pericardial effusion, tachycardia, epistaxis, anorexia, petechiae, hypotension, pain in limb, left ventricular systolic dysfunction, anxiety, constipation, edema, pain, cough, erythema, flushing, mucosal inflammation, hematuria, dizziness, bilirubin increased, jaundice, hepatomegaly, injection site pain, myalgia, respiratory distress, palmar-plantar sore throat, back pain, dyspnea, erythrodysesthesia syndrome, staphylococcal infection, oral candidiasis, appetite decreased, cellulitis, depression, irritability, arthralgia, herpes simplex, hypertension, lethargy
Occasional
Somnolence, weight gain, tremor, pleural effusion, pneumonia, systemic inflammatory response syndrome (SIRS)/capillary leak syndrome, transfusion reaction, bacteremia, creatinine increased

PRECAUTIONS AND CONTRAINDICATIONS
Hypersensitivity to clofarabine or its components
Caution:
Do not breast-feed, renal or hepatic impairment

DRUG INTERACTIONS OF CONCERN TO DENTISTRY
• CNS depressants, alcohol: may increase CNS depression and dizziness.

SERIOUS REACTIONS
! Tumor lysis syndrome may occur.
! Severe bone marrow suppression, including neutropenia, anemia, and thrombocytopenia, have been observed.

DENTAL CONSIDERATIONS
General:
• Monitor vital signs at every appointment because of cardiovascular side effects.
• Avoid NSAIDs for pain control.
• Examine for oral manifestation of opportunistic infection.
• This drug may be used in the hospital or on an outpatient basis. Confirm the patient's disease and treatment status.
• Chlorhexidine mouth rinse prior to and during chemotherapy may reduce severity of mucositis.
• Determine presence, type, and severity of blood dyscrasias prior to undertaking any dental treatment and modify therapy accordingly.
• Consider effects of drug on healing and susceptibility to infection.
• Palliative measures may be required for management of oral side effects.
Consultations:
• Consult physician to determine disease control and ability of patient to tolerate dental procedures.
• Consult physician to determine need for prophylactic antiinfectives if invasive dental procedures are needed.

• Consult physician about patient's immunologic status during cancer chemotherapy and determine safety risk, if any, posed by required dental treatment.
Teach Family/Patient to:
• Be aware of oral side effects of medication.
• Practice effective oral hygiene to prevent soft-tissue inflammation and prevent trauma when using oral hygiene aids.
• Report oral lesions, soreness, or bleeding to dentist.
• Update health and medication history if physician makes any changes in evaluation or drug regimens, including the use of OTC drugs, herbal products, and dietary supplements.

clofazimine
kloe-**faz′**-ih-meen
(Lamprene)

CATEGORY AND SCHEDULE
Pregnancy Risk Category: C

Drug Class: Leprostatic

MECHANISM OF ACTION
An antibiotic that binds to mycobacterial DNA.
Therapeutic Effect: Inhibits mycobacterial growth and produces antiinflammatory action.

USES
Treatment of lepromatous leprosy, dapsone-resistant leprosy, lepromatous leprosy complicated by erythema nodosum leprosum

PHARMACOKINETICS
Deposited in fatty tissue, reticuloendothelial system; small

amount excreted in feces, sputum, sweat. *Half-life:* 70 days.

INDICATIONS AND DOSAGES
▶ **Leprosy**
PO
Adults, Elderly. 100 mg/day in combination with dapsone and rifampin for 3 yr, then 100 mg/day as monotherapy.
Children. 1 mg/kg/day in combination with dapsone and rifampin.
▶ **Erythema Nodosum**
PO
Adults, Elderly. 100–200 mg/day for up to 3 mo, then 100 mg/day.

SIDE EFFECTS/ADVERSE REACTIONS
Frequent
Dry skin, abdominal pain, nausea, vomiting, diarrhea, skin discoloration (pink to brownish-black)
Occasional
Rash; pruritus; eye irritation; discoloration of sputum; sweat and urine

PRECAUTIONS AND CONTRAINDICATIONS
Caution:
Lactation, children, abdominal pain, diarrhea, depression

DRUG INTERACTIONS OF CONCERN TO DENTISTRY
• None reported

SERIOUS REACTIONS
! None significant

DENTAL CONSIDERATIONS

General:
• Develop awareness of the patient's disease.

Teach Patient/Family to:
• Encourage effective oral hygiene to prevent soft tissue inflammation.
• Avoid mouth rinses with high alcohol content because of drying effects.

clofibrate
kloe-**fye**′-brate
(Abitrate, Atromid-S, Claripex[CAN], Novofibrate[CAN])

CATEGORY AND SCHEDULE
Pregnancy Risk Category: C

Drug Class: Antihyperlipidemic

MECHANISM OF ACTION
An antihyperlipidemic that enhances synthesis of lipoprotein lipase and reduces triglyceride-rich lipoproteins and VLDLs.
Therapeutic Effect: Increases VLDL catabolism and reduces total plasma triglyceride levels.

USES
Treatment of hyperlipidemia (types III, IV, V)

PHARMACOKINETICS
Well absorbed from the GI tract. Protein binding: 95%–97%. Metabolized in liver. Excreted primarily in urine, lesser amount in feces. *Half-life:* 14–35 hr.

INDICATIONS AND DOSAGES
▶ **Hypercholesterolemia**
PO
Adults, Elderly. 2 g/day in divided doses. Some patients may respond to a lower dosage.

SIDE EFFECTS/ADVERSE REACTIONS
Frequent
Nausea, vomiting, loose stools, dyspepsia, flatulence, abdominal distress
Occasional
Headache, dizziness, fatigue
Rare
Muscle cramping, aching, weakness; skin rash, urticaria, pruritus; dry brittle hair, alopecia

PRECAUTIONS AND CONTRAINDICATIONS
Hypersensitivity to clofibrate, severe renal or hepatic dysfunction, pregnancy, nursing women, rhabdomyolysis, severe hyperkalemia, primary biliary cirrhosis
Caution:
Peptic ulcer

DRUG INTERACTIONS OF CONCERN TO DENTISTRY
• None reported

SERIOUS REACTIONS
! May increase excretion of cholesterol into bile, leading to cholelithiasis.
! Various cardiac arrhythmias have been reported.
! Anemia and, more frequently, leukopenia have been reported.

DENTAL CONSIDERATIONS
General:
• Consider semisupine chair position for patient comfort if GI side effects occur.
• Patients on chronic drug therapy may rarely have symptoms of blood dyscrasias, which can include infection, bleeding, and poor healing.

Consultations:
• In a patient with symptoms of blood dyscrasias, request a medical consultation for blood studies and postpone treatment until normal values are reestablished.
Teach Patient/Family to:
• Encourage effective oral hygiene to prevent soft tissue inflammation.

clomiphene
kloe′-mi-feen
(Clomhexal[AUS], Clomid, Clomid[CAN], Milophene, Milophene[CAN], Serophene, Serophene[CAN])
Do not confuse with clomipramine.

CATEGORY AND SCHEDULE
Pregnancy Risk Category: X

Drug Class: Nonsteroidal ovulatory stimulant, antiestrogen

MECHANISM OF ACTION
An ovulation stimulator that promotes release of pituitary gonadotropins.
Therapeutic Effect: Stimulates ovulation.

USES
Treatment of female infertility

PHARMACOKINETICS
Readily absorbed. Time to peak occurs within 6.5 hr. Undergoes enterohepatic recirculation. Primarily excreted in feces.
Half-life: 5–7 days.

C

INDICATIONS AND DOSAGES
▸ **Ovulatory Failure, Females**
PO
Adults. 50 mg/day for 5 days (first course); start the regimen on the fifth day of cycle. Increase dose only if unresponsive to cyclic 50 mg. Maximum: 100 mg/day for 5 days.

SIDE EFFECTS/ADVERSE REACTIONS
Frequent
Hot flashes, ovarian enlargement
Occasional
Abdominal/pelvic discomfort, bloating, nausea, vomiting, breast discomfort (females)
Rare
Vision disturbances, abnormal menstrual flow, breast enlargement (males), headache, mental depression, ovarian cyst formation, thromboembolism, uterine fibroid enlargement

PRECAUTIONS AND CONTRAINDICATIONS
Liver dysfunction, abnormal uterine bleeding, enlargement or development of ovarian cyst, uncontrolled thyroid or adrenal dysfunction in the presence of an organic intracranial lesion such as pituitary tumor, pregnancy, hypersensitivity to clomiphene
Caution:
Hypertension, depression, convulsions, diabetes mellitus

DRUG INTERACTIONS OF CONCERN TO DENTISTRY
• None reported

SERIOUS REACTIONS
‼ Thrombophlebitis, alopecia, and polyuria occurs rarely.

DENTAL CONSIDERATIONS
General:
• Consider semisupine chair position for patient comfort if GI side effects occur.
• Avoid dental light in patient's eyes; offer dark glasses for patient comfort.
• Be aware that patient may be in early stage of pregnancy.

clomipramine hydrochloride
klom-**ip′**-ra-meen
hi-droh-**klor′**-ide
(Anafranil, Apo-Clomipramine[CAN], Clopram[AUS], Novo-Clopamine[CAN], Placil[AUS])
Do not confuse clomipramine with chlorpromazine, clomiphene, or imipramine, or Anafranil with alfentanil, enalapril, or nafarelin.

CATEGORY AND SCHEDULE
Pregnancy Risk Category: C

Drug Class: Tricyclic antidepressant

MECHANISM OF ACTION
A tricyclic antidepressant that blocks the reuptake of neurotransmitters, such as norepinephrine and serotonin, at CNS presynaptic membranes, increasing their availability at postsynaptic receptor sites.
Therapeutic Effect: Reduces obsessive-compulsive behavior.

USES
Treatment of obsessive-compulsive disorder; unapproved: depression, panic disorder, narcolepsy, and neurogenic pain

PHARMACOKINETICS

Well absorbed from GI tract. Protein binding: 97%. Principally bound to albumin. Distributed into cerebrospinal fluid. Metabolized in the liver. Undergoes extensive first-pass effect. Excreted in urine and feces. *Half-life:* 19–37 hr.

INDICATIONS AND DOSAGES
▶ **Obsessive-Compulsive Disorder**
PO
Adults, Elderly. Initially, 25 mg/day. May gradually increase to 100 mg/day in the first 2 wk. Maximum: 250 mg/day.
Children 10 yr and older. Initially, 25 mg/day. May gradually increase up to maximum of 200 mg/day.

SIDE EFFECTS/ADVERSE REACTIONS
Frequent
Somnolence, fatigue, dry mouth, blurred vision, constipation, sexual dysfunction, ejaculatory failure, impotence, weight gain, delayed micturition, orthostatic hypotension, diaphoresis, impaired concentration, increased appetite, urine retention
Occasional
GI disturbances (such as nausea, GI distress, and metallic taste), asthenia, aggressiveness, muscle weakness
Rare
Paradoxical reactions (agitation, restlessness, nightmares, insomnia), extrapyramidal symptoms, (particularly fine hand tremor), laryngitis, seizures

PRECAUTIONS AND CONTRAINDICATIONS
Acute recovery period after MI, use within 14 days of MAOIs
Caution:
Seizures, suicidal patients, elderly, MAOIs, not for use in children

younger than 10 yr, renal or hepatic dysfunction

DRUG INTERACTIONS OF CONCERN TO DENTISTRY
• Increased anticholinergic effects: muscarinic blockers, antihistamines, phenothiazines
• Increased effects of direct-acting sympathomimetics (epinephrine, levonordefrin)
• Potential risk of CNS depression: alcohol, barbiturates, benzodiazepines, and other CNS depressants
• Decreased antihypertensive effects: clonidine, guanadrel, guanethidine
• Use with caution, possible reduced metabolism: drugs metabolized by CYP450 2D6 isoenzymes
• Avoid concurrent use with St. John's wort (herb)

SERIOUS REACTIONS
! Overdose may produce seizures; cardiovascular effects, such as severe orthostatic hypotension, dizziness, tachycardia, palpitations, and arrhythmias; and altered temperature regulation, including hyperpyrexia or hypothermia.
! Abrupt discontinuation after prolonged therapy may produce headache, malaise, nausea, vomiting, and vivid dreams.
! Anemia and agranulocytosis have been noted.

DENTAL CONSIDERATIONS
General:
• Take vital signs at every appointment because of cardiovascular side effects.
• Assess salivary flow as a factor in caries, periodontal disease, and candidiasis.
• Patients on chronic drug therapy may rarely have symptoms of blood

C

dyscrasias, which can include infection, bleeding, and poor healing.
• After supine positioning, have patient sit upright for at least 2 min before standing to avoid orthostatic hypotension.
• Use vasoconstrictor with caution, in low doses, and with careful aspiration. Avoid use of gingival retraction cord with epinephrine.
• Place on frequent recall because of oral side effects.
• A stress-reduction protocol may be required.

Consultations:
• In a patient with symptoms of blood dyscrasias, request a medical consultation for blood studies and postpone dental treatment until normal values are reestablished.
• Physician should be informed if significant xerostomic side effects occur (e.g., increased caries, sore tongue, problems eating or swallowing, difficulty wearing prosthesis) so that a medication change can be considered.
• Medical consultation may be required to assess disease control.

Teach Patient/Family to:
• Encourage effective oral hygiene to prevent soft tissue inflammation.
• Prevent injury when using oral hygiene aids.
• When chronic dry mouth occurs, advise patient to:
  • Avoid mouth rinses with high alcohol content because of drying effects.
  • Use daily home fluoride products for anticaries effect.
  • Use sugarless gum, frequent sips of water, or saliva substitutes.

clonazepam
kloe-**na'**-zi-pam
(Apo-Clonazepam[CAN], Clonapam[CAN], Klonopin, Paxam[AUS], Rivotril[CAN])
Do not confuse clonazepam with clonidine or lorazepam.

CATEGORY AND SCHEDULE
Pregnancy Risk Category: D
Controlled Substance Schedule IV

Drug Class: Anticonvulsant, benzodiazepine

MECHANISM OF ACTION
A benzodiazepine that depresses all levels of the CNS; inhibits nerve impulse transmission in the motor cortex and suppresses abnormal discharge in petit mal seizures.
Therapeutic Effect: Produces anxiolytic and anticonvulsant effects.

USES
Absence, atypical absence, akinetic, myoclonic seizures; unlabeled uses: Parkinson's dysarthria, adjunct in schizophrenia, neuralgias

PHARMACOKINETICS
Well absorbed from the GI tract. Protein binding: 85%. Metabolized in the liver. Excreted in urine. Not removed by hemodialysis. *Half-life:* 18–50 hr.

INDICATIONS AND DOSAGES
▸ **Adjunctive Treatment of Lennox-Gastaut Syndrome (Petit Mal Variant) and Akinetic, Myoclonic, and Absence (Petit Mal) Seizures**
PO
Adults, Elderly, Children 10 yr and older. 1.5 mg/day; may be increased in 0.5- to 1-mg increments every 3 days until seizures are controlled.

Don't exceed maintenance dosage of 20 mg/day.
Infants, Children younger than 10 yr or weighing less than 30 kg. 0.01–0.03 mg/kg/day in 2–3 divided doses; may be increased by up to 0.5 mg every 3 days until seizures are controlled. Don't exceed maintenance dosage of 0.2 mg/kg/day.

▸ **Panic Disorder**
PO
Adults, Elderly. Initially, 0.25 mg twice a day; increased in increments of 0.125–0.25 mg twice a day every 3 days. Maximum: 4 mg/day.

SIDE EFFECTS/ADVERSE REACTIONS
Frequent
Mild, transient drowsiness; ataxia; behavioral disturbances (aggression, irritability, agitation), especially in children
Occasional
Rash, ankle or facial edema, nocturia, dysuria, change in appetite or weight, dry mouth, sore gums, nausea, blurred vision
Rare
Paradoxical CNS reactions, including hyperactivity or nervousness in children and excitement or restlessness in the elderly (particularly in the presence of uncontrolled pain)

PRECAUTIONS AND CONTRAINDICATIONS
Narrow-angle glaucoma, significant hepatic disease
Caution:
Open-angle glaucoma, chronic respiratory disease, renal, hepatic disease, elderly, interferes with cognitive and motor performance, withdrawal symptoms

DRUG INTERACTIONS OF CONCERN TO DENTISTRY
• Increased sedation: alcohol, all CNS depressants, indinavir, kava (herb)
• Risk of increased serum levels: drugs that inhibit CYP3A4 isoenzymes, ketoconazole, itraconazole, fluconazole, protease inhibitor, nefazodone
• Risk of decreased effect: St. John's wort (herb)

SERIOUS REACTIONS
! Abrupt withdrawal may result in pronounced restlessness, irritability, insomnia, hand tremors, abdominal or muscle cramps, diaphoresis, vomiting, and status epilepticus.
! Overdose results in somnolence, confusion, diminished reflexes, and coma.

DENTAL CONSIDERATIONS
General:
• Patients on chronic drug therapy may rarely have symptoms of blood dyscrasias, which can include infection, bleeding, and poor healing.
• Assess salivary flow as a factor in caries, periodontal disease, and candidiasis.
• Psychologic and physical dependence may occur with chronic administration.
• Geriatric patients are more susceptible to drug effects; use lower dose.
• Ask about type of epilepsy, seizure frequency, and quality of seizure control.
Consultations:
• Medical consultation may be required to assess disease control.
• In a patient with symptoms of blood dyscrasias, request a medical

consultation for blood studies and postpone dental treatment until normal values are reestablished.

Teach Patient/Family to:
• Encourage effective oral hygiene to prevent soft tissue inflammation.
• Use caution to prevent injury when using oral hygiene aids.
• When chronic dry mouth occurs, advise patient to:
   • Avoid mouth rinses with high alcohol content because of drying effects.
   • Use daily home fluoride products for anticaries effect.
   • Use sugarless gum, frequent sips of water, or saliva substitutes.

clonidine

klon′-ih-deen

(Catapres, Catapres TTS, Dixarit[CAN], Duraclon)
Do not confuse clonidine with clomiphene, Klonopin, or quinidine, or Catapres with Cetapred.

CATEGORY AND SCHEDULE
Pregnancy Risk Category: C

Drug Class: Antihypertensive, central α-adrenergic agonist

MECHANISM OF ACTION
An antiadrenergic, sympatholytic agent that prevents pain signal transmission to the brain and produces analgesia at pre- and post-α-adrenergic receptors in the spinal cord.
Therapeutic Effect: Reduces peripheral resistance; decreases B/P and heart rate.

USES
Hypertension, severe pain in combination with opioids for cancer patients; unapproved: opioid abstinence syndrome, nicotine withdrawal, vascular headache, alcohol withdrawal, ADHD, postherpetic neuralgia

PHARMACOKINETICS

Route	Onset	Peak	Duration
PO	0.5–1 hr	2–4 hr	Up to 8 hr

Well absorbed from the GI tract. Transdermal best absorbed from the chest and upper arm; least absorbed from the thigh. Protein binding: 20%–40%. Metabolized in the liver. Primarily excreted in urine. Minimally removed by hemodialysis. *Half-life:* 12–16 hr (increased with impaired renal function).

INDICATIONS AND DOSAGES
▶ **Hypertension**
PO
Adults. Initially, 0.1 mg twice a day. Increase by 0.1–0.2 mg q2–4 days. Maintenance: 0.2–1.2 mg/day in 2–4 divided doses up to maximum of 2.4 mg/day.
Elderly. Initially, 0.1 mg at bedtime. May increase gradually.
Children. 5–25 mcg/kg/day in divided doses q6h. Increase at 5- to 7-day intervals. Maximum: 0.9 mg/day.
Transdermal
Adults, Elderly. System delivering 0.1 mg/24 hr up to 0.6 mg/24 hr q7 days.
▶ **Attention Deficit Hyperactivity Disorder (ADHD)**
PO
Children. Initially 0.05 mg/day. May increase by 0.05 mg/day q3–7 days. Maximum: 0.3–0.4 mg/day.

▶ **Severe Pain**
Epidural
Adults, Elderly. 30–40 mcg/hr.
Children. Initially, 0.5 mcg/kg/hr,
not to exceed adult dose.

SIDE EFFECTS/ADVERSE REACTIONS
Frequent
Dry mouth, somnolence, dizziness,
sedation, constipation
Occasional
Tablets, injection: Depression,
swelling of feet, loss of appetite,
decreased sexual ability, itching
eyes, dizziness, nausea, vomiting,
nervousness
Transdermal: Itching, reddening, or
darkening of skin
Rare
Nightmares, vivid dreams, cold
feeling in fingers and toes

PRECAUTIONS AND CONTRAINDICATIONS
Epidural contraindicated in those
patients with bleeding diathesis or
infection at the injection site, and in
those receiving anticoagulation
therapy
Caution:
MI (recent), cerebrovascular disease,
chronic renal failure, Raynaud's
disease, thyroid disease, depression,
COPD, children younger than 12 yr
(patches), asthma, lactation, elderly

DRUG INTERACTIONS OF CONCERN TO DENTISTRY
• Increased CNS depression:
alcohol, all CNS depressants
• Decreased hypotensive effects:
NSAIDs, sympathomimetics,
tricyclic antidepressants

SERIOUS REACTIONS
! Overdose produces profound
hypotension, irritability, bradycardia,
respiratory depression, hypothermia,
miosis (pupillary constriction),
arrhythmias, and apnea.
! Abrupt withdrawal may result in
rebound hypertension associated
with nervousness, agitation, anxiety,
insomnia, hand tingling, tremor,
flushing, and diaphoresis.

DENTAL CONSIDERATIONS
General:
• Monitor vital signs at every
appointment because of
cardiovascular side effects.
• After supine positioning, have
patient sit upright for at least 2 min
before standing to avoid orthostatic
hypotension.
• Limit use of sodium-containing
products, such as saline IV fluids,
for patients with a dietary salt
restriction.
• Observe appropriate limitations of
vasoconstrictor doses.
• Assess salivary flow as a factor in
caries, periodontal disease, and
candidiasis.
• Stress from dental procedures may
compromise cardiovascular function;
determine patient risk.
• Short appointments and a
stress-reduction protocol
may be required for anxious
patients.
• Consider drug in diagnosis of
taste alterations.
Consultations:
• Medical consultation may be
required to assess disease
control.
Teach Patient/Family:
• When chronic dry mouth occurs,
advise patient to:
  • Avoid mouth rinses with high
  alcohol content because of
  drying effects.
  • Use daily home fluoride
  products for anticaries effect.

C

• Use sugarless gum, frequent sips of water, or saliva substitutes.

clopidogrel
clo-**pid**′-oh-grill
(Iscover[AUS], Plavix)
Do not confuse Plavix with Paxil.

CATEGORY AND SCHEDULE
Pregnancy Risk Category: B

Drug Class: Platelet aggregation inhibitor

MECHANISM OF ACTION
A thienopyridine derivative that inhibits binding of the enzyme adenosine phosphate (ADP) to its platelet receptor and subsequent ADP-mediated activation of a glycoprotein complex.
Therapeutic Effect: Inhibits platelet aggregation.

USES
Adjunctive treatment in recent MI, ischemic stroke, and peripheral vascular disease in patients with atherosclerosis; treatment of acute coronary syndrome (unstable angina with non-Q wave MI)

PHARMACOKINETICS

Route	Onset	Peak	Duration
PO	1 hr	2 hr	N/A

Rapidly absorbed. Protein binding: 98%. Extensively metabolized by the liver. Eliminated equally in the urine and feces. *Half-life:* 8 hr.

INDICATIONS AND DOSAGES
▸ **MI, Stroke Reduction**
PO
Adults, Elderly. 75 mg once a day.
▸ **Acute Coronary Syndrome**
PO
Adults, Elderly. Initially, 300 mg loading dose, then 75 mg once a day (in combination with aspirin).

SIDE EFFECTS/ADVERSE REACTIONS
Frequent
Skin disorders
Occasional
Upper respiratory tract infection, chest pain, flu-like symptoms, headache, dizziness, arthralgia
Rare
Fatigue, edema, hypertension, abdominal pain, dyspepsia, diarrhea, nausea, epistaxis, dyspnea, rhinitis

PRECAUTIONS AND CONTRAINDICATIONS
Active bleeding, coagulation disorders, severe hepatic disease
Caution:
Hepatic impairment, renal impairment, hypertension, history of bleeding disorders, major surgery, safety and efficacy during lactation or use in children not established

DRUG INTERACTIONS OF CONCERN TO DENTISTRY
• Caution in use with NSAIDs

SERIOUS REACTIONS
! None known

DENTAL CONSIDERATIONS
General:
• Avoid discontinuation for dental procedures because of increased risk of thromboembolism.

• Effects on platelet aggregation return to normal in 5–7 days.
• Patients on chronic drug therapy may rarely have symptoms of blood dyscrasias, which can include infection, bleeding, and poor healing.
• Consider local hemostasis measures to prevent excessive bleeding.
• Question patient about concurrent aspirin use.
• Monitor vital signs at every appointment because of cardiovascular disease.
• Consider semisupine chair position for patient comfort if GI side effects occur.

Consultations:
• Medical consultation may be required to assess disease control and patient's ability to tolerate stress.
• Consultation should include data on bleeding time.
• In a patient with symptoms of blood dyscrasias, request a medical consultation for blood studies and postpone treatment until normal values are reestablished.

Teach Patient/Family to:
• Update health and drug history if physician makes any changes in evaluation or drug regimens.
• Use caution to prevent trauma when using oral hygiene aids.
• Report any unusual or prolonged bleeding episodes after dental treatment.

clorazepate dipotassium

klor-**az**′-e-pate di-poe-**tass**′-ee-um
(Novoclopate[CAN], Tranxene, Tranxene SD, Tranxene SD Half-Strength, T-Tab)
Do not confuse clorazepate with clofibrate.

CATEGORY AND SCHEDULE
Pregnancy Risk Category: D
Controlled Substance Schedule IV

Drug Class: Benzodiazepine

MECHANISM OF ACTION
A benzodiazepine that depresses all levels of the CNS, including limbic and reticular formation, by binding to benzodiazepine receptor sites on the gamma-aminobutyric acid (GABA) receptor complex. Modulates GABA, a major inhibitory neurotransmitter in the brain.
Therapeutic Effect: Produces anxiolytic effect, suppresses seizure activity.

USES
Anxiety, acute alcohol withdrawal, adjunctive treatment of partial seizures

PHARMACOKINETICS
Well absorbed after oral administration rapidly metabolized by liver to nordazepam, which is slowly eliminated. **Half-life:** 40–50 hr. Protein binding of nordazepam: 97%–98%. Metabolites (nordazepam, oxazepam, and glucuronide conjugates) excreted in urine.

C

INDICATIONS AND DOSAGES
▶ **Anxiety**
PO (Regular-Release)
Adults, Elderly. 7.5–15 mg 2–4 times a day.
PO (Sustained-Release)
Adults, Elderly. 11.25 mg or 22.5 mg once a day at bedtime.
▶ **Anticonvulsant**
PO
Adults, Elderly, Children older than 12 yr. Initially, 7.5 mg 2–3 times a day. May increase by 7.5 mg at weekly intervals. Maximum: 90 mg/day.
Children 9–12 yr. Initially, 3.75–7.5 mg twice a day. May increase by 2.75 mg at weekly intervals. Maximum: 60 mg/day.
▶ **Alcohol Withdrawal**
PO
Adults, Elderly. Initially, 30 mg, then 15 mg 2–4 times a day on first day. Gradually decrease dosage over subsequent days. Maximum: 90 mg/day.

SIDE EFFECTS/ADVERSE REACTIONS
Frequent
Somnolence
Occasional
Dizziness, GI disturbances, nervousness, blurred vision, dry mouth, headache, confusion, ataxia, rash, irritability, slurred speech
Rare
Paradoxical CNS reactions, such as hyperactivity or nervousness in children and excitement or restlessness in the elderly or debilitated (generally noted during first 2 wk of therapy, particularly in presence of uncontrolled pain)

PRECAUTIONS AND CONTRAINDICATIONS
Acute narrow-angle glaucoma

Caution:
Elderly, debilitated, hepatic disease, renal disease

DRUG INTERACTIONS OF CONCERN TO DENTISTRY
• Increased effects: CNS depressants, alcohol, opioid analgesics, general anesthetics, indinavir
• Increased serum levels and prolonged effect of benzodiazepines: fluconazole, ketoconazole, itraconazole, miconazole (systemic)
• Possible increase in CNS side effects: kava kava (herb)
• Contraindicated with saquinavir

SERIOUS REACTIONS
! Abrupt or too-rapid withdrawal may result in pronounced restlessness, irritability, insomnia, hand tremors, abdominal or muscle cramps, diaphoresis, vomiting, and seizures.
! Overdose results in somnolence, confusion, diminished reflexes, and coma.

DENTAL CONSIDERATIONS
General:
• Monitor vital signs at every appointment because of cardiovascular side effects.
• Assess salivary flow as a factor in caries, periodontal disease, and candidiasis.
• After supine positioning, have patient sit upright for at least 2 min to avoid orthostatic hypotension.
• Psychologic and physical dependence may occur with chronic administration.
• Geriatric patients are more susceptible to drug effects; use a lower dose.
• Short appointments and a stress-reduction protocol may be required for anxious patients.

• Seizure: Ask about type of epilepsy, seizure frequency, and degree of seizure control.
Consultations:
• Medical consultation may be required to assess disease control and the patient's ability to tolerate stress.
Teach Patient/Family:
• When chronic dry mouth occurs, advise patient to:
  • Avoid mouth rinses with high alcohol content because of drying effects.
  • Use daily home fluoride products for anticaries effect.
  • Use sugarless gum, frequent sips of water, or saliva substitutes.

clotrimazole
kloe-try´-mah-zole
(Canesten[CAN], Clotrimaderm[CAN], Mycelex, Mycelex OTC, Lotrimin, Gyne-Lotrimin, Trivagizole 3)

CATEGORY AND SCHEDULE
Pregnancy Risk Category: B (topical), C (troches)

Drug Class: Imidazole antifungal

MECHANISM OF ACTION
An antifungal that binds with phospholipids in fungal cell membrane. Damages the fungal cell membrane, altering its function.
Therapeutic Effect: Inhibits yeast growth.

USES
Treatment of tinea pedis; tinea cruris; tinea corporis; tinea versicolor; *C. albicans* infection of the vagina, vulva, throat, mouth

PHARMACOKINETICS
Poorly, erratically absorbed from GI tract. Bound to oral mucosa. Absorbed portion metabolized in liver. Eliminated in feces. Topical: Minimal systemic absorption (highest concentration in stratum corneum). Intravaginal: Small amount systemically absorbed.
Half-life: 3.5–5 hr.

INDICATIONS AND DOSAGES
▸ **Oropharyngeal Candidiasis Treatment**
PO
Adults, Elderly. 10 mg 5 times a day for 14 days.
▸ **Oropharyngeal Candidiasis Prophylaxis**
PO
Adults, Elderly. 10 mg 3 times a day.
▸ **Dermatophytosis, Cutaneous Candidiasis**
Topical
Adults, Elderly. 2 times a day. Therapeutic effect may take up to 8 wk.
▸ **Vulvovaginal Candidiasis**
Vaginal (Tablets)
Adults, Elderly. 1 tablet (100 mg) at bedtime for 7 days; 2 tablets (200 mg) at bedtime for 3 days; or 500 mg tablet one time.
Vaginal (Cream)
Adults, Elderly. 1 full applicator at bedtime for 7–14 days.

SIDE EFFECTS/ADVERSE REACTIONS
Frequent
Oral: Nausea, vomiting, diarrhea, abdominal pain

Occasional
Topical: Itching, burning, stinging, erythema, urticaria
Vaginal: Mild burning (tablets/cream); irritation, cystitis (cream)
Rare
Vaginal: Itching, rash, lower abdominal cramping, headache

PRECAUTIONS AND CONTRAINDICATIONS
Hypersensitivity to clotrimazole or any component of the formulation, children younger than 3 yr

DRUG INTERACTIONS OF CONCERN TO DENTISTRY
• None reported

SERIOUS REACTIONS
! None reported

DENTAL CONSIDERATIONS
General:
• Determine why the patient is taking the drug.
• Examine oral mucous membranes for signs of fungal infection.
Teach Patient/Family to:
• Soak full or partial dentures in an antifungal solution overnight until lesions are absent; prolonged infections may require fabrication of new prosthesis.
• Dispose of tooth brush used during oral infection after oral lesions are absent to prevent reinoculation.
• Complete entire course of medication; long-term therapy may be necessary to clear infection.

clozapine
klo′-za-peen
(Clopine[AUS], Clozaril, FazaClo)
Do not confuse clozapine with Cloxapen or clofazimine, or Clozaril with Clinoril or Colazal.

CATEGORY AND SCHEDULE
Pregnancy Risk Category: B

Drug Class: Antipsychotic, atypical

MECHANISM OF ACTION
A dibenzodiazepine derivative that interferes with the binding of dopamine at dopamine receptor sites; binds primarily at nondopamine receptor sites.
Therapeutic Effect: Diminishes schizophrenic behavior.

USES
Management of psychotic symptoms in schizophrenic patients for whom other antipsychotics have failed (available only through the Clozaril Patient Management System)

PHARMACOKINETICS
Absorbed rapidly and almost completely. Distributed rapidly and extensively. Crosses the blood-brain barrier. Protein binding: 95%. Metabolized in the liver. Excreted in urine and feces. **Half-life:** 8 hr.

INDICATIONS AND DOSAGES
▸ **Schizophrenic Disorders, Reduce Suicidal Behavior**
PO
Adults. Initially, 25 mg once or twice a day. May increase by 25–50 mg/day over 2 wk until dosage of 300–450 mg/day is achieved. May further increase by 50–100 mg/day no more than once

or twice a wk. Range: 200–600 mg/
day. Maximum: 900 mg/day.
Elderly. Initially, 25 mg/day. May
increase by 25 mg/day. Maximum:
450 mg/day.

SIDE EFFECTS/ADVERSE REACTIONS
Frequent
Somnolence, salivation, tachycardia,
dizziness, constipation
Occasional
Hypotension, headache, tremors,
syncope, diaphoresis, dry mouth,
nausea, visual disturbances,
nightmares, restlessness, akinesia,
agitation, hypertension, abdominal
discomfort or heartburn, weight gain
Rare
Rigidity, confusion, fatigue,
insomnia, diarrhea, rash

PRECAUTIONS AND CONTRAINDICATIONS
Coma, concurrent use of other drugs
that may suppress bone marrow
function, history of clozapine-
induced agranulocytosis or severe
granulocytopenia, myeloproliferative
disorders, severe CNS depression
Caution:
Lactation; children younger than
16 yr; hepatic, renal, cardiac
disease; seizures; prostatic
enlargement; elderly; increased
incidence of cardiomyopathy

DRUG INTERACTIONS OF CONCERN TO DENTISTRY
• Increased anticholinergic effects:
anticholinergics
• Increased CNS depression:
alcohol, all CNS depressant drugs
• Increased serum concentration,
leukocytosis: erythromycin base
• Possible decreased effects:
carbamazepine
• Increased plasma levels:
ciprofloxacin

SERIOUS REACTIONS
! Blood dyscrasias, particularly
agranulocytosis and mild
leukopenia, may occur.
! Seizures occur in about 3% of
patients.
! Overdose produces CNS
depression (including sedation,
coma, and delirium), respiratory
depression, and hypersalivation.

DENTAL CONSIDERATIONS
General:
• Monitor vital signs at every
appointment because of
cardiovascular and respiratory side
effects.
• Patients on chronic drug therapy
may rarely have symptoms of blood
dyscrasias, which can include
infection, bleeding, and poor
healing.
• After supine positioning, have
patient sit upright for at least 2 min
before standing to avoid orthostatic
hypotension.
• Assess salivary flow as a factor in
caries, periodontal disease, and
candidiasis.
• Determine why the patient is
taking the drug.
• Place on frequent recall because of
oral side effects.
Consultations:
• In a patient with symptoms
of blood dyscrasias, request a
medical consultation for blood
studies and postpone dental
treatment until normal values are
reestablished.
• Medical consultation may be
required to assess disease control
and stress tolerance of patient.
• Physician should be informed if
significant xerostomic side effects
occur (e.g., increased caries, sore
tongue, problems eating or
swallowing, difficulty wearing

C

prosthesis) so that a medication change can be considered.
Teach Patient/Family to:
• Encourage effective oral hygiene to prevent soft tissue inflammation.
• Use caution to prevent injury when using oral hygiene aids.
• Use powered tooth brush if patient has difficulty holding conventional devices.
• When chronic dry mouth occurs, advise patient to:
  • Avoid mouth rinses with high alcohol content because of drying effects.
  • Use daily home fluoride products for anticaries effect.
  • Use sugarless gum, frequent sips of water, or saliva substitutes.

cocaine hydrochloride
koe-**kane**′ hi-droh-**klor**′-ide
(Cocaine[CAN], Cocaine HCl)

CATEGORY AND SCHEDULE
Pregnancy Risk Category: C
Controlled Substance: Schedule II

Drug Class: Ester; topical anesthetic

MECHANISM OF ACTION
A topical anesthetic that decreases membrane permeability, increases norepinephrine at postsynaptic receptor sites, producing intense vasoconstriction.
Therapeutic Effect: Blocks conduction of nerve impulses.

USES
Topical anesthesia for mucous membranes of orolaryngeal, nasal areas; minor, uncomplicated facial lacerations

PHARMACOKINETICS
Readily absorbed from all mucous membranes. Cocaine penetrates the CNS but is rapidly metabolized. Rapidly hydrolyzed in blood by serum cholinesterases. Metabolized in liver. Excreted in urine. *Half-life:* 1–1.5 hr.

INDICATIONS AND DOSAGES
▸ **Anesthesia**
Topical
Adults, Elderly, Children. 1%–4% to mucous membranes. Maximum: 1–3 mg/kg. Dosage varies depending upon the area to be anesthetized, vascularity of the tissues, individual tolerance, and anesthetic technique. Administer lowest effective dose.

SIDE EFFECTS/ADVERSE REACTIONS
Frequent
Loss of sense of smell and taste
Occasional
Anxiety, CNS stimulation or depression

PRECAUTIONS AND CONTRAINDICATIONS
Hypersensitivity to cocaine or any component of the formulation

DRUG INTERACTIONS OF CONCERN TO DENTISTRY
• Sensitization to catecholamines, such as epinephrine; risk of serious adverse cardiovascular events
• Avoid ester-type local anesthetics in patients with allergic reactions to cocaine

SERIOUS REACTIONS
❗ Repeated nasal application may produce stuffy nose and chronic rhinitis.
❗ Early signs of overdosage are increased B/P, increased pulse, irregular heartbeat, chills or fever,

agitation, nervousness, confusion, inability to remain still, nausea, vomiting, abdominal pain, increased sweating, rapid breathing, and large pupils.

! Advanced signs of overdosage are arrhythmias, CNS hemorrhage, CHF, convulsions, delirium, hyperreflexia, loss of bladder or bowel control, and respiratory weakness.

! Late signs of overdosage are loss of reflexes, muscle paralysis, dilated pupils, LOC, cyanosis, pulmonary edema, cardiac and respiratory failure.

DENTAL CONSIDERATIONS

General:
• Acute-use drug for medical topical anesthesia (not for injection).
• Abusers of cocaine may present with oral or nasal mucosal lesions and dry mucous membranes, nervousness, and anxiety.
• Caution drug interactions in chronic abusers of cocaine.
• Determine why patient is taking the drug.
• Monitor vital signs at every appointment because of cardiovascular side effects.
• Assess salivary flow as a factor in caries, periodontal disease, and candidiasis.
• If additional analgesia is required for dental pain, consider alternative analgesics (NSAIDs) in patients taking narcotics for acute or chronic pain.
• Use vasoconstrictor with caution, in low doses, and with careful aspiration. Avoid using gingival retraction cord containing epinephrine.
• Examine for oral manifestation of opportunistic infection.

• Psychologic and physical dependence may occur with chronic administration.
• Dental local anesthetics will not interfere with urine test for cocaine abuse.

Consultations:
• Notify recovery program director if controlled substances may be required for a patient in recovery from cocaine use.

Teach Patient/Family:
• When chronic dry mouth occurs, advise patient to:
  • Avoid mouth rinses with high alcohol content because of drying effects.
  • Use daily home fluoride products for anticaries effect.
  • Use sugarless gum, frequent sips of water, or saliva substitutes.
  • Report oral lesions, soreness, or bleeding to dentist.

codeine phosphate/ codeine sulfate

koe′-deen foss′-fate/koe′-deen sull′-fate
(codeine phosphate)
Actacode[AUS], Codeine Phosphate Injection, Codeine Linctus[AUS](codeine sulfate) Contin[CAN]
Do not confuse codeine with Cardene or Lodine.

CATEGORY AND SCHEDULE

Pregnancy Risk Category: C (D if used for prolonged periods or at high dosages at term)
Controlled Substance: Schedule II (single drug), III (combination form)

Drug Class: Opioid analgesic

MECHANISM OF ACTION

An opioid agonist that binds to opioid receptors at many sites in the CNS, particularly in the medulla. This action inhibits the ascending pain pathways.
Therapeutic Effect: Alters the perception of and emotional response to pain, suppresses cough reflex.

USES

Treatment of mild-to-moderate pain, non-productive cough

PHARMACOKINETICS

Well absorbed after oral administration; rapidly metabolized by liver; 10% methylated to the active analgesic morphine. ***Half-life:*** 2.5–3 hr. Metabolites excreted in urine.

INDICATIONS AND DOSAGES
▸ **Analgesia**
PO, IM, subcutaneous
Adults, Elderly. 30 mg q4–6h.
Range: 15–60 mg.
Children. 0.5–1 mg/kg q4–6h.
Maximum: 60 mg/dose.
▸ **Cough**
PO
Adults, Elderly, Children 12 yr and older. 10–20 mg q4–6h.
Children 6–11 yr. 5–10 mg q4–6h.
Children 2–5 yr. 2.5–5 mg q4–6h.
▸ **Dosage in Renal Impairment**
Dosage is modified on the basis of creatinine clearance.

Creatinine Clearance	Dosage
10–50 ml/min	75% of usual dose
Less than 10 ml/min	50% of usual dose

SIDE EFFECTS/ADVERSE REACTIONS
Frequent
Constipation, somnolence, nausea, vomiting
Occasional
Paradoxical excitement, confusion, palpitations, facial flushing, decreased urination, blurred vision, dizziness, dry mouth, headache, hypotension (including orthostatic hypotension), decreased appetite, injection site redness, burning, or pain
Rare
Hallucinations, depression, abdominal pain, insomnia

PRECAUTIONS AND CONTRAINDICATIONS
Caution:
Elderly, cardiac dysrhythmias

DRUG INTERACTIONS OF CONCERN TO DENTISTRY
• Increased sedation with other CNS depressants and alcohol
• Increased effects of anticholinergics

SERIOUS REACTIONS
! Too-frequent use may result in paralytic ileus.
! Overdose may produce cold and clammy skin, confusion, seizures, decreased B/P, restlessness, pinpoint pupils, bradycardia, respiratory depression, decreased LOC, and severe weakness.
! The patient who uses codeine repeatedly may develop a tolerance to the drug's analgesic effect, as well as physical dependence.

DENTAL CONSIDERATIONS
General:
• Monitor vital signs at every appointment because of

cardiovascular and respiratory side
effects.
• After supine positioning, have
patient sit upright for at least 2 min
to avoid orthostatic hypotension.
• Assess salivary flow as a factor in
caries, periodontal disease, and
candidiasis.
• Psychologic and physical
dependence may occur with chronic
administration.
Teach Patient/Family:
• When chronic dry mouth occurs,
advise patient to:
   • Avoid mouth rinses with high
   alcohol content because of
   drying effects.
   • Use daily home fluoride
   products for anticaries effect.
   • Use sugarless gum, frequent
   sips of water, or saliva
   substitutes.

colchicine
kol'-chi-seen
(Colchicine, Colgout[AUS])

CATEGORY AND SCHEDULE
Pregnancy Risk Category: D

Drug Class: Antigout agent

MECHANISM OF ACTION
An alkaloid that decreases leukocyte
motility, phagocytosis, and lactic
acid production.
Therapeutic Effect: Decreases urate
crystal deposits and reduces
inflammatory process.

USES
Gout, gouty arthritis (prevention,
treatment); unlabeled uses: hepatic
cirrhosis, Behçet's disease,
scleroderma, Sweet's syndrome

PHARMACOKINETICS
Rapidly absorbed from the GI tract.
Highest concentration is in the liver,
spleen, and kidney. Protein binding:
30%–50%. Reenters the intestinal
tract by biliary secretion and is
reabsorbed from the intestines.
Partially metabolized in the liver.
Eliminated primarily in feces.

INDICATIONS AND DOSAGES
▸ **Acute Gouty Arthritis**
PO
Adults, Elderly. 0.6–1.2 mg; then
0.6 mg q1–2h or 1–1.2 mg q2h,
until pain is relieved or nausea,
vomiting, or diarrhea occurs. Total
dose: 4–8 mg.
IV
Adults, Elderly. Initially, 2 mg; then
0.5 mg q6h until satisfactory
response. Maximum: 4 mg/wk or
4 mg/one course of treatment. If
pain recurs, may give 1–2 mg/day
for several days but no sooner than
7 days after a full course of IV
therapy (total of 4 mg).
▸ **Chronic Gouty Arthritis**
PO
Adults, Elderly. 0.5–.6 mg once a
wk up to once a day, depending on
number of attacks per year.

SIDE EFFECTS/ADVERSE REACTIONS
Frequent
PO: Nausea, vomiting, abdominal
discomfort
Occasional
PO: Anorexia
Rare
Hypersensitivity reaction, including
angioedema
Parenteral: Nausea, vomiting,
diarrhea, abdominal discomfort, pain
or redness at injection site, neuritis
in injected arm

C

PRECAUTIONS AND CONTRAINDICATIONS
Blood dyscrasias; severe cardiac, GI, hepatic, or renal disorders
Caution:
Severe renal disease, blood dyscrasias, hepatic disease, elderly, lactation, children, retards B_{12} absorption

DRUG INTERACTIONS OF CONCERN TO DENTISTRY
• Increased risk of GI side effects: NSAIDs, alcohol
• Possible increased serum levels: erythromycin

SERIOUS REACTIONS
! Bone marrow depression, including aplastic anemia, agranulocytosis, and thrombocytopenia, may occur with long-term therapy.
! Overdose initially causes a burning feeling in the skin or throat, severe diarrhea, and abdominal pain. The patient then experiences fever, seizures, delirium, and renal impairment, marked by hematuria and oliguria. The third stage of overdose causes hair loss, leukocytosis, and stomatitis.

DENTAL CONSIDERATIONS
General:
• Consider drug in diagnosis of taste alteration.
• Patients on chronic drug therapy may rarely have symptoms of blood dyscrasias, which can include infection, bleeding, and poor healing.
• Avoid prescribing aspirin-containing products.
Consultations:
• Medical consultation may be required to assess disease control.

• In a patient with symptoms of blood dyscrasias, request a medical consultation for blood studies and postpone dental treatment until normal values are reestablished.
Teach Patient/Family to:
• Encourage effective oral hygiene to prevent soft tissue inflammation.
• Use caution to prevent injury when using oral hygiene aids.
• Avoid mouth rinses with high alcohol content because of drying effects.

colesevelam
ko-lee-**sev**′-a-lam
(WelChol [U.S.], Cholestagel [intl.])

CATEGORY AND SCHEDULE
Pregnancy Risk Category: B

Drug Class: Antihyperlipidemic, bile acid sequestrant, lipid-lowering agent

MECHANISM OF ACTION
Non-absorbed polymer that binds to bile acids in the intestine to prevent their absorption. As bile acid is reduced, the hepatic enzyme cholesterol 7-alpha hydroxylase is upregulated, increasing the demand for cholesterol in the liver and increasing the clearance of LDL-cholesterol from the blood. The mechanism by which blood glucose control is achieved is unknown.
Therapeutic Effect: Partially removes bile acid from enterohepatic circulation, increases clearance of LDL-cholesterol from the blood and improves glycemic control in patients with Type 2 diabetes mellitus.

USES
Adjunct to diet and exercise to reduce low-density lipoprotein cholesterol (LDL-C) in patients with primary hyperlipidemia (as monotherapy or in combination with an HMG-CoA reductase inhibitor/statin); also used to improve glycemic control in Type 2 diabetes mellitus.

PHARMACOKINETICS
Not absorbed from GI tract; not metabolized; excreted primarily in feces.

INDICATIONS AND DOSAGES
▸ **Primary Hyperlipidemia (Used as Monotherapy or in Combinations with an HMG COA Reductase Inhibitor, or "Statin")**
Adult. PO 6 tablets once daily or 3 tablets twice daily, taken with a meal and liquid.
▸ **Type 2 Diabetes Mellitus**
Adult. PO 6 tablets once daily or 3 tablets twice daily, taken with a meal and liquid.

SIDE EFFECTS/ADVERSE REACTIONS
Frequent
Constipation, nausea, vomiting, abdominal pain, dyspepsia
Occasional
Nasopharyngitis, hypoglycemia, nausea, hypertension
Rare
Myocardial infarction, aortic stenosis, bradycardia

PRECAUTIONS AND CONTRAINDICATIONS
Elevated serum triglycerides
Vitamin K or fat-soluble vitamin deficiencies (A, D, E, K)
Gastroparesis, GI tract surgery, patients at risk for bowel obstruction
Dysphagia, swallowing disorders

DRUG INTERACTIONS OF CONCERN TO DENTISTRY
• None reported

SERIOUS REACTIONS
❗ GI tract obstruction, hyperchloremic acidosis, osteoporosis secondary to excessive calcium excretion
❗ High doses may interfere with fat absorption and result in steatorrhea

DENTAL CONSIDERATIONS
General:
• Monitor vital signs at every appointment because of underlying disease and cardiovascular side effects of drug.
• Position patient for comfort if GI adverse effects occur.
• Assess glycemic control to avoid possible hypoglycemic emergency.
Consultations:
• Consult with physician to determine disease control and ability to tolerate dental procedures.
Teach Patient/Family to:
• Update medical history as changes in medication or disease status occur.

---

colestipol
koe-**les´**-ti-pole
(Colestid, Colestid[CAN])

CATEGORY AND SCHEDULE
Pregnancy Risk Category: C

Drug Class: Antihyperlipidemic

MECHANISM OF ACTION
An antihyperlipoproteinemic that binds with bile acids in the intestine, forming an insoluble complex. Binding results in partial removal of

C

bile acid from enterohepatic circulation.
Therapeutic Effect: Removes LDL and cholesterol from plasma.

USES
Adjunctive therapy to diet and exercise for the reduction of elevated serum total and LDL cholesterol in patients with primary hypercholesterolemia

PHARMACOKINETICS
Not absorbed from the GI tract. Excreted in the feces.

INDICATIONS AND DOSAGES
▸ **Primary Hypercholesterolemia**
PO, Granules
Adults, Elderly. Initially, 5 g 1–2 times a day. Range: 5–30 g/day once or in divided doses.
PO, Tablets
Adults, Elderly. Initially, 2 g 1–2 times a day. Range: 2–16 g/day.

SIDE EFFECTS/ADVERSE REACTIONS
Frequent
Constipation (may lead to fecal impaction), nausea, vomiting, stomach pain, indigestion
Occasional
Diarrhea, belching, bloating, headache, dizziness
Rare
Gallstones, peptic ulcer, malabsorption syndrome

PRECAUTIONS AND CONTRAINDICATIONS
Complete biliary obstruction, hypersensitivity to bile acid sequestering resins
Caution:
Lactation, children, bleeding disorders

DRUG INTERACTIONS OF CONCERN TO DENTISTRY
• Decreased absorption of tetracyclines, cephalexin, phenobarbital, corticosteroids, clindamycin, penicillins; administer doses several hours apart.

SERIOUS REACTIONS
! GI tract obstruction, hyperchloremic acidosis, and osteoporosis secondary to calcium excretion may occur.
! High dosage may interfere with fat absorption, resulting in steatorrhea.

DENTAL CONSIDERATIONS
General:
• Consider semisupine chair position for patient comfort because of GI side effects of disease.

conivaptan
con-ih-**vap**′-tan
(Vaprisol)

CATEGORY AND SCHEDULE
Pregnancy Risk Category: C

Drug Class: Vasopressin antagonist

MECHANISM OF ACTION
An arginine vasopressin (AVP) V1A and V2 selective antagonist that inhibits vasopressin binding V1A in the liver and V1 and V2 sites in renal collecting ducts. Results in excretion of free water.
Therapeutic Effect: Restores normal fluid and electrolyte status.

USES
Treatment of euvolemic hyponatremia in hospitalized patients

PHARMACOKINETICS

Protein binding: 99%. Metabolized in liver; CYP450 3A4 is responsible for primary metabolism. Primarily eliminated in feces (approximately 83%); minimal excretion in urine (about 12%). *Half-life:* 3.6–8.6 hr.

INDICATIONS AND DOSAGES
▸ **Hyponatremia**
IV
Adults. Initially, a loading dose of 20 mg given over 30 min. Maintenance: 20 mg/day as continuous infusion over 24 hr for an additional 1–3 days. May titrate to maximum dose of 40 mg/day; total duration should not exceed 4 days after loading dose. Safety and efficacy have not been established in children.

SIDE EFFECTS/ADVERSE REACTIONS
Frequent
Injection site reaction, headache
Occasional
Hypokalemia, thirst, vomiting, diarrhea, hypertension, orthostatic hypotension, polyuria, phlebitis, constipation, dry mouth, anemia, fever, nausea, confusion, erythema, insomnia, atrial fibrillation, hyper- or hypoglycemia, hyponatremia, pneumonia, UTI, hypomagnesemia, pain, dehydration, oral candidiasis, hematuria

PRECAUTIONS AND CONTRAINDICATIONS
Hypersensitivity to conivaptan or its components
Use with ketoconazole, itraconazole, clarithromycin, ritonavir, and indinavir is contraindicated
Caution:
Hyponatremia with underlying CHF, renal, or hepatic impairment

DRUG INTERACTIONS OF CONCERN TO DENTISTRY
• CYP3A4 inducers: may decrease the levels and effects of conivaptan.
• CYP3A4 inhibitors (e.g., erythromycin): may increase the levels and effects of conivaptan.
• CYP3A4 substrates: conivaptan may increase the levels and effects of CYP3A4 substrates.
• Digoxin: may increase the levels of digoxin.

SERIOUS REACTIONS
! Atrial fibrillation has been reported.

DENTAL CONSIDERATIONS
• Monitor vital signs at every appointment because of cardiovascular side effects.
• Avoid NSAIDs because of renal side effects.
• After supine positioning, have patient sit upright for at least 2 min before standing to avoid orthostatic hypotension.
• Patients taking this medication are treated on an inpatient basis.
Consultations:
• Consult physician to determine disease control and ability of patient to tolerate dental procedures, if needed while receiving drug.
Teach Patient/Family to:
• Report signs and symptoms of dry mouth and candidiasis.

cortisone acetate
kor′-ti-sone **ass′**-eh-tayte
(Cortate[AUS], Cortone[CAN])
Do not confuse cortisone with
Cort-Dome.

CATEGORY AND SCHEDULE
Pregnancy Risk Category: C (D if
used in the first trimester)

Drug Class: Glucocorticoid,
short-acting

MECHANISM OF ACTION
An adrenocortical steroid that
inhibits the accumulation of
inflammatory cells at inflammation
sites, phagocytosis, lysosomal
enzyme release and synthesis, and
release of mediators of
inflammation.
Therapeutic Effect: Prevents or
suppresses cell-mediated immune
reactions. Decreases or prevents
tissue response to inflammatory
process.

USES
Treatment of inflammation, severe
allergy, adrenal insufficiency,
collagen disorders, respiratory,
dermatologic disorders

PHARMACOKINETICS
Well absorbed after oral
administration. *Half-life:* 60–
90 min. Metabolized in liver and
kidneys, approximately one-third
excreted in urine as metabolites.

INDICATIONS AND DOSAGES
Dosage is dependent on the
condition being treated and patient
response.

▸ **Antiinflammation,
Immunosuppression**
PO
Adults, Elderly. 25–300 mg/day in
divided doses q12–24h.
Children. 2.5–10 mg/kg/day in
divided doses q6–8h.
▸ **Physiologic Replacement**
PO
Adults, Elderly. 25–35 mg/day.
Children. 0.5–0.75 mg/kg/day in
divided doses q8h.

SIDE EFFECTS/ADVERSE REACTIONS
Frequent
Insomnia, heartburn, anxiety,
abdominal distention, increased
diaphoresis, acne, mood swings,
increased appetite, facial flushing,
delayed wound healing, increased
susceptibility to infection, diarrhea
or constipation
Occasional
Headache, edema, change in skin
color, frequent urination
Rare
Tachycardia, allergic reaction (such
as rash and hives), psychological
changes, hallucinations, depression

PRECAUTIONS AND CONTRAINDICATIONS
Hypersensitivity to corticosteroids,
administration of live virus vaccine,
peptic ulcers (except in life-
threatening situations), systemic
fungal infection
Caution:
Diabetes mellitus, glaucoma,
osteoporosis, seizure disorders,
ulcerative colitis, CHF, myasthenia
gravis, renal disease, esophagitis,
peptic ulcer, rifampin

DRUG INTERACTIONS OF CONCERN TO DENTISTRY
• Decreased action: barbiturates,
rifabutin, rifampin

• Increased GI side effects: alcohol, salicylates, NSAIDs
• Increased action: ketoconazole, macrolide antibiotics
• Hepatotoxicity: acetaminophen (chronic, high doses)

SERIOUS REACTIONS

! Long-term therapy may cause hypocalcemia, hypokalemia, muscle wasting in arms and legs, osteoporosis, spontaneous fractures, amenorrhea, cataracts, glaucoma, peptic ulcer disease, and CHF.
! Abrupt withdrawal following long-term therapy may cause anorexia, nausea, fever, headache, joint pain, rebound inflammation, fatigue, weakness, lethargy, dizziness, and orthostatic hypotension.

DENTAL CONSIDERATIONS

General:
• Monitor vital signs at every appointment because of cardiovascular side effects.
• Patients on chronic drug therapy may rarely have symptoms of blood dyscrasias, which can include infection, bleeding, and poor healing.
• Assess salivary flow as a factor in caries, periodontal disease, and candidiasis.
• Avoid prescribing aspirin-containing products.
• Symptoms of oral infections may be masked.
• Place on frequent recall to evaluate healing response.
• Prophylactic antibiotics may be indicated to prevent infection if surgery or deep scaling is planned.
• Determine dose and duration of steroid therapy for each patient to assess risk for stress tolerance and immunosuppression.

• Patients who have been or are currently on chronic steroid therapy (>2 wk) may require supplemental steroids for dental treatment.
• Determine why the patient is taking the drug.

Consultations:
• In a patient with symptoms of blood dyscrasias, request a medical consultation for blood studies and postpone dental treatment until normal values are reestablished.
• Medical consultation may be required to assess disease control and stress tolerance of patient.
• Consultation may be required to confirm steroid dose and duration of use.

Teach Patient/Family to:
• Encourage effective oral hygiene to prevent soft tissue inflammation.
• Prevent injury when using oral hygiene aids.
• When chronic dry mouth occurs, advise patient to:
  • Avoid mouth rinses with high alcohol content because of drying effects.
  • Use daily home fluoride products for anticaries effect.
  • Use sugarless gum, frequent sips of water, or saliva substitutes.

cottonseed oil

OTHER NAMES
Numoisyn

Drug Class: Prescription nonherbal remedy

MAJOR INGREDIENTS
Hydrogenated cottonseed oil, sorbitol, polyethylene glycol, malic acid, sodium citrate, calcium

C

phosphate, citric acid, magnesium stearate, silicon dioxide in lozenge dose form

CLAIMED ACTIONS

Exerts an oral demulcent (coating) effect in the oral cavity.

USES

For oral lubrication for the relief of dry mouth (xerostomia) associated with medication use, chemotherapy, head-and-neck irradiation involving the salivary glands, or Sjögren's syndrome. It is also recommended for radiation- or chemotherapy-induced mucositis (this indication is not supported by randomized clinical trials).

ADMINISTRATION

The lozenge is dissolved slowly in the mouth as needed (not to exceed 16/day).

SIDE EFFECTS

Excessive consumption can cause minor digestive problems.

DRUG INTERACTIONS

None reported

DENTAL CONSIDERATIONS

Patients with xerostomia must be monitored carefully for periodontal inflammation and caries and treated accordingly with saliva substitutes, xylitol chewing gum, non-alcoholic mouth rinses and topical fluorides. Patients with a history of head-and-neck irradiation may develop osteoradionecrosis from invasive dental procedures, and patients with a history of the use of antineoplastic drugs should be monitored for oral signs and symptoms of recurrences of certain tumors, mucositis, and blood dyscrasias.

cromolyn sodium

kroe'-moe-lin so'-dee-um
(Apo-Cromolyn[CAN], Crolom, Gastrocom, Intal, Nasalcrom, Opticrom, Rynacrom[AUS])

CATEGORY AND SCHEDULE

Pregnancy Risk Category: B

Drug Class: Antiasthmatic, mast cell stabilizer

MECHANISM OF ACTION

An antiasthmatic and antiallergic agent that prevents mast cell release of histamine and formation of other mediators (leukotrienes) of anaphylaxis by inhibiting degranulation after contact with antigens.
Therapeutic Effect: Helps prevent symptoms of asthma, allergic rhinitis, mastocytosis, and exercise-induced bronchospasm.

USES

Treatment of allergic rhinitis, severe perennial bronchial asthma, exercise-induced bronchospasm (prevention), prevention of acute bronchospasm induced by environmental pollutants, mastocytosis

PHARMACOKINETICS

Minimal absorption after PO, inhalation, or nasal administration. Absorbed portion excreted in urine or by biliary system. *Half-life:* 80–90 min.

INDICATIONS AND DOSAGES
▶ Asthma
Inhalation (Nebulization)
Adults, Elderly, Children older than 2 yr. 20 mg 3–4 times a day.

Aerosol spray
Adults, Elderly, Children 12 yr and older. Initially, 2 sprays 4 times a day. Maintenance: 2–4 sprays 3–4 times a day.
Children 5–11 yr. Initially, 2 sprays 4 times a day, then 1–2 sprays 3–4 times a day.
▸ **Prevention of Bronchospasm**
Inhalation (Nebulization)
Adults, Elderly, Children older than 2 yr. 20 mg 1 hr before exercise or exposure to allergens.
Aerosol spray
Adults, Elderly, Children older than 5 yr. 2 sprays 1 hr before exercise or exposure to allergens.
▸ **Food Allergy, Inflammatory Bowel Disease**
PO
Adults, Elderly, Children older than 12 yr. 200–400 mg 4 times a day.
Children 2–12 yr. 100–200 mg 4 times a day. Maximum: 40 mg/kg/day.
▸ **Allergic Rhinitis**
Intranasal
Adults, Elderly, Children older than 6 yr. 1 spray each nostril 3–4 times a day. May increase up to 6 times a day.
▸ **Systemic Mastocytosis**
PO
Adults, Elderly, Children older than 12 yr. 200 mg 4 times a day.
Children 2–12 yr. 100 mg 4 times a day. Maximum: 40 mg/kg/day.
Children younger than 2 yr. 20 mg/kg/day in 4 divided doses.
Maximum: 30 mg/kg/day (children 6 mo–2 yr).
▸ **Conjunctivitis**
Ophthalmic
Adults, Elderly, Children older than 4 yr. 1–2 drops in both eyes 4–6 times a day.

SIDE EFFECTS/ADVERSE REACTIONS
Frequent
PO: Headache, diarrhea
Inhalation: Cough, dry mouth and throat, stuffy nose, throat irritation, unpleasant taste
Nasal: Nasal burning, stinging, or irritation; increased sneezing
Ophthalmic: Eye burning or stinging
Occasional
PO: Rash, abdominal pain, arthralgia, nausea, insomnia
Inhalation: Bronchospasm, hoarseness, lacrimation
Nasal: Cough, headache, unpleasant taste, postnasal drip
Ophthalmic: Lacrimation and itching of eye
Rare
Inhalation: Dizziness, painful urination, arthralgia, myalgia, rash
Nasal: Epistaxis, rash
Ophthalmic: Chemosis or edema of conjunctiva, eye irritation

PRECAUTIONS AND CONTRAINDICATIONS
Status asthmaticus
Caution:
Lactation, renal disease, hepatic disease, children younger than 5 yr

DRUG INTERACTIONS OF CONCERN TO DENTISTRY
• None reported

SERIOUS REACTIONS
! Anaphylaxis occurs rarely when cromolyn is given by the inhalation, nasal, or oral route.

DENTAL CONSIDERATIONS
General:
• Determine why patient is taking the drug.

C

• Protect patient's eyes from accidental spatter during dental treatment.
• Avoid dental light in patient's eyes; offer dark glasses for patient comfort.
• Assess salivary flow as a factor in caries, periodontal disease, and candidiasis.
• Consider semisupine chair position for patients with respiratory disease.
• A stress reduction protocol may be required.
• Midday appointments and a stress-reduction protocol may be required for anxious patients.
• Be aware that aspirin or sulfite preservatives in vasoconstrictor-containing products can exacerbate asthma.

Consultations:
• Consider drug in diagnosis of taste alteration and burning mouth syndrome.
• Medical consultation may be required to assess disease control and stress tolerance of patient.

Teach Patient/Family to:
• Rinse mouth with water after each inhaled dose to prevent dryness.
• When chronic dry mouth occurs, advise patient to:
  • Avoid mouth rinses with high alcohol content because of drying effects.
  • Use daily home fluoride products for anticaries effect.
  • Use sugarless gum, frequent sips of water, or saliva substitutes.

cyanocobalamin (vitamin B₁₂)

sye-an-oh-koe-**bal**′-ah-min
(Bedoz[CAN], Cytamen[AUS], Nascobal)

CATEGORY AND SCHEDULE

Pregnancy Risk Category: A (C if used in doses above recommended daily allowance)

Drug Class: Vitamin B₁₂, water-soluble vitamin

MECHANISM OF ACTION

Acts as a coenzyme for various metabolic functions, including fat and carbohydrate metabolism and protein synthesis.
Therapeutic Effect: Necessary for cell growth and replication, hematopoiesis, and myelin synthesis.

USES

Vitamin B₁₂ deficiency, pernicious anemia, vitamin B₁₂ malabsorption syndrome, Schilling test, increased requirements with pregnancy thyrotoxicosis, hemolytic anemia, hemorrhage, renal and hepatic disease; intranasal gel: maintaining vitamin B₁₂ levels in patients with HIV, multiple sclerosis, or Crohn's disease

PHARMACOKINETICS

In the presence of calcium, absorbed systemically in lower half of ileum. Initially, bound to intrinsic factor; this complex passes down intestine, binding to receptor sites on ileal mucosa. Protein binding: High. Metabolized in the liver. Primarily eliminated unchanged in urine.
Half-life: 6 days.

INDICATIONS AND DOSAGES
▶ **Pernicious Anemia**
IM, Subcutaneous
Adults, Elderly. 100 mcg/day for 7
days, then every other day for 7
days, then every 3–4 days for
2–3 wk. Maintenance: 100 mcg/mo
(oral 1000–2000 mcg/day).
Children. 30–50 mcg/day for 2 or
more wk. Maintenance: 100 mcg/
mo.
Neonates. 1000 mcg/day for 2 or
more wk. Maintenance: 50 mcg/mo.
Intranasal
Adults, Elderly. 500 mcg once a wk.
▶ **Uncomplicated Vitamin B₁₂
Deficiency**
PO
Adults, Elderly. 1000–2000 mcg/day.
IM, Subcutaneous
Adults, Elderly. 100 mcg/day for
5–10 days, followed by 100–
200 mcg/mo.
▶ **Complicated Vitamin B₁₂
Deficiency**
IM, Subcutaneous
Adults, Elderly. 1000 mcg (with
IM or IV folic acid 15 mg) as a
single dose, then 1000 mcg/day
plus oral folic acid 5 mg/day for 7
days.

SIDE EFFECTS/ADVERSE
REACTIONS
Occasional
Diarrhea, pruritus

PRECAUTIONS AND
CONTRAINDICATIONS
Folic acid deficiency anemia,
hereditary optic nerve atrophy,
history of allergy to cobalamins
Caution:
Lactation, children

DRUG INTERACTIONS OF
CONCERN TO DENTISTRY
• Increased absorption: prednisone

SERIOUS REACTIONS
! Impurities in preparation may
cause a rare allergic reaction.
! Peripheral vascular thrombosis,
pulmonary edema, hypokalemia, and
CHF may occur.

DENTAL CONSIDERATIONS
General:
• Deficiency in vitamin B₁₂ and
other B-complex vitamins may
cause oral symptomatology.

cyclobenzaprine
hydrochloride
sye-kloe-**ben**′-za-preen
hi-droh-**klor**′-ide
(Flexeril, Flexitec[CAN],
Novo-Cycloprine[CAN])
Do not confuse cyclobenzaprine
with cycloserine or
cyproheptadine, or Flexeril with
Floxin.

CATEGORY AND SCHEDULE
Pregnancy Risk Category: B

Drug Class: Skeletal muscle
relaxant, centrally-acting tricyclic

MECHANISM OF ACTION
A centrally-acting skeletal muscle
relaxant that reduces tonic somatic
muscle activity at the level of the
brainstem.
Therapeutic Effect: Relieves local
skeletal muscle spasm.

USES
Adjunct for relief of muscle spasm
and pain in musculoskeletal
conditions

C

PHARMACOKINETICS

Route	Onset	Peak	Duration
PO	1 hr	3–4 hr	12–24 hr

Well but slowly absorbed from the GI tract. Protein binding: 93%. Metabolized in the GI tract and the liver. Primarily excreted in urine. *Half-life:* 1–3 days.

INDICATIONS AND DOSAGES

▸ **Acute, Painful Musculoskeletal Conditions**
PO
Adults. Initially, 5 mg 3 times a day. May increase to 10 mg 3 times a day.
Elderly. 5 mg 3 times a day.
▸ **Dosage in Hepatic Impairment**
Mild. 5 mg 3 times a day.
Moderate and severe. Not recommended.

PRECAUTIONS AND CONTRAINDICATIONS

Acute recovery phase of MI, arrhythmias, CHF, heart block, conduction disturbances, hyperthyroidism, use within 14 days of MAOIs
Caution:
Renal disease, hepatic disease, addictive personality, elderly

SIDE EFFECTS/ADVERSE REACTIONS

Frequent
Somnolence, dry mouth, dizziness
Rare
Fatigue, asthenia, blurred vision, headache, nervousness, confusion, nausea, constipation, dyspepsia, unpleasant taste

PRECAUTIONS AND CONTRAINDICATIONS

Acute recovery phase of MI, dysrhythmias, heart block, CHF, hypersensitivity, children younger than 12 yr, intermittent porphyria, thyroid disease, concomitant use with or within 14 days of discontinuing MAOIs, renal disease, hepatic disease, addictive personality, elderly

DRUG INTERACTIONS OF CONCERN TO DENTISTRY

• Increased CNS depression: alcohol, narcotics, barbiturates, sedatives, hypnotics
• Increased effects of anticholinergic drugs
• Increased effects of direct-acting sympathomimetics (epinephrine, levonordefrin)

SERIOUS REACTIONS

! Overdose may result in visual hallucinations, hyperactive reflexes, muscle rigidity, vomiting, and hyperpyrexia.

DENTAL CONSIDERATIONS

General:
• Monitor vital signs at every appointment because of cardiovascular side effects.
• Assess salivary flow as a factor in caries, periodontal disease, and candidiasis.
• After supine positioning, have patient sit upright for at least 2 min to avoid orthostatic hypotension.
• Use vasoconstrictors with caution, in low doses, and with careful aspiration. Avoid use of gingival retraction cord with epinephrine.
• Place on frequent recall because of oral side effects.
• Consider drug in diagnosis of taste alterations.
Consultations:
• Medical consultation may be required to assess disease control.

Teach Patient/Family:
• When chronic dry mouth occurs, advise patient to:
    • Avoid mouth rinses with high alcohol content because of drying effects.
    • Use daily home fluoride products for anticaries effect.
    • Use sugarless gum, frequent sips of water, or saliva substitutes.

cyclopentolate hydrochloride

sye-kloe-**pen′**-toe-late hi-droh-**klor′**-ide
(AK-Pentolate, Cyclogyl, Cylate, Diopentolate[CAN], Ocu-Pentolate, Pentolair)

CATEGORY AND SCHEDULE
Pregnancy Risk Category: C

Drug Class: Cycloplegic; mydriatic

MECHANISM OF ACTION
An antimuscarinic similar to atropine that competes with acetylcholine. Blocks the responses of the sphincter muscle of the iris and the accommodative muscle of the ciliary body to cholinergic stimulation.
Therapeutic Effect: Results in mydriasis and cycloplegia.

USES
Used to dilate (enlarge) the pupil for eye examination.

PHARMACOKINETICS
Rapid systemic absorption following ophthalmic administration. Shorter duration of action than atropine. Complete recovery takes 6–24 hr.

INDICATIONS AND DOSAGES
▸ **Cycloplegia Induction, Mydriasis Induction**
Ophthalmic
Adults, Elderly, Children. Instill 1–2 drops of 0.5%–2% solution in eye(s). May repeat with 0.5% or 1% solution in 5–10 min as needed.
Neonates, infants. Instill 1 drop of 0.5%–2% solution in eye(s) followed by 1 drop of 0.5% or 1% in 5 min as needed.

SIDE EFFECTS/ADVERSE REACTIONS
Occasional
Blurred vision, burning of eye, photophobia
Rare
Conjunctivitis, increased intraocular pressure

PRECAUTIONS AND CONTRAINDICATIONS
Narrow-angle glaucoma, anatomical narrow angles, hypersensitivity to cyclopentolate or any component of the formulation

DRUG INTERACTIONS OF CONCERN TO DENTISTRY
• None reported

SERIOUS REACTIONS
! Systemic absorption, which includes signs and symptoms of confusion, psychosis, and ataxia; tachycardia and vasodilation occur rarely.

DENTAL CONSIDERATIONS
General:
• Not likely to be encountered in the dental office; used for diagnostic procedures.
• Question patient about eye health, including the presence of glaucoma.

C

cyclophosphamide

sye-kloe-**foss**′-fa-mide
(Cycloblastin[AUS], Cytoxan,
Endoxan Asta[AUS], Endoxon
Asta[AUS], Neosar,
Procytox[CAN])
Do not confuse Cytoxan with
cefoxitin, Ciloxan, cyclosporine,
or Cytotec.

CATEGORY AND SCHEDULE
Pregnancy Risk Category: D

Drug Class: Antineoplastic
alkylating agent

MECHANISM OF ACTION
An alkylating agent that inhibits
DNA and RNA protein synthesis by
cross-linking with DNA and RNA
strands, preventing cell growth. Cell
cycle-phase nonspecific.
Therapeutic Effect: Potent
immunosuppressant.

USES
Treatment of Hodgkin's disease;
lymphomas; leukemia; cancer of
female reproductive tract, lung,
prostate; multiple myeloma;
neuroblastoma, retinoblastoma;
Ewing's sarcoma; Burkitt's
lymphoma; advanced mycosis
fungoides; nephrotic syndrome
(children)

PHARMACOKINETICS
Well absorbed from the GI tract.
Protein binding: Low. Crosses the
blood-brain barrier. Metabolized in
the liver to active metabolites.
Primarily excreted in urine.
Removed by hemodialysis. *Half-life:*
3–12 hr.

INDICATIONS AND DOSAGES
▶ **Ovarian Adenocarcinoma, Breast
Carcinoma, Hodgkin's Disease,
Non-Hodgkin's Lymphoma, Multiple
Myeloma, Leukemia (Acute
Lymphoblastic, Acute Myelogenous,
Acute Monocytic, Chronic
Granulocytic, Chronic Lymphocytic),
Mycosis Fungoides, Disseminated
Neuroblastoma, Retinoblastoma**
PO
Adults. 1–5 mg/kg/day.
Children. Initially, 2–8 mg/kg/day.
Maintenance: 2–5 mg/kg twice a
wk.
IV
Adults. 40–50 mg/kg in divided
doses over 2–5 days; or 10–15 mg/
kg every 7–10 days or 3–5 mg/kg
twice a wk.
Children. 2–8 mg/kg/day for 6 days
or total dose for 7 days once a wk.
▶ **Biopsy-Proven Minimal-Change
Nephrotic Syndrome**
PO
Adults, Children. 2.5–3 mg/kg/day
for 60–90 days.

SIDE EFFECTS/ADVERSE
REACTIONS
Expected
Marked leukopenia 8–15 days after
initial therapy
Frequent
Nausea, vomiting (beginning about
6 hr after administration and lasting
about 4 hr), alopecia
Occasional
Diarrhea, darkening of skin and
fingernails, stomatitis, headache,
diaphoresis
Rare
Pain or redness at injection site

PRECAUTIONS AND
CONTRAINDICATIONS
Lactation
Caution:
Radiation therapy

DRUG INTERACTIONS OF CONCERN TO DENTISTRY

• Increased blood dyscrasia: NSAIDs, dapsone, phenothiazines, corticosteroids
• Increased metabolism: phenobarbital

SERIOUS REACTIONS

! Major toxic effect is myelosuppression resulting in blood dyscrasias, such as leukopenia, anemia, thrombocytopenia, and hypoprothrombinemia.
! Expect leukopenia to resolve in 17–28 days. Anemia generally occurs after large doses or prolonged therapy. Thrombocytopenia may occur 10–15 days after drug initiation.
! Hemorrhagic cystitis occurs commonly in long-term therapy, especially in pediatric patients.
! Pulmonary fibrosis and cardiotoxicity have been noted with high doses.
! Amenorrhea, azoospermia, and hyperkalemia may also occur.

DENTAL CONSIDERATIONS

General:
• Monitor vital signs at every appointment because of cardiovascular and respiratory side effects.
• Patients on chronic drug therapy may rarely have symptoms of blood dyscrasias, which can include infection, bleeding, and poor healing.
• Avoid prescribing aspirin-containing products.
• Prophylactic antibiotics may be indicated to prevent infection if surgery or deep scaling is planned because of leukopenic drug side effects.

• Patients receiving chemotherapy may require palliative treatment for stomatitis.
Consultations:
• In a patient with symptoms of blood dyscrasias, request a medical consultation for blood studies and postpone dental treatment until normal values are reestablished.
• Take precautions if dental surgery is anticipated and anesthesia is required.
Teach Patient/Family to:
• Encourage effective oral hygiene to prevent soft tissue inflammation.
• Prevent injury when using oral hygiene aids.

cycloserine
sye-kloe-**ser**′-een
(Closina[AUS], Seromycin)

CATEGORY AND SCHEDULE
Pregnancy Risk Category: C

Drug Class: Antitubercular

MECHANISM OF ACTION
An antitubercular that inhibits cell wall synthesis by competing with the amino acid, D-alanine, for incorporation into the bacterial cell wall.
Therapeutic Effect: Causes disruption of bacterial cell wall. Bactericidal or bacteriostatic.

USES
Treatment of pulmonary TB, extrapulmonary as adjunctive

PHARMACOKINETICS
Readily absorbed from the GI tract. No protein binding. Widely distributed (including CSF). Metabolized in liver. Primarily

excreted in urine. Removed by hemodialysis. *Half-life:* 10 hr.

INDICATIONS AND DOSAGES
▸ **TB**
Adults, Elderly. 250 mg q12h for 14 days, then 500 mg to 1g/day in 2 divided doses for 18–24 mo. Maximum: 1 g as a single daily dose.
Children. 10–20 mg/kg/day in 2 divided doses. Maximum: 1000 mg/day for 18–24 mo.
▸ **Dosage in Renal Impairment**

Creatinine Clearance	Dosage Interval
10–50 ml/min	q24h
Less than 10 ml/min	q36–48h

SIDE EFFECTS/ADVERSE REACTIONS
Occasional
Drowsiness, headache, dizziness, vertigo, seizures, confusion, psychosis, paresis, tremor, vitamin B_{12} deficiency, folate deficiency, cardiac arrhythmias, increased liver enzymes

PRECAUTIONS AND CONTRAINDICATIONS
Epilepsy, depression, severe anxiety, psychosis, severe renal insufficiency, excessive concurrent use of alcohol, history of hypersensitivity reactions with previous cycloserine therapy

DRUG INTERACTIONS OF CONCERN TO DENTISTRY
- Seizures: alcohol
- Drowsiness is a common side effect; although no drug interactions with sedatives are reported, increased drowsiness is possible

SERIOUS REACTIONS/ADVERSE REACTIONS
! Neurotoxicity, as evidenced by confusion, agitation, CNS depression, psychosis, coma, and seizures, occur rarely.
! Neurotoxic effects of cycloserine may be treated and prevented with the administration of 200–300 mg of pyridoxine daily.

DENTAL CONSIDERATIONS
General:
- Patients on chronic drug therapy may rarely have symptoms of blood dyscrasias, which can include infection, bleeding, and poor healing.
- Examine for evidence of oral signs of disease.
- Determine why the patient is taking the drug (i.e., for preventive or therapeutic therapy).
Consultation:
- Medical consultation may be required to assess patient's ability to tolerate stress.
- In a patient with symptoms of blood dyscrasias, request a medical consultation for blood studies and postpone dental treatment until normal values are reestablished.
- Determine that noninfectious status exists by ensuring that:
  - Anti-TB drugs have been taken for more than 3 wk.
  - Culture confirms antibiotic susceptibility to TB microorganism.
  - Patient has had three consecutive negative sputum smears.
  - Patient is not in the coughing stage.
Teach Patient/Family to:
- Avoid mouth rinses with high alcohol content.

• Use caution to prevent injury when using oral hygiene aids.
• Encourage effective oral hygiene to prevent soft tissue inflammation.
• Take medication for full length of prescribed therapy to ensure effectiveness of treatment and prevent the emergence of resistant forms of microbe.

cyclosporine
sye-kloe-**spor'**-in
(Cysporin[AUS], Gengraf, Neoral, Restasis, Sandimmune, Sandimmune Neoral[AUS])
Do not confuse cyclosporine with cycloserine, cyclophosphamide, or Cyklokapron.

CATEGORY AND SCHEDULE
Pregnancy Risk Category: C

Drug Class: Immunosuppressant

MECHANISM OF ACTION
A cyclic polypeptide that inhibits both cellular and humoral immune responses by inhibiting interleukin-2, a proliferative factor needed for T-cell activity.
Therapeutic Effect: Prevents organ rejection and relieves symptoms of psoriasis and arthritis.

USES
Prevent rejection of tissues/allogeneic organ transplants; severe recalcitrant psoriasis; rheumatoid arthritis (Neoral only). Note: Sandimmune and Neoral are not bioequivalent.

PHARMACOKINETICS
Variably absorbed from the GI tract. Protein binding: 90%. Widely distributed. Metabolized in the liver.

Eliminated primarily by biliary or fecal excretion. Not removed by hemodialysis. *Half-life:* Adults, 10–27 hr; children, 7–19 hr.

INDICATIONS AND DOSAGES
▶ **Transplantation, Prevention of Organ Rejection**
PO
Adults, Elderly, Children. 10–18 mg/kg/dose given 4–12 hr prior to organ transplantation.
Maintenance: 5–15 mg/kg/day in divided doses then tapered to 3–10 mg/kg/day.
IV
Adults, Elderly, Children. Initially, 5–6 mg/kg/dose given 4–12 hr prior to organ transplantation.
Maintenance: 2–10 mg/kg/day in divided doses.
▶ **Rheumatoid Arthritis**
PO
Adults, Elderly. Initially, 2.5 mg/kg a day in 2 divided doses. May increase by 0.5–0.75 mg/kg/day. Maximum: 4 mg/kg/day.
▶ **Psoriasis**
PO
Adults, Elderly. Initially, 2.5 mg/kg/day in 2 divided doses. May increase by 0.5 mg/kg/day. Maximum: 4 mg/kg/day.
▶ **Dry Eye**
Ophthalmic
Adults, Elderly. Instill 1 drip in each affected eye q12h.

SIDE EFFECTS/ADVERSE REACTIONS
Frequent
Mild-to-moderate hypertension, hirsutism, tremors
Occasional
Acne, leg cramps, gingival hyperplasia (marked by red, bleeding, and tender gums), paresthesia, diarrhea, nausea, vomiting, headache

C

Rare
Hypersensitivity reaction,
abdominal discomfort,
gynecomastia, sinusitis

PRECAUTIONS AND CONTRAINDICATIONS

History of hypersensitivity to
cyclosporine or polyoxyethylated
castor oil
Caution:
Severe renal disease, severe hepatic
disease

DRUG INTERACTIONS OF CONCERN TO DENTISTRY

Systemic Form
• Hepatotoxicity/nephrotoxicity:
erythromycin, azithromycin,
clarithromycin
• Decreased action: barbiturates,
carbamazepine
• Possibly reduced blood levels:
clindamycin
• Increased infection and
immunosuppression: corticosteroids
• Increased blood levels and risk of
toxicity: fluconazole, ketoconazole,
and itraconazole
Ophthalmic-Dose Form
• None reported

SERIOUS REACTIONS

! Mild nephrotoxicity occurs in 25%
of renal transplant patients, 38% of
cardiac transplant patients, and 37%
of liver transplant patients, generally
2 to 3 months after transplantation
(more severe toxicity generally
occurs soon after transplantation).
Hepatotoxicity occurs in 4% of renal
transplant patients, 7% of cardiac
transplant patients, and 4% of
liver transplant patients, generally
within the first month after
transplantation. Both toxicities
usually respond to dosage reduction.
! Severe hyperkalemia and
hyperuricemia occur occasionally.

DENTAL CONSIDERATIONS

Systemic Form
General:
• Monitor vital signs at every
appointment because of
cardiovascular side effects.
• Patients on chronic drug therapy
may rarely have symptoms of blood
dyscrasias, which can include
infection, bleeding, and poor
healing.
• Examine for gingival enlargement
(place on frequent recall to evaluate
gingival condition and healing
response).
• Monitor time since organ/tissue
transplant.
Consultations:
• Antibiotic prophylaxis usually
is recommended in patients with
organ transplants and
immunosuppression.
• In a patient with symptoms of
blood dyscrasias, request a medical
consultation for blood studies and
postpone dental treatment until
normal values are reestablished.
• Request baseline B/P in renal
transplant patients for patient
evaluation before dental treatment.
Teach Patient/Family to:
• Encourage effective oral
hygiene to prevent soft tissue
inflammation.
• Use caution to prevent injury when
using oral hygiene aids.

Ophthalmic-Dose Form
General:
• Determine why the patient is
taking the drug.
• Protect the patient's eyes from
accidental spatter during dental
treatment.
• Avoid dental light in the patient's
eyes; offer dark glasses for patient
comfort.
Teach Patient/Family:
• When chronic dry mouth occurs,
advise patient to:

- Avoid mouth rinses with high alcohol content because of drying effects.
- Use daily home fluoride products for anticaries effect.
- Use sugarless gum, frequent sips of water, or saliva substitutes.

cyproheptadine
si-proe-**hep**′-ta-deen
(Periactin)

CATEGORY AND SCHEDULE
Pregnancy Risk Category: B

Drug Class: Antihistamine, H_1-receptor antagonist

MECHANISM OF ACTION
An antihistamine that competes with histamine at histaminic receptor sites. Anticholinergic effects cause drying of nasal mucosa.
Therapeutic Effect: Relieves allergic conditions (urticaria, pruritus).

USES
Allergy symptoms, rhinitis, pruritus, cold urticaria

PHARMACOKINETICS
Well absorbed from GI tract. Metabolized in liver. Primarily eliminated in feces. *Half-life:* 16 hr.

INDICATIONS AND DOSAGES
▸ **Allergic Condition**
PO
Adults, Children older than 15 yr. 4 mg 3 times a day. May increase dose but do not exceed 0.5 mg/kg/day.

Children 7–14 yr. 4 mg 2–3 times a day, or 0.25 mg/kg daily in divided doses.
Children 2–6 yr. 2 mg 2–3 times a day, or 0.25 mg/kg daily in divided doses.
▸ **Usual Elderly Dosage**
PO
Initially, 4 mg 2 times a day.

SIDE EFFECTS/ADVERSE REACTIONS
Frequent
Drowsiness, dizziness, muscular weakness, dry mouth/nose/throat/lips, urinary retention, thickening of bronchial secretions
Frequent
Sedation, dizziness, hypotension
Occasional
Epigastric distress, flushing, visual disturbances, hearing disturbances, paresthesia, sweating, chills

PRECAUTIONS AND CONTRAINDICATIONS
Acute asthmatic attack, patients receiving MAOIs, history of hypersensitivity to antihistamines
Caution:
Increased intraocular pressure, renal disease, cardiac disease, hypertension, bronchial asthma, seizure disorder, stenosed peptic ulcers, hyperthyroidism, prostatic hypertrophy, bladder neck obstruction, elderly

DRUG INTERACTIONS OF CONCERN TO DENTISTRY
- Increased CNS depression: alcohol, CNS depressants
- Increased effect of anticholinergic drugs

SERIOUS REACTIONS
❗ Children may experience dominant paradoxical reaction (restlessness,

C

insomnia, euphoria, nervousness, tremors).

! Overdose in children may result in hallucinations, convulsions, death.

! Hypersensitivity reaction (eczema, pruritus, rash, cardiac disturbances, angioedema, photosensitivity) may occur.

! Overdose may vary from CNS depression (sedation, apnea, cardiovascular collapse, death) to severe paradoxical reaction (hallucinations, tremor, seizures).

DENTAL CONSIDERATIONS

General:

• Assess salivary flow as a factor in caries, periodontal disease, and candidiasis.

• Determine why the patient is taking the drug.

cysteamine bitartrate
sis-**tee**′-ah-meen bye-**tar**′-trate
(Cystagon)

CATEGORY AND SCHEDULE
Pregnancy Risk Category: C

Drug Class: Nephropathic cystinosis therapy

MECHANISM OF ACTION
An aminothiol that participates within lysosomes in a thiol-disulfide interchange reaction converting cystine into cysteine and cysteine-cysteamine mixed disulfide, both of which can exit cystinotic lysosomes.
Therapeutic Effect: Lowers the cystine content in cells.

USES
Used to prevent damage that may be caused by the buildup of cystine crystals in organs such as the kidneys.

PHARMACOKINETICS
Poorly bound to plasma proteins.
Half-life: Unknown.

INDICATIONS AND DOSAGES
▶ Cystinosis
PO
Adults. Initially, $\frac{1}{4}$–$\frac{1}{6}$ of maintenance dose. Gradually, increase dose over 4–6 wk.
Maintenance. 2 g/day in 4 divided doses.
Children older than 12 yr and weighing more than 110 lb. 2 g/day in 4 divided doses.
Children 6–12 yr. 1.30 g/m^2/day of the free base, given in 4 divided doses.

SIDE EFFECTS/ADVERSE REACTIONS
Frequent
Rash, loss of appetite, fever, vomiting, diarrhea, lethargy
Occasional
Dehydration, hypertension, nausea, abdominal pain, somnolence, nervousness, nightmares, urticaria

PRECAUTIONS AND CONTRAINDICATIONS
Hypersensitivity to cysteamine or penicillamine

DRUG INTERACTIONS OF CONCERN TO DENTISTRY
• Dental drug interactions have not been studied.

SERIOUS REACTIONS
! Leukopenia, abnormal liver function, and anemia occur rarely.
! Sudden deaths have been reported.

C

DENTAL CONSIDERATIONS

General:
• Patients taking this medication may have significant renal disease; thoroughly review medical and drug history.

Consultations:
• Specific consultation depends on type of renal disease.

Teach Patient/Family to:
• Encourage effective oral hygiene to prevent soft tissue inflammation.
• Prevent trauma when using oral hygiene aids.
• Update health and medication history if physician makes any changes in evaluation or drug regimens; include OTC, herbal, and nonherbal remedies in the update.

cytarabine

sigh-**tar**'-ah-bean
(Ara-C, Cytosar[CAN], Cytosar-U)
Do not confuse cytarabine with Cytadren, Cytovene, or vidarabine.

CATEGORY AND SCHEDULE
Pregnancy Risk Category: D

Drug Class: Antimetabolite; antineoplastic

MECHANISM OF ACTION
An antimetabolite that is converted intracellularly to a nucleotide. Cell cycle-specific for S phase of cell division.
Therapeutic Effect: May inhibit DNA synthesis. Potent immunosuppressive activity.

USES
Treatment of acute and chronic myelocytic leukemia, acute lymphocytic leukemia, meningeal leukemia, non-Hodgkin's lymphoma in children. Off label: Treatment of Hodgkin's lymphoma, myelodysplastic syndrome

PHARMACOKINETICS
Widely distributed; moderate amount crosses the blood-brain barrier. Protein binding: 15%. Primarily excreted in urine.
Half-life: 1–3 hr.

INDICATIONS AND DOSAGES
▸ **To Induce Remission in Acute Lymphocytic Leukemia, Acute and Chronic Myelocytic Leukemia, Meningeal Leukemia, or Non-Hodgkin's Lymphoma in Children**
IV
Adults, Elderly, Children. 200 mg/m^2/day for 5 days q2wk as monotherapy or 100–200 mg/m^2/day for 5- to 10-day course of therapy every q2–4wk in combination therapy.
Intrathecal
Adults, Elderly, Children. 5–7.5 mg/m^2 every 2–7 days.
▸ **To Maintain Remission in Acute Lymphocytic Leukemia, Acute and Chronic Myelocytic Leukemia, Meningeal Leukemia, or Non-Hodgkin's Lymphoma in Children**
IV
Adults, Elderly, Children. 70–200 mg/m^2/day for 2–5 days every month.
IM, Subcutaneous
Adults, Elderly, Children. 1–1.5 mg/m^2 as single dose q1–4wk.
Intrathecal
Adults, Elderly, Children. 5–7.5 mg/m^2 every 2–7 days.

SIDE EFFECTS/ADVERSE REACTIONS
Frequent
IV, Subcutaneous: Asthenia, fever, pain, altered taste and smell, nausea,

C

vomiting (risk greater with IV push than with continuous IV infusion)
Intrathecal: Headache, asthenia, altered taste and smell, confusion, somnolence, nausea, vomiting
Occasional
IV, Subcutaneous: Abnormal gait, somnolence, constipation, back pain, urinary incontinence, peripheral edema, headache, confusion
Intrathecal: Peripheral edema, back pain, constipation, abnormal gait, urinary incontinence

PRECAUTIONS AND CONTRAINDICATIONS
None known

DRUG INTERACTIONS OF CONCERN TO DENTISTRY
• Increased risk of bleeding: drugs that interfere with coagulation or platelet function, such as NSAIDs and aspirin
• Increased risk of infection; glucocorticoids

SERIOUS REACTIONS
! Myelosuppression may result in blood dyscrasias, such as leukopenia, anemia, thrombocytopenia, megaloblastosis, and reticulocytopenia, after a single IV dose.
! Leukopenia, anemia, and thrombocytopenia should be expected with daily or continuous IV therapy.
! Cytarabine syndrome, (as evidenced by fever, myalgia, rash, conjunctivitis, malaise, and chest pain) and hyperuricemia may occur.
! High-dose cytarabine therapy may produce severe CNS, GI, and pulmonary toxicity.

DENTAL CONSIDERATIONS

General:
• Determine why patient is taking the drug.
• If additional analgesia is required for dental pain, consider alternative analgesics (acetaminophen) in patients taking narcotics for acute or chronic pain.
• Avoid prescribing aspirin-containing products.
• This drug may be used in the hospital or on an outpatient basis. Confirm the patient's disease and treatment status.
• Patient on chronic drug therapy may rarely present with symptoms of blood dyscrasias, which can include infection, bleeding, and poor healing. If dyscrasia is present, caution patient to prevent oral tissue trauma when using oral hygiene aids.
• Short appointments and a stress-reduction protocol may be required for anxious patients.
• Patients may have received other chemotherapy or radiation; confirm medical and drug history.
• Patients may be at risk of infection.
• Patients may be taking a prophylactic antiinfective.
• Patients are at risk of bleeding, so check for oral signs.
• Oral infections should be eliminated and/or treated aggressively.
Consultations:
• Medical consultation should include routine blood counts including platelet counts and bleeding time.
• Consult physician; prophylactic or therapeutic antiinfectives may be indicated if surgery or periodontal treatment is required.

• Medical consultation may be required to assess immunologic status during cancer chemotherapy and determine safety risk, if any, posed by the required dental treatment.

• Medical consultation may be required to assess disease control and patient's ability to tolerate stress.

Teach Patient/Family to:

• Encourage effective oral hygiene to prevent soft tissue inflammation.

• Report oral lesions, soreness, or bleeding to dentist.

• Prevent trauma when using oral hygiene aids.

• Update health and medication history if physician makes any changes in evaluation or drug regimens; include OTC, herbal, and nonherbal remedies in the update.

D

daclizumab
day-**cly'**-zu-mab
(Zenapax)

CATEGORY AND SCHEDULE
Pregnancy Risk Category: C

Drug Class: Immunosuppressive,
IgG1 monoclonal antibody

MECHANISM OF ACTION
A monoclonal antibody that binds to
the interleukin-2 (IL-2) receptor
complex, inhibiting the IL-2-
mediated activation of T
lymphocytes, a critical pathway in
the cellular immune response
involved in allograft rejection.
Therapeutic Effect: Prevents organ
rejection.

USES
Prophylaxis of acute organ rejection
in patients with renal transplants;
used in combination with
cyclosporine and glucocorticoids.

PHARMACOKINETICS
Half-life: Adults, 20 days.

INDICATIONS AND DOSAGES
▸ **Prevention of Acute Renal
Transplant Rejection (in combination
with an immunosuppressive)**
IV
Adults, Children. 1 mg/kg over
15 min q14 days for 5 doses,
beginning no more than 24 hr before
transplantation. Maximum: 100 mg.

SIDE EFFECTS/ADVERSE
REACTIONS
Occasional
Constipation, nausea, diarrhea,
vomiting, abdominal pain, edema,
headache, dizziness, fever, pain,
fatigue, insomnia, weakness,
arthralgia, myalgia, diaphoresis

PRECAUTIONS AND
CONTRAINDICATIONS
Caution:
Risk of lymphoproliferative disease
and opportunistic infections,
anaphylaxis risk unknown,
long-term effects unknown,
lactation, children, geriatric patients

DRUG INTERACTIONS OF
CONCERN TO DENTISTRY
• None reported

SERIOUS REACTIONS
❗ Hypersensitivity reaction, which
occurs rarely, is characterized by
dyspnea, tachycardia, dysphagia,
peripheral edema, rash, and pruritus.

DENTAL CONSIDERATIONS

General:
• This is a hospital-type drug, but
because some dosing is continued,
patients may appear in the dental
office while receiving this drug.
• Transplant patients may also be
taking cyclosporine and
glucocorticoids; review each
transplant patient's medications.
• Short appointments and a stress
reduction protocol may be required
for anxious patients.
Consultations:
• Antibiotic prophylaxis usually is
recommended in patients with organ
transplants and immunosuppression.
• Medical consultation may be
required to assess disease control
and patient's ability to tolerate
stress.
Teach Patient/Family to:
• Encourage effective oral hygiene
to prevent soft tissue inflammation.
• Prevent trauma when using oral
hygiene aids.
• Update health and drug history if
physician makes any changes in
evaluation or drug regimens.

dalfampridine
dal-**fam**-pri-deen
(Ampyra)

CATEGORY AND SCHEDULE
Pregnancy Risk Category: C

Drug Class: Potassium channel blocker

MECHANISM OF ACTION
A potassium channel blocker that increases conduction of action potentials in demyelinated axons. *Therapeutic Effect:* Improved walking speed.

USES
Multiple sclerosis

PHARMACOKINETICS
Rapidly and completely absorbed after PO administration. Unbound to plasma proteins. Well distributed in saliva. Minimally metabolized in liver. Primarily excreted unchanged (90%) in urine. CYP2E1 is the major isoenzyme responsible for the 3-hydroxylation of dalfampridine. *Half-life:* 5.2–6.5 hr.

INDICATIONS AND DOSAGES
▸ **Multiple Sclerosis**
PO
Adults. 10 mg twice a day, 12 hr apart. Max: 20 mg/day.

SIDE EFFECTS/ADVERSE REACTIONS
Frequent
Nausea, vomiting, urinary tract infection
Occasional
Abdominal pain, abnormal gait, backache, asthenia, dizziness, headache, insomnia, anxiety

Rare
Constipation, indigestion, multiple sclerosis relapse, paresthesia, seizure, nasopharyngitis, pain in throat

PRECAUTIONS AND CONTRAINDICATIONS
Hypersensitivity to dalfampridine or its components
Renal impairment, moderate or severe (CrCl ≤ 50 mL/min)
History of seizures
Caution:
Concomitant use with 4-aminopyridine derivatives
Mild renal impairment

DRUG INTERACTIONS OF CONCERN TO DENTISTRY
• None reported

SERIOUS REACTIONS
! Seizures have been observed and appear to be dose related.

DENTAL CONSIDERATIONS

General:
• Consider semisupine chair position for patient comfort if GI side effects occur.
Consultations:
• Medical consultation may be required to assess disease control.
Teach Patient/Family to:
• Encourage effective oral hygiene to prevent soft tissue inflammation.
• Prevent trauma when using oral hygiene aids.
• Be alert for the possibility of secondary oral infection and the need to see dentist immediately if signs of infection occur.

D

D

dalteparin sodium
doll′-teh-pare-in so′-dee-um
(Fragmin)

CATEGORY AND SCHEDULE
Pregnancy Risk Category: B

Drug Class: Heparin-type
anticoagulant

MECHANISM OF ACTION
An antithrombin that inhibits factor
Xa and thrombin in the presence of
low-molecular-weight heparin. Only
slightly influences platelet
aggregation, PT, and aPTT.
Therapeutic Effect: Produces
anticoagulation.

USES
Prevention of deep vein thrombosis
(DVT) following abdominal surgery,
treatment of life-threatening
conditions such as unstable angina,
non–Q-wave MI; prevention of
ischemia complications caused by
blood clot formation in patients on
aspirin therapy; in combination with
warfarin in deep vein thrombosis
with or without pulmonary
embolism (PE)

PHARMACOKINETICS

Route	Onset	Peak	Duration
Subcutaneous	N/A	4 hr	N/A

Protein binding: less than 10%.
Half-life: 3–5 hr.

INDICATIONS AND DOSAGES
▸ **Low- to Moderate-Risk Abdominal
Surgery**
Subcutaneous
Adults, Elderly. 2500 international
units 1–2 hr before surgery, then
daily for 5–10 days.

▸ **High-Risk Abdominal Surgery**
Subcutaneous
Adults, Elderly. 5000 international
units 1–2 hr before surgery, then
daily for 5–10 days.
▸ **Total Hip Surgery**
Subcutaneous
Adults, Elderly. 2500 international
units 1–2 hr before surgery, then
2500 units 6 hr after surgery, then
5000 units/day for 7–10 days.
▸ **Unstable Angina, Non–Q-Wave MI**
Subcutaneous
Adults, Elderly. 120 international
units/kg q12h (maximum: 10,000
international units/dose) given with
aspirin until clinically stable.
▸ **Prevention of DVT or PE in the
Acutely Ill Patient**
Subcutaneous
Adults, Elderly. 5000 international
units once a day.

SIDE EFFECTS/ADVERSE
REACTIONS
Occasional
Hematoma at injection site
Rare
Hypersensitivity reaction (chills,
fever, pruritus, urticaria, asthma,
rhinitis, lacrimation, headache);
mild, local skin irritation

PRECAUTIONS AND
CONTRAINDICATIONS
Active major bleeding; concurrent
heparin therapy; hypersensitivity to
dalteparin, heparin, or pork
products; thrombocytopenia
associated with positive in vitro test
for antiplatelet antibody
Caution:
Hemorrhage, cannot be used
interchangeably with other forms of
heparin, lactation, children, requires
monitoring, GI bleeding

DRUG INTERACTIONS OF CONCERN TO DENTISTRY
• Avoid concurrent use of aspirin (except as noted), NSAIDs, dipyridamole, and sulfinpyrazone.

SERIOUS REACTIONS
! Overdose may lead to bleeding complications ranging from local ecchymoses to major hemorrhage.
! Thrombocytopenia occurs rarely.

DENTAL CONSIDERATIONS
General:
• Product may be used in outpatient therapy. Delay elective dental treatment until patient completes anticoagulant therapy.
• Determine why patient is taking the drug.
• Consider local hemostasis measures to prevent excessive bleeding.
• Avoid prescribing aspirin-containing products.
Consultations:
• Medical consultation should include routine blood counts, including platelet counts and bleeding time.
Teach Patient/Family to:
• Encourage effective oral hygiene to prevent soft tissue inflammation.
• Prevent trauma when using oral hygiene aids.
• Report oral lesions, soreness, or bleeding to dentist.

danaparoid
da-**nah′**-pah-roid
(Organ k)

CATEGORY AND SCHEDULE
Pregnancy Risk Category: B

Drug Class: Heparinoid-type anticoagulant

MECHANISM OF ACTION
An antithrombotic agent that inhibits thrombin formation through factor antiXa and antiIIa effects. Does not significantly influence bleeding time, PT, aPTT, or platelet function. Possesses greater antithrombotic activity than anticoagulant activity.

USES
Prevention of deep vein thrombosis (DVT) following hip or knee replacement surgery; unapproved: thromboembolism, hemodialysis, and cardiovascular surgery

PHARMACOKINETICS
Well absorbed following subcutaneous administration. Eliminated primarily in the urine. **Half-life:** 24 hr (half-life prolonged with severe renal impairment).

INDICATIONS AND DOSAGES
Note: Give initial dose as soon as possible after surgery but not more than 24 hr after surgery.
▸ **Prevention of DVT**
Subcutaneous
Adults, Elderly. 750 anti-Xa units twice daily beginning 1–4 hr preoperatively and then not sooner than 2 hr after surgery. Continue treatment throughout postoperative care until risk of DVT has diminished (average duration 7–14 days).

SIDE EFFECTS/ADVERSE REACTIONS
Frequent
Injection site pain
Occasional
Fever, pain, nausea, UTI, constipation
Rare
Rash, pruritus, infection

D

PRECAUTIONS AND CONTRAINDICATIONS

Severe hemorrhagic diathesis (hemophilia, idiopathic thrombocytopenic purpura), active major bleeding state, including hemorrhagic stroke in the acute phase, type II phase thrombocytopenia associated with positive in vitro test for antiplatelet antibody in presence of danaparoid, hypersensitivity to pork products, danaparoid, or any component of the formulation

Caution:

Cannot interchange with heparin, hemorrhage, thrombocytopenia, renal or hepatic impairment, lactation, children, antidotes not available, GI bleeding

DRUG INTERACTIONS OF CONCERN TO DENTISTRY

• Avoid concurrent use of platelet aggregation antagonist, such as aspirin; NSAIDs; dipyridamole.

SERIOUS REACTIONS

! Accidental overdosage may lead to bleeding complications ranging from minor ecchymosis to major hemorrhage. An unexplained fall in HCT or fall in B/P should lead to consideration of a hemorrhagic event. The antidote protamine sulfate only partially neutralizes danaparoid activity and is incapable of reducing severe nonsurgical bleeding during treatment. If serious bleeding occurs, discontinue danaparoid; give blood or blood product transfusions.

DENTAL CONSIDERATIONS

General:

• Determine why patient is taking the drug.

• Consider local hemostasis measures to prevent excessive bleeding if dental treatment must be performed.

• Antibiotic prophylaxis before dental treatment may be required for joint prosthesis (see section on "Medically Compromised Patients").

• Delay elective dental treatment until patient completes danaparoid therapy.

Consultations:

• Medical consultation should include routine blood counts, including platelet counts and bleeding time.

Teach Patient/Family to:

• Encourage effective oral hygiene to prevent soft tissue inflammation.

• Use caution to prevent trauma when using oral hygiene aids.

• Report oral lesions, soreness, or bleeding to dentist.

danazol
da′-na-zole
(Cyclomen[CAN], Danocrine)

CATEGORY AND SCHEDULE
Pregnancy Risk Category: X

Drug Class: Androgen, α-ethinyl testosterone derivative

MECHANISM OF ACTION
A testosterone derivative that suppresses the pituitary-ovarian axis by inhibiting the output of pituitary gonadotropins. Causes atrophy of both normal and ectopic endometrial tissue in endometriosis. Follicle-stimulating hormone (FSH) and luteinizing hormone (LH) are depressed in fibrocystic breast disease. Inhibits steroid synthesis and binding of steroids to their

receptors in breast tissues. Increases
serum levels of esterase inhibitor.
Therapeutic Effect: Produces
anovulation and amenorrhea,
reduces the production of estrogen,
corrects biochemical deficiency as
seen in hereditary angioedema.

USES
Treatment of endometriosis,
prevention of hereditary
angioedema, fibrocystic breast
disease

PHARMACOKINETICS
Well absorbed from GI tract.
Metabolized in liver, primarily to
2-hydroxymethylethisterone.
Excreted in urine. *Half-life:* 4.5 hr.

INDICATIONS AND DOSAGES
▶ **Endometriosis**
PO
Adults. 200–800 mg/day in 2 divided
doses for 3–9 mo.
▶ **Fibrocystic Breast Disease**
PO
Adults. 100–400 mg/day in 2 divided
doses.
▶ **Hereditary Angioedema**
PO
Adults. Initially, 200 mg 2–3 times a
day. Decrease dose by 50% or less
at 1–3 mo intervals. If attack occurs,
increase dose by up to 200 mg/day.

SIDE EFFECTS/ADVERSE REACTIONS
Frequent
Females: Amenorrhea, breakthrough
bleeding/spotting, decreased breast
size, increased weight, irregular
menstrual period.
Occasional
Males/females: Edema,
rhabdomyolysis (muscle cramps,
unusual fatigue), virilism (acne,
oily skin), flushed skin, altered
moods

Rare
Males/females: Hematuria,
gingivitis, carpal tunnel syndrome,
cataracts, severe headache, vomiting,
rash, photosensitivity
Females: Enlarged clitoris,
hoarseness, deepening voice, hair
growth, monilial vaginitis
Males: Decreased testicle size

PRECAUTIONS AND CONTRAINDICATIONS
Cardiac impairment, hypercalcemia,
pregnancy, prostatic or breast cancer
in males, severe liver or renal disease
Caution:
Migraine headaches, seizure
disorders

DRUG INTERACTIONS OF CONCERN TO DENTISTRY
• Increased serum concentration of
carbamazepine; consider avoiding
concurrent administration.

SERIOUS REACTIONS
! Jaundice may occur in those
receiving 400 mg/day or more. Liver
dysfunction, eosinophilia,
thrombocytopenia, pancreatitis occur
rarely.

DENTAL CONSIDERATIONS
General:
• Patients on chronic drug therapy
may rarely have symptoms of blood
dyscrasias, which can include
infection, bleeding, and poor
healing.
Consultations:
• In a patient with symptoms of
blood dyscrasias, request a medical
consultation for blood studies and
postpone dental treatment until
normal values are reestablished.
Teach Patient/Family to:
• Encourage effective oral hygiene
to prevent soft tissue inflammation.

D

• Avoid mouth rinses with high alcohol content because of drying and irritating effects.

dantrolene sodium
dan'-troe-leen so'-dee-um
(Dantrium)
Do not confuse Dantrium with Daraprim.

CATEGORY AND SCHEDULE
Pregnancy Risk Category: C

Drug Class: Skeletal muscle relaxant, direct-acting

MECHANISM OF ACTION
A skeletal muscle relaxant that reduces muscle contraction by interfering with release of calcium ion. Reduces calcium ion concentration.
Therapeutic Effect: Dissociates excitation-contraction coupling. Interferes with catabolic process associated with malignant hyperthermic crisis.

USES
Treatment of spasticity in multiple sclerosis, stroke, spinal cord injury, cerebral palsy, malignant hyperthermia

PHARMACOKINETICS
Poorly absorbed from the GI tract. Protein binding: High. Metabolized in the liver. Primarily excreted in urine. **Half-life:** IV: 4–8 hr; PO: 8.7 hr.

INDICATIONS AND DOSAGES
▶ **Spasticity**
PO
Adults, Elderly. Initially, 25 mg/day. Increase to 25 mg 2–4 times a day,
then by 25-mg increments up to 100 mg 2–4 times a day.
Children. Initially, 0.5 mg/kg twice a day. Increase to 0.5 mg/kg 3–4 times a day, then in increments of 0.5 mg/kg/day up to 3 mg/kg 2–4 times a day. Maximum: 400 mg/day.
▶ **Prevention of Malignant Hyperthermic Crisis**
PO
Adults, Elderly, Children. 4–8 mg/kg/day in 3–4 divided doses 1–2 days before surgery; give last dose 3–4 hr before surgery.
IV
Adults, Elderly, Children. 2.5 mg/kg about 1.25 hr before surgery.
▶ **Management of Malignant Hyperthermic Crisis**
IV
Adults, Elderly, Children. Initially, a minimum of 1 mg/kg rapid IV; may repeat up to total cumulative dose of 10 mg/kg. May follow with 4–8 mg/kg/day PO in 4 divided doses up to 3 days after crisis.

SIDE EFFECTS/ADVERSE REACTIONS
Frequent
Drowsiness, dizziness, weakness, general malaise, diarrhea (mild)
Occasional
Confusion, diarrhea (may be severe), headache, insomnia, constipation, urinary frequency
Rare
Paradoxical CNS excitement or restlessness, paresthesia, tinnitus, slurred speech, tremors, blurred vision, dry mouth, nocturia, impotence, rash, pruritus

PRECAUTIONS AND CONTRAINDICATIONS
Active hepatic disease
Caution:
Peptic ulcer disease, renal disease, hepatic disease, stroke, seizure

disorder, diabetes mellitus, elderly; monitor liver enzymes

DRUG INTERACTIONS OF CONCERN TO DENTISTRY
• None reported

SERIOUS REACTIONS
❗ There is a risk of liver toxicity, most notably in females, those 35 yr of age and older, and those taking other medications concurrently.
❗ Overt hepatitis noted most frequently between 3rd and 12th mo of therapy.
❗ Overdosage results in vomiting, muscular hypotonia, muscle twitching, respiratory depression, and seizures.

DENTAL CONSIDERATIONS
General:
• Monitor vital signs at every appointment because of cardiovascular and respiratory side effects.
• Patients on chronic drug therapy may rarely have symptoms of blood dyscrasias, which can include infection, bleeding, and poor healing.
• Requires proficiency in IV administration technique when used for emergency treatment of malignant hyperthermia.
Consultations:
• In a patient with symptoms of blood dyscrasias, request a medical consultation for blood studies and postpone dental treatment until normal values are reestablished.
Teach Patient/Family to:
• Encourage effective oral hygiene to prevent soft tissue inflammation.
• Avoid mouth rinses with high alcohol content because of drying effects.

dapiprazole hydrochloride
da′-pi-prah-zohl hi-droh-**klor′**-ide
(Rev-Eyes)

D

CATEGORY AND SCHEDULE
Pregnancy Risk Category: B

Drug Class: Antimydriatic

MECHANISM OF ACTION
An α-adrenergic blocker that primarily affects α-1 adrenoceptors. Does not significantly affect intraocular pressure.
Therapeutic Effect: Induces miosis via relaxation of the smooth dilator (radial) muscle of the iris, which causes papillary constriction.

USES
Reduction of pupil size after certain kinds of eye examinations

PHARMACOKINETICS
Well absorbed. Mydriasis reversal begins in 1 hr and occurs in about 6 hr.

INDICATIONS AND DOSAGES
▶ Drug-Induced Mydriasis
Ophthalmic
Adults, Elderly, Children. 2 drops applied topically to the conjunctiva of each eye. Repeat after 5 min. Do not use more than once a week.

SIDE EFFECTS/ADVERSE REACTIONS
Occasional
Burning, eyelid edema, photophobia

PRECAUTIONS AND CONTRAINDICATIONS
Acute iritis, hypersensitivity to dapiprazole or any component of the formulation

D

DRUG INTERACTIONS OF CONCERN TO DENTISTRY
- None reported

SERIOUS REACTIONS
! None reported

DENTAL CONSIDERATIONS

General:
- Used in ophthalmic examinations.
- Protect patient's eyes from accidental spatter during dental treatment.
- Avoid dental light in patient's eyes; offer dark glasses for patient comfort.

dapsone
dap′-sone
(Dapsone)

CATEGORY AND SCHEDULE
Pregnancy Risk Category: C

Drug Class: Leprostatic, antibacterial

MECHANISM OF ACTION
An antibiotic that is a competitive antagonist of para-aminobenzoic acid (PABA); it prevents normal bacterial utilization of PABA for synthesis of folic acid.
Therapeutic Effect: Inhibits bacterial growth.

USES
Treatment of leprosy (Hansen's disease); dermatitis herpetiformis; unapproved: cicatricial pemphigoid, LE, pemphigoid, malaria, *Pneumocystis carinii* pneumonia (PCP)

PHARMACOKINETICS
Rapid complete absorption; highly bound to plasma protein; metabolized in liver; excreted in urine. *Half-life:* 10–50 hr.

INDICATIONS AND DOSAGES
▶ **Leprosy**
PO
Adults, Elderly. 50–100 mg/day for 3–10 yr.
Children. 1–2 mg/kg/24 hr.
Maximum: 100 mg/day.
▶ **Dermatitis Herpetiformis**
PO
Adults, Elderly. Initially, 50 mg/day. May increase up to 300 mg/day.
▶ **PCP**
PO
Adults, Elderly. 100 mg/day in combination with trimethoprim for 21 days.
▶ **Prevention of PCP**
PO
Adults, Elderly. 100 mg/day.
Children older than 1 mo. 2 mg/kg/day. Maximum: 100 mg/day.

SIDE EFFECTS/ADVERSE REACTIONS
Frequent
Hemolytic anemia, methemoglobinemia, rash
Occasional
Hemolysis, photosensitivity reaction

PRECAUTIONS AND CONTRAINDICATIONS
Hypersensitivity to sulfones, severe anemia
Caution:
Renal disease, hepatic disease, G6PD deficiency, lactation

DRUG INTERACTIONS OF CONCERN TO DENTISTRY
- None reported

SERIOUS REACTIONS

! Agranulocytosis and blood dyscrasias may occur.

DENTAL CONSIDERATIONS

General:

• Patients on chronic drug therapy may rarely have symptoms of blood dyscrasias, which can include infection, bleeding, and poor healing.

• Avoid dental light in patient's eyes; offer dark glasses for patient comfort.

• Advise patient if dental drugs prescribed have a potential for photosensitivity.

Consultations:

• In a patient with symptoms of blood dyscrasias, request a medical consultation for blood studies and postpone dental treatment until normal values are reestablished.

Teach Patient/Family to:

• Encourage effective oral hygiene to prevent soft tissue inflammation.

• Use caution to prevent injury when using oral hygiene aids.

---

daptomycin
dap'-toe-my-sin
(Cubicin)

CATEGORY AND SCHEDULE

Pregnancy Risk Category: B

Drug Class: Antiinfective (polypeptide)

MECHANISM OF ACTION

A lipopeptide antibacterial agent that binds to bacterial membranes and causes a rapid depolarization of the membrane potential. The loss of membrane potential leads to inhibition of protein, DNA, and RNA synthesis.
Therapeutic Effect: Bactericidal.

USES

Treatment of complicated skin and skin-structure infections caused by susceptible strains of *S. aureus* (including methicillin-resistant *S. aureus*), *S. pyogenes, S. agalactiae, S. dysgalactiae, E. coli,* and *E. faecalis* (vancomycin-susceptible strains only)

PHARMACOKINETICS

Widely distributed. Protein binding: 90%. Primarily excreted unchanged in urine. Moderately removed by hemodialysis. *Half-life:* 7–8 hr (increased in impaired renal function).

INDICATIONS AND DOSAGES
▸ **Complicated Skin and Skin-Structure Infections**
IV

Adults, Elderly. 4 mg/kg every 24 hr for 7–14 days.
▸ **Dosage in Renal Impairment**
For patients with creatinine clearance of less than 30 ml/min, dosage is 4 mg/kg q48h for 7–14 days.

SIDE EFFECTS/ADVERSE REACTIONS

Frequent

Constipation, nausea, peripheral injection site reactions, headache, diarrhea

Occasional

Insomnia, rash, vomiting

Rare

Pruritus, dizziness, hypotension

PRECAUTIONS AND CONTRAINDICATIONS

Hypersensitivity

Caution:

Reduce dose in renal impairment, risk of superinfection, monitor for

D

muscle weakness, pain, and CPK levels, lactation, elderly, safety and efficacy in children younger than 18 yr not established

DRUG INTERACTIONS OF CONCERN TO DENTISTRY

• None reported

SERIOUS REACTIONS

! Skeletal muscle myopathy, characterized by muscle pain and weakness, particularly of the distal extremities, occurs rarely.
! Antibiotic-associated colitis and other superinfections may result from altered bacterial balance.

DENTAL CONSIDERATIONS

General:
• Used in the hospital environment for serious infections.
• Determine why patient is taking the drug.
• Monitor vital signs, including temperature, B/P, and respiration characteristics and rate, at every appointment.
Consultations:
• Consult with patient's physician if an acute dental infection occurs and another antiinfective is required.

darbepoetin alfa
dar-beh-**poe**′-ee-tin **al**′-fah
(Aranesp)
Do not confuse Aranesp with Aricept.

CATEGORY AND SCHEDULE
Pregnancy Risk Category: C

Drug Class: Hematopoietic agent

MECHANISM OF ACTION

A glycoprotein that stimulates formation of RBCs in bone marrow; increases serum half-life of epoetin. ***Therapeutic Effect:*** Induces erythropoiesis and release of reticulocytes from bone marrow.

USES

An erythropoiesis-stimulating protein; stimulates the division and differentiation of erythroid progenitors in bone marrow

PHARMACOKINETICS

Well absorbed after subcutaneous administration. *Half-life:* 48.5 hr.

INDICATIONS AND DOSAGES
▸ **Anemia in Chronic Renal Failure**
IV Bolus, Subcutaneous
Adults, Elderly. Initially, 0.45 mcg/kg once a wk. Adjust dosage to achieve and maintain a target Hgb not to exceed 12 g/dl. Do not increase dosage more frequently than once a mo. Limit increases in Hgb by less than 1 g/dl over any 2-wk period.
▸ **Anemia Associated with Chemotherapy**
IV, Subcutaneous
Adults, Elderly. 2.25 mcg/kg/dose once a wk.

SIDE EFFECTS/ADVERSE REACTIONS

Frequent
Myalgia, hypertension or hypotension, headache, diarrhea
Occasional
Fatigue, edema, vomiting, reaction at administration site, asthenia, dizziness

PRECAUTIONS AND CONTRAINDICATIONS

History of sensitivity to mammalian cell-derived products or human albumin, uncontrolled hypertension

Caution:
Increased risk of serious
cardiovascular events, seizures in
CRF, albumin formula has risk of
viral diseases, safety in lactation or
pediatric patients has not been
established

DRUG INTERACTIONS OF CONCERN TO DENTISTRY
• No studies reported

SERIOUS REACTIONS
! Vascular access thrombosis, CHF,
sepsis, arrhythmias, and anaphylactic
reaction occur rarely.

DENTAL CONSIDERATIONS

General:
• Monitor vital signs at every
appointment because of
cardiovascular side effects.
• Consider semisupine chair position
for patient comfort if GI side effects
occur.
• Monitor disease control and date
of last dialysis.
• Prophylactic antibiotics
may be indicated to prevent
infection if invasive procedure is
planned.
Consultations:
• Medical consultation may be
required to assess disease control
and patient's ability to tolerate
stress.
Teach Patient/Family to:
• Encourage effective oral hygiene
to prevent soft tissue inflammation,
infection.
• Update health and drug
history if physician makes any
changes in evaluation or drug
regimens.

darunavir
dar-oo'-na-veer
(Prezista)

CATEGORY AND SCHEDULE
Pregnancy Risk Category: B

Drug Class: Antiretroviral agent,
protease inhibitor

MECHANISM OF ACTION
An antiretroviral agent that inhibits
HIV-1 protease. Prevents the
cleavage of HIV encoded Gag-Pol
polyproteins in infected cells.
Therapeutic Effect: Impedes HIV
replication, slowing the progression
of HIV infection.

USES
Treatment of HIV infection

PHARMACOKENETICS
Absorption increased 30% with food.
Protein binding: 95%. Extensively
metabolized in liver, primarily by
CYP450 3A4. Primarily eliminated
in feces (about 80%, 41%
unchanged); partial excretion in
urine (approximately 14%, 8%
unchanged). *Half-life:* 15 hr.

INDICATIONS AND DOSAGES
▶ **HIV Infection (in combination with ritonavir)**
PO
Adults. 600 mg twice a day taken
with ritonavir 100 mg twice a day
with food. Safety and efficacy have
not been established in children.

SIDE EFFECTS/ADVERSE REACTIONS
Frequent
Hypertriglyceridemia, diarrhea,
nausea, increased amylase level,
headache, nasopharyngitis

Occasional
Hypercholesterolemia, rash,
hypoglycemia, hypocalcemia,
thrombocytopenia, hyponatremia,
vomiting, abdominal pain
Rare
Constipation, anxiety, acute renal
failure, fat redistribution,
confusional state, disorientation,
irritability, altered mood, nightmares,
dyspnea, cough, hiccups, night
sweats, diabetes mellitus, Stevens-
Johnson syndrome

PRECAUTIONS AND CONTRAINDICATIONS
• Hypersensitivity to darunavir or its
components
• Sulfa allergy, diabetes mellitus
• Multiple drug interactions

DRUG INTERACTIONS OF CONCERN TO DENTISTRY
• Anticonvulsants: may decrease
concentrations of darunavir
• Antihistamines: increased risk of
arrhythmias
• Benzodiazepines: may cause
increased sedation or respiratory
depression
• Clarithromycin: may increase
concentrations of clarithromycin
• Corticosteroids: may increase
levels and effects of these drugs
• CYP3A4 inducers: may
decrease levels and effects of
darunavir
• CYP3A4 substrates: may increase
levels and effects of CYP3A4
substrates
• Estrogens, oral contraceptives:
may decrease concentrations of
these drugs; may reduce
contraceptive effectiveness
• Immunosuppressants: may increase
concentrations of these drugs
• Ketoconazole: may increase levels
and effects of darunavir and
ketoconazole

• Methadone: may decrease
concentrations of methadone
• Neuroleptic agents: increased risk
of arrhythmias
• Rifampin: may decrease
concentrations of darunavir
• Sedatives/hypnotics: increased
sedation and risk of respiratory
depression
• SSRIs: may decrease the levels
and effects of SSRIs
• St. John's wort: may decrease the
levels of darunavir
• Trazodone: may increase
concentrations of trazodone

SERIOUS REACTIONS
! Protease inhibitors have been
associated with severe dermatologic
reactions, including Stevens-Johnson
syndrome.

DENTAL CONSIDERATIONS

General:
• Monitor vital signs at every
appointment because of
cardiovascular side effects.
• Examine for oral manifestation of
opportunistic infection.
• Place on frequent recall to evaluate
healing response.
• Assess salivary flow as a factor in
caries, periodontal disease, and
candidiasis.
• Consider semisupine chair position
for patient comfort because of GI
effects of drug.
Consultations:
• Medical consultation may be
required to assess disease control.
Teach Patient/Family to:
• Encourage effective oral
hygiene to prevent soft tissue
inflammation.
• See dentist immediately if
secondary oral infection occurs.
• When chronic dry mouth occurs,
advise patient to:

• Avoid mouth rinses with high alcohol content because of drying effects.
• Use daily home fluoride products for anticaries effect.
• Use sugarless gum, frequent sips of water, or saliva substitutes.

dasatinib
da-sa′-ti-nib
(Sprycel)

CATEGORY AND SCHEDULE
Pregnancy Risk Category: D

Drug Class: Antineoplastic

MECHANISM OF ACTION
Inhibits BCR-ABL tyrosine kinase, an enzyme created by the Philadelphia chromosome abnormality found in patients with chronic myeloid leukemia (CML). Also inhibits SRC family kinases.
Therapeutic Effect: Suppresses tumor growth during the three stages of CML: blast crisis, accelerated phase, and chronic phase.

USES
Treatment in CML-blast crisis, accelerated phase, and chronic phase-resistant or intolerant to prior therapy. Also used in treatment of Philadelphia chromosome-positive acute lymphoblastic leukemia (ALL) with resistance or intolerance to prior therapy.

PHARMACOKENETICS
Protein binding: 96%. Metabolized in liver, primarily by CYP450 3A4. Primarily eliminated in feces (85%, 19% as unchanged); minimal excretion in urine (4%, 0.1% unchanged). *Half-life:* 3–5 hr.

INDICATIONS AND DOSAGES
▶ ALL, Philadelphia Chromosome-Positive, Resistant or Intolerant to Prior Therapy
PO
Adults. 70 mg twice a day (morning and evening), with or without food.
▶ CML, Blast Crisis
Adults. 70 mg twice a day (morning and evening), with or without food.
▶ CML, Accelerated Phase
Adults. 70 mg twice a day (morning and evening), with or without food.
▶ CML, Chronic Phase
Adults. 70 mg twice a day (morning and evening), with or without food.
Safety and efficacy have not been established in children.

SIDE EFFECTS/ADVERSE REACTIONS (ADULT)
Frequent
Neutropenia, thrombocytopenia, diarrhea, headache, musculoskeletal pain, fatigue, fever, superficial edema, rash, nausea, dyspnea, upper respiratory infection, abdominal pain, pleural effusion, vomiting, arthralgia, asthenia, loss of appetite, inflammatory disease of mucous membrane, GI hemorrhage, constipation, weight loss, dizziness, chest pain, neuropathy, myalgia, weight increased, cardiac dysrhythmia, pruritus, pneumonia, swollen abdomen, pneumonia, shivering
Occasional
Febrile neutropenia, CHF, pericardial effusion, pulmonary edema, prolonged QT interval, anemia
Rare
Pulmonary hypertension, CNS hemorrhage, ascites

D

PRECAUTIONS AND CONTRAINDICATIONS

Hypersensitivity to dasatinib or its components, hypokalemia, hypomagnesemia, use with antiarrhythmic medication, patients at risk for fluid retention

DRUG INTERACTIONS OF CONCERN TO DENTISTRY

• NSAIDs: increased risk of bleeding
• CYP3A4 inhibitors (e.g., clarithromycin, erythromycin, azole antifungals): may increase the levels and adverse effects of dasatinib
• CYP3A4 substrates (midazolam, triazolam): increased plasma concentrations of these drugs with increased CNS depression
• Vasoconstrictors: may increase the risk of potentially fatal arrhythmias

SERIOUS REACTIONS

! Severe CNS hemorrhage, including fatalities, have been reported.
! Dasatinib may cause severe bone marrow suppression (thrombocytopenia, neutropenia, anemia).
! Fluid retention, including pleural and pericardial effusion, severe ascites, and generalized edema, has been reported.

DENTAL CONSIDERATIONS

General:
• Monitor vital signs at every appointment because of cardiovascular adverse effects.
• Determine why patient is taking drug.
• Avoid aspirin and NSAIDs.
• Consider semisupine chair position for patients with GI or respiratory adverse effects.

• Consider blood dyscrasias as factors in infection, bleeding, and poor healing.
• If blood dyscrasia present, caution patient to prevent oral tissue trauma when using oral hygiene aids.
• Examine for oral manifestations of opportunistic infection.
• Consider local hemostatic measures to prevent excessive bleeding.
• Use caution with potentially hepatotoxic drugs (e.g., telithromycin).
Consultations:
• Consult physician to determine disease control and ability of patient to tolerate dental procedures.
• Medical consultation should include routine blood counts, including platelets and bleeding time, and postpone dental therapy until values are in acceptable range.
• Consult physician to determine possible need for prophylactic antibiotics.
Teach Patient/Family to:
• Use effective, atraumatic oral hygiene to prevent soft-tissue inflammation.
• Update health and medication history if physician makes any changes in evaluation or drug regimen; include over-the-counter, herbal products, and dietary supplements.
• Report oral lesions, soreness, or bleeding to dentist.

daunorubicin citrate liposome
dawn-oh-**rue**′-bih-sin
(DaunoXome)
Do not confuse with dactinomycin or doxorubicin.

CATEGORY AND SCHEDULE
Pregnancy Risk Category: D

Drug Class: Anthracycline antibiotic; antineoplastic

MECHANISM OF ACTION
An anthracycline antibiotic that is cell cycle-phase nonspecific. Most active in S phase of cell division. Appears to bind to DNA. *Therapeutic Effect:* Inhibits DNA, DNA-dependent RNA synthesis.

USES
Treatment of advanced AIDS-associated Kaposi's sarcoma (KS), a kind of skin cancer

PHARMACOKINETICS
Widely distributed. Does not cross blood-brain barrier. Protein binding: High. Metabolized in liver to active metabolite. Excreted in urine, eliminated by biliary excretion. *Half-life:* 18.5 hr; metabolite: 26.7 hr.

INDICATIONS AND DOSAGES
▸ KS
IV
Adults. 20–40 mg/m² over 1 hr. Repeat q2wk or 100 mg/m² q3wk.

SIDE EFFECTS/ADVERSE REACTIONS
Frequent
Mild to moderate nausea, fatigue, fever
Occasional
Diarrhea, abdominal pain, esophagitis, stomatitis (redness or burning of oral mucous membranes, inflammation of gums or tongue), transverse pigmentation of fingernails and toenails
Rare
Transient fever, chills

PRECAUTIONS AND CONTRAINDICATIONS
Arrhythmias, CHF, left ventricular ejection fraction less than 40%, preexisting bone marrow suppression

DRUG INTERACTIONS OF CONCERN TO DENTISTRY
• Dental drug interactions have not been studied.

SERIOUS REACTIONS
! Bone marrow depression manifested as hematologic toxicity (severe leukopenia, anemia, and thrombocytopenia) may occur.
! Decreases in platelet and white blood cell (WBC) counts occur in 10–14 days and return to normal levels by the third wk of daunorubicin treatment.
! Cardiotoxicity noted as either acute with transient abnormal ECG findings or as chronic with cardiomyopathy manifested as CHF. The risk of cardiotoxicity increases when the cumulative dose exceeds 550 mg/m² in adults and 300 mg/m² in children older than 2 yr or when the total dosage is greater than 10 mg/kg in children younger than 2 yr.

DENTAL CONSIDERATIONS
General:
• Determine why patient is taking the drug.
• Assess salivary flow as a factor in caries, periodontal disease, and candidiasis.
• Administered in the hospital; AIDS patients will be taking many other medications; confirm medical and drug history.
Consultations:
• In a patient with symptoms of blood dyscrasias, request a medical

D

consultation for blood studies and postpone treatment until normal values are reestablished.

• Medical consultation may be required to assess disease control and patient's ability to tolerate stress.

Teach Patient/Family to:

• Encourage effective oral hygiene to prevent soft tissue inflammation.

• Prevent trauma when using oral hygiene aids.

• Report oral lesions, soreness, or bleeding to dentist.

• When chronic dry mouth occurs, advise patient to:

• Avoid mouth rinses with high alcohol content because of drying effects.

• Use daily home fluoride products for anticaries effect.

• Use sugarless gum, frequent sips of water, or saliva substitutes.

• Update health and medication history if physician makes any changes in evaluation or drug regimens; include OTC, herbal, and nonherbal remedies in the update.

decitabine
de-**sye**′-ta-been
(Dacogen)

CATEGORY AND SCHEDULE
Pregnancy Risk Category: D

Drug Class: Antineoplastic

MECHANISM OF ACTION
A pyrimidine antimetabolite that is incorporated into DNA and inhibits DNA methyltransferase causing hypomethylation and subsequent cell death.

Therapeutic Effect: Restores normal function to tumor-suppressor genes regulating cellular differentiation and proliferation.

USES
Treatment of myelodysplastic syndrome (MDS)

PHARMACOKINETICS
No information is available regarding the pharmacokinetics of decitabine.

INDICATIONS AND DOSAGES
▸ MDS
IV
Adults. 15 mg/m² over 3 hr, repeat every 8 hr for 3 days; repeat cycle every 6 wk for a minimum of 4 cycles.

SIDE EFFECTS/ADVERSE REACTIONS
Frequent

Neutropenia, thrombocytopenia, anemia, fever, nausea, cough, petechiae, constipation, diarrhea, hyperglycemia, headache, febrile neutropenia, leukopenia, insomnia, peripheral edema, hypomagnesemia, hypoalbuminemia, vomiting, pallor, bruising, hypokalemia, rigors, pneumonia, arthralgia, rash, limb pain, edema, dizziness, back pain, cardiac murmur, anorexia, pharyngitis, appetite decreased, abdominal pain, lung crackles, hyperbilirubinemia, erythema, pain, hyperkalemia, hyponatremia, oral mucosal lymphadenopathy, confusion, lethargy, cellulitis, stomatitis, dyspepsia, anxiety, hypoesthesia, lesions, pruritus, alkaline phosphatase increased, tenderness

Occasional

Candidal infection, ascites, AST increased, breath sounds diminished, hyperuricemia, hypoxia, rales, LDH increased, hemorrhoids, alopecia, catheter infection, gingival bleeding, chest discomfort, UTI, chest wall pain, loose stools, staphylococcal infection, transfusion reaction, tongue ulceration, dysphagia, oral candidiasis, dysuria, facial swelling, hypotension, musculoskeletal discomfort, blurred vision, bicarbonate increased, dehydration, hypochloremia, pulmonary edema, urticaria, malaise, hematoma, thrombocythemia, bacteremia, polyuria, hypobilirubinemia, site erythema, catheter site pain, injection site swelling, lip ulceration, abdominal distension, bicarbonate decreased, hypoproteinemia, crepitation, myalgia, gastroesophageal reflux, glossodynia, postnasal drip, sinusitis

Rare

Anaphylactic reaction, atrial fibrillation, cardiomyopathy, CHF, cholecystitis, dyspnea, fungal infection, hemorrhage, gingival pain, mental status change, mucosal inflammation, mycobacterium avium complex infection, peridiverticular abscess, pseudomonal lung infection, pulmonary embolism, renal failure, respiratory arrest, respiratory tract infection, sepsis, splenomegaly, supraventricular tachycardia, weakness

PRECAUTIONS AND CONTRAINDICATIONS

Hypersensitivity to decitabine or its components; do not breast-feed, bone marrow depression, renal or hepatic impairment

DRUG INTERACTIONS OF CONCERN TO DENTISTRY

• None reported

SERIOUS REACTIONS

! Neutropenia and thrombocytopenia are expected to occur.

DENTAL CONSIDERATIONS

General:
• Monitor vital signs at every appointment because of cardiovascular side effects.
• Avoid aspirin and NSAIDs.
• Consider immunosuppression as a factor in oral opportunistic infections.
• Consider semisupine chair position if GI or respiratory adverse effects occur.
• Chlorhexidine mouth rinse before and during chemotherapy may reduce severity of mucositis.
• Consider blood dyscrasias as a factor in infection, bleeding, and delayed healing.
• Palliative medication may be required of oral adverse effects.
• Assess salivary flow as a factor in caries, periodontal disease, and candidiasis.
• Obtain CBCs, including platelets and bleeding time, prior to initiating invasive dental procedures and postpone dental treatment as needed.

Consultations:
• Consult physician to determine why patient is taking drug.
• Consult physician to determine disease control and ability of patient to tolerate dental procedures.
• Consult physician(s) to determine if prophylactic antibiotics are required prior to dental procedures.

Teach Patient/Family to:
• Use effective atraumatic oral hygiene measures to prevent soft tissue inflammation.
• Report oral lesions, soreness, or bleeding to dentist.
• Update health history when physician changes drug regimen

and/or report use of over-the-counter medications, herbal products, and dietary supplements.
• When chronic dry mouth occurs, advise patient to:
  • Avoid mouth rinses with high alcohol content because of drying effect.
  • Use daily home fluoride products for anticaries effects.
  • Use sugarless gum, frequent sips of water, or artificial saliva substitutes.

delavirdine mesylate
deh-la′-ver-deen **mess′**-ah-late
(Rescriptor)
Do not confuse Rescriptor with Retrovir or Ritonavir.

CATEGORY AND SCHEDULE
Pregnancy Risk Category: C

Drug Class: Antiviral, nonnucleoside

MECHANISM OF ACTION
A nonnucleoside reverse transcriptase inhibitor that binds directly to HIV-1 reverse transcriptase and blocks RNA- and DNA-dependent DNA polymerase activities.
Therapeutic Effect: Interrupts HIV replication, slowing the progression of HIV infection.

USES
Treatment of HIV infection in combination with appropriate antiretroviral agents when therapy is warranted

PHARMACOKINETICS
Rapidly absorbed after PO administration. Protein binding:

98%. Primarily distributed in plasma. Metabolized in the liver. Eliminated in feces and urine.
Half-life: 2–11 hr.

INDICATIONS AND DOSAGES
▶ **HIV Infection (in combination with other antiretrovirals)**
PO
Adults. 400 mg 3 times a day.

SIDE EFFECTS/ADVERSE REACTIONS
Frequent
Rash, pruritus
Occasional
Headache, nausea, diarrhea, fatigue, anorexia

PRECAUTIONS AND CONTRAINDICATIONS
Hypersensitivity
Caution:
Modify dose in liver disease; children younger than 16 yr, lactation; rapid development of viral resistance if used as a single drug

DRUG INTERACTIONS OF CONCERN TO DENTISTRY
• Reduced absorption: antacids, cimetidine, other H₂-receptor antagonists
• Increased plasma levels of both delavirdine and clarithromycin
• Increased plasma levels of alprazolam, triazolam, midazolam
• Avoid coadministration with carbamazepine, phenobarbital, ketoconazole, fluoxetine

SERIOUS REACTIONS
! None known

DENTAL CONSIDERATIONS
General:
• Examine for oral manifestation of opportunistic infection.

• Patients on chronic drug therapy may rarely have symptoms of blood dyscrasias, which can include infection, bleeding, and poor healing.
• Assess salivary flow as a factor in caries, periodontal disease, and candidiasis.
• After supine positioning, have patient sit upright for at least 2 min before standing to avoid orthostatic hypotension.
• Do not use ingestible sodium bicarbonate products, such as the Prophy-Jet air polishing system, within 2 hr of drug use.
Consultations:
• In a patient with symptoms of blood dyscrasias, request a medical consultation for blood studies and postpone treatment until normal values are reestablished.
• Medical consultation may be required to assess disease control and patient's ability to tolerate stress.
Teach Patient/Family to:
• Encourage effective oral hygiene to prevent soft tissue inflammation.
• Use caution to prevent trauma when using oral hygiene aids.
• See dentist immediately if secondary oral infection occurs.
• When chronic dry mouth occurs, advise patient to:
  • Avoid mouth rinses with high alcohol content because of drying effects.
  • Use daily home fluoride products for anticaries effect.
  • Use sugarless gum, frequent sips of water, or saliva substitutes.

demecarium bromide
de-mi-**kare**′-ee-um **bro**′-mide
(Humorsol Ocumeter)

D

CATEGORY AND SCHEDULE
Pregnancy Risk Category: X

Drug Class: Antiglaucoma agent, ophthalmic; cyclostimulant, accommodative esotropia

MECHANISM OF ACTION
A cholinesterase inhibitor that increases the concentration of acetylcholine at cholinergic receptor sites and produces effects equivalent to excessive stimulation of cholinergic receptors.
Therapeutic Effect: Reduces intraocular pressure (IOP) because of facilitation of outflow of aqueous humor.

USES
Treatment of certain types of glaucoma and other eye conditions, such as accommodative esotropia. Also used in the diagnosis of certain eye conditions, such as accommodative esotropia.

PHARMACOKINETICS
Decreases intraocular pressure within a few hours. The duration is variable among individuals.

INDICATIONS AND DOSAGES
▸ **Glaucoma**
Ophthalmic, Topical
Adults, Elderly. 1–2 drops of the 0.125% or 0.25% solution in affected eye(s) twice a day to twice a wk.
▸ **Cyclostimulant**
Ophthalmic, Topical
Adults, Elderly. 1 drop of 0.125% or 0.25% solution in each eye daily for

D

2–3 wk, followed by 1 drop every 2 days for 4 wk.
▸ **Diagnostic Aid (accommodative esotropia)**
Ophthalmic, Topical
Adults, Elderly. 1 drop of 0.125% or 0.25% solution once a day for 2 wk, then 1 drop every 2 days for 2–3 wk.

SIDE EFFECTS/ADVERSE REACTIONS
Occasional
Brow ache, nausea, vomiting, abdominal cramps, diarrhea, hypersalivation, urinary incontinence, lid muscle twitching, redness, myopia blurred vision, increase in IOP, iris cysts, breathing difficulties, increased sweating

PRECAUTIONS AND CONTRAINDICATIONS
Pregnancy, active uveal inflammation and/or glaucoma associated with iridocyclitis, hypersensitivity to demecarium or any component of the formulation.

DRUG INTERACTIONS OF CONCERN TO DENTISTRY
• Avoid use of succinylcholine in general anesthesia
• Possible inhibition of the metabolism of ester-type local and topical anesthetics
• Avoid use of anticholinergics, such as systemic atropine or related drugs

SERIOUS REACTIONS
! Systemic absorption has been associated with demecarium resulting in anticholinesterase toxicity.
! Overdosage can produce cholinergic crisis characterized by cardiac arrhythmias, diarrhea, muscle weakness, profuse sweating, respiratory difficulties, urinary incontinence, and shock.

General:
• Determine why patient is taking the drug.
• Avoid drugs with anticholinergic activity, such as antihistamines, opioids, benzodiazepines, propantheline, atropine, and scopolamine.
• Avoid dental light in patient's eyes; offer dark glasses for patient comfort.
• Question glaucoma patient about compliance with prescribed drug regimen.
Consultations:
• Medical consultation may be required to assess disease control.
Teach Patient/Family to:
• Update health and medication history if physician makes any changes in evaluation or drug regimens; include OTC, herbal, and nonherbal remedies in the update.

demeclocycline hydrochloride
dem-eh-kloe-**sye**'-kleen
hi-droh-**klor**'-ide
(Declomycin, Ledermycin[AUS])

CATEGORY AND SCHEDULE
Pregnancy Risk Category: D

Drug Class: Tetracycline

MECHANISM OF ACTION
A tetracycline antibiotic that inhibits bacterial protein synthesis by binding to ribosomal receptor sites; also inhibits ADH-induced water reabsorption.
Therapeutic Effect: Bacteriostatic; also produces diuresis.

USES

Treatment of a wide variety of gram-positive and gram-negative bacteria, protozoa, *Rickettsia, Mycoplasma,* agents of psittacosis and ornithosis, *Actinomyces* species

PHARMACOKINETICS

PO: Peak 3–6 hr, duration 48–72 hr, *Half-life:* 10–17 hr; 36%–91% bound to serum protein; crosses placenta; excreted in urine, breast milk

INDICATIONS AND DOSAGES
▶ **Mild-to-Moderate Infections, Including Acne, Pertussis, Chronic Bronchitis, and UTIs**
PO
Adults, Elderly. 150 mg 4 times a day or 300 mg 2 times a day.
Children older than 8 yr. 8–12 mg/kg/day in 2–4 divided doses.
▶ **Uncomplicated Gonorrhea**
PO
Adults. Initially, 600 mg, then 300 mg q12h for 4 days for total of 3 g.
▶ **Syndrome of Inappropriate ADH Secretion (SIADH)**
PO
Adults, Elderly. Initially, 900–1200 mg/day in 3–4 divided doses, then decrease dose to 600–900 mg/day in divided doses.

SIDE EFFECTS/ADVERSE REACTIONS
Frequent
Anorexia, nausea, vomiting, diarrhea, dysphagia, possibly severe photosensitivity (with moderate to high demeclocycline dosage)
Occasional
Urticaria, rash; diabetes insipidus syndrome, marked by polydipsia, polyuria, and weakness (with long-term therapy)

PRECAUTIONS AND CONTRAINDICATIONS

Children 8 yr and younger, last half of pregnancy.
The use of tetracycline drugs during tooth development (last half of pregnancy, infancy, and childhood up to the age of 8 may cause permanent discoloration of the teeth (yellow-gray-brown). Enamel hypoplasia has also been reported. May also cause retardation of skeletal development and deformations.
Caution:
Renal disease, hepatic disease, lactation, nephrogenic diabetes insipidus

DRUG INTERACTIONS OF CONCERN TO DENTISTRY

• Decreased effect of penicillins, cephalosporins, oral contraceptives
• Oral contraceptives: advise patient of a potential risk for decreased contraceptive action, to maintain compliance with oral contraceptive use while using antibiotics, and to consider the use of additional nonhormonal contraception
• Contraindicated with isotretinoin (Accutane)

SERIOUS REACTIONS

! Superinfection (especially fungal), anaphylaxis, and benign intracranial hypertension occur rarely.
! Bulging fontanelles occur rarely in infants.

DENTAL CONSIDERATIONS

General:
• Examine oral cavity for side effects if on long-term drug therapy.
• Determine why the patient is taking the drug.
• Do not prescribe during pregnancy or before age 8 yr because of tooth discoloration.

• Absorption is reduced by dairy products, metals, and antacids.
• Dental staining or enamel hypoplasia may be associated with exposure to this drug before birth or up to the age of 8. Tetracycline stains may be extremely resistant to ordinary tooth-whitening procedures.
Consultations:
• Medical consultation may be required to assess disease control.
Teach Patient/Family to:
• Encourage effective oral hygiene to prevent soft tissue inflammation.
• Use caution to prevent injury when using oral hygiene aids.
• When used for dental infection, advise patient to:
   • Report sore throat, oral burning sensation, fever, and fatigue, any of which could indicate superinfection.
   • Take at prescribed intervals and complete dosage regimen.
   • Immediately notify the dentist if signs or symptoms of infection increase.

desipramine hydrochloride

dess-**ip**′-ra-meen hi-droh-**klor**′-ide
(Apo-Desipramine [CAN],
Norpramin, Novo-Desipramine
[CAN], Pertofran[AUS])
Do not confuse desipramine with clomipramine, disopyramide, imipramine, or nortriptyline.

CATEGORY AND SCHEDULE
Pregnancy Risk Category: C

Drug Class: Antidepressant, tricyclic

MECHANISM OF ACTION
A tricyclic antidepressant that blocks the reuptake of neurotransmitters, such as norepinephrine and serotonin, at presynaptic membranes, increasing their availability at postsynaptic receptor sites. Also has strong anticholinergic activity.
Therapeutic Effect: Relieves depression.

USES
Treatment of depression; unapproved: neurogenic pain

PHARMACOKINETICS
Rapidly and well absorbed from the GI tract. Protein binding: 90%. Metabolized in the liver. Primarily excreted in urine. Minimally removed by hemodialysis. **Half-life:** 12–27 hr.

INDICATIONS AND DOSAGES
▸ Depression
PO
Adults. 75 mg/day. May gradually increase to 150–200 mg/day. Maximum: 300 mg/day.
Elderly. Initially, 10–25 mg/day. May gradually increase to 75–100 mg/day. Maximum: 300 mg/ day.
Children older than 12 yr. Initially, 25–50 mg/day. May gradually increase to 100 mg/day. Maximum: 150 mg/day.
Children 6–12 yr. 1–3 mg/kg/day. Maximum: 5 mg/kg/day.

SIDE EFFECTS/ADVERSE REACTIONS
Frequent
Somnolence, fatigue, dry mouth, blurred vision, constipation, delayed micturition, orthostatic hypotension, diaphoresis, impaired concentration, increased appetite, urine retention

Occasional
GI disturbances (such as nausea, GI distress, metallic taste)
Rare
Paradoxical reactions (agitation, restlessness, nightmares, insomnia), extrapyramidal symptoms (particularly fine hand tremor)

PRECAUTIONS AND CONTRAINDICATIONS
Angle-closure glaucoma, use within 14 days of MAOIs.
Caution:
Suicidal patients, severe depression, increased intraocular pressure, narrow-angle glaucoma, elderly, MAOIs

DRUG INTERACTIONS OF CONCERN TO DENTISTRY
• Increased anticholinergic effects: muscarinic blockers, antihistamines, phenothiazines
• Increased effects of direct-acting sympathomimetics: epinephrine, levonordefrin
• Potential risk for increased CNS depression: alcohol, barbiturates, benzodiazepines, and other CNS depressants
• Decreased antihypertensive effects: clonidine, guanadrel, guanethidine
• At higher tricyclic doses, serum levels of fluconazole and ketoconazole may be elevated
• Avoid concurrent use with St. John's wort (herb)

SERIOUS REACTIONS
! Overdose may produce confusion, seizures, somnolence, arrhythmias, fever, hallucinations, dyspnea, vomiting, and unusual fatigue or weakness.
! Abrupt discontinuation after prolonged therapy may produce severe headache, malaise, nausea, vomiting, and vivid dreams.

DENTAL CONSIDERATIONS
General:
• Take vital signs at every appointment because of cardiovascular side effects.
• Assess salivary flow as a factor in caries, periodontal disease, and candidiasis.
• Patients on chronic drug therapy may rarely have symptoms of blood dyscrasias, which can include infection, bleeding, and poor healing.
• After supine positioning, have patient sit upright for at least 2 min to avoid orthostatic hypotension.
• Use vasoconstrictors with caution, in low doses, and with careful aspiration. Avoid use of gingival retraction cord with epinephrine.
• Place on frequent recall because of oral side effects.
Consultations:
• In a patient with symptoms of blood dyscrasias, request a medical consultation for blood studies and postpone dental treatment until normal values are reestablished.
• Medical consultation may be required to assess disease control.
• Physician should be informed if significant xerostomic side effects occur (e.g., increased caries, sore tongue, problems eating or swallowing, difficulty wearing prosthesis) so that a medication change can be considered.
Teach Patient/Family to:
• Encourage effective oral hygiene to prevent soft tissue inflammation.
• Use caution to prevent injury when using oral hygiene aids.
• When chronic dry mouth occurs, advise patient to:
  • Avoid mouth rinses with high alcohol content because of drying effects.
  • Use daily home fluoride products for anticaries effect.

D

- Use sugarless gum, frequent sips of water, or saliva substitutes.

desirudin
deh-**sear**'-ew-din
(Iprivask)

CATEGORY AND SCHEDULE
Pregnancy Risk Category: C

Drug Class: Anticoagulant; thrombin inhibitor

MECHANISM OF ACTION
An anticoagulant that binds specifically and directly to thrombin, inhibiting free-circulating and clot-bound thrombin.
Therapeutic Effect: Prolongs the clotting time of human plasma.

USES
Prophylaxis for deep vein thrombosis (DVT) in those undergoing hip replacement

PHARMACOKINETICS
Completely absorbed. Distributed in extracellular space. Metabolized and eliminated by the kidney. *Half-life:* 2–3 hr.

INDICATIONS AND DOSAGES
▸ **Prevention of DVT in Patients Undergoing Hip Replacement Surgery**
Subcutaneous
Adults, Elderly. Initially, 15 mg q12h given 5–15 min before surgery but following induction of regional block anesthesia, if used. May administer up to 12 days after surgery.
▸ **Moderate Renal Impairment (creatinine clearance 31–60 ml/min or higher)**

Subcutaneous
Adults, Elderly. 5 mg q12h.
▸ **Severe Renal Impairment (creatinine clearance less than 31 ml/min)**
Subcutaneous
Adults, Elderly. 1.7 mg q12h.

SIDE EFFECTS/ADVERSE REACTIONS
Frequent
Hematoma
Occasional
Injection site mass, wound secretion, nausea, hypersensitivity reaction

PRECAUTIONS AND CONTRAINDICATIONS
Hypersensitivity to natural or recombinant hirudins (anticoagulation factors), active bleeding, irreversible coagulation disorders

DRUG INTERACTIONS OF CONCERN TO DENTISTRY
- Increased risk of bleeding: salicylates, NSAIDs, or any drug that affects coagulation

SERIOUS REACTIONS
! Serious or major hemorrhage and anaphylactic reaction occur rarely.

DENTAL CONSIDERATIONS

General:
- Patients are at risk of bleeding, so check for oral signs.
- Product may be used in outpatient therapy. Delay elective dental treatment until patient completes anticoagulant therapy.
- Determine why patient is taking the drug.
- Avoid products that affect platelet function, such as aspirin and NSAIDs.

• Consider local hemostasis measures to prevent excessive bleeding.

Consultations:

• Medical consultation should include PPT or INR.

• Medical consultation may be required to assess disease control and patient's ability to tolerate stress.

Teach Patient/Family to:

• Use soft tooth brush to reduce risk of bleeding.

• Encourage effective oral hygiene to prevent soft tissue inflammation.

• Report oral lesions, soreness, or bleeding to dentist.

• Prevent trauma when using oral hygiene aids.

• Update health and medication history if physician makes any changes in evaluation or drug regimens; include OTC, herbal, and nonherbal remedies in the update.

---

desloratadine

des-loer-**at'**-ah-deen

(Aerius [CAN], Clarinex, Clarinex Redi-Tabs)

CATEGORY AND SCHEDULE

Pregnancy Risk Category: C

Do not confuse Clarinex with Claritin.

Drug Class: Antihistamine, histamine H_1-receptor antagonist

MECHANISM OF ACTION

A nonsedating antihistamine that exhibits selective peripheral histamine H_1 receptor blocking action. Competes with histamine at receptor sites.

Therapeutic Effect: Prevents allergic responses mediated by histamine, such as rhinitis and urticaria.

USES

Treatment of seasonal allergic rhinitis; chronic idiopathic urticaria

PHARMACOKINETICS

Rapidly and almost completely absorbed from the GI tract. Distributed mainly in liver, lungs, GI tract, and bile. Metabolized in the liver to active metabolite and undergoes extensive first-pass metabolism. Eliminated in urine and feces. *Half-life:* 27 hr (increased in the elderly and in renal or hepatic impairment).

INDICATIONS AND DOSAGES

▸ **Allergic Rhinitis, Urticaria**

PO

Adults, Elderly, Children older than 12 yr. 5 mg once a day.

▸ **Dosage in Hepatic or Renal Impairment**

Dosage is decreased to 5 mg every other day.

SIDE EFFECTS/ADVERSE REACTIONS

Frequent

Headache

Occasional

Dry mouth, somnolence

Rare

Fatigue, dizziness, diarrhea, nausea

PRECAUTIONS AND CONTRAINDICATIONS

Hypersensitivity to this drug or loratadine

Caution:

Distributed to breast milk (caution in nursing), incomplete dosing studies in the elderly, safety has not been established in children younger than 12 yr, dosage adjustment required in hepatic impairment

D

DRUG INTERACTIONS OF CONCERN TO DENTISTRY

• Limited studies with concurrent doses of erythromycin; ketoconazole and azithromycin show slight elevations of plasma levels but no clinically relevant changes in electrocardiographic parameters.
• One report indicated a potential for increased anticholinergic effects with other anticholinergic drugs and increased somnolence with CNS depressants; however, data are lacking.

SERIOUS REACTIONS

! None known

DENTAL CONSIDERATIONS

General:
• Assess salivary flow as a factor in caries, periodontal disease, and candidiasis.

Teach Patient/Family to:
• Encourage effective oral hygiene to prevent soft tissue inflammation.
• When chronic dry mouth occurs, advise patient to:
  • Avoid mouth rinses with high alcohol content because of drying effects.
  • Use sugarless gum, frequent sips of water, or saliva substitutes.
• Use daily home fluoride products for anticaries effect.

desmopressin

des-moe-**press**'-in
(DDAVP, Minirin[AUS], Octostim[CAN], Stimate)

CATEGORY AND SCHEDULE

Pregnancy Risk Category: B

Drug Class: Antidiuretic, central diabetes insipidus; antidiuretic, primary nocturnal enuresis; antihemorrhagic

MECHANISM OF ACTION

A synthetic pituitary hormone that increases reabsorption of water by increasing permeability of collecting ducts of the kidneys. Also serves as a plasminogen activator.
Therapeutic Effect: Increases plasma factor VIII (antihemophilic factor). Decreases urinary output.

USES

Prevents or controls the frequent urination, increased thirst, and loss of water associated with diabetes insipidus (water diabetes). It is used also to control bed-wetting and frequent urination and increased thirst associated with certain types of brain injuries or brain surgery.

PHARMACOKINETICS

Route	Onset	Peak	Duration
PO	1 hr	2–7 hr	6–8 hr
IV	15–30 min	1.5–3 hr	N/A
Intranasal	15 min–1 hr	1–5 hr	5–21 hr

Poorly absorbed after oral or nasal administration. Metabolism: Unknown. **Half-life:** Oral: 1.5–2.5 hr. Intranasal: 3.3–3.5 hr. IV: 0.4–4 hr.

INDICATIONS AND DOSAGES
▶ **Primary Nocturnal Enuresis**
PO
Children 12 yr and older. 0.2–0.6 mg once before bedtime.
Intranasal. Initially, 20 mcg (0.2 ml) at bedtime; use one-half dose in each nostril. Adjust to maximum of 40 mcg/day.
▶ **Central Cranial Diabetes Insipidus**
PO
Adults, Elderly, Children 12 yr and older. Initially, 0.05 mg twice a day. Range: 0.1–1.2 mg/day in 2–3 divided doses.

Children younger than 12 yr.
Initially, 0.05 mg; then twice a day.
Range: 0.1–0.8 mg daily.
IV, Subcutaneous
Adults, Elderly, Children 12 yr and older. 2–4 mcg/day in 2 divided doses or 1/10 of maintenance intranasal dose.
Intranasal
Adults, Elderly, Children older than 12 yr. 5–40 mcg (0.05–0.4 ml) in 1–3 doses/day.
Children 3 mo–12 yr. Initially, 5 mcg (0.05 ml)/day. Range: 5–30 mcg (0.05–0.3 ml)/day.
▶ **Hemophilia A, von Willebrand's Disease (Type I)**
IV Infusion
Adults, Elderly, Children weighing more than 10 kg. 0.3 mcg/kg diluted in 50 ml 0.9% NaCl.
Children weighing 10 kg and less. 0.3 mcg/kg diluted in 10 ml 0.9% NaCl.
Intranasal
Adults, Elderly, Children 12 yr and older weighing more than 50 kg. 300 mcg; use 1 spray in each nostril.
Adults, Elderly, Children 12 yr and older weighing 50 kg or less. 150 mcg as a single spray.

SIDE EFFECTS/ADVERSE REACTIONS

Occasional

IV: Pain, redness, or swelling at injection site; headache; abdominal cramps; vulval pain; flushed skin; mild B/P elevation; nausea with high dosages
Nasal: Rhinorrhea, nasal congestion, slight B/P elevation

PRECAUTIONS AND CONTRAINDICATIONS

Hemophilia A with factor VIII levels less than 5%; hemophilia B; severe type I, type IIB, or platelet-type von Willebrand's disease

Caution:
Lactation, hypertension

DRUG INTERACTIONS OF CONCERN TO DENTISTRY

• Decreased antidiuretic effects: demeclocycline
• Increased antidiuretic effects: carbamazepine

SERIOUS REACTIONS

! Water intoxication or hyponatremia, marked by headache, somnolence, confusion, decreased urination, rapid weight gain, seizures, and coma, may occur in overhydration. Children, elderly patients, and infants are especially at risk.

DENTAL CONSIDERATIONS

General:
• Monitor vital signs at every appointment because of cardiovascular side effects.
• Avoid prescribing aspirin-containing products if treatment is for bleeding disorder.
• Consider local hemostatic measures to prevent excessive bleeding.
• Determine why the patient is taking the drug.
• Consider semisupine chair position for patient comfort because of GI effects of disease.
Consultations:
• Medical consultation may be required to assess disease control; definite consultation for patients with chronic bleeding disorders.
• Medical consultation should include PTT or INR.
Teach Patient/Family to:
• Advise dentist if excessive bleeding occurs or continues after dental treatment.

D

desonide

dess'-oh-nide
(Delonide, Desocrot[CAN],
DesOwen, Scheinpharm
Desonide[CAN], Tridesilon)

CATEGORY AND SCHEDULE
Pregnancy Risk Category: C

Drug Class: Topical
corticosteroid, group IV low
potency

MECHANISM OF ACTION
A topical corticosteroid that has
antiinflammatory, antipruritic, and
vasoconstrictive properties. The
exact mechanism of the
antiinflammatory process is
unclear.
Therapeutic Effect: Reduces or
prevents tissue response to the
inflammatory process.

USES
Treatment of psoriasis, eczema,
contact dermatitis, pruritus

PHARMACOKINETICS
Large variation in absorption
determined by many factors.
Metabolized in the liver. Primarily
excreted by the kidneys and small
amounts in the bile.

INDICATIONS AND DOSAGES
▶ **Dermatoses**
Topical
Adults, Elderly. Apply sparingly 2–3
times a day.
▶ **Otitis Externa**
Aural
Adults, Elderly, Children. Instill
3–4 drops into the ear 3–4 times
a day.

SIDE EFFECTS/ADVERSE REACTIONS
Occasional
Burning and stinging at site of
application, dryness, skin peeling,
contact dermatitis

PRECAUTIONS AND CONTRAINDICATIONS
Perforated eardrum, history of
hypersensitivity to desonide or other
corticosteroids
Caution:
Lactation, viral infections, bacterial
infections

DRUG INTERACTIONS OF CONCERN TO DENTISTRY
• None listed

SERIOUS REACTIONS
❗ The serious reactions of long-term
therapy and the addition of occlusive
dressings are reversible
hypothalamic-pituitary-adrenal
(HPA) axis suppression,
manifestations of Cushing's
syndrome, hyperglycemia, and
glucosuria.

DENTAL CONSIDERATIONS

General:
• Determine why the patient is
taking the drug.
• Place on frequent recall to evaluate
healing response if used on chronic
basis.
• Apply lubricant to dry lips for
patient comfort before dental
procedures.

desoximetasone

des-ox-ih-**met**'-ah-sone
(Taro-Desoximetason[CAN],
Topicort, Topicort-LP)
Do not confuse with
dexamethasone.

CATEGORY AND SCHEDULE
Pregnancy Risk Category: C

Drug Class: Topical
corticosteroid, group II potency
(0.25%), group III potency
(0.05%)

MECHANISM OF ACTION
A high-potency, fluorinated topical
corticosteroid that has
antiinflammatory, antipruritic, and
vasoconstrictive properties. The exact
mechanism of the antiinflammatory
process is unclear.
Therapeutic Effect: Reduces tissue
response to the inflammatory
process.

USES
Treatment of psoriasis, eczema,
contact dermatitis, pruritus

PHARMACOKINETICS
Large variation in absorption among
sites. Protein binding in varying
degrees. Metabolized in liver.
Primarily excreted in urine.

INDICATIONS AND DOSAGES
▸ **Dermatoses**
Topical
Adults, Elderly. Apply sparingly 2
times a day.
Children. Apply sparingly 1–2 times
a day.

SIDE EFFECTS/ADVERSE REACTIONS
Frequent
Itching, redness, irritation, burning
at site of application

Occasional
Dryness, folliculitis, hypertrichosis,
acneiform eruptions,
hypopigmentation, perioral
dermatitis
Rare
Allergic contact dermatitis, adrenal
suppression, atrophy, striae, miliaria,
photosensitivity

PRECAUTIONS AND CONTRAINDICATIONS
History of hypersensitivity to
desoximetasone or other
corticosteroids
Caution:
Lactation, viral infections, bacterial
infections

SERIOUS REACTIONS
❗ Serious reactions of long-term
therapy and addition of occlusive
dressings are reversible
hypothalamic-pituitary-adrenal
(HPA) axis suppression,
manifestations of Cushing's
syndrome, hyperglycemia, and
glucosuria.
❗ Abruptly withdrawing the drug
after long-term therapy may require
supplemental systemic
corticosteroids.

DENTAL CONSIDERATIONS
General:
• Gel formulations are used in the
treatment of oral lichen planus
lesions when the diagnosis has been
confirmed by immunofluorescent
biopsy testing.
• Place on frequent recall to evaluate
healing response.
Teach Patient/Family to:
• Return for oral evaluation if
response of oral tissues has not
occurred in 7–14 days.
• Encourage effective oral hygiene
to prevent soft tissue inflammation.

D

• Not for use on oral herpetic ulcerations.
• Apply at bedtime or after meals for maximum effect.
• Apply with cotton-tipped applicator, dabbing gently, not rubbing medication on lesion.

desvenlafaxine
des-ven-la-**fax**'een
(Pristiq)

CATEGORY AND SCHEDULE
Pregnancy Risk Category: C

Drug Class: Antidepressants

MECHANISM OF ACTION
The major active metabolite of the antidepressant venlafaxine that potentiates CNS neurotransmitter activity by inhibiting the reuptake of serotonin and norepinephrine.
Therapeutic Effect: Relieves depression.

USES
Major depressive disorder

PHARMACOKINETICS
Well absorbed from the GI tract. Bioavailability: approximately 80%. Protein binding: 30%. Metabolized by conjugation (mediated by UGT isoforms); minor extent through oxidative metabolism by CYP3A4. Approximately 45% desvenlafaxine excreted unchanged in urine; approximately 19% excreted as the glucuronide metabolite, <5% as the oxidative metabolite (N,O-didesmethylvenlafaxine) in urine.
Half-life: 11 hr.

INDICATIONS AND DOSAGES
▸ **Major Depressive Disorder**
PO
Adults. 50 mg once daily with or without food. Range: 50–400 mg/day.
▸ **Dosage in Renal Impairment**
Adults, moderate impairment. 50 mg once daily with or without food.
Adults, severe impairment and end-stage renal disease (ESRD). 50 mg every other day with or without food. Do not escalate dose.
▸ **Dosage in Hepatic Impairment**
Adults. 50 mg once daily with or without food. Do not exceed 100 mg/day.

SIDE EFFECTS/ADVERSE REACTIONS
Frequent
Hypertension, nausea, dry mouth, diarrhea, fatigue, decreased appetite, dizziness, somnolence, headache, constipation, hyperhidrosis
Occasional
Palpitations, vomiting, chills, jittery, anxiety, abnormal dreams, yawning, mydriasis, irritability, tinnitus, dysgeusia, hot flush, sexual dysfunction (men), proteinuria
Rare
Tachycardia, asthenia, weight decrease, disturbed attention, nervousness, sexual dysfunction (women), mania, seizure, hyponatremia/SIADH, interstitial lung disease, eosinophilic pneumonia, abnormal bleeding, cholesterol and triglyceride elevations

PRECAUTIONS AND CONTRAINDICATIONS
Hypersensitivity to desvenlafaxine, venlafaxine or any component of the formulation
Use within 14 days of MAOIs

Caution:
Suicide risk, hypertension, abnormal
bleeding
Narrow-angle glaucoma
Renal impairment
Seizure disorder
Hyperlipidemia,
hypertriglyceridemia
Hepatic dysfunction

DRUG INTERACTIONS OF CONCERN TO DENTISTRY

• MAOIs: May cause neuroleptic
malignant syndrome, autonomic
instability (including rapid
fluctuations of vital signs), extreme
agitation, hyperthermia, mental
status changes, myoclonus, rigidity,
and coma.
• Serotonergic drugs: May increase
the risk of serotonin syndrome.
• Anticoagulants/antiplatelets,
NSAIDs: May increase the risk of
bleeding.
• CYP450 3A4 inhibitors: May
increase drug concentration levels of
desvenlafaxine.

SERIOUS REACTIONS

! Increased risk of suicidal thinking
and behavior in children,
adolescents, and young adults have
been reported.
! Seizures have been reported.
! Serotonin syndrome or neuroleptic
malignant syndrome (NMS)-like
reactions have been reported.
! When discontinuing
desvenlafaxine, plan to taper the
dosage slowly over 2 wk.
! Allow at least 14 days to elapse
before switching the patient from a
MAOI to desvenlafaxine and at least
7 days to elapse before switching
the patient from desvenlafaxine to a
MAOI.

DENTAL CONSIDERATIONS

General:
• Monitor vital signs at every
appointment because of
cardiovascular side effects.
Consultations:
• Medical consultation may be
required to assess disease control.
Teach Patient/Family to:
• Report oral lesions, soreness, or
bleeding to dentist.
• When chronic dry mouth occurs,
advise patient to:
  • Avoid mouth rinses with high
  alcohol content because of
  drying effects.
  • Use daily home fluoride
  products for anticaries effect.
  • Use sugarless gum, frequent
  sips of water, or saliva
  substitutes.

dexamethasone

dex-ah-**meth**′-ah-sone
(Decadron, Desamethasone
Intensol, Dexasone, Dexasone
LA, Dexmethsone[AUS],
Diodex[CAN], Hexadrol[CAN],
Maxidex, Solurex, Solurex LA)
Do not confuse dexamethasone
with desoximetasone or
dextromethorphan, or Maxidex
with Maxzide.

CATEGORY AND SCHEDULE

Pregnancy Risk Category: C (D if
used in the first trimester)

Drug Class: Synthetic topical
corticosteroid

MECHANISM OF ACTION

A long-acting glucocorticoid that
inhibits accumulation of
inflammatory cells at inflammation
sites, phagocytosis, lysosomal

D

enzyme release and synthesis, and release of mediators of inflammation.
Therapeutic Effect: Prevents and suppresses cell and tissue immune reactions and inflammatory process.

USES

Treatment of corticosteroid-responsive dermatoses, oral ulcerative inflammatory lesions

PHARMACOKINETICS

Rapidly, completely absorbed from the GI tract after oral administration. Widely distributed. Protein binding: High. Metabolized in the liver. Primarily excreted in urine. Minimally removed by hemodialysis.
Half-life: 3–4.5 hr.

INDICATIONS AND DOSAGES
▸ **Antiinflammatory**
PO, IV, IM
Adults, Elderly. 0.75–9 mg/day in divided doses q6–12h.
Children. 0.08–0.3 mg/kg/day in divided doses q6–12h.
▸ **Cerebral Edema**
IV
Adults, Elderly. Initially, 10 mg, then 4 mg (IV or IM) q6h.
PO, IV, IM
Children. Loading dose of 1–2 mg/kg, then 1–1.5 mg/kg/day in divided doses q4–6h.
▸ **Nausea and Vomiting in Chemotherapy Patients**
IV
Adults, Elderly. 8–20 mg once, then 4 mg (PO) q4–6h or 8 mg q8h.
Children. 10 mg/m^2/dose (Maximum: 20 mg), then 5 mg/m^2/dose q6h.
▸ **Physiologic Replacement**
PO, IV, IM
Children. 0.03–0.15 mg/kg/day in divided doses q6–12h.

▸ **Usual Ophthalmic Dosage, Ocular Inflammatory Conditions**
Ointment
Adults, Elderly, Children. Thin coating 3–4 times a day.
Suspension
Adults, Elderly, Children. Initially, 2 drops q1h while awake and q2h at night for 1 day, then reduce to 3–4 times a day.

SIDE EFFECTS/ADVERSE REACTIONS
Frequent
Inhalation: Cough, dry mouth, hoarseness, throat irritation
Intranasal: Burning, mucosal dryness
Ophthalmic: Blurred vision
Systemic: Insomnia, facial swelling or cushingoid appearance, moderate abdominal distention, indigestion, increased appetite, nervousness, facial flushing, diaphoresis
Occasional
Inhalation: Localized fungal infection, such as thrush
Intranasal: Crusting inside nose, nosebleed, sore throat, ulceration of nasal mucosa
Ophthalmic: Decreased vision, watering of eyes, eye pain, burning, stinging, redness of eyes, nausea, vomiting
Systemic: Dizziness, decreased or blurred vision
Topical: Allergic contact dermatitis, purpura or blood-containing blisters, thinning of skin with easy bruising, telangiectasia or raised dark red spots on skin
Rare
Inhalation: Increased bronchospasm, esophageal candidiasis
Intranasal: Nasal and pharyngeal candidiasis, eye pain
Systemic: General allergic reaction (such as rash and hives); pain, redness, or swelling at injection site;

psychological changes; false sense of well-being; hallucinations; depression

PRECAUTIONS AND CONTRAINDICATIONS

Active untreated infections, fungal, tuberculosis, or viral diseases of the eye

Caution:

Lactation, viral infections, bacterial infections

SERIOUS REACTIONS

! Long-term therapy may cause muscle wasting (especially in the arms and legs), osteoporosis, spontaneous fractures, amenorrhea, cataracts, glaucoma, peptic ulcer disease, and CHF.

! The ophthalmic form may cause glaucoma, ocular hypertension, and cataracts.

! Abrupt withdrawal following long-term therapy may cause severe joint pain, severe headache, anorexia, nausea, fever, rebound inflammation, fatigue, weakness, lethargy, dizziness, and orthostatic hypotension.

DENTAL CONSIDERATIONS

General:

• Monitor vital signs at every appointment because of cardiovascular side effects.

• Patients on chronic drug therapy may rarely have symptoms of blood dyscrasias, which can include infection, bleeding, and poor healing.

• Symptoms of oral infections may be masked.

• Patients who have been or are currently on chronic steroid therapy (longer than 2 wk) may require supplemental steroids for dental treatment.

• Avoid prescribing aspirin-containing products.

• Place on frequent recall to evaluate healing response.

• Prophylactic antibiotics may be indicated to prevent infection if surgery or deep scaling is planned.

Consultations:

• In a patient with symptoms of blood dyscrasias, request a medical consultation for blood studies and postpone dental treatment until normal values are reestablished.

• Medical consultation may be required to assess disease control.

• Consultation may be required to confirm steroid dose and duration of use.

Teach Patient/Family to:

• Encourage effective oral hygiene to prevent soft tissue inflammation.

• Use caution to prevent injury when using oral hygiene aids.

• Avoid mouth rinses with high alcohol content because of drug interaction.

dexamethasone sodium phosphate

dex-ah-**meth**′-ah-sone **soe**′-dee-um **foss**′-fate

(AK-Dex, Decadron Phosphate Ophthalmic, Dexamethasone Ophthalmic, Maxidex, Ocu-Dex, Diodex[CAN])

Do not confuse dexamethasone with desoximetasone, dextromethorphan, or Maxzide.

CATEGORY AND SCHEDULE

Pregnancy Risk Category: C (D if used in the first trimester)

Drug Class: Synthetic topical corticosteroid

D

MECHANISM OF ACTION

A corticosteroid that inhibits accumulation of inflammatory cells at inflammation sites, phagocytosis, lysosomal enzyme release, and synthesis and release of mediators of inflammation.
Therapeutic Effect: Prevents and suppresses cell and tissue immune reactions, inflammatory process.

USES

Treatment of corticosteroid-responsive dermatoses, oral ulcerative inflammatory lesions

PHARMACOKINETICS

Absorbed into aqueous humor, cornea, iris, choroids, ciliary body, and retina. Systemic absorption may occur and is more likely at higher doses or in pediatric therapy.

INDICATIONS AND DOSAGES
▸ Ocular Inflammatory Conditions
Ophthalmic, Ointment
Adults, Elderly. Apply thin strip 3–4 times a day.
Ophthalmic, Solution and Suspension
Adults, Elderly. Instill 1 or 2 drops up to 6 times a day.

SIDE EFFECTS/ADVERSE REACTIONS
Frequent
Blurred vision, increased intraocular pressure
Occasional
Decreased vision, watering of eyes, eye pain, burning, stinging, redness of eyes, nausea, vomiting
Rare
Optic nerve damage, posterior subcapsular cataract formation, delayed wound healing

PRECAUTIONS AND CONTRAINDICATIONS

Epithelial herpes simplex keratitis (dendritic keratitis), vaccinia, varicella or other viral diseases of the cornea and conjunctiva, mycobacterial infection of the eye, fungal diseases of ocular structures, hypersensitivity to any component of the medication
Caution:
Diabetes mellitus, glaucoma, osteoporosis, seizure disorders, ulcerative colitis, CHF, myasthenia gravis, renal disease, peptic ulcer, esophagitis

DRUG INTERACTIONS OF CONCERN TO DENTISTRY
• Decreased action: barbiturates
• Increased side effects: alcohol, salicylates, other NSAIDs
• Increased action: ketoconazole, macrolide antibiotics

SERIOUS REACTIONS
! The serious reactions of the ophthalmic form of dexamethasone sodium phosphate are glaucoma, ocular hypertension, and cataracts.
! May promote development and spread of secondary infection (usually fungal).

DENTAL CONSIDERATIONS

General:
• Place on frequent recall to evaluate healing response.
Teach Patient/Family to:
• Return for oral evaluation if response of oral tissues has not occurred in 7–14 days.
• Encourage effective oral hygiene to prevent soft tissue inflammation.
• Apply approximately 0.25 inch; measure and apply with cotton-tipped applicator by gently

dabbing, not rubbing, medication on lesion.
• Apply at bedtime or after meals for maximum effect.
• Avoid use on oral herpetic lesions.

dexchlorpheniramine
dex-klor-fen-**eer**′-ah-meen
(Polaramine, Polaramine Repetabs)

CATEGORY AND SCHEDULE
Pregnancy Risk Category: B

Drug Class: Antihistamine

MECHANISM OF ACTION
A propylamine derivative that competes with histamine for H_1-receptor sites on effector cells in the GI tract, blood vessels, and respiratory tract.
Dexchlorpheniramine is the dextro-isomer of chlorpheniramine and is approximately 2 times more active.
Therapeutic Effect: Prevents allergic response, produces mild bronchodilation, blocks histamine-induced bronchitis.

USES
Treatment of allergy symptoms, rhinitis, pruritus, contact dermatitis

PHARMACOKINETICS

Route	Onset	Peak	Duration
PO	0.5 hr	1–2 hr	3–6 hr

Well absorbed from the GI tract. Protein binding: 70%. Widely distributed. Metabolized in liver to active metabolite, undergoes extensive first-pass metabolism.

Excreted primarily in urine. Not removed by hemodialysis. *Half-life:* 20 hr.

INDICATIONS AND DOSAGES
▸ **Allergic Rhinitis, Common Cold**
PO
Adults, Elderly, Children 12 yr or older. 2 mg q4–6h or 4–6 mg timed release at bedtime or q8–10h.
Children 6–11 yr. 4 mg timed release at bedtime or 1 mg q4–6h.
Children 2–5 yr. 0.5 mg q4–6h. Do not use timed release.

SIDE EFFECTS/ADVERSE REACTIONS
Frequent
Drowsiness, dizziness, headache, dry mouth, nose, or throat, urinary retention, thickening of bronchial secretions, sedation, hypotension
Occasional
Epigastric distress, flushing, blurred vision, tinnitus, paresthesia, sweating, chills

PRECAUTIONS AND CONTRAINDICATIONS
History of hypersensitivity to antihistamines, newborn or premature infants, nursing mothers, third trimester of pregnancy
Caution:
Increased intraocular pressure, renal disease, cardiac disease, hypertension, bronchial asthma, seizure disorder, stenosed peptic ulcers, hyperthyroidism, prostatic hypertrophy, bladder neck obstruction, elderly

DRUG INTERACTIONS OF CONCERN TO DENTISTRY
• Increased CNS depression: barbiturates, narcotics, hypnotics, tricyclic antidepressants, alcohol
• Increased anticholinergic effect: anticholinergic drugs

SERIOUS REACTIONS

! Children may experience dominant paradoxical reactions, including restlessness, insomnia, euphoria, nervousness, and tremors.

! Hypersensitivity reaction, such as eczema, pruritus, rash, cardiac disturbances, and photosensitivity, may occur.

! Overdosage may vary from CNS depression, including sedation, apnea, hypotension, cardiovascular collapse, or death to severe paradoxical reaction, such as hallucinations, tremors, and seizures.

DENTAL CONSIDERATIONS

General:

• Assess salivary flow as a factor in caries, periodontal disease, and candidiasis.

• Consider semisupine chair position for patient comfort because of respiratory effects of disease.

Teach Patient/Family:

• When chronic dry mouth occurs, advise patient to:

  • Avoid mouth rinses with high alcohol content because of drying effects.

  • Use sugarless gum, frequent sips of water, or saliva substitutes.

  • Use daily home fluoride products for anticaries effect.

dexlansoprazole

dex-lan-**soe**-prah-zole
(Kapidex)
Do not confuse with dexamethasone or lansoprazole.

CATEGORY AND SCHEDULE

Pregnancy Risk Category: B

Drug Class: Antisecretory, proton pump inhibitor

MECHANISN OF ACTION

A proton pump inhibitor that selectively inhibits the parietal cell membrane enzyme system in the GI tract (hydrogen-potassium adenosine triphosphatase), or proton pump.

Therapeutic effect: Suppresses gastric acid secretion.

USES

Healing all grades of erosive esophagitis, maintenance of healing of erosive esophagitis, and treatment of heartburn due to gastroesophageal reflux disease (GERD)

PHARMACOKINETICS

Well absorbed orally, peak concentrations reached in 1–2 hr and 4–5 hr. Widely distributed. Protein binding: 96%. Extensively metabolized in the liver by oxidation (CYP 2C19 and CYP3A4).
Half-life: 1–2 hr. Metabolites excreted by the kidneys.

INDICATIONS AND DOSAGES

▶ **Erosive Esophagitis**

PO

Adult, Elderly. 60 mg once daily for up to 8 wk.

▶ **Maintenance of Healing of Erosive Esophagitis**

PO

Adult, Elderly. 30 mg once daily.

▶ **Symptomatic, Non-Erosive GERD**

PO

Adult, Elderly. 30 mg once daily for 4 wk.

SIDE EFFECTS/ADVERSE REACTIONS

Frequent

Diarrhea, abdominal pain, nausea, upper respiratory tract infections, vomiting, flatulence

PRECAUTIONS AND CONTRAINDICATIONS

Hypersensitivity to dexlansoprazole or its ingredients, children under the age of 18, pregnancy, lactation
Caution:
Symptomatic improvement with dexlansoprazole does not preclude the possibility of gastric malignancy

DRUG INTERACTIONS OF CONCERN TO DENTISTRY

• Drug interactions in dentistry not established but dexlansoprazole may interfere with the absorption of ampicillin esters, and ketoconazole.

SERIOUS REACTIONS

! None established in dental patients

DENTAL CONSIDERATIONS

General:
• Consider semisupine chair position for patient comfort because of GI effects of disease.
• Question the patient about tolerance of NSAIDs or aspirin related to GI adverse effects.
• Patients with GERD may have oral symptoms of acid reflux, including dental erosion, or TMJ dysfunction that may require appropriate dental treatment.
Teach patient/family to:
• Seek medical care for worsening or unrelieved GI symptoms.
• Use fluoridated toothpaste and effective oral hygiene measures to minimize sensitivity and caries associated with dental erosion.

dexmethylphenidate hydrochloride

dex-meth-ill-**fen**′-ih-date
hi-droh-**klor**′-ide
(Focalin)

D

CATEGORY AND SCHEDULE

Pregnancy Risk Category: C
Controlled Substance: Schedule II

Drug Class: CNS stimulant; related to the amphetamines

MECHANISM OF ACTION

A CNS stimulant that blocks the reuptake of norepinephrine and dopamine into presynaptic neurons, increasing the release of these neurotransmitters into the synaptic cleft.
Therapeutic Effect: Decreases motor restlessness and fatigue; increases motor activity, mental alertness, and attention span; elevates mood.

USES

Treatment of attention-deficit/hyperactivity disorder (ADHD)

PHARMACOKINETICS

Route	Onset	Peak	Duration
PO	N/A	N/A	4–5 hr

Readily absorbed from the GI tract. Plasma concentrations increase rapidly. Metabolized in the liver. Excreted unchanged in urine.
Half-life: 2.2 hr.

INDICATIONS AND DOSAGES
▸ ADHD
PO
Patients new to dexmethylphenidate or methylphenidate. 2.5 mg twice a

D

day (5 mg/day). May adjust dosage in 2.5- to 5-mg increments. Maximum: 20 mg/day.
Patients currently taking methylphenidate. Half the methylphenidate dosage. Maximum: 20 mg/day.

SIDE EFFECTS/ADVERSE REACTIONS

Frequent
Abdominal pain, nausea, anorexia, fever
Occasional
Tachycardia, arrhythmias, palpitations, insomnia, twitching
Rare
Blurred vision, rash, arthralgia

PRECAUTIONS AND CONTRAINDICATIONS

Diagnosis or family history of Tourette syndrome; glaucoma; history of marked agitation, anxiety, or tension; motor tics; use within 14 days of MAOIs
Caution:
Long-term effect on growth in children unknown, exacerbation of psychotic behavior, history of seizures, hypertension, heart failure, recent MI, hyperthyroidism, use in children younger than 6 yr not established, drug dependence, lactation

DRUG INTERACTIONS OF CONCERN TO DENTISTRY

• May inhibit metabolism of phenobarbital, tricyclic antidepressants, and SSRIs
• Increased effects of anticholinergics, CNS stimulants, tricyclic antidepressants, and sympathomimetics

SERIOUS REACTIONS

! Withdrawal after prolonged therapy may unmask symptoms of the underlying disorder.
! Dexmethylphenidate may lower the seizure threshold in those with a history of seizures.
! Overdose produces excessive sympathomimetic effects, including vomiting, tremor, hyperreflexia, seizures, confusion, hallucinations, and diaphoresis.
! Prolonged administration to children may delay growth.

DENTAL CONSIDERATIONS

General:
• Monitor vital signs at every appointment because of cardiovascular side effects.
• Assess salivary flow as a factor in caries, periodontal disease, and candidiasis.
• Patients on chronic drug therapy may rarely have symptoms of blood dyscrasias, which can include infection, bleeding, and poor healing.
• Use vasoconstrictor with caution, in low doses, and with careful aspiration.
• Determine why the patient is taking the drug.
Consultations:
• In a patient with symptoms of blood dyscrasias, request a medical consultation for blood studies and postpone treatment until normal values are reestablished.
• Medical consultation may be required to assess disease control.
Teach Patient/Family to:
• Encourage effective oral hygiene to prevent soft tissue inflammation, infection.
• Use caution to prevent injury when using oral hygiene aids.

• Update health and drug history if physician makes any changes in evaluation or drug regimens.
• When chronic dry mouth occurs, advise patient to:
  • Avoid mouth rinses with high alcohol content because of drying effects.
  • Use daily home fluoride products for anticaries effect.
  • Use sugarless gum, frequent sips of water, or saliva substitutes.

dextroamphetamine sulfate
dex-troe-am-fet′-ah-meen sull′-fate
(Dexamphetamine[AUS], Dexedrine, Dexedrine Spansule, DextroStat)
Do not confuse dextroamphetamine with dextromethorphan, or Dexedrine with Dextran or Excedrin.

CATEGORY AND SCHEDULE
Pregnancy Risk Category: C
Controlled Substance: Schedule II

Drug Class: Amphetamine

MECHANISM OF ACTION
An amphetamine that enhances the action of dopamine and norepinephrine by blocking their reuptake from synapses; also inhibits monoamine oxidase and facilitates the release of catecholamines.
Therapeutic Effect: Increases motor activity and mental alertness; decreases motor restlessness, drowsiness, and fatigue; suppresses appetite.

USES
Treatment of narcolepsy, attention-deficit/hyperactivity disorder (ADHD)

PHARMACOKINETICS
PO: Onset 30 min, peak 1–3 hr, duration 4–20 hr. *Half-life:* 10–30 hr; metabolized by liver; urine excretion pH dependent; crosses placenta, excreted in breast milk.

INDICATIONS AND DOSAGES
▶ **Narcolepsy**
PO
Adults, Children older than 12 yr. Initially, 10 mg/day. Increase by 10 mg/day at weekly intervals until therapeutic response is achieved.
Children 6–12 yr. Initially, 5 mg/day. Increase by 5 mg/day at weekly intervals until therapeutic response is achieved. Maximum: 60 mg/day.
▶ **ADHD**
PO
Children 6 yr and older. Initially, 5 mg once or twice a day. Increase by 5 mg/day at weekly intervals until therapeutic response is achieved.
Children 3–5 yr. Initially, 2.5 mg/day. Increase by 2.5 mg/day at weekly intervals until therapeutic response is achieved. Maximum: 40 mg/day.
▶ **Appetite Suppressant**
PO
Adults. 5–30 mg daily in divided doses of 5–10 mg each, given 30–60 min before meals; or 1 extended-release capsule in the morning.

SIDE EFFECTS/ADVERSE REACTIONS
Frequent
Irregular pulse, increased motor activity, talkativeness, nervousness, mild euphoria, insomnia

Occasional
Headache, chills, dry mouth, GI distress, worsening depression in patients who are clinically depressed, tachycardia, palpitations, chest pain, dizziness, decreased appetite

PRECAUTIONS AND CONTRAINDICATIONS
Advanced arteriosclerosis, agitated states, glaucoma, history of drug abuse, hypersensitivity to sympathomimetic amines, hyperthyroidism, moderate to severe hypertension, symptomatic cardiovascular disease, use within 14 days of MAOIs
Caution:
Gilles de la Tourette's syndrome, lactation, children younger than 3 yr

DRUG INTERACTIONS OF CONCERN TO DENTISTRY
• Increased risk of serious side effects: meperidine, propoxyphene, tricyclic antidepressants

SERIOUS REACTIONS
! Overdose may produce skin pallor or flushing, arrhythmias, and psychosis.
! Abrupt withdrawal after prolonged use of high doses may produce lethargy lasting for weeks.
! Prolonged administration to children with ADHD may inhibit growth.

DENTAL CONSIDERATIONS
General:
• Monitor vital signs at every appointment because of cardiovascular side effects.
• Assess salivary flow as a factor in caries, periodontal disease, and candidiasis.

• Psychologic and physical dependence may occur with chronic administration.
Consultations:
• Medical consultation may be required to assess disease control.
Teach Patient/Family:
• When chronic dry mouth occurs, advise patient to:
  • Avoid mouth rinses with high alcohol content because of drying effects.
  • Use daily home fluoride products for anticaries effect.
  • Use sugarless gum, frequent sips of water, or saliva substitutes.

dextromethorphan
dex-troe-meth-**or**′-fan
(Babee Cof Syrup, Benylin Adult, Benylin Pediatric, Creomulsion Cough, Creomulsion for Children, Creo-Terpin, Delsym, DexAlone, ElixSure Cough, Hold DM, PediaCare Infants' Long-Acting Cough, Robitussion[AUS], Robitussin CoughGels, Robitussin Honey Cough, Robitussin Maximum Strength Cough, Robitussin Pediatric Cough, Scot-Tussin DM Cough Chasers, Silphen DM, Simply Cough, Vicks 44 Cough Relief)

CATEGORY AND SCHEDULE
Pregnancy Risk Category: C
OTC

Drug Class: Antitussive, nonnarcotic

MECHANISM OF ACTION
A chemical relative of morphine without the narcotic properties that acts on the cough center in the

medulla oblongata by elevating the threshold for coughing.
Therapeutic Effect: Suppresses cough.

USES
Treatment of nonproductive cough

PHARMACOKINETICS
Rapidly absorbed from the GI tract. Distributed into CSF. Extensively and poorly metabolized in liver to dextrorphan (active metabolite). Excreted unchanged in urine.
Half-life: 1.4–3.9 hr (parent compound), 3.4–5.6 hr (dextrorphan).

INDICATIONS AND DOSAGES
▸ Cough
PO
Adults, Elderly, Children 12 yr and older. 10–20 mg q4h. Maximum: 120 mg/day.
Children 6–12 yr. 5–10 mg q4h. Maximum: 60 mg/day.
Children 2–5 yr. 2.5–5 mg q4h. Maximum: 30 mg/day.

SIDE EFFECTS/ADVERSE REACTIONS
Rare
Abdominal discomfort, constipation, dizziness, drowsiness, GI upset, nausea

PRECAUTIONS AND CONTRAINDICATIONS
Coadministration with MAOIs, hypersensitivity to dextromethorphan or its components
Caution:
Nausea, vomiting, increased temperature, persistent headache, drug abuse

DRUG INTERACTIONS OF CONCERN TO DENTISTRY
• Inhibition of metabolism: terbinafine

SERIOUS REACTIONS
! Overdosage may result in muscle spasticity, increase or decrease in B/P.
! Blurred vision, blue fingernails and lips, nausea, vomiting, hallucinations, and respiratory depression.

DENTAL CONSIDERATIONS
General:
• Consider semisupine chair position for patients with respiratory disease.

diazepam
dye-**az**′-eh-pam
(Antenex[AUS], Apo-Diazepam[CAN], Diastat, Diazemuls[CAN], Dizac, Ducene[AUS],Valium, Valpam[AUS], Vivol[CAN])
Do not confuse diazepam with diazoxide or Ditropan, or Valium with Valcyte.

CATEGORY AND SCHEDULE
Pregnancy Risk Category: D
Controlled Substance: Schedule IV

Drug Class: Benzodiazepine, anxiolytic

MECHANISM OF ACTION
A benzodiazepine that depresses all levels of the CNS by enhancing the action of gamma-aminobutyric acid, a major inhibitory neurotransmitter in the brain.

Therapeutic Effect: Produces anxiolytic effect, elevates the seizure threshold, produces skeletal muscle relaxation.

USES

Anxiety, acute alcohol withdrawal, adjunct in seizure disorders, skeletal muscle spasm; conscious sedation in dentistry

PHARMACOKINETICS

Route	Onset	Peak	Duration
PO	30 min	1–2 hr	2–3 hr
IV	1–5 min	15 min	15–60 min
IM	15 min	30–90 min	30–90 min

Well absorbed from the GI tract. Widely distributed. Protein binding: 98%. Metabolized in the liver to active metabolite. Excreted in urine. Minimally removed by hemodialysis. *Half-life:* 20–70 hr (increased in hepatic dysfunction and the elderly).

INDICATIONS AND DOSAGES
▶ **Anxiety, Skeletal Muscle Relaxation**
PO
Adults. 2–10 mg 2–4 times a day.
Elderly. 2.5 mg twice a day.
Children. 0.12–0.8 mg/kg/day in divided doses q6–8h.
IV, IM
Adults. 2–10 mg repeated in 3–4 hr.
Children. 0.04–0.3 mg/kg/dose q2–4h. Maximum: 0.5 mg/kg in an 8-hr period.
▶ **Preanesthesia**
IV
Adults, Elderly. 5–15 mg 5–10 min before procedure.
Children. 0.2–0.3 mg/kg. Maximum: 10 mg.

▶ **Alcohol Withdrawal**
PO
Adults, Elderly. 10 mg 3–4 times during first 24 hr, then reduced to 5–10 mg 3–4 times a day as needed.
IV, IM
Adults, Elderly. Initially, 10 mg, followed by 5–10 mg q3–4h.
▶ **Status Epilepticus**
IV
Adults, Elderly. 5–10 mg q10–15min up to 30 mg/8 hr.
Children 5 yr and older. 0.05–0.3 mg/kg/dose q15–30min. Maximum: 10 mg/dose.
Children 1 mo to younger than 5 yr. 0.05–0.3 mg/kg/dose q15–30min. Maximum: 5 mg/dose.
▶ **Control of Increased Seizure Activity in Patients with Refractory Epilepsy Who Are on Stable Regimens of Anticonvulsants**
Rectal Gel
Adults, Children 12 yr and older. 0.2 mg/kg; may be repeated in 4–12 hr.
Children 6–11 yr. 0.3 mg/kg; may be repeated in 4–12 hr.
Children 2–5 yr. 0.5 mg/kg; may be repeated in 4–12 hr.

SIDE EFFECTS/ADVERSE REACTIONS
Frequent
Pain with IM injection, somnolence, fatigue, ataxia
Occasional
Slurred speech, orthostatic hypotension, headache, hypoactivity, constipation, nausea, blurred vision
Rare
Paradoxical CNS reactions, such as hyperactivity or nervousness in children and excitement or restlessness in the elderly or debilitated (generally noted during first 2 wk of therapy, particularly in presence of uncontrolled pain)

PRECAUTIONS AND CONTRAINDICATIONS

Angle-closure glaucoma, coma, preexisting CNS depression, respiratory depression, severe, uncontrolled pain
Caution:
Elderly, debilitated, hepatic disease, renal disease

DRUG INTERACTIONS OF CONCERN TO DENTISTRY

• Increased CNS depression of diazepam: alcohol, all CNS depressants, kava kava (herb)
• Increased serum levels and prolonged effect of benzodiazepines: erythromycin, clarithromycin, ketoconazole, itraconazole, fluconazole, miconazole (systemic), cimetidine, rifamycin
• Contraindicated with saquinavir
• Possible increase in CNS side effects: kava kava (herb)

SERIOUS REACTIONS

! IV administration may produce pain, swelling, thrombophlebitis, and carpal tunnel syndrome.
! Abrupt or too-rapid withdrawal may result in pronounced restlessness, irritability, insomnia, hand tremor, abdominal or muscle cramps, diaphoresis, vomiting, and seizures.
! Abrupt withdrawal in patients with epilepsy may produce an increase in the frequency or severity of seizures.
! Overdose results in somnolence, confusion, diminished reflexes, and coma.

DENTAL CONSIDERATIONS

General:
• Assess salivary flow as a factor in caries, periodontal disease, and candidiasis.
• After supine positioning, have patient sit upright for at least 2 min before standing to avoid orthostatic hypotension.
• Psychologic and physical dependence may occur with chronic administration.
• Geriatric patients are more susceptible to drug effects; use lower dose.
• Have someone drive patient to and from dental appointment when drug used for conscious sedation.
• Provide assistance when escorting patient to and from dental chair when dizziness occurs.
• Avoid use of this drug in a patient with a history of drug abuse or alcoholism.
Teach Patient/Family to:
• Encourage effective oral hygiene to prevent soft tissue inflammation.
• When chronic dry mouth occurs, advise patient to:
  • Avoid mouth rinses with high alcohol content because of drying effects.
  • Use daily home fluoride products for anticaries effect.
  • Use sugarless gum, frequent sips of water, or saliva substitutes.

diclofenac
dye-kloe´-fen-ak
(Cataflam, Diclohexal[AUS], Diclotek[CAN], Fenac[AUS], Novo-Difenac[CAN], Solaraze, Voltaren, Voltaren Emulgel[AUS], Voltaren Ophthalmic, Voltaren Rapid[AUS], Voltaren XR)
Do not confuse diclofenac with Diflucan or Duphalac, or Voltaren with Verelan.

CATEGORY AND SCHEDULE
Pregnancy Risk Category: X

Drug Class: Nonsteroidal antiinflammatory

MECHANISM OF ACTION
An NSAID that inhibits prostaglandin synthesis, reducing the intensity of pain. Also constricts the iris sphincter. May inhibit angiogenesis (the formation of blood vessels) by inhibiting substance P or blocking the angiogenic effects of prostaglandin E. *Therapeutic Effect:* Produces analgesic and antiinflammatory effects. Prevents miosis during cataract surgery. May reduce angiogenesis in inflamed tissue.

USES
Treatment of acute, chronic rheumatoid arthritis, osteoarthritis, ankylosing spondylitis, analgesia

PHARMACOKINETICS

Route	Onset	Peak	Duration
PO	30 min	2–3 hr	Up to 8 hr

Completely absorbed from the GI tract; penetrates cornea after ophthalmic administration (may be systemically absorbed). Protein binding: greater than 99%. Widely distributed. Metabolized in the liver. Primarily excreted in urine. Minimally removed by hemodialysis. *Half-life:* 1.2–2 hr.

INDICATIONS AND DOSAGES
▸ **Osteoarthritis**
PO (Cataflam, Voltaren)
Adults, Elderly. 50 mg 2–3 times a day.
PO (Voltaren XR)
Adults, Elderly. 100 mg/day as a single dose.
▸ **Rheumatoid Arthritis**
PO (Cataflam, Voltaren)
Adults, Elderly. 50 mg 2–4 times a day. Maximum: 225 mg/day.

PO (Voltaren XR)
Adults, Elderly. 100 mg once a day. Maximum: 100 mg twice a day.
▸ **Ankylosing Spondylitis**
PO (Voltaren)
Adults, Elderly. 100–125 mg/day in 4–5 divided doses.
▸ **Analgesia, Primary Dysmenorrhea**
PO (Cataflam)
Adults, Elderly. 30 mg 3 times a day.
▸ **Usual Pediatric Dosage**
Children. 2–3 mg/kg/day in 2–4 divided doses.
▸ **Actinic Keratoses**
Topical
Adults, Adolescents. Apply twice a day to lesion for 60–90 days.
▸ **Cataract Surgery**
Ophthalmic
Adults, Elderly. Apply 1 drop to eye 4 times a day commencing 24 hr after cataract surgery. Continue for 2 wk afterward.
▸ **Pain, Relief of Photophobia in Patients Undergoing Corneal Refractive Surgery**
Ophthalmic
Adults, Elderly. Apply 1 drop to affected eye 1 hr before surgery, within 15 min after surgery, then 4 times a day for 3 days.

SIDE EFFECTS/ADVERSE REACTIONS
Frequent
PO: Headache, abdominal cramps, constipation, diarrhea, nausea, dyspepsia
Ophthalmic: Burning or stinging on instillation, ocular discomfort
Occasional
PO: Flatulence, dizziness, epigastric pain
Ophthalmic: Ocular itching or tearing
Rare
PO: Rash, peripheral edema or fluid retention, visual disturbances, vomiting, drowsiness

PRECAUTIONS AND CONTRAINDICATIONS

Hypersensitivity to aspirin, diclofenac, and other NSAIDs; porphyria

Caution:

Lactation, children, bleeding disorders, GI disorders, cardiac disorders, hypersensitivity to other antiinflammatory agents

DRUG INTERACTIONS OF CONCERN TO DENTISTRY

• Use with caution in patients with cardiovascular disease at risk of thromboembolism
• GI ulceration, bleeding: aspirin, alcohol, corticosteroids, potassium supplements
• Nephrotoxicity: acetaminophen (prolonged use)
• Possible risk of decreased renal function: cyclosporine
• When prescribed for dental pain:
• Risk of increased effects: oral anticoagulants, oral antidiabetics, lithium, methotrexate
• Decreased antihypertensive effects of diuretics, β-adrenergic blockers, and ACE inhibitors
• First-time users of SSRIs also taking NSAIDs may have a higher risk of GI side effects; until more data are available, it may be advisable to avoid use of NSAIDs in these patients (*Br J Clin Pharmacol* 55:591–595, 2003)

Diclofenac Sodium (Voltaren)
• None reported

SERIOUS REACTIONS

❗ Overdose may result in acute renal failure.
❗ Rare reactions with long-term use include peptic ulcer disease, GI bleeding, gastritis, a severe hepatic reaction (jaundice), nephrotoxicity (hematuria, dysuria, proteinuria), and a severe hypersensitivity

reaction (bronchospasm or angioedema).

DENTAL CONSIDERATIONS

General:

• Patients on chronic drug therapy may rarely have symptoms of blood dyscrasias, which can include infection, bleeding, and poor healing.
• Assess salivary flow as a factor in caries, periodontal disease, and candidiasis.
• Avoid prescribing for dental use in pregnancy.
• Avoid prescribing aspirin-containing products.
• Consider semisupine chair position for patients with rheumatic disease.
• Advise patient if dental drugs prescribed have a potential for photosensitivity.
• Severe stomach bleeding may occur in patients who regularly use NSAIDs in recommended doses, when the patient is also taking another NSAID, a blood thinning, or steroid drug, if the patient has GI or peptic ulcer disease, if they are 60 years or older, or when NSAIDs are taken longer than directed. Warn patients of the potential for severe stomach bleeding.
• Warn patient of potential risks of NSAIDs.

Consultations:

• In a patient with symptoms of blood dyscrasias, request a medical consultation for blood studies and postpone dental treatment until normal values are reestablished.
• Medical consultation may be required to assess disease control.

Teach Patient/Family to:

• Encourage effective oral hygiene to prevent soft tissue inflammation.
• Use caution to prevent injury when using oral hygiene aids.

• When chronic dry mouth occurs, advise patient to:
  • Avoid mouth rinses with high alcohol content because of drying effects.
  • Use daily home fluoride products for anticaries effect.
  • Use sugarless gum, frequent sips of water, or saliva substitutes.

Diclofenac Sodium (Voltaren)
General:
• Determine why patient is taking the drug.
• Protect patient's eyes from accidental spatter during dental treatment.
• Avoid dental light in patient's eyes; offer dark glasses for patient comfort.

dicloxacillin sodium
dye-**klox**′-ah-sill-in **soe**′-dee-um
(Dycil, Pathocil)

CATEGORY AND SCHEDULE
Pregnancy Risk Category: B

Drug Class: Penicillinase-resistant penicillin

MECHANISM OF ACTION
A penicillin that acts as a bactericidal in susceptible microorganisms.
Therapeutic Effect: Inhibits bacterial cell wall synthesis.

USES
Treatment of infections caused by penicillinase-producing *Staphylococcus*

PHARMACOKINETICS
Well absorbed from GI tract. Rate and extent reduced by food.

Distributed throughout body including CSF. Protein binding: 96%. Partially metabolized in liver. Primarily excreted in feces and urine. Not removed by hemodialysis. **Half-life:** 0.7 hr.

INDICATIONS AND DOSAGE
▶ **Respiratory Tract Infection, Staphylococcal and Streptococcal Infections**
PO
Adults, Elderly, Children weighing more than 40 kg. 125–250 mg q6h.
Children weighing less than 40 kg. 12.5–25 mg/kg/day q6h.

SIDE EFFECTS/ADVERSE REACTIONS
Frequent
GI disturbances (mild diarrhea, nausea, or vomiting), headache
Occasional
Generalized rash, urticaria

PRECAUTIONS AND CONTRAINDICATIONS
Hypersensitivity to any penicillin
Caution:
Hypersensitivity to cephalosporins

DRUG INTERACTIONS OF CONCERN TO DENTISTRY
• Tetracyclines: reduced effectiveness of dicloxacillin

SERIOUS REACTIONS
❗ Altered bacterial balance may result in potentially fatal superinfections and antibiotic-associated colitis as evidenced by abdominal cramps, watery or severe diarrhea, and fever.
❗ Severe hypersensitivity reactions, including anaphylaxis and acute interstitial nephritis, occur rarely.

D

D

DENTAL CONSIDERATIONS

General:
• Take precautions regarding allergy to medication.
• Determine why the patient is taking the drug.
Consultations:
• Concern for drug of choice if dental infection is also present.
Teach Patient/Family to:
• Encourage effective oral hygiene to prevent soft tissue inflammation.
• Use caution to prevent trauma when using oral hygiene aids.
• When used for dental infection, advise patient to:
  • Report sore throat, oral burning sensation, fever, and fatigue, any of which could indicate superinfection.
  • Take at prescribed intervals and complete dosage regimen.
  • Immediately notify the dentist if signs or symptoms of infection increase.

dicyclomine hydrochloride

dye-**sye**′-kloe-meen
hye-droe-**klor**′-ide
(Bentyl, Bentylol[CAN], Formulex[CAN], Lomine[CAN], Merbentyl[AUS])
Do not confuse dicyclomine with doxycycline or dyclonime, or Bentyl with Aventyl or Benadryl.

CATEGORY AND SCHEDULE

Pregnancy Risk Category: B

Drug Class: GI anticholinergic

MECHANISM OF ACTION

A GI antispasmodic and anticholinergic agent that directly acts as a relaxant on smooth muscle. ***Therapeutic Effect:*** Reduces tone and motility of GI tract.

USES

Treatment of irritable bowel syndrome

PHARMACOKINETICS

Route	Onset	Peak	Duration
PO	1–2 hr	N/A	4 hr

Readily absorbed from the GI tract. Widely distributed. Metabolized in the liver. ***Half-life:*** 9–10 hr.

INDICATIONS AND DOSAGES
▸ **Functional Disturbances of GI Motility**
PO
Adults. 10–20 mg 3–4 times a day up to 40 mg 4 times a day.
Children older than 2 yr. 10 mg 3–4 times a day.
Children 6 mos–2 yr. 5 mg 3–4 times a day.
Elderly. 10–20 mg 4 times a day. May increase up to 160 mg/day.
IM
20 mg q4–6h.

SIDE EFFECTS/ADVERSE REACTIONS

Frequent
Dry mouth (sometimes severe), constipation, diminished sweating ability
Occasional
Blurred vision; photophobia; urinary hesitancy; somnolence (with high dosage); agitation, excitement, confusion, or somnolence noted in elderly (even with low dosages); transient light-headedness (with IM

route), irritation at injection site
(with IM route)

Rare
Confusion, hypersensitivity reaction,
increased intraocular pressure,
nausea, vomiting, unusual fatigue

PRECAUTIONS AND CONTRAINDICATIONS

Bladder neck obstruction because of
prostatic hyperplasia, coronary
vasospasm, intestinal atony,
myasthenia gravis in patients not
treated with neostigmine, narrow-
angle glaucoma, obstructive disease
of the GI tract, paralytic ileus,
severe ulcerative colitis, tachycardia
secondary to cardiac insufficiency or
thyrotoxicosis, toxic megacolon,
unstable cardiovascular status in
acute hemorrhage

Caution:
Hyperthyroidism, CAD,
dysrhythmias, CHF, ulcerative colitis,
hypertension, hiatal hernia, hepatic
disease, renal disease, urinary
retention, prostatic hypertrophy

DRUG INTERACTIONS OF CONCERN TO DENTISTRY

• Increased anticholinergic effect:
atropine, scopolamine, other
anticholinergics, meperidine
• Decreased effect of ketoconazole

SERIOUS REACTIONS

! Overdose may produce temporary
paralysis of ciliary muscle; pupillary
dilation; tachycardia; palpitations;
hot, dry, or flushed skin; absence of
bowel sounds; hyperthermia;
increased respiratory rate; ECG
abnormalities; nausea; vomiting;
rash over face or upper trunk; CNS
stimulation; and psychosis (marked
by agitation, restlessness, rambling
speech, visual hallucinations,
paranoid behavior, and delusions,
followed by depression).

DENTAL CONSIDERATIONS

General:
• Assess salivary flow as a factor in
caries, periodontal disease, and
candidiasis.
• Avoid dental light in patient's eyes;
offer dark glasses for patient
comfort.

Consultation:
• Physician should be informed if
significant xerostomic side effects
occur (e.g., increased caries, sore
tongue, problems eating or
swallowing, difficulty wearing
prosthesis) so that a medication
change can be considered.

Teach Patient/Family to:
• Encourage effective oral hygiene
to prevent soft tissue inflammation.
• When chronic dry mouth occurs,
advise patient to:
• Avoid mouth rinses with high
alcohol content because of
drying effects.
• Use daily home fluoride
products for anticaries effect.
• Use sugarless gum, frequent
sips of water, or saliva
substitutes.

didanosine
dye-**dan**′-oh-seen
(Videx, Videx-EC)

CATEGORY AND SCHEDULE
Pregnancy Risk Category: B

Drug Class: Synthetic antiviral,
nucleoside analog

MECHANISM OF ACTION
A purine nucleoside analog that is
intracellularly converted into a
triphosphate, which interferes with
RNA-directed DNA polymerase
(reverse transcriptase).

Therapeutic Effect: Inhibits replication of retroviruses, including HIV.

USES

Treatment of advanced HIV infections in adults and children who have been unable to use zidovudine or who have not responded to treatment; used in combination with other antiretroviral drugs.

PHARMACOKINETICS

Variably absorbed from the GI tract. Protein binding: less than 5%. Rapidly metabolized intracellularly to active form. Primarily excreted in urine. Partially (20%) removed by hemodialysis. ***Half-life:*** 1.5 hr; metabolite: 8–24 hr.

INDICATIONS AND DOSAGES
▶ **HIV Infection (in combination with other antiretrovirals)**
PO (Chewable Tablets)
Adults, Children 13 yr and older weighing 60 kg or more. 200 mg q12h or 400 mg once a day.
Adults, Children 13 yr and older weighing 60 kg or less. 125 mg q12h or 250 mg once a day.
Children 3 mo to less than 13 yr. 180–300 mg/m²/day in divided doses q12h.
Children younger than 3 mo. 50 mg/m²/day in divided doses q12h.
PO (Delayed-Release Capsules)
Adults, Children 13 yr and older, weighing 60 kg or more. 400 mg once a day.
Adults, Children 13 yr and older, weighing 60 kg or less. 250 mg once a day.
PO (Oral Solution)
Adults, Children 13 yr and older weighing 60 kg or more. 250 mg q12h.

Adults, Children 13 yr and older weighing 60 kg or less. 167 mg q12h.
PO (Pediatric Powder for Oral Solution)
Children 3 mo to younger than 13 yr. 180–300 mg/m²/day in divided doses q12h.
Children younger than 3 mo. 50 mg/m²/day in divided doses q12h.
▶ **Dosage in Renal Impairment**

CrCl	Tablets	Oral Solution	Delayed Release Capsules
30–59 ml/min	75 mg twice a day	100 mg twice a day	125 mg once a day
10–29 ml/min	100 mg once a day	100 mg once a day	125 mg once a day
Less than 10 ml/min	75 mg once a day	100 mg once a day	N/A

*CrCl = creatinine clearance

Patients weighing 60 kg or more:

CrCl	Tablets	Oral Solution	Delayed Release Capsules
30–59 ml/min	100 mg twice a day	10 mg twice a day	200 mg once a day
10–29 ml/min	150 mg once a day	167 mg once a day	125 mg once a day
Less than 10 ml/min	100 mg once a day	100 mg once a day	125 mg once a day

*CrCl = creatinine clearance

SIDE EFFECTS/ADVERSE REACTIONS
Frequent
Adults: Diarrhea, neuropathy, chills and fever
Children: Chills, fever, decreased appetite, pain, malaise, nausea,

vomiting, diarrhea, abdominal pain, headache, nervousness, cough, rhinitis, dyspnea, asthenia, rash, pruritus

Occasional

Adults: Rash, pruritus, headache, abdominal pain, nausea, vomiting, pneumonia, myopathy, decreased appetite, dry mouth, dyspnea

Children: Failure to thrive, weight loss, stomatitis, oral thrush, ecchymosis, arthritis, myalgia, insomnia, epistaxis, pharyngitis

PRECAUTIONS AND CONTRAINDICATIONS

Hypersensitivity to didanosine or any of its components

Caution:

Renal disease, hepatic disease, lactation, children, sodium-restricted diets; pancreatitis (in combination with stavudine); lactic acidosis, severe hepatomegaly

DRUG INTERACTIONS OF CONCERN TO DENTISTRY

• Decreased absorption of the following drugs: ketoconazole, dapsone, itraconazole, tetracyclines, fluoroquinolone antibiotics

• Increased risk of pancreatitis: metronidazole, sulfonamides, sulindac, tetracyclines

• Increased risk of peripheral neuropathy: metronidazole, nitrous oxide

SERIOUS REACTIONS

! Pneumonia and opportunistic infections occur occasionally.

! Peripheral neuropathy, potentially fatal pancreatitis, retinal changes, and optic neuritis are the major toxic effects.

DENTAL CONSIDERATIONS

General:

• Monitor vital signs at every appointment because of cardiovascular side effects.

• Avoid dental light in patient's eyes; offer dark glasses for patient comfort.

• Patients on chronic drug therapy may rarely have symptoms of blood dyscrasias, which can include infection, bleeding, and poor healing.

Consultations:

• Medical consultation may be required to assess patient's ability to tolerate stress.

• In a patient with symptoms of blood dyscrasias, request a medical consultation for blood studies and postpone dental treatment until normal values are reestablished.

Teach Patient/Family to:

• Encourage effective oral hygiene to prevent soft tissue inflammation.

• Use caution to prevent injury when using oral hygiene aids.

• When chronic dry mouth occurs, advise patient to:

• Avoid mouth rinses with high alcohol content because of drying effects.

• Use daily home fluoride products for anticaries effect.

• Use sugarless gum, frequent sips of water, or saliva substitutes.

diethylpropion

die-ethyl-**prop**′-ion

(Tenuate, Tenuate Dospan)

CATEGORY AND SCHEDULE

Pregnancy Risk Category: B

Controlled Substance: Schedule IV

Drug Class: Anorexiant, amphetamine-like

MECHANISM OF ACTION

A sympathomimetic amine that stimulates the release of norepinephrine and dopamine. *Therapeutic Effect:* Decreases appetite.

USES

Treatment of exogenous obesity

PHARMACOKINETICS

Rapidly absorbed from the GI tract. Widely distributed. Metabolized in liver to active metabolite and undergoes extensive first-pass metabolism. Excreted in urine. Unknown if removed by hemodialysis. *Half-life:* 4–6 hr.

INDICATIONS AND DOSAGES
▶ **Obesity**
PO
Adults. 25 mg 3 times a day before meals. Extended-release: 75 mg at midmorning.

SIDE EFFECTS/ADVERSE REACTIONS

Frequent
Elevated B/P, nervousness, insomnia
Occasional
Dizziness, drowsiness, tremors, headache, nausea, stomach pain, fever, rash
Rare
Agranulocytosis, leukopenia, blurred vision, psychosis, CVA, seizure

PRECAUTIONS AND CONTRAINDICATIONS

Agitated states, use of MAOIs within 14 days, glaucoma, history of drug abuse, hyperthyroidism, advanced arteriosclerosis or severe cardiovascular disease, severe hypertension, and hypersensitivity to sympathomimetic amines
Caution:
Convulsive disorders, lactation

DRUG INTERACTIONS OF CONCERN TO DENTISTRY

• Dysrhythmia: hydrocarbon inhalation anesthetics
• Decreased effects: barbiturates, tricyclic antidepressants, phenothiazines

SERIOUS REACTIONS

! Overdose may produce agitation, tachycardia, palpitations, cardiac irregularities, chest pain, psychotic episode, seizures, and coma.
! Hypersensitivity reactions and blood dyscrasias occur rarely.

DENTAL CONSIDERATIONS

General:
• Monitor vital signs at every appointment because of cardiovascular and respiratory side effects.
• Examine for evidence of oral manifestations of blood dyscrasias (infection, bleeding, poor healing).
• Assess salivary flow as a factor in caries, periodontal disease, and candidiasis.
• Psychologic and physical dependence may occur with chronic administration.
• Consider semisupine chair position for patient comfort because of GI effects of disease.
Consultations:
• Medical consultation for blood studies (e.g., CBC); leukopenic or thrombocytopenic side effects may result in infection, delayed healing, and excessive bleeding. Postpone dental treatment until normal values are maintained.
Teach Patient/Family to:
• Encourage effective oral hygiene to prevent soft tissue inflammation.
• Use caution in use of oral hygiene aids to prevent injury.

- When chronic dry mouth occurs, advise patient to:
  - Avoid mouth rinses with high alcohol content because of drying effects.
  - Use daily home fluoride products for anticaries effect.
  - Use sugarless gum, frequent sips of water, or saliva substitutes.

diflorasone
die-**floor**'-ah-sone
(Florone[CAN], Maxiflor, Psorcon, Psorcon-e)

CATEGORY AND SCHEDULE
Pregnancy Risk Category: C

Drug Class: Topical corticosteroid, group II high potency

MECHANISM OF ACTION
A high-potency, fluorinated corticosteroid that decreases inflammation by suppression of migration of polymorphonuclear leukocytes and reversal of increased capillary permeability. The exact mechanism of the antiinflammatory process is unclear.
Therapeutic Effect: Decreases or prevents tissue response to the inflammatory process.

USES
Treatment of psoriasis, eczema, contact dermatitis, pruritus

PHARMACOKINETICS
Poor absorption; occlusive dressings increase absorption. Metabolized in liver. Primarily excreted in urine.

INDICATIONS AND DOSAGES
▶ Dermatoses
Topical
Adults, Elderly. (Cream) Apply sparingly 2–4 times a day. (Ointment) Apply sparingly 1–3 times a day.

SIDE EFFECTS/ADVERSE REACTIONS
Rare
Itching, redness, dryness, irritation, burning at site of application, arthralgia, folliculitis, maceration, muscle atrophy, secondary infection

PRECAUTIONS AND CONTRAINDICATIONS
History of hypersensitivity to diflorasone or other corticosteroids
Caution:
Lactation, viral infections, bacterial infections

SERIOUS REACTIONS
! Overdosage symptoms include moon face, central obesity, hypertension, diabetes, hyperlipidemia, peptic ulcer, increased susceptibility to infection, electrolyte and fluid imbalance, psychosis, and hallucinations.
! The serious reactions of long-term therapy and the addition of occlusive dressings are reversible hypothalamic-pituitary-adrenal (HPA) axis suppression, manifestations of Cushing's syndrome, hyperglycemia, and glucosuria.

DENTAL CONSIDERATIONS
General:
- Determine why the patient is taking the drug.

• Apply lubricant to dry lips for patient comfort before dental procedures.
• Place on frequent recall to evaluate healing response if used on chronic basis.

diflunisal
die-**floo**′-ni-sal
(Apo-Diflunisal[CAN], Dolobid, Novo-Diflunisal[CAN])
Do not confuse diflunisal with Dicarbosil or Dolobid with Slo-bid.

CATEGORY AND SCHEDULE
Pregnancy Risk Category: C

Drug Class: Salicylate derivative, nonsteroidal antiinflammatory

MECHANISM OF ACTION
A nonsteroidal antiinflammatory drug that inhibits prostaglandin synthesis, reducing inflammatory response and intensity of pain stimulus reaching sensory nerve endings.
Therapeutic Effect: Produces analgesic and antiinflammatory effect.

USES
Treatment of mild-to-moderate pain, symptoms of rheumatoid arthritis and osteoarthritis

PHARMACOKINETICS

Route	Onset	Peak	Duration
PO	1 hr	2–3 hr	8–12 hr

Completely absorbed from the GI tract. Widely distributed. Protein binding: greater than 99%.

Metabolized in liver. Primarily excreted in urine. Not removed by hemodialysis. *Half-life:* 8–12 hr.

INDICATIONS AND DOSAGES
▶ **Mild-to-Moderate Pain**
PO
Adults, Elderly. Initially, 0.5–1 g, then 250–500 mg q8–12h. Maximum: 1.5 g/day.
▶ **Rheumatoid Arthritis, Osteoarthritis**
PO
Adults, Elderly. 0.5–1 g/day in 2 divided doses. Maximum: 1.5 g/day.

SIDE EFFECTS/ADVERSE REACTIONS
Side effects are less common with short-term treatment.
Occasional
Nausea, dyspepsia (heartburn, indigestion, epigastric pain), diarrhea, headache, rash
Rare
Vomiting, constipation, flatulence, dizziness, somnolence, insomnia, fatigue, tinnitus

PRECAUTIONS AND CONTRAINDICATIONS
Active GI bleeding, factor VII or factor IX deficiencies, hypersensitivity to aspirin or NSAIDs
Caution:
Anemia, hepatic disease, renal disease, Hodgkin's disease, lactation

DRUG INTERACTIONS OF CONCERN TO DENTISTRY
• Increased risk of GI ulceration and bleeding: aspirin, steroids, alcohol, indomethacin, other NSAIDs
• Hepatotoxicity, nephrotoxicity: acetaminophen (prolonged use)
• Suspected increase in potential toxic effects: probenecid

SERIOUS REACTIONS

! Overdosage may produce drowsiness, vomiting, nausea, diarrhea, hyperventilation, tachycardia, diaphoresis, stupor, and coma.

! Peptic ulcer, GI bleeding, gastritis, and severe hepatic reaction, including cholestasis, jaundice occur rarely.

! Nephrotoxicity, including dysuria, hematuria, proteinuria, and nephrotic syndrome, and severe hypersensitivity reaction, marked by bronchospasm and angioedema, occur rarely.

DENTAL CONSIDERATIONS

General:

• Patients on chronic drug therapy may rarely have symptoms of blood dyscrasias, which can include infection, bleeding, and poor healing.

• Assess salivary flow as a factor in caries, periodontal disease, and candidiasis.

• Avoid prescribing for dental use in first and last trimester of pregnancy.

• Use with caution in patients with cardiovascular disease at risk for thromboembolism.

• Severe stomach bleeding may occur in patients who regularly use NSAIDs in recommended doses, when the patient is also taking another NSAID, anticoagulant/antiplatelet, or steroid drug, if the patient has GI or peptic ulcer disease, if they are 60 years or older, or when NSAIDs are taken longer than directed. Warn patients of the potential for severe stomach bleeding.

Consultations:

• Medical consultation may be required to assess disease control.

• In a patient with symptoms of blood dyscrasias, request a medical consultation for blood studies and postpone dental treatment until normal values are reestablished.

Teach Patient/Family to:

• Encourage effective oral hygiene to prevent soft tissue inflammation.

• Prevent injury when using oral hygiene aids.

• Warn patient of potential risks of NSAIDs.

• When chronic dry mouth occurs, advise patient to:

  • Avoid mouth rinses with high alcohol content because of drying effects.

  • Use daily home fluoride products for anticaries effect.

  • Use sugarless gum, frequent sips of water, or saliva substitutes.

digoxin

di-**jox**'-in

(Digitek, Lanoxicaps, Lanoxin, Sigmaxin[AUS])

Do not confuse digoxin with Desoxyn or doxepin, or Lanoxin with Levsinex or Lonox.

CATEGORY AND SCHEDULE

Pregnancy Risk Category: C

Drug Class: Cardiac glycoside

MECHANISM OF ACTION

A cardiac glycoside that increases the influx of calcium from extracellular to intracellular cytoplasm.

Therapeutic Effect: Potentiates the activity of the contractile cardiac muscle fibers and increases the force of myocardial contraction. Slows the heart rate by decreasing conduction through the SA and AV nodes.

USES

Treatment of CHF, atrial fibrillation, atrial flutter, paroxysmal atrial tachycardia, rapid digitalization in these disorders

PHARMACOKINETICS

Route	Onset	Peak	Duration
PO	0.5–2 hr	28 hr	3–4 days
IV	5–30 hr	1–4 hr	3–4 days

Readily absorbed from the GI tract. Widely distributed. Protein binding: 30%. Partially metabolized in the liver. Primarily excreted in urine. Minimally removed by hemodialysis. *Half-life:* 36–48 hr (increased with impaired renal function and in the elderly).

INDICATIONS AND DOSAGES
▸ **Rapid Loading Dose for the Management and Treatment of CHF; Control of Ventricular Rate in Patients with Atrial Fibrillation; Treatment and Prevention of Recurrent Paroxysmal Atrial Tachycardia**
PO
Adults, Elderly. Initially, 0.5–0.75 mg, additional doses of 0.125–0.375 mg at 6- to 8-hr intervals. Range: 0.75–1.25 mg.
Children 10 yr and older. 10–15 mcg/kg.
Children 5–9 yr. 20–35 mcg/kg.
Children 2–4 yr. 30–40 mcg/kg.
Children 1–23 mo. 35–60 mcg/kg.
Neonate, full-term. 25–35 mcg/kg.
Neonate, premature. 20–30 mcg/kg.
IV
Adults, Elderly. 0.6–1 mg.
Children 10 yr and older. 8–12 mcg/kg.
Children 5–9 yr. 15–30 mcg/kg.
Children 2–4 yr. 25–35 mcg/kg.
Children 1–23 mo. 30–50 mcg/kg.
Neonates, full-term. 20–30 mcg/kg.
Neonates, premature. 15–25 mcg/kg.
▸ **Maintenance Dosage for CHF; Control of Ventricular Rate in Patients with Atrial Fibrillation; Treatment and Prevention of Recurrent Paroxysmal Atrial Tachycardia**
PO, IV
Adults, Elderly. 0.125–0.375 mg/day.
Children. 25%–35% loading dose (20%–30% for premature neonates).
▸ **Dosage in Renal Impairment**
Dosage adjustment is based on creatinine clearance. Total digitalizing dose: decrease by 50% in end-stage renal disease.

Creatinine Clearance	Dosage
10–50 ml/min	25%–75% usual
Less than 10 ml/min	10%–25% usual

SIDE EFFECTS/ADVERSE REACTIONS

There is a very narrow margin of safety between a therapeutic and toxic result, cardiac dysrhythmias, nausea, vomiting, visual scotomas.

PRECAUTIONS AND CONTRAINDICATIONS

❗ Ventricular fibrillation, ventricular tachycardia unrelated to CHF
Caution:
Renal disease, acute MI, AV block, severe respiratory disease, hypothyroidism, elderly, sinus nodal disease, lactation, hypokalemia

DRUG INTERACTIONS OF CONCERN TO DENTISTRY

• Hypokalemia: corticosteroids
• Increased digoxin blood levels: erythromycin, clarithromycin, tetracyclines, itraconazole, propantheline

D

• Cardiac dysrhythmias: adrenergic agonists, succinylcholine

SERIOUS REACTIONS

! The most common early manifestations of digoxin toxicity are GI disturbances (anorexia, nausea, vomiting) and neurologic abnormalities (fatigue, headache, depression, weakness, drowsiness, confusion, nightmares).

! Facial pain, personality change, and ocular disturbances (photophobia, light flashes, halos around bright objects, yellow or green color perception) may be noted.

DENTAL CONSIDERATIONS

General:

• Monitor vital signs at every appointment because of cardiovascular side effects.

• After supine positioning, have patient sit upright for at least 2 min to avoid orthostatic hypotension.

• Avoid dental light in patient's eyes; offer dark glasses for patient comfort.

• An increased gag reflex may make dental procedures, such as taking radiographs or impressions, difficult.

• Use vasoconstrictors with caution, in low doses, and with careful aspiration. Avoid use of gingival retraction cord with epinephrine.

Consultations:

• Stress from dental procedures may compromise cardiovascular function; determine patient risk.

• Use stress-reduction protocol.

• Medical consultation may be required to assess disease control and patient's ability to tolerate stress.

dihydrotachysterol
dye-hye-droe-tak-ee-**ster**′-ole
(DHT, DHT Intensol, Hytakerol)

CATEGORY AND SCHEDULE
Pregnancy Risk Category: A (D if used in doses above RDA)

Drug Class: Vitamin D analog

MECHANISM OF ACTION
A fat-soluble vitamin that is essential for absorption, utilization of calcium phosphate, and normal calcification of bone.
Therapeutic Effect: Stimulates calcium and phosphate absorption from small intestine, promotes secretion of calcium from bone to blood, promotes renal tubule phosphate resorption, acts on bone cells to stimulate skeletal growth and on parathyroid gland to suppress hormone synthesis and secretion.

USES
Nutritional supplement, treatment of rickets, hypoparathyroidism, pseudo-hypoparathyroidism, postoperative tetany

PHARMACOKINETICS
Well absorbed from small intestine. Metabolized in liver. Eliminated via biliary system; excreted in urine.
Half-life: Unknown.

INDICATIONS AND DOSAGES
▶ Hypoparathyroidism
PO
Adults, Elderly, Older Children. Initially, 0.8–2.4 mg/day for several days. Maintenance: 0.2–1 mg/day.
Infants, Young Children. Initially, 1–5 mg/day for 4 days, then 0.1–0.5 mg/day.

▸ **Nutritional Rickets**
PO
Adults, Elderly, Children. 0.5 mg as a single dose or 13–50 mcg/day until healing occurs.
▸ **Renal Osteodystrophy**
PO
Adults, Elderly. 0.25–0.6 mg/24 hr adjusted as needed to achieve normal serum calcium levels and promote bone healing.

SIDE EFFECTS/ADVERSE REACTIONS
Occasional
Nausea, vomiting

PRECAUTIONS AND CONTRAINDICATIONS
Hypercalcemia, malabsorption syndrome, vitamin D toxicity, hypersensitivity to vitamin D products or analogs
Caution:
Renal calculi, lactation, cardiovascular disease

DRUG INTERACTIONS OF CONCERN TO DENTISTRY
• Decreased effect of dihydrotachysterol: prolonged use of corticosteroids, barbiturates

SERIOUS REACTIONS
! Early signs of overdosage are manifested as weakness, headache, somnolence, nausea, vomiting, dry mouth, constipation, muscle and bone pain, and metallic taste sensation.
! Later signs of overdosage are evidenced by polyuria, polydipsia, anorexia, weight loss, nocturia, photophobia, rhinorrhea, pruritus, disorientation, hallucinations, hyperthermia, hypertension, and cardiac arrhythmias.

DENTAL CONSIDERATIONS
General:
• Consider semisupine chair position for patient comfort because of GI effects of drug.
• Assess salivary flow as a factor in caries, periodontal disease, and candidiasis.
Teach Patient/Family:
• When chronic dry mouth occurs, advise patient to:
  • Avoid mouth rinses with high alcohol content because of drying effects.
  • Use daily home fluoride products for anticaries effect.
  • Use sugarless gum, frequent sips of water, or saliva substitutes.

diltiazem hydrochloride
dil-**tye**′-ah-zem hi-droh-**klor**′-ide
(Apo-Diltiaz[CAN], Auscard[AUS], Cardcal[AUS], Cardizem, Cardizem CD, Cardizem LA, Cardizem SR, Cartia, Coras[AUS], Dilacor XR, Diltahexal[AUS], Diltia XT, Diltiamax[AUS], Dilzem[AUS], Novo-Diltiazem[CAN], Taztia XT, Tiazac, Vasocardal CD[AUS])
Do not confuse Cardizem with Cardene or Cardene SR, or Tiazac with Ziac.

CATEGORY AND SCHEDULE
Pregnancy Risk Category: C

Drug Class: Calcium channel blocker

MECHANISM OF ACTION
An antianginal, antihypertensive, and antiarrhythmic agent that inhibits calcium movement across

D

cardiac and vascular smooth-muscle cell membranes. This action causes the dilation of coronary arteries, peripheral arteries, and arterioles. **Therapeutic Effect:** Decreases heart rate and myocardial contractility, slows SA and AV conduction, and decreases total peripheral vascular resistance by vasodilation.

USES

Treatment of chronic stable angina pectoris, vasospastic angina, coronary artery spasm, hypertension, supraventricular tachydysrhythmias

PHARMACOKINETICS

Route	Onset	Peak	Duration
PO	0.5–1 hr	N/A	
PO (extended release)	2–3 hr	N/A	
IV	3 min	N/A	

Well absorbed from the GI tract. Protein binding: 70%–80%. Undergoes first-pass metabolism in the liver to active metabolite. Primarily excreted in urine. Not removed by hemodialysis. *Half-life:* 3–8 hr.

INDICATIONS AND DOSAGES
▶ **Angina Related to Coronary Artery Spasm (Prinzmetal's Variant), Chronic Stable Angina (Effort-Associated)**
PO
Adults, Elderly. Initially, 30 mg 4 times a day. Increase up to 180–360 mg/day in 3–4 divided doses at 1- to 2-day intervals.
PO (Cardizem LA)
Adults, Elderly. Initially, 180 mg/day. May increase at intervals of 7–14 days up to 360 mg/day.

PO (Cardizem CD)
Adults, Elderly. Initially, 120–180 mg/day; titrate over 7–14 days. Range: Up to 480 mg/day.
▶ **Essential Hypertension**
PO (Cardizem CD, Cartia XT)
Adults, Elderly. Initially, 180–240 mg once a day. May increase at 2-wk intervals. Maintenance 240–360 mg/day. Maximum: 480 mg once a day.
PO (Cardizem SR)
Adults, Elderly. Initially, 60–120 mg twice a day. May increase at 2-wk intervals.
Maintenance: 240–360 mg/day.
PO (Cardizem LA)
Adults, Elderly. Initially, 180–240 mg once a day. May increase at 2-wk intervals. Maintenance: 120–540 mg/day.
PO (Dilacor XR)
Adults, Elderly. 180–240 mg once a day.
PO (Dilacor XT)
Adults, Elderly. Initially, 180–240 mg a day. May increase at 2-wk intervals. Maximum: 540 mg once a day.
PO (Taztia XT)
Adults, Elderly. Initially, 120–240 mg once a day. May increase at 2-wk intervals. Maximum: 540 mg once a day.
▶ **Temporary Control of Rapid Ventricular Rate in Atrial Fibrillation or Flutter, Rapid Conversion of Paroxysmal Supraventricular Tachycardia to Normal Sinus Rhythm.**
IV Push
Adults, Elderly. Initially, 0.25 mg/kg actual body weight over 2 min. May repeat in 15 min at dose of 0.35 mg/kg actual body weight. Subsequent doses individualized.
IV Infusion
Adults, Elderly. After initial bolus injection, may begin infusion at

5–10 mg/hr; may increase by 5 mg/hr up to a maximum of 15 mg/hr. Infusion duration should not exceed 24 hr.

SIDE EFFECTS/ADVERSE REACTIONS
Frequent
Peripheral edema, dizziness, light-headedness, headache, bradycardia, asthenia (loss of strength, weakness)
Occasional
Nausea, constipation, flushing, ECG changes
Rare
Rash, micturition disorder (polyuria, nocturia, dysuria, frequency of urination), abdominal discomfort, somnolence

PRECAUTIONS AND CONTRAINDICATIONS
Acute MI, pulmonary congestion, severe hypotension (less than 90 mm Hg, systolic), sick sinus syndrome, second- or third-degree AV block (except in the presence of a pacemaker)
Caution:
CHF, hypotension, hepatic injury, lactation, children, renal disease

DRUG INTERACTIONS OF CONCERN TO DENTISTRY
• Decreased effect: indomethacin, possibly other NSAIDs, phenobarbital
• Increased effect: parenteral and inhalational general anesthetics, other drugs with hypotensive actions
• Increased effects of carbamazepine, midazolam, triazolam, buspirone

SERIOUS REACTIONS
❗ Abrupt withdrawal may increase frequency or duration of angina.

❗ CHF and second- and third-degree AV block occur rarely.
❗ Overdose produces nausea, somnolence, confusion, slurred speech, and profound bradycardia.

DENTAL CONSIDERATIONS
General:
• Monitor cardiac status; take vital signs at each appointment because of cardiovascular side effects. Consider a stress-reduction protocol to prevent angina during the dental appointment.
• After supine positioning, have patient sit upright for at least 2 min to avoid orthostatic hypotension.
• Place on frequent recall to monitor possible gingival enlargement.
• Limit use of sodium-containing products, such as saline IV fluids, for patients with a dietary salt restriction.
• Assess salivary flow as a factor in caries, periodontal disease, and candidiasis.
• Consider drug in diagnosis of taste alterations.
Consultations:
• Medical consultation may be required to assess disease control.
Teach Patient/Family to:
• Encourage effective oral hygiene to prevent soft tissue inflammation and minimize gingival overgrowth.
• Schedule frequent oral prophylaxis if gingival overgrowth occurs.
• When chronic dry mouth occurs, advise patient to:
  • Avoid mouth rinses with high alcohol content because of drying effects.
  • Use daily home fluoride products for anticaries effect.
  • Use sugarless gum, frequent sips of water, or saliva substitutes.

dimenhydrinate
dye-men-**hye**´-dri-nate
(Dramamine)

CATEGORY AND SCHEDULE
Pregnancy Risk Category: B

Drug Class: H$_1$-receptor antagonist (equal parts diphenhydramine and chlorotheophylline)

MECHANISM OF ACTION
An antihistamine and anticholinergic that competes for H$_1$ receptor sites on effector cells of the GI tract, blood vessels, and respiratory tract. The anticholinergic action diminishes vestibular stimulation and depresses labyrinthine function. **Therapeutic Effect:** Prevents symptoms of motion sickness.

USES
Treatment of motion sickness, nausea, vomiting, vertigo

PHARMACOKINETICS
IM/PO: Duration 4–6 hr.

INDICATIONS AND DOSAGES
▸ Motion Sickness
PO
Adults, Elderly, Children older than 12 yr. 50–100 mg q4–6h. Maximum: 400 mg/day.
Children 6–12 yr. 25–50 mg q6–8h. Maximum: 150 mg/day.
Children 2–5 yr. 12.5–25 mg q6–8h. Maximum: 75 mg/day.

SIDE EFFECTS/ADVERSE REACTIONS
Frequent
Dry mouth
Occasional
Hypotension, palpitations, tachycardia, headache, somnolence, dizziness, paradoxical stimulation (especially in children), anorexia, constipation, dysuria, blurred vision, tinnitus, wheezing, chest tightness
Rare
Photosensitivity, rash, urticaria

PRECAUTIONS AND CONTRAINDICATIONS
Hypersensitivity to narcotics, shock
Caution:
Children, cardiac dysrhythmias, elderly, asthma, prostatic hypertrophy, bladder neck obstruction, narrow-angle glaucoma, stenosing peptic ulcer, pyloroduodenal obstruction, may mask ototoxicity of ototoxic antibiotics

DRUG INTERACTIONS OF CONCERN TO DENTISTRY
• Increased photosensitization: tetracycline
• Increased effects of alcohol, other CNS depressants, anticholinergics

SERIOUS REACTIONS
! None significant

DENTAL CONSIDERATIONS

General:
• Assess salivary flow as a factor in caries, periodontal disease, and candidiasis.
Teach Patient/Family to:
• When chronic dry mouth occurs, advise patient to:
  • Avoid mouth rinses with high alcohol content because of drying effects.
  • Use daily home fluoride products for anticaries effect.
  • Use sugarless gum, frequent sips of water, or saliva substitutes.

diphenhydramine

dye-fen-**hye**′-dra-meen
(Allerdryl[CAN], Banophen,
Benadryl, Diphen, Diphenhist,
Genahist, Nytol[CAN], Unisom
Sleepgels[AUS])
Do not confuse diphenhydramine
with dimenhydrinate or Benadryl
with benazepril, Bentyl, or
Benylin, or Banophen with
baclofen.

CATEGORY AND SCHEDULE

Pregnancy Risk Category: B
OTC (capsules, tablets, chewable
tablets, syrup, elixir, cream, spray)

Drug Class: Antihistamine,
H_1-receptor antagonist

MECHANISM OF ACTION

An ethanolamine that competitively
blocks the effects of histamine at
peripheral H_1 receptor sites.
Therapeutic Effect: Produces
anticholinergic, antipruritic,
antitussive, antiemetic,
antidyskinetic, and sedative effects.

USES

Allergy symptoms, rhinitis, motion
sickness, antiparkinsonism,
nighttime sedation, infant colic,
nonproductive cough; unlabeled use
for dental local anesthesia

PHARMACOKINETICS

Route	Onset	Peak	Duration
PO	15–30 min	1–4 hr	4–6 hr
IV, IM	Less than 15 min	1–4 hr	4–6 hr

Well absorbed after PO or parenteral
administration. Protein binding:
98%–99%. Widely distributed.

Metabolized in the liver. Primarily
excreted in urine. ***Half-life:*** 1–4 hr.

INDICATIONS AND DOSAGES
▶ **Moderate to Severe Allergic
Reaction, Dystonic Reaction**
PO, IV, IM
Adults, Elderly. 25–50 mg q4h.
Maximum: 400 mg/day.
Children. 5 mg/kg/day in divided
doses q6–8h. Maximum: 300 mg/day.
▶ **Motion Sickness, Minor Allergic
Rhinitis**
PO, IV, IM
*Adults, Elderly, Children 12 yr and
older.* 25–50 mg q4–6h. Maximum:
300 mg/day.
Children 6–11 yr. 12.5–25 mg
q4–6h. Maximum: 150 mg/day.
Children 2–5 yr. 6.25 mg q4–6h.
Maximum: 37.5 mg/day.
▶ **Antitussive**
PO
*Adults, Elderly, Children 12 yr and
older.* 25 mg q4h. Maximum:
150 mg/day.
Children 6–11 yr. 12.5 mg q4h.
Maximum: 75 mg/day.
Children 2–5 yr. 6.25 mg q4h.
Maximum: 37.5 mg/day.
▶ **Nighttime Sleep Aid**
PO
*Adults, Elderly, Children 12 yr and
older.* 50 mg at bedtime.
Children 2–11 yr. 1 mg/kg/dose.
Maximum: 50 mg.
▶ **Pruritus**
Topical
*Adults, Elderly, Children 12 yr and
older.* Apply 1% or 2% cream or
spray 3–4 times a day.
Children 2–11 yr. Apply 1% cream
or spray 3–4 times a day.

SIDE EFFECTS/ADVERSE
REACTIONS
Frequent
Somnolence, dizziness, muscle
weakness, hypotension, urine

retention, thickening of bronchial secretions, dry mouth, nose, throat, or lips; in elderly, sedation, dizziness, hypotension

Occasional

Epigastric distress, flushing, visual or hearing disturbances, paresthesia, diaphoresis, chills

PRECAUTIONS AND CONTRAINDICATIONS

Acute exacerbation of asthma, use within 14 days of MAOIs

Caution:

Increased intraocular pressure, renal disease, cardiac disease, hypertension, bronchial asthma, seizure disorder, stenosed peptic ulcers, hyperthyroidism, prostatic hypertrophy, bladder neck obstruction

DRUG INTERACTIONS OF CONCERN TO DENTISTRY

• Increased CNS depression: all CNS depressants, alcohol
• Increased anticholinergic effect: anticholinergics
• Increased plasma levels of labetalol

SERIOUS REACTIONS

❗ Hypersensitivity reactions, such as eczema, pruritus, rash, cardiac disturbances, and photosensitivity, may occur.
❗ Overdose symptoms may vary from CNS depression, including sedation, apnea, hypotension, cardiovascular collapse, and death, to severe paradoxical reactions, such as hallucinations, tremors, and seizures.
❗ Children and neonates may experience paradoxical reactions, including restlessness, insomnia, euphoria, nervousness, and tremors.

❗ Overdosage in children may result in hallucinations, seizures, and death.

DENTAL CONSIDERATIONS

General:

• Patients on chronic drug therapy may rarely have symptoms of blood dyscrasias, which can include infection, bleeding, and poor healing.
• Assess salivary flow as a factor in caries, periodontal disease, and candidiasis.
• Consider semisupine chair position for patients with respiratory disease.

Consultations:

• In a patient with symptoms of blood dyscrasias, request a medical consultation for blood studies and postpone dental treatment until normal values are reestablished.

Teach Patient/Family to:

• Encourage effective oral hygiene to prevent soft tissue inflammation.
• Use caution to prevent injury when using oral hygiene aids.
• When chronic dry mouth occurs, advise patient to:
  • Avoid mouth rinses with high alcohol content because of drying effects.
  • Use daily home fluoride products for anticaries effect.
  • Use sugarless gum, frequent sips of water, or saliva substitutes.

dipivefrin hydrochloride

die-**pih**′-ve-frin hi-droh-**klor**′-ide
(Propine)

CATEGORY AND SCHEDULE

Pregnancy Risk Category: B

Drug Class: Adrenergic agonist

MECHANISM OF ACTION

A prodrug of epinephrine that penetrates into anterior chamber of the eye through its lipophilic character.
Therapeutic Effect: Reduces intraocular pressure.

USES

Treatment of open-angle glaucoma

PHARMACOKINETICS

Onset of action occurs within 30 min and peak effect in 1 hr. Dipivefrin is more lipophilic than epinephrine. Distributed to cornea. Dipivefrin is converted to epinephrine inside the eye by enzyme hydrolysis.

INDICATIONS AND DOSAGES

▸ **Glaucoma, Open-Angle**
Ophthalmic, Topical
Adults, Elderly. Instill 1 drop of 0.1% solution in affected eye(s) q12h.

SIDE EFFECTS/ADVERSE REACTIONS

Occasional
Blurred vision, burning or stinging of eye, mydriasis, headache
Rare
Follicular conjunctivitis

PRECAUTIONS AND CONTRAINDICATIONS

Narrow-angle glaucoma, hypersensitivity to dipivefrin or any component of the formulation
Caution:
Lactation, children, aphakia

DRUG INTERACTIONS OF CONCERN TO DENTISTRY

• Avoid use of anticholinergics such as atropine, scopolamine, and propantheline; use benzodiazepines with caution.

SERIOUS REACTIONS

❗ Signs of systemic absorption include hypertension, arrhythmias, and tachycardia.
❗ Follicular conjunctivitis has been reported.

DENTAL CONSIDERATIONS

General:
• Avoid dental light in patient's eyes; offer dark glasses for patient comfort.

dipyridamole

die-peer-**id**′-ah-mole
(Apo-Dipyridamole[CAN],
Novodipiradol[CAN],
Persantin[AUS], Persantin
100[AUS], Persantin SR[AUS],
Persantine)
Do not confuse Aggrenox with Aggrastat, or dipyridamole with disopyramide, or Persantin with Periactin.

CATEGORY AND SCHEDULE

Pregnancy Risk Category: C

Drug Class: Platelet aggregation inhibitor

MECHANISM OF ACTION

A blood modifier and platelet aggregation inhibitor that inhibits the activity of adenosine deaminase and phosphodiesterase, enzymes causing accumulation of adenosine and cyclic adenosine monophosphate.
Therapeutic Effect: Inhibits platelet aggregation; may cause coronary vasodilation.

USES

Adjunctive therapy with warfarin in prosthetic heart valve replacement

D

PHARMACOKINETICS

Slowly, variably absorbed from the GI tract. Widely distributed. Protein binding: 91%–99%. Metabolized in the liver. Primarily eliminated via biliary excretion. *Half-life:* 10–15 hr.

INDICATIONS AND DOSAGES
▶ **Prevention of Thromboembolic Disorders**
PO
Adults, Elderly. 75–400 mg/day in combination with other medications.
Children. 3–6 mg/kg/day in 3 divided doses.
▶ **Diagnostic Aid**
IV
Adults, Elderly (based on weight). 0.142 mg/kg/min infused over 4 min; although a maximum hasn't been determined, doses greater than 60 mg have been determined to be unnecessary for any patient.

SIDE EFFECTS/ADVERSE REACTIONS
Frequent
Dizziness
Occasional
Abdominal distress, headache, rash
Rare
Diarrhea, vomiting, flushing, pruritus

PRECAUTIONS AND CONTRAINDICATIONS
Hypersensitivity, hypotension
Caution:
Children younger than 12 yr

DRUG INTERACTIONS OF CONCERN TO DENTISTRY
• Additive antiplatelet effects: aspirin, other NSAIDs

SERIOUS REACTIONS
! Overdose produces peripheral vasodilation, resulting in hypotension.

DENTAL CONSIDERATIONS

General:
• Monitor vital signs at every appointment because of cardiovascular side effects.
• After supine positioning, have patient sit upright for at least 2 min to avoid orthostatic hypotension.
• Avoid prescribing NSAIDs and aspirin-containing products, even though ASA/dipyridamole combination drugs are used in some patients.
• Patients with prosthetic valves require antibiotic prophylaxis.
• Evaluate for clotting ability during gingival instrumentation because inhibition of platelet aggregation may occur.
• Consider local hemostatic measures to prevent excessive bleeding during instrumentation.
Consultations:
• Medical consultation should include PTT or INR.
• Medical consultation may be required to assess disease control.
Teach Patient/Family to:
• Encourage effective oral hygiene to prevent gingival inflammation.

dirithromycin
die-rith-ro-**my**′-sin
(Dynabac)
Do not confuse Dynabac with Dynacin or DynaCirc.

CATEGORY AND SCHEDULE
Pregnancy Risk Category: C

Drug Class: Macrolide antibiotic

MECHANISM OF ACTION
A macrolide that binds to ribosomal receptor sites of susceptible

organisms, inhibiting bacterial protein synthesis.
Therapeutic Effect: Bactericidal or bacteriostatic, depending on drug dosage.

USES
Treatment of acute and secondary bacterial infection of acute bronchitis, community-acquired pneumonia, streptococcal pharyngitis, and uncomplicated skin and skin-structure infections

PHARMACOKINETICS
Rapidly absorbed from the GI tract. Protein binding: 15%–30%. Widely distributed into tissues and within cells. Eliminated primarily unchanged by biliary excretion. Not removed by hemodialysis. *Half-life:* 30–44 hr.

INDICATIONS AND DOSAGES
▶ **Pharyngitis, Tonsillitis**
PO
Adults, Elderly, Children 12 yr and older. 500 mg once a day for 10 days.
▶ **Acute or Chronic Bronchitis, Skin and Skin-Structure Infections**
PO
Adults, Elderly, Children 12 yr and older. 500 mg once a day for 7 days.
▶ **Community-Acquired Pneumonia**
PO
Adults, Elderly, Children 12 yr and older. 500 mg once a day for 14 days.

SIDE EFFECTS/ADVERSE REACTIONS
Frequent
Abdominal pain, headache, nausea, diarrhea
Occasional
Vomiting, dyspepsia, dizziness, nonspecific pain, asthenia

Rare
Increased cough, flatulence, rash, dyspnea, pruritus and urticaria, insomnia

PRECAUTIONS AND CONTRAINDICATIONS
Hypersensitivity to dirithromycin or other macrolide antibiotics
Caution:
Not for *H. influenzae* or *S. pyogenes* infections, lactation, children younger than 12 yr

DRUG INTERACTIONS OF CONCERN TO DENTISTRY
• Other drug interactions: data are limited; antacids and histamine H_2 antagonists tend to enhance absorption; refer to erythromycin for potential interacting drugs.

SERIOUS REACTIONS
! Antibiotic-associated colitis and other superinfections may result from altered bacterial balance.

DENTAL CONSIDERATIONS
General:
• Do not use in patients at risk for bacteremias caused by inadequate serum levels.
• Potential value in dental infections is unknown.
• Determine why the patient is taking the drug.
• Examine for oral manifestations of opportunistic infections.
Consultations:
• Medical consultation may be required to assess disease control.
Teach Patient/Family to:
• Be aware of the possibility of secondary oral infection and the need to see dentist immediately if infection occurs.

D

disopyramide phosphate

die-soe-**peer**′-ah-mide
(Norpace, Norpace CR,
Rythmodan[CAN])
Do not confuse disopyramide with
desipramine, dipyridamole, or
Rythmol.

CATEGORY AND SCHEDULE
Pregnancy Risk Category: C

Drug Class: Antidysrhythmic
(class Ia)

MECHANISM OF ACTION
An antiarrhythmic that prolongs the
refractory period of the cardiac cell
by direct effect, decreasing
myocardial excitability and
conduction velocity.
Therapeutic Effect: Depresses
myocardial contractility. Has
anticholinergic and negative
inotropic effects.

USES
Treatment of premature ventricular
contractions (PVCs), ventricular
tachycardia

PHARMACOKINETICS
PO: Peak 30 min–3 hr, duration
6–12 hr. *Half-life:* 4–10 hr;
metabolized in liver; excreted in
feces, urine, breast milk; crosses
placenta.

INDICATIONS AND DOSAGES
▸ **Suppression and Prevention of
Ventricular Ectopy, Unifocal or
Multifocal Premature Ventricular
Contractions, Paired Ventricular
Contractions (Couplets), and
Episodes of Ventricular
Tachycardia**

PO
*Adults, Elderly weighing 50 kg and
more.* 150 mg q6h (300 mg q12h
with extended-release).
*Adults, Elderly weighing less than
50 kg.* 100 mg q6h (200 mg q12h
with extended-release).
▸ **Rapid Control of Arrhythmias**
PO
*Adults, Elderly weighing 50 kg and
more.* Initially, 300 mg, then 150 mg
q6h or 300 mg (controlled release)
q12h.
*Adults, Elderly weighing less than
50 kg.* Initially, 200 mg, then
100 mg q6h or 200 mg (controlled
release) q12h.
▸ **Severe Refractory Arrhythmias**
PO
Adults, Elderly. Up to 400 mg q6h.
Children 12–18 yr. 6–15 mg/kg/day
in divided doses q6h.
Children 5–11 yr. 10–15 mg/kg/day
in divided doses q6h.
Children 1–4 yr. 10–20 mg/kg/day
in divided doses q6h.
Children younger than 1 yr.
10–30 mg/kg/day in divided doses
q6h.
▸ **Dosage in Renal Impairment**
With or without loading dose of
150 mg:

Creatinine Clearance	Dosage
40 ml/min and higher	100 mg q6h (extended-release 200 mg q12h)
30–39 ml/min	100 mg q8h
15–29 ml/min	100 mg q12h
Less than 15 ml/min	100 mg q24h

▸ **Dosage in Liver Impairment**
*Adults, Elderly weighing 50 kg and
more.* 100 mg q6h (200 mg q12h
with extended-release).
▸ **Dosage in Cardiomyopathy,
Cardiac Decompensation**

Adults, Elderly weighing 50 kg and more. No loading dose; 100 mg q6–8h with gradual dosage adjustments.

SIDE EFFECTS/ADVERSE REACTIONS
Frequent
Dry mouth (32%), urinary hesitancy, constipation
Occasional
Blurred vision, dry eyes, nose, or throat, urinary retention, headache, dizziness, fatigue, nausea
Rare
Impotence, hypotension, edema, weight gain, shortness of breath, syncope, chest pain, nervousness, diarrhea, vomiting, decreased appetite, rash, itching

PRECAUTIONS AND CONTRAINDICATIONS
Cardiogenic shock, narrow-angle glaucoma (unless patient is undergoing cholinergic therapy), preexisting second- or third-degree AV block, preexisting urinary retention
Caution:
Lactation, diabetes mellitus, renal disease, children, hepatic disease, myasthenia gravis, narrow-angle glaucoma, cardiomyopathy, conduction abnormalities

DRUG INTERACTIONS OF CONCERN TO DENTISTRY
• Possible increased risk of prolonged QT interval: clarithromycin, erythromycin
• Increased side effects: anticholinergics, alcohol
• Decreased effects: barbiturates, corticosteroids

SERIOUS REACTIONS
❗ May produce or aggravate CHF.

❗ May produce severe hypotension, shortness of breath, chest pain, syncope (especially in patients with primary cardiomyopathy or CHF).
❗ Hepatotoxicity occurs rarely.

DENTAL CONSIDERATIONS
General:
• Monitor vital signs at every appointment because of cardiovascular side effects.
• Consider a stress-reduction protocol.
• After supine positioning, have patient sit upright for at least 2 min before standing to avoid orthostatic hypotension.
• Patients on chronic drug therapy may rarely have symptoms of blood dyscrasias, which can include infection, bleeding, and poor healing.
• Assess salivary flow as a factor in caries, periodontal disease, and candidiasis.
Consultations:
• In a patient with symptoms of blood dyscrasias, request a medical consultation for blood studies and postpone dental treatment until normal values are reestablished.
• Medical consultation may be required to assess disease control and patient's ability to tolerate stress.
Teach Patient/Family to:
• Encourage effective oral hygiene to prevent soft tissue inflammation.
• When chronic dry mouth occurs, advise patient to:
  • Avoid mouth rinses with high alcohol content because of drying effects.
  • Use daily home fluoride products for anticaries effect.
  • Use sugarless gum, frequent sips of water, or saliva substitutes.

D

disulfiram
die-**sul'**-fi-ram
(Antabuse)

CATEGORY AND SCHEDULE
Pregnancy Risk Category: C

Drug Class: Aldehyde
dehydrogenase inhibitor

MECHANISM OF ACTION
A thiuram derivative and an
irreversible aldehyde dehydrogenase
inhibitor. When taken with alcohol,
there is an increase in serum
acetaldehyde levels.
Therapeutic Effect: Produces an
acute sensitivity to alcohol.

USES
Treatment of chronic alcoholism (as
adjunct)

PHARMACOKINETICS
Slowly absorbed from GI tract.
Metabolized in liver. Primarily
excreted in urine. Up to 20% of
dose remains in body for at least
1 wk. **Half-life:** Unknown.

INDICATIONS AND DOSAGES
▸ Adjunct in Management of
Selected Chronic Alcoholic Patients
Who Want to Remain in State of
Enforced Sobriety
PO
Adults, Elderly. Initially, administer
maximum of 500 mg daily given as
a single dose for 1–2 wk.
Maintenance: 250 mg daily (normal
range: 125–500 mg). Do not exceed
maximum daily dose of 500 mg.

SIDE EFFECTS/ADVERSE
REACTIONS
Frequent
Drowsiness

Occasional
Headache, restlessness, optic neuritis
(impaired color perception, altered
vision), peripheral neuropathy,
metallic or garlic taste, rash

PRECAUTIONS AND
CONTRAINDICATIONS
Severe heart disease, psychosis,
hypersensitivity to disulfiram or any
component of the formulation
Caution:
Hypothyroidism, hepatic disease,
diabetes mellitus, seizure disorders,
nephritis, cerebral damage

DRUG INTERACTIONS OF
CONCERN TO DENTISTRY
• Increased CNS depression:
long-acting benzodiazepines
• Increased disulfiram reaction:
alcohol
• Risk of psychosis: metronidazole
(do not use), tricyclic
antidepressants

SERIOUS REACTIONS
❗ Disulfiram-alcohol reactions to
ingestion of alcohol in any form
include flushing/throbbing in head
and neck, throbbing headache,
nausea, copious vomiting,
diaphoresis, dyspnea,
hyperventilation, tachycardia,
hypotension, marked uneasiness,
vertigo, blurred vision, confusion,
and death

DENTAL CONSIDERATIONS

General:
• Be aware of the needs of patients
who are in recovery from substance
abuse.
• Avoid other addictive drugs,
including opioids and
benzodiazepines.
Consultations:
• Medical consultation may be
required to assess disease control.

Teach Patient/Family to:
• Avoid mouth rinses with high alcohol content because of drying effects and drug-drug interaction.

dobutamine hydrochloride
doe-**bute′**-a-meen
hi-droh-**klor′**-ide
(Dobutrex)
Do not confuse dobutamine with dopamine.

CATEGORY AND SCHEDULE
Pregnancy Risk Category: B

Drug Class: Adrenergic direct-acting β_1-agonist, cardiac stimulant; Catecholamine

MECHANISM OF ACTION
A direct-acting inotropic agent acting primarily on β_1-adrenergic receptors.
Therapeutic Effect: Decreases preload and afterload, and enhances myocardial contractility, stroke volume, and cardiac output. Improves renal blood flow and urine output.

USES
Treatment of cardiac decompensation caused by organic heart disease or cardiac surgery

PHARMACOKINETICS
Metabolized in the liver. Primarily excreted in urine. Not removed by hemodialysis. *Half-life:* 2 min.

INDICATIONS AND DOSAGES
▸ Short-Term Management of Cardiac Decompensation

IV Infusion
Adults, Elderly, Children. 2.5–15 mcg/kg/min. Rarely, drug can be infused at a rate of up to 40 mcg/kg/min to increase cardiac output.
Neonates. 2–15 mcg/kg/min.

SIDE EFFECTS/ADVERSE REACTIONS
Frequent
Increased heart rate, increased B/P
Occasional
Pain at injection site
Rare
Nausea, headache, anginal pain, shortness of breath, fever

PRECAUTIONS AND CONTRAINDICATIONS
Hypovolemia patients, idiopathic hypertrophic subaortic stenosis, sulfite sensitivity

DRUG INTERACTIONS OF CONCERN TO DENTISTRY
• None reported

SERIOUS REACTIONS
! Overdose may produce a marked increase in heart rate (by 30 beats/min or higher), marked increase in B/P (by 50 mm Hg or higher), anginal pain, and premature ventricular contractions (PVCs).

DENTAL CONSIDERATIONS
General:
• Acute-use drug for use in hospitals, cardiac labs, or emergency rooms.

D

docetaxel
doe-ceh-**tax**′-el
(Taxotere)
Do not confuse docetaxel with
Taxol.

CATEGORY AND SCHEDULE
Pregnancy Risk Category: D

Drug Class: Miscellaneous
antineoplastic

MECHANISM OF ACTION
An antimitotic agent belonging to
the toxoid family that disrupts the
microtubular cell network, which is
essential for cellular function.
Therapeutic Effect: Inhibits cellular
mitosis.

USES
Locally advanced or metastatic
breast cancer, non-small-cell lung
cancer, androgen independent
metastatic prostate cancer,
post-surgery operable node-positive
breast cancer

PHARMACOKINETICS
Distributed into peripheral
compartments. Protein binding:
94%. Extensively metabolized.
Excreted primarily in feces, with
lesser amount in urine. *Half-life:*
11.1 hr.

INDICATIONS AND DOSAGES
▶ Breast Carcinoma
IV
Adults. 60–100 mg/m^2 given over
1 hr q3wk. If patient develops
febrile neutropenia, a neutrophil
count less than 500 cells/mm^3 for
longer than 1 wk, severe or
cumulative cutaneous reactions, or
severe peripheral neuropathy with
initial dose of 100 mg/m^2, dosage

should be decreased to 75 mg/m^2. If
reaction continues, dosage should be
further reduced to 55 mg/m^2 or
therapy should be discontinued.
Patients who don't experience
the above symptoms at a dose of
60 mg/m^2 may tolerate an increased
docetaxel dose.
▶ Non-Small-Cell Lung Carcinoma
IV
Adults. 75 mg/m^2 q3wk. Adjust
dosage if toxicity occurs.

SIDE EFFECTS/ADVERSE REACTIONS
Frequent
Alopecia, asthenia, hypersensitivity
reaction such as dermatitis (59%,
decreases to 16% in those pretreated
with oral corticosteroids), fluid
retention, stomatitis, nausea and
diarrhea, fever, nail changes,
vomiting, myalgia
Occasional
Hypotension, edema, anorexia,
headache, weight gain, infection
(urinary tract, injection site,
indwelling catheter tip), dizziness
Rare
Dry skin, sensory disorders (vision,
speech, taste), arthralgia, weight
loss, conjunctivitis, hematuria,
proteinuria

PRECAUTIONS AND CONTRAINDICATIONS
History of severe hypersensitivity to
docetaxel or other drugs formulated
with polysorbate 80, neutrophil
count less than 1500 cells/mm^3

DRUG INTERACTIONS OF CONCERN TO DENTISTRY
• Significant risk of increased
effects: drugs that inhibit CYP3A4
isoenzymes (including ketoconazole,
itraconazole, erythromycin)
• Caution in use of any drugs that
induce CYP3A4 isoenzymes

SERIOUS REACTIONS

! In patients with normal liver function tests, neutropenia (neutrophil count 2000 cells/mm^3) and leukopenia (WBC count less than 4000 cells/mm^3) occur in 96% of patients; anemia (hemoglobin level less than 11 g/dl) occurs in 90% of patients; thrombocytopenia (platelet count less than 100,000 cells/mm^3) occurs in 8% of patients; and infection occurs in 28% of patients.

! Neurosensory and neuromotor effects, such as distal paresthesias and weakness, occur in 54% and 13% of patients, respectively.

DENTAL CONSIDERATIONS

General:
• If additional analgesia is required for dental pain, consider alternative analgesics (NSAIDs) in patients taking narcotics for acute or chronic pain.
• Examine for oral manifestation of opportunistic infection.
• Avoid products that affect platelet function, such as aspirin and NSAIDs.
• This drug may be used in the hospital or on an outpatient basis. Confirm the patient's disease and treatment status.
• Chlorhexidine mouth rinse prior to and during chemotherapy may reduce severity of mucositis.
• Patient on chronic drug therapy may rarely present with symptoms of blood dyscrasias, which can include infection, bleeding, and poor healing. If dyscrasia is present, caution patient to prevent oral tissue trauma when using oral hygiene aids.
• Palliative medication may be required for management of oral side effects.

• Short appointments and a stress-reduction protocol may be required for anxious patients.
• Patients may be at risk of bleeding; check for oral signs.
• Oral infections should be eliminated and/or treated aggressively.
Consultations:
• Medical consultation should include routine blood counts including platelet counts and bleeding time.
• Consult physician; prophylactic or therapeutic antiinfectives may be indicated if surgery or periodontal treatment is required.
• Medical consultation may be required to assess immunologic status during cancer chemotherapy and determine safety risk, if any, posed by the required dental treatment.
• Medical consultation may be required to assess disease control and patient's ability to tolerate stress.
Teach Patient/Family to:
• Be aware of oral side effects.
• Encourage effective oral hygiene to prevent soft tissue inflammation.
• Report oral lesions, soreness, or bleeding to dentist.
• Use caution to prevent trauma when using oral hygiene aids.
• Update health and medication history if physician makes any changes in evaluation or drug regimens; include OTC, herbal, and nonherbal remedies in the update.

D

D

docosanol
do-**cos**'-ah-nole
(Abreva)

CATEGORY AND SCHEDULE
Pregnancy Risk Category: B

Drug Class: Synthetic lipophilic alcohol

MECHANISM OF ACTION
A highly lipophilic, fatty alcohol that prevents fusion of lipid-enveloped viruses with cell membranes, thereby blocking viral replication

USES
Treatment of recurrent herpes labialis (cold sores, fever blisters) on the face or lips; appears to shorten healing time by at least 1 day.

PHARMACOKINETICS
Topical: Negligible absorption.

INDICATIONS AND DOSAGES
▸ Recurrent Herpes Labialis
Topical
Adult, Children older than 12 yr.
Apply small amount to affected area on face or lips or at the first sign of lesion 5 times a day until healed.

SIDE EFFECTS/ADVERSE REACTIONS
CNS: Headache
INTEG: Site reaction, rash, pruritus, dry skin, acne

PRECAUTIONS AND CONTRAINDICATIONS
Hypersensitivity
Caution:
Avoid application to eyes, external use only (not for intraoral use), children younger than 12 yr

DRUG INTERACTIONS OF CONCERN TO DENTISTRY
• None reported

DENTAL CONSIDERATIONS

Teach Patient/Family to:
• Apply with finger cot; wash hands before and after use.
• Not share this medication to prevent potential cross contamination of virus.
• Replace tooth brush after resolution of lesion to prevent reinfection of virus.

docusate
dok'-yoo-sate
(Apo-Docusate[CAN], Colace, Colax-C[CAN], Coloxyl[AUS], Diocto, Docusoft-S, Novo-Ducosate[CAN], PMS-Docusate[CAN], Pro-Cal-Sof, Regulex[CAN], Selax[CAN], Soflax[CAN], Surfak)

CATEGORY AND SCHEDULE
Pregnancy Risk Category: C
OTC

Drug Class: Bulk-producing laxative; stool softener

MECHANISM OF ACTION
A bulk-producing laxative that decreases surface film tension by mixing liquid and bowel contents. *Therapeutic Effect:* Increases infiltration of liquid to form a softer stool.

USES
Stool softener for those who need to avoid straining during defecation; treatment of constipation associated with hard, dry stools

PHARMACOKINETICS

Minimal absorption from the GI tract. Acts in small and large intestines. Results usually occur 1–2 days after first dose, but may take 3–5 days.

INDICATIONS AND DOSAGES
▸ Stool Softener
PO
Adults, Elderly, Children 12 yr and older. 50–500 mg/day in 1–4 divided doses.
Children 6–11 yr. 40–150 mg/day in 1–4 divided doses.
Children 3–5 yr. 20–60 mg/day in 1–4 divided doses.
Children younger than 3 yr. 10–40 mg in 1–4 divided doses.

SIDE EFFECTS/ADVERSE REACTIONS
Occasional
Mild GI cramping, throat irritation (with liquid preparation)
Rare
Rash

PRECAUTIONS AND CONTRAINDICATIONS
Acute abdominal pain, concomitant use of mineral oil, intestinal obstruction, nausea, vomiting

DRUG INTERACTIONS OF CONCERN TO DENTISTRY
• None reported

SERIOUS REACTIONS
! None known

DENTAL CONSIDERATIONS
General:
• Determine why patient is taking the drug.
• Use caution when prescribing medications that may aggravate constipation.

dofetilide
doe-fet'-ill-ide
(Tikosyn)

CATEGORY AND SCHEDULE
Pregnancy Risk Category: C

Drug Class: Antidysrhythmic (class III)

MECHANISM OF ACTION
A selective potassium channel blocker that prolongs repolarization without affecting conduction velocity by blocking one or more time-dependent potassium currents. Dofetilide has no effect on sodium channels or adrenergic alpha or beta receptors.
Therapeutic Effect: Terminates reentrant tachyarrhythmias, preventing reinduction.

USES
Maintenance of normal sinus rhythm in patients with atrial fibrillation or atrial flutter longer than 1 wk duration, who have been converted to normal sinus rhythm; conversion of atrial fibrillation or atrial flutter to normal sinus rhythm

PHARMACOKINETICS
PO: Bioavailability greater than 90%, peak plasma levels 2–3 hr, steady-state levels 2–3 days, plasma protein binding 60%–70%, excreted (80%) in urine unchanged, excretion involves both glomerular filtration and active tubular secretion, limited metabolism by CYP450 3A4 isoenzymes

INDICATIONS AND DOSAGES
▸ Maintain Normal Sinus Rhythm after Conversion from Atrial Fibrillation or Flutter

PO
Adults, Elderly. Individualized using a 7-step dosing algorithm dependent upon calculated creatinine clearance and QT interval measurements.

SIDE EFFECTS/ADVERSE REACTIONS
Occasional
Headache, chest pain, dizziness, dyspnea, nausea, insomnia, back and abdominal pain, diarrhea, rash

PRECAUTIONS AND CONTRAINDICATIONS
Concurrent use of drugs that prolong the QT interval; concurrent use of amiodarone, megestrol, prochlorperazine, or verapamil; congenital or acquired prolonged QT syndrome; paroxysmal atrial fibrillation; severe renal impairment
Caution:
Requires dose adjustment in renal impairment, can cause life-threatening ventricular arrhythmias, caution in use with CYP450 3A4 isoenzyme inhibitors, hepatic impairment, abnormal serum potassium or magnesium levels, lactation, children younger than 18 yr

DRUG INTERACTIONS OF CONCERN TO DENTISTRY
• Use NSAIDs with caution in patients at risk for thromboembolism
• Decreased renal excretion: ketoconazole (contraindicated use)
• Not recommended with concurrent use of phenothiazines, tricyclic antidepressants, SSRIs, macrolide antiinfectives (erythromycin, clarithromycin), azole antifungals, or other drugs that inhibit CYP3A4 isoenzymes
• Contraindicated with cimetidine, trimethoprim, ketoconazole,

prochlorperazine, megestrol, or verapamil

SERIOUS REACTIONS
! Angioedema, bradycardia, cerebral ischemia, facial paralysis, and serious ventricular arrhythmias or various forms of heart block may be noted.

DENTAL CONSIDERATIONS

General:
• Monitor vital signs at every appointment because of cardiovascular side effects.
• Consider a stress-reduction protocol.
• Delay or avoid dental treatment if patient shows signs of cardiac symptoms or respiratory distress.
• Ensure that the patient is compliant with drug therapy.
Consultations:
• Patient's physician should be informed about use of any dental drugs.
• Medical consultation may be required to assess disease control and patient's ability to tolerate stress.
Teach Patient/Family to:
• Update health and drug history if physician makes any changes in evaluation or drug regimens.

dolasetron
doe-**lass'**-eh-tron
(Anzemet)
Do not confuse Anzemet with Aldomdet.

CATEGORY AND SCHEDULE
Pregnancy Risk Category: B

Drug Class: Antinauseant and antiemetic

MECHANISM OF ACTION

A 5-HT3 receptor antagonist that acts centrally in the chemoreceptor trigger zone and peripherally at the vagal nerve terminals.
Therapeutic Effect: Prevents nausea and vomiting.

USES

Control of nausea and vomiting associated with cancer chemotherapy and prevention of postoperative nausea and vomiting

PHARMACOKINETICS

Readily absorbed from the GI tract after PO administration. Protein binding: 69%–77%. Metabolized in the liver. Primarily excreted in urine. Unknown if removed by hemodialysis. *Half-life:* 5–10 hr.

INDICATIONS AND DOSAGES

▸ **Prevention of Chemotherapy-Induced Nausea and Vomiting**
PO
Adults. 100 mg within 1 hr of chemotherapy.
Children 2–16 yr. 1.8 mg/kg within 1 hr of chemotherapy. Maximum: 100 mg.
IV
Adults, Children 1–16 yr. 1.8 mg/kg as a single dose 30 min before chemotherapy. Maximum: 100 mg.
▸ **Treatment or Prevention of Postoperative Nausea or Vomiting**
PO
Adults. 100 mg within 2 hr of surgery.
Children 2–16 yr. 1.2 mg/kg within 2 hr of surgery. Maximum: 100 mg.
IV
Adults. 12.5 mg 15 min before cessation of anesthesia or as soon as nausea occurs.
Children 2–16 yr. 0.35 mg/kg 15 min before cessation of

anesthesia or as soon as nausea occurs. Maximum: 12.5 mg.

SIDE EFFECTS/ADVERSE REACTIONS

Frequent
Headache, diarrhea, fatigue
Occasional
Fever, dizziness, tachycardia, dyspepsia

PRECAUTIONS AND CONTRAINDICATIONS

Hypersensitivity
Caution:
Previous hypersensitivity to other 5-HT$_3$ antagonists, cardiovascular disease, seizure disorders, ECG changes, hypokalemia, hypomagnesemia, diuretics, antiarrhythmics, lactation

DRUG INTERACTIONS OF CONCERN TO DENTISTRY

• Does not influence anesthesia recovery time.

SERIOUS REACTIONS

! Overdose may produce a combination of CNS stimulant and depressant effects.

DENTAL CONSIDERATIONS

General:
• Monitor patients in recovery to avoid untoward events.
• Patients taking opioids for acute or chronic pain should be given alternative analgesics for dental pain.
• Chlorhexidine mouth rinse before and during chemotherapy may reduce severity of mucositis.
• Palliative medication may be required for management of oral side effects from chemotherapy.

Teach Patient/Family to:
• Be aware of possible oral side effects from concurrent cancer chemotherapy.
• Report to dentist excessive nausea and vomiting in patients recovering from anesthesia after dental treatment.

donepezil hydrochloride
dah-**nep**′-eh-zil hi-droh-**klor**′-ide
(Aricept)
Do not confuse Aricept with AcipHex or Ascriptin.

CATEGORY AND SCHEDULE
Pregnancy Risk Category: C

Drug Class: Cholinesterase inhibitor

MECHANISM OF ACTION
A cholinesterase inhibitor that inhibits the enzyme acetyl-cholinesterase, thus increasing the concentration of acetylcholine at cholinergic synapses and enhancing cholinergic function in the CNS.
Therapeutic Effect: Slows the progression of Alzheimer's disease.

USES
Treatment of mild-to-moderate dementia associated with Alzheimer's disease

PHARMACOKINETICS
Well absorbed after PO administration. Protein binding: 96%. Extensively metabolized. Eliminated in urine and feces.
Half-life: 70 hr. Tablets (Orally Disintegrating): 5 mg, 10 mg.

INDICATIONS AND DOSAGES
▸ **Alzheimer's Disease**
PO
Adults, Elderly. 5–10 mg/day as a single dose. If initial dose is 5 mg, do not increase to 10 mg for 4–6 wk.

SIDE EFFECTS/ADVERSE REACTIONS
Frequent
Nausea, diarrhea, headache, insomnia, nonspecific pain, dizziness
Occasional
Mild muscle cramps, fatigue, vomiting, anorexia, ecchymosis
Rare
Depression, abnormal dreams, weight loss, arthritis, somnolence, syncope, frequent urination

PRECAUTIONS AND CONTRAINDICATIONS
History of hypersensitivity to donepezil or piperidine derivatives
Caution:
Bradycardia, sick sinus syndrome, GI ulcer disease, bladder obstruction, seizures, asthma, obstructive pulmonary disease, lactation, children, hepatic impairment

DRUG INTERACTIONS OF CONCERN TO DENTISTRY
• Enhanced succinylcholine muscle relaxation during anesthesia
• Risk of GI side effects: NSAIDs
• Action may be inhibited by anticholinergic drugs or enhanced by cholinergic agonists
• Increased blood levels: ketoconazole, paroxetine
• Use with caution drugs that inhibit CYP3A4 or CYP2D6 isoenzymes

SERIOUS REACTIONS
! Overdose may result in cholinergic crisis, characterized by severe nausea, increased salivation,

diaphoresis, bradycardia, hypotension, flushed skin, abdominal pain, respiratory depression, seizures, and cardiorespiratory collapse. Increasing muscle weakness may result in death if respiratory muscles are involved. ! The antidote is 1–2 mg IV atropine sulfate with subsequent doses based on therapeutic response.

DENTAL CONSIDERATIONS

General:
• Determine why patient is taking the drug.
• Monitor vital signs at every appointment because of cardiovascular side effects.
• After supine positioning, have patient sit upright for at least 2 min before standing to avoid orthostatic hypotension.
• Use caution if sedation or general anesthesia is required.
• Patients on chronic drug therapy may rarely have symptoms of blood dyscrasias, which can include infection, bleeding, and poor healing.
• Drug is used early in the disease; ensure that patient or caregiver understands informed consent.
• Place on frequent recall because early attention to dental health is important for Alzheimer's patients.
• Assess salivary flow as factor in caries, periodontal disease, and candidiasis.
• Consider semisupine chair position for patient comfort if GI side effects occur.
Consultations:
• Consultation with physician may be necessary if sedation or general anesthesia is required.
• Medical consultation may be required to assess disease control and patient's ability to tolerate stress.

• In a patient with symptoms of blood dyscrasias, request a medical consultation for blood studies and postpone treatment until normal values are reestablished.
Teach Patient/Family to:
• Encourage effective oral hygiene to prevent soft tissue inflammation.
• Prevent trauma when using oral hygiene aids.
• Use powered tooth brush if patient has difficulty holding conventional devices.
• When chronic dry mouth occurs, advise patient to:
    • Avoid mouth rinses with high alcohol content because of drying effects.
    • Use daily home fluoride products for anticaries effect.
    • Use sugarless gum, frequent sips of water, or saliva substitutes.

doripenem
(door-eh-pee′-nam)
(Doribax [U.S.], Finibax [JAPAN])

CATEGORY AND SCHEDULE
Pregnancy Risk Category: B

Drug Class: Broad-spectrum, carbapenem antibiotic

MECHANISM OF ACTION
Beta-lactam that binds to and inhibits bacterial cell wall synthesis. Doripenem inactivates multiple penicillin-binding proteins (PBPs), resulting in defective cell walls and bacterial death.
Therapeutic Effect: Broad-spectrum, bactericidal action treats complicated intraabdominal and urinary infections (including pyelonephritis).

USES
Serious systemic infections, particularly those caused by susceptible strains of *Pseudomonas aeruginosa* and *E. coli*

PHARMACOKINETICS
Completely absorbed after parenteral administration. Protein binding: 8%. Metabolized by non-hepatic pathways (dehydropeptidase-I). Excreted primarily in unchanged form by the kidneys.

INDICATIONS AND DOSAGES
▸ **Complicated Intraabdominal Infection**
Adult. 500 mg IV q8h over 1 hr, for 5–14 days.
▸ **Complicated Urinary Tract Infection, Including Pyelonephritis**
Adult. 500 mg IV q8h over 1 hr, for 10 days.

SIDE EFFECTS/ADVERSE REACTIONS
Frequent
Headache, nausea, diarrhea, rash, phlebitis
Occasional
Anemia, renal impairment, pruritus, rash, hepatic enzyme elevations, oral and vaginal fungal infections
Rare
Anaphylaxis

PRECAUTIONS
• Hypersensitivity
• Reductions of blood levels of sodium valproate (with possible loss of seizure control)
• *Clostridium difficile*–associated diarrhea and colitis
• Development of drug-resistant bacteria

DRUG INTERACTIONS OF CONCERN TO DENTISTRY
• Bacteriostatic antibiotics can theoretically reduce the effectiveness of doripenem.

SERIOUS REACTIONS
! Hypersensitivity, anaphylaxis

DENTAL CONSIDERATIONS
General:
• Determine why patient is receiving drug.
• Avoid administration of antibiotics that could reduce effectiveness of doripenem.
Consultations:
• Consult with physician to determine disease control and ability to tolerate dental procedures.
Teach Patient/Family to:
• Update medical history as changes in disease or drug regimen occur.

dornase alfa
door'-nace al'-fa
(Pulmozyme)

CATEGORY AND SCHEDULE
Pregnancy Risk Category: B

Drug Class: Recombinant human deoxyribonuclease (rh DNase)

MECHANISM OF ACTION
An enzyme that selectively splits and hydrolyzes DNA in sputum.
Therapeutic Effect: Reduces sputum viscosity and elasticity.

USES
Treatment of cystic fibrosis; reduces incidence of pulmonary infections; improves pulmonary function.

PHARMACOKINETICS
Inhalation: Peak sputum levels
15 min

INDICATIONS AND DOSAGES
▶ **To Improve Management of Pulmonary Function in Patients with Cystic Fibrosis**
Nebulization
Adults, Children older than 5 yr.
2.5 mg (1 ampule) once daily by recommended nebulizer. May increase to 2.5 mg twice daily.

SIDE EFFECTS/ADVERSE REACTIONS
Frequent
Pharyngitis, chest pain or discomfort, voice changes
Occasional
Conjunctivitis, hoarseness, rash

PRECAUTIONS AND CONTRAINDICATIONS
Sensitivity to dornase alfa or epoetin alfa
Caution:
Lactation, children younger than 5 yr

DRUG INTERACTIONS OF CONCERN TO DENTISTRY
• None documented

SERIOUS REACTIONS
! None significant

DENTAL CONSIDERATIONS
General:
• Consider semisupine chair position for patients with respiratory disease.
• Monitor vital signs at every appointment because of respiratory and cardiovascular side effects.
• Stress-reduction protocol may be required.

Consultations:
• Medical consultation may be required to assess disease control.
Teach Patient/Family to:
• Encourage effective oral hygiene to prevent soft tissue inflammation.

D

dorzolamide hydrochloride
door-**zol´**-ah-mide
hi-droh-**klor´**-ide
(Trusopt)

CATEGORY AND SCHEDULE
Pregnancy Risk Category: C

Drug Class: Carbonic anhydrase inhibitor

MECHANISM OF ACTION
An ophthalmic agent that inhibits carbonic anhydrase.
Therapeutic Effect: Reduces intraocular pressure (IOP).

USES
Treatment of ocular hypertension, open-angle glaucoma

PHARMACOKINETICS
Peak response occurs in 2 hr and the duration of action is 8–12 hr. Systemically absorbed to some degree. Protein binding: 33%. Distributed in red blood cells. Sites of metabolism have not been established. Metabolized to active metabolite, N-desethyldorzolamide. Excreted in urine. *Half-life:* Unknown; 147 days (terminal red blood cell).

INDICATIONS AND DOSAGES
▶ **Glaucoma, Ocular Hypertension**
Ophthalmic
Adults, Elderly. 1 drop in affected eye(s) 3 times a day.

SIDE EFFECTS/ADVERSE REACTIONS

Frequent
Ocular burning, bitter taste

Occasional
Superficial punctuate keratitis, ocular allergic reaction

PRECAUTIONS AND CONTRAINDICATIONS

Hypersensitivity to dorzolamide or any other component of the formulation

Caution:
Allergy to sulfonamides, renal or hepatic impairment, lactation, children, oral carbonic anhydrase inhibitors, contact lenses

DRUG INTERACTIONS OF CONCERN TO DENTISTRY

• Avoid drugs that may exacerbate glaucoma (anticholinergic drugs)
• High-dose salicylates to avoid systemic toxicity

SERIOUS REACTIONS

! Iridocyclitis, skin rash, and urolithiasis occur rarely.
! Electrolyte imbalance, development of an acidotic state, and possible CNS effects may occur.

DENTAL CONSIDERATIONS

General:
• Avoid dental light in patient's eyes; offer dark glasses for patient comfort.
• Protect patient's eyes from accidental spatter during dental treatment.
• Check patient's compliance with prescribed drug regimen for glaucoma.

Consultations:
• Medical consultation may be required to assess disease control.

doxazosin mesylate

dox-**ay**'-zoe-sin **mess**'-ah-late
(Apo-Doxazosin[CAN], Cardura)
Do not confuse doxazosin with doxapram, doxepin, or doxorubicin, or Cardura with Cardene, Cordarone, Coumadin, K-Dur, or Ridaura.

CATEGORY AND SCHEDULE
Pregnancy Risk Category: C

Drug Class: α-adrenergic blocker

MECHANISM OF ACTION
An antihypertensive that selectively blocks α_1-adrenergic receptors, decreasing peripheral vascular resistance.
Therapeutic Effect: Causes peripheral vasodilation and lowers of B/P. Also relaxes smooth muscle of bladder and prostate.

USES
Treatment of benign prostatic hyperplasia (BPH)

PHARMACOKINETICS
54%–59% absorbed; peak blood levels 8–9 hr. 99% protein binding. Primarily metabolized in the liver by the CYP 3A4 isoenzyme. 63% excreted in feces, 9% in urine.

Route	Onset	Peak	Duration
PO	N/A	2–6 hr	24 hr

Well absorbed from the GI tract. Protein binding: 98%–99%. Metabolized in the liver. Primarily eliminated in feces. Not removed by hemodialysis. ***Half-life:*** 19–22 hr.

INDICATIONS AND DOSAGES
▶ **Mild-to-Moderate Hypertension**
PO
Adults. Initially, 1 mg once a day. May increase to a maximum of 16 mg/day.
Elderly. Initially, 0.5 mg once a day.
▶ **Benign Prostatic Hyperplasia, Alone or in Combination with Finasteride (Proscar)**
PO
Adults, Elderly. Initially, 1 mg/day. May increase q1–2 wk. Maximum: 8 mg/day.

SIDE EFFECTS/ADVERSE REACTIONS
Frequent
Dizziness, asthenia, headache, edema
Occasional
Nausea, pharyngitis, rhinitis, pain in extremities, somnolence
Rare
Palpitations, diarrhea, constipation, dyspnea, myalgia, altered vision, dizziness, nervousness

PRECAUTIONS AND CONTRAINDICATIONS
Hypersensitivity to other quinazolines
Caution:
Children, lactation, hepatic disease

DRUG INTERACTIONS OF CONCERN TO DENTISTRY
• Increased hypotensive effects: all CNS depressants
• Reduced effects with indomethacin, NSAIDs, sympathomimetics
• Caution in use of drugs that may cause urinary retention: anticholinergics, opioids

SERIOUS REACTIONS
! First-dose syncope (hypotension with sudden loss of consciousness) may occur 30–90 min following initial dose of 2 mg or greater, a too-rapid increase in dosage, or addition of another antihypertensive agent to therapy. First-dose syncope may be preceded by tachycardia (pulse rate of 120–160 beats/min).

DENTAL CONSIDERATIONS
General:
• Monitor vital signs at every appointment because of cardiovascular side effects.
• After supine positioning, have patient sit upright for at least 2 min before standing to avoid orthostatic hypotension.
• Consider a stress-reduction protocol.
• Assess salivary flow as a factor in caries, periodontal disease, and candidiasis.
Consultations:
• Medical consultation may be required to assess disease control and patient's ability to tolerate stress.
Teach Patient/Family to:
• When chronic dry mouth occurs, advise patient to:
  • Avoid mouth rinses with high alcohol content because of drying effects.
  • Use daily home fluoride products for anticaries effect.
  • Use sugarless gum, frequent sips of water, or saliva substitutes.

D

doxepin hydrochloride

dox′-eh-pin hye-droe-**klor′**-ide
(Apo-Doxepin[CAN],
Deptran[AUS], Novo-
Doxepin[CAN], Prudoxin,
Sinequan, Zonalon)
Do not confuse doxepin with
doxapram, doxazosin, or Doxidan,
or Sinequan with saquinavir.

CATEGORY AND SCHEDULE

Pregnancy Risk Category: C (B
for topical form)

Drug Class: Antidepressant,
tricyclic

MECHANISM OF ACTION

A tricyclic antidepressant,
antianxiety agent, antineuralgic
agent, antipruritic, and antiulcer
agent that increases synaptic
concentrations of norepinephrine
and serotonin.
Therapeutic Effect: Produces
antidepressant and anxiolytic
effects.

USES

Treatment of major depression,
anxiety; unapproved: panic
disorders

PHARMACOKINETICS

Rapidly and well absorbed from
the GI tract. Protein binding:
80%–85%. Metabolized in the liver
to active metabolite. Primarily
excreted in urine. Not removed by
hemodialysis. *Half-life:* 6–8 hr.
Topical: Absorbed through the skin.
Distributed to body tissues.
Metabolized to active metabolite.
Excreted in urine.

INDICATIONS AND DOSAGES

▸ **Depression, Anxiety**
PO
Adults. 30–150 mg/day at bedtime
or in 2–3 divided doses. May
increase to 300 mg/day.
Elderly. Initially, 10–25 mg at
bedtime. May increase by 10–
25 mg/day every 3–7 days.
Maximum: 75 mg/day.
Adolescents. Initially, 25–50 mg/day
as a single dose or in divided doses.
May increase to 100 mg/day.
Children 12 yr and younger.
1–3 mg/kg/day.
▸ **Pruritus Associated with Eczema**
Topical
Adults, Elderly. Apply thin film 4
times a day.

SIDE EFFECTS/ADVERSE REACTIONS

Frequent
Oral: Orthostatic hypotension,
somnolence, dry mouth, headache,
increased appetite, weight gain,
nausea, unusual fatigue, unpleasant
taste
Topical: Edema; increased pruritus
and eczema; burning, tingling, or
stinging at application site; altered
taste; dizziness; drowsiness; dry
skin; dry mouth; fatigue; headache;
thirst
Occasional
Oral: Blurred vision, confusion,
constipation, hallucinations, difficult
urination, eye pain, irregular
heartbeat, fine muscle tremors,
nervousness, impaired sexual
function, diarrhea, diaphoresis,
heartburn, insomnia
Topical: Anxiety, skin irritation or
cracking, nausea
Rare
Oral: Allergic reaction, alopecia,
tinnitus, breast enlargement
Topical: Fever, photosensitivity

PRECAUTIONS AND CONTRAINDICATIONS

Angle-closure glaucoma, hypersensitivity to other tricyclic antidepressants, urine retention
Caution:
Suicidal patients, elderly, MAOIs

DRUG INTERACTIONS OF CONCERN TO DENTISTRY FOR TOPICAL FORM

• Potential for interactions depends on how much drug is absorbed and duration of use (longer than 8 days)
• Increased anticholinergic effects: anticholinergics, antihistamines, phenothiazines, other tricyclic antidepressants
• Potential risk for increased CNS depression: all CNS depressants
• Increased effects of direct-acting sympathomimetics: epinephrine, levonordefrin
• Avoid concurrent use with St. John's wort (herb)

DRUG INTERACTIONS OF CONCERN TO DENTISTRY FOR SYSTEMIC-DOSE FORM

• Increased anticholinergic effects: anticholinergic blockers, antihistamines, phenothiazines
• Increased effects of direct-acting sympathomimetics (epinephrine, levonordefrin)
• Potential risk of increased CNS depression: alcohol, barbiturates, benzodiazepines, other CNS depressants
• Decreased antihypertensive effects: clonidine, guanadrel, guanethidine

SERIOUS REACTIONS

! Abrupt or too-rapid withdrawal may result in headache, malaise, nausea, vomiting, and vivid dreams.
! Overdose may produce seizures, dizziness, and cardiovascular effects, such as severe orthostatic

hypotension, tachycardia, palpitations, and arrhythmias.

DENTAL CONSIDERATIONS

▶ Topical Form
General:
• Doxepin may be absorbed and produce typical systemic side effects of tricyclic drugs.
• Monitor vital signs at every appointment because of cardiovascular side effects.
• Use vasoconstrictors with caution, in low doses, and with careful aspiration.
• Place on frequent recall because of oral side effects.
• Apply lubricant to dry lips for patient comfort before dental procedures.
• Assess salivary flow as a factor in caries, periodontal disease, and candidiasis.
Consultations:
• Medical consultation may be required to assess disease control.
Teach Patient/Family to:
• Avoid mouth rinses with high alcohol content because of interaction with alcohol (see precautions) and drying effects.
• When chronic dry mouth occurs, advise patient to:
  • Use daily home fluoride products for anticaries effect.
  • Use sugarless gum, frequent sips of water, or saliva substitutes.
▶ Systemic-Dose Form
General:
• Monitor vital signs at every appointment because of cardiovascular side effects.
• Assess salivary flow as a factor in caries, periodontal disease, and candidiasis.
• Patients on chronic drug therapy may rarely have symptoms of blood

dyscrasias, which can include infection, bleeding, and poor healing.
• After supine positioning, have patient sit upright for at least 2 min before standing to avoid orthostatic hypotension.
• Use vasoconstrictors with caution, in low doses, and with careful aspiration. Avoid use of gingival retraction cord with epinephrine.
• Place on frequent recall because of oral side effects.

Consultations:
• In a patient with symptoms of blood dyscrasias, request a medical consultation for blood studies and postpone dental treatment until normal values are reestablished.
• Medical consultation may be required to assess disease control.
• Physician should be informed if significant xerostomic side effects occur (e.g., increased caries, sore tongue, problems eating or swallowing, difficulty wearing prosthesis) so that a medication change can be considered.

Teach Patient/Family to:
• Encourage effective oral hygiene to prevent soft tissue inflammation.
• When chronic dry mouth occurs, advise patient to:
  • Avoid mouth rinses with high alcohol content because of drying effects.
  • Use daily home fluoride products for anticaries effect.
  • Use sugarless gum, frequent sips of water, or saliva substitutes.

doxorubicin

dox-oh-**roo**′-bi-sin
(Doxil)
Do not confuse doxorubicin with Daunorubicin, Idamycin, or Idarubicin.

CATEGORY AND SCHEDULE
Pregnancy Risk Category: D

Drug Class: Anthracycline antibiotic; antineoplastic

MECHANISM OF ACTION
An anthracycline antibiotic that inhibits DNA and DNA-dependent RNA synthesis by binding with DNA strands. Liposomal encapsulation increases uptake by tumors, prolongs action, and may decrease toxicity.
Therapeutic Effect: Prevents cellular division.

USES
Treatment of some kinds of cancer

PHARMACOKINETICS
Widely distributed. Protein binding: Unknown. Metabolized in liver. Minimal excretion in urine.
Half-life: 45–55 hr.

INDICATIONS AND DOSAGES
▶ **AIDS-Related Kaposi's Sarcoma**
IV Infusion
Adults. 20 mg/m^2 over 30 min q3wk.
▶ **Ovarian Cancer**
IV Infusion
Adults. 50 mg/m^2 q4wk.
▶ **Dosage in Liver Impairment**

Serum Bilirubin Concentration	Dosage
1.2–3 mg/dl	50% usual dose
More than 3 mg/dl	25% usual dose

SIDE EFFECTS/ADVERSE REACTIONS
Frequent
Nausea
Occasional
Anorexia, diarrhea, hyperpigmentation of nailbeds, phalangeal and dermal creases
Rare
Fever, chills, conjunctivitis, lacrimation

PRECAUTIONS AND CONTRAINDICATIONS
Nursing mothers, hypersensitivity to doxorubicin compounds or daunorubicin

DRUG INTERACTIONS OF CONCERN TO DENTISTRY
• None reported

SERIOUS REACTIONS
! Bone marrow depression manifested as hematologic toxicity (principally leukopenia and, to lesser extent, anemia, thrombocytopenia) may occur.
! Cardiotoxicity noted as either acute, transient abnormal ECG findings or cardiomyopathy manifested as CHF may occur.

DENTAL CONSIDERATIONS
General:
• If additional analgesia is required for dental pain, consider alternative analgesics (NSAIDs) in patients taking narcotics for acute or chronic pain.
• Avoid prescribing aspirin-containing products.
• Examine for oral manifestation of opportunistic infection.
• This drug usually is administered in a hospital, a cancer treatment center, or possibly a home IV service. Dentists are involved in the management of oral mucositis associated with the chemotherapy.
• Chlorhexidine mouth rinse prior to and during chemotherapy may reduce severity of mucositis.
• Patient on chronic drug therapy may rarely present with symptoms of blood dyscrasias, which can include infection, bleeding, and poor healing. If dyscrasia is present, caution patient to prevent oral tissue trauma when using oral hygiene aids.
• Palliative medication may be required for management of oral side effects.
• Consider local hemostasis measures to prevent excessive bleeding.
• Patient may be at risk of bleeding; check oral signs.
Consultations:
• Medical consultation should include routine blood counts including platelet counts and bleeding time.
• Consult physician; prophylactic or therapeutic antiinfectives may be indicated if surgery or periodontal treatment is required.
• Medical consultation may be required to assess immunologic status during cancer chemotherapy and determine safety risk, if any, posed by the required dental treatment.
• Medical consultation may be required to assess disease control and patient's ability to tolerate stress.
• In a patient with symptoms of blood dyscrasias, request a medical consultation for blood studies and postpone treatment until normal values are reestablished.
Teach Patient/Family to:
• Be aware of oral side effects.
• Encourage effective oral hygiene to prevent soft tissue inflammation.

D

• See dentist immediately if signs of secondary oral infection occur.
• Prevent trauma when using oral hygiene aids.
• Update health and medication history if physician makes any changes in evaluation or drug regimens; include OTC, herbal, and nonherbal remedies in the update.

doxycycline

dox-ih-sye′-kleen
(Adoxa, Apo-Doxy[CAN], Doryx, Doxsig[AUS], Doxy-100, Doxycin[CAN], Doxyhexal[AUS], Doxylin[AUS], Monodox, Vibramycin, Vibra-Tabs)
Do not confuse doxycycline with Dicyclomine or doxylamine, or Monodox with Monopril.

CATEGORY AND SCHEDULE
Pregnancy Risk Category: D

Drug Class: Tetracycline, broad-spectrum antiinfective

MECHANISM OF ACTION
A tetracycline antibiotic that inhibits bacterial protein synthesis by binding to ribosomes.
Therapeutic Effect: Bacteriostatic.

USES
Treatment of syphilis, *C. trachomatis,* gonorrhea, lymphogranuloma venereum, uncommon gram-negative and gram-positive organisms, necrotizing ulcerative gingivostomatitis; cutaneous or inhalational anthrax exposure

PHARMACOKINETICS
PO: Peak 1.5–4 hr, *Half-life:* 15–22 hr; 25%–93% protein bound; excreted in bile.

INDICATIONS AND DOSAGES
▸ **Respiratory, Skin, and Soft-Tissue Infections; UTIs; Pelvic Inflammatory Disease (PID); Brucellosis; Trachoma; Rocky Mountain Spotted Fever; Typhus; Q Fever; Rickettsia; Severe Acne (Adoxa); Smallpox; Psittacosis; Ornithosis; Granuloma Inguinale; Lymphogranuloma Venereum; Intestinal Amebiasis (Adjunctive Treatment); Prevention of Rheumatic Fever**
PO
Adults, Elderly. Initially, 100 mg q12h, then 100 mg/day as single dose or 50 mg q12h for severe infections.
Children 8 yr and older and weighing more than 45 kg. 2–4 mg/ kg/day divided q12–24h. Maximum: 200 mg/day.
IV
Adults, Elderly. Initially, 200 mg as 1–2 infusions; then 100–200 mg/day in 1–2 divided doses.
Children 8 yr and older. 2–4 mg/kg/ day divided q12–24h. Maximum: 200 mg/day.
▸ **Acute Gonococcal Infections**
PO
Adults. Initially, 200 mg, then 100 mg at bedtime on first day; then 100 mg twice a day for 14 days.
▸ **Syphilis**
PO, IV
Adults. 200 mg/day in divided doses for 14–28 days.
▸ **Traveler's Diarrhea**
PO
Adults, Elderly. 100 mg/day during a period of risk (up to 14 days) and for 2 days after returning home.
▸ **Periodontitis**
PO
Adults. 20 mg twice a day as an adjunct to scaling and root planning; may be administered for up to 9 mo; exceeding the recommended dosage may increase risk of side effects,

including the development of resistant organisms.

SIDE EFFECTS/ADVERSE REACTIONS
Frequent
Anorexia, nausea, vomiting, diarrhea, dysphagia, possibly severe photosensitivity
Occasional
Rash, urticaria

PRECAUTIONS AND CONTRAINDICATIONS
Children 8 yr and younger, hypersensitivity to tetracyclines or sulfites, last half of pregnancy, severe hepatic dysfunction.
The use of tetracycline drugs during tooth development (last half of pregnancy, infancy and childhood up to the age of 8 may cause permanent discoloration of the teeth (yellow-gray-brown). Enamel hypoplasia has also been reported. May also cause retardation of skeletal development and deformations.
Caution:
Hepatic disease, lactation

DRUG INTERACTIONS OF CONCERN TO DENTISTRY
• No data reported for this dose form; see doxycycline hyclate monograph for drug interactions reported with tetracyclines.

DRUG INTERACTIONS OF CONCERN TO DENTISTRY FOR SYSTEMIC FORM
• Decreased absorption: NaHCO$_3$, other antacids
• Increased rate of metabolism: barbiturates, carbamazepine, hydantoins
• Decreased effect of penicillins, cephalosporins

• May increase the effectiveness of anticoagulants, methotrexate, digoxin
• Contraindicated with isotretinoin (Accutane)

SERIOUS REACTIONS
! Superinfection (especially fungal) and benign intracranial hypertension (headache, visual changes) may occur.
! Hepatotoxicity, fatty degeneration of the liver, and pancreatitis occur rarely.

DENTAL CONSIDERATIONS
▶ **Doxycycline Hyclate (Dental-Systemic)**
General:
• Examine for oral manifestation of opportunistic infection.
• Should be administered at least 1 hr before or 2 hr after morning or evening meals.
Teach Patient/Family to:
• Avoid using ingestible sodium bicarbonate products, such as the Prophy-Jet air polishing system, within 2 hr of drug use.
▶ **Doxycycline Hyclate/Doxycycline Calcium (Systemic Form)**
General:
• Determine why the patient is taking tetracycline.
• Broad-spectrum antibiotics may promote oral or vaginal *Candida* infection.
• Dental staining or enamel hypoplasia may be associated with exposure to this drug before birth or up to the age of 8. Tetracycline stains may be extremely resistant to ordinary tooth-whitening procedures.
Consultations:
• Medical consultation may be required to assess disease control.

Teach Patient/Family:
• That tetracycline can be taken with milk, food; take with a full glass of water.
• To take tetracycline doses 1 hr before or 2 hr after air polishing device (Prophy-Jet), if used.
• When used for dental infection, advise patient:
  • To report sore throat, oral burning sensation, fever, and fatigue, any of which could indicate superinfection.
  • To take at prescribed intervals and complete dosage regimen.
  • To immediately notify the dentist if signs or symptoms of infection increase.

doxycycline hyclate (dental-systemic)
dox-ih-**sye**′-kleen
(Periostat)

CATEGORY AND SCHEDULE
Pregnancy Risk Category: D

Drug Class: Tetracycline derivative for nonantibacterial use

MECHANISM OF ACTION
Reduces elevated collagenase activity in gingival crevicular fluid of patients with adult periodontitis; no antibacterial effect reported at this dose.

USES
Adjunct to scaling and root planing to promote attachment level gain and reduce pocket depth in adult periodontitis

PHARMACOKINETICS
No data available.

INDICATIONS AND DOSAGES
PO
Adult. 20 mg twice daily as an adjunct to scaling and root planing; may be administered for up to 9 mo; exceeding the recommended dosage may increase risk of side effects, including the development of resistant organisms.

SIDE EFFECTS/ADVERSE REACTIONS
Note: In a clinical study of 428 patients, there was little to no difference in the incidence of side effects reported between this drug and a placebo. See doxycycline hyclate monograph for typical side effects associated with oral administration. Whether these side effects would occur at doses used in this product is unknown.

PRECAUTIONS AND CONTRAINDICATIONS
Hypersensitivity to tetracyclines
Caution:
Children younger than 8 yr, pregnant and nursing mothers, predisposition to oral or vaginal candidiasis; not to be used for antimicrobial effect in periodontitis

DRUG INTERACTIONS OF CONCERN TO DENTISTRY
• No data reported for this dose form; see doxycycline hyclate monograph for drug interactions reported with tetracyclines.

SERIOUS REACTIONS
! Pregnancy (permanent tooth discoloration), fetal toxicity

DENTAL CONSIDERATIONS

General:
• Examine for oral manifestation of opportunistic infection.
• Should be administered at least 1 hr before or 2 hr after morning or evening meals.
Teach Patient/Family to:
• Avoid using ingestible sodium bicarbonate products, such as the air polishing system Prophy Jet, within 2 hr of drug use.

doxycycline hyclate gel
dox-ih-**sye**′-kleen
(Atridox)

CATEGORY AND SCHEDULE
Pregnancy Risk Category: D

Drug Class: Tetracycline, antiinfective

MECHANISM OF ACTION
Inhibits bacterial protein synthesis by disruption of transfer RNA and messenger RNA.

USES
Adjunctive treatment of chronic adult periodontitis to increase clinical attachment, reduce probing depth, and reduce bleeding on probing

PHARMACOKINETICS
Gingival crevicular fluid levels peak at 2 hr, sustained levels up to 18 hr and decline over 7 days; low serum levels not exceeding 0.1 g/ml.

INDICATIONS AND DOSAGES
Topical
Adult. Mix contents of syringes according to detailed instructions, completing 100 cycles; attach blunt cannula to syringe A and fill the pocket; after it becomes firm, the mixture may be packed further into the pocket with a dental instrument.

SIDE EFFECTS/ADVERSE REACTIONS
Oral: Gingival discomfort, pain, loss of attachment, toothache, periodontal abscess, exudate, infection, drainage, swelling, thermal tooth sensitivity, extreme mobility, localized allergic reaction
CNS: Headache
CV: High B/P
GI: Diarrhea
GU: PMS
EENT: Skin infection, photosensitivity
MS: Muscle aches, backache

PRECAUTIONS AND CONTRAINDICATIONS
Hypersensitivity
Caution:
Children (tooth staining), lactation, photosensitivity, predisposition to candidiasis

DRUG INTERACTIONS OF CONCERN TO DENTISTRY
• None specifically identified for this product; unknown whether typical tetracycline interactions occur.

SERIOUS REACTIONS
! Pregnancy (permanent tooth discoloration), fetal toxicity

DENTAL CONSIDERATONS

General:
• Examine for oral manifestation of opportunistic infection.
Teach Patient/Family to:
• Be alert to the possibility of secondary oral infection and the

need to see dentist immediately if signs of infection occur.
• Avoid oral hygiene procedures in treated areas of mouth for 7 days to avoid dislodging product.

dronabinol
droe-**nab**′-ih-nol
(Marinol)
Do not confuse dronabinol with droperidol.

CATEGORY AND SCHEDULE
Pregnancy Risk Category: C
Controlled Substance Schedule: III

Drug Class: Antiemetic, appetite stimulant

MECHANISM OF ACTION
An antiemetic and appetite stimulant that may act by inhibiting vomiting control mechanisms in the medulla oblongata.
Therapeutic Effect: Inhibits vomiting and stimulates appetite.

USES
Control of nausea, vomiting in selected patients receiving emetogenic cancer chemotherapy; stimulate appetite in AIDS-associated anorexia

PHARMACOKINETICS
Well absorbed after PO administration. Protein binding: 97%. Undergoes first-pass metabolism. Is highly lipid soluble. Primarily excreted in feces.
Half-life: 4 hr.

INDICATIONS AND DOSAGES
▸ **Prevention of Chemotherapy-Induced Nausea and Vomiting**

PO
Adults, Children. Initially, 5 mg/m^2 1–3 hr before chemotherapy, then q2–4h after chemotherapy for total of 4–6 doses a day. May increase by 2.5 mg/m^2 up to 15 mg/m^2 per dose.
▸ **Appetite Stimulant**
PO
Adults. Initially, 2.5 mg twice a day (before lunch and dinner). Range: 2.5–20 mg/day.

SIDE EFFECTS/ADVERSE REACTIONS
Frequent
Euphoria, dizziness, paranoid reaction, somnolence
Occasional
Asthenia, ataxia, confusion, abnormal thinking, depersonalization
Rare
Diarrhea, depression, nightmares, speech difficulties, headache, anxiety, tinnitus, flushed skin

PRECAUTIONS AND CONTRAINDICATIONS
Treatment of nausea and vomiting not caused by chemotherapy, hypersensitivity to sesame oil or tetrahydrocannabinol products
Caution:
Lactation, children, elderly, cardiac disorders, drug abuse, alcoholism, hypertension, manic or depressive state, schizophrenia

DRUG INTERACTIONS OF CONCERN TO DENTISTRY
• Increased CNS depression: alcohol, CNS depressants, tricyclic antidepressants
• Additive hypertension, tachycardia, possible cardiotoxicity: tricyclic antidepressants, amphetamines, other sympathomimetics
• Additive tachycardia, drowsiness: atropine, scopolamine, antihistamines, anticholinergic drugs

SERIOUS REACTIONS

! Mild intoxication may produce increased sensory awareness (including taste, smell, and sound), altered time perception, reddened conjunctiva, dry mouth, and tachycardia.

! Moderate intoxication may produce memory impairment and urine retention.

! Severe intoxication may produce lethargy, decreased motor coordination, slurred speech, and orthostatic hypotension.

DENTAL CONSIDERATIONS

General:

• Monitor vital signs at every appointment because of cardiovascular side effects.

• After supine positioning, have patient sit upright for at least 2 min to avoid orthostatic hypotension.

• Patients taking opioids for acute or chronic pain should be given alternative analgesics for dental pain.

• Assess salivary flow as a factor in caries, periodontal disease, and candidiasis.

• Consider semisupine chair position for patient comfort if GI side effects occur.

Teach Patient/Family to:

• When chronic dry mouth occurs, advise patient to:

  • Avoid mouth rinses with high alcohol content because of drying effects.

  • Use daily home fluoride products for anticaries effect.

  • Use sugarless gum, frequent sips of water, or saliva substitutes.

dronedarone
droe-**ne**-da-rone
(Multaq)

CATEGORY AND SCHEDULE
Pregnancy Risk Category: X

Drug Class: Antiarrhythmic agents

MECHANISM OF ACTION
A non-iodinated amiodarone analogue with unknown mechanism of action. Properties of all four Vaughan-Williams classes; inhibits calcium, sodium, and potassium channels; α- and β-adrenergic receptor antagonist.

Therapeutic Effect: Suppresses atrial fibrillation or atrial flutter.

USES
Atrial fibrillation
Atrial flutter

PHARMACOKINETICS

Route	Onset	Peak	Duration
PO	Unknown	3–6 hr	12 hr

Poor bioavailability. Protein binding: >98%. Extensive first pass hepatic metabolism, mostly by CYP3A. Primarily excreted in feces; minimal excretion in urine. Food increases bioavailability. *Half-life:* 13–19 hr.

INDICATIONS AND DOSAGES
▸ **Atrial Fibrillation**
PO

Adults. 400 mg twice a day, with morning and evening meals.

▸ **Atrial Flutter**
PO

Adults. 400 mg twice a day, with morning and evening meals.

SIDE EFFECTS/ADVERSE REACTIONS

Frequent

Prolonged QT interval, elevated serum creatinine

Occasional

Dermatitis, eczema, pruritus, rash, diarrhea, nausea, asthenia

Rare

Bradyarrhythmia, photosensitivity, hypokalemia, hypomagnesemia, abdominal pain, indigestion, altered taste, vomiting

PRECAUTIONS AND CONTRAINDICATIONS

Hypersensitivity to dronedarone or its components

Bradycardia (<50 bpm)

Concomitant use of strong CYP3A inhibitors

Heart failure, Class II or III, with recent decompensation requiring hospitalization

Heart failure, Class IV

Severe hepatic impairment

Pregnancy

Nursing mothers

Concomitant use of QT prolonging agents

QTc Bazett interval ≥ 500 ms

Second- or third-degree atrioventricular block or sick sinus syndrome

Caution:

• Concurrent use with CYP450 3A inducers, antiarrhythmic agents, or β-blockers

• Women of childbearing potential

• New or worsening heart failure

• Hypokalemia or hypomagnesemia

• QT prolongation (discontinue dronedarone if QTc Bazett ≥ 500 ms)

• Moderate hepatic impairment

• Patients of Asian decent

DRUG INTERACTIONS OF CONCERN TO DENTISTRY

• QT prolonging agents: May increase the risk of QT prolongation.

• CYP450 3A4 inhibitors: May increase dronedarone levels and risk of adverse effects.

• CYP450 3A4 substrates: May increase drug concentrations of CYP3A4 substrates and risk of adverse effects.

• CYP450 3A4 inducers: May decrease dronedarone levels and effectiveness.

• Antiarrhythmics: May increase the risk of adverse cardiovascular effects.

• β-blocker: May increase risk of bradycardia.

• Digoxin: May increase digoxin levels and risk of toxicity; discontinue or reduce dose by 50%.

• Grapefruit juice: May increase dronedarone levels and risk of toxicity.

• HMG-CoA reductase inhibitors: May increase the drug levels of HMG-CoA reductase inhibitors and risk of toxicity.

• Calcium channel blockers: May increase the drug levels of dronedarone and/or calcium channel blockers and risk of toxicity.

• Photosensitizers: May increase the risk of photosensitivity.

• Potassium-depleting agents: May increase the risk of hypokalemia.

• SSRIs, TCA antidepressants: May increase drug levels of SSRIs and TCA antidepressants and effects.

SERIOUS REACTIONS

! Black box warning: patients with NYHA Class IV heart failure or NYHA Class II-III heart failure with recent decompensation require hospitalization or referral to specialized clinic.

! QT prolongation may occur.

! Heart failure may develop;
existing heart failure may worsen
during treatment.
! Raised serum creatinine may
occur.

DENTAL CONSIDERATIONS

General:
• Monitor vital signs at every
appointment because of
cardiovascular side effects.
• Consider semisupine chair position
for patient if GI side effects occur.
Consultations:
• Medical consultation may be
required to assess disease control.
Teach Patient/Family to:
• Encourage effective oral hygiene
to prevent soft tissue inflammation.
• Prevent trauma when using oral
hygiene aids.
• Be alert for the possibility of
secondary oral infection and the
need to see dentist immediately if
signs of infection occur.
• Women of childbearing potential
should avoid pregnancy.

droperidol
droe-**pear**′-ih-dall
(Inapsine)

CATEGORY AND SCHEDULE
Pregnancy Risk Category: C

Drug Class: General anesthetic;
anesthesia adjunct, antiemetic

MECHANISM OF ACTION
A general anesthetic and antiemetic
agent that antagonizes dopamine
neurotransmission at synapses by
blocking postsynaptic dopamine
receptor sites; partially blocks
adrenergic receptor binding sites.
Therapeutic Effect: Produces
tranquilization, antiemetic effect.

USES
Treatment of nausea and vomiting
associated with surgical and
diagnostic procedures.

PHARMACOKINETICS
Onset of action occurs within
30 min. Well absorbed. Metabolized
in liver. Excreted in urine and feces.
Half-life: 2.3 hr.

INDICATIONS AND DOSAGES
▸ **Preoperative**
IM/IV
*Adults, Elderly, Children 12 yr
and older.* 2.5–10 mg 30–60 min
before induction of general
anesthesia.
Children 2–12 yr. 0.088–0.165 mg/
kg.
▸ **Adjunct for Induction of General
Anesthesia**
IV
*Adults, Elderly, Children 12 yr and
older.* 0.22–0.275 mg/kg.
Children 2–12 yr. 0.088–0.165 mg/
kg.
▸ **Adjunct for Maintenance of
General Anesthesia**
IV
Adults, Elderly. 1.25–2.5 mg.
▸ **Diagnostic Procedures without
General Anesthesia**
IM
Adults, Elderly. 2.5–10 mg
30–60 min before procedure. If
needed, may give additional doses of
1.25–2.5 mg (usually by IV
injection).

SIDE EFFECTS/ADVERSE
REACTIONS
Frequent
Mild-to-moderate hypotension
Occasional
Tachycardia, postoperative
drowsiness, dizziness, chills,
shivering

Rare
Postoperative nightmares, facial sweating, bronchospasm

PRECAUTIONS AND CONTRAINDICATIONS
Known or suspected QT prolongation, hypersensitivity to droperidol or any component of the formulation

DRUG INTERACTIONS OF CONCERN TO DENTISTRY
• Increased frequency of nausea/vomiting: propofol
• Increased CNS depression: all CNS depressants
• Prolonged QT interval: intravenous narcotics
• Increased hypotension: anesthetics, systemic or local
• Risk of hypotension: epinephrine
• Orthostatic hypotension: antihypertensive medications

SERIOUS REACTIONS
❗ Extrapyramidal symptoms may appear as akathisia (motor restlessness) and dystonias: torticollis (neck muscle spasm), opisthotonos (rigidity of back muscles), and oculogyric crisis (rolling back of eyes).
❗ Overdosage includes symptoms of hypotension, tachycardia, hallucinations, and extrapyramidal symptoms.
❗ Prolonged QT interval, seizures, and arrhythmias have been reported.

DENTAL CONSIDERATIONS

General:
• Used in a hospital, emergency room, or cancer treatment center for acute need.
• Caution in the use of drugs that prolong the QT interval.

• Use caution if sedation or general anesthesia is required; risk of hypotensive episode.
• After supine positioning, have patient sit upright for at least 2 min before standing to avoid orthostatic hypotension.
• Monitor vital signs at every appointment because of cardiovascular side effects.

Consultations:
• Consultation with physician may be necessary if sedation or general anesthesia is required.
• Medical consultation may be required to assess disease control.

duloxetine
doo-**lox**´-eh-teen
(Cymbalta)

CATEGORY AND SCHEDULE
Pregnancy Risk Category: C

Drug Class: Antidepressant

MECHANISM OF ACTION
Selectively inhibits the reuptake of serotonin (5-HT) and norepinephrine in the brain.

USES
Treatment of major depressive disorder; diabetic peripheral neuropathic pain

PHARMACOKINETICS
Peak 6 hr, plasma protein binding greater than 90%; metabolized in liver by CYP2D6 and CYP1A2 isoenzymes; excreted in urine (70%) and feces (30%) **Half-life:** 8–17 hr.

INDICATIONS AND DOSAGES
▸ **Depression**
PO
Adult. 40 mg per day (20 mg twice daily) to 60 mg/day (once daily or 30 mg twice daily).
▸ **Diabetic Peripheral Neuropathic Pain**
PO
Adult. Up to a total dose of 60 mg per day (once a day).
Available forms include Caplets 20, 30, and 60 mg.

SIDE EFFECTS/ADVERSE REACTIONS
Oral: Dry mouth
CNS: Insomnia, anxiety, decreased appetite, dizziness, somnolence, tremors, fatigue, decreased libido
CV: Hot flushes, elevated B/P
GI: Nausea, constipation, diarrhea, vomiting, dyspepsia
RESP: Cough, nasopharyngitis
GU: Erectile and ejaculation dysfunction, polyuria
EENT: Blurred vision, pharyngolaryngeal pain
INTEG: Sweating
MS: Muscle cramps, myalgia
SYST: Fatigue, asthenia, pyrexia

PRECAUTIONS AND CONTRAINDICATIONS
Hypersensitivity, MAOIs, uncontrolled narrow-angle glaucoma, hepatotoxicity, elevated B/P, psychiatric changes, seizures, glaucoma, physical and psychological symptoms of withdrawal, renal impairment

DRUG INTERACTIONS OF CONCERN TO DENTISTRY
• Potentiation of anticholinergic effects by antisialagogues used in dentistry (e.g., atropine, glycopyrrolate)
• Increased fluoxetine blood levels and toxicity with some fluoroquinolone antibacterials
• Centrally acting drugs (e.g., sedatives) may enhance CNS adverse effects
• Caution: can inhibit CYP2D6 isoenzymes, use phenothiazines with caution (see Appendix I)
• Avoid administration with alcohol or alcohol-containing agents (e.g., elixirs)

SERIOUS REACTIONS
! Hepatotoxicity
! Worsening of suicide risk
! Activation of mania seizures
! Increased intraocular pressure
! Withdrawal symptoms if abruptly discontinued

DENTAL CONSIDERATIONS
General:
• Monitor vital signs at every appointment because of cardiovascular side effects.
• Assess salivary flow as a factor in caries, periodontal disease, candidiasis, denture sore mouth.
• Assess salivary flow as a factor in reduced retention and/or increased irritation of removable prostheses.
Consultations:
• Medical consultation may be required to assess disease control and patient's ability to tolerate stress.
• Inform physician of potential adverse effects of dry mouth and possible need to change medications if severe.
Teach Patient/Family to:
• Encourage effective oral hygiene measures to minimize effects of reduced salivary flow.
• Avoid mouth rinses with high alcohol content because of drying effects.

D

• Use daily home fluoride products for anticaries effect.
• Use sugarless or xylitol chewing gums, frequent sips of water, and/or saliva substitutes if dry mouth occurs.

dutasteride
do-tah-**stir'**-eyed
(Avodart)

CATEGORY AND SCHEDULE
Pregnancy Risk Category: X

Drug Class: Synthetic steroid

MECHANISM OF ACTION
An androgen hormone inhibitor that inhibits 5-alpha reductase, an intracellular enzyme that converts testosterone into dihydrotestosterone (DHT) in the prostate gland, reducing the serum DHT level.
Therapeutic Effect: Reduces size of the prostate gland.

USES
Treatment of benign prostate hyperplasia (BPH) in men to improve symptoms, reduce the risk of urinary retention, and reduce the need for BPH-related surgery

PHARMACOKINETICS

Route	Onset	Peak	Duration
PO	24 hr	N/A	3–8 wk

Moderately absorbed after PO administration. Widely distributed. Protein binding: 99%. Metabolized in the liver. Primarily excreted in feces. **Half-life:** Up to 5 wk.

INDICATIONS AND DOSAGES
▶ BPH
PO
Adults, Elderly. 0.5 mg once a day.

SIDE EFFECTS/ADVERSE REACTIONS
Occasional
Gynecomastia, sexual dysfunction (decreased libido, impotence, and decreased volume of ejaculate)

PRECAUTIONS AND CONTRAINDICATIONS
Females, physical handling of tablets by those who are or may be pregnant
Caution:
Hepatic impairment, men cannot donate blood until at least 6 mo after last dose, drug also found in semen, no data on use in patients younger than 18 yr or in renal impairment, nursing mothers (not used in women)

DRUG INTERACTIONS OF CONCERN TO DENTISTRY
• No drug interaction studies have been conducted; however, caution should be observed when used in combination with potent and chronically used CYP3A4 inhibitors.
• Opioids and anticholinergic drugs may enhance urinary retention; use alternative analgesics (NSAIDs).

SERIOUS REACTIONS
! Toxicity may be manifested as rash, diarrhea, and abdominal pain.

DENTAL CONSIDERATIONS

General:
• Determine why patient is taking the drug.
Consultations:
• Medical consultation may be required to assess disease control.

Teach Patient/Family to:
• Update health and drug history if physician makes any changes in evaluation or drug regimens.

dyphylline
die´-fih-lin
(Dilor, Lufyllin)
Do not confuse with Dilacor.

CATEGORY AND SCHEDULE
Pregnancy Risk Category: C

Drug Class: Xanthine derivative

MECHANISM OF ACTION
A xanthine derivative that acts as a bronchodilator by directly relaxing smooth muscle of the bronchial airway and pulmonary blood vessels similar to theophylline.
Therapeutic Effect: Relieves bronchospasm, increases vital capacity, produces cardiac arrhythmias, and skeletal muscle stimulation.

USES
Treatment of bronchial asthma, bronchospasm in chronic bronchitis, COPD, emphysema

PHARMACOKINETICS
Rapid absorption after PO administration. Excreted in urine.
Half-life: 2 hr.

INDICATIONS AND DOSAGES
▸ **Chronic Bronchospasm, Asthma**
PO
Adults, Elderly. 15 mg/kg 4 times a day.
IM
Adults, Elderly. 250–500 mg.
Maximum: 15 mg/kg q6h.
Children. 4.4–6.6 mg/kg/day in divided doses.

▸ **Dosage in Renal Impairment**

Creatinine Clearance	Dosage Percent
50–80 ml/min	Administer 75% of dose
10–50 ml/min	Administer 50% of dose
Less than 10 ml/min	Administer 25% of dose

SIDE EFFECTS/ADVERSE REACTIONS
Frequent
Tachycardia, nervousness, restlessness
Occasional
Heartburn, vomiting, headache, mild diuresis, insomnia, nausea

PRECAUTIONS AND CONTRAINDICATIONS
Uncontrolled arrhythmias, hyperthyroidism, history of hypersensitivity to dyphylline, related xanthine derivatives, or any component of the formulation
Caution:
Elderly, CHF, cor pulmonale, hepatic disease, active peptic ulcer disease, diabetes mellitus, hyperthyroidism, hypertension, children, renal disease, glaucoma

DRUG INTERACTIONS OF CONCERN TO DENTISTRY
• Increased action: erythromycin, ciprofloxacin, tetracyclines
• Increased risk of cardiac dysrhythmia: halothane-inhalation anesthesia, CNS stimulants
• Decreased effect: barbiturates, carbamazepine, ketoconazole
• May decrease sedative effects of benzodiazepines

SERIOUS REACTIONS
! Ventricular arrhythmias, hypotension, circulatory failure, seizures, hyperglycemia, and

syndrome of inappropriate antidiuretic hormone (SIADH) have been reported.

cardiovascular and respiratory side effects.
• Consider semisupine chair position for patients with respiratory disease.

DENTAL CONSIDERATIONS

General:
• Monitor vital signs at every appointment because of

echothiophate iodide

ek-oh-**thye**′-oh-fate **eye**′-oh-dide
(Phospholine iodide)

CATEGORY AND SCHEDULE
Pregnancy Risk Category: C

Drug Class: Antiglaucoma agent, ophthalmic; cyclostimulant, accommodative esotropia; diagnostic aid, accommodative esotropia

MECHANISM OF ACTION
A cholinesterase inhibitor that causes acetylcholine to accumulate at cholinergic receptor sites and produce effects like excessive stimulation of cholinergic receptors. *Therapeutic Effect:* Causes conjunctival hyperemia and constriction of the sphincter pupillae and ciliary muscles, which results in miosis and paralysis of accommodation.

USES
Treatment of certain types of glaucoma and other eye conditions, such as accommodative esotropia. They may also be used in the diagnosis of certain eye conditions, such as accommodative esotropia.

PHARMACOKINETICS
None reported

INDICATIONS AND DOSAGES
▸ **Glaucoma**
Ophthalmic
Adults, Elderly. Instill 1 drop twice daily into eyes with 1 dose prior to bedtime.

▸ **Accommodative Esotropia, Diagnosis**
Ophthalmic
Children. Instill 1 drop once daily into both eyes at bedtime for 2–3 wk.
▸ **Accommodative Esotropia, Treatment**
Ophthalmic
Children. Instill 1 drop once daily.

SIDE EFFECTS/ADVERSE REACTIONS
Occasional
Headache, brow ache, blurred vision, burning and stinging of eyes, decreased night vision, intraocular pressure changes, iritis, uveitis

PRECAUTIONS AND CONTRAINDICATIONS
Active uveal inflammation, angle-closure glaucoma, hypersensitivity to echothiophate products

DRUG INTERACTIONS OF CONCERN TO DENTISTRY
• Avoid use of succinylcholine in general anesthesia
• Possible inhibition of the metabolism of ester-type local and topical anesthetics
• Avoid use of anticholinergics, such as systemic atropine or related drugs, benzodiazepine sedatives

SERIOUS REACTIONS
! Cardiac irregularities have been reported.

DENTAL CONSIDERATIONS
General:
• Determine why patient is taking the drug.
• Avoid drugs with anticholinergic activity, such as antihistamines,

E

opioids, benzodiazepines, propantheline, atropine, and scopolamine.
• Avoid dental light in patient's eyes; offer dark glasses for patient comfort.
• Question glaucoma patient about compliance with prescribed drug regimen.
Consultations:
• Medical consultation may be required to assess disease control.
Teach Patient/Family to:
• Update health and medication history if physician makes any changes in evaluation or drug regimens; include OTC, herbal, and nonherbal remedies in the update.

efalizumab
ef-ah-**liz**′-yoo-mab
(Raptiva)

CATEGORY AND SCHEDULE
Pregnancy Risk Category: C

Drug Class: Monoclonal antibody

MECHANISM OF ACTION
A monoclonal antibody that interferes with lymphocyte activation by binding to the lymphocyte antigen, inhibiting the adhesion of leukocytes to other cell types. ***Therapeutic Effect:*** Prevents the release of cytokines and the growth and migration of circulating total lymphocytes, predominant in psoriatic lesions.

USES
Treatment of chronic moderate to severe plaque psoriasis in patients (older than 18 yr) who are candidates for systemic therapy or phototherapy

PHARMACOKINETICS
Clearance is affected by body weight, not by gender or race, after subcutaneous injection. Serum concentration reaches steady state at 4 wk. Mean time to elimination: 25 days.

INDICATIONS AND DOSAGES
▸ Psoriasis
Subcutaneous
Adults, Elderly. Initially, 0.7 mg/kg followed by weekly doses of 1 mg/kg. Maximum: 200 mg (single dose).

SIDE EFFECTS/ADVERSE REACTIONS
Frequent
Headache, chills, nausea, injection site pain
Occasional
Myalgia, flu-like symptoms, fever
Rare
Back pain, acne

PRECAUTIONS AND CONTRAINDICATIONS
Concurrent use of immunosuppressive agents
Caution:
Increased risk of infections, malignancies, worsening of psoriasis, use in elderly, safety and efficacy have not been established in lactation or children

DRUG INTERACTIONS OF CONCERN TO DENTISTRY
• None reported

SERIOUS REACTIONS
! Hypersensitivity reaction, malignancies, serious infections (abscess, cellulitis, postoperative wound infection, pneumonia),

thrombocytopenia and worsening of psoriasis occur rarely.

General:
• Understand the disease and the patient's need to use this drug.
• Rarely, oral lesions and geographic tongue may occur in patients with psoriasis.

efavirenz
eh-fahv′-er-ins
(Stocrin[AUS], Sustiva)
Do not confuse Sustiva with Survanta.

CATEGORY AND SCHEDULE
Pregnancy Risk Category: C.

Drug Class: Antiviral (nonnucleoside)

MECHANISM OF ACTION
A nonnucleoside reverse transcriptase inhibitor that inhibits the activity of HIV reverse transcriptase of HIV-1 and the transcription of HIV-1 RNA to DNA.
Therapeutic Effect: Interrupts HIV replication, slowing the progression of HIV infection.

USES
Treatment in HIV-1 infection, only in combination with other HIV-1 antiretroviral agents

PHARMACOKINETICS
Rapidly absorbed after PO administration. Protein binding: 99%. Metabolized to major isoenzymes in the liver. Eliminated

in urine and feces. *Half-life:* 40-55 hr.

INDICATIONS AND DOSAGES
▶ HIV Infection (in Combination with Other Antiretrovirals)
PO
Adults, Elderly, Children 3 yr and older weighing 40 kg or more.
600 mg once a day at bedtime.
Children 3 yr and older weighing 32.5 kg to less than 40 kg. 400 mg once a day.
Children 3 yr and older weighing 25 kg to less than 32.5 kg. 350 mg once a day.
Children 3 yr and older weighing 20 kg to less than 25 kg. 300 mg once a day.
Children 3 yr and older weighing 15 kg to less than 20 kg. 250 mg once a day.
Children 3 yr and older weighing 10 kg to less than 15 kg. 200 mg once a day.

SIDE EFFECTS/ADVERSE REACTIONS
Frequent
Mild to severe: Dizziness, vivid dreams, insomnia, confusion, impaired concentration, amnesia, agitation, depersonalization, hallucinations, euphoria, somnolence (mild symptoms don't interfere with daily activities; severe symptoms interrupt daily activities)
Occasional
Mild to moderate: Maculopapular rash; nausea, fatigue, headache, diarrhea, fever, cough (moderate symptoms may interfere with daily activities)

PRECAUTIONS AND CONTRAINDICATIONS
Concurrent use with ergot derivatives, midazolam, or triazolam;

E

efavirenz as monotherapy; hypersensitivity to efavirenz
Caution:
Must not be used as a single agent for HIV, avoid pregnancy with use, lactation, mental illness, substance abuse, caution with alcohol or psychotropic drugs, driving or other hazardous tasks, monitor cholesterol, hepatic impairment

DRUG INTERACTIONS OF CONCERN TO DENTISTRY
• Contraindicated drugs: midazolam, triazolam
• Decreased plasma levels of clarithromycin, carbamazepine, St. John's wort (herb)
• Potential for increased levels with ketoconazole, itraconazole (no studies)
• Increased risk of CNS side effects with CNS depressants

SERIOUS REACTIONS
! None known

DENTAL CONSIDERATIONS

General:
• Examine for oral manifestations of opportunistic infection.
• Monitor vital signs at every appointment because of cardiovascular and respiratory side effects.
• Consider semisupine chair position for patient comfort because of GI side effects of drug.
• Assess salivary flow as a factor in caries, periodontal disease, and candidiasis.
• Short appointments and a stress-reduction protocol may be required for anxious patients.
Consultations:
• Medical consultation may be required to assess disease control.

Teach Patient/Family to:
• Prevent trauma when using oral hygiene aids.
• Encourage effective oral hygiene to prevent soft tissue inflammation.
• Be alert for the possibility of secondary oral infection and to see dentist immediately if signs of infection occur.
• When chronic dry mouth occurs, advise patient to:
  • Avoid mouth rinses with high alcohol content because of drying effects.
  • Use daily home fluoride products for anticaries effect.
  • Use sugarless gum, frequent sips of water, or saliva substitutes.

eletriptan
el-eh-trip′-tan
(Relpax)

CATEGORY AND SCHEDULE
Pregnancy Risk Category: C

Drug Class: Serotonin receptor agonist

MECHANISM OF ACTION
A serotonin receptor agonist that binds selectively to vascular receptors, producing a vasoconstrictive effect on cranial blood vessels.
Therapeutic Effect: Relieves migraine headache.

USES
Treatment of acute migraine with or without aura in adults

PHARMACOKINETICS
Well absorbed after PO administration. Metabolized by the

liver to inactive metabolite. Eliminated in urine. *Half-life:* 4.4 hr (increased in hepatic impairment and the elderly [older than 65 yr]).

INDICATIONS AND DOSAGES
▸ **Acute Migraine Headache**
PO
Adults, Elderly. 20–40 mg. If headache improves but then returns, dose may be repeated after 2 hr. Maximum: 80 mg/day.

SIDE EFFECTS/ADVERSE REACTIONS
Occasional
Dizziness, somnolence, asthenia, nausea
Rare
Paresthesia, headache, dry mouth, warm or hot sensation, dyspepsia, dysphagia

PRECAUTIONS AND CONTRAINDICATIONS
Arrhythmias associated with conduction disorders, coronary artery disease, ischemic heart disease, severe hepatic impairment, uncontrolled hypertension
Caution:
Do not use within 72 hr of treatment with CYP3A4 enzyme inhibitors, caution in lactation, safety and use in children younger than 18 yr has not been established

DRUG INTERACTIONS OF CONCERN TO DENTISTRY
• Avoid use of CYP3A4 inhibitors concurrently or within 72 hr of use of eletriptan: ketoconazole, itraconazole, erythromycin, clarithromycin, others

SERIOUS REACTIONS
! Cardiac reactions (including ischemia, coronary artery vasospasm and MI) and noncardiac vasospasm-related reactions (such as hemorrhage and CVA) occur rarely, particularly in patients with hypertension, diabetes, or a strong family history of coronary artery disease; obese patients; smokers; males older than 40 yr; and postmenopausal women.

DENTAL CONSIDERATIONS
General:
• This is an acute-use drug; it is doubtful that patients will seek dental treatment during acute migraine attacks.
• Be aware of the patient's disease, its severity and its frequency, when known.
• Monitor vital signs at every appointment because of cardiovascular side effects.
• Assess salivary flow as a factor in caries, periodontal disease, and candidiasis.
• Consider semisupine chair position for patient comfort if GI side effects occur.
Consultations:
• If treating chronic orofacial pain, consult with patient's physician.
Teach Patient/Family to:
• Be aware that oral symptoms will disappear when drug is discontinued.

emedastine
eh-**med**′-ah-steen
(Emadine)

CATEGORY AND SCHEDULE
Pregnancy Risk Category: B

Drug Class: Ophthalmic antihistamine

MECHANISM OF ACTION
An ophthalmic H_1-receptor antagonist that inhibits histamine-stimulated vascular permeability in the conjunctiva.
Therapeutic Effect: Relieves ocular itching associated with allergic conjunctivitis.

USES
Temporary relief of signs and symptoms of allergic conjunctivitis

PHARMACOKINETICS
Negligible absorption after ophthalmic administration. Metabolized into inactive metabolites. Excreted in urine.
Half-life: 6.6 hr.

INDICATIONS AND DOSAGES
▸ **Allergic Conjunctivitis**
Ophthalmic
Adults, Elderly, Children 3 yr and older. 1–2 drops in affected eye(s) twice daily.

SIDE EFFECTS/ADVERSE REACTIONS
Frequent
Headache
Occasional
Abnormal dreams, asthenia (loss of strength, energy), bad taste, blurred vision, burning or stinging, dry eyes, foreign body sensation, tearing

PRECAUTIONS AND CONTRAINDICATIONS
Hypersensitivity to emedastine or any other component of the formulation
Caution:
Avoid wearing contact lens if eye is red, wait at least 10 min after application to insert contact lens, lactation, no data for use in children younger than 3 yr

DRUG INTERACTIONS OF CONCERN TO DENTISTRY
• None reported

SERIOUS REACTIONS
! Somnolence and malaise occurs rarely.

emtricitabine
em-trih-**sit′**-ah-bean
(Emtriva)

CATEGORY AND SCHEDULE
Pregnancy Risk Category: B

Drug Class: Antiviral, nucleoside reverse transcriptase inhibitor

MECHANISM OF ACTION
An antiretroviral that inhibits HIV-1 reverse transcriptase by incorporating itself into viral DNA, resulting in chain termination.
Therapeutic Effect: Interrupts HIV replication, slowing the progression of HIV infection.

USES
Treatment of HIV-1 infection in adults; used in combination with other antiretroviral medications

PHARMACOKINETICS
Rapidly and extensively absorbed from the GI tract. Excreted primarily in urine (86%) and, to a lesser extent, in feces (14%); 30% removed by hemodialysis. Unknown if removed by peritoneal dialysis.
Half-life: 10 hr.

INDICATIONS AND DOSAGES
▶ **HIV Infection (in Combination with Other Antiretrovirals)**
PO
Adults, Elderly. 200 mg once a day.
▶ **Dosage in Renal Impairment**
Dosage and frequency are modified on the basis of creatinine clearance.

Creatinine Clearance	Dosage
30–49 ml/min	200 mg q48h
15–29 ml/min	200 mg q72h
Less than 15 ml/min, hemodialysis patients	200 mg q96h

SIDE EFFECTS/ADVERSE REACTIONS
Frequent
Headache, rhinitis, rash, diarrhea, nausea
Occasional
Cough, vomiting, abdominal pain, insomnia, depression, paresthesia, dizziness, peripheral neuropathy, dyspepsia, myalgia
Rare
Arthralgia, abnormal dreams

PRECAUTIONS AND CONTRAINDICATIONS
Hypersensitivity
Caution:
Possible risk of lactic acidosis, severe hepatomegaly with steatosis, use not established in HIV/HBV infections, renal impairment (dose reduction required), avoid nursing when taking this drug, safety and efficacy in pediatric patients have not been established

DRUG INTERACTIONS OF CONCERN TO DENTISTRY
• None reported

SERIOUS REACTIONS
! Lactic acidosis and hepatomegaly with steatosis occur rarely and may be severe.

DENTAL CONSIDERATIONS
General:
• Examine for oral manifestations of opportunistic infection.
• Consider semisupine chair position for patient comfort if GI side effects occur.
• Patient history should include all medications and herbal or nonherbal remedies taken by the patient.
Consultations:
• Medical consultation may be required to assess disease control and patient's ability to tolerate stress.
Teach Patient/Family to:
• Encourage effective oral hygiene to prevent soft tissue inflammation, infection.
• Prevent trauma when using oral hygiene aids.
• Update health and drug history, reporting changes in health status, drug regimen changes or disease/treatment status.

enalapril maleate
en-**al′**-ah-pril **ma′**-lee-ate
(Alphapril[AUS], Amprace[AUS], Apo-Enalapril[CAN], Auspril[AUS], Renitec[AUS], Vasotec)
Do not confuse enalapril with Anafranil, Eldepryl, or ramipril.

CATEGORY AND SCHEDULE
Pregnancy Risk Category: D (C if used in first trimester)

Drug Class: Angiotensin-converting enzyme (ACE) inhibitor

E

MECHANISM OF ACTION

This ACE inhibitor suppresses the renin-angiotensin-aldosterone system and prevents conversion of angiotensin I to angiotensin II, a potent vasoconstrictor; may inhibit angiotensin II at local vascular, renal sites. Decreases plasma angiotensin II, increases plasma renin activity, decreases aldosterone secretion. *Therapeutic Effect:* In hypertension, reduces peripheral arterial resistance. In CHF, increases cardiac output; decreases peripheral vascular resistance, B/P, pulmonary capillary wedge pressure, heart size.

USES

Treatment of hypertension, heart failure adjunct, asymptomatic left ventricular dysfunction

PHARMACOKINETICS

Route	Onset	Peak	Duration
PO	1 hr	4–6 hr	24 hr
IV	15 min	1–4 hr	6 hr

Readily absorbed from the GI tract (not affected by food). Protein binding: 50%–60%. Converted to active metabolite. Primarily excreted in urine. Removed by hemodialysis. *Half-life:* 11 hr (half-life is increased with impaired renal function).

INDICATIONS AND DOSAGES

▶ **Hypertension Alone or in Combination with Other Antihypertensives**
PO
Adults, Elderly. Initially, 2.5–5 mg/day. Range: 10–40 mg/day in 1–2 divided doses.
Children. 0.1 mg/kg/day in 1–2 divided doses. Maximum: 0.5 mg/kg/day.
Neonates. 0.1 mg/kg/day q24h.

IV
Adults, Elderly. 0.625–1.25 mg q6h up to 5 mg q6h.
Children, Neonates. 5–10 mcg/kg/dose q8–24h.
▶ **Adjunctive Therapy for CHF**
PO
Adults, Elderly. Initially, 2.5–5 mg/day. Range: 5–20 mg/day in 2 divided doses.
▶ **Dosage in Renal Impairment**
Dosage is modified on the basis of creatinine clearance.

Creatinine Clearance	% of Usual Dose
10–50 ml/min	75–100
Less than 10 ml/min	50

SIDE EFFECTS/ADVERSE REACTIONS

Frequent
Headache, dizziness
Occasional
Orthostatic hypotension, fatigue, diarrhea, cough, syncope
Rare
Angina, abdominal pain, vomiting, nausea, rash, asthenia (loss of strength, energy), syncope

PRECAUTIONS AND CONTRAINDICATIONS

History of angioedema from previous treatment with ACE inhibitors
Caution:
Renal disease, hyperkalemia

DRUG INTERACTIONS OF CONCERN TO DENTISTRY

• Increased hypotension: alcohol, phenothiazines
• Decreased hypotensive effects: indomethacin, possibly other NSAIDs, sympathomimetics
• Suspected reduction in the antihypertensive and vasodilator

effects by salicylates; monitor B/P if used concurrently

SERIOUS REACTIONS

! Excessive hypotension ("first-dose syncope") may occur in patients with CHF and in those who are severely salt or volume depleted.
! Angioedema (swelling of face, lips) and hyperkalemia occur rarely.
! Agranulocytosis and neutropenia may be noted in patients with collagen vascular diseases, including scleroderma and systemic lupus erythematosus and impaired renal function.
! Nephrotic syndrome may be noted in those with history of renal disease.

DENTAL CONSIDERATIONS

General:
• Monitor vital signs at every appointment because of cardiovascular side effects.
• After supine positioning, have patient sit upright for at least 2 min before standing to avoid orthostatic hypotension.
• Patients on chronic drug therapy may rarely have symptoms of blood dyscrasias, which can include infection, bleeding, and poor healing.
• Assess salivary flow as a factor in caries, periodontal disease, and candidiasis.
• Limit use of sodium-containing products, such as saline IV fluids, for those patients with a dietary salt restriction.
• Use vasoconstrictors with caution, in low doses and with careful aspiration.
• Stress from dental procedures may compromise cardiovascular function; determine patient risk.

• Short appointments and a stress-reduction protocol may be required for anxious patients.
Consultations:
• Medical consultation may be required to assess patient's ability to tolerate stress.
• In a patient with symptoms of blood dyscrasias, request a medical consultation for blood studies and postpone dental treatment until normal values are reestablished.
• Take precautions if dental surgery is anticipated and sedation or general anesthesia is required; risk of hypotensive episode.
Teach Patient/Family to:
• Encourage effective oral hygiene to prevent soft tissue inflammation.
• When chronic dry mouth occurs, advise patient to:
  • Avoid mouth rinses with high alcohol content because of drying effects.
  • Use daily home fluoride products for anticaries effect.
  • Use sugarless gum, frequent sips of water, or saliva substitutes.

E

enfuvirtide

en-**few**'-vir-tide
(Fuzeon)
Do not confuse Fuzeon with Furoxone.

CATEGORY AND SCHEDULE

Pregnancy Risk Category: B

Drug Class: Antiviral

MECHANISM OF ACTION

A fusion inhibitor that interferes with the entry of HIV-1 into CD4+ cells by inhibiting the fusion of viral and cellular membranes. *Therapeutic Effect:* Impairs HIV replication, slowing the progression of HIV infection.

USES

Treatment, in combination with other antiretroviral agents, of HIV-1 infection in treatment-experienced patients with HIV-1 replication despite ongoing antiretroviral therapy

PHARMACOKINETICS

Comparable absorption when injected into subcutaneous tissue of abdomen, arm, or thigh. Protein binding: 92%. Undergoes catabolism to amino acids. *Half-life:* 3.8 hr.

INDICATIONS AND DOSAGES
▸ **HIV Infection (in combination with other antiretrovirals)**
Subcutaneous
Adults, Elderly. 90 mg (1 ml) twice a day.
Children 6–16 yr. 2 mg/kg twice a day. Maximum 90 mg twice a day.
Pediatric dosing guidelines

Weight: lb (kg)	Dose: mg (ml)
11–15.5 (24–34)	27 (0.3)
15.6–20 (35–44)	36 (0.4)
20.1–24.5 (45–54)	45 (0.5)
24.6–29 (55–64)	54 (0.6)
29.1–33.5 (65–74)	63 (0.7)
33.6–38 (75–84)	72 (0.8)
38.1–42.5 (85–94)	81 (0.9)
Greater than 42.5 (greater than 94)	90 (1)

SIDE EFFECTS/ADVERSE REACTIONS

Expected
Local injection site reactions (pain, discomfort, induration, erythema, nodules, cysts, pruritus, ecchymosis)
Frequent
Diarrhea, nausea, fatigue
Occasional
Insomnia, peripheral neuropathy, depression, cough, decreased appetite or weight loss, sinusitis, anxiety, asthenia, myalgia, cold sores
Rare
Constipation, influenza, upper abdominal pain, anorexia, conjunctivitis

PRECAUTIONS AND CONTRAINDICATIONS

Hypersensitivity; patients should be instructed in recognizing local injection site reactions and trained in aseptic technique, HIV-infected mothers must not nurse, use in children younger than 6 yr has not been established

DRUG INTERACTIONS OF CONCERN TO DENTISTRY
• None reported

SERIOUS REACTIONS
! Enfuvirtide use may potentiate bacterial pneumonia.
! Hypersensitivity (rash, fever, chills, rigors, hypotension), thrombocytopenia, neutropenia, and renal insufficiency or failure may occur rarely.

DENTAL CONSIDERATIONS

General:
• Patients taking this drug will be taking other antiviral drugs that may interact with some dental drugs. Be sure to take a complete drug history.

• Patients on chronic drug therapy may rarely have symptoms of blood dyscrasias, which can include infection, bleeding, and poor healing.
• Examine for oral manifestation of opportunistic infection.
Consultations:
• Medical consultation may be required to assess disease control in the patient.
• In a patient with symptoms of blood dyscrasias, request a medical consultation for blood studies and postpone treatment until normal values are reestablished.
Teach Patient/Family to:
• Encourage effective oral hygiene to prevent soft tissue inflammation.
• Prevent trauma when using oral hygiene aids.
• Update health and drug history if physician makes any changes in evaluation or drug regimens.

enoxaparin sodium
eh-nox-ah-**pair'**-in **soe'**-dee-um
(Clexane[AUS], Klexane[CAN], Lovenox)
Do not confuse Lovenox with Lotronex.

CATEGORY AND SCHEDULE
Pregnancy Risk Category: B

Drug Class: Heparin-type anticoagulant

MECHANISM OF ACTION
A low-molecular-weight heparin that potentiates the action of antithrombin III and inactivates coagulation factor Xa.
Therapeutic Effect: Produces anticoagulation. Does not significantly influence bleeding time, PT, or aPTT.

USES
Prevention and treatment of deep vein thrombosis (DVT) following hip or knee replacement surgery; also used in abdominal and gynecologic surgery; with aspirin in the prevention of ischemic complications of unstable angina and non–Q-wave MI; in combination with warfarin for DVT, with or without pulmonary embolism

PHARMACOKINETICS

Route	Onset	Peak	Duration
Subcutaneous	N/A	3–5 hr	12 hr

Well absorbed after subcutaneous administration. Eliminated primarily in urine. Not removed by hemodialysis. *Half-life:* 4.5 hr.

INDICATIONS AND DOSAGES
▸ **Prevention of DVT after Hip and Knee Surgery**
Subcutaneous
Adults, Elderly. 30 mg twice a day, generally for 7–10 days.
▸ **Prevention of DVT after Abdominal Surgery**
Subcutaneous
Adults, Elderly. 40 mg a day for 7–10 days.
▸ **Prevention of Long-Term DVT in Nonsurgical Acute Illness**
Subcutaneous
Adults, Elderly. 40 mg once a day for 3 wk.
▸ **Prevention of Ischemic Complications of Unstable Angina and Non–Q-Wave MI (with Oral Aspirin Therapy)**
Subcutaneous
Adults, Elderly. 1 mg/kg q12h.

▸ **Acute DVT**
Subcutaneous
Adults, Elderly. 1 mg/kg q12h or
1.5 mg/kg once daily.
▸ **Usual Pediatric Dosage**
Subcutaneous
Children. 0.5 mg/kg q12h
(prophylaxis); 1 mg/kg q12h
(treatment).
▸ **Dosage in Renal Impairment**
Clearance of enoxaparin is
decreased when creatinine clearance
is less than 30 ml/min. Monitor
patient and adjust dosage as
necessary. When enoxaparin is used
in abdominal, hip, or knee surgery
or acute illness, the dosage in renal
impairment is 30 mg once a day.
When enoxaparin is used to treat
DVT, angina, or MI the dosage in
renal impairment is 1 mg/kg once
a day.

SIDE EFFECTS/ADVERSE REACTIONS
Occasional
Injection site hematoma, nausea,
peripheral edema

PRECAUTIONS AND CONTRAINDICATIONS
Active major bleeding, concurrent
heparin therapy, hypersensitivity to
heparin or pork products,
thrombocytopenia associated with
positive in vitro test for antiplatelet
antibodies
Caution:
Hemorrhage, thrombocytopenia,
renal impairment, elderly, lactation,
children, requires monitoring, GI
bleeding

DRUG INTERACTIONS OF CONCERN TO DENTISTRY
• Avoid concurrent use of aspirin,
NSAIDs, dipyridamole,
sulfinpyrazone

• Use with caution in patients taking
olanzapine

SERIOUS REACTIONS
! Overdose may lead to bleeding
complications ranging from local
ecchymoses to major hemorrhage.
Antidote: Protamine sulfate (1%
solution) equal to the dose of
enoxaparin injected. 1 mg protamine
sulfate neutralizes 1 mg enoxaparin.
A second dose of 0.5 mg protamine
sulfate per 1 mg enoxaparin may be
given if aPTT tested 2–4 hr after
first injection remains prolonged.

DENTAL CONSIDERATIONS
General:
• Determine why patient is taking
the drug.
• Product may be used in outpatient
therapy. Delay elective dental
treatment until patient completes
enoxaparin therapy.
• Consider local hemostasis
measures to prevent excessive
bleeding if dental treatment must be
performed.
• Avoid products that affect platelet
function, such as aspirin and
NSAIDs.
• Antibiotic prophylaxis before
dental treatment required for joint
prosthesis.
Consultations:
• Medical consultation should
include routine blood counts,
including platelet counts and
bleeding time.
Teach Patient/Family to:
• Encourage effective oral hygiene
to prevent soft tissue inflammation.
• Use caution to prevent trauma
when using oral hygiene aids.
• Report oral lesions, soreness, or
bleeding to dentist.

entacapone
en-**tak**′-ah-pone
(Comtan)

CATEGORY AND SCHEDULE
Pregnancy Risk Category: C

Drug Class: Antiparkinsonian

MECHANISM OF ACTION
An antiparkinson agent that inhibits the enzyme, catechol-O-methyltransferase (COMT), potentiating dopamine activity and increasing the duration of action of levodopa.
Therapeutic Effect: Decreases signs and symptoms of Parkinson's disease.

USES
Adjunct to levodopa/carbidopa in the treatment of Parkinson's disease, not used alone

PHARMACOKINETICS
Rapidly absorbed after PO administration. Protein binding: 98%. Metabolized in the liver. Primarily eliminated by biliary excretion. Not removed by hemodialysis. *Half-life:* 2.4 hr.

INDICATIONS AND DOSAGES
▶ **Adjunctive Treatment of Parkinson's Disease**
PO
Adults, Elderly. 200 mg concomitantly with each dose of carbidopa and levodopa up to a maximum of 8 times a day (1600 mg).

SIDE EFFECTS/ADVERSE REACTIONS
Frequent
Dyskinesia, nausea, dark yellow or orange urine and sweat, diarrhea
Occasional
Abdominal pain, vomiting, constipation, dry mouth, fatigue, back pain
Rare
Anxiety, somnolence, agitation, dyspepsia, flatulence, diaphoresis, asthenia, dyspnea

PRECAUTIONS AND CONTRAINDICATIONS
Hypersensitivity, use within 14 days of MAOIs
Caution:
Enhanced orthostatic hypotension with levodopa and carbidopa, hepatic impairment, caution in driving, lactation, children

DRUG INTERACTIONS OF CONCERN TO DENTISTRY
• Increased heart rate, arrhythmias, hypertension: epinephrine, norepinephrine, levonordefrin, other sympathomimetics metabolized by COMT
• Possible decrease in urinary excretion: erythromycin

SERIOUS REACTIONS
! None known

DENTAL CONSIDERATIONS
General:
• Monitor vital signs at every appointment because of cardiovascular side effects.
• Short appointments and a stress-reduction protocol may be required for anxious patients.
• Consider semisupine chair position for patient comfort if GI side effects occur.

E

• Use vasoconstrictor with caution, in low doses and with careful aspiration. Avoid using gingival retraction cord containing epinephrine.

• Assess for presence of extrapyramidal motor symptoms, such as tardive dyskinesia and akathisia. Extrapyramidal motor activity may complicate dental treatment.

• After supine positioning, have patient sit upright for at least 2 min to avoid orthostatic hypotension.

• Assess salivary flow as a factor in caries, periodontal disease and candidiasis.

Consultations:

• Medical consultation may be required to assess disease control and patient's ability to tolerate stress.

Teach Patient/Family to:

• Use powered tooth brush if patient has difficulty holding conventional devices.

• Update health and drug history if physician makes any changes in evaluation or drug regimens.

• When chronic dry mouth occurs, advise patient to:

   • Avoid mouth rinses with high alcohol content because of drying effects.

   • Use daily home fluoride products for anticaries effect.

   • Use sugarless gum, frequent sips of water, or saliva substitutes.

ephedrine
eh-**fed**′-rin
(Pretz-D)
Do not confuse ephedrine with epinephrine.

CATEGORY AND SCHEDULE
Pregnancy Risk Category: C

Drug Class: Adrenergic, mixed direct and indirect effects

MECHANISM OF ACTION
An adrenergic agonist that stimulates alpha-adrenergic receptors causing vasoconstriction and pressor effects, β_1-adrenergic receptors, resulting in cardiac stimulation, and β_2-adrenergic receptors, resulting in bronchial dilation and vasodilation. *Therapeutic Effect:* Increases B/P and pulse rate, reduces nasal congestion.

USES
Treatment of shock, increased perfusion, hypotension, bronchodilation, nasal decongestant

PHARMACOKINETICS
Well absorbed after nasal and parenteral absorption. Metabolized in liver. Excreted in urine. *Half-life:* 3–6 hr.

INDICATIONS AND DOSAGES
▶ **Asthma**
PO
Adults. 25–50 mg q3–4h as needed.
Children. 3 mg/kg/day in 4 divided doses.
▶ **Hypotension**
IM
Adults. 25–50 mg as a single dose. Maximum 150 mg/day.
Children. 0.2–0.3 mg/kg/dose q4–6h.

IV
Adults. 5 mg/dose slow IVP as
prevention. 10–25 mg/dose slow
IVP repeated q5–10 min as
treatment. Maximum: 150 mg/day.
Children. 0.2–0.3 mg/kg/dose slow
IVP q4–6h.
Subcutaneous
Adults. 25–50 q4–6h. Maximum
150 mg/day.
Children. 3 mg/kg/day q4–6h.
▸ **Nasal Congestion**
PO
Adults. 25–50 mg q6h as needed.
Children. 3 mg/kg/day in 4 divided
doses.
Nasal
Adults, Children 12 yr and older.
2–3 sprays into each nostril q4h.
Children 6–12 yr. 1–2 sprays into
each nostril q4h.

SIDE EFFECTS/ADVERSE REACTIONS
Frequent
Hypertension, anxiety
Occasional
Nausea, vomiting, palpitations,
tremor
Nasal: Burning, stinging, runny nose
Rare
Psychosis, decreased urination,
necrosis at injection site from
repeated injections

PRECAUTIONS AND CONTRAINDICATIONS
Anesthesia with cyclopropane or
halothane, diabetes (ephedrine
injection), hypersensitivity to
ephedrine or other sympathomimetic
amines, hypertension or other
cardiovascular disorders, pregnancy
with maternal B/P above 130/80,
thyrotoxicosis

Caution:
Cardiac disorders, hyperthyroidism,
diabetes mellitus, prostatic
hypertrophy

DRUG INTERACTIONS OF CONCERN TO DENTISTRY
• Decreased pressor effect:
haloperidol, phenothiazines,
thioxanthenes
• Dysrhythmia: halogenated general
anesthetics

SERIOUS REACTIONS
❗ Excessive doses may cause
hypertension, intracranial
hemorrhage, anginal pain, and fatal
arrhythmias.
❗ Prolonged or excessive use may
result in metabolic acidosis due to
increased serum lactic acid
concentrations.
❗ Observe for disorientation,
weakness, hyperventilation,
headache, nausea, vomiting, and
diarrhea.

DENTAL CONSIDERATIONS
General:
• Monitor vital signs at every
appointment because of
cardiovascular side effects.
• Avoid or limit dose of
vasoconstrictor.
• Assess salivary flow as a factor in
caries, periodontal disease, and
candidiasis.
• Consider semisupine chair
position for patients with respiratory
disease.
• Consider short appointments and a
stress-reduction protocol for anxious
patients.
Consultations:
• Medical consultation may be
required to assess disease control
and patient's tolerance for stress.

E

Teach Patient/Family:
• When chronic dry mouth occurs, advise patient to:
  • Avoid mouth rinses with high alcohol content because of drying effects.
  • Use daily home fluoride products for anticaries effect.
  • Use sugarless gum, frequent sips of water, or saliva substitutes.

epinastine
eh-pin-**ass**′-teen
(Elestat)

CATEGORY AND SCHEDULE
Pregnancy Risk Category: C

Drug Class: Ophthalmic antihistamine

MECHANISM OF ACTION
An ophthalmic H_1 receptor antagonist that inhibits the release of histamine from the mast cell.
Therapeutic Effect: Prevents pruritus associated with allergic conjunctivitis.

USES
Prevention of itching associated with allergic conjunctivitis

PHARMACOKINETICS
Low systemic exposure. Protein binding: 64%. Less than 10% is metabolized. Excreted primarily in urine and, to a lesser extent, in feces. *Half-life:* 12 hr.

INDICATIONS AND DOSAGES
▸ **Allergic Conjunctivitis**
Ophthalmic
Adults, Elderly, Children 3 yr and older. 1 drop in each eye twice a

day. Continue treatment until period of exposure (pollen season, exposure to offending allergen) is over.

SIDE EFFECTS/ADVERSE REACTIONS
Occasional
Ocular (10%–1%): Burning sensation in the eye, hyperemia, pruritus
Nonocular (10%): Cold symptoms, upper respiratory tract infection
Rare
Headache, rhinitis, sinusitis, increased cough, pharyngitis

PRECAUTIONS AND CONTRAINDICATIONS
Hypersensitivity
Caution:
Do not wear contact lens if the eye is red, otherwise contact may be placed in eye 10 min after dosing; use in nursing and in children younger than 3 yr has not been established

DRUG INTERACTIONS OF CONCERN TO DENTISTRY
• None reported

SERIOUS REACTIONS
! None known

DENTAL CONSIDERATIONS

General:
• Avoid dental light in patient's eyes; offer dark glasses for patient comfort.

epinephrine
ep-ih-**nef**′-rin
(Adrenalin, Adrenaline
Injection[AUS], EpiPen, EpiPen Jr.
0.15 Adrenaline
Autoinjector[AUS], Primatene)
Do not confuse epinephrine with
ephedrine.

CATEGORY AND SCHEDULE
Pregnancy Risk Category: C

Drug Class: Adrenergic agonist,
catecholamine

MECHANISM OF ACTION
A sympathomimetic, adrenergic
agonist that stimulates alpha-
adrenergic receptors causing
vasoconstriction and pressor effects,
β_1-adrenergic receptors, resulting in
cardiac stimulation, and β_2-
adrenergic receptors, resulting in
bronchial dilation and vasodilation.
With ophthalmic form, increases
outflow of aqueous humor from
anterior eye chamber.
Therapeutic Effect: Relaxes smooth
muscle of the bronchial tree,
produces cardiac stimulation and
dilates skeletal muscle vasculature.
The ophthalmic form dilates pupils
and constricts conjunctival blood
vessels.

USES
Treatment of acute asthmatic
attacks, hemostasis, bronchospasm,
anaphylaxis, allergic reactions,
cardiac arrest, vasopressor,
open-angle glaucoma, nasal
congestion

PHARMACOKINETICS

Route	Onset	Peak	Duration
IM	5–10 min	20 min	1–4 hr
Subcutaneous	5–10 min	20 min	1–4 hr
Inhalation	3–5 min	20 min	1–3 hr
Ophthalmic	1 hr	4–8 hr	12–24 hr

Well absorbed after parenteral
administration; minimally absorbed
after inhalation. Metabolized in the
liver, other tissues and sympathetic
nerve endings. Excreted in urine.
The ophthalmic form may be
systemically absorbed as a result of
drainage into nasal pharyngeal
passages. Mydriasis occurs within
several min and persists several hr;
vasoconstriction occurs within 5 min
and lasts less than 1 hr.

INDICATIONS AND DOSAGES
▶ **Asystole**
IV
Adults, Elderly. 1 mg q3–5 min up
to 0.1 mg/kg q3–5 min.
Children. 0.01 mg/kg (0.1 ml/kg of
1:10,000 solution). May repeat
q3–5 min. Subsequent doses of
0.1 mg/kg (0.1 ml/kg) of a 1:1000
solution q3–5 min.
▶ **Bradycardia**
IV Infusion
Adults, Elderly. 1–10 mcg/min
titrated to desired effect.
IV
Children. 0.01 mg/kg (0.1 mg/kg of
1:10,000 solution) q3–5 min.
Maximum: 1 mg/10 ml.
▶ **Bronchodilation**
IM, Subcutaneous
Adults, Elderly. 0.3 mg (1:1000)
q10–15 min to 4 hr.
Subcutaneous
Children. 10 mcg/kg (0.01 ml/kg of
1:1,000) Maximum: 0.5 mg or
suspension (1:200) 0.005 ml/kg/dose

E

E

(0.025 mg/kg/dose) to a maximum of 0.15 ml (0.75 mg for single dose) q8–12h.

▸ **Hypersensitivity Reaction**
IM, Subcutaneous
Adults, Elderly. 0.3 mg q15–20 min.
Subcutaneous
Children. 0.01 mg/kg q15 min for 2 doses, then q4h. Maximum single dose: 0.5 mg.
Inhalation
Adults, Elderly, Children 4 yr and older. 1 inhalation, may repeat in at least 1 min. Give subsequent doses no sooner than 3 hr.
Nebulizer
Adults, Elderly, Children 4 yr and older. 1–3 deep inhalations. Give subsequent doses no sooner than 3 hr.

▸ **Glaucoma**
Ophthalmic
Adults, Elderly. 1–2 drops 1–2 times a day.

SIDE EFFECTS/ADVERSE REACTIONS

Frequent
Systemic: Tachycardia, palpitations, nervousness
Ophthalmic: Headache, eye irritation, watering of eyes
Occasional
Systemic: Dizziness, light-headedness, facial flushing, headache, diaphoresis, increased B/P, nausea, trembling, insomnia, vomiting, fatigue
Ophthalmic: Blurred or decreased vision, eye pain
Rare
Systemic: Chest discomfort or pain, arrhythmias, bronchospasm, dry mouth or throat

PRECAUTIONS AND CONTRAINDICATIONS

Cardiac arrhythmias, cerebrovascular insufficiency, hypertension, hyperthyroidism, ischemic heart disease, narrow-angle glaucoma, shock
Caution:
Cardiac disorders, hyperthyroidism, diabetes mellitus, prostatic hypertrophy

DRUG INTERACTIONS OF CONCERN TO DENTISTRY

• Hypotension, tachycardia: haloperidol, loxapine, phenothiazines, thioxanthenes
• Ventricular dysrhythmia: hydrocarbon-inhalation anesthetics, CNS stimulants, tricyclic antidepressants
• With larger doses of epinephrine, risk of hypertension followed by bradycardia with non-cardioselective β-adrenergic antagonists

SERIOUS REACTIONS

! Excessive doses may cause acute hypertension or arrhythmias.
! Prolonged or excessive use may result in metabolic acidosis because of increased serum lactic acid concentrations. Metabolic acidosis may cause disorientation, fatigue, hyperventilation, headache, nausea, vomiting, and diarrhea.

DENTAL CONSIDERATIONS

General:
• Monitor vital signs at every appointment because of cardiovascular side effects.
• Assess salivary flow as a factor in caries, periodontal disease, and candidiasis.
• Consider semisupine chair position for patients with respiratory disease.

• Acute asthmatic episodes may be precipitated in the dental office. Sympathomimetic inhalants should be available for emergency use; a stress-reduction protocol may be required.

epinephryl borate
ep-ih-**nef**′-rill **bor**′-ate
(Epifrin, Epinal, Eppy/N)

CATEGORY AND SCHEDULE
Pregnancy Risk Category: C

Drug Class: Antiglaucoma agent, ophthalmic; surgical aid, ophthalmic

MECHANISM OF ACTION
A direct-acting sympathomimetic amine whose mechanism of action is unknown.
Therapeutic Effect: Increases outflow of aqueous humor from anterior eye chamber.

USES
Treatment of certain types of glaucoma. It may also be used in eye surgery.

PHARMACOKINETICS
May have systemic absorption from drainage into nasal pharyngeal passages. Mydriasis occurs within several min, persists several hr; vasoconstriction occurs within 5 min, lasts less than 1 hr.

INDICATIONS AND DOSAGES
▸ **Glaucoma**
Ophthalmic
Adults, Elderly. Instill 1 drop 1–2 times a day.

SIDE EFFECTS/ADVERSE REACTIONS
Frequent
Headache, stinging, burning or other eye irritation, watering of eyes
Occasional
Blurred or decreased vision, eye pain

PRECAUTIONS AND CONTRAINDICATIONS
Cardiac arrhythmias, cerebrovascular insufficiency, hypertension, hyperthyroidism, ischemic heart disease, narrow-angle glaucoma, shock, hypersensitivity to epinephryl borate or any component of the formulation

DRUG INTERACTIONS OF CONCERN TO DENTISTRY
• Risk of arrhythmias: halogenated hydrocarbon anesthetics, tricyclic antidepressants, amphetamine-like drugs

SERIOUS REACTIONS
! Systemic absorption occurs rarely. These effects include fast, irregular, or pounding heartbeat, feeling faint, increased sweating, paleness, trembling and increased B/P.

DENTAL CONSIDERATIONS
General:
• Determine why patient is taking the drug.
• Avoid drugs with anticholinergic activity, such as antihistamines, opioids, benzodiazepines, propantheline, atropine, and scopolamine.
• Avoid dental light in patient's eyes; offer dark glasses for patient comfort.
• Question glaucoma patient about compliance with prescribed drug regimen.

E

Consultations:
• Medical consultation may be required to assess disease control.
Teach Patient/Family to:
• Update health and medication history if physician makes any changes in evaluation or drug regimens; include OTC, herbal, and nonherbal remedies in the update.

epirubicin
eh-pea-**rew**′-bih-sin
(Ellence, Pharm Rubicin)

CATEGORY AND SCHEDULE
Pregnancy Risk Category: D

Drug Class: Anthracycline antibiotic; antineoplastic

MECHANISM OF ACTION
An anthracycline antibiotic whose exact mechanism is unknown but may include formation of a complex with DNA and subsequent inhibition of DNA, RNA, and protein synthesis. Also inhibits DNA helicase activity, preventing enzymatic separation of double-stranded DNA and interfering with replication and transcription.
Therapeutic Effect: Produces antiproliferative and cytotoxic activity.

USES
Treatment of some kinds of cancers of the breast, lung, lymph system, stomach, and ovaries

PHARMACOKINETICS
Widely distributed into tissues. Protein binding: 77%. Metabolized in the liver and RBCs. Primarily eliminated through biliary excretion.

Not removed by hemodialysis.
Half-life: 33 hr.

INDICATIONS AND DOSAGES
▸ **Breast Cancer**
IV
Adults. Initially, 100–120 mg/m^2 in repeated cycles of 3–4 wk, in combination with fluorouracil (5-FU) and Cytoxan. Total dose may be given on day 1 of each cycle or in equally divided doses on days 1 and 8 of each cycle.

SIDE EFFECTS/ADVERSE REACTIONS
Frequent
Nausea, vomiting, alopecia, amenorrhea
Occasional
Stomatitis, diarrhea, hot flashes
Rare
Rash, pruritus, fever, lethargy, conjunctivitis

PRECAUTIONS AND CONTRAINDICATIONS
Baseline neutrophil count less than 1500/mm^3, hypersensitivity to epirubicin, previous treatment with anthracyclines up to maximum cumulative dose, recent MI, severe hepatic impairment, severe myocardial insufficiency

DRUG INTERACTIONS OF CONCERN TO DENTISTRY
• None reported

SERIOUS REACTIONS
! The risk of cardiotoxicity (either acute, manifested as transient ECG abnormalities, or chronic, manifested as CHF) increases when the total cumulative dose exceeds 900 mg/m^2.
! Extravasation during administration may result in severe local tissue necrosis.

! Myelosuppression may cause hematologic toxicity, manifested principally as leukopenia and, to a lesser extent, anemia and thrombocytopenia.

DENTAL CONSIDERATIONS

General:
• If additional analgesia is required for dental pain, consider alternative analgesics (NSAIDs) in patients taking opioids for acute or chronic pain.
• Examine for oral manifestations of opportunistic infection.
• This drug may be used in the hospital or on an outpatient basis. Confirm the patient's disease and treatment status.
• Chlorhexidine mouth rinse prior to and during chemotherapy may reduce severity of mucositis.
• Patient on chronic drug therapy may rarely present with symptoms of blood dyscrasias, which can include infection, bleeding, and poor healing. If dyscrasia is present, caution patient to prevent oral tissue trauma when using oral hygiene aids.
• Palliative medication may be required for management of oral side effects.
• Patient may be at risk of bleeding; check oral signs.
• Patient may be at risk of infection.
Consultations:
• Medical consultation should include routine blood counts including platelet counts and bleeding time.
• In a patient with symptoms of blood dyscrasias, request a medical consultation for blood studies and postpone treatment until normal values are reestablished.
• Consult physician; prophylactic or therapeutic antiinfectives may be

indicated if surgery or periodontal treatment is required.
• Medical consultation may be required to assess immunologic status during cancer chemotherapy and determine safety risk, if any, posed by the required dental treatment.
• Medical consultation may be required to assess disease control and patient's ability to tolerate stress.
Teach Patient/Family to:
• Be aware of oral side effects.
• Encourage effective oral hygiene to prevent soft tissue inflammation.
• Report oral lesions, soreness, or bleeding to dentist.
• Prevent trauma when using oral hygiene aids.
• Update health and medication history if physician makes any changes in evaluation or drug regimens; include OTC, herbal, and nonherbal remedies in the update.

eplerenone
eh-**plear′**-ah-nown
(Inspra)

CATEGORY AND SCHEDULE
Pregnancy Risk Category: B

Drug Class: Antihypertensive, aldosterone antagonist

MECHANISM OF ACTION
An aldosterone receptor antagonist that binds to the mineralocorticoid receptors in the kidney, heart, blood vessels and brain, blocking the binding of aldosterone.
Therapeutic Effect: Reduces B/P.

USES
Treatment of hypertension as a single drug or in combination with other antihypertensive drugs; improved survival of CHF patients following an acute heart attack

PHARMACOKINETICS
Absorption unaffected by food. Protein binding: 50%. No active metabolites. Excreted in the urine with a lesser amount eliminated in the feces. Not removed by hemodialysis. *Half-life:* 4–6 hr.

INDICATIONS AND DOSAGES
▶ **Hypertension**
PO
Adults, Elderly. 50 mg once a day. If 50 mg once a day produces an inadequate B/P response, may increase dosage to 50 mg twice a day. If patient is concurrently receiving erythromycin, saquinavir, verapamil, or fluconazole, reduce initial dose to 25 mg once a day.
▶ **CHF Following MI**
PO
Adults, Elderly. Initially, 25 mg once a day. If tolerated, titrate up to 50 mg once a day within 4 wk.

SIDE EFFECTS/ADVERSE REACTIONS
Rare
Dizziness, diarrhea, cough, fatigue, flu-like symptoms, abdominal pain

PRECAUTIONS AND CONTRAINDICATIONS
Concurrent use of potassium supplements or potassium-sparing diuretics (such as amiloride, spironolactone and triamterene), or inhibitors of the cytochrome P450 3A4 enzyme system (including erythromycin, ketoconazole and itraconazole), creatinine clearance less than 50 ml/min, serum creatinine level greater than 2 mg/dl in males or 1.8 mg/dl in females, serum potassium level greater than 5.5 mEq/L, type 2 diabetes mellitus with microalbuminuria
Caution:
Hyperkalemia, monitor serum potassium periodically, impaired hepatic or renal function, angiotensin-converting enzyme (ACE) inhibitors, angiotensin II antagonists, lactation, use in children has not been established

DRUG INTERACTIONS OF CONCERN TO DENTISTRY
• See contraindications; use with caution in patients taking strong inhibitors of CYP3A4 isoenzymes (erythromycin)
• Monitor blood pressure if NSAIDs are required

SERIOUS REACTIONS
❗ Hyperkalemia may occur, particularly in patients with Type 2 diabetes mellitus and microalbuminuria.

DENTAL CONSIDERATIONS
General:
• Monitor vital signs at every appointment because of cardiovascular side effects.
• Avoid or limit dose of vasoconstrictor.
• Short appointments and a stress-reduction protocol may be required for anxious patients.
• Take precautions if dental surgery is anticipated and general anesthesia is required.
Consultations:
• Medical consultation may be required to assess disease control and patient's ability to tolerate stress.

- Consultation with physician may be necessary if sedation or general anesthesia is required.

Teach Patient/Family to:
- Update health and drug history if physician makes any changes in evaluation or drug regimens.

epoetin alfa
eh-**poh´**-ee-tin **al´**-fa
(Epogen, Eprex[CAN], Procrit)
Do not confuse Epogen with Neupogen.

CATEGORY AND SCHEDULE
Pregnancy Risk Category: C

Drug Class: Hematinic, antianemic

MECHANISM OF ACTION
A glycoprotein that stimulates division and differentiation of erythroid progenitor cells in bone marrow.
Therapeutic Effect: Induces erythropoiesis and releases reticulocytes from bone marrow.

USES
Anemia of chronic renal failure, end-stage renal disease, anemia in zidovudine-treated HIV patients, anemia in cancer patients on chemotherapy, reduction of allogenic blood transfusion in surgery patients

PHARMACOKINETICS
Well absorbed after subcutaneous administration. Following administration, an increase in reticulocyte count occurs within 10 days and increases in Hgb, Hct, and RBC count are seen within 2–6 wk.
Half-life: 4–13 hr.

INDICATIONS AND DOSAGES
▸ **Treatment of Anemia in Chemotherapy Patients**
IV, Subcutaneous
Adults, Elderly, Children. 150 units/kg/dose 3 times a wk. Maximum: 1200 units/kg/wk.
▸ **Reduction of Allogenic Blood Transfusions in Elective Surgery**
Subcutaneous
Adults, Elderly. 300 units/kg/day 10 days before day of and 4 days after surgery.
▸ **Chronic Renal Failure**
IV Bolus, Subcutaneous
Adults, Elderly. Initially, 50–100 units/kg 3 times a wk. Target Hct range: 30%–36%. Adjust dosage no earlier than 1-mo intervals unless prescribed. Decrease dosage if Hct is increasing and approaching 36%. Plan to temporarily withhold doses if Hct continues to rise and to reinstate lower dosage when Hct begins to decrease. If Hct increases by more than 4 points in 2 wk, monitor Hct twice a wk for 2–6 wk. Increase dose if Hct does not increase 5–6 points after 8 wk (with adequate iron stores) and if Hct is below target range. Maintenance: For patients on dialysis: 75 units/kg 3 times a wk. Range: 12.5–525 units/kg. For patients not on dialysis: 75–150 units/kg/wk.
▸ **HIV Infection in Patients Treated with AZT**
IV, Subcutaneous
Adults. Initially, 100 units/kg 3 times a wk for 8 wk; may increase by 50–100 units/kg 3 times a wk. Evaluate response q4–8wk thereafter. Adjust dosage by 50–100 units/kg 3 times a wk. If dosages larger than 300 units/kg 3 times a wk are not eliciting response, it is unlikely patient will respond. Maintenance: Titrate to maintain desired Hct.

E

SIDE EFFECTS/ADVERSE REACTIONS

▶ **Patients Receiving Chemotherapy**

Frequent

Fever, diarrhea, nausea, vomiting, edema

Occasional

Asthenia, shortness of breath, paresthesia

Rare

Dizziness, trunk pain

▶ **Patients with Chronic Renal Failure**

Frequent

Hypertension, headache, nausea, arthralgia

Occasional

Fatigue, edema, diarrhea, vomiting, chest pain, skin reactions at administration site, asthenia, dizziness

▶ **Patients with HIV Infection Treated with AZT**

Frequent

Fever, fatigue, headache, cough, diarrhea, rash, nausea

Occasional

Shortness of breath, asthenia, skin reaction at injection site, dizziness

PRECAUTIONS AND CONTRAINDICATIONS

History of sensitivity to mammalian cell-derived products or human albumin, uncontrolled hypertension

Caution:

Contains benzyl alcohol (risk of complications in premature infants), increased thrombosis risk in CHF, ischemic heart disease, coronary artery bypass, pure red cell aplasia, monitor and control B/P, seizures in CRF, thrombosis during hemodialysis, porphyria, lactation, safety and efficacy in children younger than 1 mo have not been established, monitor renal function, monitor hematocrit

DRUG INTERACTIONS OF CONCERN TO DENTISTRY

• None reported

SERIOUS REACTIONS

! Hypertensive encephalopathy, thrombosis, cerebrovascular accident, MI, and seizures have occurred rarely.

! Hyperkalemia occurs occasionally in patients with chronic renal failure, usually in those who do not conform to medication regimen, dietary guidelines, and frequency of dialysis regimen.

DENTAL CONSIDERATIONS

General:

• Patient's disease, treatment history, and use of other drugs will affect patient evaluation and management.

• Determine why patient is taking the drug.

• Monitor vital signs at every appointment because of cardiovascular and respiratory side effects.

• Take precautions if dental surgery is anticipated and general anesthesia is required.

• Patient history should include all medications and herbal or nonherbal remedies taken by the patient.

• Consider semisupine chair position for patient comfort if GI side effects occur.

• Place on frequent recall because of oral side effects, depending on chemotherapy regimen or HIV immunologic status.

Consultations:

• Medical consultation should include hematocrit and routine blood counts, including platelet counts and bleeding time.

• Consultation with physician may be necessary if sedation or general anesthesia is required.

• Medical consultation may be required to assess disease control and patient's ability to tolerate stress.
Teach Patient/Family to:
• Encourage effective oral hygiene to prevent soft tissue inflammation, infection.

epoprostenol sodium, prostacyclin

eh-poe-pros'-ten-ol soe'-dee-um, pros-ta-sih'-klin
(Flolan)

CATEGORY AND SCHEDULE
Pregnancy Risk Category: B

Drug Class: Vasodilator; antihypertensive

MECHANISM OF ACTION
An antihypertensive that directly dilates pulmonary and systemic arterial vascular beds and inhibits platelet aggregation.
Therapeutic Effect: Reduces right and left ventricular afterload; increases cardiac output and stroke volume.

USES
Treatment of the symptoms of primary pulmonary hypertension, or the high B/P that occurs in the main artery that carries blood from the right side of the heart (the ventricle) to the lungs

INDICATIONS AND DOSAGES
▶ **Long-Term Treatment of New York Heart Association Class III and IV Primary Pulmonary Hypertension**
IV Infusion
Adults, Elderly. Procedure to determine dose range: Initially, 2 ng/kg/min, increased in increments of 2 ng/kg/min q15 min until dose-limiting adverse effects occur. Chronic infusion: Start at 4 ng/kg/min less than the maximum dose rate tolerated during acute dose ranging (or one-half of the maximum rate if rate was less than 5 ng/kg/min).

SIDE EFFECTS/ADVERSE REACTIONS
Frequent
Acute phase: Flushing, headache, nausea, vomiting, hypotension, anxiety, chest pain, dizziness
Chronic phase: Dyspnea, asthenia, dizziness, headache, chest pain, nausea, vomiting, palpitations, edema, jaw pain, tachycardia, flushing, myalgia, nonspecific muscle pain, paresthesia, diarrhea, anxiety, chills, fever, or flu-like symptoms
Occasional
Acute phase: Bradycardia, abdominal pain, muscle pain, dyspnea, back pain
Chronic phase: Rash, depression, hypotension, pallor, syncope, bradycardia, ascites
Rare
Acute phase: Paresthesia
Chronic phase: Diaphoresis, dyspepsia, tachycardia

PRECAUTIONS AND CONTRAINDICATIONS
Long-term use in patients with CHF (severe ventricular systolic dysfunction)

DRUG INTERACTIONS OF CONCERN TO DENTISTRY

• Increased risk of bleeding: drugs which interfere with coagulation or platelet function; such as NSAIDs and aspirin

SERIOUS REACTIONS

! Overdose may cause hyperglycemia or ketoacidosis manifested as increased urination, thirst, and fruit-like breath odor.
! Angina, MI, and thrombocytopenia occur rarely.
! Abrupt withdrawal, including a large reduction in dosage or interruption in drug delivery, may produce rebound pulmonary hypertension as evidenced by dyspnea, dizziness, and asthenia.

DENTAL CONSIDERATIONS

General:
• Continuous-use drug for patients with severe cardiovascular disease. Provide palliative emergency dental care as required.
• Determine why patient is taking the drug.
• Monitor vital signs at every appointment because of cardiovascular side effects.
• Avoid products that affect platelet function, such as aspirin and NSAIDs.
• Stress from dental procedures may compromise cardiovascular function, determine patient risk.
• Postpone elective dental treatment if patient shows signs of cardiac symptoms or respiratory distress.
• Use vasoconstrictor with caution, in low doses and with careful aspiration. Avoid using gingival retraction cord containing epinephrine.

Consultations:
• Medical consultation may be required to assess disease control and patient's ability to tolerate stress.
• Medical consultation should include routine blood counts including platelet counts and bleeding time.
Teach Patient/Family to:
• Encourage effective oral hygiene to prevent soft tissue inflammation.
• Prevent trauma when using oral hygiene aids.
• Update health and medication history if physician makes any changes in evaluation or drug regimens; include OTC, herbal, and nonherbal remedies in the update.

---

eprosartan
eh-pro-**sar′**-tan
(Teveten)

CATEGORY AND SCHEDULE
Pregnancy Risk Category: C (D if used in second or third trimester)

Drug Class: Antihypertensive, angiotensin II receptor (AT_1) antagonist

MECHANISM OF ACTION
An angiotensin II receptor antagonist that blocks the vasoconstrictor and aldosterone-secreting effects of angiotensin II, inhibiting the binding of angiotensin II to the AT_1 receptors.
Therapeutic Effect: Causes vasodilation, decreases peripheral resistance, and decreases B/P.

USES
Treatment of hypertension as a single drug or in combination with other antihypertensive drugs

PHARMACOKINETICS
Rapidly absorbed after PO administration. Protein binding: 98%. Undergoes first-pass metabolism in the liver to active metabolites. Excreted in urine and biliary system. Minimally removed by hemodialysis. *Half-life:* 5–9 hr.

INDICATIONS AND DOSAGES
▸ **Hypertension**
PO
Adults, Elderly. Initially, 600 mg/day. Range: 400–800 mg/day.

SIDE EFFECTS/ADVERSE REACTIONS
Occasional
Headache, cough, dizziness
Rare
Muscle pain, fatigue, diarrhea, upper respiratory tract infection, dyspepsia

PRECAUTIONS AND CONTRAINDICATIONS
Bilateral renal artery stenosis, hyperaldosteronism
Caution:
Renal impairment maximum daily dose is 600 mg, risk of renal impairment, pregnancy category C (first trimester) and pregnancy category D (second and third trimesters); safety and efficacy in lactation and patients younger than 18 yr have not been established

DRUG INTERACTIONS OF CONCERN TO DENTISTRY
• None reported

SERIOUS REACTIONS
! Overdosage may manifest as hypotension and tachycardia. Bradycardia occurs less often.

DENTAL CONSIDERATIONS

E

General:
• Monitor vital signs at every appointment because of cardiovascular side effects.
• Avoid or limit dose of vasoconstrictor.
• Stress from dental procedures may compromise cardiovascular function; determine patient risk.
• Limit use of sodium-containing products, such as saline IV fluids, for those patients with a dietary salt restriction.
• Short appointments and a stress-reduction protocol may be required for anxious patients.
• Use precaution if sedation or general anesthesia is required; risk of hypotensive episode.
• Assess salivary flow as a factor in caries, periodontal disease, and candidiasis.
• After supine positioning, have patient sit upright for at least 2 min before standing to avoid orthostatic hypotension.
Consultations:
• Medical consultation may be required to assess disease control and patient's ability to tolerate stress.
Teach Patient/Family to:
• Update health and drug history if physician makes any changes in evaluation or drug regimens.
• When chronic dry mouth occurs, advise patient to:
  • Avoid mouth rinses with high alcohol content because of drying effects.
  • Use daily home fluoride products for anticaries effect.

• Use sugarless gum, frequent sips of water, or saliva substitutes.

eptifibatide
ep-tih-**fib**′-ah-tide
(Integrilin)

CATEGORY AND SCHEDULE
Pregnancy Risk Category: B

Drug Class: Glycoprotein IIb/ IIIa inhibitor; antiplatelet, antithrombotic

MECHANISM OF ACTION
A glycoprotein IIb/IIIa inhibitor that rapidly inhibits platelet aggregation by preventing binding of fibrinogen to receptor sites on platelets. *Therapeutic Effect:* Prevents closure of treated coronary arteries. Also prevents acute cardiac ischemic complications.

USES
Treatment of patients with acute coronary syndrome (ACS), including those managed medically and those undergoing percutaneous coronary intervention (PCI)

PHARMACOKINETICS
Half-life 2.5 hr, steady state 4–6 hr, metabolism limited, excretion via kidneys.

INDICATIONS AND DOSAGES
▶Adjunct to Percutaneous Coronary Intervention
IV Bolus, IV Infusion
Adults, Elderly. 180 mcg/kg before PCI initiation; then continuous drip of 2 mcg/kg/min and a second 180 mcg/kg bolus 10 min after the first. Maximum: 15 mg/h. Continue until hospital discharge or for up to 18–24 hr. Minimum 12 hr is recommended. Concurrent aspirin and heparin therapy is recommended.
▶ Acute Coronary Syndrome
IV Bolus, IV Infusion
Adults, Elderly. 180 mcg/kg bolus then 2 mcg/kg/min until discharge or coronary artery bypass graft, up to 72 hr. Maximum: 15 mg/hr. Concurrent aspirin and heparin therapy is recommended.
▶ Dosage in Renal Impairment
Creatinine clearance less than 50 ml/ min. Use 180 mcg/kg bolus (maximum 22.6 mg) and 1 mcg/kg/ min infusion (maximum: 7.5 mg/hr).

SIDE EFFECTS/ADVERSE REACTIONS
Occasional
Hypotension

PRECAUTIONS AND CONTRAINDICATIONS
Active internal bleeding, AV malformation or aneurysm, history of cerebrovascular accident (CVA) within 2 yr or CVA with residual neurologic defect, history of vasculitis, intracranial neoplasm, oral anticoagulant use within last 7 days unless PT is less than 1.22 times the control, recent (6 wk) GI or GU bleeding, recent (6 wk) surgery or trauma, prior IV dextran use before or during PTCA, severe uncontrolled hypertension, thrombocytopenia (fewer than 100,000 cells/mcl)

DRUG INTERACTIONS OF CONCERN TO DENTISTRY
• Increased risk of bleeding: drugs that interfere with coagulation or

platelet function, such as NSAIDs and aspirin

SERIOUS REACTIONS

! Minor to major bleeding complications may occur, most commonly at arterial access site for cardiac catheterization.

DENTAL CONSIDERATIONS

General:
• Monitor vital signs at every appointment because of cardiovascular side effects.
• Avoid products that affect platelet function, such as aspirin and NSAIDs.
• Consider local hemostasis measures to prevent excessive bleeding.
• For acute use in emergency rooms or hospitals.
• Provide palliative emergency dental care only during drug use.
• Patients may be at risk of bleeding; check for oral signs.
• Confirm patient's medical and drug history.
Consultations:
• Medical consultation may be required to assess disease control and patient's ability to tolerate stress.
• Medical consultation should include routine blood counts including platelet counts and bleeding time.
• Medical consultation should include PPT or INR.
Teach Patient/Family to:
• Encourage effective oral hygiene to prevent soft tissue inflammation.
• Prevent trauma when using oral hygiene aids.
• Report oral lesions, soreness, or bleeding to dentist.

• Update health and medication history if physician makes any changes in evaluation or drug regimens; include OTC, herbal, and nonherbal remedies in the update.
• Use soft tooth brush to reduce risk of bleeding.

E

ergoloid mesylates
ur′-go-loyd mess′-ah-lates
(Gerimal, Hydergine, Hydergine[CAN])

CATEGORY AND SCHEDULE
Pregnancy Risk Category: C

Drug Class: Ergot alkaloids

MECHANISM OF ACTION
An ergot alkaloid that centrally acts on and decreases vascular tone, slows heart rate. Peripheral action blocks alpha adrenergic receptors. *Therapeutic Effect:* Improved O_2 uptake and improves cerebral metabolism.

USES
Senile dementia, Alzheimer's dementia, multiinfarct dementia, primary progressive dementia

PHARMACOKINETICS
Rapidly, incompletely absorbed from GI tract. Metabolized in liver. Eliminated primarily in feces. *Half-life:* 2–5 hr.

INDICATIONS AND DOSAGES
▶ **Age-Related Decline in Mental Capacity**
PO
Adults, Elderly. Initially, 1 mg 3 times a day. Range: 1.5–12 mg/day.

SIDE EFFECTS/ADVERSE REACTIONS

Occasional

GI distress, transient nausea, sublingual irritation

PRECAUTIONS AND CONTRAINDICATIONS

Acute or chronic psychosis (regardless or etiology), hypersensitivity to ergoloid mesylates or any component of the formulation.

Caution:

Acute intermittent porphyria

SERIOUS REACTIONS

! Overdose may produce blurred vision, dizziness, syncope, headache, flushed face, nausea, vomiting, decreased appetite, stomach cramps, and stuffy nose.

DENTAL CONSIDERATIONS

General:

• Monitor vital signs at every appointment because of cardiovascular side effects.

• After supine positioning, have patient sit upright for at least 2 min before standing to avoid orthostatic hypotension.

• Consider semisupine chair position for patient comfort because of GI effects of drug.

• Emphasize preventive oral home care.

Teach Patient/Family to:

• Use powered tooth brush if patient is unable to carry out oral hygiene procedures.

---

ergotamine tartrate/ dihydroergotamine

er-**got′**-ah-meen **tahr′**-treyt/ dahy-hahy-droh-ur-**got′**-uh-meen ergotamine tartrate (Cafergot[CAN], Ergodryl Mono[AUS], Ergomar, Ergostat, Gynergen) dihydroergotamine: (D.H.E. 45, Dihydergot[AUS], Dihydroergotamine Sandoz[CAN], Migranal)

CATEGORY AND SCHEDULE

Pregnancy Risk Category: X

Drug Class: α-Adrenergic blocker

MECHANISM OF ACTION

An ergotamine derivative that directly stimulates vascular smooth muscle, resulting in peripheral and cerebral vasoconstriction. May also have antagonist effects on serotonin. *Therapeutic Effect:* Suppresses vascular headaches.

USES

Treatment of vascular headache (migraine or histamine), cluster headache

PHARMACOKINETICS

Slowly and incompletely absorbed from the GI tract; rapidly and extensively absorbed after rectal administration. Protein binding: greater than 90%. Undergoes extensive first-pass metabolism in the liver to active metabolite. Eliminated in feces by the biliary system. *Half-life:* 21 hr.

INDICATIONS AND DOSAGES
▸ **Vascular Headaches**
PO (Cafergot [Fixed-Combination of Ergotamine and Caffeine])
Adults, Elderly. 2 mg at onset of headache, then 1–2 mg q30 min. Maximum: 6 mg/episode; 10 mg/wk.
PO, Sublingual
Children. 1 mg at onset of headache, then 1 mg q30 min. Maximum: 3 mg/episode.
IV
Adults, Elderly. 1 mg at onset of headache; may repeat hourly. Maximum: 2 mg/day; 6 mg/wk.
Sublingual
Adults, Elderly. 1 tablet at onset of headache, then 1 tablet q30 min. Maximum: 3 tablets/24 hr; 5 tablets/wk.
IM, Subcutaneous
(Dihydroergotamine)
Adults, Elderly. 1 mg at onset of headache; may repeat hourly. Maximum: 3 mg/day; 6 mg/wk.
Intranasal
Adults, Elderly. 1 spray (0.5 mg) into each nostril; may repeat in 15 min. Maximum: 4 sprays/day; 8 sprays/wk.
Rectal
Adults, Elderly. 1 suppository at onset of headache; may repeat dose in 1 hr. Maximum: 2 suppositories/episode; 5 suppositories/wk.

SIDE EFFECTS/ADVERSE REACTIONS
Occasional
Cough, dizziness
Rare
Myalgia, fatigue, diarrhea, upper respiratory tract infection, dyspepsia

PRECAUTIONS AND CONTRAINDICATIONS
Coronary artery disease, hypertension, impaired hepatic or renal function, malnutrition, peripheral vascular diseases (such as thromboangiitis obliterans, syphilitic arteritis, severe arteriosclerosis, thrombophlebitis, and Raynaud's disease), sepsis, severe pruritus
Caution:
Lactation, children, anemia

DRUG INTERACTIONS OF CONCERN TO DENTISTRY
• Vasoconstrictor in local anesthetics
• Suspected increased risk of ergotism: erythromycin, clarithromycin, troleandomycin
• Use anticholinergics with caution in the elderly

SERIOUS REACTIONS
! Prolonged administration or excessive dosage may produce ergotamine poisoning, manifested as nausea and vomiting; paresthesia, muscle pain or weakness; precordial pain; tachycardia or bradycardia; and hypertension or hypotension. Vasoconstriction of peripheral arteries and arterioles may result in localized edema and pruritus. Muscle pain will occur when walking and later, even at rest. Other rare effects include confusion, depression, drowsiness, seizures, and gangrene.

DENTAL CONSIDERATIONS
General:
• This is an acute-use drug; patients are unlikely to seek dental treatment while using this drug.
• Monitor vital signs at every appointment because of cardiovascular side effects.
Teach Patient/Family to:
• Use powered tooth brush if patient has difficulty holding conventional devices.

E

erlotinib
er-**low**′-tih-nib
(Tarceva)

CATEGORY AND SCHEDULE
Pregnancy Risk Category: D

Drug Class: Antineoplastic

MECHANISM OF ACTION
A human epidermal growth factor that inhibits tyrosine kinases (TK) associated with transmembrane cell surface receptors found on both normal and cancer cells. One such receptor is epidermal growth factor receptor (EGFR).
Therapeutic Effect: TK activity appears to be vitally important to cell proliferation and survival.

USES
Treatment of non–small-cell lung cancer after the failure of other chemotherapy treatment. It is also used together with another medicine called gemcitabine (e.g., Gemzar) to treat cancer of the pancreas

PHARMACOKINETICS
Slowly absorbed, peak 3–7 hr, excreted in feces (86%), urine (less than 4%), metabolized by CYP3A4.
Terminal Half-Life: 36 hr.

INDICATIONS AND DOSAGES
▶ Non–Small-Cell Lung Pancreatic Cancer
PO
Adults, Elderly. Initially, 7.5 mg once a day. If response is not adequate after a minimum of 2 wk, dosage may be increased to 15 mg once a day. Do not exceed 7.5 mg once a day in patients with moderate hepatic impairment.

SIDE EFFECTS/ADVERSE REACTIONS
Frequent
Dry mouth, constipation
Occasional
Dyspepsia, headache, nausea, abdominal pain
Rare
Asthenia, diarrhea, dizziness, ocular dryness

PRECAUTIONS AND CONTRAINDICATIONS
Pregnancy

DRUG INTERACTIONS OF CONCERN TO DENTISTRY
• Increased blood levels and effects: potent inhibitors of CYP3A4 isoenzymes (ketoconazole, itraconazole, erythromycin, clarithromycin, diclofenac, doxycycline, protease inhibitors)
• Decreased effects: potent inducers of CYP3A4 isoenzymes (carbamazepine, phenobarbital, St. John's wort [herb])

SERIOUS REACTIONS
! UTI occurs occasionally.

DENTAL CONSIDERATIONS

General:
• For longer dental appointments, offer patient frequent breaks.
• Consider semisupine chair position for patient comfort if GI side effects occur.
• Avoid dental light in patient's eyes; offer dark glasses for patient comfort.
• Examine for oral manifestation of opportunistic infection.
• Assess salivary flow as a factor in caries, periodontal disease, and candidiasis.
• Place on frequent recall because of oral side effects.

Consultations:
• Physician should be informed if significant xerostomic side effects occur (increased caries, sore tongue, problems eating or swallowing, difficulty wearing prosthesis) so that a medication change can be considered.

Teach Patient/Family to:
• Encourage effective oral hygiene to prevent soft tissue inflammation.
• Update health and medication history if physician makes any changes in evaluation or drug regimens; include OTC, herbal, and nonherbal remedies in the update.
• When chronic dry mouth occurs advise patient to:
 • Avoid mouth rinses with high alcohol content because of drying effects.
 • Use daily home fluoride products for anticaries effect.
 • Use sugarless gum, frequent sips of water, or saliva substitutes.

---

ertapenem
er-ta-**pen**′-em
(Invanz)

CATEGORY AND SCHEDULE
Pregnancy Risk Category: B

Drug Class: Antiinfective-miscellaneous; carbapenem

MECHANISM OF ACTION
A carbapenem that penetrates the bacterial cell wall of microorganisms and binds to penicillin-binding proteins, inhibiting cell wall synthesis.

Therapeutic Effect: Produces bacterial cell death.

USES
Treatment of infections caused by bacteria

PHARMACOKINETICS
Almost completely absorbed after IM administration. Protein binding: 85%–95%. Widely distributed. Primarily excreted in urine with smaller amount eliminated in feces. Removed by hemodialysis. ***Half-life:*** 4 hr.

INDICATIONS AND DOSAGES
▸ **Intraabdominal Infection**
IV, IM
Adults, Elderly. 1 g/day for 5–14 days.
▸ **Skin and Skin Structure Infection**
IV, IM
Adults, Elderly. 1 g/day for 7–14 days.
▸ **Pneumonia, UTI**
IV, IM
Adults, Elderly. 1 g/day for 10–14 days.
▸ **Pelvic Infection**
IV, IM
Adults, Elderly. 1 g/day for 3–10 days.
▸ **Dosage in Renal Impairment**
For adults and elderly patients with creatinine clearance less than 30 ml/min, dosage is 500 mg once a day.

SIDE EFFECTS/ADVERSE REACTIONS
Frequent
Diarrhea, nausea, headache
Occasional
Altered mental status, insomnia, rash, abdominal pain, constipation, vomiting, edema, fever

E

Rare
Dizziness, cough, oral candidiasis, anxiety, tachycardia, phlebitis at IV site

PRECAUTIONS AND CONTRAINDICATIONS
History of hypersensitivity to beta-lactams (imipenem and cilastin, meropenem), hypersensitivity to amide-type local anesthetics (IM)

DRUG INTERACTIONS OF CONCERN TO DENTISTRY
• Increased or prolonged plasma levels: probenecid
• Dental drug interactions have not been studied

SERIOUS REACTIONS
! Antibiotic-associated colitis and other superinfections may occur.
! Anaphylactic reactions have been reported.
! Seizures may occur in those with CNS disorders (including patients with brain lesions or a history of seizures), bacterial meningitis, or severe renal impairment.

DENTAL CONSIDERATIONS

General:
• For selected infections in the hospital setting; provide palliative emergency dental treatment only.
• Examine for oral manifestation of opportunistic infection.
• Determine why patient is taking the drug.
• Caution regarding allergy to medication.

Consultations:
• Medical consultation may be required to assess disease control and patient's ability to tolerate stress.

Teach Patient/Family to:
• Encourage effective oral hygiene to prevent soft tissue inflammation.
• Report sore throat, oral burning sensation, fever, or fatigue, any of which could indicate presence of a superinfection.

erythromycin
er-ith-roe-**mye**′-sin
(A/T/S, Akne-Mycin, Apo-Erythro Base[CAN], EES, Emgel, Eryacne[AUS], Erybid[CAN], Eryc, Eryc LD[AUS], EryDerm, Erygel, EryPed, Ery-Tab, Erythra-Derm, Erythrocin, Erythromid[CAN], PCE)
Do not confuse erythromycin with azithromycin or Ethmozine, or Eryc with Emct.

CATEGORY AND SCHEDULE
Pregnancy Risk Category: B

Drug Class: Antiinfective

MECHANISM OF ACTION
A macrolide that reversibly binds to bacterial ribosomes, inhibiting bacterial protein synthesis.
Therapeutic Effect: Bacteriostatic.

USES
Treatment of infection of external eye, prophylaxis of neonatal conjunctivitis and ophthalmia neonatorum; acne vulgaris; infections caused by *N. gonorrhoeae;* mild-to-moderate respiratory tract, skin, soft tissue infections caused by *S. pneumoniae, M. pneumoniae, C. diphtheriae, B. pertussis, L. monocytogenes, S. pyogenes;* syphilis; legionnaires' disease; *C. trachomatis; H. influenzae;* endocarditis prophylaxis

PHARMACOKINETICS

Variably absorbed from the GI tract (depending on dosage form used). Protein binding: 70%–90%. Widely distributed. Metabolized in the liver. Primarily eliminated in feces by bile. Not removed by hemodialysis. *Half-life:* 1.4–2 hr (increased in impaired renal function).

INDICATIONS AND DOSAGES

▸ **Mild-to-Moderate Infections of the Upper and Lower Respiratory Tract, Pharyngitis, Skin Infections**
PO
Adults, Elderly. 500 mg q6h, or 333 mg q8h. Maximum: 2 g/day.
Children. 30–50 mg/kg/day in divided doses up to 60–100 mg/kg/day for severe infections.
Neonates. 20–40 mg/kg/day in divided doses q6–12h.
IV
Adults, Elderly, Children. 15–20 mg/kg/day in divided doses. Maximum: 4 g/day.
▸ **Preoperative Intestinal Antisepsis**
PO
Adults, Elderly. 1 g at 1 PM, 2 PM, and 11 PM on day before surgery (with neomycin).
Children. 20 mg/kg at 1 PM, 2 PM, and 11 PM on day before surgery (with neomycin).
▸ **Acne Vulgaris**
Topical
Adults. Apply thin layer to affected area twice a day.
▸ **Gonococcal Ophthalmia Neonatorum**
Ophthalmic
Neonates. 0.5–2 cm no later than 1 hr after delivery.

SIDE EFFECTS/ADVERSE REACTIONS

Frequent
IV: Abdominal cramping or discomfort, phlebitis or thrombophlebitis
Topical: Dry skin
Occasional
Nausea, vomiting, diarrhea, rash, urticaria
Rare
Ophthalmic: Sensitivity reaction with increased irritation, burning, itching, and inflammation
Topical: Urticaria

PRECAUTIONS AND CONTRAINDICATIONS

Administration of fixed-combination product, Pediazole, to infants younger than 2 mo; history of hepatitis because of macrolides; hypersensitivity to macrolides; preexisting hepatic disease.
Caution:
Hepatic disease, lactation

DRUG INTERACTIONS OF CONCERN TO DENTISTRY

• Increased duration of alfentanil, cyclosporine
• Increased serum levels: indinavir, digoxin
• Decreased action of clindamycin, penicillins, lincomycin
• Increased serum levels of alfentanil, carbamazepine, theophylline (and other methylxanthines) and felodipine (possibly with other calcium blockers in the dihydropyridine class), ergot alkaloids, oral anticoagulants, buspirone, tacrolimus
• Risk of rhabdomyolysis: HMG-CoA reductase inhibitors
• May increase the effects of certain benzodiazepines (e.g., midazolam, triazolam)

E

E

• Risk of prolonged QT interval; use with caution in patients taking gatifloxacin, moxifloxacin, pimozide, disopyramide
• Possible serotonin syndrome with SSRIs
• Suspected increase in plasma levels of repaglinide

SERIOUS REACTIONS

! Antibiotic-associated colitis and other superinfections may occur.
! High dosages in patients with renal impairment may lead to reversible hearing loss.
! Anaphylaxis and hepatotoxicity occur rarely.
! Ventricular arrhythmias and prolonged QT interval occur rarely with the IV drug form.

DENTAL CONSIDERATIONS

▸ **Erythromycin (Ophthalmic)**
General:
• Avoid dental light in patient's eyes; offer dark glasses for patient comfort.
▸ **Erythromycin (Topical)**
• None indicated
▸ **Erythromycin Base/Erythromycin Estolate/Erythromycin Ethylsuccinate/Erythromycin Glucceptate/Erythromycin Lactobionate/Erythromycin Stearate**
General:
• Alternative drug of choice for mild infection caused by a susceptible organism in patients who are allergic to penicillin.
• Determine why the patient is taking the drug.
• Estolate salt form is not indicated because of risk of cholestatic jaundice.

Teach Patient/Family to:
• Take oral drug with full glass of water.
• When used for dental infection, advise patient to:
 • Report sore throat, oral burning sensation, fever and fatigue, any of which could indicate superinfection.
 • Take at prescribed intervals and complete dosage regimen.
 • Immediately notify the dentist if signs or symptoms of infection increase.

escitalopram
es-sy-**tal**′-oh-pram
(Lexapro)

CATEGORY AND SCHEDULE
Pregnancy Risk Category: C

Drug Class: Antidepressant, selective serotonin reuptake inhibitor

MECHANISM OF ACTION
A selective serotonin reuptake inhibitor that blocks the uptake of the neurotransmitter serotonin at neuronal presynaptic membranes, increasing its availability at postsynaptic receptor sites.
Therapeutic Effect: Relieves depression.

USES
Treatment of major depressive disorder; maintenance treatment of major depressive disorder

PHARMACOKINETICS

Well absorbed after PO administration. Primarily metabolized in the liver. Primarily excreted in feces with a lesser amount eliminated in urine.
Half-life: 35 hr.

INDICATIONS AND DOSAGES

▶ **Depression, General Anxiety Disorder (GAD)**

PO

Adults. Initially, 10 mg once a day in the morning or evening. May increase to 20 mg after a minimum of 1 wk.

Elderly. Patients with hepatic impairment. 10 mg/day.

SIDE EFFECTS/ADVERSE REACTIONS

Frequent

Nausea, dry mouth, somnolence, insomnia, diaphoresis

Occasional

Tremor, diarrhea, abnormal ejaculation, dyspepsia, fatigue, anxiety, vomiting, anorexia

Rare

Sinusitis, sexual dysfunction, menstrual disorder, abdominal pain, agitation, decreased libido

PRECAUTIONS AND CONTRAINDICATIONS

Breast-feeding, use within 14 days of MAOIs

Caution:

Hyponatremia, activation of mania/hypomania, seizures, suicide, hepatic impairment, renal impairment, concurrent use of citalopram, lactation; use in children has not been established

DRUG INTERACTIONS OF CONCERN TO DENTISTRY

• Increased sedation: alcohol, other CNS depressants

• Drugs that inhibit CYP3A4 or other CYP isoenzymes may or may not affect plasma levels; should be used with observation and caution
• Modest inhibitor of CYP2D6
• NSAIDs may have a higher risk of GI side effects

SERIOUS REACTIONS

! Overdose is manifested as dizziness, drowsiness, tachycardia, somnolence, confusion, and seizures.

DENTAL CONSIDERATIONS

General:

• Assess salivary flow as a factor in caries, periodontal disease, and candidiasis.
• Consider semisupine chair position for patient comfort if GI side effects occur.
• Question patient about tolerance of NSAIDs or aspirin related to GI disease.
• Evaluate respiration characteristics and rate.

Consultations:

• Medical consultation may be required to assess disease control and patient's ability to tolerate stress.
• Physician should be informed if significant xerostomia occurs (e.g., increased caries, sore tongue, problems eating or swallowing, difficulty wearing prosthesis) so that a medication change can be considered.

Teach Patient/Family to:

• Encourage effective oral hygiene to prevent soft tissue inflammation, infection.
• When chronic dry mouth occurs, advise patient to:
  • Avoid mouth rinses with high alcohol content because of drying effects.

E

• Use daily home fluoride products for anticaries effect.
• Use sugarless gum, frequent sips of water, or saliva substitutes.
• Comply with recommended regimens for oral care.

esomeprazole
es-oh-**me**′-pray-zole
(Nexium, Nexium IV)

CATEGORY AND SCHEDULE
Pregnancy Risk Category: B

Drug Class: Antisecretory, proton pump inhibitor

MECHANISM OF ACTION
A proton pump inhibitor that is converted to active metabolites that irreversibly bind to and inhibit hydrogen-potassium adenosine triphosphates, an enzyme on the surface of gastric parietal cells. Inhibits hydrogen ion transport into gastric lumen.
Therapeutic Effect: Increases gastric pH, reducing gastric acid production.

USES
Treatment of gastroesophageal reflux disease (GERD), healing and maintenance of erosive esophagitis and *H. pylori* eradication in combination with antibiotics

PHARMACOKINETICS
Well absorbed after oral administration. Protein binding: 97%. Extensively metabolized by the liver. Primarily excreted in urine.
Half-life: 1–1.5 hr.

INDICATIONS AND DOSAGES
▸ **Erosive Esophagitis**
PO
Adults, Elderly. 20–40 mg once daily for 4–8 wk.
IV
Adults, Elderly. 20 or 40 mg once daily by IV injection over at least 3 min or IV infusion over 10–30 min.
▸ **To Maintain Healing of Erosive Esophagitis**
PO
Adults, Elderly. 20 mg/day.
▸ **GERD, to Reduce the Risk of NSAID-Induced Gastric Ulcer**
PO
Adults, Elderly. 20 mg once a day for 4 wk.
▸ **Duodenal Ulcer Caused by *H. pylori***
PO
Adults, Elderly. 40 mg (esomeprazole) once a day, with amoxicillin 1000 mg and clarithromycin 500 mg twice a day for 10 days.

SIDE EFFECTS/ADVERSE REACTIONS
Frequent
Headache
Occasional
Diarrhea, abdominal pain, nausea
Rare
Dizziness, asthenia or loss of strength, vomiting, constipation, rash, cough

PRECAUTIONS AND CONTRAINDICATIONS
Hypersensitivity to benzimidazoles
Caution:
Presence of gastric malignancy, atrophic gastritis, lactation, use in pediatric patients has not been studied, severe hepatic impairment,

Estazolam

allergic reactions to related proton pump inhibitors

DRUG INTERACTIONS OF CONCERN TO DENTISTRY
• May interfere with absorption of drugs where gastric pH is an important factor in bioavailability (e.g., iron products, ketoconazole, trovafloxacin, ampicillin)

SERIOUS REACTIONS
! None known

DENTAL CONSIDERATIONS
General:
• Assess salivary flow as a factor in caries, periodontal disease, and candidiasis.
• Question patient about tolerance of NSAIDs or aspirin related to GI disease.
• Consider semisupine chair position for patient comfort because of GI side effects of disease.
• Patients on chronic drug therapy may rarely have symptoms of blood dyscrasias, which can include infection, bleeding, and poor healing.
• Place on frequent recall because of oral side effects and oral effects of reflux disease.
Consultations:
• In a patient with symptoms of blood dyscrasias, request a medical consult for blood studies and postpone treatment until normal values are reestablished.
Teach Patient/Family to:
• Be aware of oral side effects and potential sequelae.
• Prevent trauma when using oral hygiene aids.
• Encourage effective oral hygiene to prevent soft tissue inflammation, infection.

• When chronic dry mouth occurs, advise patient to:
  • Avoid mouth rinses with high alcohol content because of drying effects.
  • Use daily home fluoride products for anticaries effect.
  • Use sugarless gum, frequent sips of water, or saliva substitutes.

estazolam
es-**tay'**-zoe-lam
(ProSom)

CATEGORY AND SCHEDULE
Pregnancy Risk Category: X
Controlled Substance: Schedule IV

Drug Class: Benzodiazepine, sedative hypnotic

MECHANISM OF ACTION
A benzodiazepine that enhances action of gamma-aminobutyric acid (GABA) neurotransmission in the CNS.
Therapeutic Effect: Produces depressant effect at all levels of CNS, relieves insomnia.

USES
Treatment of insomnia

PHARMACOKINETICS
Rapidly absorbed from GI tract. Protein binding: 93%. Metabolized in liver. Primarily excreted in urine, minimal in feces. *Half-life:* 10–24 hr.

INDICATIONS AND DOSAGES

▸ **Insomnia**

PO

Adults (older than 18 yr). 1–2 mg at bedtime.

Elderly, debilitated, liver disease, low serum albumin. 0.5–1 mg at bedtime.

SIDE EFFECTS/ADVERSE REACTIONS

Frequent

Drowsiness, sedation, rebound insomnia (may occur for 1–2 nights after drug is discontinued), dizziness, confusion, euphoria

Occasional

Weakness, anorexia, diarrhea

Rare

Paradoxical CNS excitement, restlessness (particularly noted in elderly/debilitated)

PRECAUTIONS AND CONTRAINDICATIONS

Pregnancy, hypersensitivity to other benzodiazepines

Caution:

Hepatic disease, renal disease, suicidal individuals, drug abuse, elderly, psychosis, children younger than 18 yr, lactation, depression, pulmonary insufficiency, narrow-angle glaucoma

DRUG INTERACTIONS OF CONCERN TO DENTISTRY

• Increased CNS depression: alcohol, all CNS depressants

• Increased serum levels and prolonged effect of benzodiazepines: ketoconazole, itraconazole, fluconazole, miconazole (systemic), indinavir

• Contraindicated with saquinavir

• Possible increase in CNS side effects: kava kava (herb)

• Decreased plasma levels: St. John's wort (herb)

SERIOUS REACTIONS

! Overdosage results in somnolence, confusion, diminished reflexes, and coma.

DENTAL CONSIDERATIONS

General:

• Psychologic and physical dependence may occur with chronic administration.

• Geriatric patients are more susceptible to drug effects; use lower dose.

• Avoid the use of this drug in a patient with a history of drug abuse or alcoholism.

Teach Patient/Family to:

• Avoid mouth rinses with high alcohol content because of drying effects.

estradiol

ess-tra-**dye′**-ole

(Aerodil[AUS], Alora, Climara, Delestrogen, Depo-Estradiol, Esclim, Estrace, Estraderm, Estraderm MX[AUS], Estradot[CAN], Estrasorb, EstroGel, Estring, Evamist, Femring, Kliovance[AUS], Menostar, Oesclim[CAN], Primogyn Depot[AUS], Progynova[AUS], Sandrena Gel[AUS], Vagifem, Vivelle, Vivelle Dot, Zumenon[AUS])

Do not confuse Estraderm with Testoderm.

CATEGORY AND SCHEDULE

Pregnancy Risk Category: X

Drug Class: Estrogen

MECHANISM OF ACTION

An estrogen that increases synthesis of DNA, RNA, and proteins in target tissues; reduces release of gonadotropin-releasing hormone from the hypothalamus; and reduces follicle-stimulating hormone and luteinizing hormone (LH) release from the pituitary.
Therapeutic Effect: Promotes normal growth, promotes development of female sex organs and maintains GU function and vasomotor stability. Prevents accelerated bone loss by inhibiting bone resorption, restoring balance of bone resorption and formation. Inhibits LH and decreases serum testosterone concentration.

USES

Treatment of menopause, breast cancer, prostatic cancer, atrophic vaginitis, kraurosis vulvae, hypogonadism, ovariectomy, primary ovarian failure, prevention of osteoporosis, and menopause-related vasomotor symptoms

PHARMACOKINETICS

Well absorbed from the GI tract. Widely distributed. Protein binding: 50%–80%. Metabolized in the liver. Primarily excreted in urine.
Half-life: Unknown.

INDICATIONS AND DOSAGES
▶ **Prostate Cancer**
IM (Estradiol Valerate)
Adults, Elderly. 30 mg or more q1–2wk.
PO
Adults, Elderly. 10 mg 3 times a day for at least 3 mo.
▶ **Breast Cancer**
PO
Adults, Elderly. 10 mg 3 times a day for at least 3 mo.

▶ **Osteoporosis Prophylaxis in Postmenopausal Females**
PO
Adults, Elderly. 0.5 mg/day cyclically (3 wk on, 1 wk off).
Transdermal (Climara)
Adults, Elderly. Initially, 0.025 mg/wk, adjust dose as needed.
Transdermal (Alora, Vivelle, Vivelle-Dot)
Adults, Elderly. Initially, 0.025 mg patch twice a wk, adjust dose as needed.
Transdermal (Estraderm)
Adults, Elderly. 0.05 mg twice a wk.
Transdermal (Menostar)
Adults, Elderly. 1 mg a wk.
▶ **Female Hypoestrogenism**
PO
Adults, Elderly. 1–2 mg/day, adjust dose as needed.
IM (Cypionate)
Adults, Elderly. 1.5–2 mg/mo.
IM (Estradiol Valerate)
Adults, Elderly. 10–20 mg q4wk.
▶ **Vasomotor Symptoms Associated with Menopause**
PO
Adults, Elderly. 1–2 mg/day cyclically (3 wk on, 1 wk off), adjust dose as needed.
IM (Estradiol Cypionate)
Adults, Elderly. 1–5 mg q3–4wk.
IM (Estradiol Valerate)
Adults, Elderly. 10–20 mg q4wk.
Topical Emulsion (Estrasorb)
Adults, Elderly. 3.84 g once a day in the morning.
Topical Gel (EstroGel)
Adults, Elderly. 1.25 g/day.
Transdermal (Climara)
Adults, Elderly. 0.025 mg/wk. Adjust dose as needed.
Transdermal (Alora, Esclim, Estraderm, Vivelle-Dot)
Adults, Elderly. 0.05 mg twice a wk.
Transdermal (Vivelle)
Adults, Elderly. 0.0375 mg twice a wk.

E

Vaginal Ring (Femring)
Adults, Elderly. 0.05 mg. May increase to 0.1 mg if needed.

▸ **Vaginal Atrophy**
Vaginal Ring (Estring)
Adults, Elderly. 2 mg.

▸ **Atrophic Vaginitis**
Vaginal Tablet (Vagifem)
Adults, Elderly. Initially, 1 tablet/day for 2 wk. Maintenance: 1 tablet twice a wk.

SIDE EFFECTS/ADVERSE REACTIONS

Frequent
Anorexia, nausea, swelling of breasts, peripheral edema marked by swollen ankles and feet
Transdermal: Skin irritation, redness
Occasional
Vomiting, especially with high doses; headache that may be severe; intolerance to contact lenses; hypertension; glucose intolerance; brown spots on exposed skin
Vaginal: Local irritation, vaginal discharge, changes in vaginal bleeding, including spotting and breakthrough or prolonged bleeding
Rare
Chorea or involuntary movements, hirsutism or abnormal hairiness, loss of scalp hair, depression

PRECAUTIONS AND CONTRAINDICATIONS

Abnormal vaginal bleeding, active arterial thrombosis, blood dyscrasias, estrogen-dependent cancer, known or suspected breast cancer, pregnancy, thrombophlebitis or thromboembolic disorders, thyroid dysfunction
Caution:
Hypertension, asthma, blood dyscrasias, gallbladder disease, CHF, diabetes mellitus, bone disease, depression, migraine headache, convulsive disorders, hepatic

disease, renal disease, family history of cancer of breast or reproductive tract

DRUG INTERACTIONS OF CONCERN TO DENTISTRY

• Increased action of corticosteroids

SERIOUS REACTIONS

! Estrogen therapy may increase the risk of developing coronary artery disease, hypercalcemia, gallbladder disease, cerebrovascular disease, and breast cancer.
! Prolonged administration increases the risk of gallbladder disease, thromboembolic disease and breast, cervical, vaginal, endometrial, and hepatic carcinoma.
! Cholestatic jaundice occurs rarely.

DENTAL CONSIDERATIONS

General:
• Place on frequent recall to evaluate gingival condition.
• Monitor vital signs because of cardiovascular side effects.
Teach Patient/Family to:
• Encourage effective oral hygiene to prevent gingival inflammation.

estramustine phosphate sodium
es-trah-**mew**'-steen **foss**'-fate **soe**'-dee-um
(Emcyt)
Do not confuse Emcyt with Eryc.

CATEGORY AND SCHEDULE
Pregnancy Risk Category: C

Drug Class: Antineoplastic

MECHANISM OF ACTION

An alkylating agent, estrogen and nitrogen mustard that binds to microtubule-associated proteins, causing their disassembly. *Therapeutic Effect:* Reduces serum testosterone concentration.

USES

Treatment of metastatic prostate cancer

PHARMACOKINETICS

Well absorbed from the GI tract. Highly localized in prostatic tissue. Rapidly dephosphorylated during absorption into peripheral circulation. Metabolized in the liver. Primarily eliminated in feces by biliary system. *Half-life:* 20 hr.

INDICATIONS AND DOSAGES
▸ **Prostatic Carcinoma**
PO
Adults, Elderly. 10–16 mg/kg/day or 140 mg 4 times a day.

SIDE EFFECTS/ADVERSE REACTIONS

Frequent
Peripheral edema of lower extremities, breast tenderness or enlargement, diarrhea, flatulence, nausea
Occasional
Increase in B/P, thirst, dry skin, ecchymosis, flushing, alopecia, night sweats
Rare
Headache, rash, fatigue, insomnia, vomiting

PRECAUTIONS AND CONTRAINDICATIONS

Active thrombophlebitis or thromboembolic disorders (unless the tumor is the cause of the thromboembolic disorder and the benefits outweigh the risk), hypersensitivity to estradiol or nitrogen mustard

DRUG INTERACTIONS OF CONCERN TO DENTISTRY

• Increased risk of hepatotoxicity: hepatotoxic drugs
• Impaired absorption: calcium-containing products

SERIOUS REACTIONS

! Estramustine use may exacerbate CHF and increase the risk of pulmonary emboli, thrombophlebitis and cerebrovascular accident.

DENTAL CONSIDERATIONS

General:
• Patients with prostate disease may experience urinary retention; caution with use of anticholinergic drugs that could aggravate urinary retention.
• Patients may have received other chemotherapy or radiation; confirm medical and drug history.
• Determine why patient is taking the drug.
• Monitor vital signs at every appointment because of cardiovascular side effects.
• Consider semisupine chair position for patient comfort if GI side effects occur.
• Patient may need assistance in getting into and out of dental chair. Adjust chair position for patient comfort.
• Short appointments and a stress-reduction protocol may be required for anxious patients.
Consultations:
• Consultation with physician may be needed if sedation or general anesthesia is required.
• Medical consultation may be required to assess disease control.

Teach Patient/Family to:
• Encourage effective oral hygiene to prevent soft tissue inflammation.
• Update health and medication history if physician makes any changes in evaluation or drug regimens; include OTC, herbal, and nonherbal remedies in the update.

estrogens, conjugated; medroxyprogesterone acetate

ess'-troe-jens, kon'-joo-gay-ted; me-**drox**'-ee-proe-**jes**'-ter-rone ass'-eh-tayte
(Premphase, Prempro, Prempro Low Dose)

CATEGORY AND SCHEDULE
Pregnancy Risk Category: X

Drug Class: Estrogens

MECHANISM OF ACTION
Conjugated estrogens are estrogens that increase synthesis of DNA, RNA and various proteins in responsive tissues; reduces release of gonadotropin-releasing hormone, reducing follicle-stimulating hormone (FSH) and leuteinizing hormone (LH). Medroxyprogesterone acetate is a hormone that transforms endometrium from proliferative to secretory in an estrogen-primed endometrium; inhibits secretion of pituitary gonadotropins.
Therapeutic Effect: Conjugated estrogens promote vasomotor stability, maintain GU function, normal growth, development of female sex organs; prevents accelerated bone loss by inhibiting bone resorption, restoring balance of bone resorption and formation; inhibits LH, decreases serum concentration of testosterone. Medroxyprogesterone acetate prevents follicular maturation and ovulation; stimulates growth of mammary alveolar tissue; relaxes uterine smooth muscle; restores hormonal imbalance.

USES
Treatment of symptoms associated with menopause, inoperable breast cancer, prostatic cancer, abnormal uterine bleeding, hypogonadism, primary ovarian failure, prevention of osteoporosis

PHARMACOKINETICS
Conjugated estrogens are well absorbed from the GI tract. Widely distributed. Protein binding: 50%–80%. Metabolized in liver. Primarily excreted in urine.
Half-life: 4–10 hr.
Medroxyprogesterone's absorption varies depending on the patient but is generally low. Binds mainly to albumin or other plasma proteins. Metabolized in liver. Primarily excreted in urine. **Half-life:** 2–4 hr.

INDICATIONS AND DOSAGES
▸ **Menopausal Symptoms, Osteoporosis, Vulvar/Vaginal Atrophy**
PO
(Prempro) Adults, Elderly. 1 tablet once daily.
▸ **Menopausal Symptoms, Osteoporosis, Vulvar/Vaginal Atrophy**
PO
(Premphase) Adults, Elderly. 1 maroon conjugated estrogen tablet on days 1–14 and 1 light blue conjugated estrogens/medroxyprogesterone tablet on days 15–28.

SIDE EFFECTS/ADVERSE REACTIONS

Frequent

Change in vaginal bleeding, such as spotting or breakthrough bleeding, breast pain or tenderness, gynecomastia

Occasional

Headache, increased B/P, intolerance to contact lenses, nausea, edema, weight change, breast tenderness, nervousness, insomnia, fatigue, dizziness

Rare

Loss of scalp hair, mental depression, dermatologic changes, headache, fever

PRECAUTIONS AND CONTRAINDICATIONS

Breast cancer with some exceptions, liver disease, thrombophlebitis, undiagnosed vaginal bleeding, estrogen-dependent neoplasia (known or suspected), pregnancy (known or suspected), hypersensitivity to conjugated estrogens, medroxyprogesterone acetate, or any component of the formulation

Caution:

Hypertension, asthma, blood dyscrasias, gallbladder disease, CHF, diabetes mellitus, bone disease, depression, migraine headache, convulsive disorders, hepatic disease, renal disease, family history of cancer of breast or reproductive tract

DRUG INTERACTIONS OF CONCERN TO DENTISTRY

• Increased action of corticosteroids

SERIOUS REACTIONS

Estrogens A, Conjugated Synthetic

! Prolonged administration may increase risk of gallbladder, thromboembolic disease, or breast, cervical, vaginal, endometrial, and liver carcinoma.

DENTAL CONSIDERATIONS

▸ **Estrogens A, Conjugated Synthetic**

General:

• Place on frequent recall to evaluate gingival condition.
• Monitor vital signs because of cardiovascular side effects.
• Consider semisupine chair position for patient comfort if GI side effects occur.

Teach Patient/Family to:

• Encourage effective oral hygiene to prevent gingival soft tissue inflammation.

E

---

estropipate

es-tro-**pip**´-ate

(Genoral[AUS], Ogen, Ortho-Est)

CATEGORY AND SCHEDULE

Pregnancy Risk Category: X

Drug Class: Estrogen (piperazine estrone sulfate)

MECHANISM OF ACTION

An estrogen that increases synthesis of DNA, RNA, and proteins in target tissues; reduces release of gonadotropin-releasing hormone from the hypothalamus; and reduces follicle-stimulating hormone (FSH) and luteinizing hormone (LH) from the pituitary.

Therapeutic Effect: Promotes normal growth, promotes development of female sex organs and maintains GU function and vasomotor stability. Prevents accelerated bone loss by inhibiting bone resorption, restoring balance of bone resorption and formation.

Inhibits LH and decreases serum testosterone concentration.

USES

Treatment of vasomotor symptoms of menopause, atrophic vaginitis, primary female hypogonadism, primary ovarian failure, estrogen imbalance, ovariectomy

PHARMACOKINETICS

PO: Well absorbed; moderate-to-high protein binding; hepatic metabolism with primary renal excretion

INDICATIONS AND DOSAGES

▶ **Vasomotor Symptoms, Atrophic Vaginitis, Kraurosis Vulvae**
PO
Adults, Elderly. 0.625–5 mg/day cyclically.
▶ **Atrophic Vaginitis, Kraurosis Vulvae**
Intravaginal
Adults, Elderly. 2–4 g/day cyclically.
▶ **Female Hypogonadism, Castration, Primary Ovarian Failure**
PO
Adults, Elderly. 1.25–7.5 mg/day for 21 days; then off for 8–10 days. Repeat if bleeding does not occur by end of off cycle.
▶ **Prevention of Osteoporosis**
PO
Adults, Elderly. 0.625 mg/day (25 days of 31-day cycle/mo).

SIDE EFFECTS/ADVERSE REACTIONS

Frequent
Anorexia, nausea, swelling of breasts, peripheral edema marked by swollen ankles and feet
Occasional
Vomiting, especially with high doses; headache that may be severe; intolerance to contact lenses; hypertension; glucose intolerance; brown spots on exposed skin
Vaginal: Local irritation, vaginal discharge, changes in vaginal bleeding, including spotting and breakthrough or prolonged bleeding
Rare
Chorea or involuntary movements, hirsutism or abnormal hairiness, loss of scalp hair, depression

PRECAUTIONS AND CONTRAINDICATIONS

Abnormal vaginal bleeding, active arterial thrombosis, blood dyscrasias, estrogen-dependent cancer, known or suspected breast cancer, pregnancy, thrombophlebitis or thromboembolic disorders, thyroid dysfunction
Caution:
Hypertension, asthma, blood dyscrasias, gallbladder disease, CHF, diabetes mellitus, bone disease, depression, migraine headache, convulsive disorders, hepatic disease, renal disease, family history of cancer of breast or reproductive tract

DRUG INTERACTIONS OF CONCERN TO DENTISTRY

• Increased action of corticosteroids

SERIOUS REACTIONS

! Prolonged administration increases the risk of gallbladder disease, thromboembolic disease and breast, cervical, vaginal, endometrial, and hepatic carcinoma.
! Cholestatic jaundice occurs rarely.

DENTAL CONSIDERATIONS

General:
• Place on frequent recall to evaluate gingival condition.
• Monitor vital signs because of cardiovascular side effects.

Teach Patient/Family to:
• Encourage effective oral hygiene to prevent gingival inflammation.

eszopiclone
es-**zoe**′-pih-clone
(Lunesta)

CATEGORY AND SCHEDULE
Pregnancy Risk Category: C
Controlled Substance: Schedule IV

Drug Class: Sedative-hypnotic

MECHANISM OF ACTION
A nonbenzodiazepine that enhances the action of the inhibitory neurotransmitter gamma-aminobutyric acid (GABA).

USES
Treatment of insomnia

PHARMACOKINETICS
Rapidly absorbed, peak 1 hr.
Half-life: 6 hr, metabolized in liver by CYP3A4 and CYP 2E1, weak protein binding (52%–59%), unchanged drug (10%) and metabolites (75%) excreted in urine.

INDICATIONS AND DOSAGES
▸ **Insomnia**
PO
Adult. 2 mg per day at bedtime.

SIDE EFFECTS/ADVERSE REACTIONS
ORAL: Dry mouth, taste alterations
CNS: Somnolence, nervousness, anxiety, confusion, depression, dizziness, hallucinations, decreased libido
GI: Dyspepsia, nausea, vomiting
RESP: Infection
GU: Dysmenorrhea (females), gynecomastia (males)
INTEG: Rash
SYST: Headache, chest pain, viral infection

PRECAUTIONS AND CONTRAINDICATIONS
Mental impairment, behavior and mood changes (depression), use lower doses in elderly and patients with renal/hepatic impairment

DRUG INTERACTIONS OF CONCERN TO DENTISTRY
• Increased CNS depression: all CNS depressants, alcohol
• Inhibitors of CYP 3A4 (azole antifungals, macrolide antibiotics, e.g., erythromycin/clarithromycin): increased blood levels and CNS depression
• Food: Effects delayed by taking with or immediately after heavy/fatty meal

DENTAL CONSIDERATIONS
General:
• Assess salivary flow as a factor in caries, periodontal disease, and candidiasis.
• Differentiate taste changes because of drug from those associated with restorative materials.
• Use all appropriate precautions if prescribing for preoperative sedation.
• After supine positioning, allow patient to sit upright for 2 min before standing to avoid dizziness.
Consultations:
• Medical consultation may be required to assess disease control.

Teach Patient/Family to:
• Avoid mouth rinses with high alcohol content because of drying effect.
• Use home fluoride products to prevent caries.
• Use sugarless chewing gum, frequent sips of water, or saliva substitutes if dry mouth occurs.

etanercept
eh-**tan**′-er-cept
(Enbrel)

CATEGORY AND SCHEDULE
Pregnancy Risk Category: B

Drug Class: Antiinflammatory and immunomodulator; biologic response modifier

MECHANISM OF ACTION
A protein that binds to tumor necrosis factor (TNF), blocking its interaction with cell surface receptors. Elevated levels of TNF, which is involved in inflammatory and immune responses, are found in the synovial fluid of rheumatoid arthritis patients.
Therapeutic Effect: Relieves symptoms of rheumatoid arthritis.

USES
Reduction in signs and symptoms of moderately to severely active rheumatoid arthritis in patients with an inadequate response to one or more disease-modifying antirheumatic drugs; polyarticular-course juvenile rheumatoid arthritis; psoriatic arthritis; also approved for initial therapy

PHARMACOKINETICS
Well absorbed after subcutaneous administration. *Half-life:* 115 hr.

INDICATIONS AND DOSAGES
▸ **Rheumatoid Arthritis, Psoriatic Arthritis, Ankylosing Spondylitis**
Subcutaneous
Adults, Elderly. 25 mg twice weekly, given 72–96 hr apart. Alternative weekly dosing: 0.8 mg/kg/dose once a wk. Maximum: 50 mg/wk. Maximum: 25 mg/dose.
▸ **Juvenile Rheumatoid Arthritis**
Subcutaneous
Children 4–17 yr. 0.4 mg/kg (Maximum: 25 mg dose) twice a wk given 72–96 hr apart. Alternative weekly dosing: 50 mg once a wk. Maximum: 25 mg/dose.
▸ **Plaque Psoriasis**
Subcutaneous
Adults, Elderly. 50 mg twice a wk (give 3–4 days apart) for 3 mo. Maintenance: 50 mg once a wk.

SIDE EFFECTS/ADVERSE REACTIONS
Frequent
Injection site erythema, pruritus, pain, and swelling; abdominal pain, vomiting (more common in children than adults)
Occasional
Headache, rhinitis, dizziness, pharyngitis, cough, asthenia, abdominal pain, dyspepsia
Rare
Sinusitis, allergic reaction

PRECAUTIONS AND CONTRAINDICATIONS
Serious active infection or sepsis
Caution:
Risk of new malignancies and infrequent severe cardiovascular events, discontinue if serious infection occurs, immunosuppression risk, caution with preexisting

demyelinating disorders, lactation, viral infections, children younger than 4 yr

DRUG INTERACTIONS OF CONCERN TO DENTISTRY
No studies have been conducted.

SERIOUS REACTIONS
! Infections (such as pyelonephritis, cellulitis, osteomyelitis, wound infection, leg ulcer, septic arthritis, diarrhea, bronchitis, and pneumonia), occur in 29%–38% of patients.
! Rare adverse effects include heart failure, hypertension, hypotension, pancreatitis, GI hemorrhage, and dyspnea.
! The patient also may develop autoimmune antibodies.

DENTAL CONSIDERATIONS
General:
• Monitor vital signs at every appointment because of potential cardiovascular side effects.
• Consider semisupine chair position for patient comfort because of GI side effects of drug.
• If acute oral infection occurs, inform physician.
• Note elevated antinuclear antibody (ANA) levels if diagnosing Sjögren's syndrome.
Consultations:
• Medical consultation if needed.
Teach Patient/Family to:
• Encourage effective oral hygiene to prevent soft tissue inflammation.
• Use powered tooth brush if patient has difficulty holding conventional devices.

ethambutol
eh-**tham'**-byoo-tole
(Etibi[CAN], Myambutol)
Do not confuse ethambutol or Myambutol with Nembutal.

CATEGORY AND SCHEDULE
Pregnancy Risk Category: B

Drug Class: Antitubercular

MECHANISM OF ACTION
An isonicotinic acid derivative that interferes with RNA synthesis.
Therapeutic Effect: Suppresses the multiplication of mycobacteria.

USES
Treatment of pulmonary tuberculosis (TB), as an adjunct

PHARMACOKINETICS
Rapidly and well absorbed from the GI tract. Protein binding: 20%–30%. Widely distributed. Metabolized in the liver. Primarily excreted in urine. Removed by hemodialysis. *Half-life:* 3–4 hr (increased in impaired renal function).

INDICATIONS AND DOSAGES
▸ TB
PO
Adults, Elderly, Children. 15–25 mg/kg/day as a single dose or 50 mg/kg 2 times a wk. Maximum: 2.5 g/dose.
▸ Atypical Mycobacterial Infections
PO
Adults, Elderly, Children. 15 mg/kg/day. Maximum: 1 g/day.
▸ Dosage in Renal Impairment
Dosage interval is modified on the basis of creatinine clearance.

Creatinine Clearance	Dosage Interval
10–50 ml/ min	q24–36h
Less than 10 ml/min	q48h

SIDE EFFECTS/ADVERSE REACTIONS

Occasional

Acute gouty arthritis (chills, pain, swelling of joints with hot skin), confusion, abdominal pain, nausea, vomiting, anorexia, headache

Rare

Rash, fever, blurred vision, eye pain, red-green color blindness

PRECAUTIONS AND CONTRAINDICATIONS

Optic neuritis

Caution:

Renal disease, diabetic retinopathy, cataracts, ocular defects, hepatic disorders, hematopoietic disorders

DRUG INTERACTIONS OF CONCERN TO DENTISTRY

• None reported

SERIOUS REACTIONS

! Optic neuritis (more common with high-dosage or long-term ethambutol therapy), peripheral neuritis, thrombocytopenia, and an anaphylactoid reaction occur rarely.

DENTAL CONSIDERATIONS

General:

• Examine for evidence of oral signs of disease.

• Avoid dental light in patient's eyes; offer dark glasses for patient comfort.

• Determine why the patient is taking the drug.

• Do not treat patients with active tuberculosis.

Consultations:

• Medical consultation is required to assess patient's current status; avoid elective dental procedures in active infections.

• Determine that noninfectious status exists by ensuring the following:

  • Anti-TB drugs have been taken for longer than 3 wk.

  • Culture confirms antibiotic susceptibility to TB microorganisms.

  • Patient has had three consecutive negative sputum smears.

  • Patient is not in the coughing stage.

Teach Patient/Family to:

• Take medication for full length of prescribed therapy to ensure effectiveness of treatment and to prevent the emergence of resistant forms of microbes.

ethionamide

eh-thye-**on**′-am-ide

(Trecator)

Do not confuse with TriCor.

CATEGORY AND SCHEDULE

Pregnancy Risk Category: C

Drug Class: Antitubercular

MECHANISM OF ACTION

An antitubercular agent that inhibits peptide synthesis.

Therapeutic Effect: Suppresses mycobacterial multiplication. Bactericidal.

USES

Treatment of pulmonary, extrapulmonary tuberculosis (TB)

when other antitubercular drugs have failed

PHARMACOKINETICS

Rapidly absorbed from the GI tract. Widely distributed. Protein binding: 10%. Metabolized in liver. Primarily excreted in urine. Removed by hemodialysis. *Half-life:* 2–3 hr (half-life is increased with impaired renal function).

INDICATIONS AND DOSAGES

▸ **TB**
PO
Adults, Elderly. 500–1000 mg/day as a single to 3 divided doses.
Children. 15–20 mg/kg/day.
Maximum 1 g/day.
▸ **Dosage in Renal Impairment**
Creatinine clearance less than 50 ml/min. Reduce dose by 50%.

SIDE EFFECTS/ADVERSE REACTIONS

Occasional
Abdominal pain, nausea, vomiting, weakness, postural hypotension, psychiatric disturbances, drowsiness, dizziness, headache, confusion, metallic taste, anorexia, diarrhea, stomatitis, peripheral neuritis
Rare
Rash, fever, blurred vision, optic neuritis, seizures, hypothyroidism, hypoglycemia, gynecomastia, thrombocytopenia, jaundice

PRECAUTIONS AND CONTRAINDICATIONS

Severe hepatic impairment, hypersensitivity to ethionamide
Caution:
Lactation, renal disease, diabetic retinopathy, cataracts, ocular defects, children younger than 12 yr; pyridoxine concurrent use is recommended, resistance may develop

DRUG INTERACTIONS OF CONCERN TO DENTISTRY

• None reported

SERIOUS REACTIONS

! Peripheral neuropathy, anorexia, and joint pain rarely occur.

E

DENTAL CONSIDERATIONS

General:
• Monitor vital signs at every appointment because of cardiovascular side effects.
• After supine positioning, have patient sit upright for at least 2 min before standing to avoid orthostatic hypotension.
• Consider semisupine chair position for patient comfort because of GI effects of disease.
• Evaluate for clotting ability during gingival instrumentation.
• Examine for evidence of oral manifestations of blood dyscrasias (infection, bleeding, poor healing).
• Palliative treatment may be required for oral side effects.
• Examine for evidence of oral signs of disease.
Consultations:
• Medical consultation for blood studies (CBC); leukopenic or thrombocytopenic side effects may result in infection, delayed healing, and excessive bleeding. Postpone elective dental treatment until normal values are maintained. Instruct patient to take with meals to decrease GI symptoms.
• Medical consultation may be required to assess disease control and determine infectious nature of disease.
• Confirm that patient is non-infectious prior to dental treatment.
Teach Patient/Family to:
• Encourage effective oral hygiene to prevent soft tissue inflammation.

• Use caution in use of oral hygiene aids to prevent injury.

ethosuximide
eth-oh-**sux**'-ih-mide
(Zarontin)
Do not confuse with Zaroxolyn or Neurontin.

CATEGORY AND SCHEDULE
Pregnancy Risk Category: C

Drug Class: Anticonvulsant

MECHANISM OF ACTION
An anticonvulsant that increases the seizure threshold and suppresses paroxysmal spike-and-wave pattern in absence seizures; depresses nerve transmission in the motor cortex.
Therapeutic Effect: Produces anticonvulsant activity.

USES
Treatment of absence seizures (petit mal); unapproved: complex partial seizures

PHARMACOKINETICS
Well absorbed from the GI tract. Metabolized in liver. Excreted in urine. Removed by hemodialysis.
Half-life: 50–60 hr (in adults); 30 hr (in children).

INDICATIONS AND DOSAGES
▸ Absence Seizures
PO
Adults, Elderly, Children older than 6 yr. Initially, 250 mg/day or 15 mg/kg/day in 2 divided doses.
Maintenance: 15–40 mg/kg/day in 2 divided doses.
Children 3–6 yr. Initially, 250 mg in 2 divided doses, increased by 250 mg as needed every 4–7 days.

Maintenance: 20–40 mg/kg/day in 2 divided doses. Use with caution in patients with renal impairment.

SIDE EFFECTS/ADVERSE REACTIONS
Occasional
Dizziness, drowsiness, double vision, headache, ataxia, nausea, diarrhea, vomiting, somnolence, urticaria
Rare
Agranulocytosis, gum hypertrophy, leucopenia, myopia, swelling of the tongue, systemic lupus erythematosus, vaginal bleeding

PRECAUTIONS AND CONTRAINDICATIONS
Hypersensitivity to succinimides
Caution:
Lactation, hepatic disease, renal disease

DRUG INTERACTIONS OF CONCERN TO DENTISTRY
• Enhanced CNS depression
• CNS depressants, alcohol

SERIOUS REACTIONS
! Abrupt withdrawal may increase seizure frequency.
! Overdosage results in nausea, vomiting, and CNS depression including coma with respiratory depression.

DENTAL CONSIDERATIONS

General:
• Patients on chronic drug therapy may rarely have symptoms of blood dyscrasias, which can include infection, bleeding, and poor healing.
• Talk with patient to ascertain seizure frequency and how well seizures are controlled. A stress reduction protocol may be required.

E

Consultations:
• In a patient with symptoms of blood dyscrasias, request a medical consultation for blood studies, and postpone dental treatment until normal values are reestablished.
• Medical consultation may be required to assess disease control and patient's ability to tolerate stress.

Teach Patient/Family to:
• Encourage effective oral hygiene to prevent gingival inflammation.
• Avoid mouth rinses with high alcohol content because of drying effects.

etidronate disodium
ee-**tid**'-roe-nate die-**soe**'-dee-um
(Didronel)
Do not confuse etidronate with etidocaine or etomidate.

CATEGORY AND SCHEDULE
Pregnancy Risk Category: C (parenteral), B (oral)

Drug Class: Antihypercalcemic

MECHANISM OF ACTION
A bisphosphonate that decreases mineral release and matrix in bone and inhibits osteocytic osteolysis. **Therapeutic Effect:** Decreases bone resorption.

USES
Treatment of Paget's disease, heterotopic ossification, hypercalcemia of malignancy

PHARMACOKINETICS
Therapeutic response: 1–3 mo; not metabolized; excreted in urine.

INDICATIONS AND DOSAGES
▶ **Paget's Disease**
PO
Adults, Elderly. Initially, 5–10 mg/kg/day not to exceed 6 mo, or 11–20 mg/kg/day not to exceed 3 mo. Repeat only after drug-free period of at least 90 days.
▶ **Heterotopic Ossification Caused by Spinal Cord Injury**
PO
Adult, Elderly. 20 mg/kg/day for 2 wk; then 10 mg/kg/day for 10 wk.
▶ **Heterotopic Ossification Complicating Total Hip Replacement**
PO
Adults, Elderly. 20 mg/kg/day for 1 mo before surgery; then 20 mg/kg/day for 3 mo after surgery.
▶ **Hypercalcemia Associated with Malignancy**
IV
Adults, Elderly. 7.5 mg/kg/day for 3 days. For retreatment, allow 7 days between treatment courses. Follow with oral therapy on day after last infusion. Begin with 20 mg/kg/day for 30 days; may extend up to 90 days.

SIDE EFFECTS/ADVERSE REACTIONS
Frequent
Nausea; diarrhea; continuing or more frequent bone pain in patients with Paget's disease
Occasional
Bone fractures, especially of the femur
Parenteral: Metallic, altered taste
Rare
Hypersensitivity reaction

PRECAUTIONS AND CONTRAINDICATIONS
Clinically overt osteomalacia
Caution:
Renal disease, lactation, adequate intake of vitamin D and calcium,

safety and efficacy in children have not been established

DRUG INTERACTIONS OF CONCERN TO DENTISTRY

• Possible increased risk of gastric ulceration: NSAIDs

SERIOUS REACTIONS

‼ Nephrotoxicity, including hematuria, dysuria, and proteinuria, has occurred with parenteral route.
‼ Osteonecrosis of the jaw

DENTAL CONSIDERATIONS

General:
• Evaluate for signs and symptoms of osteonecrosis.
• Be aware of oral manifestations of Paget's disease (macrognathia, alveolar pain).
• Emphasize atraumatic and effective oral hygiene.
Consultations:
• Medical consultation may be required to assess disease control.

---

etodolac
eh-toe-**doe′**-lak
(Apo-Etodolac[CAN], Lodine, Lodine XL, Ultradol[CAN])
Do not confuse Lodine with codeine or iodine.

CATEGORY AND SCHEDULE

Pregnancy Risk Category: C (D if used in third trimester or near delivery)

Drug Class: Nonsteroidal antiinflammatory

MECHANISM OF ACTION

An NSAID that produces analgesic and antiinflammatory effects by inhibiting prostaglandin synthesis. **Therapeutic Effect:** Reduces the inflammatory response and intensity of pain.

USES

Mild-to-moderate pain, osteoarthritis, rheumatoid arthritis

PHARMACOKINETICS

Route	Onset	Peak	Duration
PO (analgesic)	30 min	N/A	4–12 hr

Completely absorbed from the GI tract. Protein binding: greater than 99%. Widely distributed. Metabolized in the liver. Primarily excreted in urine. Not removed by hemodialysis. **Half-life:** 6–7 hr.

INDICATIONS AND DOSAGES
▸ **Osteoarthritis, Rheumatoid Arthritis**
PO (Immediate-Release)
Adults, Elderly. Initially, 300 mg 2–3 times a day or 400–500 mg twice a day. Maintenance: 600–1000 mg/day in 2–4 divided doses.
PO (Extended-Release)
Adults, Elderly. 400–1000 mg once daily. Maximum: 1200 mg/day.
▸ **Juvenile Rheumatoid Arthritis**
PO (Extended-Release)
Children 6–16 yr. 1000 mg in children weighing more than 60 kg, 800 mg once daily in children weighing 46–60 kg, 600 mg once daily in children weighing 31–45 kg, 400 mg once daily in children weighing 20–30 kg.

E

Analgesia

PO

Adults, Elderly. 200–400 mg q6–8h as needed. Maximum: 1200 mg/day.

SIDE EFFECTS/ADVERSE REACTIONS

Occasional

Dizziness, headache, abdominal pain or cramps, bloated feeling, diarrhea, nausea, indigestion

Rare

Constipation, rash, pruritus, visual disturbances, tinnitus

PRECAUTIONS AND CONTRAINDICATIONS

Active peptic ulcer disease, chronic inflammation of GI tract, GI bleeding or ulceration, history of hypersensitivity to aspirin or NSAIDs

Caution:

Lactation, children, bleeding disorders, GI disorders, cardiac disorders, elderly, renal, hepatic disorders

DRUG INTERACTIONS OF CONCERN TO DENTISTRY

• GI ulceration, bleeding: aspirin, alcohol, corticosteroids, bisphosphonates
• Decreased action: salicylates
• Nephrotoxicity: acetaminophen (prolonged use)
• Possible risk of decreased renal function: cyclosporine
• NSAIDs may have a higher risk of GI side effects
• When prescribed for dental pain:
  • Risk of increased effects: oral anticoagulants, oral antidiabetics, lithium, methotrexate
  • Decreased effects of diuretics
  • Increased risk of methotrexate toxicity

SERIOUS REACTIONS

! Overdose may result in acute renal failure.
! There is an increased risk of cardiovascular events (including MI and CVA) and serious and potentially life-threatening GI bleeding.
! Rare reactions with long-term use include peptic ulcer disease, GI bleeding, gastritis, severe hepatic reactions (jaundice), nephrotoxicity (hematuria, dysuria, proteinuria), and a severe hypersensitivity reaction (bronchospasm, angioedema).

DENTAL CONSIDERATIONS

General:

• Possible increase in adverse cardiovascular events in patients at risk for thromboembolism.
• Patients on chronic drug therapy may rarely have symptoms of blood dyscrasias, which can include infection, bleeding, and poor healing.
• Assess salivary flow as a factor in caries, periodontal disease, and candidiasis.
• Avoid prescribing in pregnancy.
• Avoid prescribing with aspirin-containing products.
• Consider semisupine chair position for patients with arthritic disease.
• Severe stomach bleeding may occur in patients who regularly use NSAIDs in recommended doses, when the patient is also taking another NSAID, a blood thinning, or steroid drug, if the patient has GI or peptic ulcer disease, if they are 60 yr or older, or when NSAIDs are taken longer than directed. Warn patients of the potential for severe stomach bleeding.

Consultations:
• In a patient with symptoms of blood dyscrasias, request a medical consultation for blood studies and postpone dental treatment until normal values are reestablished.
• Medical consultation may be required to assess disease control.
Teach Patient/Family to:
• Avoid mouth rinses with high alcohol content because of drying effects.
• Warn patient of potential risks of NSAIDs.

etoposide, VP-16

eh-**toe'**-poe-side
(Etopophos, Toposar, VePesid)
Do not confuse VePesid with Pepcid or Versed.

CATEGORY AND SCHEDULE

Pregnancy Risk Category: D

Drug Class: Antineoplastic-miscellaneous; semisynthetic podophyllotoxin

MECHANISM OF ACTION

An epipodophyllotoxin that induces single-and double-stranded breaks in DNA. Cell cycle–dependent and phase-specific; most effective in the S and G2 phases of cell division.
Therapeutic Effect: Inhibits or alters DNA synthesis.

USES

Leukemias, testicular cancer, lymphomas, small cell carcinoma of the lung

PHARMACOKINETICS

Variably absorbed from the GI tract. Rapidly distributed, low concentrations in CSF. Protein binding: 97%. Metabolized in the liver. Primarily excreted in urine. Not removed by hemodialysis.
Half-life: 3–12 hr.

INDICATIONS AND DOSAGES
▸ **Refractory Testicular Tumors**
IV
Adults. 50–100 mg/m^2/day on days 1–5, or 100 mg/m^2/day on days 1, 3, and 5 (as combination therapy).
▸ **Acute Myelocytic Leukemia**
IV
Children. 150 mg/m^2/day for 2–3 days and 2–3 cycles.
▸ **Brain Tumor**
IV
Children. 150 mg/m^2/day on days 2 and 3 of treatment course.
▸ **Neuroblastoma**
IV
Children. 100 mg/m^2/day on days 1–5 of treatment course; repeated q4wk.
▸ **Small-Cell Lung Carcinoma**
PO
Adults. Twice the IV dose rounded to nearest 50 mg. Give once a day for doses 400 mg or less, in divided doses for dosages greater than 400 mg.
IV
Adults. 35 mg/m^2/day for 4 consecutive days up to 50 mg/m^2/day for 5 consecutive days (as combination therapy).
Children. 60–150 mg/m^2/day for 2–5 days q3–6wk.
▸ **Dosage in Renal Impairment**
Creatinine clearance 10–50 ml/min. 75% of normal dose. Creatinine clearance less than 10 ml/min. 50% of normal dose.

SIDE EFFECTS/ADVERSE REACTIONS

Frequent

Mild to moderate nausea and vomiting, alopecia

Occasional

Diarrhea, anorexia, stomatitis

Rare

Hypotension, peripheral neuropathy

PRECAUTIONS AND CONTRAINDICATIONS

Pregnancy

DRUG INTERACTIONS OF CONCERN TO DENTISTRY

• None reported

SERIOUS REACTIONS

❗ Myelosuppression may result in hematologic toxicity, manifested as anemia, leukopenia (occurring 7–14 days after drug administration), thrombocytopenia (occurring 9–16 days after administration) and, to a lesser extent, pancytopenia. Bone marrow recovery occurs by day 20.

❗ Hepatotoxicity occurs occasionally.

DENTAL CONSIDERATIONS

General:

• Determine why patient is taking the drug.

• If additional analgesia is required for dental pain, consider alternative analgesics (NSAIDs) in patients taking narcotics for acute or chronic pain.

• Examine for oral manifestations of opportunistic infection.

• Avoid products that affect platelet function, such as aspirin and NSAIDs.

• This drug may be used in the hospital or on an outpatient basis. Confirm the patient's disease and treatment status.

• Chlorhexidine mouth rinse prior to and during chemotherapy may reduce severity of mucositis.

• Patient on chronic drug therapy may rarely present with symptoms of blood dyscrasias, which can include infection, bleeding, and poor healing. If dyscrasia is present, caution patient to prevent oral tissue trauma when using oral hygiene aids.

• Palliative medication may be required for management of oral side effects.

• Short appointments and a stress-reduction protocol may be required for anxious patients.

• Consider semisupine chair position for patient comfort if GI side effects occur.

• Patients may be at risk of bleeding; check for oral signs.

• Oral infections should be eliminated and/or treated aggressively.

Consultations:

• Medical consultation should include routine blood counts including platelet counts and bleeding time.

• Consult physician; prophylactic or therapeutic antiinfectives may be indicated if surgery or periodontal treatment is required.

• Medical consultation may be required to assess immunologic status during cancer chemotherapy and determine safety risk, if any, posed by the required dental treatment.

• Medical consultation may be required to assess disease control and patient's ability to tolerate stress.

Teach Patient/Family to:

• Encourage effective oral hygiene to prevent soft tissue inflammation.

• Report oral lesions, soreness, or bleeding to dentist.

E

• Prevent trauma when using oral hygiene aids.
• Update health and medication history if physician makes any changes in evaluation or drug regimens; include OTC, herbal, and nonherbal remedies in the update.

etravirine
et-ra-**vir**´-een
(Intelence)

CATEGORY AND SCHEDULE
Pregnancy Risk Category: B

Drug Class: Antiretroviral agent, reverse transcriptase inhibitor

MECHANISM OF ACTION
Non-nucleoside reverse transcriptase inhibitor (NNRTI) of human immunodeficiency virus type 1 (HIV-1). Binds directly to reverse transcriptase and blocks the RNA-dependent and DNA-dependent DNA polymerase activities. Does not inhibit the human DNA polymerases alpha, beta, and gamma.

USES
HIV-1 infection in combination with at least two additional antiretroviral agents in treatment-experienced patients exhibiting viral replication.

PHARMACOKINETICS
Food increases systemic exposure by 50%. Protein binding 99.9%. Metabolized by the liver via CYP 3A4, 2C9, and 2C19. Primarily excreted in feces (94%, up to 86% as unchanged drug), urine (1%). **Half-life:** 41 hr.

INDICATIONS AND DOSAGES
PO
Adult. HIV-1 infection: 200 mg twice daily after meals.
Renal Impairment: No dose adjustment necessary.
Hepatic Impairment: No dose adjustment necessary for mild-to-moderate impairment.

SIDE EFFECTS/ADVERSE REACTIONS
Frequent
Rash, nausea, hyperglycemia
Occasional
Peripheral neuropathy, hypertension, abdominal pain

PRECAUTIONS AND CONTRAINDICATIONS
Contraindications have not been determined.
Skin reactions (severe and life threatening, including Stevens-Johnson syndrome), opportunistic infections, inflammatory response (immune reconstitution syndrome) and redistribution of fat may occur. Coadministration with other non-nucleoside reverse transcriptase inhibitors is not recommended. Coadministration of protease inhibitors administered without ritonavir is not recommended.

DRUG INTERACTIONS OF CONCERN TO DENTISTRY
• CYP3A4, 2C9, and 2C19 substrates (e.g., triazolam): Etravirine may increase the levels and effects of these drugs.
• CYP3A4, 2C9, and 2C19 inducers: May decrease the levels and effects of etravirine.
• Avoid use.
• Macrolides: Etravirine may decrease the levels and effects of clarithromycin.

• Methadone: Etravirine may decrease the levels and effects of methadone. Monitor for opioid withdrawal symptoms.

SERIOUS REACTIONS

! Rash including Stevens-Johnson syndrome (blisters, peeling of the skin, loosening of skin and mucous membranes, and fever may occur) and hypersensitivity reaction may occur.

! Immune reconstitution syndrome may occur.

! Fat redistribution has been reported.

DENTAL CONSIDERATIONS

General:
• Examine for oral manifestations of opportunistic infection.
• Patient on chronic drug therapy may rarely have symptoms of blood dyscrasias, which include infection and poor healing.
• Place on frequent recall because of oral side effects.
• Consider semisupine chair position for patient comfort if GI side effects occur.
• Palliative medication may be required for management of oral side effects.
• Stomatitis as an adverse effect with relation to dental treatment.
Consultations:
• In a patient with symptoms of blood dyscrasias, request a medical consultation for blood studies and postpone treatment until normal values are reestablished.
• Medical consultation may be required to assess disease control and patient's ability to tolerate stress.
Teach Patient/Family to:
• Encourage effective oral hygiene to prevent soft tissue inflammation.

• Prevent trauma when using oral hygiene aids.
• Update health and drug history if physician makes any changes in evaluation or drug regimens.
• See dentist immediately if secondary oral infection occurs.
• Stomatitis and the need to see dentist as soon as symptoms occur.

everolimus
eh-**vier**-oh-lee-mus
(Afinitor, Certican, Zortress)

CATEGORY AND SCHEDULE
Pregnancy Risk Category: C (Zortress); D (Afinitor)

Drug Class: Immunosuppressant, antineoplastic agents, mTOR kinase inhibitor

MECHANISM OF ACTION
A macrolide antibiotic that suppresses the immune system by inhibiting the autophosphorylation and activation of an enzyme known as mTOR (mammalian target of rapamycin), a key regulatory kinase in cell cycle progression. Curtails the proliferation of T cells and B cells (essential components of immune response).
Therapeutic Effect: Reduces risk of acute organ rejection and thickening of grafts that restricts blood supply. Reduces cell proliferation, angiogenesis, and glucose uptake by tumors thereby assisting in tumor death.

USES
Prophylaxis of organ rejection in patients following renal transplant in

combination with cyclosporine and corticosteroids
Advanced renal cell carcinoma (RCC) after failure of treatment with sunitinib or sorafenib
Treatment also used in reducing the severity and incidence of serious complications in heart transplant patients
Kidney transplant rejection prophylaxis in patients at low-moderate immunologic risk

PHARMACOKINETICS

Route	Onset	Peak	Duration
PO	Unknown	1–2 hr	24 hr

Well and rapidly absorbed following oral administration. Bioavailability: about 30%. Distributed in plasma. Protein binding: 74%. Primarily metabolized by liver and other systems. CYP450 3A4 substrate and multidrug efflux transporter P-glycoprotein substrate; and competitive inhibitor of CYP3A4 and a mixed inhibitor of CYP2D6. Excreted primarily in feces; minimal excretion in urine. *Half-life:* 30 hr ± 11 hr.

INDICATIONS AND DOSAGES
▶**Prophylaxis of Organ Rejection**
PO (Certican)
Adults, elderly. 1–4 mg daily in combination with cyclosporine and corticosteroids. Drug should be administered twice a day.
▶ **Hepatic Impairment**
PO
For mild to moderate impairment: Reduce initial dose by one-half if laboratory parameters are met.

▶ **Advanced Renal Cell Cancer Who Have Failed Treatment with Sunitinib or Sorafenib**
PO (Afinitor)
Adults, Elderly. Initially, 10 mg/day, can increase by 5-mg increments to 20 mg/day. Dose increase to 20 mg/day is indicated for patients on strong 3A4 inducers.
▶ **Kidney Transplant Rejection Prophylaxis in Patients at Low-Moderate Immunologic Risk**
PO (Zortress)
Adults, Elderly. Initially, 0.75 mg q12h (1.5 mg/day) in combination with basiliximab induction and concurrently with reduced doses of cyclosporine, and corticosteroids. Adjust maintenance dose if needed at 4-to 5-day intervals.

SIDE EFFECTS/ADVERSE REACTIONS
Frequent
Stomatitis, infections, asthenia, fatigue, cough, diarrhea, anemia, anorexia, hyperglycemia, hyperlipidemia, hypertriglyceridemia, mouth ulcers, rash, peripheral edema, hypertension, nausea, infection
Occasional
Dyspnea, fatigue, stomatitis, dehydration, pneumonitis, abdominal pain, asthenias, pulmonary toxicity, dysuria, urinary tract infection
Rare
Acute respiratory failure, acute renal failure, chest pain, tachycardia, chills, depression, anxiety, hypotension, gout, hypoglycemia, diabetes mellitus

PRECAUTIONS AND CONTRAINDICATIONS
Hypersensitivity to everolimus or any component of the formulation
Severe hepatic impairment
Immunosuppression

Renal impairment
Renal artery/vein thrombosis
Children
Caution:
Prior hypersensitivity to sirolimus,
tacrolimus
History of allergies
Angioedema
Diabetes mellitus
Coronary artery disease
Moderate hepatic impairment
Elderly
Breast-feeding

DRUG INTERACTIONS OF CONCERN TO DENTISTRY

• CYP3A4 inhibitors, P-glycoprotein inhibitors: May increase the blood concentration and risk of toxicity of everolimus.
• CYP3A4 inducers: May decrease the blood concentration and effects of everolimus.
• Live-virus vaccines: May potentiate virus replication, increase vaccine side effects, and decrease the patient's antibody response to the vaccine.
• Other immunosuppressants: May increase the risk of infection or lymphomas.

SERIOUS REACTIONS

! Black box warning: Increase susceptibility to infections and possibility of developing lymphoma and other malignancies.
! Leukopenia, thrombocytopenia, pneumonitis, and infection may occur.
! Anemia occurs rarely.

DENTAL CONSIDERATIONS

General:
• Mucositis, stomatitis, and taste disturbances may occur as key adverse effects with relation to dental treatment.

• Examine for oral manifestation of infections, stomatitis, oral mucositis, and mouth ulcers.
• Consider semisupine chair position for patient comfort if GI side effects occur.
• Assess for symptoms of non-infectious pneumonitis.
• May experience poor wound healing.
• Assess medication list at each appointment.
Consultations:
• Medical consultation may be required to assess disease control.
• Review patient's medical and drug history.
• Renal function, liver function, glucose, and lipid profile should be monitored.
Teach Patient/Family to:
• Be alert for the possibility of mucositis, stomatitis, and taste disturbances and the need to be consulted by a dentist if any signs and symptoms occur.
• Practice good oral hygiene to prevent soft tissue inflammation.
• Prevent trauma when using oral hygiene aids.

exemestane
ex-eh-**mess**′-tane
(Aromasin)

CATEGORY AND SCHEDULE
Pregnancy Risk Category: D

Drug Class: Antineoplastic; aromatase inhibitor

MECHANISM OF ACTION
Inactivates aromatase, the principal enzyme that converts androgens to estrogens in both premenopausal and postmenopausal women, thereby

E

lowering the circulating estrogen level.
Therapeutic Effect: Inhibits the growth of breast cancers that are stimulated by estrogens.

USES

Treatment of advanced breast carcinoma not responsive to other therapy (postmenopausal)

PHARMACOKINETICS

Rapidly absorbed after PO administration. Protein binding: 90%. Distributed extensively into tissues. Metabolized in the liver; eliminated in urine and feces.
Half-life: 24 hr.

INDICATIONS AND DOSAGES
▶ **Breast Cancer**
PO
Adults, Elderly. 25 mg once a day after a meal.

SIDE EFFECTS/ADVERSE REACTIONS

Frequent
Fatigue, nausea, depression, hot flashes, pain, insomnia, anxiety, dyspnea
Occasional
Headache, dizziness, vomiting, peripheral edema, abdominal pain, anorexia, flu-like symptoms, diaphoresis, constipation, hypertension
Rare
Diarrhea

PRECAUTIONS AND CONTRAINDICATIONS

Hypersensitivity to exemestane

DRUG INTERACTIONS OF CONCERN TO DENTISTRY

• Data not available; however, possible reduction in plasma levels by inducers of CYP3A4 isoenzymes

SERIOUS REACTIONS

! None known

DENTAL CONSIDERATIONS

General:
• Monitor vital signs at every appointment because of cardiovascular side effects.
• If additional analgesia is required for dental pain, consider alternative analgesics (NSAIDs) in patients taking narcotics for acute or chronic pain.
• Product may be used in outpatient therapy.
• If used in prostate cancer, consider urinary retention concern and avoid anticholinergic drugs that may aggravate retention.
Consultations:
• Medical consultation may be required to assess disease control and patient's ability to tolerate stress.
Teach Patient/Family to:
• Encourage effective oral hygiene to prevent soft tissue inflammation.
• Prevent trauma when using oral hygiene aids.
• Update health and medication history if physician makes any changes in evaluation or drug regimens; include OTC, herbal, and nonherbal remedies in the update.

---

exenatide
ex-**en**′-a-tide
(Byetta)

CATEGORY AND SCHEDULE
Pregnancy Risk Category: C

Drug Class: Antidiabetic agent, incretin mimetic

MECHANISM OF ACTION
An analog of the hormone incretin (glucagon-like peptide 1 or GLP-1) which enhances insulin secretion; suppresses elevated glucagon secretion; slows gastric emptying; decreases food intake.
Therapeutic Effect: Improves glycemic control; decreases hemoglobin A_{1c}.

USES
Treatment of Type 2 diabetes mellitus (noninsulin dependent, NIDDM), adjunct or monotherapy

PHARMACOKINETICS
Bioavailability: 65%–76%. Minimal systemic metabolism. Primarily excreted in urine. *Half-life:* 2.4 hr.

INDICATIONS AND DOSAGES
▸ **Treatment of Type 2 Diabetes Mellitus (NIDDM), Adjunct or Monotherapy**
SC
Adults. Initially, 5 mcg twice a day for 1 month. Maintenance: 10 mcg twice a day after one month of therapy. Administer within 60 min prior to a meal in upper arm, thigh, or abdomen.

SIDE EFFECTS/ADVERSE REACTIONS
Frequent
Hypoglycemia, nausea, vomiting, diarrhea, anti-exenatide antibodies
Occasional
Dizziness, headache, hyperhidrosis, reduced appetite, dyspepsia, GERD, weakness, feeling jittery

PRECAUTIONS AND CONTRAINDICATIONS
Hypersensitivity to exenatide or its components
Renal insufficiency (Cl_{cr} <30 ml/min), end-stage renal disease
Type 1 diabetes
Caution:
Renal transplantation, moderate renal impairment (Cl_{cr} 30–50 ml/min)
Gastrointestinal disease
Pancreatitis
Diabetic patients with gastroparesis

DRUG INTERACTIONS OF CONCERN TO DENTISTRY
• Insulin secretagogues (e.g., sulfonylurea, meglitinide): May increase the risk of hypoglycemia.
• Oral medications: May reduce the rate and extent of absorption of orally administered drugs.
• Ethanol: May increase the risk of hypoglycemia.
• Warfarin: May increase the risk of bleeding.

SERIOUS REACTIONS
! Altered renal function, including renal insufficiency, acute renal failure, and worsening chronic renal failure may occur.
! Acute pancreatitis has been reported.
! Severe hypersensitivity (e.g., anaphylaxis, angioedema) has been reported.

DENTAL CONSIDERATIONS
General:
• Short appointments and a stress-reduction protocol may be required for anxious patients.
• Patients with diabetes may be more susceptible to infection and have delayed wound healing.
• Question the patient about self-monitoring of drug's antidiabetic effect including blood glucose values or finger-stick records.
• Avoid prescribing aspirin-containing products.

- Consider semisupine chair position for patient comfort if GI side effects occur.
Consultations:
- Medical consultation may include data from patient's blood glucose monitoring, including glycosylated hemoglobin or HbA$_{1c}$ testing.
- Medical consultation may be required to assess disease control.
Teach Patient/Family to:
- Encourage effective oral hygiene to prevent soft tissue inflammation.
- Prevent trauma when using oral hygiene aids.
- Avoid mouth rinses with high alcohol content because of drying effects.
- Instruct patients to take antibiotics at least 1 hr prior to administering exenatide.

ezetimibe
eh-**zet**-eh-mibe
(Zetia)
Do not confuse Zetia with Zestril.

CATEGORY AND SCHEDULE
Pregnancy Risk Category: C

Drug Class: Antihyperlipidemics

MECHANISM OF ACTION
An antihyperlipidemic that inhibits cholesterol absorption in the small intestine, leading to a decrease in the delivery of intestinal cholesterol to the liver.
Therapeutic Effect: Reduces total serum cholesterol, LDL cholesterol, and triglyceride levels; and increases HDL cholesterol concentration.

USES
Hypercholesterolemia

PHARMACOKINETICS
Well absorbed following oral administration. Protein binding: greater than 90%. Metabolized in the small intestine and liver. Excreted by the kidneys and bile.
Half-life: 22 hr.

INDICATIONS AND DOSAGES
▶ Hypercholesterolemia
PO
Adults, Elderly. 10 mg once a day, given with or without food. If the patient is also receiving a bile acid sequestrant, give ezetimibe at least 2 hr before or at least 4 hr after the bile acid sequestrant.

SIDE EFFECTS/ADVERSE REACTIONS
Occasional
Back pain, diarrhea, arthralgia, sinusitis, abdominal pain, nasopharyngitis, myalgia, upper respiratory tract infection, pain in extremities, cough, fatigue

PRECAUTIONS AND CONTRAINDICATIONS
Hypersensitivity to ezetimibe or any component of the formulation
Concurrent use of an HMG-CoA reductase inhibitor (atorvastatin, fluvastatin, lovastatin, pravastatin, or simvastatin) in patients with active liver disease, pregnancy, or nursing mothers
Active hepatic disease or unexplained persistent elevations in serum transaminase levels
Caution:
Moderate or severe hepatic insufficiency
Chronic renal failure; CrCl ≤ 30ml/min
Diabetes
Hypothyroidism
Concurrent use with cyclosporine

DRUG INTERACTIONS OF CONCERN TO DENTISTRY

• Aluminum and magnesium-containing antacids: Increase ezetimibe plasma concentration.
• Bile acid sequestrants: Decreases drug effectiveness.
• Cyclosporine: Combination significantly increases exposure of ezetimibe and cyclosporine.
• Fenofibrate: Combination increases exposure of ezetimibe. Use with other fibrates is not recommended.

SERIOUS REACTIONS

! Elevations in liver transaminases and hepatitis were reported.
! Hypersensitivity reactions, including angioedema and rash, have been reported.
! Myopathy and rhabdomyolysis occur rarely.

DENTAL CONSIDERATIONS

General:
• Consider semisupine chair position for patient comfort if GI side effects occur.
• Monitor vital signs at every appointment due to cardiovascular side effects.

Consultations:
• Update health and drug history if physician makes any changes in evaluation or drug regimens.

Teach Patient/Family to:
• Encourage effective oral hygiene to prevent soft tissue inflammation.
• Use soft tooth brush to reduce risk of bleeding.
• Immediately report any sign of infection to the dentist.

E

famciclovir
fam-si′-klo-veer
(Famvir)
Do not confuse Famvir with
Femhrt.

CATEGORY AND SCHEDULE
Pregnancy Risk Category: B

Drug Class: Antiviral

MECHANISM OF ACTION
A synthetic nucleoside that inhibits
viral DNA synthesis.
Therapeutic Effect: Suppresses
replication of herpes simplex virus
and varicella-zoster virus.

USES
Treatment of acute herpes zoster
(shingles) infection; recurrent
genital herpes; recurrent herpes
simplex virus infections in
HIV-infected patients

PHARMACOKINETICS
Rapidly and extensively absorbed
after PO administration. Protein
binding: 20%–25%. Rapidly
metabolized to penciclovir by
enzymes in the GI wall, liver, and
plasma. Eliminated unchanged in
urine. Removed by hemodialysis.
Half-life: 2 hr.

INDICATIONS AND DOSAGES
▶ **Herpes Zoster**
PO
Adults. 500 mg q8h for 7 days.
▶ **Recurrent Genital Herpes**
PO
Adults. 125 mg twice a day for 5
days.
▶ **Suppression of Recurrent Genital
Herpes**
PO
Adults. 250 mg twice a day for up to
1 yr.

▶ **Recurrent Herpes Simplex**
PO
Adults. 500 mg twice a day for 7 days.
▶ **Dosage in Renal Impairment**
Dosage and frequency are modified
on the basis of creatinine clearance.

Creatinine Clearance	Herpes Zoster	Genital Herpes
40–59 ml/min	500 mg q12h	125 mg q12h
20–39 ml/min	500 mg q24h	125 mg q24h
Less than 20 ml/min	250 mg q24h	125 mg q24h

▶ **Dosage in Hemodialysis Patients**
For adults with herpes zoster, give
250 mg after each dialysis treatment;
for adults with genital herpes, give
125 mg after each dialysis treatment.

SIDE EFFECTS/ADVERSE REACTIONS
Frequent
Headache, nausea
Occasional
Dizziness, somnolence, numbness of
feet, diarrhea, vomiting,
constipation, decreased appetite,
fatigue, fever, pharyngitis, sinusitis,
pruritus
Rare
Insomnia, abdominal pain,
dyspepsia, flatulence, back pain,
arthralgia

PRECAUTIONS AND CONTRAINDICATIONS
Hypersensitivity
Caution:
Children younger than 18 yr,
lactation, elderly, hepatic and renal
function impairment

DRUG INTERACTIONS OF CONCERN TO DENTISTRY
• None reported in otherwise
uncompromised patients

SERIOUS REACTIONS
! None known

DENTAL CONSIDERATIONS

General:
• Determine why the patient is taking the drug.
• Consider semisupine chair position for patient comfort because of GI effects of drug.
• Be aware of general discomfort associated with shingles; acute symptoms may preclude patient's routine dental visit or mandate short appointments.

Consultations:
• Medical consultation may be required to assess disease control and patient's ability to tolerate stress.

famotidine
fam-oh′-tah-deen
(Amfamox[AUS], Novo-Famotidine[CAN] Pepcid, Pepcid AC, Pepcidine[AUS], Ulcidine[CAN])

CATEGORY AND SCHEDULE
Pregnancy Risk Category: B
OTC (10 mg tablets)

Drug Class: Histamine H_2-receptor antagonist

MECHANISM OF ACTION
An antiulcer agent and gastric acid secretion inhibitor that inhibits histamine action at H_2 receptors of parietal cells.
Therapeutic Effect: Inhibits gastric acid secretion when fasting, at night, or when stimulated by food, caffeine, or insulin.

USES
Short-term treatment of active duodenal ulcer, maintenance therapy for duodenal ulcer, Zollinger-Ellison syndrome, multiple endocrine adenomas, benign gastric ulcers, gastroesophageal reflux disease (GERD); OTC: heartburn, acid indigestion

PHARMACOKINETICS

Route	Onset	Peak	Duration
PO	1 hr	1–4 hr	10–12 hr
IV	1 hr	0.5–3 hr	10–12 hr

Rapidly, incompletely absorbed from the GI tract. Protein binding: 15%–20%. Partially metabolized in the liver. Primarily excreted in urine. Not removed by hemodialysis.
Half-life: 2.5–3.5 hr (increased with impaired renal function).

INDICATIONS AND DOSAGES
▶ **Acute Treatment of Duodenal and Gastric Ulcers**
PO
Adults, Elderly, Children 12 yr and older. 40 mg/day at bedtime.
Children 1–11 yr. 0.5 mg/kg/day at bedtime. Maximum: 40 mg/day.
▶ **Duodenal Ulcer Maintenance**
PO
Adults, Elderly. 20 mg/day at bedtime.
▶ **GERD**
PO
Adults, Elderly, Children 12 yr and older. 20 mg twice a day.
Children 1–11 yr. 1 mg/kg/day in 2 divided doses.
Children 3–11 mo. 0.5 mg/kg/dose twice a day.
Children younger than 3 mo. 0.5 mg/kg/dose once a day.

F

▸ **Esophagitis**
PO
Adults, Elderly, Children 12 yr and older. 2–40 mg twice a day.
▸ **Hypersecretory Conditions**
PO
Adults, Elderly, Children 12 yr and older. Initially, 20 mg q6h. May increase up to 160 mg q6h.
▸ **Acid Indigestion, Heartburn (OTC)**
PO
Adults, Elderly, Children 12 yr and older. 10–20 mg 15–60 min before eating. Maximum: 2 doses per day.
▸ **Usual Parenteral Dosage**
IV
Adults, Elderly, Children 12 yr and older. 20 mg q12h.
▸ **Dosage in Renal Impairment**
Dosing frequency is modified on the basis of creatinine clearance.

Creatinine Clearance	Dosage Interval
10–50 ml/min	q24h
Less than 10 ml/min	q36–48h

SIDE EFFECTS/ADVERSE REACTIONS
Occasional
Headache
Rare
Constipation, diarrhea, dizziness

PRECAUTIONS AND CONTRAINDICATIONS
Hypersensitivity
Caution:
Lactation, children, severe renal disease, severe hepatic function, elderly, RPD tablets contain aspartame (caution: phenylketonuria)

DRUG INTERACTIONS OF CONCERN TO DENTISTRY
• Decreased absorption of ketoconazole or itraconazole (take doses 2 hr apart)

SERIOUS REACTIONS
! None known

DENTAL CONSIDERATIONS

General:
• Avoid prescribing aspirin-containing products in patients with active GI disease.
• Consider semisupine chair position for patient comfort because of GI effects of disease.
• Assess salivary flow as a factor in caries, periodontal disease, and candidiasis.
Teach Patient/Family to:
• Encourage effective oral hygiene to prevent gingival inflammation.
• When chronic dry mouth occurs, advise patient to:
  • Avoid mouth rinses with high alcohol content because of drying effects.
  • Use daily home fluoride products for anticaries effect.
  • Use sugarless gum, frequent sips of water, or saliva substitutes.

---

febuxostat
feb-**ux**′-oh-stat
(Uloric)

CATEGORY AND SCHEDULE
Pregnancy Risk Category: C

Drug Class: Xanthine oxidase inhibitor

MECHANISM OF ACTION

A non-purine, selective inhibitor of xanthine oxidase.
Therapeutic Effect: Decreases serum uric acid.

USES

Hyperuricemia in patients with gout

PHARMACOKINETICS

Partially absorbed. Protein binding: 99.2%. Extensively metabolized by both conjugation via uridine diphosphate glucuronosyltransferase enzymes and oxidation via CYP enzymes, including CYP1A2, 2C8, and 2C9. Partially excreted in urine; partially excreted in feces. *Half-life:* 5–8 hr.

INDICATIONS AND DOSAGES

▸ **Hyperuricemia in Patients with Gout**

PO

Adults. 40 mg a day. May increase to 80 mg/day in patients who do not achieve serum uric acid < 6 mg/dl after 2 wk of 40-mg treatment.

SIDE EFFECTS/ADVERSE REACTIONS

Rare (≤1%)

Dizziness, rash, nausea, abnormal liver function tests (LFTs), arthralgia

PRECAUTIONS AND CONTRAINDICATIONS

Hypersensitivity to febuxostat or its components
Drugs metabolized by xanthine oxidase (e.g., azathioprine, mercaptopurine, theophylline)
Caution:
Hepatic impairment
Renal impairment

Pregnancy
Cardiovascular disease

DRUG INTERACTIONS OF CONCERN TO DENTISTRY

• Drugs metabolized by xanthine oxidase (e.g., azathioprine, mercaptopurine, theophylline): May increase plasma concentrations of these agents.

SERIOUS REACTIONS

! Elevated transaminases have been reported.
! Cardiovascular thromboembolic events (cardiovascular deaths, non-fatal myocardial infarctions, and non-fatal strokes) may occur.
! Gout flares may occur during the initiation of treatment.

DENTAL CONSIDERATIONS

General:
• Patient on chronic drug therapy may rarely have symptoms of blood dyscrasias, which include infection, bleeding, and poor healing.
Consultations:
• In a patient with symptoms of blood dyscrasias, request a medical consultation for blood studies and postpone treatment until normal values are reestablished.
• Medical consultation may be required to assess disease control.
Teach Patient/Family to:
• Encourage effective oral hygiene to prevent soft tissue inflammation.
• Avoid mouth rinses with high alcohol content because of drying effects.

F

felbamate
fel'-ba-mate
(Felbatol)

CATEGORY AND SCHEDULE
Pregnancy Risk Category: C

Drug Class: Anticonvulsant
(carbamate derivative)

MECHANISM OF ACTION
An anticonvulsant, structurally
similar to meprobamate, that weakly
blocks repetitive, sustained firing of
neurons by enhancing the ability of
γ-aminobutyric acid (GABA) and
antagonizes the strychnine-
insensitive glycine recognition site
of the N-methyl-D-aspartate
receptor-ionophore complex.
Therapeutic Effect: Decreases
seizure activity.

USES
Used alone or as adjunct therapy in
partial seizures; also for partial
seizures associated with Lennox-
Gastaut syndrome in children;
because of severe side effects use
only for severe seizures when other
therapy is inadequate

PHARMACOKINETICS
Rapidly and almost completely
absorbed after PO administration.
Protein binding: 22%–25%,
primarily to albumin. Partially
excreted unchanged in the urine.
Half-life: 20–23 hr.

INDICATIONS AND DOSAGES
▸ **Monotherapy or Adjunctive
Therapy in the Treatment of Partial
Seizures, with and without
Generalization**
PO
Adults, Children older than 14 yr.
Initially, 1200 mg/day in divided

doses 3–4 times a day. At week 2,
increase the felbamate dosage to
2400 mg/day while reducing the
dosage of other antiepileptic drugs
(AEDs) up to an additional one-third
of their original dosage. At week 3,
increase the felbamate dosage up to
3600 mg/day and continue to reduce
the dosage of other AEDs as
clinically indicated.
▸ **Adjunctive Therapy in the
Treatment of Partial Seizures, with
and without Generalization**
PO
Adults, Children older than 14 yr.
Add 1200 mg/day in divided doses
3–4 times a day while reducing
present AEDs by 20% in order;
control plasma concentrations of
concurrent phenytoin, valproic acid,
and carbamazepine and its
metabolites. Increase dosage by
1200 mg/day increments at weekly
intervals to 3600 mg/day.

SIDE EFFECTS/ADVERSE REACTIONS
Frequent
Somnolence, dizziness, headache,
fatigue, nausea, anorexia, vomiting,
constipation
Occasional
Chest pain, palpitations, tachycardia,
depression and behavioral changes,
anxiety, nervousness, ataxia,
malaise, agitation, rash, acne,
pruritus, diarrhea, weight gain,
tremors, abnormal vision, diplopia,
sinusitis, difficulty with
coordination, taste perversion
Rare
Delusion, bradycardia,
hallucinations, urinary retention,
acute renal failure

PRECAUTIONS AND CONTRAINDICATIONS
History of any blood dyscrasia or
hepatic dysfunction, hypersensitivity

to felbamate, its ingredients, or known sensitivity to other carbamates
Caution:
Lactation, warning of increased risk of aplastic anemia, hepatic failure; safety and efficacy in children with other types of seizures has not been established

DRUG INTERACTIONS OF CONCERN TO DENTISTRY
• Decreased effects of carbamazepine
• Increased photosensitization: drugs causing photosensitivity (e.g., tetracyclines)

SERIOUS REACTIONS
Alert
! Aplastic anemia has been reported during felbamate therapy.
! Hepatic failure resulting in death has been reported.

DENTAL CONSIDERATIONS
General:
• Examine for evidence of oral manifestations of blood dyscrasia (infection, bleeding, poor healing).
• Short appointments and a stress reduction protocol may be required for anxious patients.
• Determine type of epilepsy, seizure frequency, and quality of seizure control. A stress reduction protocol may be required.
• Assess salivary flow as a factor in caries, periodontal disease, and candidiasis.
• Monitor vital signs at every appointment because of cardiovascular side effects.
• Advise patient if dental drugs prescribed have a potential for photosensitivity.
Consultations:
• Medical consultation may be required to assess disease control and patient's ability to tolerate stress.

Teach Patient/Family to:
• Encourage effective oral hygiene to prevent soft tissue inflammation.
• Use caution to prevent injury when using oral hygiene aids.
• Use powered tooth brush if patient has difficulty holding conventional devices.
• When chronic dry mouth occurs, advise patient to:
  • Avoid mouth rinses with high alcohol content because of drying effects.
  • Use daily home fluoride products for anticaries effect.
  • Use sugarless gum, frequent sips of water, or saliva substitutes.

felodipine
fell-oh′-da-peen
(AGON SR[AUS], Felodur ER[AUS], Plendil, Plendil ER[AUS], Renedil[CAN])
Do not confuse Plendil with Pletal, or Renedil with Prinivil.

CATEGORY AND SCHEDULE
Pregnancy Risk Category: C

Drug Class: Calcium channel blocker

MECHANISM OF ACTION
An antihypertensive and antianginal agent that inhibits calcium movement across cardiac and vascular smooth-muscle cell membranes. Potent peripheral vasodilator (does not depress SA or AV nodes).
Therapeutic Effect: Increases myocardial contractility, heart rate, and cardiac output; decreases peripheral vascular resistance and B/P.

F

USES
Essential hypertension, alone or with other antihypertensives, chronic angina pectoris

PHARMACOKINETICS

Route	Onset	Peak	Duration
PO	2–5 hr	N/A	N/A

Rapidly, completely absorbed from the GI tract. Protein binding: greater than 99%. Undergoes first-pass metabolism in the liver. Primarily excreted in urine. Not removed by hemodialysis. *Half-life:* 11–16 hr.

INDICATIONS AND DOSAGES
▸ **Hypertension**
PO
Adults. Initially, 5 mg/day as single dose.
Elderly, Patients with impaired hepatic function. Initially, 2.5 mg/day. Adjust dosage at no less than 2-wk intervals. Maintenance: 2.5–10 mg/day.

SIDE EFFECTS/ADVERSE REACTIONS
Frequent
Headache, peripheral edema
Occasional
Flushing, respiratory infection, dizziness, light-headedness, asthenia (loss of strength, weakness), gingival enlargement
Rare
Paresthesia, abdominal discomfort, nervousness, muscle cramping, cough, diarrhea, constipation

PRECAUTIONS AND CONTRAINDICATIONS
Hypersensitivity, sick sinus syndrome, second- or third-degree heart block

Caution:
CHF, hypotension less than 90 mm Hg systolic, hepatic injury, lactation, children, renal disease, elderly

DRUG INTERACTIONS OF CONCERN TO DENTISTRY
• Decreased effect: NSAIDs, phenobarbital, carbamazepine
• Increased effect: parenteral and inhalational general anesthetics, other drugs with hypotensive actions
• Increased effects of nondepolarizing muscle relaxants, diazepam, midazolam
• Increased plasma levels: itraconazole, erythromycin, carbamazepine

SERIOUS REACTIONS
! Overdose produces nausea, somnolence, confusion, slurred speech, hypotension and bradycardia.

DENTAL CONSIDERATIONS

General:
• Monitor cardiac status; take vital signs at each appointment because of cardiovascular side effects. Consider a stress reduction protocol to prevent stress-induced angina during the dental appointment.
• After supine positioning, have patient sit upright for at least 2 min before standing to avoid orthostatic hypotension at dismissal.
• Place on frequent recall to monitor gingival condition.
• Limit use of sodium-containing products, such as saline IV fluids, for patients with a dietary salt restriction.
• Assess salivary flow as a factor in caries, periodontal disease, and candidiasis.
• Use vasoconstrictors with caution, in low doses and with careful

aspiration. Avoid use of gingival retraction cord with epinephrine.
• Use precaution if sedation or general anesthesia is required; risk of hypotensive episode.
Consultations:
• Medical consultation may be required to assess disease control.
• Consultation with physician may be necessary if sedation or general anesthesia is required.
Teach Patient/Family to:
• Encourage effective oral hygiene to prevent gingival inflammation and minimize enlargement.
• Schedule frequent oral prophylaxis if enlargement occurs.
• When chronic dry mouth occurs, advise patient to:
  • Avoid mouth rinses with high alcohol content because of drying effects.
  • Use daily home fluoride products for anticaries effect.
  • Use sugarless gum, frequent sips of water, or saliva substitutes.

fenofibrate

fee-no-fye′-brate
(Apo-Fenofibrate[CAN], Lofibra, TriCor)
Do not confuse TriCor with Tracleer.

CATEGORY AND SCHEDULE
Pregnancy Risk Category: C

Drug Class: Antihyperlipidemic

MECHANISM OF ACTION
An antihyperlipidemic that enhances synthesis of lipoprotein lipase and reduces triglyceride-rich lipoproteins and VLDLs.

Therapeutic Effect: Increases VLDL catabolism and reduces total plasma triglyceride levels.

USES
Treatment of hyperlipidemia, types IV and V, as an adjunct to diet therapy

PHARMACOKINETICS
Well absorbed from the GI tract. Absorption increased when given with food. Protein binding: 99%. Rapidly metabolized in the liver to active metabolite. Excreted primarily in urine; lesser amount in feces. Not removed by hemodialysis. *Half-life:* 20 hr.

INDICATIONS AND DOSAGES
▸ **Reduction of Very High Serum Triglyceride Levels in Patients at Risk for Pancreatitis**
PO
Adults, Elderly. Initially, 67 mg/day (capsule); may increase to 200 mg/day. Or initially, 48 mg/day (tablet); may increase to 145 mg/day.
▸ **Hypercholesterolemia**
PO
Adults, Elderly. 200 mg/day (capsule) with meals. Or 145 mg/day (tablet) with meals.

SIDE EFFECTS/ADVERSE REACTIONS
Frequent
Pain, rash, headache, asthenia or fatigue, flu symptoms, dyspepsia, nausea or vomiting, rhinitis
Occasional
Diarrhea, abdominal pain, constipation, flatulence, arthralgia, decreased libido, dizziness, pruritus
Rare
Increased appetite, insomnia, polyuria, cough, blurred vision, eye floaters, earache

PRECAUTIONS AND CONTRAINDICATIONS

Gallbladder disease, hypersensitivity to fenofibrate, severe renal or hepatic dysfunction (including primary biliary cirrhosis, unexplained persistent liver function abnormality)

Caution:

Monitor liver function; may lead to cholelithiasis; can be associated with myositis, myopathy, or rhabdomyolysis; avoid if lactating; safe use in children unknown; discontinue use if no response in 2 mo; increased anticoagulant effect with oral anticoagulants

DRUG INTERACTIONS OF CONCERN TO DENTISTRY

• None reported

SERIOUS REACTIONS

! Fenofibrate may increase excretion of cholesterol into bile, leading to cholelithiasis.

! Pancreatitis, hepatitis, thrombocytopenia, and agranulocytosis occur rarely.

DENTAL CONSIDERATIONS

General:

• Monitor vital signs at every appointment because of cardiovascular and respiratory side effects.

• Consider semisupine chair position for patient comfort because of GI side effects of drug.

• Patients on chronic drug therapy may rarely have symptoms of blood dyscrasias, which can include infection, bleeding, and poor healing.

• Avoid dental light in patient's eyes; offer dark glasses for patient comfort.

Consultations:

• In a patient with symptoms of blood dyscrasias, request a medical consultation for blood studies and postpone treatment until normal values are reestablished.

Teach Patient/Family to:

• Use powered tooth brush if patient has difficulty holding conventional devices.

• Prevent trauma when using oral hygiene aids.

fenoprofen calcium
fen-oh-proe'-fen
(Nalfon)
Do not confuse Nalfon with Naldecon.

CATEGORY AND SCHEDULE

Pregnancy Risk Category: B (D if used in third trimester or near delivery)

Drug Class: Nonsteroidal antiinflammatory, propionic acid derivative

MECHANISM OF ACTION

An NSAID that produces analgesic and antiinflammatory effects by inhibiting prostaglandin synthesis.

Therapeutic Effect: Reduces the inflammatory response and intensity of pain.

USES

Treatment of mild-to-moderate pain, osteoarthritis, rheumatoid arthritis, acute gout, arthritis, ankylosing spondylitis, nonrheumatic inflammation, dysmenorrhea

PHARMACOKINETICS

PO: Peak 2 hr. **Half-life:** 3–3.5 hr; 99% plasma protein binding;

metabolized in liver; excreted in urine (metabolites), breast milk.

INDICATIONS AND DOSAGES
▸ **Mild-to-Moderate Pain**
PO
Adults, Elderly. 200 mg q4–6h as needed.
▸ **Rheumatoid Arthritis, Osteoarthritis**
PO
Adults, Elderly. 300–600 mg 3–4 times a day.

SIDE EFFECTS/ADVERSE REACTIONS
Frequent
Headache, somnolence, dyspepsia, nausea, vomiting, constipation
Occasional
Dizziness, pruritus, nervousness, asthenia, diarrhea, abdominal cramps, flatulence, tinnitus, blurred vision, peripheral edema and fluid retention

PRECAUTIONS AND CONTRAINDICATIONS
Active peptic ulcer disease, chronic inflammation of GI tract, GI bleeding or ulceration, history of hypersensitivity to aspirin or NSAIDs, significant renal impairment
Caution:
Lactation, children, bleeding disorders, GI disorders, cardiac disorders, hypersensitivity to other antiinflammatory agents

DRUG INTERACTIONS OF CONCERN TO DENTISTRY
• GI bleeding, ulceration: salicylates, alcohol, corticosteroids, other NSAIDs, bisphosphonates
• May decrease effects of fenoprofen: phenobarbital
• Nephrotoxicity: acetaminophen (prolonged use)

• Possible risk of decreased renal function: cyclosporine
• Probable increased bleeding risk: warfarin
• Suspected increased risk for methotrexate toxicity
• First-time users of SSRIs also taking NSAIDs may have a higher risk of GI side effects; avoid use of NSAIDs in these patients

SERIOUS REACTIONS
❗ Overdose may result in acute hypotension and tachycardia.
❗ Rare reactions with long-term use include peptic ulcer disease, GI bleeding, gastritis, severe hepatic reaction (jaundice), nephrotoxicity (hematuria, dysuria, proteinuria) and a severe hypersensitivity reaction (bronchospasm, angioedema).

DENTAL CONSIDERATIONS
General:
• Assess salivary flow as a factor in caries, periodontal disease, and candidiasis.
• Avoid prescribing in pregnancy.
• Possibility of cross-allergenicity when patient is allergic to aspirin.
• Severe stomach bleeding may occur in patients who regularly use NSAIDs in recommended doses, when the patient is also taking another NSAID, a blood thinning, or steroid drug, if the patient has GI or peptic ulcer disease, if they are 60 years or older, or when NSAIDs are taken longer than directed. Warn patients of the potential for severe stomach bleeding.
Consultations:
• Medical consultation may be required to assess disease control.
Teach Patient/Family to:
• Encourage effective oral hygiene to prevent gingival inflammation.

F

- Use caution to prevent injury when using oral hygiene aids.
  - Warn patient of potential risks of NSAIDs.
- When chronic dry mouth occurs, advise patient to:
  - Avoid mouth rinses with high alcohol content because of drying effects.
  - Use daily home fluoride products for anticaries effect.
  - Use sugarless gum, frequent sips of water, or saliva substitutes.

fentanyl transdermal system

fen′-ta-nil trans-derr′-mal sis′-tem
(Duragesic 25, 50, 75, 100
Transdermal Patches, Fentanyl
Oralet oral: transmucosal fentanyl
citrate: Actiq [lozenges])

CATEGORY AND SCHEDULE
Pregnancy Risk Category: C
Controlled Substance Schedule II

Drug Class: Narcotic analgesics

MECHANISM OF ACTION
Interacts with opioid receptors in the CNS to alter pain perception.

USES
Management of chronic pain when opioids are necessary; transmucosal form: only for management of breakthrough cancer pain in patients with malignancies who are using or tolerant to opioids; not appropriate for acute postoperative pain

PHARMACOKINETICS
Transdermal: Dosage adjusted according to opioid tolerance if patient has been taking opioids

(2.5 mg of transdermal fentanyl is equivalent to approximately 90 mg of oral morphine in 24 hr); peak serum levels take up to 24 hr after applied; liver metabolism; renal excretion of metabolites.

INDICATIONS AND DOSAGES
▸ **Chronic Pain**
Topical
Adult only. One patch every 72 hr; dose depends on need for pain control; titrate as required.
Transmucosal Form
Adult only. (Patch and lozenge on a stick only [Actiq].) Dose must be titrated starting with lowest dose size (must be kept secure from children).
Conscious Sedation or Anesthesia (Oralet Only) in Hospital Setting
Adult. Doses must match patient, usually no more than 5 mcg/kg (400 mcg); doses for children must be adjusted for weight; see package insert directions for use.

SIDE EFFECTS/ADVERSE REACTIONS
ORAL: Dry mouth
CNS: Dizziness, delirium, euphoria
CV: Bradycardia, arrest, hypotension, or hypertension
GI: Nausea, vomiting
RESP: Respiratory depression, arrest, laryngospasm
EENT: Blurred vision, miosis
MS: Muscle rigidity

PRECAUTIONS AND CONTRAINDICATIONS
Hypersensitivity to opiates, myasthenia gravis
Caution:
Elderly, respiratory depression, increased intracranial pressure, seizure disorders, severe respiratory disorders, cardiac dysrhythmias

DRUG INTERACTIONS OF CONCERN TO DENTISTRY

• Effects may be increased with other CNS depressants: alcohol, narcotics, sedative/hypnotics, skeletal muscle relaxants, chlorpromazine
• Additive hypotension: nitrous oxide, benzodiazepines, phenothiazines
• Increased anticholinergic effect: anticholinergics
• Contraindication: MAOIs

SERIOUS REACTIONS

! Life-threatening respiratory depression, cardiorespiratory arrest, generalized CNS depression, coma, death

DENTAL CONSIDERATIONS

General:
• Monitor vital signs at every appointment because of cardiovascular and respiratory side effects.
• After supine positioning, have patient sit upright for at least 2 min before standing to avoid orthostatic hypotension.
• Assess salivary flow as a factor in caries, periodontal disease, and candidiasis.
• Psychologic and physical dependence may occur with chronic administration.
• Determine why the patient is taking the drug.
• Consider alternative drugs to opioids and NSAIDs for management of dental pain.
Consultations:
• Medical consultation may be required to assess disease control.
Teach Patient/Family to:
• Encourage effective oral hygiene to prevent gingival inflammation.
• Avoid mouth rinses with high alcohol content because of drying effects.

ferrous fumarate/ ferrous gluconate/ ferrous sulfate

fer′-us fume′-ah-rate/fer′-us glue′-kuh-nate/fer′-us sul′-fate
ferrous fumarate
(Feostat, Femiron, Ferro-Sequels, Nephro-Fer, Palafer[CAN])
ferrous gluconate
(Apo-Ferrous Gluconate[CAN], Fergon)
ferrous sulfate
(Apo-Ferrous Sulfate[CAN], Fer-In-Sol, Fer-Iron, Ferro-Gradumet[AUS], Slow-Fe)

CATEGORY AND SCHEDULE

Pregnancy Risk Category: A
OTC

Drug Class: Hematinic, iron preparation

MECHANISM OF ACTION

An enzymatic mineral that is an essential component in the formation of Hgb, myoglobin and enzymes. Promotes effective erythropoiesis and transport and utilization of oxygen (O_2).
Therapeutic Effect: Prevents iron deficiency.

USES

Treatment of iron deficiency anemia, prophylaxis for iron deficiency in pregnancy

PHARMACOKINETICS

Absorbed in the duodenum and upper jejunum. Ten percent absorbed in patients with normal iron stores; increased to 20%–30% in those with inadequate iron stores. Primarily bound to serum transferrin. Excreted in urine, sweat and sloughing of intestinal mucosa and by menses.
Half-life: 6 hr.

F

INDICATIONS AND DOSAGES
▶ **Iron Deficiency Anemia**
Dosage is expressed in terms of milligrams of elemental iron, degree of anemia, patient weight and presence of any bleeding. Expect to use periodic hematologic determinations as guide to therapy.
PO (Ferrous Fumarate)
Adults, Elderly. 60–100 mg twice a day.
Children. 3–6 mg/kg/day in 2–3 divided doses.
PO (Ferrous Gluconate)
Adults, Elderly. 60 mg 2–4 times a day.
Children. 3–6 mg/kg/day in 2–3 divided doses.
PO (Ferrous Sulfate)
Adults, Elderly. 325 mg 2–4 times a day.
Children. 3–6 mg/kg/day in 2–3 divided doses.
▶ **Prevention of Iron Deficiency**
PO (Ferrous Fumarate)
Adults, Elderly. 60–100 mg/day.
Children. 1–2 mg/kg/day.
PO (Ferrous Gluconate)
Adults, Elderly. 60 mg/day.
Children. 1–2 mg/kg/day.
PO (Ferrous Sulfate)
Adults, Elderly. 325 mg/day.
Children. 1–2 mg/kg/day.

SIDE EFFECTS/ADVERSE REACTIONS
Occasional
Mild, transient nausea, extrinsic stain on teeth (liquid form)
Rare
Heartburn, anorexia, constipation, diarrhea

PRECAUTIONS AND CONTRAINDICATIONS
Hemochromatosis, hemosiderosis, hemolytic anemias, peptic ulcer disease, regional enteritis, ulcerative colitis

Caution:
Long-term anemia

DRUG INTERACTIONS OF CONCERN TO DENTISTRY
• Decreased absorption of tetracycline, zinc, ciprofloxacin

SERIOUS REACTIONS
! Large doses may aggravate existing GI tract disease, such as peptic ulcer disease, regional enteritis and ulcerative colitis.
! Severe iron poisoning occurs most often in children and is manifested as vomiting, severe abdominal pain, diarrhea, and dehydration, followed by hyperventilation, pallor or cyanosis, and cardiovascular collapse.

DENTAL CONSIDERATIONS
Teach Patient/Family to:
• Avoid frequent use if patient is using hydrogen peroxide as a dentifrice to remove extrinsic stain so that peroxide-related soft tissue injury does not occur.
• Take through straw followed by rinsing mouth to reduce staining.

fesoterodine
fes′-oh-**ter′**-oh-deen
(Toviaz)

CATEGORY AND SCHEDULE
Pregnancy Risk Category: C

Drug Class: Urinary antispasmodics

MECHANISM OF ACTION
An anticholinergic that antagonizes acetylcholine at muscarinic receptors and relaxes the detrusor smooth muscle of the bladder.

Therapeutic Effect: Reduces urinary frequency and urgency.

USES
Overactive bladder

PHARMACOKINETICS
Well absorbed following PO administration. Protein binding: 50%. Rapidly and extensively metabolized to its active metabolite, 5-hydroxymethyl derivative (5-HMT). 5-HMT is metabolized by CYP450 2D6 and 3A4. Primarily excreted in urine and smaller amounts in feces. *Half-life:* 7 hr (active metabolite).

INDICATIONS AND DOSAGES
▸ **Overactive Bladder**
PO
Adults. 4 mg a day. May increase to 8 mg a day, based upon individual response and tolerability.
Patients with severe renal insufficiency or those taking potent CYP3A4 inhibitors should not use doses greater than 4 mg a day.
Not recommended in patients with hepatic impairment.

SIDE EFFECTS/ADVERSE REACTIONS
Frequent
Dry mouth, dry eye, constipation, dysuria
Occasional
Dizziness, headache, dry throat, abdominal pain, diarrhea, dyspepsia, nausea, insomnia

PRECAUTIONS AND CONTRAINDICATIONS
Hypersensitivity to fesoterodine or its components
Urinary retention
Gastric retention
Uncontrolled narrow-angle glaucoma

Caution:
Bladder outlet obstruction
Decreased gastrointestinal motility
Controlled narrow-angle glaucoma
Myasthenia gravis
Severe hepatic impairment

DRUG INTERACTIONS OF CONCERN TO DENTISTRY
• Anticholinergic agents: Increased effects of anticholinergics.
• CYP3A4 inhibitors (e.g., ketoconazole, itraconazole, clarithromycin): May increase levels of fesoterodine; increased risk of adverse effects.
• CYP3A4 inducers (rifampin, carbamazepine): May decrease levels of fesoterodine.
• Orally administered drugs: May alter the GI absorption of concomitantly administered drug due to anticholinergic effects on GI motility.

SERIOUS REACTIONS
❗ None reported

DENTAL CONSIDERATIONS

General:
• Monitor vital signs at every appointment because of cardiovascular side effects.
• Assess salivary flow as a factor in caries, periodontal disease, and candidiasis.
• Avoid dental light in patient's eyes; offer dark glasses for patient comfort.
• Consider semisupine chair position for patient comfort if GI side effects occur.
Consultations:
• Physician should be informed if significant xerostomic side effects occur (e.g., increased caries, sore tongue, problems eating or swallowing, difficulty wearing

F

prosthesis) so that medication change can be considered.
• Medical consultation may be required to assess disease control.

Teach Patient/Family to:
• Encourage effective oral hygiene to prevent soft tissue inflammation.
• When chronic dry mouth occurs, advise patient to:
  • Avoid mouth rinses with high alcohol content because of drying effects.
  • Use daily home fluoride products for anticaries effect.
  • Use sugarless gum, frequent sips of water, or saliva substitutes.

fexofenadine hydrochloride
fex-oh-fen′-eh-deen
hi-droh-klor′-ide
(Allegra, Telfast[AUS])

CATEGORY AND SCHEDULE
Pregnancy Risk Category: C

Drug Class: Antihistamine, nonsedating

MECHANISM OF ACTION
A piperidine that competes with histamine for H_1-receptor sites on effector cells.
Therapeutic Effect: Relieves allergic rhinitis symptoms.

USES
Treatment of seasonal allergic rhinitis, chronic idiopathic urticaria

PHARMACOKINETICS
Rapidly absorbed after PO administration. Protein binding: 60%–70%. Does not cross the blood-brain barrier. Minimally

metabolized. Eliminated in feces and urine. Not removed by hemodialysis.
Half-life: 14.4 hr (increased in renal impairment).

INDICATIONS AND DOSAGES
▶ **Allergic Rhinitis, Urticaria**
PO
Adults, Elderly, Children 12 yr and older. 60 mg twice a day or 180 mg once a day.
Children 6–11 yr. 30 mg twice a day.
▶ **Dosage in Renal Impairment**
Adults, Elderly and Children 12 yr and older. Dosage is reduced to 60 mg once a day.
Children 6–11 yr. Dosage is reduced to 30 mg once a day.

SIDE EFFECTS/ADVERSE REACTIONS
Rare
Somnolence, headache, fatigue, nausea, vomiting, abdominal distress, dysmenorrhea

PRECAUTIONS AND CONTRAINDICATIONS
Hypersensitivity; troglitazone
Caution:
Reduce dose in elderly, renally impaired, lactation, children younger than 12 yr

DRUG INTERACTIONS OF CONCERN TO DENTISTRY
• Elevated plasma levels with erythromycin, ketoconazole
• Decreased absorption: grapefruit juice
• Suspected decreased antihistaminic effects: rifampin

SERIOUS REACTIONS
! None known

DENTAL CONSIDERATIONS

General:
• Consider semisupine chair position for patient comfort because of GI effects of drug.

filgrastim

fill-grass'-tim
(Neupogen)
Do not confuse Neupogen with Epogen or Nutramigen.

CATEGORY AND SCHEDULE

Pregnancy Risk Category: C

Drug Class: Biologic modifier; granulocyte colony-stimulating factor

MECHANISM OF ACTION

A biologic modifier that stimulates production, maturation, and activation of neutrophils to increase their migration and cytotoxicity.
Therapeutic Effect: Decreases incidence of infection.

USES

Stimulates the bone marrow to make new white blood cells

PHARMACOKINETICS

Readily absorbed after subcutaneous administration. Not removed by hemodialysis. *Half-life:* 3.5 hr.

INDICATIONS AND DOSAGES

▸ **Myelosuppression**
IV or Subcutaneous Infusion, Subcutaneous Injection
Adults, Elderly. Initially, 5 mcg/kg/day. May increase by 5 mcg/kg for each chemotherapy cycle on the basis of duration or severity of absolute neutrophil count nadir.

▸ **Bone Marrow Transplant**
IV or Subcutaneous Infusion
Adults, Elderly. 5–10 mcg/kg/day. Adjust dosage daily during period of neutrophil recovery on the basis of neutrophil response.

▸ **Mobilization Progenitor Cells**
IV or Subcutaneous Infusion
Adults. 10 mcg/kg/day beginning at least 4 days before first leukapheresis and continuing until last leukapheresis.

▸ **Chronic Neutropenia, Congenital Neutropenia**
Subcutaneous
Adults, Children. 6 mcg/kg/dose twice a day.

▸ **Idiopathic or Cyclic Neutropenia**
Subcutaneous
Adults, Children. 5 mcg/kg/dose once a day.

SIDE EFFECTS/ADVERSE REACTIONS

Frequent
Nausea or vomiting, mild to severe bone pain that occurs more frequently with high-dose IV form and less frequently with low-dose subcutaneous form; alopecia, diarrhea, fever, fatigue
Occasional
Anorexia, dyspnea, headache, cough, rash
Rare
Psoriasis, hematuria or proteinuria, osteoporosis

PRECAUTIONS AND CONTRAINDICATIONS

Hypersensitivity to *Escherichia coli*–derived proteins, 24 hr before or after cytotoxic chemotherapy, concurrent use of other drugs that may result in lowered platelet count

DRUG INTERACTIONS OF CONCERN TO DENTISTRY

• Dental drug interactions have not been studied.

SERIOUS REACTIONS

! Long-term administration occasionally produces chronic neutropenia and splenomegaly.
! Thrombocytopenia, MI, and arrhythmias occur rarely.
! Adult respiratory distress syndrome may occur in patients with sepsis.

F

DENTAL CONSIDERATIONS

General:
• Determine why patient is taking the drug.
• Examine for oral manifestations of opportunistic infection.
• Monitor vital signs at every appointment because of cardiovascular side effects.
• Patient may need assistance in getting into and out of dental chair. Adjust chair position for patient comfort.
• Patients are at risk for infection.
• Oral infections should be eliminated and/or treated aggressively.
• Patients may have been treated with radiation and/or chemotherapy; confirm medical and drug history.
Consultations:
• Medical consultation may be required to assess disease control and patient's ability to tolerate stress.
• In a patient with symptoms of blood dyscrasias, request a medical consultation for blood studies and postpone treatment until normal values are reestablished.
• Medical consultation should include routine blood counts including platelet counts and bleeding time.
Teach Patient/Family to:
• Encourage effective oral hygiene to prevent soft tissue inflammation.
• Prevent trauma when using oral hygiene aids.

• Update health and medication history if physician makes any changes in evaluation or drug regimens; include OTC, herbal, and nonherbal remedies in the update.

finasteride
feen-as′-ter-ide
(Propecia, Proscar)
Do not confuse Proscar with Posicor, ProSom, Prozac, or Psorcon.

CATEGORY AND SCHEDULE
Pregnancy Risk Category: X

Drug Class: Synthetic steroid

MECHANISM OF ACTION
An androgen hormone inhibitor that inhibits 5-alpha reductase, an intracellular enzyme that converts testosterone into dihydrotestosterone (DHT) in the prostate gland, resulting in a decreased serum DHT level.
Therapeutic Effect: Reduces size of the prostate gland.

USES
Proscar: Treatment of symptomatic benign prostatic hyperplasia (BPH), reduce risk for acute urinary retention and surgery
Propecia: Treatment of male pattern baldness (androgenic alopecia) in men 18–41 yr

PHARMACOKINETICS

Route	Onset	Peak	Duration
PO	24 hr	1–2 days	5–7 days

Rapidly absorbed from the GI tract. Protein binding: 90%. Widely distributed. Metabolized in the liver.

Half-life: 6–8 hr. Onset of clinical effect: 3–6 mo of continued therapy.

INDICATIONS AND DOSAGES
▶ **BPH**
PO
Adults, Elderly. 5 mg once a day (for a minimum of 6 mo).
▶ **Hair Loss**
PO
Adults. 1 mg/day.

SIDE EFFECTS/ADVERSE REACTIONS
Rare

Gynecomastia, sexual dysfunction (impotence, decreased libido, decreased volume of ejaculate)

PRECAUTIONS AND CONTRAINDICATIONS
Exposure to the patient's semen or handling of finasteride tablets by those who are or may be pregnant
Caution:
Lactation, lower PSA levels do not suggest absence of prostate cancer; women should avoid drug or semen contact, hepatic impairment

DRUG INTERACTIONS OF CONCERN TO DENTISTRY
• Opioids and anticholinergic drugs may enhance urinary retention; use alternative analgesics (NSAIDs)

SERIOUS REACTIONS
! None known

DENTAL CONSIDERATIONS
Consultations:
• Determine why patient is taking the drug (for prostatic hyperplasia or male pattern baldness).
• Medical consultation may be required to assess disease control.

flavocoxid
flay-**voh-cox′**-id
(Limbrel)

CATEGORY AND SCHEDULE
Pregnancy Risk Category: Not classified.

Drug Class: Oral nutritional supplement

MECHANISM OF ACTION
An oral nutritional supplement that inhibits prostaglandin synthesis and arachidonic acid metabolism, reducing the production of leukotrienes. Also acts through an antioxidant mechanism.
Therapeutic Effect: Produces antiinflammatory and analgesic effects and increases mobility.

USES
Dietary management of osteoarthritis

PHARMACOKINETICS
Undergoes hydrolysis at the gut mucosal border. Food decreases absorption. Little hepatic metabolism.

INDICATIONS AND DOSAGES
▶ **Osteoarthritis**
PO
Adults 18 yr and older, Elderly. One 250-mg capsule q12h.

SIDE EFFECTS/ADVERSE REACTIONS
Rare

Increase in varicose veins, psoriasis, mild hypertension

F

PRECAUTIONS AND CONTRAINDICATIONS
History of peptic ulcer

DRUG INTERACTIONS OF CONCERN TO DENTISTRY
• None reported

SERIOUS REACTIONS
! GI bleeding, perforation, and ulceration occur rarely in patients currently or previously treated with NSAIDs or COX-2 inhibitors.

DENTAL CONSIDERATIONS

General:
• Determine why patient is taking the drug.
• Patient may need assistance in getting into and out of dental chair. Adjust chair position for patient comfort.
• Patients presenting with a history of osteoarthritis will be taking other agents; confirm medical and drug/herbal and nonherbal history.
Consultations:
• Medical consultation may be required to assess disease control and patient's ability to tolerate stress.
Teach Patient/Family to:
• Use powered tooth brush if patient has difficulty holding conventional devices.
• Encourage effective oral hygiene to prevent soft tissue inflammation.
• Prevent trauma when using oral hygiene aids.
• Update health and medication history if physician makes any changes in evaluation or drug regimens; include OTC, herbal, and nonherbal remedies in the update.

---

flavoxate
fla-vox´-ate
(Urispas)
Do not confuse Urispas with Urised.

CATEGORY AND SCHEDULE
Pregnancy Risk Category: B

Drug Class: Antispasmodic

MECHANISM OF ACTION
An anticholinergic that relaxes detrusor and other smooth muscle by cholinergic blockade, counteracting muscle spasm in the urinary tract.
Therapeutic Effect: Produces anticholinergic, local anesthetic and analgesic effects, relieving urinary symptoms.

USES
Relief of nocturia, incontinence, suprapubic pain, dysuria, frequency associated with urologic conditions (symptomatic only)

PHARMACOKINETICS
Excreted in urine.

INDICATIONS AND DOSAGES
▶ To Relieve Symptoms of Cystitis, Prostatitis, Urethritis, Urethrocystitis, or Urethrotrigonitis
PO
Adults, Elderly, Adolescents.
100–200 mg 3–4 times a day.

SIDE EFFECTS/ADVERSE REACTIONS
Frequent
Somnolence, dry mouth and throat
Occasional
Constipation, difficult urination, blurred vision, dizziness, headache,

increased light sensitivity, nausea,
vomiting, abdominal pain
Rare
Confusion (primarily in elderly),
hypersensitivity, increased
intraocular pressure, leukopenia

PRECAUTIONS AND CONTRAINDICATIONS
Duodenal or pyloric obstruction, GI
hemorrhage or obstruction, ileus,
lower urinary tract obstruction
Caution:
Lactation, suspected glaucoma,
children younger than 12 yr

DRUG INTERACTIONS OF CONCERN TO DENTISTRY
• Increased anticholinergic effect:
anticholinergic drugs
• Drug may cause drowsiness or
blurred vision: advise patients
when other CNS depressants
are used

SERIOUS REACTIONS
! Overdose may produce
anticholinergic effects, including
unsteadiness, severe dizziness,
somnolence, fever, facial flushing,
dyspnea, nervousness, and
irritability.

DENTAL CONSIDERATIONS
General:
• Assess salivary flow as a factor in
caries, periodontal disease, and
candidiasis.
Teach Patient/Family to:
• Encourage effective oral hygiene
to prevent gingival inflammation.
• Avoid mouth rinses with high
alcohol content because of drying
effects.

flecainide
fle′-kah-nide
(Flecatab[AUS], Tambocor)

CATEGORY AND SCHEDULE
Pregnancy Risk Category: C

Drug Class: Antidysrhythmic
(Class IC)

MECHANISM OF ACTION
An antiarrhythmic that slows atrial,
AV, His-Purkinje, and
intraventricular conduction.
Decreases excitability, conduction
velocity, and automaticity.
Therapeutic Effect: Controls atrial,
supraventricular, and ventricular
arrhythmias.

USES
Prevention of life-threatening
ventricular dysrhythmias, sustained
supraventricular tachycardia;
prevention of paroxysmal atrial
flutter (PAF), fibrillation, or
paroxysmal atrial tachycardia

PHARMACOKINETICS
PO: Peak 3 hr. **Half-life:** 12–27 hr;
metabolized by liver; excreted
unchanged by kidneys (10%);
excreted in breast milk.

INDICATIONS AND DOSAGES
▶ Life-Threatening Ventricular
Arrhythmias, Sustained Ventricular
Tachycardia
PO
Adults, Elderly. Initially, 100 mg
q12h, increased by 100 mg (50 mg
twice a day) every 4 days until
effective dose or maximum of
400 mg/day is attained.

▸ **Paroxysmal Supraventricular Tachycardias (PSVT), PAF**

PO

Adults, Elderly. Initially, 50 mg q12h, increased by 100 mg (50 mg twice a day) every 4 days until effective dose or maximum of 300 mg/day is attained.

SIDE EFFECTS/ADVERSE REACTIONS

Frequent

Dizziness, dyspnea, headache

Occasional

Nausea, fatigue, palpitations, chest pain, asthenia (loss of strength, energy), tremors, constipation

PRECAUTIONS AND CONTRAINDICATIONS

Cardiogenic shock, preexisting second- or third-degree AV block, right bundle-branch block (without presence of a pacemaker)

Caution:

Lactation, children, renal disease, liver disease, CHF, respiratory depression, myasthenia gravis

DRUG INTERACTIONS OF CONCERN TO DENTISTRY

• No specific interactions are reported with dental drugs; however, any drug that could affect the cardiac action of flecainide (e.g., other local anesthetics, vasoconstrictors, anticholinergics) should be used in the lowest effective dose.

SERIOUS REACTIONS

! Flecainide may worsen existing arrhythmias or produce new ones.
! CHF may occur or existing CHF may worsen.
! Overdose may increase QRS duration, prolong QT interval, cause conduction disturbances, reduce myocardial contractility and cause hypotension.

DENTAL CONSIDERATIONS

General:

• Monitor vital signs at every appointment because of cardiovascular and respiratory side effects.
• Assess salivary flow as a factor in caries, periodontal disease, and candidiasis.
• Stress from dental procedures may compromise cardiovascular function; determine patient risk, use a stress-reduction protocol.
• Use vasoconstrictors with caution, in low doses and with careful aspiration. Avoid use of gingival retraction cord with epinephrine.

Consultations:

• Medical consultation may be required to assess disease control and patient's ability to tolerate stress.

Teach Patient/Family to:

• Encourage effective oral hygiene to prevent gingival inflammation.
• Avoid mouth rinses with high alcohol content because of drying effects.

---

fluconazole

floo-con'-ah-zole

(Apo-Fluconazole[CAN], Diflucan)

Do not confuse Diflucan with diclofenac.

CATEGORY AND SCHEDULE

Pregnancy Risk Category: C

Drug Class: Antifungal

MECHANISM OF ACTION

A fungistatic antifungal that interferes with cytochrome P-450, an enzyme necessary for ergosterol formation.

Therapeutic Effect: Directly damages fungal membrane, altering its function.

USES

Treatment of oropharyngeal candidiasis, chronic mucocutaneous candidiasis, vaginal candidiasis, cryptococcal meningitis, esophageal candidiasis and prophylaxis in patients receiving bone marrow transplants with chemotherapy or radiation

PHARMACOKINETICS

Well absorbed from GI tract. Widely distributed, including to CSF. Protein binding: 11%. Partially metabolized in liver. Excreted unchanged primarily in urine. Partially removed by hemodialysis. *Half-life:* 20–30 hr (increased in impaired renal function).

INDICATIONS AND DOSAGES
▸ **Oropharyngeal Candidiasis**
PO, IV

Adults, Elderly. 200 mg once, then 100 mg/day for at least 14 days.
Children. 6 mg/kg/day once, then 3 mg/kg/day.
▸ **Esophageal Candidiasis**
PO, IV

Adults, Elderly. 200 mg once, then 100 mg/day (up to 400 mg/day) for 21 days and at least 14 days following resolution of symptoms.
Children. 6 mg/kg/day once, then 3 mg/kg/day (up to 12 mg/kg/day) for 21 days at least 14 days following resolution of symptoms.
▸ **Vaginal Candidiasis**
PO

Adults. 150 mg once.

▸ **Prevention of Candidiasis in Patients Undergoing Bone Marrow Transplantation**
PO

Adults. 400 mg/day.
▸ **Systemic Candidiasis**
PO, IV

Adults, Elderly. 400 mg once, then 200 mg/day (up to 400 mg/day) for at least 28 days and at least 14 days following resolution of symptoms.
Children. 6–12 mg/kg/day.
▸ **Cryptococcal Meningitis**
PO, IV

Adults, Elderly. 400 mg once, then 200 mg/day (up to 800 mg/day) for 10–12 wk after CSF becomes negative (200 mg/day for suppression of relapse in patients with AIDS).
Children. 12 mg/kg/day once, then 6–12 mg/kg/day (6 mg/kg/day for suppression of relapse in patients with AIDS).
▸ **Onychomycosis**
PO

Adults. 150 mg/wk.
▸ **Dosage in Renal Impairment**
After a loading dose of 400 mg, the daily dosage is based on creatinine clearance.

Creatinine Clearance	% of Recommended Dose
Greater than 50 ml/min	100
21–50 ml/min	50
11–20 ml/min	25
Dialysis	Dose after dialysis

SIDE EFFECTS/ADVERSE REACTIONS
Occasional

Hypersensitivity reaction (including chills, fever, pruritus, and rash), dizziness, drowsiness, headache,

constipation, diarrhea, nausea,
vomiting, abdominal pain

PRECAUTIONS AND CONTRAINDICATIONS
Hypersensitivity
Caution:
Renal disease

DRUG INTERACTIONS OF CONCERN TO DENTISTRY
• Caution: potent inhibitor of
cytochrome P450 3A4 isoenzymes
• Increased plasma levels of oral
hypoglycemics: theophylline,
cyclosporine, tacrolimus,
corticosteroids
• Inhibits metabolism of
benzodiazepines: alprazolam,
chlordiazepoxide, clonazepam,
clorazepate, diazepam, estazolam,
flurazepam, halazepam, midazolam,
triazolam, quazepam, zolpidem
• Increased anticoagulant effect:
may inhibit metabolism of warfarin
• Suspected risk of increased
neurologic side effects: haloperidol,
tricyclic antidepressants
• May increase levels and side
effects of HMG-CoA reductase
inhibitors
• Suspected increase in
antihypertensive effects of losartan;
monitor blood pressure if used
concurrently
• Decreased renal clearance:
hydrochlorothiazide
• Suspected decrease in oral
contraceptive effectiveness; may
want to suggest additional
contraception

SERIOUS REACTIONS
! Exfoliative skin disorders, serious
hepatic effects and blood dyscrasias
(such as eosinophilia,
thrombocytopenia, anemia, and
leukopenia) have been reported
rarely.

DENTAL CONSIDERATIONS
General:
• Culture may be required to
confirm fungal organism.
• Patients on chronic drug therapy
may rarely have symptoms of blood
dyscrasias, which can include
infection, bleeding, and poor
healing.
Consultations:
• In a patient with symptoms of
blood dyscrasias, request a medical
consultation for blood studies and
postpone treatment until normal
values are reestablished.
Teach Patient/Family to:
• Be aware that long-term therapy
may be necessary to clear infection.
• Prevent reinoculation of *Candida*
infection by disposing of tooth brush
or other contaminated oral hygiene
devices used during period of
infection.

flucytosine
floo-sye´- toe-seen
(Ancobon)

CATEGORY AND SCHEDULE
Pregnancy Risk Category: C

Drug Class: Antifungal

MECHANISM OF ACTION
An antifungal that penetrates fungal
cells and is converted to fluorouracil
which competes with uracil
interfering with fungal RNA and
protein synthesis.
Therapeutic Effect: Damages fungal
membrane.

USES

Treatment of *Candida* infections (septicemia, endocarditis, pulmonary and UTIs), *Cryptococcus* (meningitis, pulmonary and urinary tract infections)

PHARMACOKINETICS

Well absorbed from GI tract. Widely distributed, including CSF. Protein binding: 2%–4%. Metabolized in liver. Partially removed by hemodialysis. *Half-life:* 3–8 hr (half-life is increased with impaired renal function).

INDICATIONS AND DOSAGES

▶ **Fungal Infections, Candidiasis, Cryptococcosis**
PO
Adults, Elderly, Children. 50–150 mg/kg/day in 4 equally divided doses.
▶ **Dosage in Renal Function Impairment**
Based on creatinine clearance:

Creatinine Clearance	Dosage Interval
20–40 ml/min	q12h
10–20 ml/min	q24h
0–10 ml/min	q24–48h

SIDE EFFECTS/ADVERSE REACTIONS

Occasional
Pruritus, rash, photosensitivity, dizziness, drowsiness, headache, diarrhea, nausea, vomiting, abdominal pain, increased liver enzymes, jaundice, increased BUN and creatinine, weakness, hearing loss

PRECAUTIONS AND CONTRAINDICATIONS

Hypersensitivity to flucytosine
Caution:
Renal disease, bone marrow depression, blood dyscrasias, radiation therapy, or chemotherapy

DRUG INTERACTIONS OF CONCERN TO DENTISTRY

• None reported

SERIOUS REACTIONS

! Hepatic dysfunction and severe bone marrow suppression occur rarely.

DENTAL CONSIDERATIONS

General:
• Patients on chronic drug therapy may rarely have symptoms of blood dyscrasias, which can include infection, bleeding, and poor healing.
• Examine for evidence of oral *Candida* infection.
Consultations:
• Medical consultation may be required to assess disease control.
• In a patient with symptoms of blood dyscrasias, request a medical consultation for blood studies and postpone dental treatment until normal values are reestablished.
Teach Patient/Family to:
• Encourage effective oral hygiene to prevent gingival inflammation.

fludarabine phosphate

flew-dare'-ah-been foss'-fate
(Fludara)
Do not confuse Fludara with
FUDR.

CATEGORY AND SCHEDULE
Pregnancy Risk Category: D

Drug Class: Antineoplastic,
antimetabolite

MECHANISM OF ACTION
An antimetabolite that inhibits DNA
synthesis by interfering with DNA
polymerase alpha, ribonucleotide
reductase and DNA primase.
Therapeutic Effect: Induces cell
death.

USES
Treatment of chronic lymphocyte
leukemia, non-Hodgkin's lymphoma

PHARMACOKINETICS
Rapidly dephosphorylated in serum,
then phosphorylated intracellularly
to active triphosphate. Primarily
excreted in urine. *Half-life:* 7–20 hr.

INDICATIONS AND DOSAGES
▸ **Chronic Lymphocytic Leukemia**
IV
Adults. 25 mg/m^2 daily for 5
consecutive days. Continue for up to
3 additional cycles. Begin each
course of treatment every 28 days.
▸ **Non-Hodgkin's Lymphoma**
IV
Adults, Elderly. Initially, 20 mg/m^2,
then 30 mg/m^2/day for 48 hr.

▸ **Dosage in Renal Impairment**

Creatinine Clearance	Dosage
30–70 ml/min	Decrease dose by 20%
Less than 30 ml/min	Not recommended

SIDE EFFECTS/ADVERSE REACTIONS
Frequent
Fever, nausea and vomiting
Occasional
Chills, fatigue, generalized pain,
rash, diarrhea, cough, asthenia,
stomatitis, dyspnea, peripheral
edema
Rare
Anorexia, sinusitis, dysuria, myalgia,
paresthesia, headaches, visual
disturbances

PRECAUTIONS AND CONTRAINDICATIONS
Concurrent use with pentostatin

DRUG INTERACTIONS OF CONCERN TO DENTISTRY
• None reported

SERIOUS REACTIONS
! Pneumonia occurs frequently.
! Severe hematologic toxicity (as
evidenced by anemia,
thrombocytopenia, and neutropenia)
and GI bleeding may occur.
! Tumor lysis syndrome may start
with flank pain and hematuria and
may include hypercalcemia,
hyperphosphatemia, hyperuricemia,
and renal failure.
! High-dosage therapy may produce
acute leukemia, blindness, and
coma.

DENTAL CONSIDERATIONS

General:

• Monitor vital signs at every appointment because of cardiovascular side effects.

• If additional analgesia is required for dental pain, consider alternative analgesics in patients taking narcotics for acute or chronic pain.

• Examine for oral manifestation of opportunistic infection.

• Avoid products that affect platelet function, such as aspirin and NSAIDs.

• This drug may be used in the hospital or on an outpatient basis. Confirm the patient's disease and treatment status.

• Chlorhexidine mouth rinse prior to and during chemotherapy may reduce severity of mucositis.

• Patient on chronic drug therapy may rarely present with symptoms of blood dyscrasias, which can include infection, bleeding, and poor healing. If dyscrasia is present, caution patient to prevent oral tissue trauma when using oral hygiene aids.

• Palliative medication may be required for management of oral side effects.

• Patients may be at risk of infection.

• Patients may be at risk of bleeding; check for oral signs.

• Oral infections should be eliminated and/or treated aggressively.

Consultations:

• Medical consultation should include routine blood counts including platelet counts and bleeding time.

• Consult physician; prophylactic or therapeutic antiinfectives may be indicated if surgery or periodontal treatment is required.

• Medical consultation may be required to assess immunologic status during cancer chemotherapy and determine safety risk, if any, posed by the required dental treatment.

• Medical consultation may be required to assess disease control and patient's ability to tolerate stress.

Teach Patient/Family to:

• Be aware of oral side effects.

• Encourage effective oral hygiene to prevent soft tissue inflammation.

• Report oral lesions, soreness, or bleeding to dentist.

• Prevent trauma when using oral hygiene aids.

• Update health and medication history if physician makes any changes in evaluation or drug regimens; include OTC, herbal, and nonherbal remedies in the update.

---

fludrocortisone

floo-droe-kor′-ti-sone
(Florinef)
Do not confuse Florinef with Fioricet or Florinal.

CATEGORY AND SCHEDULE

Pregnancy Risk Category: C

Drug Class: Glucocorticoid and mineralocorticoid

MECHANISM OF ACTION

A mineralocorticoid that acts at distal renal tubules.

Therapeutic Effect: Increases potassium and hydrogen ion excretion. Replaces sodium loss and raises blood pressure (with low dosages). Inhibits endogenous adrenal cortical secretion, thymic activity, and secretion of corticotropin by pituitary gland (with higher dosages).

USES

Treatment of adrenal insufficiency (Addison's disease), salt-losing adrenogenital syndrome

PHARMACOKINETICS

Well absorbed from the GI tract. Protein binding: 42%. Widely distributed. Metabolized in the liver and kidney. Primarily excreted in urine. *Half-life:* 3.5 hr.

INDICATIONS AND DOSAGES

▶ **Addison's Disease**
PO
Adults, Elderly. 0.05–0.1 mg/day. Range: 0.1 mg 3 times a wk to 0.2 mg/day. Administration with cortisone or hydrocortisone preferred.
▶ **Salt-Losing Adrenogenital Syndrome**
PO
Adults, Elderly. 0.1–0.2 mg/day.
Usual Pediatric Dosage
Children. 0.05–0.1 mg/day.

SIDE EFFECTS/ADVERSE REACTIONS

Frequent
Increased appetite, exaggerated sense of well-being, abdominal distention, weight gain, insomnia, mood swings
High dosages, prolonged therapy, too rapid withdrawal: Increased susceptibility to infection with masked signs and symptoms, delayed wound healing, hypokalemia, hypocalcemia, GI distress, diarrhea or constipation, hypertension
Occasional
Headache, dizziness, menstrual difficulty or amenorrhea, gastric ulcer development

Rare
Hypersensitivity reaction

PRECAUTIONS AND CONTRAINDICATIONS

CHF, systemic fungal infection
Caution:
Lactation, osteoporosis, CHF, safety and use in children has not been established

DRUG INTERACTIONS OF CONCERN TO DENTISTRY

• Decreased action: barbiturates
• Increased side effects: sodium-containing food, sodium-containing polishing devices
• Decreased effects of salicylates

SERIOUS REACTIONS

! Long-term therapy may cause muscle wasting (especially in the arms and legs), osteoporosis, spontaneous fractures, amenorrhea, cataracts, glaucoma, peptic ulcer disease, and CHF.
! Abruptly withdrawing the drug after long-term therapy may cause anorexia, nausea, fever, headache, joint pain, rebound inflammation, fatigue, weakness, lethargy, dizziness, and orthostatic hypotension.

DENTAL CONSIDERATIONS

General:
• Patients with Addison's disease are more susceptible to stress and may require supplemental systemic glucocorticoids before dental treatment.
• Patients who have been or are currently on chronic steroid therapy (longer than 2 wk) may require supplemental steroids for dental treatment.
• Monitor vital signs at every appointment because of nature of disease.

• Short appointments and a stress-reduction protocol may be required for anxious patients.
• Patients with Addison's disease must be evaluated closely for presence of oral infection.
• Do not use ingestible sodium bicarbonate products, such as the Prophy-Jet air polishing system, or IV saline fluids for patients on a salt-restricted regimen.
• Use precautions if dental surgery is anticipated and conscious sedation or general anesthesia is required.
• Monitor patient for any signs of inadequate management of disease, such as potassium depletion, muscle weakness, paresthesia, fatigue, nausea, depression, polyuria, and edema.
Consultations:
• Medical consultation is required to assess disease control and patient's ability to tolerate stress.
• Consultation may be required to confirm steroid dose and duration of use.
Teach Patient/Family to:
• Carry identification as a steroid user.
• Report to the dental office any signs that might indicate an oral infection.

flumazenil
flew-maz′-ah-nil
(Anexate[CAN], Romazicon)

CATEGORY AND SCHEDULE
Pregnancy Risk Category: C

Drug Class: Benzodiazepine receptor antagonist

MECHANISM OF ACTION
An antidote that antagonizes the effect of benzodiazepines on the gamma-aminobutyric acid receptor complex in the CNS.
Therapeutic Effect: Reverses sedative effect of benzodiazepines.

USES
Reversal of the sedative effects of benzodiazepines

PHARMACOKINETICS

Route	Onset	Peak	Duration
IV	1–2 min	6–10 min	Less than 1 hr

Duration and degree of benzodiazepine reversal depend on dosage and plasma concentration. Protein binding: 50%. Metabolized by the liver; excreted in urine.

INDICATIONS AND DOSAGES
▶ **Reversal of Conscious Sedation or General Anesthesia**
IV
Adults, Elderly. Initially, 0.2 mg (2 ml) over 15 sec; may repeat dose in 45 sec; then at 60-sec intervals. Maximum: 1 mg (10-ml) total dose.
Children, Neonates. Initially, 0.01 mg/kg; may repeat in 45 sec, then at 60-sec intervals. Maximum: 0.2 mg single dose; 0.05 mg/kg or 1 mg cumulative dose.
▶ **Benzodiazepine Overdose**
IV
Adults, Elderly. Initially, 0.2 mg (2 ml) over 30 sec; if desired LOC is not achieved after 30 sec, 0.3 mg (3 ml) may be given over 30 sec. Further doses of 0.5 mg (5 ml) may be administered over 30 sec at 60-sec intervals. Maximum: 3 mg (30 ml) total dose.

Children, Neonates. Initially, 0.01 mg/kg; may repeat in 45 sec, then at 60-sec intervals. Maximum: 0.2 mg single dose; 1 mg cumulative dose.

SIDE EFFECTS/ADVERSE REACTIONS

Frequent

Agitation, anxiety, dry mouth, dyspnea, insomnia, palpitations, tremors, headache, blurred vision, dizziness, ataxia, nausea, vomiting, pain at injection site, diaphoresis

Occasional

Fatigue, flushing, auditory disturbances, thrombophlebitis, rash

Rare

Urticaria, pruritus, hallucinations

PRECAUTIONS AND CONTRAINDICATIONS

Anticholinergic signs (such as mydriasis, dry mucosa, and hypoperistalsis), arrhythmias, cardiovascular collapse, history of hypersensitivity to benzodiazepines, patients with signs of serious cyclic antidepressant overdose (such as motor abnormalities), patients who have been given a benzodiazepine for control of a potentially life-threatening condition (such as control of status epilepticus or increased intracranial pressure)

Caution:

Lactation, elderly, renal disease, seizure disorders, head injury, labor and delivery, hepatic disease, hypoventilation, panic disorder, drug and alcohol dependency, ambulatory patients; no risk-benefits have been established for children

DRUG INTERACTIONS OF CONCERN TO DENTISTRY

• May not be effective: mixed drug overdosage

SERIOUS REACTIONS

! Toxic effects, such as seizures and arrhythmias, of other drugs taken in overdose, especially tricyclic antidepressants, may emerge with reversal of sedative effect of benzodiazepines.

! Flumazenil may provoke a panic attack in those with a history of panic disorder.

DENTAL CONSIDERATIONS

General:

• Monitor vital signs at every appointment because of cardiovascular side effects.

• Monitor for resedation; duration of antagonism is short compared with benzodiazepines.

• IM administration delays onset of effect.

Teach Patient/Family to:

• Be alert for possible resedation when discharged from office.

flunisolide

floo-niss'-oh-lide

(AeroBid, Nasalide, Nasarel, Rhinalar[CAN])

Do not confuse flunisolide with fluocinonide, or Nasalide with NasalCrom.

CATEGORY AND SCHEDULE

Pregnancy Risk Category: C

Drug Class: Synthetic glucocorticoid

MECHANISM OF ACTION

An adrenocorticosteroid that controls the rate of protein synthesis, depresses migration of polymorphonuclear leukocytes, reverses capillary permeability, and stabilizes lysosomal membranes.

Therapeutic Effect: Prevents or
controls inflammation.

USES
Oral inhalation for prophylaxis or
maintenance treatment of chronic
asthma; nasal solution for seasonal
or perennial rhinitis

PHARMACOKINETICS
Aerosol: Effective response time
1–4 wk; metabolized in liver;
excreted in urine and feces.

INDICATIONS AND DOSAGES
▸ **Long-Term Control of Bronchial
Asthma, Assists in Reducing or
Discontinuing Oral Corticosteroid
Therapy**
Inhalation
Adults, Elderly. 2 inhalations twice a
day, morning and evening.
Maximum: 4 inhalations twice a day.
Children 6–15 yr. 2 inhalations
twice a day.
▸ **Relief of Symptoms of Perennial
and Seasonal Rhinitis**
Intranasal
Adults, Elderly. Initially, 2 sprays
each nostril twice a day, may
increase at 4–7 day intervals to 2
sprays 3 times a day. Maximum: 8
sprays in each nostril daily.
Children 6–14 yr. Initially, 1 spray 3
times a day or 2 sprays twice a day.
Maximum: 4 sprays in each nostril
daily. Maintenance: 1 spray into
each nostril each day.

SIDE EFFECTS/ADVERSE
REACTIONS
Frequent
Inhalation: Unpleasant taste, nausea,
vomiting, sore throat, diarrhea, upset
stomach, cold symptoms, nasal
congestion
Occasional
Inhalation: Dizziness, irritability,
nervousness, tremors, abdominal

pain, heartburn, oropharynx
candidiasis, edema
Nasal: Mild nasopharyngeal
irritation or dryness, rebound
congestion, bronchial asthma,
rhinorrhea, altered taste

PRECAUTIONS AND
CONTRAINDICATIONS
Hypersensitivity to any
corticosteroid, persistently positive
sputum cultures for *C. albicans,*
primary treatment of status
asthmaticus, systemic fungal
infections
Caution:
Lactation; warning: switching
patients from systemic steroids to
inhalation must be done carefully to
avoid severe adrenal insufficiency

SERIOUS REACTIONS
❗ An acute hypersensitivity reaction,
marked by urticaria, angioedema
and severe bronchospasm, occurs
rarely.
❗ A transfer from systemic to local
steroid therapy may unmask
previously suppressed bronchial
asthma condition.

DENTAL CONSIDERATIONS
General:
• Examine oral cavity for evidence
of drug side effects.
• Assess salivary flow as a factor in
caries, periodontal disease, and
candidiasis.
• Evaluate respiration characteristics
and rate.
• Consider semisupine chair position
for patients with respiratory disease.
• Determine dose and duration of
steroid therapy for each patient to
assess risk for stress tolerance and
immunosuppression.
• Acute asthmatic episodes may be
precipitated in the dental office.

Sympathomimetic inhalants should be available for emergency use. A stress reduction protocol may be required.

• Consider the drug in the diagnosis of taste alterations.

Consultations:

• Medical consultation may be required to assess disease control.

Teach Patient/Family to:

• Encourage effective oral hygiene to prevent soft tissue inflammation.

• Use caution to prevent injury when using oral hygiene aids.

• Gargle, rinse mouth with water and expectorate after each aerosol dose.

• When chronic dry mouth occurs, advise patient to:

  • Use daily home fluoride products for anticaries effect.

  • Avoid mouth rinses with high alcohol content because of drying effects.

  • Use sugarless gum, frequent sips of water, or saliva substitutes.

fluocinolone acetonide

floo-oh-sin′-oh-lone
ah-seat′-oh-nide
(Capex, Derma-Smooth/FS, Fluoderm[CAN], Synalar)

CATEGORY AND SCHEDULE

Pregnancy Risk Category: C

Drug Class: Antiinflammatory, steroidal, topical; corticosteroid, topical

MECHANISM OF ACTION

A fluorinated topical corticosteroid that controls the rate of protein synthesis; depresses migration of polymorphonuclear leukocytes and fibroblasts; reduces capillary permeability; prevents or controls inflammation.

Therapeutic Effect: Decreases tissue response to inflammatory process.

USES

Relief of redness, swelling, itching, and discomfort of inflammatory skin problems

PHARMACOKINETICS

Use of occlusive dressings may increase percutaneous absorption. Protein binding: more than 90%. Excreted in urine. ***Half-life:*** Unknown.

INDICATIONS AND DOSAGES

▸ **Atopic Dermatitis**

Topical

Adults, Elderly. Apply 3 times a day. *Children 2 yr and older.* Apply 2 times a day.

▸ **Scalp Psoriasis**

Topical

Adults, Elderly. Apply to damp or wet hair and leave on overnight or for at least 4 hr. Remove by washing hair with shampoo.

▸ **Seborrheic Dermatitis, Scalp**

Shampoo

Adults, Elderly. Apply once daily; allow to remain on scalp for at least 5 min.

SIDE EFFECTS/ADVERSE REACTIONS

Occasional

Burning, dryness, itching, stinging

Rare

Allergic contact dermatitis, purpura or blood-containing blisters, thinning of skin with easy bruising, telangiectasis or raised dark red spots on skin

PRECAUTIONS AND CONTRAINDICATIONS

Hypersensitivity to fluocinolone or other corticosteroids

DRUG INTERACTIONS OF CONCERN TO DENTISTRY

• None reported

SERIOUS REACTIONS

❗ When taken in excessive quantities, systemic hypercorticism and adrenal suppression may occur.

DENTAL CONSIDERATIONS

General:
• Determine why patient is taking the drug.
Teach Patient/Family to:
• Avoid use on oral herpetic ulcerations.

---

fluocinonide
floo-oh-sin′-oh-nide
(Lidex, Lidex-E)

CATEGORY AND SCHEDULE

Pregnancy Risk Category: C

Drug Class: Topical corticosteroid, synthetic fluorinated agent, group II potency

MECHANISM OF ACTION

A topical corticosteroid that has antiinflammatory, antipruritic, and vasoconstrictive properties. The exact mechanism of the antiinflammatory process is unclear. *Therapeutic Effect:* Reduces or prevents tissue response to the inflammatory process.

USES

Treatment of psoriasis, eczema, contact dermatitis, pruritus, oral lichen planus lesions

PHARMACOKINETICS

Well absorbed systemically. Large variation in absorption among sites. Protein binding: varies. Metabolized in liver. Primarily excreted in urine.

INDICATIONS AND DOSAGES

▸ **Dermatoses**
Topical
Adults, Elderly. Apply sparingly 2–4 times a day.

SIDE EFFECTS/ADVERSE REACTIONS

Occasional
Itching, redness, irritation, burning at site of application, dryness, folliculitis, acneiform eruptions, hypopigmentation
Rare
Allergic contact dermatitis, maceration of the skin, secondary infection, skin atrophy

PRECAUTIONS AND CONTRAINDICATIONS

History of hypersensitivity to fluocinonide or other corticosteroids
Caution:
Lactation, viral infections, bacterial infections

DRUG INTERACTIONS OF CONCERN TO DENTISTRY

• None reported

SERIOUS REACTIONS

❗ The serious reactions of long-term therapy and the addition of occlusive dressings are reversible hypothalamic-pituitary-adrenal (HPA) axis suppression,

F

manifestations of Cushing's syndrome, hyperglycemia, and glucosuria.

DENTAL CONSIDERATIONS

General:
• Place on frequent recall to evaluate healing response.
Teach Patient/Family to:
• Return for oral evaluation if response of oral tissues has not occurred in 7–14 days.
• Avoid use on oral herpetic ulcerations.
• Encourage effective oral hygiene to prevent soft tissue inflammation.
• Apply at bedtime or after meals for maximum effect.
• Apply with cotton-tipped applicator by pressing, not rubbing, paste on lesion.

---

fluorometholone
flure-oh-meth′-oh-lone
(Eflone, Flarex, Fluor-Op, FML Forte Liquifilm, FML Liquifilm, FML S.O.P.)

CATEGORY AND SCHEDULE
Pregnancy Risk Category: C

Drug Class: Antiinflammatory, steroidal, ophthalmic; corticosteroid, ophthalmic

MECHANISM OF ACTION
An ophthalmic corticosteroid that decreases inflammation by suppression of migration of polymorphonuclear leukocytes and reversal of increased capillary permeability.
Therapeutic Effect: Decreased ocular inflammation.

USES
Prevention of permanent damage to the eye, which may occur with certain eye problems. They also provide relief from redness, irritation, and other discomfort.

PHARMACOKINETICS
Absorbed into aqueous humor with slight systemic absorption.

INDICATIONS AND DOSAGES
▸ **Treatment of Steroid-Responsive Inflammatory Conditions of the Eye**
Ophthalmic Ointment
Adults, Elderly. Apply thin strip to conjunctival sac every 4 hr in severe cases or 1–3 times a day in mild to moderate cases.
Ophthalmic Solution
Adults, Elderly, Children 2 yr and older. Instill 1–2 drops into conjunctival sac every hour during the day, every 2 hr at night until favorable response is obtained. Then use 1 drop every 4 hr. For mild to moderate inflammation, instill 1–2 drops into conjunctival sac 2–4 times a day.

SIDE EFFECTS/ADVERSE REACTIONS
Occasional
Burning, tearing, itching, blurred vision
Rare
Cataract formation, corneal ulcers, glaucoma with optic nerve damage

PRECAUTIONS AND CONTRAINDICATIONS
Viral diseases of the cornea and conjunctiva, mycobacterial or fungal infections of the eye, untreated eye infections that may be masked or enhanced by steroids, hypersensitivity to fluorometholone or any component of the formulation

DRUG INTERACTIONS OF CONCERN TO DENTISTRY
• None reported

SERIOUS REACTIONS
! Hypercorticoidism and taste perversion occurs rarely.
! Superinfections, particularly with fungi, may result from bacterial imbalance via any route of administration.

DENTAL CONSIDERATIONS

General:
• Determine why patient is taking the drug.
• Avoid dental light in patient's eyes; offer dark glasses for patient comfort.
• Protect patient's eyes from accidental spatter during dental treatment.

fluorouracil, 5FU
flure-oh-yoor'-ah-sill
(Adrucil, Carac, Efudex, Efudex[AUS], Fluoroplex)
Do not confuse Efudex with Efidac.

CATEGORY AND SCHEDULE
Pregnancy Risk Category: D

Drug Class: Topical antineoplastic

MECHANISM OF ACTION
An antimetabolite that blocks formation of thymidylic acid. Cell cycle–specific for S phase of cell division.
Therapeutic Effect: Inhibits DNA and RNA synthesis. Topical form destroys rapidly proliferating cells.

USES
Treatment of keratosis (multiple/actinic), basal cell carcinoma; unapproved: condyloma acuminatum

PHARMACOKINETICS
Widely distributed. Crosses the blood-brain barrier. Rapidly metabolized in tissues to active metabolite, which is localized intracellularly. Primarily excreted by lungs as carbon dioxide. Removed by hemodialysis. *Half-life:* 20 hr.

INDICATIONS AND DOSAGES
▸ **Carcinoma of Breast, Colon, Pancreas, Rectum, and Stomach; in Combination with Levamisole after Surgical Resection in Patients with Duke's Stage C Colon Cancer**
IV
Adults, Elderly, Children. Initially, 12 mg/kg/day for 4–5 days. Maximum: 800 mg/day. Maintenance: 6 mg/kg every other day for 4 doses repeated in 4 wk; or 15 mg/kg as a single bolus dose; or 5–15 mg/kg/wk as a single dose, not to exceed 1 g.
▸ **Multiple Actinic or Solar Keratoses**
Topical (Carac)
Adults, Elderly. Apply once a day.
Topical (Efudex, Fluoroplex)
Adults, Elderly. Apply twice a day.
▸ **Basal Cell Carcinoma**
Topical (Efudex)
Adults, Elderly. Apply twice a day.

SIDE EFFECTS/ADVERSE REACTIONS
Occasional
Parenteral: Anorexia, diarrhea, minimal alopecia, fever, dry skin, skin fissures, scaling, erythema
Topical: Pain, pruritus, hyperpigmentation, irritation, inflammation, and burning at application site; photosensitivity

F

Rare
Nausea, vomiting, anemia, esophagitis, proctitis, GI ulcer, confusion, headache, lacrimation, visual disturbances, angina, allergic reactions

PRECAUTIONS AND CONTRAINDICATIONS
Major surgery within previous month, myelosuppression, poor nutritional status, potentially serious infections
Caution:
Occlusive dressings, lactation, children, excessive exposure to sunlight

DRUG INTERACTIONS OF CONCERN TO DENTISTRY
• None reported, but limit drugs that may also produce photosensitivity reaction.

SERIOUS REACTIONS
! The earliest sign of toxicity, which may occur 4–8 days after beginning therapy, is stomatitis (as evidenced by dry mouth, burning sensation, mucosal erythema, and ulceration at inner margin of lips).
! Hematologic toxicity may be manifested as leukopenia (generally within 9–14 days after drug administration but possibly as late as the 25th day), thrombocytopenia (within 7–17 days after administration), pancytopenia, or agranulocytosis.
! The most common dermatologic toxicity is a pruritic rash on the extremities or, less frequently, the trunk.

DENTAL CONSIDERATIONS

General:
• Be aware of patient's disease and avoid treated areas to prevent further irritation.

fluoxetine hydrochloride
floo-ox′-eh-teen hi-droh-klor′-ide
(Auscap[AUS], Fluohexal[AUS], Lovan[AUS], Novo-Fluoxetine [CAN], Prozac, Prozac Weekly, Sarafem, Zactin[AUS])
Do not confuse fluoxetine with fluvastatin, Prozac with Prilosec, Proscar, or ProSom; or Sarafem with Serophene.

CATEGORY AND SCHEDULE
Pregnancy Risk Category: C

Drug Class: Antidepressant

MECHANISM OF ACTION
A psychotherapeutic agent that selectively inhibits serotonin uptake in the CNS, enhancing serotonergic function. Selective serotonin reuptake inhibitor (SSRI).
Therapeutic Effect: Relieves depression; reduces obsessive-compulsive and bulimic behavior.

USES
Treatment of major depressive disorder, bulimia, obsessive-compulsive disorder, premenstrual tension, geriatric depression in patients older than 65 yr, panic disorder with or without agoraphobia; premenstrual dysphoric disorder (Sarafem)

PHARMACOKINETICS
Well absorbed from the GI tract. Crosses the blood-brain barrier. Protein binding: 94%. Metabolized in the liver to active metabolite. Primarily excreted in urine. Not removed by hemodialysis. ***Half-life:*** 2–3 days; metabolite 7–9 days.

INDICATIONS AND DOSAGES
▸ **Depression, Obsessive-Compulsive Disorder**
PO
Adults. Initially, 20 mg each morning. If therapeutic improvement does not occur after 2 wk, gradually increase to maximum of 80 mg/day in 2 equally divided doses in morning and at noon. Prozac Weekly: 90 mg/wk, begin 7 days after last dose of 20 mg.
Elderly. Initially, 10 mg/day. May increase by 10–20 mg q2wk.
Children 7–17 yr. Initially, 5–10 mg/day. Titrate upward as needed. Usual dosage is 20 mg/day.
▸ **Panic Disorder**
PO
Adults, Elderly. Initially, 10 mg/day. May increase to 20 mg/day after 1 wk. Maximum: 60 mg/day.
▸ **Bulimia Nervosa**
PO
Adults. 60 mg each morning.
▸ **Premenstrual Dysphoric Disorder**
PO
Adults. 20 mg/day.

SIDE EFFECTS/ADVERSE REACTIONS
Frequent
Headache, asthenia, insomnia, anxiety, nervousness, somnolence, nausea, diarrhea, decreased appetite
Occasional
Dizziness, tremors, fatigue, vomiting, constipation, dry mouth, abdominal pain, nasal congestion, diaphoresis, rash
Rare
Flushed skin, light-headedness, impaired concentration

PRECAUTIONS AND CONTRAINDICATIONS
Use within 14 days of MAOIs

Caution:
Lactation, children, elderly; treatment-emergent adverse effects, hepatic impairment, interference with cognitive or motor performance

DRUG INTERACTIONS OF CONCERN TO DENTISTRY
• Increased CNS depression: alcohol, all CNS depressants, tricyclic antidepressants, benzodiazepines, St. John's wort (herb)
• Increased side effects: highly protein-bound drugs (aspirin)
• Caution: can inhibit cytochrome P4502D6 isoenzymes
• Increased serum levels of carbamazepine
• Possible "serotonin syndrome" with macrolide antibiotics
• NSAIDs: increased risk of GI side effects

SERIOUS REACTIONS
! Overdose may produce seizures, nausea, vomiting, agitation, and restlessness.

DENTAL CONSIDERATIONS
General:
• Monitor vital signs at every appointment because of cardiovascular side effects.
• Assess salivary flow as a factor in caries, periodontal disease, and candidiasis.
Consultations:
• Medical consultation may be required to assess disease control and patient's ability to tolerate stress.
• Physician should be informed if significant xerostomic side effects occur (e.g., increased caries, sore tongue, problems eating or swallowing, difficulty wearing

prosthesis) so that a medication change can be considered.
Teach Patient/Family to:
• Use powered tooth brush if patient has difficulty holding conventional devices.
• When chronic dry mouth occurs, advise patient to:
  • Avoid mouth rinses with high alcohol content because of drying effects.
  • Use daily home fluoride products for anticaries effect.
  • Use sugarless gum, frequent sips of water, or saliva substitutes.

fluoxymesterone

floo-ox-ih-mes′-teh-rone
(Android-F, Halotestin, Halotestin[CAN])

CATEGORY AND SCHEDULE
Pregnancy Risk Category: X
Controlled substance: Schedule III

Drug Class: Androgenic anabolic steroid

MECHANISM OF ACTION
An androgen that suppresses gonadotropin-releasing hormone, luteinizing hormone (LH) and follicle-stimulating hormone (FSH).
Therapeutic Effect: Stimulates spermatogenesis, development of male secondary sex characteristics, and sexual maturation at puberty. Stimulates production of red blood cells (RBCs).

USES
Treatment of impotence from testicular deficiency, hypogonadism, palliative treatment of female breast cancer

PHARMACOKINETICS
Rapidly absorbed from the GI tract. Protein binding: 98%. Metabolized in liver. Excreted in urine. **Half-life:** 9.2 hr.

INDICATIONS AND DOSAGES
▸ **Males (Hypogonadism)**
PO
Adults. 5–20 mg/day.
▸ **Males (Delayed Puberty)**
PO
Adults. 2.5–20 mg/day for 4–6 mo.
▸ **Females (Inoperable Breast Cancer)**
PO
Adults. 10–40 mg/day in divided doses for 1–3 mo.
▸ **Females (Prevent Postpartum Breast Pain/Engorgement)**
PO
Adults. Initially, 2.5 mg shortly after delivery, then 5–10 mg/day in divided doses for 4–5 days.

SIDE EFFECTS/ADVERSE REACTIONS
Frequent
Females: Amenorrhea, virilism (e.g., acne, decreased breast size, enlarged clitoris, male pattern baldness), deepening voice
Males: UTI, breast soreness, gynecomastia, priapism, virilism (e.g., acne, early pubic hair growth)
Occasional
Females: Edema, nausea, vomiting, mild acne, diarrhea, stomach pain
Males: Impotence, testicular atrophy

PRECAUTIONS AND CONTRAINDICATIONS
Serious cardiac, renal, or hepatic dysfunction, men with carcinomas of the breast or prostate, hypersensitivity to fluoxymesterone or any component of the formulation including tartrazine

Caution:
Diabetes mellitus, CV disease, MI

DRUG INTERACTIONS OF CONCERN TO DENTISTRY

• Edema: corticosteroids

SERIOUS REACTIONS

! Peliosis hepatitis (liver, spleen replaced with blood-filled cysts), hepatic neoplasms, and hepatocellular carcinoma have been associated with prolonged high dosage.

DENTAL CONSIDERATIONS

General:
• Monitor vital signs at every appointment because of cardiovascular side effects.
• Patients receiving chemotherapy may require palliative treatment for stomatitis.
Teach Patient/Family to:
• Encourage effective oral hygiene to prevent soft tissue inflammation.
• Prevent trauma when using oral hygiene aids.

fluphenazine decanoate

floo-fen′-ah-zeen
(Apo-Fluphenazine[CAN], Modecate[AUS], Prolixin); fluphenazine enanthate (Moditen[CAN], Prolixin); fluphenazine hydrochloride (Prolixin, Permitil)

CATEGORY AND SCHEDULE

Pregnancy Risk Category: C

Drug Class: Phenothiazine antipsychotic

MECHANISM OF ACTION

A phenothiazine that blocks dopamine at postsynaptic receptor sites. Possesses weak anticholinergic, sedative and antemetic effects, and strong extrapyramidal activity.
Therapeutic Effect: Decreases psychotic behavior.

USES

Treatment of psychotic disorders, schizophrenia

PHARMACOKINETICS

Erratic and variable absorption from the GI tract. Widely distributed. Metabolized in liver. Primarily excreted in urine. *Half-life:* 16.3–23.2 hr.

INDICATIONS AND DOSAGES
▸ **Psychotic Disorders**
PO
Adults. Initially, 0.5–10 mg/day fluphenazine HCl in divided doses q6–8h. Increase gradually until therapeutic response is achieved (usually under 20 mg daily); decrease gradually to maintenance level (1–5 mg/day).
Elderly. Initially, 1–2.5 mg/day.
IM
Adults. Initially, 1.25 mg, followed by 2.5–10 mg/day in divided doses q6–8h.
▸ **Chronic Schizophrenic Disorder**
IM
Adults. Initially, 12.5–25 mg of fluphenazine decanoate q1–6wk, or 25 mg fluphenazine enanthate q2wk.
▸ **Usual Elderly Dosage (Nonpsychotic)**
PO
Initially, 1–2.5 mg/day. May increase by 1–2.5 mg/day q4–7 days. Maximum: 20 mg/day.

F

SIDE EFFECTS/ADVERSE REACTIONS

Frequent
Hypotension, dizziness, and fainting occur frequently after first injection, occasionally after subsequent injections, and rarely with oral dosage
Occasional
Drowsiness during early therapy, dry mouth, blurred vision, lethargy, constipation or diarrhea, nasal congestion, peripheral edema, urinary retention
Rare
Ocular changes, skin pigmentation (those on high doses for prolonged periods)

PRECAUTIONS AND CONTRAINDICATIONS

Severe CNS depression, comatose states, severe cardiovascular disease, bone marrow depression, subcortical brain damage, hypersensitivity to fluphenazine or any component of the formulation including tartrazine
Caution:
Lactation, seizure disorders, hypertension, hepatic disease, cardiac disease

DRUG INTERACTIONS OF CONCERN TO DENTISTRY

• Increased sedation: other CNS depressants, alcohol, barbiturate anesthetics, opioid analgesics
• Hypotension, tachycardia: epinephrine
• Increased extrapyramidal effects: phenothiazines and related drugs (haloperidol, droperidol), metoclopramide
• Additive photosensitization: tetracyclines
• Increased anticholinergic effects: anticholinergics

SERIOUS REACTIONS

‼ Extrapyramidal symptoms appear dose related (particularly high dosage), divided into 3 categories: akathisia (inability to sit still, tapping of feet, urge to move around); parkinsonian symptoms (mask-like face, tremors, shuffling gait, hypersalivation); and acute dystonias: torticollis (neck muscle spasm), opisthotonos (rigidity of back muscles), and oculogyric crisis (rolling back of eyes).
‼ Dystonic reaction may also produce profuse sweating and pallor.
‼ Tardive dyskinesia (protrusion of tongue, puffing of cheeks, chewing/puckering of the mouth) occurs rarely (may be irreversible).
‼ Abrupt withdrawal after long-term therapy may precipitate nausea, vomiting, gastritis, dizziness, and tremors.
‼ Blood dyscrasias, particularly agranulocytosis, or mild leukopenia (sore mouth/gums/throat) may occur.
‼ May lower seizure threshold.

DENTAL CONSIDERATIONS

General:
• Monitor vital signs at every appointment because of cardiovascular side effects.
• Patients on chronic drug therapy may rarely have symptoms of blood dyscrasias, which can include infection, bleeding, and poor healing.
• After supine positioning, have patient sit upright for at least 2 min before standing to avoid orthostatic hypotension.
• Assess salivary flow as a factor in caries, periodontal disease, and candidiasis.
• Avoid dental light in patient's eyes; offer dark glasses for patient comfort.

• Assess for presence of extrapyramidal motor symptoms, such as tardive dyskinesia and akathisia. Extrapyramidal motor activity may complicate dental treatment.
• Geriatric patients are more susceptible to drug effects; use a lower dose.
• Use vasoconstrictors with caution, in low doses and with careful aspiration.
Consultations:
• In a patient with symptoms of blood dyscrasias, request a medical consultation for blood studies and postpone dental treatment until normal values are reestablished.
• Take precautions if dental surgery is anticipated and anesthesia is required.
• If signs of tardive dyskinesia or akathisia are present, refer to physician.
• Physician should be informed if significant xerostomic side effects occur (e.g., increased caries, sore tongue, problems eating or swallowing, difficulty wearing prosthesis) so that a medication change can be considered.
Teach Patient/Family to:
• Encourage effective oral hygiene to prevent soft tissue inflammation.
• Prevent injury when using oral hygiene aids.
• Use powered tooth brush if patient has difficulty holding conventional devices.
• When chronic dry mouth occurs, advise patient to:
  • Avoid mouth rinses with high alcohol content because of drying effects.
  • Use daily home fluoride products for anticaries effect.
  • Use sugarless gum, frequent sips of water, or saliva substitutes.

flurandrenolide
flure-an-dren'-oh-lide
(Cordran, Cordran SP)

CATEGORY AND SCHEDULE
Pregnancy Risk Category: C

Drug Class: Topical corticosteroid, group III medium potency

MECHANISM OF ACTION
A fluorinated corticosteroid that decreases inflammation by suppressing the migration of polymorphonuclear leukocytes and reversal of increased capillary permeability.
Therapeutic Effect: Decreases tissue response to inflammatory process.

USES
Treatment of corticosteroid-responsive dermatoses, pruritus

PHARMACOKINETICS
Repeated applications may lead to percutaneous absorption. Absorption is about 36% from scrotal area, 7% from the forehead, 4% from scalp, and 1% from forearm. Metabolized in liver. Excreted in urine. *Half-life:* Unknown.

INDICATIONS AND DOSAGES
▸ **Antiinflammatory, Immunosuppressant, Corticosteroid Replacement Therapy**
Topical
Adults, Elderly. Apply 2–3 times a day.
Children. Apply 1–2 times a day.

SIDE EFFECTS/ADVERSE REACTIONS

Occasional
Itching, dry skin, folliculitis
Rare
Intracranial hemorrhage, acne, striae, miliaria, allergic contact dermatitis, telangiectasis or raised dark red spots on skin

PRECAUTIONS AND CONTRAINDICATIONS

Hypersensitivity to flurandrenolide or any component of the formulation, viral, fungal, or tubercular skin lesions
Caution:
Lactation, viral infections, bacterial infections

DRUG INTERACTIONS OF CONCERN TO DENTISTRY

• None reported

SERIOUS REACTIONS

! When taken in excessive quantities, systemic hypercorticism and adrenal suppression may occur.

DENTAL CONSIDERATIONS

General:
• Determine why the patient is taking the drug.
• Apply lubricant to dry lips for patient comfort before dental procedures.
• Place on frequent recall to evaluate healing response when used on chronic basis.

flurazepam hydrochloride

flure-az′-eh-pam hi-droh-klor′-ide
(Apo-Flurazepam[Can], Dalmane)
Do not confuse Dalmane with Dialume.

CATEGORY AND SCHEDULE

Pregnancy Risk Category: X
Controlled Substance: Schedule IV

Drug Class: Benzodiazepine, sedative-hypnotic

MECHANISM OF ACTION

A benzodiazepine that enhances action of inhibitory neurotransmitter gamma-aminobutyric acid (GABA).
Therapeutic Effect: Produces hypnotic effect because of CNS depression.

USES

Treatment of insomnia

PHARMACOKINETICS

Route	Onset	Peak	Duration
PO	15–20 min	3–6 hr	7–8 hr

Well absorbed from the GI tract. Protein binding: 97%. Crosses the blood-brain barrier. Widely distributed. Metabolized in liver to active metabolite. Primarily excreted in urine. Not removed by hemodialysis. *Half-life:* 2.3 hr; metabolite: 40–114 hr.

INDICATIONS AND DOSAGES

▸ **Insomnia**
PO
Adults. 15–30 mg at bedtime.
Elderly, debilitated, liver disease, low serum albumin, Children 15 yr and older. 15 mg at bedtime.

SIDE EFFECTS/ADVERSE REACTIONS
Frequent
Drowsiness, dizziness, ataxia, sedation
Morning drowsiness may occur initially
Occasional
GI disturbances, nervousness, blurred vision, dry mouth, headache, confusion, skin rash, irritability, slurred speech
Rare
Paradoxical CNS excitement or restlessness, particularly noted in elderly or debilitated

PRECAUTIONS AND CONTRAINDICATIONS
Acute alcohol intoxication, acute angle-closure glaucoma, pregnancy or breast-feeding
Caution:
Anemia, hepatic disease, renal disease, suicidal individuals, drug abuse, elderly, psychosis, children younger than 15 yr

DRUG INTERACTIONS OF CONCERN TO DENTISTRY
• Increased sedation: alcohol, CNS depressants
• Increased serum levels and prolonged effect of benzodiazepines: ketoconazole, itraconazole, fluconazole, miconazole (systemic), indinavir, macrolide antibiotics
• Contraindicated with saquinavir
• Possible increase in CNS side effects: kava kava (herb)

SERIOUS REACTIONS
! Abrupt or too-rapid withdrawal after long-term use may result in pronounced restlessness and irritability, insomnia, hand tremors, abdominal or muscle cramps, vomiting, diaphoresis, and seizures.

! Overdose results in somnolence, confusion, diminished reflexes, and coma.

DENTAL CONSIDERATIONS
General:
• Assess salivary flow as a factor in caries, periodontal disease, and candidiasis.
• Psychologic and physical dependence may occur with chronic administration.
• Geriatric patients are more susceptible to drug effects; use lower dose.
Consultations:
• Medical consultation may be required to assess disease control.
Teach Patient/Family to:
• Avoid mouth rinses with high alcohol content because of drying effects.

flurbiprofen
flure-bi′-proe-fen
(Ansaid, Froben[CAN], Ocufen, Strepfen[AUS])
Do not confuse Ocufen with Ocuflox.

CATEGORY AND SCHEDULE
Pregnancy Risk Category: B (D if used in third trimester or near delivery; C for ophthalmic solution)

Drug Class: Nonsteroidal antiinflammatory

MECHANISM OF ACTION
A phenylalkanoic acid that produces analgesic and antiinflammatory effect by inhibiting prostaglandin synthesis. Also relaxes the iris sphincter.

Therapeutic Effect: Reduces the inflammatory response and intensity of pain. Prevents or decreases miosis during cataract surgery.

USES

Acute, long-term treatment of rheumatoid arthritis, osteoarthritis

PHARMACOKINETICS

Well absorbed from the GI tract; ophthalmic solution penetrates cornea after administration, and may be systemically absorbed. Protein binding: 99%. Widely distributed. Metabolized in the liver. Primarily excreted in urine. *Half-life:* 3–4 hr.

INDICATIONS AND DOSAGES
▸ **Rheumatoid Arthritis, Osteoarthritis**
PO
Adults, Elderly. 200–300 mg/day in 2–4 divided doses. Maximum: 100 mg/dose or 300 mg/day.
▸ **Dysmenorrhea, Pain**
PO
Adults. 50 mg 4 times a day
▸ **Usual Ophthalmic Dosage**
Adults, Elderly, Children. Apply 1 drop q30min starting 2 hr before surgery for total of 4 doses.

SIDE EFFECTS/ADVERSE REACTIONS
Occasional
PO: Headache, abdominal pain, diarrhea, indigestion, nausea, fluid retention
Ophthalmic: Burning or stinging on instillation, keratitis, elevated intraocular pressure
Rare
PO: Blurred vision, flushed skin, dizziness, somnolence, nervousness, insomnia, unusual fatigue, constipation, decreased appetite, vomiting, confusion

PRECAUTIONS AND CONTRAINDICATIONS

Active peptic ulcer, chronic inflammation of GI tract, GI bleeding or ulceration, history of hypersensitivity to aspirin or NSAIDs
Caution:
Lactation, children, bleeding disorders, GI disorders, cardiac disorders, severe renal disease, severe hepatic disease

DRUG INTERACTIONS OF CONCERN TO DENTISTRY
• GI ulceration, bleeding: aspirin, alcohol, corticosteroids
• Decreased action: salicylates
• Nephrotoxicity: acetaminophen (prolonged use)
• When prescribed for dental pain:
  • Risk of increased effects: oral anticoagulants, oral antidiabetics, lithium, methotrexate
  • Decreased effects of diuretics
  • SSRIs: increased risk of GI side effects

SERIOUS REACTIONS
❗ Overdose may result in acute renal failure.
❗ Rare reactions with long-term use include peptic ulcer disease, GI bleeding, gastritis, severe hepatic reaction (jaundice), nephrotoxicity (hematuria, dysuria, proteinuria), a severe hypersensitivity reaction (angioedema, bronchospasm), and cardiac arrhythmias.

DENTAL CONSIDERATIONS

General:
• Patients on chronic drug therapy may rarely have symptoms of blood dyscrasias, which can include infection, bleeding, and poor healing.

• Assess salivary flow as a factor in caries, periodontal disease, and candidiasis.
• Avoid prescribing for dental use in last trimester of pregnancy.
• Avoid prescribing aspirin-containing products.
• Consider semisupine chair position for patients with arthritic disease.
• Severe stomach bleeding may occur in patients who regularly use NSAIDs in recommended doses, when the patient is also taking another NSAID, anticoagulant/antiplatelet, or steroid drug, if the patient has GI or peptic ulcer disease, if they are 60 years or older, or when NSAIDs are taken longer than directed. Warn patients of the potential for severe stomach bleeding.

Consultations:
• Medical consultation may be required to assess disease control.
• In a patient with symptoms of blood dyscrasias, request a medical consultation for blood studies and postpone dental treatment until normal values are reestablished.

Teach Patient/Family to:
• Encourage effective oral hygiene to prevent soft tissue inflammation.
• Prevent injury when using oral hygiene aids.
• Warn patient of potential risks of NSAIDs.
• When chronic dry mouth occurs, advise patient to:
  • Avoid mouth rinses with high alcohol content because of drying effects.
  • Use daily home fluoride products for anticaries effect.
  • Use sugarless gum, frequent sips of water, or saliva substitutes.

flutamide
flew'-tah-myd
(Euflex[CAN], Eulexin, Flugerel[AUS], Flutamin[AUS], Fugerel[AUS], Novo-Flutamide[CAN])
Do not confuse flutamide with Flumadine.

CATEGORY AND SCHEDULE
Pregnancy Risk Category: D

Drug Class: Antineoplastic

MECHANISM OF ACTION
An antiandrogen hormone that inhibits androgen uptake and prevents androgen from binding to androgen receptors in target tissue. Used in conjunction with leuprolide to inhibit the stimulant effects of flutamide on serum testosterone levels.
Therapeutic Effect: Suppresses testicular androgen production and decreases growth of prostate carcinoma.

USES
Treatment of metastatic prostatic carcinoma, stage D2; early-stage prostate cancer, stages B2 and C, in combination with LHRH agonist analogs (leuprolide) and radiation

PHARMACOKINETICS
Completely absorbed from the GI tract. Protein binding: 94%–96%. Metabolized in the liver to active metabolite. Primarily excreted in urine. Not removed by hemodialysis.
Half-life: 6 hr (increased in elderly).

INDICATIONS AND DOSAGES
▸ **Prostatic Carcinoma (in Combination with Leuprolide)**
PO
Adults, Elderly. 250 mg q8h.

F

SIDE EFFECTS/ADVERSE REACTIONS
Frequent
Hot flashes; decreased libido, diarrhea; generalized pain; asthenia; constipation; nausea, nocturia
Occasional
Dizziness, paresthesia, insomnia, impotence, peripheral edema, gynecomastia
Rare
Rash, diaphoresis, hypertension, hematuria, vomiting, urinary incontinence, headache, flu-like syndromes, photosensitivity

PRECAUTIONS AND CONTRAINDICATIONS
Severe hepatic impairment
Caution:
Liver toxicity, monitoring requirements for hepatic injury, women

SERIOUS REACTIONS
! Hepatotoxicity, including hepatic encephalopathy and hemolytic anemia may be noted.

DENTAL CONSIDERATIONS

General:
• Possible increase in adverse cardiovascular events in patients at risk for thromboembolism.
• Talk with patient about any pain medication being taken.
• Avoid drugs (anticholinergics) that could exacerbate urinary retention (if present).

fluticasone propionate
flu-tic′-ah-zone proh′-pee-uh-neyt
(Beconase Allergy 24 Hour[AUS], Beconase Hayfever[AUS], Cutivate, Flixotide Disks[AUS], Flixotide Inhaler[AUS], Flonase, Flovent, Flovent Diskus, Flovent HFA, Veramyst)

CATEGORY AND SCHEDULE
Pregnancy Risk Category: C

Drug Class: Synthetic corticosteroid, medium potency

MECHANISM OF ACTION
A corticosteroid that controls the rate of protein synthesis, depresses migration of polymorphonuclear leukocytes, reverses capillary permeability, and stabilizes lysosomal membranes.
Therapeutic Effect: Prevents or controls inflammation.

USES
Nasal spray: Management of nasal symptoms of seasonal and perennial allergic and nonallergic rhinitis in adults and pediatric patient 4 yr and older
Oral: inhalation: For maintenance treatment of asthma as prophylactic therapy; also indicated for patients requiring oral glucocorticoid therapy

PHARMACOKINETICS
Inhalation/intranasal: Protein binding: 91%. Undergoes extensive first-pass metabolism in liver. Excreted in urine. **Half-life:** 3–7.8 hr. **Topical:** Amount absorbed depends on affected area and skin condition (absorption increased with fever, hydration, inflamed or denuded skin).

INDICATIONS AND DOSAGES
▶ Allergic Rhinitis
Intranasal
Adults, Elderly. Initially, 200 mcg (2 sprays in each nostril once daily or 1 spray in each nostril q12h).
Maintenance: 1 spray in each nostril once daily. Maximum: 200 mcg/day.
Children 4 yr and older. Initially, 100 mcg (1 spray in each nostril once daily). Maximum: 200 mcg/day.

▶ Relief of Inflammation and Pruritus associated with Steroid-Responsive Disorders, such as Contact Dermatitis and Eczema
Topical
Adults, Elderly, Children 3 mo and older. Apply sparingly to affected area once or twice a day.

▶ Maintenance Treatment for Asthma for Those Previously Treated with Bronchodilators
Inhalation Powder (Flovent Diskus)
Adults, Elderly, Children 12 yr and older. Initially, 100 mcg q12h.
Maximum: 500 mcg/day.
Inhalation (Oral [Flovent])
Adults, Elderly, Children 12 yr and older. 88 mcg twice a day.
Maximum: 440 mcg twice a day.

▶ Maintenance Treatment for Asthma for Those Previously Treated with Inhaled Steroids
Inhalation Powder (Flovent Diskus)
Adults, Elderly, Children 12 yr and older. Initially, 100–250 mcg q12h.
Maximum: 500 mcg q12h.
Inhalation (Oral [Flovent])
Adults, Elderly, Children 12 yr and older. 88–220 mcg twice a day.
Maximum: 440 mcg twice a day.

▶ Maintenance Treatment for Asthma for Those Previously Treated with Oral Steroids
Inhalation Powder (Flovent Diskus)
Adults, Elderly, Children 12 yr and older. 500–1000 mcg twice a day.

Inhalation (Oral [Flovent])
Adults, Elderly, Children 12 yr and older. 88 mcg twice a day.

SIDE EFFECTS/ADVERSE REACTIONS
Frequent
Inhalation: Throat irritation, hoarseness, dry mouth, cough, temporary wheezing, oropharyngeal candidiasis (particularly if mouth is not rinsed with water after each administration)
Intranasal: Mild nasopharyngeal irritation; nasal burning, stinging, or dryness; rebound congestion; rhinorrhea; loss of taste
Occasional
Inhalation: Oral candidiasis
Intranasal: Nasal and pharyngeal candidiasis, headache
Topical: Skin burning, pruritus

PRECAUTIONS AND CONTRAINDICATIONS
Primary treatment of status asthmaticus or other acute asthma episodes (inhalation); untreated localized infection of nasal mucosa
Caution:
Suppression of hypothalamic-pituitary-adrenal (HPA) axis, warning of manifestation of HPA suppression when switching drug from oral to inhaled steroids, suppression of growth in children younger than 4 yr; use is restricted for some dose forms to children older than 12 yr; lactation

DRUG INTERACTIONS OF CONCERN TO DENTISTRY
• No specific interactions reported

SERIOUS REACTIONS
! Deaths because of adrenal insufficiency have occurred in asthma patients during and after transfer from use of long-term systemic corticosteroids to less

systemically available inhaled corticosteroids.

DENTAL CONSIDERATIONS

General:
• Examine oral cavity for evidence of opportunistic candidiasis in patients using the inhaler.
• Allergic rhinitis may be a factor in mouth breathing and drying of oral tissues.
• Be aware that aspirin or sulfite preservatives in vasoconstrictor-containing products can exacerbate asthma.
• Acute asthmatic episodes may be precipitated in the dental office. Rapid-acting sympathomimetic inhalants should be available for emergency use. A stress reduction protocol may be required.
• Consider semisupine chair position for patients with respiratory disease.

Consultations:
• Consultation may be required to confirm steroid dose and duration of use.

Teach Patient/Family to:
• Update health and drug history if physician makes any changes in drug regimens.
• Gargle, rinse mouth with water, and expectorate after each aerosol use.
• Avoid use of topical preparations on fungal or herpetic lesions.

fluvastatin

floo′-va-sta-tin

(Lescol, Lescol XL, Vastin[Aus])
Do not confuse fluvastatin with fluoxetine.

CATEGORY AND SCHEDULE

Pregnancy Risk Category: X

Drug Class: Cholesterol-lowering agent, antihyperlipidemic

MECHANISM OF ACTION

An antihyperlipidemic that inhibits HMG-CoA reductase, the enzyme that catalyzes the early step in cholesterol synthesis.
Therapeutic Effect: Decreases low-density lipoprotein (LDL) cholesterol, very low-density lipoproteins (VLDLs), and plasma triglyceride levels. Slightly increases high-density lipoprotein (HDL) cholesterol concentration.

USES

As an adjunct in homozygous familial hypercholesterolemia, mixed hyperlipidemia, elevated serum triglyceride levels, and type IV hyperproteinemia, also reduces total cholesterol LDL-C, apo B, and triglyceride levels; patient should first be placed on cholesterol-lowering diet; to reduce risk in coronary artery revascularization procedures; prevention of secondary coronary events

PHARMACOKINETICS

Well absorbed from the GI tract and is unaffected by food. Does not cross the blood-brain barrier. Protein binding: greater than 98%. Primarily eliminated in feces. ***Half-life:*** 1.2 hr. Tablets (Extended-Release [Lescol XL]): 80 mg.

INDICATIONS AND DOSAGES

▸ **Hyperlipoproteinemia**
PO
Adults, Elderly. Initially, 20 mg/day (capsule) in the evening. May increase up to 40 mg/day. Maintenance: 20–40 mg/day in a single dose or divided doses.
Patients requiring more than a 25% decrease in LDL cholesterol. 40 mg (capsule) 1–2 times a day, or 80 mg tablet once a day.

SIDE EFFECTS/ADVERSE REACTIONS

Frequent
Headache, dyspepsia, back pain, myalgia, arthralgia, diarrhea, abdominal cramping, rhinitis
Occasional
Nausea, vomiting, insomnia, constipation, flatulence, rash, pruritus, fatigue, cough, dizziness

PRECAUTIONS AND CONTRAINDICATIONS

Active hepatic disease, unexplained increased serum transaminase levels
Caution:
Liver dysfunction; alcoholism; severe acute infection; metabolic, endocrine, or electrolyte disorders; uncontrolled seizures; alterations in liver function tests may be observed with use

DRUG INTERACTIONS OF CONCERN TO DENTISTRY

• Increased plasma levels: alcohol, fluconazole, itraconazole, ketoconazole, erythromycin

SERIOUS REACTIONS

❗ Myositis (inflammation of voluntary muscle) with or without increased CK and muscle weakness, occur rarely. These conditions may progress to frank rhabdomyolysis and renal impairment.

DENTAL CONSIDERATIONS

General:
• Consider semisupine chair position for patient comfort because of GI, musculoskeletal, and respiratory side effects.

---

fluvoxamine maleate
floo-vox'-ah-meen mal'-ee-ate
(Faverin[AUS], Luvox)

CATEGORY AND SCHEDULE
Pregnancy Risk Category: C

Drug Class: Selective serotonin reuptake inhibitor, antidepressant

MECHANISM OF ACTION

An antidepressant and antiobsessive agent that selectively inhibits neuronal reuptake of serotonin (SSRI).
Therapeutic Effect: Relieves depression and symptoms of obsessive-compulsive disorder.

USES

Obsessive-compulsive disorder and panic disorder

PHARMACOKINETICS

PO: Rapid absorption, peak plasma levels 5 hr; plasma protein binding 77%; hepatic metabolism; urinary excretion.

INDICATIONS AND DOSAGES

▸ **Obsessive-Compulsive Disorder**
PO
Adults. 50 mg at bedtime; may increase by 50 mg every 4–7 days. Dosages greater than 100 mg/day given in 2 divided doses. Maximum: 300 mg/day.
Children 8–17 yr. 25 mg at bedtime; may increase by 25 mg every 4–7 days. Dosages greater than 50 mg/day given in 2 divided doses. Maximum: 200 mg/day.

SIDE EFFECTS/ADVERSE REACTIONS

Frequent
Nausea, headache, somnolence, insomnia

F

Occasional
Dizziness, diarrhea, dry mouth,
asthenia, weakness, dyspepsia,
constipation, abnormal ejaculation
Rare
Anorexia, anxiety, tremors,
vomiting, flatulence, urinary
frequency, sexual dysfunction,
altered taste

PRECAUTIONS AND CONTRAINDICATIONS

Use within 14 days of MAOIs
Caution:
Lactation, renal and hepatic
impairment, epilepsy, elderly

DRUG INTERACTIONS OF CONCERN TO DENTISTRY

• Increased plasma levels of tricyclic
antidepressants, carbamazepine,
benzodiazepine; reduce doses of
alprazolam, diazepam, midazolam,
triazolam by half
• Risk of serotonin syndrome:
SSRIs
• NSAIDs: increased risk of GI side
effects

SERIOUS REACTIONS

! Overdose may produce seizures,
nausea, vomiting, and extreme
agitation and restlessness.

DENTAL CONSIDERATIONS

General:
• After supine positioning, have
patient sit upright for at least 2 min
to avoid orthostatic hypotension.
• Assess salivary flow as a factor in
caries, periodontal disease, and
candidiasis.
• Consider semisupine chair position
for patient comfort because of GI
effects of drug.
Consultations:
• Medical consultation may be
required to assess patient's ability to
tolerate stress.

• Physician should be informed if
significant xerostomic side effects
occur (e.g., increased caries, sore
tongue, problems eating or
swallowing, difficulty wearing
prosthesis) so that a medication
change can be considered.
Teach Patient/Family:
• When chronic dry mouth occurs,
advise patient to:
  • Avoid mouth rinses with high
  alcohol content because of
  drying effects.
  • Use daily home fluoride
  products for anticaries effect.
  • Use sugarless gum, frequent
  sips of water, or saliva
  substitutes.

folic acid/sodium folate (vitamin B$_9$)

foe'-lik ass'-id/soe'-dee-um
foe'-late
folic acid
(Apo-Folic[CAN], Folvite,
Megafol[AUS])
sodium folate
(Folvite-parenteral)
Do not confuse Folvite with
Florvite.

CATEGORY AND SCHEDULE

Pregnancy Risk Category: A (C if
used in doses above the
recommended daily allowance)
OTC (0.4- and 0.8-mg tablets
only)

Drug Class: Water-soluble B
vitamin

MECHANISM OF ACTION

A coenzyme that stimulates
production of platelets, RBCs, and
WBCs.

Therapeutic Effect: Essential for nucleoprotein synthesis and maintenance of normal erythropoiesis.

USES

Treatment of megaloblastic or macrocytic anemia caused by folic acid deficiency, liver disease, alcoholism, hemolysis, intestinal obstruction, pregnancy

PHARMACOKINETICS

PO form almost completely absorbed from the GI tract (upper duodenum). Protein binding: High. Metabolized in the liver and plasma to active form. Excreted in urine. Removed by hemodialysis.

INDICATIONS AND DOSAGES

▸ **Vitamin B₉ Deficiency**
PO, IV, IM, Subcutaneous
Adults, Elderly, Children 12 yr and older. Initially, 1 mg/day.
Maintenance: 0.5 mg/day.
Children 1–11 yr. Initially 1 mg/day.
Maintenance: 0.1–0.4 mg/day.
Infants. 50 mcg/day.
▸ **Dietary Supplement**
PO, IV, IM, Subcutaneous
Adults, Elderly, Children 4 yr and older. 0.4 mg/day.
Children at least 1 yr and younger than 4 yr. 0.3 mg/day.
Children younger than 1 yr. 0.1 mg/day.
Pregnant women. 0.8 mg/day.

SIDE EFFECTS/ADVERSE REACTIONS

None known

PRECAUTIONS AND CONTRAINDICATIONS

Anemias (aplastic, normocytic, pernicious, refractory)

DRUG INTERACTIONS OF CONCERN TO DENTISTRY

• Increased metabolism of phenobarbital

SERIOUS REACTIONS

! Allergic hypersensitivity occurs rarely with parenteral form. Oral folic acid is nontoxic.

DENTAL CONSIDERATIONS

General:
• Deficiency in folic acid; glossitis may be a symptom of folic acid deficiency.

formoterol fumarate
for-moe′-ter-ol fyoo′-muh-ate
(Foradil Aerolizer, Foradile[AUS], Oxis[AUS])

CATEGORY AND SCHEDULE
Pregnancy Risk Category: C

Drug Class: Selective β₂-adrenergic bronchodilator

MECHANISM OF ACTION

A long-acting bronchodilator that stimulates β₂-adrenergic receptors in the lungs, resulting in relaxation of bronchial smooth muscle. Also inhibits release of mediators from various cells in the lungs, including mast cells, with little effect on heart rate.
Therapeutic Effect: Relieves bronchospasm, reduces airway resistance. Improves bronchodilation, nighttime asthma control, and peak flow rates.

USES

Long-term treatment of asthma and prevention of bronchospasm in adults and children older than 5 yr;

prevention of exercise-induced bronchospasm in adults and children older than 12 yr; maintenance treatment of COPD

PHARMACOKINETICS

Route	Onset	Peak	Duration
Inhalation	1–3 min	0.5–1 hr	12 hr

Absorbed from bronchi after inhalation. Metabolized in the liver. Primarily excreted in urine. Unknown if removed by hemodialysis. *Half-life:* 10 hr.

INDICATIONS AND DOSAGES
▸ **Asthma, COPD**
Inhalation
Adults, Elderly, Children 5 yr and older. 12 mcg capsule q12h.
▸ **Exercise-Induced Bronchospasm**
Inhalation
Adults, Elderly, Children 5 yr and older. 12 mcg capsule at least 15 min before exercise. Do not repeat for another 12 hr.

SIDE EFFECTS/ADVERSE REACTIONS
Occasional
Tremors, muscle cramps, tachycardia, insomnia, headache, irritability, irritation of mouth or throat

PRECAUTIONS AND CONTRAINDICATIONS
Hypersensitivity
Caution:
Not for acute asthma symptoms, not for use in life-threatening situations; paradoxic bronchospasm may occur with use; not a substitute for corticosteroids; cardiovascular disease (coronary insufficiency, cardiac arrhythmias, hypertension), hyperthyroidism, seizures, hypokalemia, lactation

DRUG INTERACTIONS OF CONCERN TO DENTISTRY
• Avoid MAOIs, tricyclic antidepressants, and drugs that prolong the QT interval (phenothiazines, procainamide).
• Adrenergic agents/sympathomimetics may potentiate effects.
• β-Adrenergic blockers may antagonize sympathomimetic effects.

SERIOUS REACTIONS
! Excessive sympathomimetic stimulation may produce palpitations, extrasystole, and chest pain.

DENTAL CONSIDERATIONS

General:
• Monitor vital signs at every appointment because of cardiovascular side effects.
• Assess salivary flow as a factor in caries, periodontal disease, and candidiasis.
• Consider semisupine chair position for patient comfort because of respiratory side effects of disease.
• Short midday appointments and a stress-reduction protocol may be required for anxious patients.
• Have patient bring personal short-acting bronchodilator to appointment for use in emergency.
• Acute asthmatic episodes may be precipitated in the dental office. Rapid-acting sympathomimetic inhalants should be available for emergency use.
• Avoid prescribing aspirin-containing products.
Consultations:
• Medical consultation may be required to assess disease control and patient's ability to tolerate stress.

Teach Patient/Family to:
• Gargle, rinse mouth with water, and expectorate after each aerosol dose.
• When chronic dry mouth occurs, advise patient to:
  • Avoid mouth rinses with high alcohol content because of drying effects.
  • Use daily home fluoride products for anticaries effect.
  • Use sugarless gum, frequent sips of water, or saliva substitutes.

fosamprenavir
foss-am-pren'-ah-vur
(Lexiva)

CATEGORY AND SCHEDULE
Pregnancy Risk Category: C

Drug Class: Antiretroviral; protease inhibitor

MECHANISM OF ACTION
An antiretroviral that is rapidly converted to amprenavir, which inhibits HIV-1 protease by binding to the enzyme's active site, thus preventing the processing of viral precursors and resulting in the formation of immature, noninfectious viral particles.
Therapeutic Effect: Impairs HIV replication and proliferation.

USES
Treatment of HIV-1 infection in combination with antiretrovirals

PHARMACOKINETICS
Rapidly absorbed after PO administration. Protein binding: 90%. Metabolized in the liver. Excreted in urine and feces.
Half-life: 7.7 hr.

INDICATIONS AND DOSAGES
▶ **HIV Infection in Patients Who Have Not Had Previous Protease Inhibitor Therapy**
PO
Adults, Elderly. 1400 mg twice daily without ritonavir; or 1400 mg twice daily plus ritonavir 200 mg once daily; or 700 mg twice daily plus ritonavir 100 mg twice daily.
▶ **HIV Infection in Patients Who Have Had Previous Protease Inhibitor Therapy**
PO
Adults, Elderly. 700 mg twice daily plus ritonavir 100 mg twice daily.
▶ **Concurrent Therapy with Efavirenz**
PO
Adults, Elderly. In patients receiving fosamprenavir plus once-daily ritonavir in combination with efavirenz, an additional 100 mg/day ritonavir (300 mg total/day) should be given.

SIDE EFFECTS/ADVERSE REACTIONS
Frequent
Nausea, rash, diarrhea
Occasional
Headache, vomiting, fatigue, depression
Rare
Pruritus, abdominal pain, perioral paresthesia

PRECAUTIONS AND CONTRAINDICATIONS
Concurrent use of amprenavir, dihydroergotamine, ergonovine, ergotamine, methylergonovine, pimozide, midazolam, or triazolam. If fosamprenavir is given concurrently with ritonavir, flecainide and propafenone are also contraindicated.

DRUG INTERACTIONS OF CONCERN TO DENTISTRY

• Contraindicated with midazolam, triazolam
• Increased plasma levels of: tricyclic antidepressants, lidocaine, alprazolam, clorazepate, diazepam, flurazepam, ketoconazole, itraconazole, sildenafil, vardenafil
• Reduced absorption: antacids, carbamazepine, phenobarbital, St. John's wort (herb)

SERIOUS REACTIONS

❗ Severe and possibly life-threatening dermatologic reactions occur rarely.

DENTAL CONSIDERATIONS

General:
• Caution significant drug interactions with drugs used in dentistry.
• Question patient about other drugs or herbals they may be taking.
• Patient on chronic drug therapy may rarely present with symptoms of blood dyscrasias, which can include infection, bleeding, and poor healing. If dyscrasia is present, caution patient to prevent oral tissue trauma when using oral hygiene aids.
• Consider semisupine chair position for patient comfort if GI side effects occur.
Consultations:
• In a patient with symptoms of blood dyscrasias, request a medical consultation for blood studies and postpone treatment until normal values are reestablished.
• Medical consultation may be required to assess disease control and patient's ability to tolerate stress.
Teach Patient/Family to:
• Encourage effective oral hygiene to prevent soft tissue inflammation.

• Prevent trauma when using oral hygiene aids.
• Update health and medication history if physician makes any changes in evaluation or drug regimens; include OTC, herbal, and nonherbal remedies in the update.

foscarnet sodium
foss-car′-net soe′-dee-um
(Foscavir)

CATEGORY AND SCHEDULE
Pregnancy Risk Category: C

Drug Class: Antiviral

MECHANISM OF ACTION

An antiviral that selectively inhibits binding sites on virus-specific DNA polymerase and reverse transcriptase.
Therapeutic Effect: Inhibits replication of herpes virus.

USES

Treatment of cytomegalovirus (CMV) retinitis in AIDS, acyclovir-resistant herpes simplex I mucocutaneous diseases, and acyclovir-resistant HSV in immunocompromised patients

PHARMACOKINETICS

Sequestered into bone and cartilage. Protein binding: 14%–17%. Primarily excreted unchanged in urine. Removed by hemodialysis.
Half-life: 3.3–6.8 hr (increased in impaired renal function).

INDICATIONS AND DOSAGES
▸ **CMV Retinitis**
IV
Adults, Elderly. Initially, 60 mg/kg q8h or 100 mg/kg q12h for 2–3 wk.

Maintenance: 90–120 mg/kg/day as
a single IV infusion.
▶ **Herpes Infection**
IV
Adults. 40 mg/kg q8–12h for
2–3 wk or until healed.
▶ **Dosage in Renal Impairment**
Dosages are individualized on the
basis of creatinine clearance. Refer
to the dosing guide provided by the
manufacturer.

SIDE EFFECTS/ADVERSE REACTIONS

Frequent
Fever, nausea, vomiting, diarrhea
Occasional
Anorexia, pain and inflammation at
injection site, fever, rigors, malaise,
headache, paresthesia, dizziness,
rash, diaphoresis, abdominal pain
Rare
Back or chest pain, edema, flushing,
pruritus, constipation, dry mouth

PRECAUTIONS AND CONTRAINDICATIONS

Hypersensitivity
Caution:
Lactation, children, elderly, renal
disease, seizure disorders,
electrolyte/mineral imbalances,
severe anemia; monitor for renal
impairment

DRUG INTERACTIONS OF CONCERN TO DENTISTRY

• Avoid nephrotoxic drugs
(amphotericin B)
• Possible increased risk of seizures:
fluoroquinolones

SERIOUS REACTIONS

! Nephrotoxicity occurs to some
extent in most patients.
! Seizures and serum mineral or
electrolyte imbalances may be
life-threatening.

DENTAL CONSIDERATIONS

General:
• Examine for oral manifestations of
opportunistic infections.
• Examine for evidence of oral
manifestations of blood dyscrasias
(infection, bleeding, poor healing).
• Consider local hemostasis
measures to prevent excessive
bleeding.
• Assess salivary flow as a factor in
caries, periodontal disease, and
candidiasis.
• Monitor vital signs at every
appointment because of
cardiovascular and respiratory side
effects.
• Place on frequent recall to evaluate
healing response.
Consultations:
• Medical consultation for blood
studies (CBC); leukopenic or
thrombocytopenic side effects may
result in infection, delayed healing,
and excessive bleeding. Postpone
elective dental treatment until
normal values are maintained.
• Medical consultation may be
required to assess disease control.
Teach Patient/Family to:
• Use oral hygiene aids carefully to
prevent injury.
• See dentist immediately if
secondary oral infection occurs.
• Encourage effective oral hygiene
to prevent soft tissue inflammation.
• Use powered tooth brush if patient
has difficulty holding conventional
devices because of extrapyramidal
side effects.
• When chronic dry mouth occurs,
advise patient to:
  • Avoid mouth rinses with high
  alcohol content because of
  drying effects.
  • Use daily home fluoride
  products for anticaries effect.

F

• Use sugarless gum, frequent sips of water, or saliva substitutes.

fosfomycin tromethamine

foss-fo-mye'-sin
troe-meth'-a-mine
(Monurol)
Do not confuse Monurol with Monopril.

CATEGORY AND SCHEDULE
Pregnancy Risk Category: B

Drug Class: Antiinfective (phosphonic acid derivative)

MECHANISM OF ACTION
An antibiotic that prevents bacterial cell wall formation by inhibiting the synthesis of peptidoglycan.
Therapeutic Effect: Bactericidal.

USES
Treatment of uncomplicated UTIs in women caused by susceptible strains of *E. coli* and *Enterococcus faecalis*

PHARMACOKINETICS
PO: Peak plasma levels after 2 hr; not plasma protein bound; widely distributed to GU tissues; excreted unchanged in urine and feces.

INDICATIONS AND DOSAGES
▸ **Uncomplicated UTIs**
PO
Females. 3 g mixed in 4 oz water as a single dose.
Males. 3 g/day for 2–3 days.

SIDE EFFECTS/ADVERSE REACTIONS
Occasional
Diarrhea, nausea, headache, back pain
Rare
Dysmenorrhea, pharyngitis, abdominal pain, rash

PRECAUTIONS AND CONTRAINDICATIONS
Hypersensitivity
Caution:
Renal impairment, one dose per single episode of cystitis, lactation, children younger than 12 yr

DRUG INTERACTIONS OF CONCERN TO DENTISTRY
• Lowered serum concentrations: metoclopramide

SERIOUS REACTIONS
! None known

DENTAL CONSIDERATIONS

General:
• Determine why patient is taking the drug.
• Consider semisupine chair position for patient comfort if GI side effects occur.
Teach Patient/Family:
• When chronic dry mouth occurs, advise patient to:
  • Avoid mouth rinses with high alcohol content because of drying effects.
  • Use daily home fluoride products for anticaries effect.
  • Use sugarless gum, frequent sips of water, or saliva substitutes.

fosinopril
fo-sin'-oh-pril
(Monopril)
Do not confuse Monopril with
Monurol.

CATEGORY AND SCHEDULE
Pregnancy Risk Category: C (D if
used in second or third trimester)

Drug Class: Angiotensin-
converting enzyme (ACE)
inhibitor

MECHANISM OF ACTION
An ACE inhibitor that suppresses
the renin-angiotensin-aldosterone
system and prevents conversion of
angiotensin I to angiotensin II, a
potent vasoconstrictor; may also
inhibit angiotensin II at local
vascular and renal sites. Decreases
plasma angiotensin II, increases
plasma renin activity and decreases
aldosterone secretion.
Therapeutic Effect: Reduces
peripheral arterial resistance,
pulmonary capillary wedge pressure;
improves cardiac output and exercise
tolerance.

USES
Treatment of hypertension, alone or
in combination with thiazide
diuretics, management of heart
failure

PHARMACOKINETICS

Route	Onset	Peak	Duration
PO	1 hr	2–6 hr	24 hr

Slowly absorbed from the GI tract.
Protein binding: 97%–98%.
Metabolized in the liver and GI
mucosa to active metabolite.

Primarily excreted in urine. Minimal
removal by hemodialysis. *Half-life:*
11.5 hr.

INDICATIONS AND DOSAGES
▶ **Hypertension (Monotherapy)**
PO
Adults, Elderly. Initially, 10 mg/day.
Maintenance: 20–40 mg/day.
Maximum: 80 mg/day.
▶ **Hypertension (with Diuretic)**
PO
Adults, Elderly. Initially, 10 mg/day
titrated to patient's needs.
▶ **Heart Failure**
PO
Adults, Elderly. Initially, 5–10 mg.
Maintenance: 20–40 mg/day.

SIDE EFFECTS/ADVERSE
REACTIONS
Frequent
Dizziness, cough
Occasional
Hypotension, nausea, vomiting,
upper respiratory tract infection

PRECAUTIONS AND
CONTRAINDICATIONS
History of angioedema from
previous treatment with ACE
inhibitors
Caution:
Impaired liver function,
hypovolemia, blood dyscrasias, CHF,
COPD, asthma, elderly

DRUG INTERACTIONS OF
CONCERN TO DENTISTRY
• Increased hypotension: alcohol,
phenothiazines
• Decreased hypotensive effects:
indomethacin, possibly other
NSAIDs, sympathomimetics
• Suspected reduction in the
antihypertensive and vasodilator
effects by salicylates; monitor B/P if
used concurrently

F

SERIOUS REACTIONS

❗ Excessive hypotension ("first-dose syncope") may occur in patients with CHF and in those who are severely salt and volume depleted.

❗ Angioedema (swelling of face and lips) and hyperkalemia occur rarely.

❗ Agranulocytosis and neutropenia may be noted in those with collagen vascular disease, including scleroderma and systemic lupus erythematosus and impaired renal function.

❗ Nephrotic syndrome may be noted in those with history of renal disease.

DENTAL CONSIDERATIONS

General:

• Monitor vital signs at every appointment because of cardiovascular and respiratory side effects.

• After supine positioning, have patient sit upright for at least 2 min before standing to avoid orthostatic hypotension.

• Patients on chronic drug therapy may rarely have symptoms of blood dyscrasias, which can include infection, bleeding, and poor healing.

• Assess salivary flow as a factor in caries, periodontal disease, and candidiasis.

• Limit use of sodium-containing products, such as saline IV fluids, for patients with a dietary salt restriction.

• Stress from dental procedures may compromise cardiovascular function; determine patient risk.

• Short appointments and a stress-reduction protocol may be required for anxious patients.

Consultations:

• Medical consultation may be required to assess disease control and patient's ability to tolerate stress.

• In a patient with symptoms of blood dyscrasias, request a medical consultation for blood studies and postpone dental treatment until normal values are reestablished.

• Take precautions if dental surgery is anticipated and sedation or general anesthesia is required; risk of hypotensive episode.

Teach Patient/Family to:

• Encourage effective oral hygiene to prevent soft tissue inflammation.

• Use caution to prevent injury when using oral hygiene aids.

• When chronic dry mouth occurs, advise patient to:

  • Avoid mouth rinses with high alcohol content because of drying effects.

  • Use daily home fluoride products for anticaries effect.

  • Use sugarless gum, frequent sips of water, or saliva substitutes.

fosphenytoin

fos-phen'-ih- toyn
(Cerebyx)
Do not confuse Cerebyx with Celebrex or Celexa.

CATEGORY AND SCHEDULE

Pregnancy Risk Category: D

Drug Class:
Hydantoin-anticonvulsant

MECHANISM OF ACTION

A hydantoin-anticonvulsant that stabilizes neuronal membranes by decreasing sodium and calcium ion influx into the neurons. Also decreases post-tetanic potentiation and repetitive discharge.

Therapeutic Effect: Decreases seizure activity.

USES

Control of generalized convulsive status epilepticus; prevention and treatment of seizures during neurosurgery; short-term substitute for oral phenytoin

PHARMACOKINETICS

Completely absorbed after IM administration. Protein binding: 95%–99%. Rapidly and completely hydrolyzed to phenytoin after IM or IV administration. Time of complete conversion to phenytoin: 4 hr after IM injection; 2 hr after IV infusion. *Half-life:* 8–15 min (for conversion to phenytoin).

INDICATIONS AND DOSAGES
▸ **Status Epilepticus**
IV

Adults. Loading dose: 15–20 mg phenytoin equivalent (PE)/kg infused at rate of 100–150 mg PE/min.
▸ **Nonemergent Seizures**
IV, IM

Adults. Loading dose: 10–20 mg PE/kg. Maintenance: 4–6 mg PE/kg/day.
▸ **Short-Term Substitution for Oral Phenytoin**
IV, IM

Adults. May substitute for oral phenytoin at same total daily dose.

SIDE EFFECTS/ADVERSE REACTIONS
Frequent
Dizziness, paresthesia, tinnitus, pruritus, headache, somnolence
Occasional
Morbilliform rash

PRECAUTIONS AND CONTRAINDICATIONS
Adams-Stokes syndrome, hypersensitivity to fosphenytoin or phenytoin, second- or third-degree AV block, severe bradycardia, sinoatrial block
Caution:
IV: Do not exceed injection rate of 150 mg PE/min, risk of seizures with abrupt withdrawal; hypotension, severe myocardial insufficiency, phosphate restriction; thyroid, renal, or hepatic disease; elderly, lactation, pediatric use

DRUG INTERACTIONS OF CONCERN TO DENTISTRY
• Increased phenytoin levels: benzodiazepines (chlordiazepoxide, diazepam), halothane, salicylates
• Increased CNS depression: benzodiazepines, H_1-blocker antihistamines, opiate agonists
• Decreased phenytoin levels: carbamazepine, ciprofloxacin
• Decreased effectiveness of corticosteroids
• Suspected risk of hepatic toxicity: chronic use of acetaminophen and phosphenytoin

SERIOUS REACTIONS
❗ An elevated fosphenytoin blood concentration may produce ataxia, nystagmus, diplopia, lethargy, slurred speech, nausea, vomiting, and hypotension. As the drug level increases, extreme lethargy may progress to coma.

DENTAL CONSIDERATIONS

General:
• This drug is intended for short-term use in an emergency department or hospital setting. Patient probably will return to oral phenytoin or other anticonvulsant after hospital care.
• Use precaution if sedation or general anesthesia is required; risk of hypotensive episode.

F

Consultations:
• Determine type of epilepsy, seizure frequency and quality of seizure control. A stress reduction protocol may be required.
• Medical consultation may be required to assess disease control and patient's ability to tolerate stress.
Teach Patient/Family to:
• Update health and drug history if physician makes any changes in evaluation or drug regimens.

frovatriptan
fro-va-trip′-tan
(Frovan)

CATEGORY AND SCHEDULE
Pregnancy Risk Category: C

Drug Class: Antimigraine agent; $5HT_1$-receptor agonist

MECHANISM OF ACTION
A serotonin receptor agonist that binds selectively to vascular receptors, producing a vasoconstrictive effect on cranial blood vessels.
Therapeutic Effect: Relieves migraine headache.

USES
Acute treatment of migraine with or without aura

PHARMACOKINETICS
Well absorbed after PO administration. Metabolized by the liver to inactive metabolite. Eliminated in urine. *Half-life:* 26 hr (increased in hepatic impairment).

INDICATIONS AND DOSAGES
▸ **Acute Migraine Attack**
PO
Adults, Elderly. Initially 2.5 mg. If headache improves but then returns, dose may be repeated after 2 hr. Maximum: 7.5 mg/day.

SIDE EFFECTS/ADVERSE REACTIONS
Occasional
Dizziness, paresthesia, fatigue, flushing
Rare
Hot or cold sensation, dry mouth, dyspepsia

PRECAUTIONS AND CONTRAINDICATIONS
Basilar or hemiplegic migraine, cerebrovascular or peripheral vascular disease, coronary artery disease, ischemic heart disease (including angina pectoris, history of MI, silent ischemia, and Prinzmetal's angina), severe hepatic impairment (Child-Pugh grade C), uncontrolled hypertension, use within 24 hr of ergotamine-containing preparations or another serotonin receptor agonist, use within 14 days of MAOIs

DRUG INTERACTIONS OF CONCERN TO DENTISTRY
• Potential serotonin crisis: SSRIs, ergot-containing drugs (avoid use within 24 hr of taking this drug)
• Decreased plasma levels: cimetidine

SERIOUS REACTIONS
! Cardiac reactions (including ischemia, coronary artery vasospasm and MI) and noncardiac vasospasm-related reactions (such as hemorrhage and CVA) occur rarely, particularly in patients with hypertension, diabetes, or a strong family history of coronary artery

disease; obese patients; smokers; males older than 40 yr; and postmenopausal women.

DENTAL CONSIDERATIONS

General:

• This is an acute-use drug; it is doubtful that patients will seek dental treatment during acute migraine attacks.

• Be aware of patient's disease, its severity and its frequency, when known.

• Advise patient if dental drugs prescribed have a potential for photosensitivity.

Consultations:

• If treating chronic orofacial pain, consult with physician of record.

• Medical consultation may be required to assess disease control and patient's ability to tolerate stress.

Teach Patient/Family to:

• Avoid mouth rinses with high alcohol content because of additional drying effects.

• Update health and drug history if physician makes any changes in evaluation or drug regimens.

furosemide

fur-oh'-se-mide

(Apo-Furosemide[CAN], Frusehexal[AUS], Frusid[AUS], Lasix, Uremide[AUS], Urex-M[AUS])

Do not confuse Lasix with Lidex, Luvox, or Luxiq, or furosemide with Torsemide.

CATEGORY AND SCHEDULE

Pregnancy Risk Category: C (D if used in pregnancy-induced hypertension)

Drug Class: Loop diuretic

MECHANISM OF ACTION

A loop diuretic that enhances excretion of sodium, chloride, and potassium by direct action at the ascending limb of the loop of Henle.

Therapeutic Effect: Produces diuresis and lowers B/P.

USES

Pulmonary edema, edema in CHF, liver disease, nephrotic syndrome, ascites, hypertension

PHARMACOKINETICS

Route	Onset	Peak	Duration
PO	30–60 min	1–2 hr	6–8 hr
IV	5 min	20–60 min	2 hr
IM	30 min	N/A	N/A

Well absorbed from the GI tract. Protein binding: 91%–97%. Partially metabolized in the liver. Primarily excreted in urine (nonrenal clearance increases in severe renal impairment). Not removed by hemodialysis. *Half-life:* 30–90 min (increased in renal or hepatic impairment and in neonates).

INDICATIONS AND DOSAGES

▸ **Edema, Hypertension**

PO

Adults, Elderly. Initially, 20–80 mg/dose; may increase by 20–40 mg/dose q6–8h. May titrate up to 600 mg/day in severe edematous states.

Children. 1–6 mg/kg/day in divided doses q6–12h.

IV, IM

Adults, Elderly. 20–40 mg/dose; may increase by 20 mg/dose q1–2h.

Children. 1–2 mg/kg/dose q6–12h.

Neonates. 1–2 mg/kg/dose q12–24h.

IV infusion
Adults, Elderly. Bolus of 0.1 mg/kg, followed by infusion of 0.1 mg/kg/hr; may double q2h. Maximum: 0.4 mg/kg/hr.
Children. 0.05 mg/kg/hr; titrate to desired effect.

SIDE EFFECTS/ADVERSE REACTIONS

Expected
Increased urinary frequency and urine volume
Frequent
Nausea, dyspepsia, abdominal cramps, diarrhea or constipation, electrolyte disturbances
Occasional
Dizziness, light-headedness, headache, blurred vision, paresthesia, photosensitivity, rash, fatigue, bladder spasm, restlessness, diaphoresis
Rare
Flank pain

PRECAUTIONS AND CONTRAINDICATIONS

Anuria, hepatic coma, severe electrolyte depletion
Caution:
Diabetes mellitus, dehydration, ascites, severe renal disease

DRUG INTERACTIONS OF CONCERN TO DENTISTRY

• Increased electrolyte imbalance: corticosteroids
• Masked ototoxicity: phenothiazines
• Decreased antihypertensive effect: NSAIDs, especially indomethacin

SERIOUS REACTIONS

! Vigorous diuresis may lead to profound water loss and electrolyte depletion, resulting in hypokalemia, hyponatremia, and dehydration.

! Sudden volume depletion may result in increased risk of thrombosis, circulatory collapse, and sudden death.
! Acute hypotensive episodes may occur, sometimes several days after beginning therapy.
! Ototoxicity—manifested as deafness, vertigo, or tinnitus—may occur, especially in patients with severe renal impairment.
! Furosemide use can exacerbate diabetes mellitus, systemic lupus erythematosus, gout, and pancreatitis.
! Blood dyscrasias have been reported.

DENTAL CONSIDERATIONS

General:
• Monitor vital signs at every appointment because of cardiovascular side effects.
• Patients on chronic drug therapy may rarely have symptoms of blood dyscrasias, which can include infection, bleeding, and poor healing.
• Assess salivary flow as a factor in caries, periodontal disease, and candidiasis.
• After supine positioning, have patient sit upright for at least 2 min before standing to avoid orthostatic hypotension.
• Patients on high-potency diuretics should be monitored for serum K levels.
Consultations:
• In a patient with symptoms of blood dyscrasias, request a medical consultation for blood studies and postpone dental treatment until normal values are reestablished.
• Medical consultation may be required to assess disease control.
Teach Patient/Family to:
• Encourage effective oral hygiene to prevent soft tissue inflammation.

• Use caution to prevent injury when using oral hygiene aids.
• When chronic dry mouth occurs, advise patient to:
  • Use daily home fluoride products for anticaries effect.

• Avoid mouth rinses with high alcohol content because of drying effects.
• Use sugarless gum, frequent sips of water, or saliva substitutes.

F

gabapentin
ga´-ba-pen-tin
(Neurontin, Pendine[AUS])
Do not confuse Neurontin with
Noroxin.

CATEGORY AND SCHEDULE
Pregnancy Risk Category: C

G

Drug Class: Anticonvulsant,
analgesic

MECHANISM OF ACTION
An anticonvulsant and antineuralgic
agent whose exact mechanism
unknown. May increase the
synthesis or accumulation of
gamma-aminobutyric acid (GABA)
by binding to as-yet-undefined
receptor sites in brain tissue.
Therapeutic Effect: Reduces seizure
activity and neuropathic pain.

USES
Adjunctive therapy in patients 12 yr
or older with partial seizures with or
without secondary generalization
and as adjunctive therapy for partial
seizures in children 3–12 yr;
postherpetic neuralgia in adults

PHARMACOKINETICS
Well absorbed from the GI tract (not
affected by food). Protein binding:
less than 5%. Widely distributed.
Crosses the blood-brain barrier.
Primarily excreted unchanged in
urine. Removed by hemodialysis.
Half-life: 5–7 hr (increased in
impaired renal function and the
elderly).

INDICATIONS AND DOSAGES
▸ **Adjunctive Therapy for Seizure
Control**
PO
*Adults, Elderly, Children older than
12 yr.* Initially, 300 mg 3 times a
day. May titrate dosage. Range:
900–1800 mg/day in 3 divided
doses. Maximum: 3600 mg/day.
Children 3–12 yr. Initially,
10–15 mg/kg/day in 3 divided doses.
May titrate up to 25–35 mg/kg/day
(for children 5–12 yr) and 40 mg/
kg/day (for children 3–4 yr).
Maximum: 50 mg/kg/day.
▸ **Adjunctive Therapy for
Neuropathic Pain**
PO
Adults, Elderly. Initially, 100 mg 3
times a day; may increase by
300 mg/day at weekly intervals.
Maximum: 3600 mg/day in 3
divided doses.
Children. Initially, 5 mg/kg/dose at
bedtime, followed by 5 mg/kg/dose
for 2 doses on day 2, then 5 mg/kg/
dose for 3 doses on day 3. Range:
8–35 mg/kg/day in 3 divided doses.
▸ **Postherpetic Neuralgia**
PO
Adults, Elderly. 300 mg on day
1300 mg twice a day on day 2 and
300 mg 3 times a day on day 3.
Titrate up to 1800 mg/day.
▸ **Dosage in Renal Impairment**
Dosage and frequency are modified
on the basis of creatinine clearance:

Creatinine Clearance	Dosage
60 ml/min or higher	400 mg q8h
30–59 ml/min	300 mg q12h
16–29 ml/min	300 mg daily
Less than 16 ml/min	300 mg every other day
Hemodialysis	200–300 mg after each 4-hr hemodialysis session

SIDE EFFECTS/ADVERSE REACTIONS

Frequent
Fatigue, somnolence, dizziness, ataxia
Occasional
Nystagmus, tremors, diplopia, rhinitis, weight gain
Rare
Nervousness, dysarthria, memory loss, dyspepsia, pharyngitis, myalgia

PRECAUTIONS AND CONTRAINDICATIONS

Hypersensitivity
Caution:
Lactation, renal function impairment, children younger than 12 yr, elderly

DRUG INTERACTIONS OF CONCERN TO DENTISTRY

• None reported at this time, but, because CNS side effects are common, the use of anxiolytic sedative drugs may potentially increase the CNS side effects.

SERIOUS REACTIONS

! Abrupt withdrawal may increase seizure frequency.
! Overdosage may result in diplopia, slurred speech, drowsiness, lethargy, and diarrhea.

DENTAL CONSIDERATIONS

General:
• Early-morning appointments and a stress-reduction protocol may be required for anxious patients.
• Place on frequent recall because of oral side effects.
• Monitor vital signs at every appointment because of cardiovascular side effects.
• Assess salivary flow as a factor in caries, periodontal disease, and candidiasis.

• Determine type of epilepsy and quality of seizure control.
Consultations:
• Medical consultation may be required to assess disease control and patient's ability to tolerate stress.
Teach Patient/Family to:
• Encourage effective oral hygiene to prevent soft tissue inflammation.
• Use caution with oral hygiene aids to prevent injury.
• When chronic dry mouth occurs, advise patient to:
  • Avoid mouth rinses with high alcohol content because of drying effects.
  • Use daily home fluoride products for anticaries effect.
  • Use sugarless gum, frequent sips of water, or saliva substitutes.

galantamine
ga-**lan**'-ta-mene
(Reminyl)
Do not confuse Reminyl with Remeron, Remicade, or Robinul.

CATEGORY AND SCHEDULE
Pregnancy Risk Category: B

Drug Class: Cholinesterase inhibitor

MECHANISM OF ACTION
A cholinesterase inhibitor that inhibits the enzyme acetylcholinesterase, thus increasing the concentration of acetylcholine at cholinergic synapses and enhancing cholinergic function in the CNS.
Therapeutic Effect: Slows the progression of Alzheimer's disease.

USES
Treatment of mild-to-moderate dementia of Alzheimer's disease

PHARMACOKINETICS
Rapidly absorbed from the GI tract. Protein binding: 18%. Distributed to blood cells; binds to plasma proteins, mainly albumin. Metabolized in the liver. Excreted in urine. *Half-life:* 7 hr.

INDICATIONS AND DOSAGES
▶ **Alzheimer's Disease**
PO
Adults, Elderly. Initially, 4 mg twice a day (8 mg/day). After a minimum of 4 wk (if well tolerated), may increase to 8 mg twice a day (16 mg/day). After another 4 wk, may increase to 12 mg twice daily (24 mg/day). Range: 16–24 mg/day in 2 divided doses.
▶ **Dosage in Renal Impairment**
For moderate impairment, maximum dosage is 16 mg/day. Drug is not recommended for patients with severe impairment.

SIDE EFFECTS/ADVERSE REACTIONS
Frequent
Nausea, vomiting, diarrhea, anorexia, weight loss
Occasional
Abdominal pain, insomnia, depression, headache, dizziness, fatigue, rhinitis
Rare
Tremors, constipation, confusion, cough, anxiety, urinary incontinence

PRECAUTIONS AND CONTRAINDICATIONS
Severe hepatic or renal impairment
Caution:
Potentiation of succinylcholine-like neuromuscular blocking drugs, obstructive GI disease, Parkinson's disease, epilepsy, cardiac conduction disorders, AV block, bradycardia, history of GI ulcer, hypersecretory disorders (gastric), bladder outflow obstruction, COPD, asthma, moderate hepatic impairment, moderate renal impairment, lactation, pediatric use

DRUG INTERACTIONS OF CONCERN TO DENTISTRY
• Increased plasma levels: ketoconazole
• Increased bioavailability: cimetidine, paroxetine
• Enhanced succinylcholine muscle relaxation during anesthesia
• Action may be inhibited by anticholinergic drugs or enhanced by cholinergic agonists

SERIOUS REACTIONS
❗ Overdose may cause cholinergic crisis, characterized by increased salivation, lacrimation, severe nausea and vomiting, bradycardia, respiratory depression, hypotension, and increased muscle weakness. Treatment usually consists of supportive measures and an anticholinergic such as atropine.

DENTAL CONSIDERATIONS

General:
• Monitor vital signs at every appointment because of cardiovascular side effects.
• After supine positioning, have patient sit upright for at least 2 min to avoid orthostatic hypotension.
• Drug is used early in the disease; ensure that patient or caregiver understands informed consent.
• Place on frequent recall because early attention to dental health is important for Alzheimer's patients.
• Consider semisupine chair position for patient comfort if GI side effects occur.

Consultations:
• Consultation with physician may be necessary if sedation or general anesthesia is required.
• Medical consultation may be required to assess disease control and patient's ability to tolerate stress.

Teach Patient/Family to:
• Encourage effective oral hygiene to prevent soft tissue inflammation.
• Have caregiver assist patient with oral home-care regimen as cognitive ability declines.
• Use powered tooth brush if patient has difficulty holding conventional devices.
• Update health and drug history if physician makes any changes in evaluation or drug regimens.

galsulfase
gal-**sul**′-face
(Naglazyme)

CATEGORY AND SCHEDULE
Pregnancy Risk Category: B

Drug Class: Enzyme

MECHANISM OF ACTION
A recombinant normal variant form of a polymorphic enzyme (*N*-acetylgalactosamine 4-sulfatase), produced in Chinese hamster cells, that is taken up into lysosomes and increases the catabolism of glycosaminoglycans.
Therapeutic Effect: Replaces enzyme (*N*-acetylgalactosamine 4-sulfatase).

USES
Treatment of Maroteaux-Lamy syndrome

PHARMACOKINETICS
Half-life: wk 1: 6–21 hr; wk 24: 8–40 hr.

INDICATIONS AND DOSAGES
▶ **Maroteaux-Lamy Syndrome**
IV
Adults. 1 mg/kg once a wk.
Children (5 yr and older). 1 mg/kg once a wk.

SIDE EFFECTS/ADVERSE REACTIONS
Frequent
Antibody development, abdominal pain, ear pain, headache, fever, arthralgia, vomiting, upper respiratory infections, diarrhea, cough, otitis media, infusion-related reactions, pain, rigors, conjunctivitis, dyspnea, chest pain, pharyngitis, facial edema, hypertension, malaise, gastroenteritis, areflexia, corneal opacification, nasal congestion, umbilical hernia
Less frequent adverse effects were not described

PRECAUTIONS AND CONTRAINDICATIONS
Hypersensitivity to galsulfase or its components
Caution:
Respiratory illness

DRUG INTERACTIONS OF CONCERN TO DENTISTRY
• None reported

SERIOUS REACTIONS
! Respiratory distress has been reported.

DENTAL CONSIDERATIONS
General
• Monitor vital signs at every appointment because of cardiovascular side effects.

• Consider semisupine chair position for patient comfort because of respiratory complications.
• Avoid aspirin and NSAIDs.
• Consider visual disturbances when presenting instructions to patients.
Consultations:
• Consult physician to determine disease control and ability of patient to tolerate dental procedures.
Teach Patient/Family to:
• Update medication/health history whenever symptoms of disease or medication regimen is changed.
• Use effective, atraumatic oral hygiene measures to reduce soft tissue inflammation.
• Use home fluoride products for anticaries effect.

ganciclovir sodium

gan-**sy′**-clo-ver **soe′**-dee-um
(Cymevene[AUS], Cytovene, Vitrasert)
Do not confuse Cytovene with Cytosar.

CATEGORY AND SCHEDULE

Pregnancy Risk Category: C

Drug Class: Antiviral, nucleoside analog

MECHANISM OF ACTION

This synthetic nucleoside competes with viral DNA polymerase and is incorporated into growing viral DNA chains.
Therapeutic Effect: Interferes with synthesis and replication of viral DNA.

USES

Prevention and treatment of cytomegalovirus (CMV) retinitis in patients with AIDS or organ transplants; life-threatening CMV disease

PHARMACOKINETICS

Widely distributed. Protein binding: 1%–2%. Undergoes minimal metabolism. Excreted unchanged primarily in urine. Removed by hemodialysis. *Half-life:* 2.5–3.6 hr (increased in impaired renal function).

INDICATIONS AND DOSAGES
▶ **CMV Retinitis**
IV
Adults, Children 3 mo and older.
10 mg/kg/day in divided doses q12h for 14–21 days, then 5 mg/kg/day as a single daily dose.
▶ **Prevention of CMV Disease in Transplant Patients**
IV
Adults, Children. 10 mg/kg/day in divided doses q12h for 7–14 days, then 5 mg/kg/day as a single daily dose.
▶ **Other CMV Infections**
IV
Adults. Initially, 10 mg/kg/day in divided doses q12h for 14–21 days, then 5 mg/kg/day as a single daily dose. Maintenance: 1000 mg 3 times a day or 500 mg q3h (6 times a day).
Children. Initially, 10 mg/kg/day in divided doses q12h for 14–21 days, then 5 mg/kg/day as a single daily dose. Maintenance: 30 mg/kg/dose q8h.
▶ **Intravitreal Implant**
Adults. 1 implant q6–9mo plus oral ganciclovir.
Children 9 yr and older. 1 implant q6–9mo plus oral ganciclovir (30 mg/dose q8h).
▶ **Adult Dosage in Renal Impairment**
Dosage and frequency are modified on the basis of CrCl.

CrCl	Induction Dosage	Mainte- nance Dosage	Oral
50–69 ml/min	2.5 mg/kg q12h	2.5 mg/kg q24h	1500 mg/day
25–49 ml/min	2.5 mg/kg q24h	1.25 mg/kg q24h	1000 mg/day
10–24 ml/min	1.25 mg/kg q24h	0.625 mg/kg q24h	500 mg/day
Less than 10 ml/min	1.25 mg/kg 3 times a wk	0.625 mg/kg 3 times a wk	500 mg 3 times a wk

CrCl = creatinine clearance

SIDE EFFECTS/ADVERSE REACTIONS
Frequent
Diarrhea, fever, nausea, abdominal pain, vomiting
Occasional
Diaphoresis, infection, paresthesia, flatulence, pruritus
Rare
Headache, stomatitis, dyspepsia, phlebitis

PRECAUTIONS AND CONTRAINDICATIONS
Hypersensitivity to acyclovir or ganciclovir
Caution:
Preexisting cytopenia, renal function impairment, lactation, children younger than 6 mo, elderly, platelet count less than 25,000/mm^3

DRUG INTERACTIONS OF CONCERN TO DENTISTRY
• Increased risk of blood dyscrasias: dapsone, carbamazepine, phenothiazines
• Increased risk of seizures: imipenem/cilastatin (Primaxin)
• Low platelet counts may prevent the use of aspirin, NSAIDs

SERIOUS REACTIONS
! Hematologic toxicity occurs commonly: leukopenia in 29%–41% of patients and anemia in 19%–25%.
! Intraocular insertion occasionally results in visual acuity loss, vitreous hemorrhage, and retinal detachment.
! GI hemorrhage occurs rarely.

DENTAL CONSIDERATIONS
General:
• Examine for oral manifestations of opportunistic infection.
• Examine for evidence of oral manifestations of blood dyscrasias (infection, bleeding, poor healing).
• Place on frequent recall to evaluate healing response.
• Consider local hemostasis measures to prevent excessive bleeding.
• Monitor vital signs at every appointment because of cardiovascular and respiratory side effects.
Consultations:
• Medical consultation for blood studies (CBC); leukopenic or thrombocytopenic side effects may result in infection, delayed healing, and excessive bleeding. Postpone elective dental treatment until normal values are maintained.
• Medical consultation may be required to assess disease control.
Teach Patient/Family to:
• Use caution in use of oral hygiene aids to prevent injury.
• See dentist immediately if secondary oral infection occurs.
• Encourage effective oral hygiene to prevent soft tissue inflammation.

G

gatifloxacin
gah-tee-**floks**'-ah-sin
(Tequin, Zymar)

CATEGORY AND SCHEDULE
Pregnancy Risk Category: C

Drug Class: Fluoroquinolone
antiinfective

MECHANISM OF ACTION
A fluoroquinolone that inhibits two
enzymes, topoisomerase II and IV,
in susceptible microorganisms.
Therapeutic Effect: Interferes with
bacterial DNA replication. Prevents
or delays resistance emergence.
Bactericidal.

USES
Treatment of acute bacterial
exacerbation of chronic bronchitis
caused by *S. pneumoniae, H.
influenzae, H. parainfluenzae, M.
catarrhalis,* or *S. aureus;* acute
sinusitis (*S. pneumoniae, H.
influenzae*); community-acquired
pneumonia (*S. pneumoniae, H.
influenzae, H. para-influenzae, M.
catarrhalis, M. pneumoniae, C.
pneumoniae, L. pneumoniae,* or *S.
aureus;* complicated or
uncomplicated UTI (*E. coli, K.
pneumoniae, P. mirabilis*);
pyelonephritis (*E. coli*), acute
uncomplicated rectal infections in
women or uncomplicated urethral or
cervical gonorrhea (*N.
gonorrhoeae*); uncomplicated skin
and skin-structure infections

PHARMACOKINETICS
Well absorbed from the GI tract
after PO administration. Protein
binding: 20%. Widely distributed.
Metabolized in liver. Primarily
excreted in urine. *Half-life:* 7–14 hr.

INDICATIONS AND DOSAGES
▶ **Chronic Bronchitis, Complicated
UTIs, Pyelonephritis, Skin Infections**
PO, IV
Adults, Elderly. 400 mg/day for
7–10 days (5 days for chronic
bronchitis).
▶ **Sinusitis**
PO, IV
Adults, Elderly. 400 mg/day for 10
days.
▶ **Pneumonia**
PO, IV
Adults, Elderly. 400 mg/day for
7–14 days.
▶ **Cystitis**
PO, IV
Adults, Elderly. 400 mg as a single
dose or 200 mg/day for 3 days.
▶ **Urethral Gonorrhea in Men and
Women, Endocervical and Rectal
Gonorrhea in Women**
PO, IV
Adults, Elderly. 400 mg as a single
dose.
▶ **Topical Treatment of Bacterial
Conjunctivitis Caused by
Susceptible Strains of Bacteria**
Ophthalmic
*Adults, Elderly, Children 1 yr and
older.* 1 drop q2h while awake for 2
days, then 1 drop up to 4 times a
day for days 3–7.
▶ **Dosage in Renal Impairment**

Creatinine Clearance	Dosage
40 ml/min	400 mg/day
Less than 40 ml/min	Initially, 400 mg/day, then 200 mg/day
Hemodialysis	Initially, 400 mg/day, then 200 mg/day
Peritoneal dialysis	Initially, 400 mg/day, then 200 mg/day

SIDE EFFECTS/ADVERSE REACTIONS

Occasional
Nausea, vaginitis, diarrhea, headache, dizziness
Ophthalmic: conjunctival irritation, increased tearing, corneal inflammation
Rare
Abdominal pain, constipation, dyspepsia, stomatitis, edema, insomnia, abnormal dreams, diaphoresis, altered taste, rash
Ophthalmic: corneal swelling, dry eye, eye pain, eyelid swelling, headache, red eye, reduced visual acuity, altered taste

PRECAUTIONS AND CONTRAINDICATIONS

Hypersensitivity to quinolones
Caution:
Reduce dose with creatinine clearance less than 40 ml/min; probenecid increases half-life; children younger than 18 yr, lactation, seizure history, avoid use with class IA and III antiarrhythmics; many prolong QT interval; cross resistance with other fluoroquinolones, monitor blood glucose in diabetes

DRUG INTERACTIONS OF CONCERN TO DENTISTRY

• Use caution with erythromycin and tricyclic antidepressants (no data, risk of prolonged QT interval)
• Decreased absorption: divalent and trivalent cations, iron and zinc salts
• Increased risk of CNS stimulation and seizures: NSAIDs

SERIOUS REACTIONS

‼ Pseudomembranous colitis as evidenced by severe abdominal pain and cramps, severe watery diarrhea, and fever may occur.

‼ Superinfection manifested as genital or anal pruritus, ulceration, or changes in oral mucosa and moderate to severe diarrhea may occur.

DENTAL CONSIDERATIONS

General:
• Determine why patient is taking the drug.
• Monitor vital signs at every appointment because of cardiovascular side effects.
• Examine for oral manifestation of opportunistic infection.
• Advise patient if dental drugs prescribed have a potential for photosensitivity.
• Ruptures of the shoulder, hand, and Achilles tendons requiring surgical repair or resulting in prolonged disability have been reported with use of fluoroquinolones. Question patient about history of side effects associated with fluoroquinolone use.
Consultations:
• Physician consultation is advised in the presence of an acute dental infection requiring another antibiotic.
Teach Patient/Family to:
• Minimize exposure to sunlight and wear sunscreen if sun exposure is planned.
• Discontinue treatment and inform dentist immediately if patient experiences pain or inflammation of a tendon and to rest and refrain from exercise.

Gatifloxacin Ophthalmic

General:
• Avoid dental light in patient's eyes; offer dark glasses for patient comfort.

G

gefitinib
geh-**fih**′-tih-nib
(Iressa)

CATEGORY AND SCHEDULE
Pregnancy Risk Category: D

Drug Class: Antineoplastic-
miscellaneous; epidermal growth
factor receptor inhibitor

G

MECHANISM OF ACTION
Blocks the signaling pathway that
binds to the epidermal growth factor
receptor (EGFR) on the surface of
normal and cancer cells. EGFR
activates the enzyme tyrosine kinase,
which sends signals instructing the
cells to grow.
Therapeutic Effect: Inhibits the
growth of cancer cells.

USES
Treatment of advanced/metastatic
non–small-cell lung cancer in those
who have not responded to platinum
or docetaxel products

PHARMACOKINETICS
Slowly absorbed and extensively
distributed throughout the body.
Protein binding: 90%. Undergoes
extensive metabolism in the liver.
Excreted in the feces. *Half-life:*
48 hr.

INDICATIONS AND DOSAGES
▸ Non–Small-Cell Lung Cancer
PO
Adults, Elderly. 250 mg/day; may
increase to 500 mg/day for patients
receiving drugs that may decrease
gefitinib blood concentrations, such
as rifampin and phenytoin

SIDE EFFECTS/ADVERSE REACTIONS
Frequent
Diarrhea, rash, acne
Occasional
Dry skin, nausea, vomiting, pruritus
Rare
Anorexia, asthenia, weight loss,
peripheral edema, eye pain

PRECAUTIONS AND CONTRAINDICATIONS
None known

DRUG INTERACTIONS OF CONCERN TO DENTISTRY
• Decreased plasma levels: sodium
bicarbonate
• Decreased metabolism: potent
inhibitors of CYP3A4 isoenzymes
(ketoconazole, itraconazole,
erythromycin, clarithromycin)

SERIOUS REACTIONS
❗ Pancreatitis and ocular hemorrhage
occur rarely.
❗ Hypersensitivity reaction produces
angioedema and urticaria.

DENTAL CONSIDERATIONS

General:
• If additional analgesia is required
for dental pain, consider alternative
analgesics (NSAIDs) in patients
taking narcotics for acute or chronic
pain.
• This drug may be used in the
hospital or on an outpatient basis.
Confirm the patient's disease and
treatment status.
• Consider semisupine chair position
for patients with respiratory disease.
• Examine for oral manifestation of
opportunistic infection.
• Patients may have received other
chemotherapy or radiation: confirm
medical and drug history.

• Caution: drug interactions with drugs used in dentistry.

Consultations:

• Medical consultation may be required to assess disease control and patient's ability to tolerate stress.

• Medical consultation may be required to assess immunologic status during cancer chemotherapy and determine safety risk, if any, posed by the required dental treatment.

Teach Patient/Family to:

• Encourage effective oral hygiene to prevent soft tissue inflammation.

• Use caution to prevent trauma when using oral hygiene aids.

• Update health and medication history if physician makes any changes in evaluation or drug regimens; include OTC, herbal, and nonherbal remedies in the update.

gemcitabine hydrochloride
jem-**cih**′-tah-bean
hi-droh-**klor**′-ide
(Gemzar)

CATEGORY AND SCHEDULE
Pregnancy Risk Category: D

Drug Class: Antineoplastic-miscellaneous; nucleoside analog

MECHANISM OF ACTION
An antimetabolite that inhibits ribonucleotide reductase, the enzyme necessary for catalyzing DNA synthesis.
Therapeutic Effect: Produces death in cells undergoing DNA synthesis.

USES
Treatment of cancer of the breast, pancreas, and lung

PHARMACOKINETICS
Not extensively distributed after IV infusion (increased with length of infusion). Protein binding: less than 10%. Excreted primarily in urine as metabolite. *Half-life:* 42–94 min (influenced by gender of patient and duration of infusion).

INDICATIONS AND DOSAGES
▸ **Non–Small-Cell Lung Cancer (in Combination with Cisplatin)**
IV

Adults, Elderly, Children. 1000 mg/m^2 on days 1, 8 and 15, repeated every 28 days; or 1250 mg/m^2 on days 1 and 8. Repeat every 21 days.
▸ **Pancreatic Cancer**
IV

Adults. 1000 mg/m^2 once weekly for up to 7 wk or until toxicity necessitates decreasing dosage or withholding the dose, followed by 1 wk of rest. Subsequent cycles should consist of once-weekly dose for 3 consecutive wk out of every 4 wk. For patients completing cycles at 1000 mg/m^2, increase dose to 1250 mg/m^2 as tolerated. Dose for next cycle may be increased to 1500 mg/m^2.

▸ **Dosage Reduction Guidelines**
Dosage adjustments should be on the basis of granulocyte count and platelet count, as follows:

Absolute Granulocyte Counts (cells/mm^3)	Platelet Count (cells/mm^3)	% of Full Dose
1000	100,000	100
500–999	50,000–99,999	75
Fewer than 500	Fewer than 50,000	Hold

G

G

SIDE EFFECTS/ADVERSE REACTIONS

Frequent

Nausea and vomiting, generalized pain, fever, mild to moderate pruritic rash, mild to moderate dyspnea, constipation, peripheral edema

Occasional

Diarrhea, petechiae, alopecia, stomatitis, infection, somnolence, paresthesia

Rare

Diaphoresis, rhinitis, insomnia, malaise

PRECAUTIONS AND CONTRAINDICATIONS

None known

DRUG INTERACTIONS OF CONCERN TO DENTISTRY

• None reported

SERIOUS REACTIONS

! Severe myelosuppression, as evidenced by anemia, thrombocytopenia, and leukopenia, is a common reaction.

DENTAL CONSIDERATIONS

General:

• Monitor vital signs at every appointment because of cardiovascular side effects.

• Consider semisupine chair position for patients with respiratory disease.

• If additional analgesia is required for dental pain, consider alternative analgesics in patients taking narcotics for acute or chronic pain.

• Examine for oral manifestation of opportunistic infection.

• Avoid products that affect platelet function, such as aspirin and NSAIDs.

• This drug may be used in the hospital or on an outpatient basis. Confirm the patient's disease and treatment status.

• Chlorhexidine mouth rinse prior to and during chemotherapy may reduce severity of mucositis.

• Patient on chronic drug therapy may rarely present with symptoms of blood dyscrasias, which can include infection, bleeding, and poor healing. If dyscrasia is present, caution patient to prevent oral tissue trauma when using oral hygiene aids.

• Palliative medication may be required for management of oral side effects.

• Short appointments and a stress-reduction protocol may be required for anxious patients.

• Patients may be at risk of bleeding; check for oral signs.

• Oral infections should be eliminated and/or treated aggressively.

Consultations:

• Medical consultation should include routine blood counts including platelet counts and bleeding time.

• Consult physician; prophylactic or therapeutic antiinfectives may be indicated if surgery or periodontal treatment is required.

• Medical consultation may be required to assess immunologic status during cancer chemotherapy and determine safety risk, if any, posed by the required dental treatment.

• Medical consultation may be required to assess disease control and patient's ability to tolerate stress.

Teach Patient/Family to:

• Be aware of oral side effects.

• Use effective, atraumatic oral hygiene to prevent soft tissue inflammation.

• Report oral lesions, soreness, or bleeding to dentist.

• Prevent trauma when using oral hygiene aids.

• Update health and medication history if physician makes any changes in evaluation or drug regimens; include OTC, herbal, and nonherbal remedies in the update.

gemfibrozil
jem-**fi**′-broe-zil
(Apo-Gemfibrozil[CAN],
Ausgem[AUS],
Gemfibromax[AUS], Jezil[AUS],
Lipazil[AUS], Lopid,
Novo-Gemfibrozil[CAN])
Do not confuse Lopid with
Lorabid or Levbid.

CATEGORY AND SCHEDULE
Pregnancy Risk Category: C

Drug Class: Antihyperlipidemic

MECHANISM OF ACTION
A fibric acid derivative that inhibits lipolysis of fat in adipose tissue; decreases liver uptake of free fatty acids and reduces hepatic triglyceride production. Inhibits synthesis of very low-density lipoproteins (VLDLs) carrier apolipoprotein B.
Therapeutic Effect: Lowers serum cholesterol and triglycerides (decreases VLDL, low-density lipoproteins [LDLs]; increases high-density lipoproteins [HDLs]).

USES
Treatment of type IIb, IV, and V hyperlipidemia

PHARMACOKINETICS
Well absorbed from the GI tract. Protein binding: 99%. Metabolized in liver. Primarily excreted in urine. Not removed by hemodialysis.
Half-life: 1.5 hr.

INDICATIONS AND DOSAGES
▶ **Hyperlipidemia**
PO
Adults, Elderly. 1200 mg/day in 2 divided doses 30 min before breakfast and dinner.

SIDE EFFECTS/ADVERSE REACTIONS
Frequent
Dyspepsia
Occasional
Abdominal pain, diarrhea, nausea, vomiting, fatigue
Rare
Constipation, acute appendicitis, vertigo, headache, rash, pruritus, altered taste

PRECAUTIONS AND CONTRAINDICATIONS
Liver dysfunction (including primary biliary cirrhosis), preexisting gallbladder disease, severe renal dysfunction
Caution:
Monitor hematologic and hepatic function, lactation

DRUG INTERACTIONS OF CONCERN TO DENTISTRY
• None reported

SERIOUS REACTIONS
! Cholelithiasis, cholecystitis, acute appendicitis, pancreatitis, and malignancy occur rarely.

DENTAL CONSIDERATIONS
General:
• Patients on chronic drug therapy may rarely have symptoms of blood dyscrasias, which can include infection, bleeding, and poor healing.
Consultations:
• In a patient with symptoms of blood dyscrasias, request a medical consultation for blood studies and

postpone dental treatment until normal values are reestablished.

gemifloxacin mesylate

jem-ih-**flocks**'-ah-sin **mess**'-ah-late
(Factive)

CATEGORY AND SCHEDULE
Pregnancy Risk Category: C

Drug Class: Fluoroquinolone antiinfective

MECHANISM OF ACTION
A fluoroquinolone that inhibits the enzyme DNA gyrase in susceptible microorganisms, interfering with bacterial cell replication and repair. *Therapeutic Effect:* Bactericidal.

USES
Treatment of acute bacterial exacerbation of chronic bronchitis caused by susceptible strains of *S. pneumoniae, H. influenzae, H. parainfluenzae,* or *M. catarrhalis;* community-acquired pneumonia caused by susceptible strains of *S. pneumoniae* (except drug-resistant strains), *H. influenzae, M. catarrhalis, M. pneumoniae, C. pneumoniae,* or *K. pneumoniae*

PHARMACOKINETICS
Rapidly and well absorbed from the GI tract. Protein binding: 70%. Widely distributed. Penetrates well into lung tissue and fluid. Undergoes limited metabolism in the liver. Primarily excreted in feces; lesser amount eliminated in urine. Partially removed by hemodialysis. *Half-life:* 4–12 hr.

INDICATIONS AND DOSAGES
▸ **Acute Bacterial Exacerbation of Chronic Bronchitis**
PO
Adults, Elderly. 320 mg once a day for 5 days.
▸ **Community-Acquired Pneumonia**
PO
Adults, Elderly. 320 mg once a day for 7 days.
▸ **Dosage in Renal Impairment**
Dosage and frequency are modified on the basis of creatinine clearance.

Creatinine Clearance	Dosage
Greater than 40 ml/min	320 mg once a day
40 ml/min or less	160 mg once a day

SIDE EFFECTS/ADVERSE REACTION
Occasional
Diarrhea, rash, nausea
Rare
Headache, abdominal pain, dizziness, tendon ruptures

PRECAUTIONS AND CONTRAINDICATIONS
Concurrent use of amiodarone, quinidine, procainamide, or sotalol; history of prolonged QT interval; hypersensitivity to fluoroquinolones; uncorrected electrolyte disorders (such as hypokalemia and hypomagnesemia)
Caution:
Safety and efficacy in children younger than 18 yr, pregnancy and nursing not established; may prolong QT interval, risk of tendinitis and tendon rupture, epilepsy, cerebral arteriosclerosis, renal dysfunction

DRUG INTERACTIONS OF CONCERN TO DENTISTRY
• Decreased absorption: divalent or trivalent antacids, iron or zinc salts
• Use with caution or avoid drugs that affect QT interval: erythromycin, antipsychotics, tricyclic antidepressants

SERIOUS REACTIONS
! Antibiotic-associated colitis may result from altered bacterial balance. Hypersensitivity reactions, including photosensitivity (as evidenced by rash, pruritus, blisters, edema, and burning skin), have occurred in patients receiving fluoroquinolones.

DENTAL CONSIDERATIONS

General:
• Determine why patient is taking the drug.
• Avoid dental light in patient's eyes; offer dark glasses for patient comfort.
• Examine for oral manifestation of opportunistic infection.
• Advise patient if dental drugs prescribed have a potential for photosensitivity.
• As with other fluoroquinolones there is a risk of tendinitis and tendon rupture.
• Consider semisupine chair position for patient comfort if GI side effects occur.
Consultations:
• Consult with patient's physician if an acute dental infection occurs and another antiinfective is required.
Teach Patient/Family:
• When chronic dry mouth occurs, advise patient to:
  • Avoid mouth rinses with high alcohol content because of drying effects.
  • Use daily home fluoride products for anticaries effect.

• Use sugarless gum, frequent sips of water, or saliva substitutes.

gentamicin sulfate
jen-ta-**mye'**-sin **suhl'**-fate
(Alcomicin[CAN], Cidomycin[CAN], Garamycin, Genoptic, Gentak, Gentacidin)

CATEGORY AND SCHEDULE
Pregnancy Risk Category: C

Drug Class: Aminoglycoside antiinfective ophthalmic

MECHANISM OF ACTION
An aminoglycoside antibiotic that irreversibly binds to the protein of bacterial ribosomes.
Therapeutic Effect: Interferes with protein synthesis of susceptible microorganisms. Bacteriostatic.

USES
Treatment of external eye infection

PHARMACOKINETICS
Rapid, complete absorption after IM administration. Protein binding: less than 30%. Widely distributed (does not cross the blood-brain barrier, low concentrations in CSF). Excreted unchanged in urine. Removed by hemodialysis. *Half-life:* 2–4 hr (increased in impaired renal function and neonates; decreased in cystic fibrosis and burn or febrile patients).

G

INDICATIONS AND DOSAGES

▸ **Acute Pelvic, Bone, Intraabdominal, Joint, Respiratory Tract, Burn Wound, Postoperative and Skin or Skin-Structure Infections; Complicated UTIs; Septicemia; Meningitis**

IV, IM

Adults, Elderly. Usual dosage, 3–6 mg/kg/day in divided doses q8h or 4–6.6 mg/kg once a day.
Children 5–12 yr. Usual dosage 2–2.5 mg/kg/dose q8h.
Children younger than 5 yr. Usual dosage, 2.5 mg/kg/dose q8h.
Neonates. Usual dosage 2.5–3.5 mg/kg/dose q8–12h.

▸ **Hemodialysis**

IV, IM

Adults, Elderly. 0.5–0.7 mg/kg/dose after dialysis.
Children. 1.25–1.75 mg/kg/dose after dialysis.

Intrathecal

Adults. 4–8 mg/day.
Children 3 mo–12 yr. 1–2 mg/day.
Neonates. 1 mg/day.

▸ **Superficial Eye Infections**

Ophthalmic Ointment

Adults, Elderly. Usual dosage, apply thin strip to conjunctiva 2–3 times a day.

Ophthalmic Solution

Adults, Elderly, Children. Usual dosage, 1–2 drops q2–4h up to 2 drops/hr.

▸ **Superficial Skin Infections**

Topical

Adults, Elderly. Usual dosage, apply 3–4 times a day.

▸ **Dosage in Renal Impairment**

Creatinine clearance greater than 41–60 ml/min. Dosage interval q12h.
Creatinine clearance 20–40 ml/min. Dosage interval q24h.
Creatinine clearance less than 20 ml/min. Monitor levels to determine dosage interval.

SIDE EFFECTS/ADVERSE REACTIONS

Occasional
IM: Pain, induration
IV: Phlebitis, thrombophlebitis, hypersensitivity reactions (fever, pruritus, rash, urticaria)
Ophthalmic: Burning, tearing, itching, blurred vision
Topical: Redness, itching
Rare
Alopecia, hypertension, weakness
EENT: Poor corneal wound healing, temporary visual haze, overgrowth of nonsusceptible organisms

PRECAUTIONS AND CONTRAINDICATIONS

Hypersensitivity to gentamicin, other aminoglycosides (cross-sensitivity), or their components; sulfite sensitivity may result in anaphylaxis, especially in asthmatic patients.
Caution:
Antibiotic hypersensitivity

DRUG INTERACTIONS OF CONCERN TO DENTISTRY

• Increased risk of nephrotoxicity: cephalosporins, vancomycin, enflurane
• Increased neuromuscular blockade: neuromuscular-blocking drugs

SERIOUS REACTIONS

! Nephrotoxicity (as evidenced by increased BUN and serum creatinine levels and decreased creatinine clearance) may be reversible if the drug is stopped at the first sign of symptoms.
! Irreversible ototoxicity (manifested as tinnitus, dizziness, ringing or roaring in the ears, and diminished hearing) and neurotoxicity (as evidenced by headache, dizziness, lethargy, tremors, and visual disturbances) occur occasionally. The risk of these effects increases

with higher dosages or prolonged therapy and when the solution is applied directly to the mucosa.
! Suprainfections, particularly with fungal infections, may result from bacterial imbalance no matter which administration route is used.
! Ophthalmic application may cause paresthesia of conjunctiva or mydriasis.

DENTAL CONSIDERATIONS

General:
• For selected infections in the hospital setting; provide emergency dental treatment only.
• Examine for oral manifestation of opportunistic infection.
• Determine why patient is taking the drug.
• Caution patient regarding allergy to medication.
Consultations:
• Medical consultation may be required to assess disease control and patient's ability to tolerate stress.
Teach Patient/Family to:
• Encourage effective oral hygiene to prevent soft tissue inflammation.
• Prevent trauma when using oral hygiene aids.
• Report oral lesions, soreness, or bleeding to dentist.

gentamicin sulfate; prednisolone acetate
jen-ta-**mye**′sin **suhl**′-feyt;
pred-**nis**′-oh-lone **ass**′-eh-tayte
(Pred-G, Pred-G S.O.P.)

CATEGORY AND SCHEDULE
Pregnancy Risk Category: C

Drug Class: Aminoglycoside antiinfective ophthalmic

MECHANISM OF ACTION
Gentamicin is an aminoglycoside that irreversibly binds to the protein of bacterial ribosomes. Prednisolone is an adrenal corticosteroid that inhibits accumulation of inflammatory cells at inflammation sites, phagocytosis, lysosomal enzyme release, and synthesis and release of mediators of inflammation.
Therapeutic Effect: Interferes in protein synthesis of susceptible microorganisms. Prevents or suppresses cell-mediated immune reactions; decreases or prevents tissue response to inflammatory process.

USES
Treatment of external eye infection

PHARMACOKINETICS
None reported

INDICATIONS AND DOSAGES
▸ **Treatment of Steroid Responsive Inflammatory Conditions, Superficial Ocular Infections**
Ophthalmic Ointment
Adults, Elderly. Apply ½ inch ribbon in the conjunctival sac 1–3 times a day.
Ophthalmic Suspension
Adults, Elderly. Instill 1 drop 2–4 times a day. During the initial 24–48 hr, the dosing frequency may be increased if necessary up to 1 drop/hr.

SIDE EFFECTS/ADVERSE REACTIONS
Occasional
Burning, tearing, itching, blurred vision
Rare
Delayed wound healing, secondary infection, intraocular pressure increased, glaucoma

PRECAUTIONS AND CONTRAINDICATIONS

Viral disease of the cornea and conjunctiva (including epithelia herpes simplex keratitis, vaccinia, varicella), mycobacterial or fungal infection of the eye, uncomplicated removal of a corneal foreign body, hypersensitivity to gentamicin, prednisolone, other aminoglycosides, or corticosteroids, or any component of the formulation

SERIOUS REACTIONS

! Optic nerve damage occurs rarely.

DENTAL CONSIDERATIONS

General:
• Avoid dental light in patient's eyes; offer dark glasses for patient comfort.

glatiramer
gla-**teer**′-ah-mer
(Copaxone)
Do not confuse Copaxone with Compazine.

CATEGORY AND SCHEDULE
Pregnancy Risk Category: B

Drug Class: Multiple sclerosis agent

MECHANISM OF ACTION

An immunosuppressive whose exact mechanism is unknown. May act by modifying immune processes thought to be responsible for the pathogenesis of multiple sclerosis. *Therapeutic Effect:* Slows progression of multiple sclerosis.

USES

Reduction of the frequency of relapses in patients with relapsing-remitting multiple sclerosis

PHARMACOKINETICS

Substantial fraction of glatiramer is hydrolyzed locally. Some fraction of injected material enters lymphatic circulation, reaching regional lymph nodes; some may enter systemic circulation intact.

INDICATIONS AND DOSAGES
▸ **Multiple Sclerosis**
Subcutaneous
Adults, Elderly. 20 mg once a day.

SIDE EFFECTS/ADVERSE REACTIONS

Expected
Pain, erythema, inflammation, or pruritus at injection site; asthenia
Frequent
Arthralgia, vasodilation, anxiety, hypertonia, nausea, transient chest pain, dyspnea, flu-like symptoms, rash, pruritus
Occasional
Palpitations, back pain, diaphoresis, rhinitis, diarrhea, urinary urgency
Rare
Anorexia, fever, neck pain, peripheral edema, ear pain, facial edema, vertigo, vomiting

PRECAUTIONS AND CONTRAINDICATIONS

Hypersensitivity to glatiramer or mannitol

DRUG INTERACTIONS OF CONCERN TO DENTISTRY

• Dental drug interactions have not been studied.

SERIOUS REACTIONS

! Infection is a common effect.
! Lymphadenopathy occurs occasionally.

DENTAL CONSIDERATIONS

General:
• Monitor vital signs at every appointment because of cardiovascular side effects.
• Protect patient's eyes from accidental spatter during dental treatment.
• Avoid dental light in patient's eyes; offer dark glasses for patient comfort.
• Short appointments may be required because of effects of disease on musculature.
• Short appointments and a stress-reduction protocol may be required for anxious patients.
• Advise patient if dental drugs prescribed have a potential for photosensitivity.
• Inquire about history of disease, any physical limitations, and other drugs the patient may be taking.
• For longer dental appointments, offer patient frequent breaks.

Consultations:
• Consultation with physician may be necessary if sedation or general anesthesia is required.
• Medical consultation may be required to assess disease control and patient's ability to tolerate stress.

Teach Patient/Family to:
• Encourage effective oral hygiene to prevent soft tissue inflammation.
• Prevent trauma when using oral hygiene aids.
• Update health and medication history if physician makes any changes in evaluation or drug regimens; include OTC, herbal, and nonherbal remedies in the update.

glimepiride
gly-**mep**′-er-ide
(Amaryl)
Do not confuse glimepiride with glipizide or glyburide.

CATEGORY AND SCHEDULE
Pregnancy Risk Category: C

Drug Class: Oral antidiabetic (second generation)

MECHANISM OF ACTION
A second-generation sulfonylurea that promotes release of insulin from beta cells of the pancreas and increases insulin sensitivity at peripheral sites.
Therapeutic Effect: Lowers blood glucose concentration.

USES
Stable adult-onset diabetes mellitus (type II); may also be used with insulin or metformin where diet and exercise are not effective in controlling hyperglycemia.

PHARMACOKINETICS

Route	Onset	Peak	Duration
PO	N/A	2–3 hr	24 hr

Completely absorbed from the GI tract. Protein binding: greater than 99%. Metabolized in the liver. Excreted in urine and eliminated in feces. *Half-life:* 5–9.2 hr.

INDICATIONS AND DOSAGES
▶ **Diabetes Mellitus**
PO
Adults, Elderly. Initially, 1–2 mg once a day, with breakfast or first main meal. Maintenance: 1–4 mg once a day. After dose of 2 mg is

reached, dosage should be increased in increments of up to 2 mg q1–2wk, on the basis of blood glucose response. Maximum: 8 mg/day.

▸ **Dosage in Renal Impairment**
PO
Adults. 1 mg once a day.

SIDE EFFECTS/ADVERSE REACTIONS
Frequent
Altered taste sensation, dizziness, somnolence, weight gain, constipation, diarrhea, heartburn, nausea, vomiting, stomach fullness, headache
Occasional
Increased sensitivity of skin to sunlight, peeling of skin, itching, rash

PRECAUTIONS AND CONTRAINDICATIONS
Diabetic complications, such as ketosis, acidosis and diabetic coma; severe hepatic or renal impairment; monotherapy for type 1 diabetes mellitus; stress situations, including severe infection, trauma, and surgery
Caution:
Malnourished; adrenal, pituitary, or hepatic insufficiency; hypoglycemia recognition in elderly or in those taking β-blockers; increased risk of cardiovascular mortality has been reported in patients using oral hypoglycemics; alcohol use; lactation; children

DRUG INTERACTIONS OF CONCERN TO DENTISTRY
• Risk of potentiation of hypoglycemic effects: NSAIDs, salicylates, sulfonamides, β-adrenergic blockers, ketoconazole

SERIOUS REACTIONS
❗ Overdose or insufficient food intake may produce hypoglycemia, especially with increased glucose demands.
❗ GI hemorrhage, cholestatic hepatic jaundice, leukopenia, thrombocytopenia, pancytopenia, agranulocytosis, and aplastic or hemolytic anemia occur rarely.

DENTAL CONSIDERATIONS
General:
• Short appointments and a stress-reduction protocol may be required for anxious patients.
• Question patient about self-monitoring of drug's antidiabetic effect, including blood glucose values or finger-stick records.
• Ensure that patient is following prescribed diet and regularly takes medication.
• Patients on chronic drug therapy may rarely have symptoms of blood dyscrasias, which can include infection, bleeding, and poor healing.
• Diabetics may be more susceptible to infection and have delayed wound healing.
• Place on frequent recall to evaluate healing response.
• Advise patient if dental drugs prescribed have a potential for photosensitivity.
Consultations:
• Medical consultation may be required to assess disease control.
• In a patient with symptoms of blood dyscrasias, request a medical consultation for blood studies and postpone treatment until normal values are reestablished.
• Medical consultation may include data from patient's blood glucose monitoring, including glycosylated hemoglobin or HbA$_{1c}$ testing.

Teach Patient/Family to:
• Encourage effective oral hygiene to prevent soft tissue inflammation.
• Use caution to prevent trauma when using oral hygiene aids.
• Update health and drug history if physician makes any changes in evaluation or drug regimens.

glipizide
glip′-ih-zide
(Glucotrol, Glucotrol XL, Melizide[AUS], Mini DiaB[AUS])
Do not confuse glipizide with glimepiride or glyburide.

CATEGORY AND SCHEDULE
Pregnancy Risk Category: C

Drug Class: Oral antidiabetic (second generation)

MECHANISM OF ACTION
A second-generation sulfonylurea that promotes the release of insulin from beta cells of the pancreas and increases insulin sensitivity at peripheral sites.
Therapeutic Effect: Lowers blood glucose concentration.

USES
Stable adult-onset diabetes mellitus (Type 2)

PHARMACOKINETICS

Route	Onset	Peak	Duration
PO	15–30 min	2–3 hr	12–24 hr
Extended	2–3 hr	6–12 hr	24 hr

Well absorbed from the GI tract. Protein binding: 99%. Metabolized in the liver. Excreted in urine.
Half-life: 2–4 hr.

INDICATIONS AND DOSAGES
▶ Diabetes Mellitus
PO
Adults. Initially, 5 mg/day or 2.5 mg in the elderly or those with hepatic disease. Adjust dosage in 2.5- to 5-mg increments at intervals of several days. Maximum single dose: 15 mg. Maximum dose/day: 40 mg. Maintenance (extended-release tablet): 20 mg/day.
Elderly. Initially, 2.5–5 mg/day. May increase by 2.5–5 mg/day q1–2wk.

SIDE EFFECTS/ADVERSE REACTIONS
Frequent
Altered taste sensation, dizziness, somnolence, weight gain, constipation, diarrhea, heartburn, nausea, vomiting, stomach fullness, headache
Occasional
Increased sensitivity of skin to sunlight, peeling of skin, itching, rash

PRECAUTIONS AND CONTRAINDICATIONS
Diabetic ketoacidosis with or without coma, type 1 diabetes mellitus
Caution:
Elderly, cardiac disease, severe renal disease, severe hepatic disease, thyroid disease

DRUG INTERACTIONS OF CONCERN TO DENTISTRY
• Increased hypoglycemic effects: salicylates, ketoconazole
• Decreased action of glipizide: corticosteroids
• Disulfiram-like reaction: alcohol

SERIOUS REACTIONS
! Overdose or insufficient food intake may produce hypoglycemia, especially with increased glucose demands.

G

G

! GI hemorrhage, cholestatic hepatic jaundice, leukopenia, thrombocytopenia, pancytopenia, agranulocytosis, and aplastic or hemolytic anemia occurs rarely.

DENTAL CONSIDERATIONS

General:
• Monitor vital signs at every appointment because of cardiovascular side effects.
• Patients on chronic drug therapy may rarely have symptoms of blood dyscrasias, which can include infection, bleeding, and poor healing.
• Short appointments and a stress-reduction protocol may be required for anxious patients.
• Place on frequent recall to evaluate healing response.
• Diabetics may be more susceptible to infection and have delayed wound healing.
• Question patient about self-monitoring of drug's antidiabetic effect, including blood glucose values or finger-stick records.
• Ensure that patient is following prescribed diet and regularly takes medication.
• Avoid prescribing aspirin-containing products.
Consultations:
• In a patient with symptoms of blood dyscrasias, request a medical consultation for blood studies and postpone dental treatment until normal values are reestablished.
• Medical consultation may be required to assess disease control.
• Medical consultation may include data from patient's blood glucose monitoring, including glycosylated hemoglobin or HbA_{1c} testing.
Teach Patient/Family to:
• Encourage effective oral hygiene to prevent soft tissue inflammation.

• Use caution to prevent injury when using oral hygiene aids.
• Avoid mouth rinses with high alcohol content because of drying effects.

glucagon hydrochloride

glue′-ka-gon hi-droh-**klor**′-ide
(GlucaGen, GlucaGen Diagnostic Kit, GlucaGen[AUS], Glucagon, Glucagon Diagnostic Kit, Glucagon Emergency Kit)
Do not confuse glucagon with Glaucon.

CATEGORY AND SCHEDULE
Pregnancy Risk Category: B

Drug Class: Antihypoglycemic, hormone

MECHANISM OF ACTION
A glucose-elevating agent that promotes hepatic glycogenolysis, gluconeogenesis. Stimulates production of cyclic adenosine monophosphate (cAMP), which results in increased plasma glucose concentration, smooth muscle relaxation, and an inotropic myocardial effect.
Therapeutic Effect: Increases plasma glucose level.

USES
Severe hypoglycemia; as a diagnostic aid to facilitate in the radiologic examination of the GI tract by relaxing smooth muscle

PHARMACOKINETICS
Parenteral: Peak levels in 20 min (subcutaneous) or 13 min (IM); extensively metabolized in liver, kidney, and plasma.

INDICATIONS AND DOSAGES
▸ **Hypoglycemia**

IV, IM, Subcutaneous
Adults, Elderly, Children weighing more than 20 kg. 0.5–1 mg. May give 1 or 2 additional doses if response is delayed.
Children weighing 20 kg or less. 0.5 mg.

▸ **Diagnostic Aid**

IV, IM
Adults, Elderly. 0.25–2 mg 10 min prior to procedure.

SIDE EFFECTS/ADVERSE REACTIONS

Occasional
Nausea, vomiting
Rare
Allergic reaction, such as urticaria, respiratory distress, and hypotension

PRECAUTIONS AND CONTRAINDICATIONS

Hypersensitivity to glucagon or beef or pork proteins, known pheochromocytoma
Caution:
For hypoglycemia in type 1 diabetes give supplemental carbohydrates as soon as possible; insulinoma, starvation, glycogen depletion, adrenal insufficiency, chronic hypoglycemia, lactation

DRUG INTERACTIONS OF CONCERN TO DENTISTRY

• Patients taking β-adrenergic blockers: may be expected to have a transient but greater increase in B/P and pulse

SERIOUS REACTIONS

! Overdose may produce persistent nausea and vomiting and hypokalemia, marked by severe weakness, decreased appetite, irregular heartbeat, and muscle cramps.

DENTAL CONSIDERATIONS

General:
• Glucagon may be used as an emergency drug for severe hypoglycemia. Patients should be closely monitored and referred immediately for evaluation.
• IV glucose may be required for patients nonresponsive to glucagon.
• Unconscious patients should awaken within 15 min or less.

G

---

glyburide
glye′-byoor-ide
(Daonil[CAN], DiaBeta, Euglucon[CAN], Glimel[AUS], Glynase, Micronase, Semi-Daonil[AUS], Semi-Euglucon[AUS])
Do not confuse glyburide with glimepiride or glipizide, or Micronase with Micro-K or Micronor.

CATEGORY AND SCHEDULE
Pregnancy Risk Category: C

Drug Class: Oral antidiabetic (second-generation)

MECHANISM OF ACTION
A second-generation sulfonylurea that promotes release of insulin from beta cells of the pancreas and increases insulin sensitivity at peripheral sites.
Therapeutic Effect: Lowers blood glucose concentration.

USES
Treatment of stable adult-onset diabetes mellitus (Type 2)

PHARMACOKINETICS

Route	Onset	Peak	Duration
PO	0.25–1 hr	1–2 hr	12–24 hr

Well absorbed from the GI tract. Protein binding: 99%. Metabolized in the liver to weakly active metabolite. Primarily excreted in urine. Not removed by hemodialysis. *Half-life:* 1.4–1.8 hr.

INDICATIONS AND DOSAGES
▸ **Diabetes Mellitus**
PO
Adults. Initially, 2.5–5 mg. May increase by 2.5 mg/day at weekly intervals. Maintenance: 1.25–20 mg/day. Maximum: 20 mg/day.
Elderly. Initially, 1.25–2.5 mg/day. May increase by 1.25–2.5 mg/day at 1- to 3-wk intervals.
PO (Micronized Tablets [Glynase])
Adults, Elderly. Initially, 0.75–3 mg/day. May increase by 1.5 mg/day at weekly intervals. Maintenance: 0.75–12 mg/day as a single dose or in divided doses.
▸ **Dosage in Renal Impairment**
Glyburide is not recommended in patients with creatinine clearance less than 50 ml/min.

SIDE EFFECTS/ADVERSE REACTIONS
Frequent
Altered taste sensation, dizziness, somnolence, weight gain, constipation, diarrhea, heartburn, nausea, vomiting, stomach fullness, headache
Occasional
Increased sensitivity of skin to sunlight, peeling of skin, itching, rash

PRECAUTIONS AND CONTRAINDICATIONS
Diabetic ketoacidosis with or without coma, monotherapy for type 1 diabetes mellitus

Caution:
Elderly, cardiac disease, severe renal disease, severe hepatic disease, thyroid disease, severe hypoglycemia reactions

DRUG INTERACTIONS OF CONCERN TO DENTISTRY
• Increased hypoglycemic effects: NSAIDs, salicylates, ketoconazole
• Decreased action of glyburide: corticosteroids
• Disulfiram-like reaction: alcohol

SERIOUS REACTIONS
❗ Overdose or insufficient food intake may produce hypoglycemia, especially in patients with increased glucose demands.
❗ Cholestatic jaundice, leukopenia, thrombocytopenia, pancytopenia, agranulocytosis, and aplastic or hemolytic anemia occur rarely.

DENTAL CONSIDERATIONS
General:
• Monitor vital signs at every appointment because of cardiovascular side effects.
• Patients on chronic drug therapy may rarely have symptoms of blood dyscrasias, which can include infection, bleeding, and poor healing.
• Place on frequent recall to evaluate healing response.
• Ensure that patient is following prescribed diet and regularly takes medication.
• Short appointments and stress-reduction protocol may be required for anxious patients.
• Patients with diabetes may be more susceptible to infection and have delayed wound healing.
• Question patient about self-monitoring of drug's antidiabetic

effect, including blood glucose values or finger-stick records.
• Avoid prescribing aspirin-containing products.
Consultations:
• In a patient with symptoms of blood dyscrasias, request a medical consultation for blood studies and postpone dental treatment until normal values are reestablished.
• Medical consultation may be required to assess disease control.
• Medical consultation may include data from patient's blood glucose monitoring, including glycosylated hemoglobin or HbA$_{1c}$ testing.
Teach Patient/Family to:
• Encourage effective oral hygiene to prevent soft tissue inflammation.
• Use caution to prevent injury when using oral hygiene aids.
• Avoid mouth rinses with high alcohol content because of drying effects.

glycopyrrolate
glye-koe-**pye**′-roe-late
(Robinul, Robinul Forte, Robinul Injection[AUS])
Do not confuse Robinul with Reminyl.

CATEGORY AND SCHEDULE
Pregnancy Risk Category: B

Drug Class: Anticholinergic

MECHANISM OF ACTION
A quaternary anticholinergic that inhibits action of acetylcholine at postganglionic parasympathetic sites in smooth muscle, secretory glands, and CNS.
Therapeutic Effect: Reduces salivation and excessive secretions of respiratory tract; reduces gastric secretions and acidity.

USES
Decreased secretions before surgery, reversal of neuromuscular blockade, peptic ulcer disease, irritable bowel syndrome

PHARMACOKINETICS
Poorly and irregularly absorbed from GI tract after oral administration. Metabolized in the liver. Primarily excreted in urine. *Half-life:* 1.7 hr.

INDICATIONS AND DOSAGES
▸ **Preoperative Inhibition of Salivation and Excessive Respiratory Tract Secretions**
IM
Adults, Elderly. 4 mcg/kg 30–60 min before procedure.
Children 2 yr and older. 4 mcg/kg.
Children younger than 2 yr. 4–9 mcg/kg.
▸ **To Block Effects of Anticholinesterase Agents**
IV
Adults, Elderly. 0.2 mg for each 1 mg neostigmine or 5 mg pyridostigmine.
▸ **Peptic Ulcer Disease, Adjunct**
IV, IM
Adults, Elderly. 0.1 mg IV or IM 3–4 times a day.
PO
Adults, Elderly. 1–2 mg 2–3 times a day. Maximum: 8 mg/day.

SIDE EFFECTS/ADVERSE REACTIONS
Frequent
Dry mouth, decreased sweating, constipation
Occasional
Blurred vision, gastric bloating, urinary hesitancy, somnolence (with high dosage), headache, intolerance to light, loss of taste, nervousness, flushing, insomnia, impotence, mental confusion or excitement

G

(particularly in the elderly and children), temporary light-headedness (with parenteral form), local irritation (with parenteral form)

Rare

Dizziness, faintness

PRECAUTIONS AND CONTRAINDICATIONS

Acute hemorrhage, myasthenia gravis, narrow-angle glaucoma, obstructive uropathy, paralytic ileus, tachycardia, ulcerative colitis

Caution:

Elderly, lactation, prostatic hypertrophy, renal disease, CHF, pulmonary disease, hyperthyroidism

DRUG INTERACTIONS OF CONCERN TO DENTISTRY

• Increased anticholinergic effect: antihistamines, phenothiazines, meperidine, haloperidol, scopolamine, atropine
• Do not mix with diazepam, pentobarbital, in syringe or solution
• Constipation, urinary retention: opioid analgesics
• Reduced absorption of ketoconazole

SERIOUS REACTIONS

! Overdose may produce temporary paralysis of ciliary muscle; pupillary dilation; tachycardia; palpitations; hot, dry, or flushed skin; absence of bowel sounds; hyperthermia; increased respiratory rate; ECG abnormalities; nausea; vomiting; rash over face or upper trunk; CNS stimulation; and psychosis (marked by agitation, restlessness, rambling speech, visual hallucinations, paranoid behavior, and delusions, followed by depression).

DENTAL CONSIDERATIONS

General:

• May be useful to control salivation in adults during dental procedures.
• Avoid dental light in patient's eyes; offer dark glasses for patient comfort.
• Assess salivary flow as a factor in caries, periodontal disease, and candidiasis.

Consultation:

• Physician should be informed if significant xerostomic side effects occur (e.g., increased caries, sore tongue, problems eating or swallowing, difficulty wearing prosthesis) so that a medication change can be considered.

Teach Patient/Family:

• When chronic dry mouth occurs, advise patient to:
  • Avoid mouth rinses with high alcohol content because of drying effects.
  • Use daily home fluoride products for anticaries effect.
  • Use sugarless gum, frequent sips of water, or saliva substitutes.

goserelin acetate

gos-er′-ah-lin ass′-eh-tayte
(Zoladex, Zoladex Implant[AUS], Zoladex LA)

CATEGORY AND SCHEDULE

Pregnancy Risk Category: D (advanced breast cancer), X (endometriosis, endometrial thinning)

Drug Class: Gonadotropin-releasing hormone, antineoplastic (hormone); synthetic decapeptide analog of LHRH

MECHANISM OF ACTION

A gonadotropin-releasing hormone analog and antineoplastic agent that stimulates the release of luteinizing hormone (LH) and follicle-stimulating hormone (FSH) from the anterior pituitary gland. In males, increases testosterone concentrations initially, and then suppresses secretion of LH and FSH, resulting in decreased testosterone levels. *Therapeutic Effect:* In females, causes a reduction in ovarian size and function, reduction in uterine and mammary gland size and regression of sex-hormone–responsive tumors. In males, produces pharmacologic castration and decreases the growth of abnormal prostate tissue.

USES

Treatment of advanced prostate cancer stage B2-C (10.8 mg), endometriosis, advanced breast cancer, endometrial thinning (3.6 mg)

PHARMACOKINETICS

Peak serum concentrations in 14–28 days. *Half-life:* 4.5 hr.

INDICATIONS AND DOSAGES
▸ **Prostatic Carcinoma**
Implant
Adults older than 18 yr, Elderly. 3.6 mg every 28 days or 10.8 mg q12wk subcutaneously into upper abdominal wall.
▸ **Breast Carcinoma, Endometriosis**
Implant
Adults. 3.6 mg every 28 days subcutaneously into upper abdominal wall.
▸ **Endometrial Thinning**

Implant
Adults. 3.6 mg subcutaneously into upper abdominal wall as a single dose or in 2 doses 4 wk apart.

SIDE EFFECTS/ADVERSE REACTIONS
Frequent
Headache, hot flashes, depression, diaphoresis, sexual dysfunction, decreased erection, lower urinary tract symptoms
Occasional
Pain, lethargy, dizziness, insomnia, anorexia, nausea, rash, upper respiratory tract infection, hirsutism, abdominal pain
Rare
Pruritus

PRECAUTIONS AND CONTRAINDICATIONS
Pregnancy

DRUG INTERACTIONS OF CONCERN TO DENTISTRY
• None reported

SERIOUS REACTIONS

❗ Arrhythmias, CHF and hypertension occur rarely.
❗ Ureteral obstruction and spinal cord compression have been observed. An immediate orchiectomy may be necessary if these conditions occur.

DENTAL CONSIDERATIONS

General:
• Monitor vital signs at every appointment because of cardiovascular side effects.
• Determine why patient is taking the drug.
• If additional analgesia is required for dental pain, consider alternative analgesics (NSAIDs) in patients taking narcotics for acute or chronic pain.

G

• Consider semisupine chair position for patient comfort if GI side effects occur.
• Assess salivary flow as a factor in caries, periodontal disease, and candidiasis.
• If used in prostate cancer, consider urinary retention concern and avoid anticholinergic drugs that may aggravate retention.
• Patients may be taking other medications; see complete drug and herbal history.

Consultations:
• Medical consultation may be required to assess immunologic status during cancer chemotherapy and determine safety risk, if any, posed by the required dental treatment.
• Medical consultation may be required to assess disease control and patient's ability to tolerate stress.

Teach Patient/Family to:
• When chronic dry mouth occurs advise patient to:
  • Avoid mouth rinses with high alcohol content because of drying effects.
  • Use daily home fluoride products for anticaries effect.
  • Use sugarless gum, frequent sips of water, or saliva substitutes.
• Encourage effective oral hygiene to prevent soft tissue inflammation.
• Report oral lesions, soreness, or bleeding to dentist.
• Prevent trauma when using oral hygiene aids.
• Update health and medication history if physician makes any changes in evaluation or drug regimens; include OTC, herbal, and nonherbal remedies in the update.

granisetron
gra-**ni**'se-tron
(Kytril, Sancuso)

CATEGORY AND SCHEDULE
Pregnancy Risk Category: B

Drug Class: Antiemetics, 5-HT₃ receptor antagonists

MECHANISM OF ACTION
A 5-HT3 receptor antagonist that acts centrally in the chemoreceptor trigger zone of the area postrema, in the brain, and peripherally at the vagal nerve terminals in the intestines.
Therapeutic Effect: Prevents nausea and vomiting.

USES
Prevention of chemotherapy-induced nausea and vomiting
Prevention of radiation-induced nausea and vomiting
Postoperative nausea or vomiting (PONV)

PHARMACOKINETICS

Route	Onset	Peak	Duration
IV	1–3 min	N/A	24 hr
Oral	N/A	N/A	Generally up to 24 hr
Topical	N/A	48 hr	N/A

Rapidly and widely distributed to tissues. Protein binding: 65%. Metabolized in the liver to both active and inactive metabolites. Granisetron is metabolized via CYP3A4 and CYP1A1. Eliminated in urine and feces. Topical: slowly absorbed. *Half-life:* 6 hr (oral), 9 hr (IV), 36 hr (transdermal).

INDICATIONS AND DOSAGES
▶ **Prevention of Chemotherapy-Induced Nausea and Vomiting**
PO
Adults, Elderly. 1 mg 1 hr before chemotherapy, followed by second tablet 12 hr later on the days of chemotherapy or 2 mg as a single dose any time within 1 hr prior to chemotherapy.
IV
Adults, Elderly, Children 2 yr and older. 10 mcg/kg/dose (or 1 mg/dose) within 30 min before chemotherapy.
Transdermal Patch
Adults, 18 yr and older. Apply one patch to clean, dry, intact healthy skin on upper outer arm 24 to 48 hr before chemotherapy; remove at least 24 hr after chemotherapy is completed. May wear patch for up to 7 days. Do not cut patch. Each patch contains 34.3 mg of granisetron; it releases 3.1 mg of granisetron per 24 hr for up to 7 days.
▶ **Prevention of Radiation-Induced Nausea and Vomiting**
PO
Adults, Elderly. 2 mg once a day, given 1 hr before radiation therapy.
▶ **Postoperative Nausea or Vomiting**
PO
Adults, Elderly, Children 4 yr and older. 0–40 mcg/kg as a single postoperative dose.
IV
Adults, Elderly. 1 mg IV push as a single postoperative dose.
Children, 4 yr and older. 20–40 mcg/kg. Maximum: 1 mg.

SIDE EFFECTS/ADVERSE REACTIONS
Frequent
Headache, constipation, asthenia
Occasional
Diarrhea, abdominal pain, somnolence, dyspepsia,
hypertension, fever, dizziness, anxiety, insomnia
Rare
Altered taste, hypersensitivity reaction, QT prolongation

PRECAUTIONS AND CONTRAINDICATIONS
Hypersensitivity to granisetron, benzyl alcohol, or any component of the formulation
Cardiac arrhythmias
Breast-feeding
Caution:
Topical: direct sun or UV light

DRUG INTERACTIONS OF CONCERN TO DENTISTRY
• CYP450 3A4 and 1A1 inducers and inhibitors: May alter granisetron concentrations.
• Apomorphine: May cause profound hypotension and altered consciousness.
• Phenobarbital: May increase plasma clearance.

SERIOUS REACTIONS
❗ Hypertension, hypotension, QT prolongation, arrhythmias such as sinus bradycardia, atrial fibrillation, varying degrees of A-V block, ventricular ectopy including non-sustained tachycardia, and ECG abnormalities have been observed.
❗ Rare cases of hypersensitivity reactions, sometimes severe (e.g., anaphylaxis, shortness of breath, hypotension, urticaria), have been reported.

DENTAL CONSIDERATIONS
General:
• Assess the patient for nausea and vomiting.
Consultations:
• Medical consultation may be required to assess disease control.

G

G

Teach Patient/Family to:
• Inform the patient that granisetron is effective shortly after administration in preventing nausea and vomiting.
• Explain to the patient that the drug may affect the sense of taste temporarily.
• Teach the patient other methods of reducing nausea and vomiting, such as lying quietly and avoiding strong odors.
• Instruct the patient not to apply transdermal patch to red, damaged, or irritated skin. The transdermal system should not be cut.

griseofulvin
griz-ee-oh-**full**'-vin
(Fulvicin P/G, Fulvicin U/F, Grifulvin V, Gris-PEG, Grisovin[AUS])

CATEGORY AND SCHEDULE
Pregnancy Risk Category: C

Drug Class: Antifungal

MECHANISM OF ACTION
An antifungal that inhibits fungal cell mitosis by disrupting mitotic spindle structure.
Therapeutic Effect: Fungistatic.

USES
Mycotic infections: tinea corporis, tinea pedis, tinea cruris, tinea barbae, tinea capitis, tinea unguium if caused by *Epidermophyton, Microsporum,* or *Trichophyton*

PHARMACOKINETICS
Variable GI absorption after oral administration; fatty meals may enhance absorption. Peak blood levels: 4 hr. Deposited in keratinized cells.

INDICATIONS AND DOSAGES
▸ **Tinea Capitis, Tinea Corporis, Tinea Cruris, Tinea Pedis, Tinea Unguium**
PO (Microsize Tablets, Oral Suspension)
Adults. Usual dosage, 500–1000 mg as a single dose or in divided doses.
Children 2 yr and older. Usual dosage, 10–20 mg/kg/day.
PO (Ultramicrosize Tablets)
Adults. Usual dosage, 330–750 mg/day as a single dose or in divided doses.
Children 2 yr and older. 5–10 mg/kg/day.

SIDE EFFECTS/ADVERSE REACTIONS
Occasional
Hypersensitivity reaction (including pruritus, rash and urticaria), headache, nausea, diarrhea, excessive thirst, flatulence, oral thrush, dizziness, insomnia
Rare
Paresthesia of hands or feet, proteinuria, photosensitivity reaction

PRECAUTIONS AND CONTRAINDICATIONS
Hepatocellular failure, porphyria

DRUG INTERACTIONS OF CONCERN TO DENTISTRY
• Possible decreased effects: phenobarbital

SERIOUS REACTIONS
! Granulocytopenia occurs rarely.

DENTAL CONSIDERATIONS

General:
• Determine why patient is taking the drug.
• Assess salivary flow as a factor in caries, periodontal disease, and candidiasis.

• Examine for oral manifestation of opportunistic infection.
• Advise patient if dental drugs prescribed have a potential for photosensitivity.

Teach Patient/Family to:
• Report oral lesions, soreness, or bleeding to dentist.
• Encourage effective oral hygiene to prevent soft tissue inflammation.
• Report sore throat, oral burning sensation, fever, or fatigue, any of which could indicate presence of a superinfection.
• Update health and medication history if physician makes any changes in evaluation or drug regimens; include OTC, herbal, and nonherbal remedies in the update.
• Avoid concurrent use of alcohol.
• When chronic dry mouth occurs advise patient to:
  • Avoid mouth rinses with high alcohol content because of drying effects.
  • Use daily home fluoride products for anticaries effect.
  • Use sugarless gum, frequent sips of water, or saliva substitutes.

guaifenesin

gwye-**fen′**-eh-sin
(Balminil[CAN], Benylin E[CAN], Guiatuss, Humibid LA, Mucinex, Organidin, Robitussin, Tussin)
Do not confuse guaifenesin with guanfacine.

CATEGORY AND SCHEDULE
Pregnancy Risk Category: C
OTC

Drug Class: Expectorant, glyceryl guaiacolate

MECHANISM OF ACTION
An expectorant that stimulates respiratory tract secretions by decreasing adhesiveness and viscosity of phlegm.
Therapeutic Effect: Promotes removal of viscous mucus.

USES
Treatment of dry, nonproductive cough

PHARMACOKINETICS
Well absorbed from the GI tract. Metabolized in the liver. Excreted in urine.

INDICATIONS AND DOSAGES
▸ **Expectorant**
PO
Adults, Elderly, Children older than 12 yr. 200–400 mg q4h.
Children 6–12 yr. 100–200 mg q4h.
Maximum: 1.2 g/day.
Children 2–5 yr. 50–100 mg q4h.
Children younger than 2 yr. 12 mg/kg/day in 6 divided doses.
PO (Extended-Release)
Adults, Elderly, Children older than 12 yr. 600–1200 mg q12h.
Maximum: 2.4 g/day.
Children 2–5 yr. 600 mg q12h.
Maximum: 600 mg/day.

SIDE EFFECTS/ADVERSE REACTIONS
Rare
Dizziness, headache, rash, diarrhea, nausea, vomiting, abdominal pain

PRECAUTIONS AND CONTRAINDICATIONS
Hypersensitivity, persistent cough

SERIOUS REACTIONS
❗ Overdose may produce nausea and vomiting.

G

DENTAL CONSIDERATIONS

General:
• Consider semisupine chair position for patients with respiratory disease.
• Elective dental treatment may be precluded by significant coughing episodes.

guanabenz
gwan′-ah-benz
(Wytensin)

CATEGORY AND SCHEDULE
Pregnancy Risk Category: C

Drug Class: Centrally acting antihypertensive

MECHANISM OF ACTION
An α-adrenergic agonist that stimulates α_2-adrenergic receptors. Inhibits sympathetic CNS cardioaccelerator and vasoconstrictor center impulses to heart, kidneys, peripheral vasculature.
Therapeutic Effect: Decreases systolic, diastolic B/P. Chronic use decreases peripheral vascular resistance.

USES
Treatment of hypertension

PHARMACOKINETICS
Well absorbed from GI tract. Widely distributed. Protein binding: 90%. Metabolized in liver. Excreted in urine and feces. Not removed by hemodialysis. **Half-life:** 6 hr.

INDICATIONS AND DOSAGES
▸ Hypertension
PO
Adults. Initially, 4 mg 2 times a day. Increase by 4–8 mg at 1–2 wk intervals.

Elderly. Initially, 4 mg/day. May increase q1–2 wk. Maintenance: 8–16 mg/day. Maximum: 32 mg/day.

SIDE EFFECTS/ADVERSE REACTIONS
Frequent
Drowsiness, dry mouth, dizziness
Occasional
Weakness, headache, nausea, decreased sexual ability
Rare
Ataxia, sleep disturbances, rash, itching, diarrhea, constipation, altered taste, muscle aches

PRECAUTIONS AND CONTRAINDICATIONS
History of hypersensitivity to guanabenz or any component of the formulation
Caution:
Lactation, children younger than 12 yr, severe coronary insufficiency, recent MI, cerebrovascular disease, severe hepatic or renal failure

DRUG INTERACTIONS OF CONCERN TO DENTISTRY
• Increased CNS depression: alcohol, all CNS depressants
• Decreased hypotensive effects: NSAIDs, especially indomethacin, sympathomimetics

SERIOUS REACTIONS
! Abrupt withdrawal may result in rebound hypertension manifested as nervousness, agitation, anxiety, insomnia, hand tingling, tremors, flushing, and sweating.
! Overdosage produces hypotension, somnolence, lethargy, irritability, bradycardia, and miosis (pupillary constriction).

DENTAL CONSIDERATIONS

General:
• Monitor vital signs at every appointment because of cardiovascular side effects.
• Limit use of sodium-containing products, such as saline IV fluids, for patients with a dietary salt restriction.
• Assess salivary flow as a factor in caries, periodontal disease, and candidiasis.
• Stress from dental procedures may compromise cardiovascular function; determine patient risk.
• Short appointments and a stress-reduction protocol may be required for anxious patients.

Consultations:
• Medical consultation may be required to assess disease control and patient's ability to tolerate stress.

Teach Patient/Family:
• When chronic dry mouth occurs, advise patient to:
  • Avoid mouth rinses with high alcohol content because of drying effects.
  • Use daily home fluoride products for anticaries effect.
  • Use sugarless gum, frequent sips of water, or saliva substitutes.

guanadrel sulfate
gwahn'-ah-drel sull'-fate
(Hylorel)

CATEGORY AND SCHEDULE
Pregnancy Risk Category: C

Drug Class: Antihypertensive

MECHANISM OF ACTION
An adrenergic blocking agent that depletes norepinephrine from adrenergic nerve endings. Prevents release of norepinephrine normally produced by nerve stimulation.
Therapeutic Effect: Reduces B/P.

USES
Treatment of hypertension

PHARMACOKINETICS
Rapidly and well absorbed from GI tract. Widely distributed. Protein binding: 20%. Primarily excreted in urine. *Half-life:* 10 hr.

INDICATIONS AND DOSAGES
▸ Hypertension
PO
Adults. Initially, 5 mg 2 times a day. Increase at 1–4 wk intervals. Maintenance: 20–75 mg/day in 2 divided doses. Maximum: 400 mg/day.
Elderly. Initially, 5 mg/day. May gradually increase at 1–4 wk intervals. Maintenance: 20–75 mg/day in 2 divided doses.

SIDE EFFECTS/ADVERSE REACTIONS
Frequent
Fatigue, headache, faintness, drowsiness, nocturia, urinary frequency, change in weight, aching limbs, shortness of breath (resting)
Occasional
Cough, change in vision, paresthesia, confusion, indigestion, constipation, anorexia, peripheral edema, leg cramps
Rare
Depression, altered sleep, nausea, vomiting, dry mouth, throat, impotence, backache

G

PRECAUTIONS AND CONTRAINDICATIONS

Frank CHF, pheochromocytoma, hypersensitivity to guanadrel or any component of the formulation

Caution:

Elderly, bronchial asthma, peptic ulcer, electrolyte imbalances, vascular disease

DRUG INTERACTIONS OF CONCERN TO DENTISTRY

• Increased orthostatic hypotension: alcohol, opioid analgesics, barbiturates, phenothiazines, haloperidol

• Decreased hypotensive effect: ephedrine, sympathomimetics, NSAIDs, indomethacin, tricyclic antidepressants

SERIOUS REACTIONS

! Overdose may produce blurred vision, severe dizziness/faintness.

DENTAL CONSIDERATIONS

General:

• Monitor vital signs at every appointment because of cardiovascular side effects.

• After supine positioning, have patient sit upright for at least 2 min before standing to avoid orthostatic hypotension.

• Limit use of sodium-containing products, such as saline IV fluids, for patients with a dietary salt restriction.

• Stress from dental procedures may compromise cardiovascular function; determine patient risk.

• Short appointments and a stress-reduction protocol may be required for anxious patients.

• Assess salivary flow as a factor in caries, periodontal disease, and candidiasis.

Consultations:

• Medical consultation may be required to assess disease control and patient's ability to tolerate stress.

Teach Patient/Family:

• When chronic dry mouth occurs, advise patient to:

  • Avoid mouth rinses with high alcohol content because of drying effects.

  • Use daily home fluoride products for anticaries effect.

  • Use sugarless gum, frequent sips of water, or saliva substitutes.

---

guanethidine monosulfate

gwahn-**eth'**-ih-deen mah-no-**sull'**-fate
(Ismelin)

CATEGORY AND SCHEDULE

Pregnancy Risk Category: C

Drug Class: Antihypertensive

MECHANISM OF ACTION

An adrenergic blocker that inhibits the release of catecholamines produced by sympathetic nerve stimulation, thus suppressing peripheral sympathetic vasoconstriction.

Therapeutic Effect: Decreases B/P.

USES

Treatment of moderate-to-severe hypertension

PHARMACOKINETICS

Absorption is highly variable among patients. Protein binding: 26%. Metabolized in liver. Excreted in urine and feces. **Half-life:** 5–10 days.

INDICATIONS AND DOSAGES
▶ **Hypertension**
PO
Adults. Initially, 10 mg/day. May increase in 10–25 mg increments at 5–7 day intervals. Maximum: 100 mg/day. Lower initial doses are recommended for the elderly.

SIDE EFFECTS/ADVERSE REACTIONS
Frequent
Bradycardia, dizziness, blurred vision, orthostatic hypotension, fluid retention
Occasional
Impotence, inhibition of ejaculation, nasal stuffiness
Rare
Apnea, hypertension, renal dysfunction

PRECAUTIONS AND CONTRAINDICATIONS
MAOI therapy within 1 wk, overt CHF, pheochromocytoma, hypersensitivity to guanethidine or any component of the formulation
Caution:
Lactation, children; peptic ulcer, asthma, frequent orthostatic hypotension, fever, renal impairment

DRUG INTERACTIONS OF CONCERN TO DENTISTRY
• Increased orthostatic hypotension: alcohol, opioid analgesics, barbiturates, phenothiazines, haloperidol
• Decreased hypotensive effect: ephedrine, NSAIDs, indomethacin, sympathomimetics, tricyclic antidepressants

SERIOUS REACTIONS
! Arrhythmias, angina, and pulmonary edema have been reported.

! Overdosage may produce bradycardia, diarrhea, nausea, orthostatic hypotension, and shock.

DENTAL CONSIDERATIONS
General:
• Monitor vital signs at every appointment because of cardiovascular and respiratory side effects.
• Patients on chronic drug therapy may rarely have symptoms of blood dyscrasias, which can include infection, bleeding, and poor healing.
• Assess salivary flow as a factor in caries, periodontal disease, and candidiasis.
• After supine positioning, have patient sit upright for at least 2 min before standing to avoid orthostatic hypotension.
• Limit use of sodium-containing products, such as saline IV fluids, for patients with a dietary salt restriction.
• Stress from dental procedures may compromise cardiovascular function; determine patient risk.
• Short appointments and a stress-reduction protocol may be required for anxious patients.
• Use vasoconstrictors with caution, in low doses and with careful aspiration. Avoid using gingival retraction cord with epinephrine.
• Consider semisupine chair position for patients with respiratory distress.
Consultations:
• Medical consultation may be required to assess disease control and patient's ability to tolerate stress.
• In a patient with symptoms of blood dyscrasias, request a medical consultation for blood studies and postpone dental treatment until normal values are reestablished.

G

G

Teach Patient/Family to:
• Encourage effective oral hygiene to prevent soft tissue inflammation.
• Use caution to prevent injury when using oral hygiene aids.
• When chronic dry mouth occurs, advise patient to:
  • Avoid mouth rinses with high alcohol content because of drying effects.
  • Use daily home fluoride products for anticaries effect.
  • Use sugarless gum, frequent sips of water, or saliva substitutes.

guanfacine
gwan′-fa-seen
(Tenex)

CATEGORY AND SCHEDULE
Pregnancy Risk Category: B

Drug Class: Antihypertensive

MECHANISM OF ACTION
An α-adrenergic agonist that stimulates α_2-adrenergic receptors and inhibits sympathetic cardioaccelerator and vasoconstrictor center to heart, kidneys, peripheral vasculature.
Therapeutic Effect: Decreases systolic, diastolic B/P. Chronic use decreases peripheral vascular resistance.

USES
Treatment of hypertension in individual using a thiazide diuretic or other antihypertensive

PHARMACOKINETICS
Well absorbed from GI tract. Widely distributed. Protein binding: 71%. Metabolized in liver. Excreted in urine and feces. Not removed by hemodialysis. *Half-life:* 17 hr.

INDICATIONS AND DOSAGES
▶ **Hypertension**
PO
Adults, Elderly. Initially, 1 mg/day. Increase by 1 mg/day at intervals of 3–4 wk up to 3 mg/day in single or divided doses.

SIDE EFFECTS/ADVERSE REACTIONS
Frequent
Dry mouth, somnolence
Occasional
Fatigue, headache, asthenia (loss of strength, energy), dizziness

PRECAUTIONS AND CONTRAINDICATIONS
History of hypersensitivity to guanfacine or any component of the formulation

DRUG INTERACTIONS OF CONCERN TO DENTISTRY
• Possible increase in CNS depression: alcohol and all CNS depressants
• Possible reduced antihypertensive effect: indomethacin and perhaps other NSAIDs
• Possible increase in antihypertensive effects: other antihypertensive drugs

SERIOUS REACTIONS
! Overdosage may produce difficult breathing, dizziness, faintness, severe drowsiness, bradycardia.

DENTAL CONSIDERATIONS

General:
• Monitor vital signs at every appointment because of cardiovascular side effects.

• After supine positioning, have patient sit upright for at least 2 min before standing to avoid orthostatic hypotension.
• Limit use of sodium-containing products, such as saline IV fluids, for patients with a dietary salt restriction.
• Assess salivary flow as a factor in caries, periodontal disease, and candidiasis.
• Short appointments and a stress-reduction protocol may be required for anxious patients.
• Stress from dental procedures may compromise cardiovascular function; determine patient risk.
• Use precaution if sedation or general anesthesia is required; risk of hypotensive episode.

Consultations:
• Medical consultation may be required to assess disease control and patient's ability to tolerate stress.

Teach Patient/Family to:
• Update health and medication history if physician makes any changes in evaluation or drug regimens; include OTC, herbal, and nonherbal remedies in the update.
• Use caution when driving or performing other tasks requiring mental alertness; avoid if drowsiness occurs.
• When chronic dry mouth occurs advise patient to:
  • Avoid mouth rinses with high alcohol content because of drying effects.
  • Use daily home fluoride products for anticaries effect.
  • Use sugarless gum, frequent sips of water, or saliva substitutes.

G

halcinonide
hal-**sin**′-oh-nide
(Halog, Halog-E)

CATEGORY AND SCHEDULE
Pregnancy Risk Category: C

Drug Class: Corticosteroid, synthetic topical

MECHANISM OF ACTION
A topical corticosteroid that has antiinflammatory, antipruritic, and vasoconstrictive properties. The exact mechanism of the antiinflammatory process is unclear. *Therapeutic Effect:* Reduces or prevents tissue response to the inflammatory process.

USES
Treatment of inflammation of corticosteroid-responsive dermatoses

PHARMACOKINETICS
Well absorbed systemically. Large variation in absorption among sites. Protein binding: varies. Metabolized in liver. Primarily excreted in urine.

INDICATIONS AND DOSAGES
▸ **Dermatoses**
Topical
Adults, Elderly. Apply sparingly 1–3 times a day.

SIDE EFFECTS/ADVERSE REACTIONS
Occasional
Itching, redness, irritation, burning at site of application, dryness, folliculitis, acneiform eruptions, hypopigmentation
Rare
Allergic contact dermatitis, maceration of the skin, secondary infection, skin atrophy

PRECAUTIONS AND CONTRAINDICATIONS
History of hypersensitivity to halcinonide or other corticosteroids

SERIOUS REACTIONS
! The serious reactions of long-term therapy and the addition of occlusive dressings are reversible hypothalamic-pituitary-adrenal (HPA) axis suppression, manifestations of Cushing's syndrome, hyperglycemia, and glucosuria.

DENTAL CONSIDERATIONS

General:
• Place on frequent recall to evaluate healing response when used on chronic basis.
Teach Patient/Family to:
• Encourage effective oral hygiene to prevent soft tissue inflammation.
• Return for oral evaluation if response of oral tissues has not occurred in 7–14 days.
• Apply at bedtime or after meals for maximum effect.
• Apply with cotton-tipped applicator by pressing, not rubbing, paste on lesion.
• Avoid use on oral herpetic ulcerations.

halobetasol
hal-oh-**bay**′-ta-sol
(Ultravate)

CATEGORY AND SCHEDULE
Pregnancy Risk Category: C

Drug Class: Topical corticosteroid, group VI potency

MECHANISM OF ACTION
A corticosteroid that inhibits accumulation of inflammatory cells at inflammation sites, phagocytosis, lysosomal enzyme release, and synthesis or release of mediators of inflammation.
Therapeutic Effect: Decreases or prevents tissue response to inflammatory process.

USES
Treatment of psoriasis, eczema, contact dermatitis, pruritus

PHARMACOKINETICS
Variation in absorption among individuals and sites: scrotum 36%, forehead 7%, scalp 4%, forearm 1%.

INDICATIONS AND DOSAGES
▸ **Dermatoses,**
Corticosteroid-Unresponsive
Topical
Adults, Elderly, Children 12 yr and older. Apply 1–2 times a day.
Maximum: 50 g for 2 wk.

SIDE EFFECTS/ADVERSE REACTIONS
Frequent
Burning, stinging, pruritus
Rare
Cushing's syndrome, hyperglycemia, glucosuria, hypothalamic-pituitary-adrenal axis suppression

PRECAUTIONS AND CONTRAINDICATIONS
Hypersensitivity to halobetasol or other corticosteroids
Caution:
Lactation, viral infections, bacterial infections

SERIOUS REACTIONS
! Overdosage can occur from topically applied halobetasol

absorbed in sufficient amounts to produce systemic effects producing reversible adrenal suppression, manifestations of Cushing's syndrome, hyperglycemia, and glucosuria in some patients.

DENTAL CONSIDERATIONS
Teach Patient/Family to:
• Avoid use on oral herpetic ulcerations.

H

haloperidol
ha-loe-**per′**-ih-dole
(Apo-Haloperidol[CAN], Haldol, Haldol Decanoate, Novo-Peridol[CAN], Peridol[CAN], Serenace[AUS])
Do not confuse Haldol with Halcion, Halog or Stadol.

CATEGORY AND SCHEDULE
Pregnancy Risk Category: C

Drug Class: Antipsychotic/butyrophenone

MECHANISM OF ACTION
An antipsychotic, antiemetic, and antidyskinetic agent that competitively blocks postsynaptic dopamine receptors, interrupts nerve impulse movement, and increases turnover of dopamine in the brain. Has strong extrapyramidal and antiemetic effects; weak anticholinergic and sedative effects.
Therapeutic Effect: Produces tranquilizing effect.

USES
Treatment of psychotic disorders, control of tics and vocal utterances in Tourette's syndrome, short-term

treatment of hyperactive children showing excessive motor activity

PHARMACOKINETICS

Readily absorbed from the GI tract. Protein binding: 92%. Extensively metabolized in the liver. Primarily excreted in urine. Not removed by hemodialysis. *Half-life:* 12–37 hr PO; 10–19 hr IV; 17–25 hr IM.

INDICATIONS AND DOSAGES

▸ **Treatment of Psychotic Disorders**
PO
Adults, Children 12 yr and older.
Initially, 0.5–5 mg 2–3 times a day. Dosage gradually adjusted as needed.
Elderly. 0.5–2 mg 2–3 times a day. Dosage gradually adjusted as needed.
Children 3–12 yr or weighing 15–40 kg. Initially, 0.05 mg/kg/day in 2–3 divided doses. May increase by 0.5 mg increments at 5–7 day intervals. Maximum: 0.15 mg/kg/day in divided doses.
IM
Adults, Elderly, Children 12 yr and older. Initially, 2–5. May repeat at 1-hr intervals as needed. Maximum: 100 mg/day.
IM (Decanoate)
Adults, Elderly, Children 12 yr and older. Initially, 10–15 times previous daily oral dose up to maximum initial dose of 100 mg. Maximum: 300 mg/mo.
▸ **Treatment of Nonpsychotic Disorders, Tourette's Syndrome**
PO
Children 3–12 yr or weighing 15–40 kg. Initially, 0.05 mg/kg/day in 2–3 divided doses. May increase by 0.5 mg at 5–7 day intervals. Maximum: 0.075 mg/kg/day.

SIDE EFFECTS/ADVERSE REACTIONS

Frequent
Blurred vision, constipation, orthostatic hypotension, dry mouth, swelling or soreness of female breasts, peripheral edema
Occasional
Allergic reaction, difficulty urinating, decreased thirst, dizziness, decreased sexual function, drowsiness, nausea, vomiting, photosensitivity, lethargy

PRECAUTIONS AND CONTRAINDICATIONS

Angle-closure glaucoma, CNS depression, myelosuppression, Parkinson's disease, severe cardiac or hepatic disease
Caution:
Lactation, seizure disorders, hypertension, hepatic disease, cardiac disease

DRUG INTERACTIONS OF CONCERN TO DENTISTRY

• Increased sedation: other CNS depressants, alcohol, barbiturate anesthetics, opioid analgesics
• Hypotension, tachycardia: epinephrine
• Increased extrapyramidal effects: phenothiazines and related drugs (haloperidol, droperidol), metoclopramide
• Additive photosensitization: tetracyclines
• Increased anticholinergic effects: anticholinergics
• Suspected increase in neurologic side effects: fluconazole, itraconazole, ketoconazole

SERIOUS REACTIONS

❗ Extrapyramidal symptoms appear to be dose related and typically occur in the first few days of therapy. Marked drowsiness and lethargy, excessive salivation, and fixed stare occur frequently.

! Less common reactions include severe akathisia (motor restlessness) and acute dystonias (such as torticollis, opisthotonos, and oculogyric crisis).

! Tardive dyskinesia (tongue protrusion, puffing of the cheeks, chewing or puckering of the mouth) may occur during long-term therapy or after discontinuing the drug and may be irreversible. Elderly female patients have a greater risk of developing this reaction.

DENTAL CONSIDERATIONS

General:
• Monitor vital signs at every appointment because of cardiovascular side effects.
• After supine positioning, have patient sit upright for at least 2 min before standing to avoid orthostatic hypotension.
• Assess salivary flow as a factor in caries, periodontal disease, and candidiasis.
• Avoid dental light in patient's eyes; offer dark glasses for patient comfort.
• Assess for presence of extrapyramidal motor symptoms, such as tardive dyskinesia and akathisia. Extrapyramidal motor activity may complicate dental treatment.
• Geriatric patients are more susceptible to drug effects; use lower dose.
• Use vasoconstrictors with caution, in low doses and with careful aspiration. Avoid use of gingival retraction cord with epinephrine.
Consultations:
• Take precautions if dental surgery is anticipated and anesthesia is required.

• Confirm patient's mental ability to give informed consent.
• Refer to physician if signs of tardive dyskinesia or akathisia are present.
• Physician should be informed if significant xerostomic side effects occur (e.g., increased caries, sore tongue, problems eating or swallowing, difficulty wearing prosthesis) so that a medication change can be considered.
Teach Patient/Family to:
• Encourage effective oral hygiene to prevent soft tissue inflammation.
• Use caution to prevent injury when using oral hygiene aids.
• Use powered tooth brush if patient has difficulty holding conventional devices.
• When chronic dry mouth occurs, advise patient to:
  • Avoid mouth rinses with high alcohol content because of drying effects.
  • Use daily home fluoride products for anticaries effect.
  • Use sugarless gum, frequent sips of water, or saliva substitutes.

histrelin
his-**trel**'-in
(Supprelin LA)

CATEGORY AND SCHEDULE
Pregnancy Risk Category: X
Controlled substance: Schedule IV

Drug Class: Gonadotropin releasing hormone agonist

MECHANISM OF ACTION
Inhibits gonadotropin secretion. It increases level of luteinizing

H

hormone (LH) and follicle-stimulating hormone (FSH) upon initiation of treatment but after continuous administration will decrease LH, FSH, testosterone, and estrogen.
Therapeutic Effect: Histrelin slows prostate cancer growth by lowering testosterone levels, decreasing estrogen levels in females, and decreasing testosterone levels in males.

USES

Palliative treatment of advanced prostate cancer and children with central precocious puberty (CPP).

PHARMACOKINETICS

Rapidly absorbed after injection (92%). Protein binding: 70%. Metabolism in liver via C-terminal dealkylation and hydrolysis.
Half-life: ~4 hr.

INDICATIONS AND DOSAGES

Adult. Palliative treatment of advanced prostate cancer: one 50-mg implant (releases 65 mcg per day over 12 months) inserted subcutaneously for 12 months.
Pediatric. CPP: one 50-mg implant inserted subcutaneously every 12 months. Discontinue at the appropriate time for the onset of puberty.
Safety and efficacy in children younger than 2 yr have not been established.

SIDE EFFECTS/ADVERSE REACTIONS

Frequent
Hot sweats, headache, fatigue, implant site reaction (bruising, discomfort, itching, pain, soreness, swelling, and tingling)

Occasional
Erectile dysfunction, insomnia, abdominal discomfort, constipation, weight gain, keloid scar, postprocedural pain, pain at the application site, menorrhagia

PRECAUTIONS AND CONTRAINDICATIONS

Contraindicated in patients with a history of hypersensitivity to GnRH, GnRH agonist analogs, histrelin acetate, or any component of the product; pregnancy (may cause fetal harm and spontaneous abortion). Not recommended in pediatric patients (<2 yr of age).
Initial agonistic action can occur; there is an initial transient increase of estrogen in females and testosterone in both males and females, which may temporarily worsen symptoms.

DRUG INTERACTIONS OF CONCERN TO DENTISTRY

• Insufficient evidence available

SERIOUS REACTIONS

! Pituitary adenoma, pituitary apoplexy (frequently secondary to pituitary adenoma), urinary tract obstruction, and spinal cord compression may occur in rare cases.

DENTAL CONSIDERATIONS

• Avoid bright dental light directly into patient's eyes; use sunglasses for patient's comfort.
Consultations:
• Medical consultation may be required to assess disease control.
• Review patient's medical and drug history, including over the counter and herbal.
• If additional analgesia is required for dental pain, consider alternative

analgesics (NSAIDs) in patient taking opioids for acute or chronic pain.

Teach Patient/Family to:
• Encourage effective oral hygiene to prevent soft tissue inflammation.
• Use caution to prevent injury when using oral hygiene aids.

homatropine hydrobromide
hoe-**ma**′-troe-peen
high-droh-**broh**′-mide
(Isopto Homatropine, Minims Homatropine[CAN])

CATEGORY AND SCHEDULE
Pregnancy Risk Category: C

Drug Class: Mydriatic (topical)

MECHANISM OF ACTION
An ophthalmic agent that blocks response of iris sphincter muscle and the accommodative muscle of the ciliary body to cholinergic stimulation, resulting in dilation and loss of accommodation.
Therapeutic Effect: Produces cycloplegia and mydriasis for refraction.

USES
Treatment of cycloplegic refraction, uveitis, mydriatic lens opacities

PHARMACOKINETICS
Maximum mydriatic effect occurs within 10–30 min; maximum cycloplegic effect occurs within 30–90 min. Duration of mydriasis is 6 hr–4 days; duration of cycloplegia is 10–48 hr.

INDICATIONS AND DOSAGES
▸ **Mydriasis and Cycloplegia for Refraction**
Ophthalmic
Adults, Elderly. Instill 1–2 drops of 2% solution or 1 drop of 5% solution before the procedure. Repeat at 5- to 10-min intervals as needed. Maximum: 3 doses for refraction.
Children. Instill 1 drop of 2% solution immediately before the procedure. Repeat at 10-min intervals as needed.
▸ **Uveitis**
Ophthalmic
Adults, Elderly. Instill 1–2 drops of 2% or 5% solution 2–3 times a day up to every 3–4 hr as needed.
Children. Instill 1 drop of 2% solution 2–3 times a day.

SIDE EFFECTS/ADVERSE REACTIONS
Frequent
Blurred vision, photophobia
Occasional
Irritation, increased intraocular pressure, congestion
Rare
Eczematoid dermatitis, edema, exudates, follicular conjunctivitis, somnolence, vascular congestion

PRECAUTIONS AND CONTRAINDICATIONS
Narrow-angle glaucoma, acute hemorrhage, hypersensitivity to homatropine or any component of the formulation
Caution:
Children, elderly, hypertension, hyperthyroidism, diabetes

H

DRUG INTERACTIONS OF CONCERN TO DENTISTRY

• Avoid concurrent use with pilocarpine
• Increased anticholinergic effects with other anticholinergic drugs (when significant absorption from the eye occurs)

SERIOUS REACTIONS

! Overdosage may produce symptoms of blurred vision, urinary retention, and tachycardia.
! Anticholinergic toxicity is caused by strong binding of the drug to cholinergic receptors.

DENTAL CONSIDERATIONS

General:
• Avoid dental light in patient's eyes; offer dark glasses for patient comfort.

hydralazine hydrochloride

high-**dral**'-ah-zeen
high-droh-**klor**'-ide
(Alphapress[AUS], Apresoline, Novo-Hylazin[CAN])
Do not confuse hydralazine with hydroxyzine.

CATEGORY AND SCHEDULE

Pregnancy Risk Category: C

Drug Class: Antihypertensive, direct-acting peripheral vasodilator

MECHANISM OF ACTION

An antihypertensive with direct vasodilating effects on arterioles. ***Therapeutic Effect:*** Decreases B/P and systemic resistance.

USES

Treatment of essential hypertension; parenteral: treatment of severe essential hypertension

PHARMACOKINETICS

Route	Onset	Peak	Duration
PO	20–30 min	N/A	2–4 hr
IV	5–20 min	N/A	2–6 hr

Well absorbed from the GI tract. Widely distributed. Protein binding: 85%–90%. Metabolized in the liver to active metabolite. Primarily excreted in urine. Not removed by hemodialysis. ***Half-life:*** 3–7 hr (increased with impaired renal function).

INDICATIONS AND DOSAGES
▸ **Moderate to Severe Hypertension**
PO
Adults. Initially, 10 mg 4 times a day. May increase by 10–25 mg/dose q2–5 days. Maximum: 300 mg/day.
Children. Initially, 0.75–1 mg/kg/day in 2–4 divided doses, not to exceed 25 mg/dose. May increase over 3–4 wk. Maximum: 7.5 mg/kg/day (5 mg/kg/day in infants).
IV, IM
Adults, Elderly. Initially, 10–20 mg/dose q4–6h. May increase to 40 mg/dose.
Children. Initially, 0.1–0.2 mg/kg/dose (maximum: 20 mg) q4–6h, as needed, up to 1.7–3.5 mg/kg/day in divided doses q4–6h.
▸ **Dosage in Renal Impairment**
Dosage interval is based on creatinine clearance.

Creatinine Clearance	Dosage Interval
10–50 ml/min	q8h
Less than 10 ml/min	q8–24h

SIDE EFFECTS/ADVERSE REACTIONS
Frequent
Headache, palpitations, tachycardia (generally disappears in 7–10 days)
Occasional
GI disturbance (nausea, vomiting, diarrhea), paraesthesia, fluid retention, peripheral edema, dizziness, flushed face, nasal congestion

PRECAUTIONS AND CONTRAINDICATIONS
Coronary artery disease, lupus erythematosus, rheumatic heart disease
Caution:
CVA, advanced renal disease

DRUG INTERACTIONS OF CONCERN TO DENTISTRY
• Reduced effects: NSAIDs, indomethacin, sympathomimetics

SERIOUS REACTIONS
! High dosage may produce lupus erythematosus-like reaction, including fever, facial rash, muscle and joint aches and splenomegaly.
! Severe orthostatic hypotension, skin flushing, severe headache, myocardial ischemia, and cardiac arrhythmias may develop.
! Profound shock may occur with severe overdosage.

DENTAL CONSIDERATIONS

General:
• Monitor vital signs at every appointment because of cardiovascular side effects.
• Limit dose or avoid vasoconstrictor.
• Patients on chronic drug therapy may rarely have symptoms of blood dyscrasias, which can include

infection, bleeding, and poor healing.
• Limit use of sodium-containing products, such as saline IV fluids, for patients with a dietary salt restriction.
• After supine positioning, have patient sit upright for at least 2 min to avoid orthostatic hypotension.
Consultations:
• In a patient with symptoms of blood dyscrasias, request a medical consultation for blood studies and postpone dental treatment until normal values are reestablished.
• Medical consultation may be required to assess disease control and patient's ability to tolerate stress.
Teach Patient/Family to:
• Encourage effective oral hygiene to prevent soft tissue inflammation.
• Use caution to prevent injury when using oral hygiene aids.

hydrochlorothiazide
high-droe-klor-oh-**thye′**-ah-zide
(Apo-Hydro[CAN], Aquazide H, Dichlotride[AUS], Dithiazide[AUS], Esidrix, HydroDIURIL, Microzide, Oretic)

CATEGORY AND SCHEDULE
Pregnancy Risk Category: B (D if used in pregnancy-induced hypertension)

Drug Class: Thiazide diuretic

MECHANISM OF ACTION
A sulfonamide derivative that acts as a thiazide diuretic and antihypertensive. As a diuretic, blocks reabsorption of water, sodium, and potassium at the

cortical diluting segment of the distal tubule. As an antihypertensive reduces plasma, extracellular fluid volume, and peripheral vascular resistance by direct effect on blood vessels.
Therapeutic Effect: Promotes diuresis; reduces B/P.

USES
Treatment of edema, hypertension, diuresis, CHF

PHARMACOKINETICS

Route	Onset	Peak	Duration
PO (diuretic)	2 hr	4–6 hr	6–12 hr

Variably absorbed from the GI tract. Primarily excreted unchanged in urine. Not removed by hemodialysis.
Half-life: 5.6–14.8 hr.

INDICATIONS AND DOSAGES
▶ **Edema, Hypertension**
PO
Adults. 12.5–100 mg/day. Maximum: 200 mg/day.
▶ **Usual Pediatric Dosage**
PO
Children 6 mo–12 yr. 2 mg/kg/day in 2 divided doses. Maximum: 200 mg/day.
Children younger than 6 mo. 2–4 mg/kg/day in 2 divided doses. Maximum: 37.5 mg/day.

SIDE EFFECTS/ADVERSE REACTIONS
Expected
Increase in urinary frequency and urine volume
Frequent
Potassium depletion
Occasional
Orthostatic hypotension, headache, GI disturbances, photosensitivity

PRECAUTIONS AND CONTRAINDICATIONS
Anuria, history of hypersensitivity to sulfonamides or thiazide diuretics, renal decompensation
Caution:
Hypokalemia, renal disease, hepatic disease, gout, COPD, lupus erythematosus, diabetes mellitus

DRUG INTERACTIONS OF CONCERN TO DENTISTRY
• Decreased hypotensive response: NSAIDs, especially indomethacin

SERIOUS REACTIONS
! Vigorous diuresis may lead to profound water and electrolyte depletion, resulting in hypokalemia, hyponatremia, and dehydration.
! Acute hypotensive episodes may occur.
! Hyperglycemia may occur during prolonged therapy.
! Pancreatitis, blood dyscrasias, pulmonary edema, allergic pneumonitis, and dermatologic reactions occur rarely.
! Overdose can lead to lethargy and coma without changes in electrolytes or hydration.

DENTAL CONSIDERATIONS
General:
• Monitor vital signs at every appointment because of cardiovascular side effects.
• Limit dose or avoid vasoconstrictor.
• Patients on chronic drug therapy may rarely have symptoms of blood dyscrasias, which can include infection, bleeding, and poor healing.
• After supine positioning, have patient sit upright for at least 2 min before standing to avoid orthostatic hypotension.

• Assess salivary flow as a factor in caries, periodontal disease, and candidiasis.

• Limit use of sodium-containing products, such as saline IV fluids, for patients with a dietary salt restriction.

• Stress from dental procedures may compromise cardiovascular function; determine patient risk.

• Short appointments and a stress-reduction protocol may be required for anxious patients.

• Patients taking diuretics should be monitored for serum K levels.

Consultations:

• In a patient with symptoms of blood dyscrasias, request a medical consultation for blood studies and postpone dental treatment until normal values are reestablished.

• Medical consultation may be required to assess disease control and patient's ability to tolerate stress.

• Physician should be informed if significant xerostomic side effects occur (e.g., increased caries, sore tongue, problems eating or swallowing, difficulty wearing prosthesis) so that a medication change can be considered.

Teach Patient/Family to:

• Encourage effective oral hygiene to prevent soft tissue inflammation.

• Use caution to prevent injury when using oral hygiene aids.

• When chronic dry mouth occurs, advise patient to:

• Avoid mouth rinses with high alcohol content because of drying effects.

• Use daily home fluoride products for anticaries effect.

• Use sugarless gum, frequent sips of water, or saliva substitutes.

hydrocodone bitartrate

high-drough-**koe′**-doan
bye-**tar′**-trate
(Hycodan[CAN], Robidone[CAN])

CATEGORY AND SCHEDULE

Pregnancy Risk Category: C
Controlled Substance: Schedule III

Drug Class: Opioid analgesic

H

MECHANISM OF ACTION

An opioid analgesic and antitussive that binds with opioid receptors in the CNS.

Therapeutic Effect: Alters the perception of and emotional response to pain; suppresses cough reflex.

USES

Treatment of hyperactive and nonproductive cough; mild-to-moderate pain; normally used in combination with aspirin or acetaminophen for post-treatment pain control.

PHARMACOKINETICS

Route	Onset	Peak	Duration
PO (analgesic)	10–20 min	30–60 min	4–6 hr
PO (antitussive)	N/A	N/A	4–6 hr

Well absorbed from the GI tract. Metabolized in the liver. Primarily excreted in urine. *Half-life:* 3.8 hr (increased in elderly).

INDICATIONS AND DOSAGES
▸ **Analgesia**
PO
Adults, Children older than 12 yr.
5–10 mg q4–6h.
Elderly. 2.5–5 mg q4–6h.
▸ **Cough**
PO
Adults. 5–10 mg q4–6h as needed.
Maximum: 15 mg/dose.
Children. 0.6 mg/kg/day in 3–4
divided doses at intervals of at least
4 hr. Maximum single dose: 5 mg
(children 2–12 yr), 1.25 mg
(children younger than 2 yr).
PO (Extended-Release)
Adults. 10 mg q12h.
Children 6–12 yr. 5 mg q12h.

SIDE EFFECTS/ADVERSE REACTIONS
Frequent
Sedation, hypotension, diaphoresis,
facial flushing, dizziness,
somnolence
Occasional
Urine retention, blurred vision,
constipation, dry mouth, headache,
nausea, vomiting, difficult or
painful urination, euphoria,
dysphoria

PRECAUTIONS AND CONTRAINDICATIONS
Hypersensitivity, addiction (narcotic)
Caution:
Addictive personality, lactation,
increased intracranial pressure, MI
(acute), severe heart disease,
respiratory depression, hepatic
disease, renal disease, children
younger than 18 yr

DRUG INTERACTIONS OF CONCERN TO DENTISTRY
• Increased CNS depression:
alcohol, other opioids,
phenothiazines, sedative/hypnotics,
skeletal muscle relaxants, general
anesthetics
• Contraindication: MAOIs
• Increased effects of
anticholinergics

SERIOUS REACTIONS
! Overdose results in respiratory
depression, skeletal muscle
flaccidity, cold or clammy skin,
cyanosis and extreme somnolence
progressing to seizures, stupor, and
coma.
! The patient who uses hydrocodone
repeatedly may develop a tolerance
to the drug's analgesic effect, as well
as physical dependence.
! The drug may have a prolonged
duration of action and cumulative
effect in patients with hepatic or
renal impairment.

DENTAL CONSIDERATIONS

General:
• Monitor vital signs at every
appointment because of
cardiovascular and respiratory side
effects.
• After supine positioning, have
patient sit upright for at least
2 min to avoid orthostatic
hypotension.
• Psychologic and physical
dependence may occur with chronic
administration.
• Determine why the patient is
taking the drug.
Teach Patient/Family to:
• Avoid mouth rinses with high
alcohol content because of drying
effects.

hydrocodone

high-droe-**koe'**-done
Hydrocodone and acetaminophen
(Anexsia, Bancap HC, Ceta-Plus,
Co-Gesic, Hydrocet, Hydrogesic,
Ibudone, Lorcet 10/650,
Lorcet-HD Lorcet Plus, Lortab,
Margesic H, Maxidone, Norco,
Reprexain, Stagesic, Vicodin,
Vicodin ES, Vicodin HP, Zydone);
hydrocodone and aspirin
(Damason-P); hydrocodone and
chlorpheniramine (Tussionex);
hydrocodone and guaifenesin
(Codiclear DH, Hycosin,
Hycotuss, Kwelcof,
Pneumotussin, Vicodin Tuss,
Vitussin); hydrocodone and
homatropine (Hycodan and
Hydromet, Hydropane, Tussigon);
hydrocodone and ibuprofen,
(Vicoprofen); hydrocodone and
pseudoephedrine (Detussin,
Histussin D, P-V Tussin);
hydrocodone, chlorpheniramine,
phenylephrine, acetaminophen
and caffeine (Hycomine
Compound)

CATEGORY AND SCHEDULE
Pregnancy Risk Category: C
Controlled substance: Schedule III

Drug Class: Antitussive opioid
analgesic, nonopioid analgesic

MECHANISM OF ACTION
Hydrocodone blocks pain perception
in the cerebral cortex by binding to
specific opiate receptors (μ and κ) at
neuronal membranes of synapses.
This binding results in a decreased
synaptic chemical transmission
throughout the CNS, thus inhibiting
the flow of pain sensations into the
higher centers and causing
analgesia.

Therapeutic Effect: Alters
perception of pain and produces
analgesic effect.

USES
Treatment of hyperactive and
nonproductive cough, mild pain

PHARMACOKINETICS
Well absorbed. Metabolized in liver.
Excreted in urine. *Half-life:*
3.3–3.4 hr.

INDICATIONS AND DOSAGES
Analgesia
▶ **Hydrocodone and Acetaminophen**
PO
*Adults, Children older than 13 yr or
weighing more than 50 kg.* 2.5–
10 mg q4–6h. Maximum: 60 mg/day
hydrocodone. Maximum dose of
acetaminophen: 4 g/day.
Elderly. 2.5–5 mg hydrocodone
q4–6h. Titrate dose to appropriate
analgesic effect. Maximum: 4 g/day
acetaminophen.
*Children 2–13 yr or weighing less
than 50 kg.* 0.135 mg/kg/dose
hydrocodone q4–6h. Maximum: 6
doses/day of hydrocodone or
maximum recommended dose of
acetaminophen.
Hydrocodone and Aspirin
PO
Adults. 2.5–10 mg q4–6h.
Maximum: 60 mg/day hydrocodone.
Elderly. 2.5–5 mg hydrocodone
q4–6h. Titrate dose to appropriate
analgesic effect.
*Children 2–13 yr or weighing less
than 50 kg.* 0.135 mg/kg/dose
hydrocodone q4–6h.
Hydrocodone and
Chlorpheniramine
*Adults, Elderly, Children 12 yr and
older.* 5 ml q12h. Maximum:
10 ml/24h.
Children 6–12 yr. 2.5 ml q12h.
Maximum: 5 ml/24h.

Hydrocodone and Guaifenesin
Adults, Elderly, Children 12 yr and older. 5 ml q4h. Maximum: 30 ml/24h.
Children 2–12 yr. 2.5 ml q4h.
Children younger than 2 yr. 0.3 mg/kg/day (hydrocodone) in 4 divided doses.
Hydrocodone and Homatropine
Adults, Elderly. 10 mg (hydrocodone) q4–6h. A single dose should not exceed 15 mg and should not be administered more frequently than q4h.
Children. 0.6 mg/kg/day (hydrocodone) in 3–4 divided doses. Do not administer more frequently than q4h.
Hydrocodone and Ibuprofen
Adults. 7.5–15 mg (hydrocodone) q4–6h as needed for pain. Maximum: 5 tablets/day.
Hydrocodone and Pseudoephedrine
Adults, Elderly. 5 ml 4 times a day.
Hydrocodone, Chlorpheniramine, Phenylephrine, Acetaminophen, and Caffeine
Adults, Elderly. 1 tablet q4h up to 4 times a day.

SIDE EFFECTS/ADVERSE REACTIONS

Frequent
Dizziness, sedation, drowsiness, bradycardia
Occasional
Anxiety, dysphoria, euphoria, fear, lethargy, light-headedness, malaise, mental clouding, mental impairment, mood changes, physiological dependence, sedation, somnolence, constipation, bradycardia, heartburn, nausea, vomiting
Rare
Hypersensitivity reaction, rash

PRECAUTIONS AND CONTRAINDICATIONS

CNS depression, severe respiratory depression, hypersensitivity to hydrocodone, or any component of the formulation

DRUG INTERACTIONS OF CONCERN TO DENTISTRY

• Increased CNS depression: alcohol, local anesthetics, other opioids, phenothiazines, sedative/hypnotics, skeletal muscle relaxants, general anesthetics
• Contraindication: MAOIs
• Increased effects of anticholinergics

SERIOUS REACTIONS

! Cardiac arrest, circulatory collapse, coma, hypotension, hypoglycemic coma, ureteral spasm, urinary retention, vesical sphincter spasm, agranulocytosis, bleeding time prolonged, hemolytic anemia, iron deficiency anemia, occult blood loss, thrombocytopenia, hepatic necrosis, hepatitis, skeletal muscle rigidity, renal toxicity, renal tubular necrosis have been reported.
! Hearing impairment or loss have been reported with chronic overdose.
! Acute airway obstruction, apnea, dyspnea, and respiratory depression occur rarely and are usually dose related.

DENTAL CONSIDERATIONS

General:
• Monitor vital signs at every appointment because of cardiovascular and respiratory side effects.
• After supine positioning, have patient sit upright for at least 2 min to avoid orthostatic hypotension.
• Psychologic and physical dependence may occur with chronic administration.

• Determine why the patient is taking the drug.
Teach Patient/Family to:
• Avoid mouth rinses with high alcohol content because of drying effects.

hydrocortisone
high-droh-**kor′**-tih-sone
(A-Hydrocort, Anusol-HC, Colifoam[AUS], Cortaid, Cortef cream[AUS], Cortic cream[AUS], Cortic DS[AUS], Cortifoam, Cortizone-5, Cortizone-10, Derm-Aid cream[AUS], Dermaide[AUS], Dermaide soft cream[AUS], Ego Cort cream[AUS], Emcort, HICOR[AUS], HICOR Eye Ointment[AUS], Hysone[AUS], Hytone, Locoid, Nupercainal Hydrocortisone Cream, Preparation H Hydrocortisone, Proctocort, Sequent HICOR[AUS], Solu-Cortef, Squibb HC[AUS], Westcort)

CATEGORY AND SCHEDULE
Pregnancy Risk Category: C
OTC (Hydrocortisone 0.5% and 1% Cream, Gel, and Ointment)

Drug Class: Topical corticosteroid

MECHANISM OF ACTION
An adrenocortical steroid that inhibits accumulation of inflammatory cells at inflammation sites, phagocytosis, lysosomal enzyme release, and synthesis and release of mediators of inflammation.
Therapeutic Effect: Prevents or suppresses cell-mediated immune reactions. Decreases or prevents

tissue response to inflammatory process.

USES
Treatment of psoriasis, eczema, contact dermatitis, pruritus

PHARMACOKINETICS

Route	Onset	Peak	Duration
IV	N/A	4–6 hr	8–12 hr

Well absorbed after IM administration. Widely distributed. Metabolized in the liver. *Half-life:* Plasma, 1.5–2 hr; biologic, 8–12 hr.

INDICATIONS AND DOSAGES
▸ **Acute Adrenal Insufficiency**
IV
Adults, Elderly. 100 mg IV bolus; then 300 mg/day in divided doses q8h.
Children. 1–2 mg/kg IV bolus; then 150–250 mg/day in divided doses q6–8h.
Infants. 1–2 mg/kg/dose IV bolus; then 25–150 mg/day in divided doses q6–8h.
▸ **Antiinflammation, Immunosuppression**
IV, IM
Adults, Elderly. 15–240 mg q12h.
Children. 1–5 mg/kg/day in divided doses q12h.
▸ **Physiologic Replacement**
PO
Children. 0.5–0.75 mg/kg/day in divided doses q8h.
IM
Children. 0.25–0.35 mg/kg/day as a single dose.
▸ **Status Asthmaticus**
IV
Adults, Elderly. 100–500 mg q6h.
Children. 2 mg/kg/dose q6h.

▶ **Shock**

IV

Adults, Elderly, Children 12 yr and older. 100–500 mg q6h.

Children younger than 12 yr. 50 mg/kg. May repeat in 4 hr, then q24h as needed.

▶ **Adjunctive Treatment of Ulcerative Colitis**

Rectal

Adults, Elderly. 100 mg at bedtime for 21 nights or until clinical and proctologic remission occurs (may require 2–3 mo of therapy).

Rectal (Cortifoam)

Adults, Elderly. 1 applicator 1–2 times a day for 2–3 wk, then every second day until therapy ends.

Topical

Adults, Elderly. Apply sparingly 2–4 times a day.

SIDE EFFECTS/ADVERSE REACTIONS

Frequent

Insomnia, heartburn, nervousness, abdominal distention, diaphoresis, acne, mood swings, increased appetite, facial flushing, delayed wound healing, increased susceptibility to infection, diarrhea or constipation

Occasional

Headache, edema, change in skin color, frequent urination

Topical: Itching, redness, irritation

Rare

Tachycardia, allergic reaction (such as rash and hives), psychological changes, hallucinations, depression

Topical: Allergic contact dermatitis, purpura

Systemic: Absorption more likely with use of occlusive dressings or extensive application in young children

PRECAUTIONS AND CONTRAINDICATIONS

Fungal, tuberculosis, or viral skin lesions; serious infections

Caution:

Lactation, viral infections, bacterial infections

DRUG INTERACTIONS OF CONCERN TO DENTISTRY

• Inhibitors of CYP hepatic isoenzymes (e.g., azole antifungals, macrolide antibiotics): potential increased blood levels of hydrocortisone and increased hydrocortisone toxicity

• Aspirin, salicylates: potentially increased salicylate GI irritation and toxicity

• Anticoagulants: variable effects on coagulation levels, potentially increased bleeding

SERIOUS REACTIONS

! Long-term therapy may cause hypocalcemia, hypokalemia, muscle wasting (especially in arms and legs), osteoporosis, spontaneous fractures, amenorrhea, cataracts, glaucoma, peptic ulcer disease, and CHF.

! Abruptly withdrawing the drug after long-term therapy may cause anorexia, nausea, fever, headache, sudden severe joint pain, rebound inflammation, fatigue, weakness, lethargy, dizziness, and orthostatic hypotension.

DENTAL CONSIDERATIONS

Topical Form

General:

• Place on frequent recall to evaluate healing response if used on a chronic basis.

Teach Patient/Family to:

• Encourage effective oral hygiene to prevent soft tissue inflammation.

- Apply at bedtime or after meals for maximum effect.
- Avoid use on oral herpetic ulcerations.
- Apply with cotton-tipped applicator by pressing, not rubbing, paste on lesion.
- Return for oral evaluation if response of oral tissues has not occurred in 7–14 days.

hydroflumethiazide
high-droh-floo-meth-**eye**'-ah-zide
(Diucardin, Saluron)

CATEGORY AND SCHEDULE
Pregnancy Risk Category: C, D if used in pregnancy-induced hypertension

Drug Class: Antidiuretic, central and nephrogenic diabetes insipidus; antihypertensive; antiurolithic, calcium calculi; diuretic

MECHANISM OF ACTION
A diuretic that blocks reabsorption of water and the electrolytes sodium and potassium at cortical diluting segment of distal tubule. As an antihypertensive, it reduces plasma and extracellular fluid volume and decreases peripheral vascular resistance (PVR) by direct effect on blood vessels.
Therapeutic Effect: Promotes diuresis, reduces B/P.

USES
Treatment of high B/P (hypertension)

PHARMACOKINETICS
Rapidly but incompletely absorbed from the GI tract. Metabolized to metabolite that is extensively bound to red blood cells and has a longer half-life than parent compound. Primarily excreted in urine. Not removed by hemodialysis. *Half-life:* 2–17 hr.

INDICATIONS AND DOSAGES
▶ **Edema**
PO
Adults, Elderly. Initially, 50 mg 2 times a day. Maintenance: 25–200 mg/day.
▶ **Hypertension**
Adults, Elderly, Children. 1 mg/kg/day. Initially, 50 mg 2 times a day. Maintenance: 50–100 mg/day.

SIDE EFFECTS/ADVERSE REACTIONS
Expected
Increase in urine frequency and volume
Frequent
Potassium depletion
Occasional
Postural hypotension, headache, GI disturbances, photosensitivity reaction

PRECAUTIONS AND CONTRAINDICATIONS
Anuria, history of hypersensitivity to sulfonamides or thiazide diuretics, renal decompensation, pregnancy

DRUG INTERACTIONS OF CONCERN TO DENTISTRY
- Decreased hypotensive response: NSAIDs

SERIOUS REACTIONS
! Vigorous diuresis may lead to profound water loss and electrolyte depletion, resulting in hypokalemia, hyponatremia, and dehydration.
! Acute hypotensive episodes may occur.
! Hyperglycemia may be noted during prolonged therapy.

H

! GI upset, pancreatitis, dizziness, paresthesias, headache, blood dyscrasias, pulmonary edema, allergic pneumonitis, and dermatologic reactions occur rarely.
! Overdosage can lead to lethargy and coma without changes in electrolytes or hydration.

DENTAL CONSIDERATIONS

General:
• Monitor vital signs at every appointment due to cardiovascular side effects.
• Limit dose or avoid vasoconstrictor.
• Patient on chronic drug therapy may rarely present with symptoms of blood dyscrasias, which can include infection, bleeding, and poor healing. If dyscrasia is present, caution patient to prevent oral tissue trauma when using oral hygiene aids.
• After supine positioning, have patient sit upright for at least 2 min before standing to avoid orthostatic hypotension.
• Assess salivary flow as a factor in caries, periodontal disease, and candidiasis.
• Limit use of sodium-containing products, such as saline IV fluids, for patients with a dietary salt restriction.
• Stress from dental procedures may compromise cardiovascular function, determine patient risk.
• Patients taking diuretics should be monitored for serum K levels.
Consultations:
• In a patient with symptoms of blood dyscrasias, request a medical consultation for blood studies and postpone treatment until normal values are reestablished.
• Medical consultation may be required to assess disease control

and patient's ability to tolerate stress.
• Physician should be informed if significant xerostomic side effects occur (increased caries, sore tongue, problems eating or swallowing, difficulty wearing prosthesis) so that a medication change can be considered.
Teach Patient/Family to:
• Encourage effective oral hygiene to prevent soft tissue inflammation.
• Prevent trauma when using oral hygiene aids.
• When chronic dry mouth occurs advise patient to:
  • Avoid mouth rinses with high alcohol content due to drying effects.
  • Use daily home fluoride products for anticaries effect.
  • Use sugarless gum, frequent sips of water, or saliva substitutes.
• Update health and medication history if physician makes any changes in evaluation or drug regimens; include OTC, herbal, and nonherbal remedies in the update.

hydromorphone hydrochloride

high-droe-**mor**′-fone
high-droh-**klor**′-ide
(Dilaudid, Dilaudid HP, Hydromorph Contin[CAN], Palladone)
Do not confuse with morphine or Dilantin.

CATEGORY AND SCHEDULE
Pregnancy Risk Category: C
Controlled Substance: Schedule II

Drug Class: Synthetic opioid analgesic

MECHANISM OF ACTION

An opioid agonist that binds to opioid receptors in the CNS, reducing the intensity of pain stimuli from sensory nerve endings. *Therapeutic Effect:* Alters the perception of and emotional response to pain; suppresses cough reflex.

USES

Treatment of moderate-to-severe pain

PHARMACOKINETICS

Route	Onset	Peak	Duration
PO	30 min	90–120 min	4 hr
IV	10–15 min	15–30 min	2–3 hr
IM	15 min	30–60 min	4–5 hr
Subcutaneous	15 min	30–90 min	4 hr
Rectal	15–30 min	N/A	N/A

Well absorbed from the GI tract after IM administration. Widely distributed. Metabolized in the liver. Excreted in urine. *Half-life:* 1–3 hr.

INDICATIONS AND DOSAGES
▸ **Analgesia**
PO
Adults, Elderly, Children weighing 50 kg and more. 2–4 mg q3–4h. Range: 2–8 mg/dose.
Children older than 6 mo and weighing less than 50 kg. 0.03–0.08 mg/kg/dose q3–4h.
PO (Extended-Release)
Adults, Elderly. 12–32 mg once a day.
IV
Adults, Elderly, Children weighing more than 50 kg. 0.2–0.6 mg q2–3h.

Children weighing 50 kg or less. 0.015 mg/kg/dose q3–6h as needed.
Rectal
Adults, Elderly. 3 mg q4–8h.
▸ **Patient-Controlled Analgesia (PCA)**
IV
Adults, Elderly. 0.05–0.5 mg at 5–15 min lockout. Maximum (4 hr): 4–6 mg.
Epidural
Adults, Elderly. Bolus dose of 1–1.5 mg at rate of 0.04–0.4 mg/hr. DEM and dose of 0.15 mg at 30-min lockout.
▸ **Cough**
PO
Adults, Elderly, Children older than 12 yr. 1 mg q3–4h.
Children 6–12 yr. 0.5 mg q3–4h.

SIDE EFFECTS/ADVERSE REACTIONS
Frequent
Somnolence, dizziness, hypotension (including orthostatic hypotension), decreased appetite
Occasional
Confusion, diaphoresis, facial flushing, urine retention, constipation, dry mouth, nausea, vomiting, headache, pain at injection site
Rare
Allergic reaction, depression

PRECAUTIONS AND CONTRAINDICATIONS
Hypersensitivity, addiction (narcotic), MAOIs
Caution:
Addictive personality, lactation, increased intracranial pressure, MI (acute), severe heart disease, respiratory depression, hepatic disease, renal disease, children younger than 18 yr

DRUG INTERACTIONS OF CONCERN TO DENTISTRY

• Effects may be increased with other CNS depressants: alcohol, narcotics, sedative/hypnotics, skeletal muscle relaxants
• Increased effects of anticholinergic drugs

SERIOUS REACTIONS

! Overdose results in respiratory depression, skeletal muscle flaccidity, cold or clammy skin, cyanosis and extreme somnolence progressing to seizures, stupor, and coma.
! The patient who uses hydromorphone repeatedly may develop a tolerance to the drug's analgesic effect, as well as physical dependence.
! This drug may have a prolonged duration of action and cumulative effect in patients with hepatic or renal impairment.

DENTAL CONSIDERATIONS

General:

• Monitor vital signs at every appointment because of cardiovascular and respiratory side effects.
• After supine positioning, have patient sit upright for at least 2 min to avoid orthostatic hypotension.
• Assess salivary flow as a factor in caries, periodontal disease, and candidiasis.
• Psychologic and physical dependence may occur with chronic administration.
• Determine why the patient is taking the drug.
• Avoid use in patients with chronic obstructive pulmonary disease.

Teach Patient/Family to:
• Avoid mouth rinses with high alcohol content because of drying effects.

hydroxychloroquine sulfate

high-drox-ee-**klor**′-oh-kwin
sull′-fate
(Apo-Hydroxyquine[CAN],
Plaquenil)
Do not confuse
hydroxychloroquine with
hydrocortisone or hydroxyzine.

CATEGORY AND SCHEDULE

Pregnancy Risk Category: C

Drug Class: Antimalarial

MECHANISM OF ACTION

An antimalarial and antirheumatic that concentrates in parasite acid vesicles, increasing the pH of the vesicles and interfering with parasite protein synthesis. Antirheumatic action may involve suppressing formation of antigens responsible for hypersensitivity reactions. ***Therapeutic Effect:*** Inhibits parasite growth.

USES

Treatment of malaria caused by *P. vivax, P. malariae, P. ovale, P. falciparum* (some strains); lupus erythematosus; rheumatoid arthritis

PHARMACOKINETICS

PO: Peak 1–2 hr. ***Half-life:*** 3–5 days; metabolized in liver; excreted in urine, feces, breast milk; crosses placenta.

INDICATIONS AND DOSAGES

▶ **Treatment of Acute Attack of Malaria (Dosage in mg Base)**
PO

Dose	Times	Adult	Children
Initial	Day 1	620 mg	10 mg/kg
Second	6 hr later	310 mg	5 mg/kg
Third	Day 2	310 mg	5 mg/kg
Fourth	Day 3	310 mg	5 mg/kg

▶ **Suppression of Malaria**
PO
Adults. 310 mg base weekly on same day each wk, beginning 2 wk before entering an endemic area and continuing for 4–6 wk after leaving the area.
Children. 5 mg base/kg/wk, beginning 2 wk before entering an endemic area and continuing for 4–6 wk after leaving the area. If therapy is not begun before exposure, administer a loading dose of 10 mg base/kg in 2 equally divided doses 6 hr apart, followed by the usual dosage regimen.
▶ **Rheumatoid Arthritis**
PO
Adults. Initially, 400–600 mg (310–465 mg base) daily for 5–10 days, gradually increased to optimum response level. Maintenance (usually within 4–12 wk): Dosage decreased by 50% and then continued at maintenance dose of 200–400 mg/day. Maximum effect may not be seen for several months.
▶ **Lupus Erythematosus**
PO
Adults. Initially, 400 mg once or twice a day for several wk or mo. Maintenance: 200–400 mg/day.

SIDE EFFECTS/ADVERSE REACTIONS

Frequent
Mild, transient headache; anorexia; nausea; vomiting
Occasional
Visual disturbances, nervousness, fatigue, pruritus (especially of palms, soles, and scalp), irritability, personality changes, diarrhea
Rare
Stomatitis, dermatitis, impaired hearing

PRECAUTIONS AND CONTRAINDICATIONS

Long-term therapy for children, porphyria, psoriasis, retinal or visual field changes
Caution:
Blood dyscrasias, severe GI disease, neurologic disease, alcoholism, hepatic disease, G6PD deficiency, psoriasis, eczema

DRUG INTERACTIONS OF CONCERN TO DENTISTRY

• None reported

SERIOUS REACTIONS

! Ocular toxicity, especially retinopathy, may occur and may progress even after drug is discontinued.
! Prolonged therapy may result in peripheral neuritis, neuromyopathy, hypotension, ECG changes, agranulocytosis, aplastic anemia, thrombocytopenia, seizures, and psychosis.
! Overdosage may result in headache, vomiting, visual disturbances, drowsiness, seizures, and hypokalemia followed by cardiovascular collapse and death.

DENTAL CONSIDERATIONS

General:
• Patients on chronic drug therapy may rarely have symptoms of blood dyscrasias, which can include infection, bleeding, and poor healing.
• Avoid dental light in patient's eyes; offer dark glasses for patient comfort.
• Determine why the patient is taking the drug.

Consultations:
• In a patient with symptoms of blood dyscrasias, request a medical consultation for blood studies and postpone dental treatment until normal values are reestablished.

Teach Patient/Family to:
• Encourage effective oral hygiene to prevent soft tissue inflammation.
• Avoid mouth rinses with high alcohol content because of drying effects.

hydroxyurea
high-**drocks'**-ee-your-**ee'**-ah
(Droxia, Hydrea, Mylocel)

CATEGORY AND SCHEDULE
Pregnancy Risk Category: D

Drug Class: Antineoplastic

MECHANISM OF ACTION
A synthetic urea analog that inhibits DNA synthesis without interfering with RNA synthesis or protein.
Therapeutic Effect: Interferes with the normal repair process of cancer cells damaged by irradiation.

USES
Treatment of melanoma, chronic myelocytic leukemia (CML),

recurrent or metastatic ovarian cancer, in combination with irradiation therapy for carcinomas of the head and neck (except the lip); sickle cell anemia

PHARMACOKINETICS
PO: Readily absorbed with PO use, peak level in 2 hr; 80% excreted in urine.

INDICATIONS AND DOSAGES
▶ **Melanoma; Recurrent, Metastatic, or Inoperable Ovarian Carcinoma**
PO
Adults, Elderly. 80 mg/kg every 3 days or 20–30 mg/kg/day as a single dose.
▶ **Control of Primary Squamous Cell Carcinoma of the Head and Neck, Excluding Lips (in Combination with Radiation Therapy)**
PO
Adults, Elderly. 80 mg/kg every 3 days, beginning at least 7 days before starting radiation therapy.
▶ **Resistant CML**
PO
Adults, Elderly. 20–30 mg/kg once a day.
Children. 10–20 mg/kg once a day.
▶ **HIV Infection**
PO
Adults, Elderly. 500 mg twice a day with didanosine.
▶ **Sickle Cell Anemia**
PO
Adults, Elderly, Children. Initially, 15 mg/kg once a day. May increase by 5 mg/kg/day. Maximum: 35 mg/kg/day.

SIDE EFFECTS/ADVERSE REACTIONS
Frequent
Nausea, vomiting, anorexia, constipation, or diarrhea

Occasional

Mild, reversible rash; facial flushing; pruritus; fever; chills; malaise

Rare

Alopecia, headache, drowsiness, dizziness, disorientation

PRECAUTIONS AND CONTRAINDICATIONS

WBC count less than 2500/mm³ or platelet count less than 100,000/mm³

Caution:

Monitor blood counts and hemoglobin, renal impairment, elderly

DRUG INTERACTIONS OF CONCERN TO DENTISTRY

• None reported

SERIOUS REACTIONS

! Myelosuppression may cause hematologic toxicity (manifested as leukopenia and, to a lesser extent, thrombocytopenia and anemia).

DENTAL CONSIDERATIONS

General:

• Patients receiving chemotherapy may be taking chronic opioids for pain. Consider NSAIDs for dental pain management.

• Patients receiving chemotherapy may require palliative therapy for stomatitis.

• Patients on chronic drug therapy may rarely have symptoms of blood dyscrasias, which can include infection, bleeding, and poor healing.

Consultations:

• Medical consultation may be required to assess disease control.

• In a patient with symptoms of blood dyscrasias, request a medical consultation for blood studies and postpone dental treatment until normal values are reestablished.

Teach Patient/Family to:

• See dentist immediately if secondary oral infection occurs.

• When chronic dry mouth occurs, advise patient to:

  • Avoid mouth rinses with high alcohol content because of drying effects.

  • Use sugarless gum, frequent sips of water, or saliva substitutes.

  • Use daily home fluoride products for anticaries effect.

H

hydroxyzine

high-**drox**′-ih-zeen

(Apo-Hydroxyzine[CAN], Atarax, Novo-Hydroxyzin[CAN], Vistaril)

Do not confuse hydroxyzine with hydralazine or hydroxyurea.

CATEGORY AND SCHEDULE

Pregnancy Risk Category: C

Drug Class: Antianxiety, antihistamine

MECHANISM OF ACTION

A piperazine derivative that competes with histamine for H_1 receptor sites in the GI tract, blood vessels, and respiratory tract. May exert CNS depressant activity in subcortical areas. Diminishes vestibular stimulation and depresses labyrinthine function.

Therapeutic Effect: Produces anxiolytic, anticholinergic, antihistaminic, and analgesic effects; relaxes skeletal muscle; controls nausea and vomiting.

USES

Treatment of anxiety, preoperatively or postoperatively to prevent nausea and vomiting, to potentiate narcotic analgesics, sedation, pruritus

PHARMACOKINETICS

Route	Onset	Peak	Duration
PO	15–30 min	N/A	4–6 hr

Well absorbed from the GI tract and after parenteral administration. Metabolized in the liver. Primarily excreted in urine. Not removed by hemodialysis. *Half-life:* 20–25 hr (increased in the elderly).

INDICATIONS AND DOSAGES
▸ **Anxiety**
PO
Adults, Elderly. 25–100 mg 4 times a day. Maximum: 600 mg/day.
▸ **Nausea and Vomiting**
IM
Adults, Elderly. 25–100 mg/dose q4–6h.
▸ **Pruritus**
PO
Adults, Elderly. 25 mg 3–4 times a day.
▸ **Preoperative Sedation**
PO
Adults, Elderly. 50–100 mg.
IM
Adults, Elderly. 25–100 mg.
▸ **Usual Pediatric Dosage**
PO
Children. 2 mg/kg/day in divided doses q6–8h.
IM
Children. 0.5–1 mg/kg/dose q4–6h.

SIDE EFFECTS/ADVERSE REACTIONS
Side effects are generally mild and transient.
Frequent
Somnolence, dry mouth, marked discomfort with IM injection

Occasional
Dizziness, ataxia, asthenia, slurred speech, headache, agitation, increased anxiety
Rare
Paradoxical CNS reactions, such as hyperactivity or nervousness in children and excitement or restlessness in elderly or debilitated patients (generally noted during first 2 wk of therapy, particularly in presence of uncontrolled pain)

PRECAUTIONS AND CONTRAINDICATIONS
Hypersensitivity, avoid in pregnancy
Caution:
Elderly, debilitated, hepatic disease, renal disease

DRUG INTERACTIONS OF CONCERN TO DENTISTRY
• Increased CNS depressant effect: alcohol, all CNS depressants
• Increased anticholinergic effects: other antihistamines, anticholinergics, opioid analgesics

SERIOUS REACTIONS
! A hypersensitivity reaction, including wheezing, dyspnea, and chest tightness, may occur.

DENTAL CONSIDERATIONS

General:
• Potentiates other CNS depressant drugs. When used in combination, the dose of other CNS depressants should be reduced by half.
• Assess salivary flow as a factor in caries, periodontal disease, and candidiasis.
• Geriatric patients are more susceptible to drug effects; use lower dose.
• Have someone drive patient to and from dental appointment if the drug is prescribed for sedation during dental therapy.

Teach Patient/Family:
• When chronic dry mouth occurs, advise patient to:
  • Avoid mouth rinses with high alcohol content because of drying effects.
  • Use sugarless gum, frequent sips of water, or saliva substitutes.
  • Use daily home fluoride products for anticaries effect.

hyoscyamine
high-oh-**sye′**-ah-meen
(Anaspaz, Buscopan[CAN], Cystospaz, Cystospaz-M, Hyoscine, Levbid, Levsin, Levsin S/L, Levsinex, NuLev, Spacol, Spacol T/S, Symax SL, Symax SR)
Do not confuse Anaspaz with Anaprox.

CATEGORY AND SCHEDULE
Pregnancy Risk Category: C

Drug Class: Anticholinergic

MECHANISM OF ACTION
A GI antispasmodic and anticholinergic agent that inhibits the action of acetylcholine at post-ganglionic (muscarinic) receptor sites.
Therapeutic Effect: Decreases secretions (bronchial, salivary, sweat gland) and gastric juices and reduces motility of GI and urinary tract.

USES
Treatment of peptic ulcer disease in combination with other drugs, other GI disorders, other spastic disorders such as parkinsonism, preoperatively to reduce secretions, GU disorders

(cystitis, renal colic), partial heart block

PHARMACOKINETICS
PO: Duration 4–6 hr; metabolized by liver, excreted in urine. ***Half-life:*** 3.5 hr.

INDICATIONS AND DOSAGES
▸ **GI Tract Disorders**
PO
Adults, Elderly, Children 12 yr and older. 0.125–0.25 mg q4h as needed. Extended-release: 0.375–0.75 mg q12h. Maximum: 1.5 mg/day.
Children 2–11 yr. 0.0625–0.125 mg q4h as needed. Extended-release: 0.375 mg q12h. Maximum: 0.75 mg/day.
IV, IM
Adults, Elderly, Children 12 yr and older. 0.25–0.5 mg q4h for 1–4 doses.
▸ **Hypermotility of Lower Urinary Tract**
PO, Sublingual
Adults, Elderly. 0.15–0.3 mg 4 times a day; or extended-release 0.375 mg q12h.
▸ **Infant Colic**
PO
Infants. Individualized drops dosed q4h as needed.

SIDE EFFECTS/ADVERSE REACTIONS
Frequent
Dry mouth (sometimes severe), decreased sweating, constipation
Occasional
Blurred vision, bloated feeling, urinary hesitancy, somnolence (with high dosage), headache, intolerance to light, loss of taste, nervousness, flushing, insomnia, impotence, mental confusion or excitement (particularly in the elderly and children), temporary

light-headedness (with parenteral form), local irritation (with parenteral form)
Rare
Dizziness, faintness

PRECAUTIONS AND CONTRAINDICATIONS
GI or GU obstruction, myasthenia gravis, narrow-angle glaucoma, paralytic ileus, severe ulcerative colitis
Caution:
Hyperthyroidism, CAD, dysrhythmias, CHF, ulcerative colitis, hypertension, hiatal hernia, hepatic disease, renal disease, urinary retention

DRUG INTERACTIONS OF CONCERN TO DENTISTRY
- Increased anticholinergic effect: other anticholinergics, opioid analgesics
- Decreased effect of phenothiazines

SERIOUS REACTIONS
! Overdose may produce temporary paralysis of ciliary muscle; pupillary dilation; tachycardia; palpitations; hot, dry, or flushed skin; absence of bowel sounds; hyperthermia; increased respiratory rate; ECG abnormalities; nausea; vomiting; rash over face or upper trunk; CNS stimulation; and psychosis (marked by agitation, restlessness, rambling speech, visual hallucinations, paranoid behavior, and delusions, followed by depression).

DENTAL CONSIDERATIONS

General:
- After supine positioning, have patient sit upright for at least 2 min to avoid orthostatic hypotension.
- Assess salivary flow as a factor in caries, periodontal disease, and candidiasis.
- Avoid dental light in patient's eyes; offer dark glasses for patient comfort.

Consultation:
- Physician should be informed if significant xerostomic side effects occur (e.g., increased caries, sore tongue, problems eating or swallowing, difficulty wearing prosthesis) so that a medication change can be considered.

Teach Patient/Family to:
- Encourage effective oral hygiene to prevent soft tissue inflammation.
- When chronic dry mouth occurs, advise patient to:
  - Avoid mouth rinses with high alcohol content because of drying effects.
  - Use sugarless gum, frequent sips of water, or artificial saliva substitutes.
- Use daily home fluoride products for anticaries effect.

ibandronate sodium
eye-**band**'-droh-nate **soe**'-dee-um
(Boniva)

CATEGORY AND SCHEDULE
Pregnancy Risk Category: C

Drug Class: Bisphosphonate;
calcium regulator

MECHANISM OF ACTION
A bisphosphonate that binds to bone
hydroxyapatite (part of the mineral
matrix of bone) and inhibits
osteoclast activity.
Therapeutic Effect: Reduces rate of
bone turnover and bone resorption,
resulting in a net gain in bone mass.

USES
Treatment and prevention of
osteoporosis in postmenopausal
women

PHARMACOKINETICS
Absorbed in the upper GI tract.
Extent of absorption impaired by
food or beverages (other than plain
water). Rapidly binds to bone.
Unabsorbed portion is eliminated in
urine. Protein binding: 90%.
Half-life: 10–60 hr.

INDICATIONS AND DOSAGES
▸ Osteoporosis
PO
Adults, Elderly. 2.5 mg daily.

SIDE EFFECTS/ADVERSE REACTIONS
Frequent
Back pain; dyspepsia, including
epigastric distress and heartburn;
peripheral discomfort; diarrhea;
headache; myalgia
Occasional
Dizziness, arthralgia, asthenia

Rare
Vomiting, hypersensitivity reaction,
osteonecrosis of the jaw

PRECAUTIONS AND CONTRAINDICATIONS
Hypersensitivity to other
bisphosphonates, including
alendronate, etidronate, pamidronate,
risedronate, and tiludronate; inability
to stand or sit upright for at least
60 min; severe renal impairment
with creatinine clearance less than
30 ml/min; uncorrected
hypocalcemia

DRUG INTERACTIONS OF CONCERN TO DENTISTRY
• Decreased absorption: antacids
containing aluminum, calcium, or
magnesium salts, vitamin D
• Use with monitoring, risk of
increased GI side effects: aspirin
and NSAIDs

SERIOUS REACTIONS
❗ Upper respiratory tract infection
occurs occasionally.
❗ Overdose causes hypocalcemia,
hypophosphatemia, and significant
GI disturbances.

DENTAL CONSIDERATIONS
General:
• Bisphosphonates may increase the
risk for osteonecrosis of the jaw (see
section on "Medically Compromised
Patients" for management
considerations).
• Consider semisupine chair position
for patient comfort if GI side effects
occur.
• Patient may need assistance in
getting into and out of dental chair.
Adjust chair position for patient
comfort.
• Emphasize importance of caries
prevention.

Consultations:
• Medical consultation may be required to assess disease control and patient's ability to tolerate stress.
Teach Patient/Family to:
• Observe regular recall schedule and practice effective oral hygiene to minimize risk of osteonecrosis of the jaw.
• Update health and medication history if physician makes any changes in evaluation or drug regimens; include OTC, herbal, and nonherbal remedies in the update.

ibuprofen

eye-byoo-**pro'**-fen
(Act-3[AUS], Advil, Apo-Ibuprofen, Brufen[AUS], Codral Period Pain[AUS], Ibudone, Motrin, Novoprofen[CAN], Nurofen[AUS], Rafen[AUS], Reprexain)

CATEGORY AND SCHEDULE

Pregnancy Risk Category: B (D if used in third trimester or near delivery)
OTC (Tablets: 200 mg, Oral Suspension: 100 mg/5 ml)

Drug Class: Nonsteroidal antiinflammatory

MECHANISM OF ACTION

An NSAID that inhibits prostaglandin synthesis. Also produces vasodilation by acting centrally on the heat-regulating center of the hypothalamus.
Therapeutic Effect: Produces analgesic and antiinflammatory effects and decreases fever.

USES

Treatment of rheumatoid arthritis, osteoarthritis, primary dysmenorrhea, gout, mild to moderate pain, fever

PHARMACOKINETICS

Route	Onset	Peak	Duration
PO (analgesic)	0.5 hr	N/A	4–6 hr
PO (antirheumatic)	2 days	1–2 wk	N/A

Rapidly absorbed from the GI tract. Protein binding: greater than 90%. Metabolized in the liver. Primarily excreted in urine. Not removed by hemodialysis. *Half-life:* 2–4 hr.

INDICATIONS AND DOSAGES

▶ **Acute or Chronic Rheumatoid Arthritis, Osteoarthritis, Migraine Pain, Gouty Arthritis**
PO
Adults, Elderly. 400–800 mg 3–4 times a day. Maximum: 3.2 g/day.
▶ **Mild-to-Moderate Pain, Primary Dysmenorrhea**
PO
Adults, Elderly. 200–400 mg q4–6h as needed. Maximum: 1.6 g/day.
▶ **Fever, Minor Aches, or Pain**
PO
Adults, Elderly. 200–400 mg q4–6h. Maximum: 1.6 g/day.
Children. 5–10 mg/kg/dose q6–8h. Maximum: 40 mg/kg/day. OTC: 7.5 mg/kg/dose q6–8h. Maximum: 30 mg/kg/day.
▶ **Juvenile Arthritis**
PO
Children. 30–70 mg/kg/day in 3–4 divided doses. Maximum: 400 mg/day in children weighing less than 20 kg, 600 mg/day in children weighing 20–30 kg, 800 mg/day in

children weighing greater than 30–40 kg.

SIDE EFFECTS/ADVERSE REACTIONS

Occasional

Nausea with or without vomiting, dyspepsia, dizziness, rash

Rare

Diarrhea or constipation, flatulence, abdominal cramps or pain, pruritus

PRECAUTIONS AND CONTRAINDICATIONS

Active peptic ulcer, chronic inflammation of GI tract, GI bleeding disorders or ulceration, history of hypersensitivity to aspirin or NSAIDs

Possible increased risk for adverse cardiovascular events in patients at risk for thromboembolism

Caution:

Lactation, children, bleeding disorders, GI disorders, cardiac disorders, hypersensitivity to other antiinflammatory agents

DRUG INTERACTIONS OF CONCERN TO DENTISTRY

- GI ulceration, bleeding: aspirin, alcohol (three or more drinks per day), corticosteroids
- Decreased action: salicylates
- Nephrotoxicity: acetaminophen (prolonged use)
- Possible risk of decreased renal function: cyclosporine
- SSRIs: NSAIDs increase risk of GI side effects
- When prescribed for dental pain:
  - Risk of increased effects: oral anticoagulants, oral antidiabetics, lithium, methotrexate
  - Decreased antihypertensive effects of diuretics, β-adrenergic blockers, and ACE inhibitors

SERIOUS REACTIONS

! Acute overdose may result in metabolic acidosis.

! Rare reactions with long-term use include peptic ulcer disease, GI bleeding, gastritis, a severe hepatic reaction (cholestasis, jaundice), nephrotoxicity (dysuria, hematuria, proteinuria, nephrotic syndrome), and a severe hypersensitivity reaction (particularly in patients with systemic lupus erythematosus or other collagen diseases).

DENTAL CONSIDERATIONS

General:

- Patients on chronic drug therapy may rarely have symptoms of blood dyscrasias, which can include infection, bleeding, and poor healing.
- Assess salivary flow as a factor in caries, periodontal disease, and candidiasis.
- Avoid prescribing aspirin-containing products.
- Consider semisupine chair position for patients with arthritic disease.
- Severe stomach bleeding may occur in patients who regularly use NSAIDs in recommended doses, when the patient is also taking another NSAID, anticoagulant/antiplatelet drug, or steroid drug, if the patient has GI or peptic ulcer disease, if they are 60 years or older, or when NSAIDs are taken longer than directed. Warn patients of the potential for severe stomach bleeding.

Consultations:

- In a patient with symptoms of blood dyscrasias, request a medical consultation for blood studies and postpone dental treatment until normal values are reestablished.
- Medical consultation may be required to assess disease control.

Teach Patient/Family to:
• Follow labeled directions for OTC products.
• Encourage effective oral hygiene to prevent soft tissue inflammation.
• Use caution to prevent injury when using oral hygiene aids.
• Warn patient of potential risks of NSAIDs.
• When chronic dry mouth occurs, advise patient to:
  • Avoid mouth rinses with high alcohol content because of drying effects.
  • Use sugarless gum, frequent sips of water, or saliva substitutes.
  • Use daily home fluoride products for anticaries effect.

ibutilide fumarate
eye-byoo′-ti-lide **fyoo′**-muh-reyt
(Corvert)

CATEGORY AND SCHEDULE
Pregnancy Risk Category: C

Drug Class: Antidysrhythmic

MECHANISM OF ACTION
An antiarrhythmic that prolongs both atrial and ventricular action potential duration and increases the atrial and ventricular refractory period. Activates slow, inward current (mostly of sodium), produces mild slowing of sinus node rate and AV conduction, and causes dose-related prolongation of QT interval.
Therapeutic Effect: Converts arrhythmias to sinus rhythm.

USES
For rapid conversion of atrial fibrillation/flutter occurring within 1 wk of coronary artery bypass or valve surgery

PHARMACOKINETICS
After IV administration, highly distributed, rapidly cleared. Protein binding: 40%. Primarily excreted in urine as metabolite. *Half-life:* 2–12 hr (average: 6 hr).

INDICATIONS AND DOSAGES
▶ **Rapid Conversion of Atrial Fibrillation or Flutter of Recent Onset to Normal Sinus Rhythm**
IV Infusion
Adults, Elderly weighing 60 kg and more. One vial (1 mg) given over 10 min. If arrhythmia does not stop within 10 min after end of initial infusion, a second 1 mg/10-min infusion may be given.
Adults, Elderly weighing less than 60 kg. 0.01 mg/kg given over 10 min. If arrhythmia does not stop within 10 min after end of initial infusion, a second 0.01 mg/kg, 10-min infusion may be given.

SIDE EFFECTS/ADVERSE REACTIONS
Ibutilide is generally well tolerated.
Occasional
Ventricular extrasystoles (5.1%), ventricular tachycardia (4.9%), headache (3.6%), hypotension, orthostatic hypotension (2%)
Rare
Bundle-branch block, AV block, bradycardia, hypertension

PRECAUTIONS AND CONTRAINDICATIONS
None known

DRUG INTERACTIONS OF CONCERN TO DENTISTRY
• Potential for arrhythmia: drugs that prolong the QT interval, such as antidepressants

SERIOUS REACTIONS

! Sustained polymorphic ventricular tachycardia, occasionally with QT prolongation (torsades de pointes) occurs rarely.

! Overdose results in CNS toxicity, including CNS depression, rapid and gasping breathing, and seizures.

! Expect prolongation of repolarization may be exaggerated.

! Existing arrhythmias may worsen or new arrhythmias may develop.

DENTAL CONSIDERATIONS

General:

• Acute-use drug for use in hospitals, emergency rooms, or cardiac labs.

• Patients who have received this drug for arrhythmias may be at risk when it is combined with other drugs that prolong the QT interval.

Consultations:

• Medical consultation may be required to assess disease control and patient's ability to tolerate stress.

Teach Patient/Family to:

• Update health and medication history if physician makes any changes in evaluation or drug regimens; include OTC, herbal, and nonherbal remedies in the update.

idarubicin hydrochloride

eye-dah-**roo**′-bi-sin
high-droh-**klor**′-ide
(Idamycin PFS, Zavedos)
Do not confuse idarubicin with doxorubicin, or Idamycin with Adriamycin.

CATEGORY AND SCHEDULE

Pregnancy Risk Category: D

Drug Class: Anthracycline antibiotic; antineoplastic

MECHANISM OF ACTION

An anthracycline antibiotic that inhibits nucleic acid synthesis by interacting with the enzyme topoisomerase II, which promotes DNA strand supercoiling.
Therapeutic Effect: Causes death of rapidly dividing cells.

USES

Treatment of acute myeloid leukemia (AML)

PHARMACOKINETICS

Widely distributed. Protein binding: 97%. Rapidly metabolized in the liver to active metabolite. Primarily eliminated by biliary excretion. Not removed by hemodialysis. *Half-life:* 4–46 hr; metabolite: 8–92 hr.

INDICATIONS AND DOSAGES

▸ **AML**
IV
Adults. 8–12 mg/m^2/day for 3 days in combination with Ara-C.
Children (solid tumor). 5 mg/m^2 once a day for 3 days.
Children (leukemia). 10–12 mg/m^2 once a day for 3 days.
▸ **Dosage in Hepatic or Renal Impairment**
Dosage is modified on the basis of serum creatinine or bilirubin level.

Serum Level	Dose Reduction
Serum creatinine 2 mg/dl or more	25%
Serum bilirubin greater than 2.5 mg/dl	50%
Serum bilirubin greater than 5 mg/dl	Do not give

SIDE EFFECTS/ADVERSE REACTIONS

Frequent
Nausea, vomiting, complete alopecia (scalp, axillary, pubic hair), abdominal cramping, diarrhea, mucositis
Occasional
Hyperpigmentation of nail beds, phalangeal and dermal creases, fever, headache
Rare
Conjunctivitis, neuropathy

PRECAUTIONS AND CONTRAINDICATIONS

Preexisting arrhythmias, cardiomyopathy, myelosuppression, pregnancy, severe CHF

DRUG INTERACTIONS OF CONCERN TO DENTISTRY

• Dental drug interactions have not been studied.

SERIOUS REACTIONS

! Myelosuppression may cause hematologic toxicity (manifested principally as leukopenia and, to a lesser extent, anemia and thrombocytopenia), usually within 10–15 days of starting therapy.
! Blood counts typically return to normal levels by the third week.
! Cardiotoxicity (either acute, manifested as transient ECG abnormalities, or chronic, manifested as CHF) may occur.

DENTAL CONSIDERATIONS

General:
• If additional analgesia is required for dental pain, consider alternative analgesics (acetaminophen) in patients taking opioids for acute or chronic pain.
• Examine for oral manifestation of opportunistic infection.

• This drug may be used in the hospital or on an outpatient basis. Confirm the patient's disease and treatment status.
• Chlorhexidine mouth rinse prior to and during chemotherapy may reduce severity of mucositis.
• Patient on chronic drug therapy may rarely present with symptoms of blood dyscrasias, which can include infection, bleeding, and poor healing. If dyscrasia is present, caution patient to prevent oral tissue trauma when using oral hygiene aids.
• Palliative medication may be required for management of oral side effects.
Consultations:
• Consult physician; prophylactic or therapeutic antiinfectives may be indicated if surgery or periodontal treatment is required.
• Medical consultation may be required to assess immunologic status during cancer chemotherapy and determine safety risk, if any, posed by the required dental treatment.
• Medical consultation may be required to assess disease control and patient's ability to tolerate stress.
Teach Patient/Family to:
• Be aware of oral side effects.
• Encourage effective oral hygiene to prevent soft tissue inflammation.
• Report oral lesions, soreness, or bleeding to dentist.
• Prevent trauma when using oral hygiene aids.
• Update health and medication history if physician makes any changes in evaluation or drug regimens; include OTC, herbal, and nonherbal remedies in the update.

idursulfase
eye-dur-**sul**′-face
(Elaprase)

CATEGORY AND SCHEDULE
Pregnancy Risk Category: C

Drug Class: Enzyme

MECHANISM OF ACTION
A recombinant form of iduronate-2-sulfatase that allows for catabolism of glycosaminoglycans. Hunter syndrome is a disease caused by insufficient levels of this lysosomal enzyme, iduronate-2-sulfate.
Therapeutic Effect: Replaces enzyme (iduronate-2-sulfatase).

USES
Treatment of Hunter syndrome

PHARMACOKINETICS
Half-life: 44–48 min.

INDICATIONS AND DOSAGES
▸ Hunter Syndrome
IV
Adults. 0.5 mg/kg once a wk.
Children (5 yr and older). 0.5 mg/kg once a wk.

SIDE EFFECTS/ADVERSE REACTIONS
Frequent
Fever, headache, antibody development, arthralgia, limb pain, pruritus, hypertension, malaise, visual disturbance, wheezing, musculoskeletal pain, musculoskeletal dysfunction, chest wall, urticaria, abscess, pruritic rash, skin disorder, atrial abnormality, anxiety, irritability, dyspepsia, infusion-site edema, superficial injury

Rare
Angioedema, cardiac arrhythmia, cyanosis, hypotension, infection, pulmonary embolism, respiratory distress, respiratory failure, seizure

PRECAUTIONS AND CONTRAINDICATIONS
Hypersensitivity to idursulfase or its components
Caution:
Impaired respiratory function, fever

DRUG INTERACTIONS OF CONCERN TO DENTISTRY
• None reported

SERIOUS REACTIONS
! Anaphylactic reactions have been reported.

DENTAL CONSIDERATIONS
General:
• Monitor vital signs at every appointment because of cardiovascular side effects.
• Consider semisupine chair position for patient comfort because of respiratory complications.
• Avoid aspirin and NSAIDs.
• Consider visual disturbances when presenting instructions to patients.
Consultations:
• Consult physician to determine disease control and ability of patient to tolerate dental procedures.
Teach Patient/Family to:
• Update medication/health history whenever symptoms of disease or medication regimen is changed.
• Use effective, atraumatic oral hygiene measures to reduce soft tissue inflammation.
• Use home fluoride products for anticaries effect.

ifosfamide
eye-**fos′**-fah-mide
(Holoxan[AUS], Ifex)

CATEGORY AND SCHEDULE
Pregnancy Risk Category: D

Drug Class: Alkylating agent;
antineoplastic

MECHANISM OF ACTION
An alkylating agent that inhibits
DNA and RNA protein synthesis by
cross-linking with DNA and RNA
strands, preventing cell growth. Cell
cycle-phase nonspecific.
Therapeutic Effect: Interferes with
DNA and RNA function.

USES
Treatment of cancer of the testicles
as well as some other kinds of
cancer

PHARMACOKINETICS
Metabolized in the liver to active
metabolite. Crosses the blood-brain
barrier (to a limited extent).
Primarily excreted in urine.
Removed by hemodialysis. ***Half-life:***
15 hr.

INDICATIONS AND DOSAGES
▸ **Germ Cell Testicular Carcinoma**
IV
Adults. 700–2000 mg/m^2/day for 5
consecutive days. Repeat every 3 wk
or after recovery from hematologic
toxicity. Administer with mesna.
Children. 1200–1800 mg/m^2/day for
5 days every 21–28 days.

SIDE EFFECTS/ADVERSE
REACTIONS
Frequent
Alopecia, nausea, vomiting

Occasional
Confusion, somnolence,
hallucinations, infection
Rare
Dizziness, seizures, disorientation,
fever, malaise, stomatitis

PRECAUTIONS AND
CONTRAINDICATIONS
Pregnancy, severe myelosuppression

DRUG INTERACTIONS OF
CONCERN TO DENTISTRY
• Dental drug interactions have not
been studied.

SERIOUS REACTIONS
❗ Hemorrhagic cystitis with
hematuria and dysuria occurs
frequently if a protective agent
(mesna) is not used.
❗ Myelosuppression, characterized
by leukopenia and, to a lesser extent,
thrombocytopenia occurs frequently.
❗ Pulmonary toxicity, hepatotoxicity,
nephrotoxicity, cardiotoxicity, and
CNS toxicity (manifested as
confusion, hallucinations,
somnolence, and coma) may require
discontinuation of therapy.

DENTAL CONSIDERATIONS

General:
• Determine why patient is taking
the drug.
• If additional analgesia is required
for dental pain, consider alternative
analgesics (NSAIDs) in patients
taking narcotics for acute or chronic
pain.
• Examine for oral manifestation of
opportunistic infection.
• Avoid products that affect platelet
function, such as aspirin and NSAIDs.
• This drug may be used in the
hospital or on an outpatient basis.
Confirm the patient's disease and
treatment status.

- Chlorhexidine mouth rinse prior to and during chemotherapy may reduce severity of mucositis.
- Patient on chronic drug therapy may rarely present with symptoms of blood dyscrasias, which can include infection, bleeding, and poor healing. If dyscrasia is present, caution patient to prevent oral tissue trauma when using oral hygiene aids.
- Palliative medication may be required for management of oral side effects.
- Short appointments and a stress-reduction protocol may be required for anxious patients.
- Patients may be at risk of bleeding; check for oral signs.
- Oral infections should be eliminated and/or treated aggressively.

Consultations:
- Medical consultation should include routine blood counts including platelet counts and bleeding time.
- Consult physician; prophylactic or therapeutic antiinfectives may be indicated if surgery or periodontal treatment is required.
- Medical consultation may be required to assess immunologic status during cancer chemotherapy and determine safety risk, if any, posed by the required dental treatment.
- Medical consultation may be required to assess disease control and patient's ability to tolerate stress.

Teach Patient/Family to:
- Be aware of oral side effects.
- Encourage effective oral hygiene to prevent soft tissue inflammation.
- Report oral lesions, soreness, or bleeding to dentist.
- Prevent trauma when using oral hygiene aids.

- Update health and medication history if physician makes any changes in evaluation or drug regimens; include OTC, herbal, and nonherbal remedies in the update.

iloperidone
ilo-**per'**-i-done
(Fanapt)

CATEGORY AND SCHEDULE
Pregnancy Risk Category: C

Drug Class: Antipsychotic agent, atypical; dopamine and serotonin antagonist

MECHANISM OF ACTION
A piperidinyl-benzisoxazole derivative that antagonizes dopamine Type 2 and serotonin Type 2 receptors. *Therapeutic Effect:* Diminishes symptoms of schizophrenia.

USES
Schizophrenia

PHARMACOKINETICS
Well absorbed following PO administration. Bioavailability: 96%. Protein binding: 95%. Primarily metabolized by CYP2D6 and CYP3A4 to active metabolites P95 and P88. Partially excreted in urine; partially excreted in feces. *Half-life:* 18–37 hr; for iloperidone. P88 and P95 in CYP2D6 extensive metabolizers: 18, 26, and 23 hr, respectively; poor metabolizers: 33, 37, and 31 hr, respectively.

INDICATIONS AND DOSAGES
▸ **Schizophrenia**
PO
Adults. Initially, 1 mg twice a day. Maintenance dose: 12–24 mg a day. May titrate dose as needed

according to the following dosing schedule: 2 mg twice a day on day 2; 4 mg twice a day on day 3; 6 mg twice on day 4; 8 mg twice a day on day 5; 10 mg twice a day on day 6; 12 mg twice a day on day 7. Max dose: 12 mg twice a day.

SIDE EFFECTS/ADVERSE REACTIONS

Frequent
Tachycardia, dry mouth, nausea, dizziness, somnolence

Occasional
Orthostatic hypotension, hypotension, diarrhea, abdominal discomfort, ejaculation failure, weight gain, blurred vision, nasal congestion, nasopharyngitis, upper respiratory tract infection, dyspnea, arthralgia, musculoskeletal stiffness, rash

Rare
Palpitation, erectile dysfunction, urinary incontinence, weight loss, muscle spasm, myalgia, conjunctivitis, low hematocrit

PRECAUTIONS AND CONTRAINDICATIONS

Hypersensitivity to iloperidone or its components

Caution:
Elderly with dementia-related psychosis (increased mortality)—black box warning
Hepatic impairment
Neuroleptic malignant syndrome
Tardive dyskinesia
Seizures
Leukopenia, neutropenia, agranulocytosis
Patients at risk for suicide
Cognitive and motor impairment
Hyperglycemia, diabetes, patients should be monitored for signs and symptoms of hyperglycemia
QT prolongation; electrolyte disturbances; serum potassium and

magnesium should be monitored as hypokalemia and hypomagnesemia may increase the risk of QT prolongation

DRUG INTERACTIONS OF CONCERN TO DENTISTRY

• CNS depressants, alcohol: Additive CNS depressant effects
• Antihypertensive agents: May enhance the hypotensive effects
• CYP2D6 inhibitors: May increase iloperidone concentrations
• CYP3A4 inhibitors: May increase iloperidone concentrations
• QT-interval prolonging drugs: May cause additive effects

SERIOUS REACTIONS

! Prolongation of QT interval may produce torsades de pointes. Patients with bradycardia, hypokalemia, hypomagnesemia are at increased risk.
! Priapism has been reported.
! Orthostatic hypotension including dizziness, tachycardia, and syncope with standing may occur.
! Cerebrovascular accident and transient ischemic attack can occur.
! Monitor for thoughts of suicide.

DENTAL CONSIDERATIONS

General:
• Monitor vital signs at every appointment because of cardiovascular side effects.
• After supine positioning, have patient sit upright for at least 2 min before standing to avoid orthostatic hypotension.
• Assess salivary flow as a factor in caries, periodontal disease, and candidiasis.
• Assess for presence of extrapyramidal motor symptoms such as tardive dyskinesia and akathisia. Extrapyramidal motor

activity may complicate dental treatment.

• Consider semisupine chair position for patient comfort if GI side effects occur.

Consultations:

• In a patient with symptoms of blood dyscrasias, request a medical consultation for blood studies and postpone treatment until normal values are reestablished.

• Medical consultation may be required to assess disease control.

• Physician should be informed if significant xerostomic side effects occur (e.g., increased caries, sore tongue, problems eating or swallowing, difficulty wearing prosthesis) so that medication change can be considered.

• Consultation with physician may be necessary if sedation or general anesthesia is required.

Teach Patient/Family to:

• Encourage effective oral hygiene to prevent soft tissue inflammation.

• Prevent trauma when using oral hygiene aids.

• When chronic dry mouth occurs, advise patient to:

• Avoid mouth rinses with high alcohol content because of drying effects.

• Use daily home fluoride products for anticaries effect.

• Use sugarless gum, frequent sips of water, or saliva substitutes

iloprost
eye-low-prost
(Ventavis)

CATEGORY AND SCHEDULE
Pregnancy Risk Category: C

Drug Class: Agents for pulmonary hypertension

MECHANISM OF ACTION
A prostaglandin that dilates systemic and pulmonary arterial vascular beds, alters pulmonary vascular resistance, and suppresses vascular smooth muscle proliferation. Inhibits platelet aggregation.

Therapeutic Effect: Improves symptoms and exercise tolerance in patients with pulmonary hypertension; delays deterioration of condition.

USES
Pulmonary hypertension in patients with NYHA Class III or IV symptoms

PHARMACOKINETICS
Protein binding: 60%. Metabolized in liver; primarily by beta-oxidation of the carboxyl side chain to tetranoriloprost. Primarily excreted in urine; minimal elimination in feces. **Half-life:** 20–30 min.

INDICATIONS AND DOSAGES
▶ **Pulmonary Hypertension in Patients with NYHA Class III or IV Symptoms**
Oral Inhalation
Adults, Elderly. Initially, 2.5 mcg/dose; if tolerated, increased to 5 mcg/dose. Administer 6–9 times a day at intervals of 2 hr or longer while patient is awake. Maintenance: 5 mcg/dose. Maximum daily dose: 45 mcg.

SIDE EFFECTS/ADVERSE REACTIONS
Frequent
Increased cough, headache, flushing (vasodilation)
Occasional
Flu-like symptoms, nausea, trismus, jaw pain, hypotension

Rare
Insomnia, syncope, palpitations, vomiting, back pain, muscle cramps, GGT increased, CHF

PRECAUTIONS AND CONTRAINDICATIONS
Hypersensitivity to iloprost or any component of the formulation. If signs of pulmonary edema occur when inhaled iloprost is administered in patients with pulmonary hypertension, treatment should be stopped immediately; may be a sign of pulmonary venous hypertension.
Caution:
Hepatic impairment
Renal impairment
Elderly
Pregnancy
Bleeding disorders
Hypotension (systolic B/P <85 mm Hg)
Respiratory disease (COPD, severe asthma, acute pulmonary infections)

DRUG INTERACTIONS OF CONCERN TO DENTISTRY
• Anticoagulants, antiplatelet agents: May increased the risk of bleeding
• Antihypertensives, other vasodilators: May increase the hypotensive effects of iloprost
• Monoamine oxidase inhibitors (MAOIs): Additive hypotensive effects

SERIOUS REACTIONS
! Hemoptysis and pneumonia occur occasionally.
! CHF, renal failure, dyspnea, and chest pain occur rarely.

DENTAL CONSIDERATIONS
General:
• Monitor vital signs at every appointment due to cardiovascular side effects.

• After supine positioning, have patient sit upright for at least 2 min before standing to avoid orthostatic hypotension.
• Assess for signs of pulmonary venous hypertension (pulmonary edema).
Consultations:
• Medical consultation may be required to assess disease control.
Teach Patient/Family to:
• Encourage effective oral hygiene to prevent soft tissue inflammation.
• Use soft tooth brush to reduce risk of bleeding.
• Immediately report any sign of infection to the dentist.

---

imatinib mesylate
im'-ah-tin-ib
(Gleevec, Glivec[AUS])

CATEGORY AND SCHEDULE
Pregnancy Risk Category: D

Drug Class: Antineoplastic

MECHANISM OF ACTION
Inhibits Bcr-Abl tyrosine kinase, an enzyme created by the Philadelphia chromosome abnormality found in patients with chronic myeloid leukemia (CML).
Therapeutic Effect: Suppresses tumor growth during the three stages of CML; blast crisis, accelerated phase, and chronic phase.

USES
Treatment of CML in blast crisis, accelerated phase or chronic phase after failure of interferon-α therapy; GI stromal tumors

PHARMACOKINETICS
Well absorbed after PO administration. Binds to plasma

proteins, particularly albumin. Metabolized in the liver. Eliminated mainly in the feces as metabolites. *Half-life:* 18 hr.

INDICATIONS AND DOSAGES
▸ CML
PO
Adults, Elderly. 400 mg/day for patients in chronic-phase CML; 600 mg/day for patients in accelerated phase or blast crisis. May increase dosage from 400 to 600 mg/day for patients in chronic phase or from 600 to 800 mg (given as 300–400 mg twice a day) for patients in accelerated phase or blast crisis in the absence of a severe drug reaction or severe neutropenia or thrombocytopenia in the following circumstances: progression of the disease, failure to achieve a satisfactory hematologic response after 3 mo or more of treatment, or loss of a previously achieved hematologic response.
Children. 260 mg/m^2 a day as a single daily dose or in 2 divided doses.

SIDE EFFECTS/ADVERSE REACTIONS
Frequent
Nausea, diarrhea, vomiting, headache, fluid retention (periorbital, lower extremities), rash, musculoskeletal pain, muscle cramps, arthralgia
Occasional
Abdominal pain, cough, myalgia, fatigue, fever, anorexia, dyspepsia, constipation, night sweats, pruritus
Rare
Nasopharyngitis, petechiae, asthenia, epistaxis

PRECAUTIONS AND CONTRAINDICATIONS
Known hypersensitivity to imatinib

Caution:
Fluid retention, edema risk; neutropenia, thrombocytopenia, GI irritation, liver function abnormalities; safety in lactation or pediatric patients has not been studied

DRUG INTERACTIONS OF CONCERN TO DENTISTRY
• Increased plasma levels with CYP3A4 isoenzyme inhibitors: ketoconazole; possibly macrolide antibiotics, itraconazole, benzodiazepines
• Use acetaminophen with caution or avoid if hepatotoxicity is present
• Possible decrease in plasma concentrations: dexamethasone, carbamazepine, St. John's wort (herb)

SERIOUS REACTIONS
! Severe fluid retention (manifested as pleural effusion, pericardial effusion, pulmonary edema, and ascites) and hepatotoxicity occur rarely.
! Neutropenia and thrombocytopenia are expected responses to the drug.
! Respiratory toxicity, manifested as dyspnea and pneumonia, may occur.

DENTAL CONSIDERATIONS
General:
• Prophylactic or therapeutic antibiotics may be indicated to prevent or treat infection if surgery or periodontal debridement is required.
• Patients taking opioids for acute or chronic pain should be given alternative analgesics for dental pain.
• Short appointments and a stress reduction protocol may be required for anxious patients.

- Consider local hemostasis measures to control excessive bleeding.
- Patients on chronic drug therapy may rarely have symptoms of blood dyscrasias, which can include infection, bleeding, and poor healing.
- Consider semisupine chair position for patient comfort if GI side effects occur.

Consultations:
- In a patient with symptoms of blood dyscrasias, request a medical consultation for blood studies and postpone treatment until normal values are reestablished.
- Consultation with physician may be necessary if sedation or general anesthesia is required.
- Medical consultation should include routine blood counts, including platelet counts and bleeding time.

Teach Patient/Family to:
- Encourage effective oral hygiene to prevent soft tissue inflammation, infection.
- Inform dentist of unusual bleeding episodes following dental treatment.

imipramine
ih-**mih′**-prah-meen
(Apo-Imipramine[CAN], Melipramine[AUS], Tofranil, Tofranil-PM)
Do not confuse imipramine with desipramine.

CATEGORY AND SCHEDULE
Pregnancy Risk Category: D

Drug Class: Antidepressant (tricyclic)

MECHANISM OF ACTION
A tricyclic antidepressant, antibulimic, anticataleptic, antinarcoleptic, antineuralgic, antineuritic, and antipanic agent that blocks the reuptake of neurotransmitters, such as norepinephrine and serotonin, at presynaptic membranes, increasing their concentration at postsynaptic receptor sites.
Therapeutic Effect: Relieves depression and controls nocturnal enuresis.

USES
Treatment of depression, enuresis in children

PHARMACOKINETICS
PO: Steady state 2–5 days.
Half-life: 6–20 hr; metabolized by liver; excreted by kidneys, feces; crosses placenta; excreted in breast milk.

INDICATIONS AND DOSAGES
▶ **Depression**
PO
Adults. Initially, 75–100 mg/day. May gradually increase to 300 mg/day for hospitalized patients, or 200 mg/day for outpatients; then reduce dosage to effective maintenance level, 50–150 mg/day.
Elderly. Initially, 10–25 mg/day at bedtime. May increase by 10–25 mg every 3–7 days. Range: 50–150 mg/day.
Children. 1.5 mg/kg/day. May increase by 1 mg/kg every 3–4 days. Maximum: 5 mg/kg/day.
▶ **Enuresis**
PO
Children older than 6 yr. Initially, 10–25 mg at bedtime. May increase by 25 mg/day. Maximum: 50 mg for children older than 12 yr.

SIDE EFFECTS/ADVERSE REACTIONS

Frequent

Somnolence, fatigue, dry mouth, blurred vision, constipation, delayed micturition, orthostatic hypotension, diaphoresis, impaired concentration, increased appetite, urine retention, photosensitivity

Occasional

GI disturbances (nausea, metallic taste)

Rare

Paradoxical reactions, (agitation, restlessness, nightmares, insomnia), extrapyramidal symptoms (particularly fine hand tremors)

PRECAUTIONS AND CONTRAINDICATIONS

Acute recovery period after MI, use within 14 days of MAOIs.

Caution:

Suicidal patients, severe depression, increased intraocular pressure, narrow-angle glaucoma, urinary retention, cardiac disease, hepatic disease, hyperthyroidism, electroshock therapy, elective surgery, elderly, MAOIs

DRUG INTERACTIONS OF CONCERN TO DENTISTRY

• Increased anticholinergic effects: muscarinic blockers, antihistamines, phenothiazines
• Increased effects of direct-acting sympathomimetics (epinephrine, levonordefrin)
• Potential risk of increased CNS depression: alcohol, barbiturates, benzodiazepines, other CNS depressants
• Decreased antihypertensive effects: clonidine, guanadrel, guanethidine
• Avoid concurrent use with St. John's wort (herb)

• Suspected increased tricyclic antidepressant effects: fluconazole, ketoconazole
• Increased serum levels of carbamazepine
• Caution in using drugs metabolized by CYP2D6: increased effects

SERIOUS REACTIONS

❗ Overdose may produce seizures; cardiovascular effects, such as severe orthostatic hypotension, dizziness, tachycardia, palpitations, and arrhythmias; and altered temperature regulation, including hyperpyrexia or hypothermia.
❗ Abrupt discontinuation after prolonged therapy may produce headache, malaise, nausea, vomiting, and vivid dreams.

DENTAL CONSIDERATIONS

General:

• Monitor vital signs at every appointment because of cardiovascular side effects.
• Limit dose or avoid vasoconstrictor.
• Assess salivary flow as a factor in caries, periodontal disease, and candidiasis.
• Patients on chronic drug therapy may rarely have symptoms of blood dyscrasias, which can include infection, bleeding, and poor healing.
• After supine positioning, have patient sit upright for at least 2 min to avoid orthostatic hypotension.
• Use vasoconstrictors with caution, in low doses, and with careful aspiration. Avoid use of gingival retraction cord with epinephrine.
• Place on frequent recall because of oral side effects.

Consultations:

• In a patient with symptoms of blood dyscrasias, request a medical

consultation for blood studies and postpone dental treatment until normal values are reestablished.
• Medical consultation may be required to assess disease control.
• Physician should be informed if significant xerostomic side effects occur (e.g., increased caries, sore tongue, problems eating or swallowing, difficulty wearing prosthesis) so that a medication change can be considered.

Teach Patient/Family to:
• Encourage effective oral hygiene to prevent soft tissue inflammation.
• Prevent injury when using oral hygiene aids.
• When chronic dry mouth occurs, advise patient to:
    • Avoid mouth rinses with high alcohol content because of drying effects.
    • Use sugarless gum, frequent sips of water, or saliva substitutes.
    • Use daily home fluoride products for anticaries effect.

imiquimod
im-**ick**′-wih-mod
(Aldara)

CATEGORY AND SCHEDULE
Pregnancy Risk Category: C

Drug Class: Immune response modifier

MECHANISM OF ACTION
An immune response modifier whose mechanism of action is unknown.
Therapeutic Effect: Reduces genital and perianal warts.

USES
Treatment of external genital and perianal warts, condylomata acuminata

PHARMACOKINETICS
Minimal absorption after topical administration. Minimal excretion in urine and feces.

INDICATIONS AND DOSAGES
▶ **Warts/Condyloma Acuminata**
Topical
Adults, Elderly, Children 12 yr and older. Apply 3 times a wk before normal sleeping hours; leave on skin 6–10 hr. Remove following treatment period. Continue therapy for maximum of 16 wk.

SIDE EFFECTS/ADVERSE REACTIONS
Frequent
Local skin reactions: erythema, itching, burning, erosion, excoriation/flaking, fungal infections (women)
Occasional
Pain, induration, ulceration, scabbing, soreness, headache, flu-like symptoms

PRECAUTIONS AND CONTRAINDICATIONS
History of hypersensitivity to imiquimod
Caution:
Has not been evaluated in papilloma viral diseases, cream may weaken condoms and diaphragms, external use only, lactation, children younger 18 yr

DRUG INTERACTIONS OF CONCERN TO DENTISTRY
• None reported

SERIOUS REACTIONS
❗ None reported

DENTAL CONSIDERATIONS

General:
• Oral manifestations of the disease may occur in the oral mucosa.

• Patient may have history of other sexually transmitted diseases (STDs).
Consultations:
• Medical consultation may be required to assess disease control.
Teach Patient/Family to:
• Report oral lesions to the dentist.
• Update health and drug history if physician makes any changes in evaluation or drug regimens.

indapamide
in-**dap**′-ah-mide
(Dapa-tabs[AUS], Indahexal[AUS], Insig[AUS], Lozide[CAN], Lozol, Natrilix[AUS], Natrilix SR[AUS])
Do not confuse indapamide with iodamide or iopamidol.

CATEGORY AND SCHEDULE
Pregnancy Risk Category: B (D if used in pregnancy-induced hypertension)

Drug Class: Diuretic, thiazide-like

MECHANISM OF ACTION
A thiazide-like diuretic that blocks reabsorption of water, sodium, and potassium at the cortical diluting segment of the distal tubule; also reduces plasma and extracellular fluid volume and peripheral vascular resistance by direct effect on blood vessels.
Therapeutic Effect: Promotes diuresis and reduces B/P.

USES
Treatment of edema, hypertension

PHARMACOKINETICS
PO: Onset 1–2 hr, peak 2 hr, duration up to 36 hr. *Half-life:* 14–18 hr; excreted in urine, feces.

INDICATIONS AND DOSAGES
▸ **Edema**
PO
Adults. Initially, 2.5 mg/day, may increase to 5 mg/day after 1 wk.
▸ **Hypertension**
PO
Adults, Elderly. Initially, 1.25 mg, may increase to 2.5 mg/day after 4 wk or 5 mg/day after additional 4 wk.

SIDE EFFECTS/ADVERSE REACTIONS
Frequent
Fatigue, numbness of extremities, tension, irritability, agitation, headache, dizziness, light-headedness, insomnia, muscle cramps
Occasional
Tingling of extremities, urinary frequency, urticaria, rhinorrhea, flushing, weight loss, orthostatic hypotension, depression, blurred vision, nausea, vomiting, diarrhea or constipation, dry mouth, impotence, rash, pruritus

PRECAUTIONS AND CONTRAINDICATIONS
Hypersensitivity, anuria
Caution:
Hypokalemia, dehydration, ascites, hepatic disease, severe renal disease

DRUG INTERACTIONS OF CONCERN TO DENTISTRY
• Decreased hypotensive response: NSAIDs, especially indomethacin

SERIOUS REACTIONS
❗ Vigorous diuresis may lead to profound water and electrolyte depletion, resulting in hypokalemia, hyponatremia, and dehydration.
❗ Acute hypotensive episodes may occur.
❗ Hyperglycemia may occur during prolonged therapy.

! Pancreatitis, blood dyscrasias, pulmonary edema, allergic pneumonitis, and dermatologic reactions occur rarely.

! Overdose can lead to lethargy and coma without changes in electrolytes or hydration.

DENTAL CONSIDERATIONS

General:

• Monitor vital signs at every appointment because of cardiovascular side effects.

• Patients on chronic drug therapy may rarely have symptoms of blood dyscrasias, which can include infection, bleeding, and poor healing.

• After supine positioning, have patient sit upright for at least 2 min before standing to avoid orthostatic hypotension.

• Assess salivary flow as a factor in caries, periodontal disease, and candidiasis.

• Limit use of sodium-containing products, such as saline IV fluids, for patients with a dietary salt restriction.

• Stress from dental procedures may compromise cardiovascular function; determine patient risk.

• Short appointments and a stress-reduction protocol may be required for anxious patients.

• Patients on diuretic therapy should be monitored for serum K levels.

Consultations:

• In a patient with symptoms of blood dyscrasias, request a medical consultation for blood studies and postpone dental treatment until normal values are reestablished.

• Medical consultation may be required to assess disease control and patient's ability to tolerate stress.

Teach Patient/Family to:

• Encourage effective oral hygiene to prevent soft tissue inflammation.

• Use caution to prevent injury when using oral hygiene aids.

• When chronic dry mouth occurs, advise patient to:

  • Avoid mouth rinses with high alcohol content because of drying effects.

  • Use sugarless gum, frequent sips of water, or saliva substitutes.

  • Use daily home fluoride products for anticaries effect.

indinavir
in-**din**′-ah-veer
(Crixivan)
Do not confuse indinavir with Denavir.

CATEGORY AND SCHEDULE
Pregnancy Risk Category: C

Drug Class: Antiviral

MECHANISM OF ACTION
A protease inhibitor that suppresses HIV protease, an enzyme necessary for splitting viral polyprotein precursors into mature and infectious viral particles.
Therapeutic Effect: Interrupts HIV replication, slowing the progression of HIV infection.

USES
Treatment of HIV infection; prophylaxis after needle stick with AZT and lamivudine within 2 hr of needle stick

PHARMACOKINETICS
Rapidly absorbed after PO administration. Protein binding: 60%. Metabolized in the liver. Primarily excreted in urine. Unknown if removed by

hemodialysis. *Half-life:* 1.8 hr (increased in impaired hepatic function).

INDICATIONS AND DOSAGES
▶ **HIV Infection (in Combination with Other Antiretrovirals)**
PO
Adults. 800 mg (two 400-mg capsules) q8h.
▶ **HIV Infection in Patients with Hepatic Insufficiency**
PO
Adults. 600 mg q8h.

SIDE EFFECTS/ADVERSE REACTIONS
Frequent
Nausea, abdominal pain, headache, diarrhea
Occasional
Vomiting, asthenia, fatigue, insomnia, accumulation of fat in waist, abdomen, or back of neck
Rare
Abnormal taste sensation, heartburn, symptomatic urinary tract disease, transient renal dysfunction

PRECAUTIONS AND CONTRAINDICATIONS
Hypersensitivity to indinavir; nephrolithiasis
Caution:
Nephrolithiasis (requires adequate hydration), hyperbilirubinemia, serum transaminase elevation, hepatic impairment, dose reduction of rifabutin required, lactation, children

DRUG INTERACTIONS OF CONCERN TO DENTISTRY
• Contraindicated with triazolam, midazolam
• Reduce dose when given with ketoconazole

SERIOUS REACTIONS
! Nephrolithiasis (flank pain with or without hematuria) occurs in 4% of patients.

DENTAL CONSIDERATIONS
General:
• Consider semisupine chair position when GI side effects occur.
• Assess salivary flow as a factor in caries, periodontal disease, and candidiasis.
• Monitor vital signs at every appointment because of cardiovascular side effects.
• Examine for oral manifestation of opportunistic infection.
• Patients with gastroesophageal reflux may have oral symptoms, including burning mouth, secondary candidiasis, and signs of tooth erosion.
Consultations:
• Medical consultation may be required to assess disease control.
Teach Patient/Family to:
• Encourage effective oral hygiene to prevent soft tissue inflammation.
• Report oral lesions, soreness, or bleeding to dentist.
• Update health history/drug record if physician makes any changes in evaluation or drug regimens.
• When chronic dry mouth occurs, advise patient to:
  • Avoid mouth rinses with high alcohol content because of drying effects.
  • Use daily home fluoride products for anticaries effect.
  • Use sugarless gum, frequent sips of water, or saliva substitutes.

indomethacin

in-doe-**meth'**-ah-sin
(Apo-Indomethacin[CAN],
Arthrexin[AUS], Indocid[CAN],
Indocin, Indocin-IV, Indocin-SR,
Novomethacin[CAN])
Do not confuse Indocin with
Imodium or Vicodin.

CATEGORY AND SCHEDULE

Pregnancy Risk Category: B (D if
used after 34 wk gestation, close
to delivery, or for longer than
48 hr)

Drug Class: Nonsteroidal
antiinflammatory

MECHANISM OF ACTION

An NSAID that produces analgesic
and antiinflammatory effects by
inhibiting prostaglandin synthesis.
Also increases the sensitivity of the
premature ductus to the dilating
effects of prostaglandins.
Therapeutic Effect: Reduces the
inflammatory response and intensity
of pain. Closure of the patent ductus
arteriosus.

USES

Treatment of rheumatoid arthritis,
osteoarthritis, ankylosing rheumatoid
spondylitis, acute gouty arthritis

PHARMACOKINETICS

PO: Onset 1–2 hr, peak 3 hr,
duration 4–6 hr; 99% plasma-protein
binding; metabolized in liver,
kidneys; excreted in urine, bile,
feces, breast milk; crosses placenta

INDICATIONS AND DOSAGES
▸ **Moderate-to-Severe Rheumatoid
Arthritis, Osteoarthritis, Ankylosing
Spondylitis**
PO
Adults, Elderly. Initially, 25 mg 2–3
times a day; increased by 25–50 mg/
wk up to 150–200 mg/day, or
75 mg/day (extended-release) up to
75 mg twice a day.
Children. 1–2 mg/kg/day. Maximum:
150–200 mg/day.
▸ **Acute Gouty Arthritis**
PO
Adults, Elderly. Initially, 100 mg,
then 50 mg 3 times a day.
▸ **Acute Shoulder Pain**
PO
Adults, Elderly. 75–150 mg/day in
3–4 divided doses.
▸ **Usual Rectal Dosage**
Adults, Elderly. 50 mg 4 times a day.
Children. Initially, 1.5–2.5 mg/kg/
day, increased up to 4 mg/kg/day.
Maximum: 150–200 mg/day.
▸ **Patent Ductus Arteriosus**
IV
Neonates. Initially, 0.2 mg/kg.
Subsequent doses are on the basis of
age, as follows:
Neonates older than 7 days.
0.25 mg/kg for second and third
doses.
Neonates 2–7 days. 0.2 mg/kg for
second and third doses.
Neonates less than 48 hr. 0.1 mg/kg
for second and third doses.

SIDE EFFECTS/ADVERSE
REACTIONS
Frequent
Headache, nausea, vomiting,
dyspepsia, dizziness
Occasional
Depression, tinnitus, diaphoresis,
somnolence, constipation, diarrhea,
bleeding disturbances in patent
ductus arteriosus

Rare
Hypertension, confusion, urticaria, pruritus, rash, blurred vision

PRECAUTIONS AND CONTRAINDICATIONS
Active GI bleeding or ulcerations; hypersensitivity to aspirin, indomethacin, or other NSAIDs; renal impairment, thrombocytopenia.
Caution:
Lactation, children, bleeding disorders, GI disorders, cardiac disorders, hypersensitivity to other antiinflammatory agents, depression

DRUG INTERACTIONS OF CONCERN TO DENTISTRY
• Increased GI bleeding, ulceration: corticosteroids, alcohol, aspirin, other NSAIDs
• Renal toxicity: acetaminophen (high doses, prolonged use)
• Possible risk of decreased renal function: cyclosporine
• When prescribed for dental pain:
  • Risk of increased effects: oral anticoagulants, oral antidiabetics, lithium, methotrexate
  • Decreased antihypertensive effects of diuretics, β-adrenergic blockers, ACE inhibitors
  • Increased toxicity of zidovudine
  • SSRIs: increased risk of GI side effects

SERIOUS REACTIONS
! Paralytic ileus and ulceration of the esophagus, stomach, duodenum, or small intestine may occur.
! Patients with impaired renal function may develop hyperkalemia and worsening of renal impairment.
! Indomethacin use may aggravate epilepsy, parkinsonism, and depression or other psychiatric disturbances.

! Nephrotoxicity, including dysuria, hematuria, proteinuria, and nephrotic syndrome, occurs rarely.
! Metabolic acidosis or alkalosis, apnea, and bradycardia occur rarely in patients with patent ductus arteriosus.

DENTAL CONSIDERATIONS
General:
• Avoid prescribing aspirin-containing products.
• Patients on chronic drug therapy may rarely have symptoms of blood dyscrasias, which can include infection, bleeding, and poor healing.
• Assess salivary flow as a factor in caries, periodontal disease, and candidiasis.
• Consider semisupine chair position for patients with arthritic disease.
• Severe stomach bleeding may occur in patients who regularly use NSAIDs in recommended doses, when the patient is also taking another NSAID, an anticoagulant/antiplatelet drug, or steroid drug, if the patient has GI or peptic ulcer disease, if they are 60 years or older, or when NSAIDs are taken longer than directed. Warn patients of the potential for severe stomach bleeding.
Consultations:
• In a patient with symptoms of blood dyscrasias, request a medical consultation for blood studies and postpone dental treatment until normal values are reestablished.
• Medical consultation may be required to assess disease control.
Teach Patient/Family to:
• Encourage effective oral hygiene to prevent soft tissue inflammation.
• Use caution to prevent injury when using oral hygiene aids.

• When chronic dry mouth occurs, advise patient to:
  • Avoid mouth rinses with high alcohol content because of drying effects.
  • Use sugarless gum, frequent sips of water, or saliva substitutes.
  • Use daily home fluoride products for anticaries effect.
• Warn patient of potential risks of NSAIDs.

infliximab
in-**flicks**′-ih-mab
(Remicade)
Do not confuse Remicade with Reminyl.

CATEGORY AND SCHEDULE
Pregnancy Risk Category: C

Drug Class: Antiinflammatory

MECHANISM OF ACTION
A monoclonal antibody that binds to tumor necrosis factor (TNF), inhibiting functional activity of TNF. Reduces infiltration of inflammatory cells.
Therapeutic Effect: Decreases inflamed areas of the intestine.

USES
Reduces signs and symptoms, progression of structural damage in rheumatoid arthritis in combination with methotrexate; improvement of physical function in moderate-to-severe rheumatoid arthritis in combination with methotrexate; reduction in signs and symptoms in patients with Crohn's disease with inadequate response to conventional therapy, long-term control of remission-level Crohn's disease;

reduces and maintains fistulas in Crohn's disease

PHARMACOKINETICS

Route	Onset	Peak	Duration
IV (Crohn's disease)	1–2 wk	N/A	8–48 wk
IV (rheumatoid arthritis)	3–7 days	N/A	6–12 wk

Absorbed into the GI tissue; primarily distributed in the vascular compartment. **Half-life:** 9.5 days.

INDICATIONS AND DOSAGES
▶ **Moderate-to-Severe Crohn's Disease**
IV Infusion
Adults, Elderly. 5 mg/kg as a single IV infusion.
▶ **Fistulizing Crohn's Disease**
IV Infusion
Adults, Elderly. Initially, 5 mg/kg followed by additional 5-mg/kg doses at 2 and 6 wk after first infusion.
▶ **Rheumatoid Arthritis**
IV Infusion
Adults, Elderly. 3 mg/kg; followed by additional doses at 2 and 6 wk after first infusion. Then q8wk.

SIDE EFFECTS/ADVERSE REACTIONS
Frequent
Headache, nausea, fatigue, fever
Occasional
Fever or chills during infusion, pharyngitis, vomiting, pain, dizziness, bronchitis, rash, rhinitis, cough, pruritus, sinusitis, myalgia, back pain
Rare
Hypotension or hypertension, paresthesia, anxiety, depression, insomnia, diarrhea, urinary tract infection

PRECAUTIONS AND CONTRAINDICATIONS
Sensitivity to infliximab or murine proteins, sepsis, serious active infection
Caution:
Risk of serious infections, risk of autoimmunity, chronic use increases risk of lymphoma, do not give live vaccines to patients taking this drug, patients should be tested for tuberculosis before starting therapy, no data on lactation or pediatric use

DRUG INTERACTIONS OF CONCERN TO DENTISTRY
• No drug interaction studies conducted

SERIOUS REACTIONS
! Hypersensitivity reaction, lupus-like syndrome, and severe hepatic reactions may occur.

DENTAL CONSIDERATIONS
General:
• Determine why patient is taking the drug.
• Avoid drugs that irritate the GI tract.
• Question patient about other drugs being taken.
• Examine for oral manifestation of opportunistic infection.
• Report oral infections to patient's physician; treat infections aggressively.
Consultations:
• Medical consultation may be required to assess disease control and patient's ability to tolerate stress.
Teach Patient/Family to:
• Encourage effective oral hygiene to prevent soft tissue inflammation, infection.
• Immediately report any signs or symptoms of oral infection.

insulin
in'-su-lin
Rapid acting: Insulin Lispro (Humalog); Insulin Aspart (Novolog, NovoMix 30[AUS], Novorapid[AUS]); Regular Insulin (Actrapid[AUS], Humulin R, Novolin R, Regular Iletin II); Intermediate acting: NPH (Humulin N, Novolin N, NPH Iletin II); Lente: (Humulin L, Lente Iletin II, Monotard[AUS], Novolin L); Long acting: Insulin Glargine (Lantus)

CATEGORY AND SCHEDULE
Pregnancy Risk Category: B

Drug Class: Hormone, antidiabetic

MECHANISM OF ACTION
An exogenous insulin that facilitates passage of glucose, potassium, and magnesium across the cellular membranes of skeletal and cardiac muscle and adipose tissue. Controls storage and metabolism of carbohydrates, protein, and fats. Promotes conversion of glucose to glycogen in the liver.
Therapeutic Effect: Controls glucose levels in diabetic patients.

USES
Treatment of severe ketoacidosis, type 1 (IDDM) and type 2 (NIDDM; when diet, weight control, exercise, or oral hypoglycemics are not sufficient); hyperkalemia, hyperalimentation

PHARMACOKINETICS

Drug Form	Onset (hr)	Peak (hr)	Duration (hr)
Lispro	0.25	0.5–1.5	4–5
Insulin aspart	1/6	1–3	3–5
Regular	0.5–1	2–4	5–7
NPH	1–2	6–14	24
Lente	1–3	6–14	24
Insulin glargine	N/A	N/A	24

Long Acting: Lantus.

INDICATIONS AND DOSAGES

▶ **Treatment of Insulin-Dependent Type 1 Diabetes Mellitus and Non–Insulin-Dependent Type 2 Diabetes Mellitus When Diet or Weight Control Has Failed to Maintain Satisfactory Blood Glucose Levels or in Event of Fever, Infection, Pregnancy, Surgery, or Trauma, or Severe Endocrine, Hepatic or Renal Dysfunction; Emergency Treatment of Ketoacidosis (Regular Insulin); to Promote Passage of Glucose Across Cell Membrane in Hyperalimentation (Regular Insulin): to Facilitate Intracellular Shift of Potassium in Hyperkalemia (Regular Insulin)**

Subcutaneous
Adults, Elderly, Children. 0.5–1 unit/kg/day.
Adolescents (during growth spurt). 0.8–1.2 unit/kg/day.

SIDE EFFECTS/ADVERSE REACTIONS

Occasional
Localized redness, swelling, and itching caused by improper injection technique or allergy to cleansing solution or insulin

Infrequent
Somogyi effect, including rebound hyperglycemia with chronically excessive insulin dosages: systemic allergic reaction, marked by rash, angioedema, and anaphylaxis; lipodystrophy or depression at injection site because of breakdown of adipose tissue; lipohypertrophy or accumulation of subcutaneous tissue at injection site because of inadequate site rotation

Rare
Insulin resistance

PRECAUTIONS AND CONTRAINDICATIONS

Hypersensitivity or insulin resistance may require change of type or species source of insulin

DRUG INTERACTIONS OF CONCERN TO DENTISTRY

• Increased hypoglycemia: salicylates, NSAIDs (large doses and chronic use), alcohol
• Hyperglycemia: corticosteroids, epinephrine

SERIOUS REACTIONS

❗ Severe hypoglycemia caused by hyperinsulinism may occur with insulin overdose, decrease or delay of food intake, or excessive exercise and in those with brittle diabetes.
❗ Diabetic ketoacidosis may result from stress, illness, omission of insulin dose, or long-term poor insulin control.

DENTAL CONSIDERATIONS

General:
• Monitor vital signs at every appointment.
• Potential for hypoglycemia.
• Place on frequent recall to evaluate healing response.

• Diabetics may be more susceptible to infection and have delayed wound healing.

• Assess salivary flow as a factor in caries, periodontal disease, and candidiasis.

• Prophylactic antibiotics may be indicated in uncontrolled diabetics to prevent infection if surgery or deep scaling is planned.

• Ensure that patient is following prescribed diet and regularly takes medication.

• Question patient about self-monitoring of drug's antidiabetic effect, including blood glucose values or finger-stick records.

• Keep a readily available source of sugar or fruit juice in case of insulin overdose.

Consultations:

• Medical consultation may be required to assess disease control and patient's ability to tolerate stress.

• Medical consultation may include data from patient's blood glucose monitoring, including glycosylated hemoglobin or HbA$_{1c}$ testing.

Teach Patient/Family to:

• Encourage effective oral hygiene to prevent soft tissue inflammation.

• Use caution to prevent injury when using oral hygiene aids.

• Avoid mouth rinses with high alcohol content because of drying effects.

insulin glargine
in′-su-lin **glare′**-jeen
(Lantus)

CATEGORY AND SCHEDULE
Pregnancy Risk Category: C

Drug Class: Hormone, antidiabetic

MECHANISM OF ACTION
An exogenous insulin that facilitates passage of glucose, potassium, magnesium across cellular membranes of skeletal and cardiac muscle, adipose tissue; controls storage and metabolism of carbohydrates, protein, fats. Promotes conversion of glucose to glycogen in liver.
Therapeutic Effect: Controls glucose levels in diabetic patients.

USES
Treatment of severe ketoacidosis, Type 1 (IDDM) and Type 2 (NIDDM; when diet, weight control, exercise, or oral hypoglycemics are not sufficient); hyperkalemia, hyperalimentation

PHARMACOKINETICS

Drug Form	Onset (hr)	Peak (hr)	Duration (hr)
Insulin glargine	N/A	N/A	24

Metabolized at the carboxyl terminus of the B chain in the subcutaneous depot to form two active metabolites. Unchanged drug and degradation products are present throughout circulation.

INDICATIONS AND DOSAGES
▸ **Treatment of Insulin-Dependent Type 1 Diabetes Mellitus, Non–Insulin-Dependent Type 2 Diabetes Mellitus When Diet or Weight Control Therapy Has Failed to Maintain Satisfactory Blood Glucose Levels or in Event of Fever, Infection, Pregnancy, Severe Endocrine, Liver or Renal Dysfunction, Surgery, or Trauma, Regular Insulin Used in Emergency Treatment of Ketoacidosis, to**

Promote Passage of Glucose Across Cell Membrane in Hyperalimentation, to Facilitate Intracellular Shift of Potassium in Hyperkalemia

Subcutaneous
Adults, Elderly, Children. 10 units once daily, preferably at bedtime, adjusted according to patient response.

SIDE EFFECTS/ADVERSE REACTIONS

Frequent
Hypoglycemia
Occasional
Local redness, swelling, itching, caused by improper injection technique or allergy to cleansing solution or insulin
Infrequent
Systemic allergic reaction, marked by rash, angioedema, and anaphylaxis, lipodystrophy, or depression at injection site because of breakdown of adipose tissue, lipohypertrophy, or accumulation of subcutaneous tissue at injection site because of lack of adequate site rotation
Rare
Insulin resistance

PRECAUTIONS AND CONTRAINDICATIONS

Hypersensitivity or insulin resistance may require change of type or species source of insulin

DRUG INTERACTIONS OF CONCERN TO DENTISTRY

• Increased hypoglycemia: salicylates, NSAIDs (large doses and chronic use), alcohol
• Hyperglycemia: corticosteroids, epinephrine

SERIOUS REACTIONS

❗ Severe hypoglycemia caused by hyperinsulinism may occur in overdose of insulin, decrease or delay of food intake, excessive exercise, or those with brittle diabetes.
❗ Diabetic ketoacidosis may result from stress, illness, omission of insulin dose, or long-term poor insulin control.

DENTAL CONSIDERATIONS

General:
• Monitor vital signs at every appointment.
• Potential for hypoglycemia.
• Place on frequent recall to evaluate healing response.
• Diabetics may be more susceptible to infection and have delayed wound healing.
• Assess salivary flow as a factor in caries, periodontal disease, and candidiasis.
• Prophylactic antibiotics may be indicated in uncontrolled diabetics to prevent infection if invasive procedures are planned.
• Ensure that patient is following prescribed diet and regularly takes medication.
• Question patient about self-monitoring of drug's antidiabetic effect, including blood glucose values or finger-stick records.
• Keep a readily available source of glucose in case of insulin overdose.
Consultations:
• Medical consultation may be required to assess disease control and patient's ability to tolerate stress.
• Medical consultation may include data from patient's blood glucose monitoring, including glycosylated hemoglobin or HbA$_{1c}$ testing.
Teach Patient/Family to:
• Encourage effective oral hygiene to prevent soft tissue inflammation.

• Use caution to prevent injury when using oral hygiene aids.
• Avoid mouth rinses with high alcohol content because of drying effects.

insulin glulisine
in'-su-lin gluh'-lih-seen
(Apidra)

CATEGORY AND SCHEDULE
Pregnancy Risk Category: C

Drug Class: Hormone, antidiabetic

MECHANISM OF ACTION
A recombinant, rapid-acting insulin analog that facilitates passage of glucose, potassium, magnesium across cellular membranes of skeletal and cardiac muscle, adipose tissue; controls storage and metabolism of carbohydrates, protein, fats. Promotes conversion of glucose to glycogen in liver.
Therapeutic Effect: Controls glucose levels in diabetic patients.

USES
Treatment of severe ketoacidosis, Type 1 (IDDM) and Type 2 (NIDDM; when diet, weight control, exercise, or oral hypoglycemics are not sufficient); hyperkalemia, hyperalimentation

PHARMACOKINETICS

Drug Form	Onset (hr)	Peak (min)	Duration (hr)
Insulin Glulisine	20 min	55 min	5 hr

INDICATIONS AND DOSAGES
▶ **Diabetes Mellitus (Type 1 and Type 2)**
Subcutaneous, Infusion Pump
Adults, Elderly, Children.
Individualize per patient needs.

SIDE EFFECTS/ADVERSE REACTIONS
Occasional
Local redness, swelling, itching, caused by improper injection technique or allergy to cleansing solution or insulin
Infrequent
Somogyi effect, including rebound hyperglycemia, with chronically excessive insulin doses. Systemic allergic reaction, marked by rash, angioedema, and anaphylaxis, lipodystrophy or depression at injection site because of breakdown of adipose tissue, lipohypertrophy or accumulation of subcutaneous tissue at injection site because of lack of adequate site rotation
Rare
Insulin resistance

PRECAUTIONS AND CONTRAINDICATIONS
Current hypoglycemic episode, hypersensitivity, or insulin resistance may require change of type or species source of insulin

DRUG INTERACTIONS OF CONCERN TO DENTISTRY
• Increased hypoglycemia: salicylates, NSAIDs (large doses and chronic use), alcohol
• Hyperglycemia: corticosteroids, epinephrine

SERIOUS REACTIONS
❗ Severe hypoglycemia caused by hyperinsulinism may occur in overdose of insulin, decrease or delay of food intake, excessive

exercise, or those with brittle diabetes.

! Diabetic ketoacidosis may result from stress, illness, omission of insulin dose, or long-term poor insulin control.

DENTAL CONSIDERATIONS

General:

• Monitor vital signs at every appointment.
• Potential for hypoglycemia.
• Place on frequent recall to evaluate healing response.
• Diabetics may be more susceptible to infection and have delayed wound healing.
• Assess salivary flow as a factor in caries, periodontal disease, and candidiasis.
• Prophylactic antibiotics may be indicated in uncontrolled diabetics to prevent infection if surgery or deep scaling is planned.
• Ensure that patient is following prescribed diet and regularly takes medication.
• Question patient about self-monitoring of drug's antidiabetic effect, including blood glucose values or finger-stick records.
• Keep a readily available source of glucose in case of insulin overdose.

Consultations:

• Medical consultation may be required to assess disease control and patient's ability to tolerate stress.
• Medical consultation may include data from patient's blood glucose monitoring, including glycosylated hemoglobin or HbA_{1c} testing.

Teach Patient/Family to:

• Encourage effective oral hygiene to prevent soft tissue inflammation.
• Use caution to prevent injury when using oral hygiene aids.

• Avoid mouth rinses with high alcohol content because of drying effects.

interferon alfa-2a
in-ter-**fear**′-on **al**′-fa
(Roferon-A)
Do not confuse interferon alfa-2a with interferon alfa-2b.

CATEGORY AND SCHEDULE
Pregnancy Risk Category: C

Drug Class: Biologic response modifier

MECHANISM OF ACTION
A biological response modifier that inhibits viral replication in virus-infected cells, suppresses cell proliferation, increases phagocytic action of macrophage, and augments specific lymphocytic cell toxicity.
Therapeutic Effect: Prevents rapid growth of malignant cells; inhibits hepatitis virus.

USES
Treatment of hairy-cell leukemia in patients older than 18 yr, AIDS-related Kaposi's sarcoma (KS), chronic hepatitis C, chronic myelogenous leukemia

PHARMACOKINETICS
Well absorbed after IM and subcutaneous administration. Undergoes proteolytic degradation during reabsorption in kidneys.
Half-life: 2 hr (IM); 3 hr (subcutaneous).

INDICATIONS AND DOSAGES
▶ Hairy Cell Leukemia
IM, Subcutaneous
Adults. Initially, 3 million units/day for 16–24 wk. Maintenance: 3

million units 3 times a wk. Do not use 36-million-unit vial.

▸ **Chronic Myelocytic Leukemia**
IM, Subcutaneous
Adults. 9 million units/day.

▸ **Melanoma**
IM, Subcutaneous
Adults, Elderly. 12 million units/m² 3 times a wk for 3 mo.

▸ **AIDS-Related KS**
IM, Subcutaneous
Adults. Initially, 36 million units/day for 10–12 wk, may give 3 million units on day 1, 9 million units on day 2, 18 million units on day 3, then 36 million units/day for remaining 10–12 wk. Maintenance: 36 million units/day 3 times a wk.

▸ **Chronic Hepatitis C**
IM, Subcutaneous
Adults, Elderly. 6 million units 3 times a wk for 3 mo, then 3 million units 3 times a wk for 9 mo.

SIDE EFFECTS/ADVERSE REACTIONS
Frequent
Flu-like symptoms, nausea, vomiting, cough, dyspnea, hypotension, edema, chest pain, dizziness, diarrhea, weight loss, altered taste, abdominal discomfort, confusion, paresthesia, depression, visual and visual disturbances, diaphoresis, lethargy
Occasional
Alopecia (partial), rash, dry throat or skin, pruritus, flatulence, constipation, hypertension, palpitations, sinusitis
Rare
Hot flashes, hypermotility, Raynaud's syndrome, bronchospasm, earache, ecchymosis

PRECAUTIONS AND CONTRAINDICATIONS
Autoimmune hepatitis

Caution:
Severe hypotension, dysrhythmia, tachycardia, lactation, children younger than 18 yr, severe renal or hepatic disease, convulsion disorder, thrombophlebitis, coagulation disorders, hemophilia, GI bleeding; closely monitor patients; severe, life-threatening neuropsychiatric, autoimmune, ischemic, or infectious disorders may cause or aggravate these conditions

DRUG INTERACTIONS OF CONCERN TO DENTISTRY
• Risk of hepatotoxicity in severe liver disease: acetaminophen

SERIOUS REACTIONS
! Arrhythmias, CVA, transient ischemic attacks, CHF, pulmonary edema, and MI occur rarely.

DENTAL CONSIDERATIONS
General:
• Determine why the patient is taking the drug.
• Monitor vital signs at every appointment because of cardiovascular side effects.
• Patients on chronic drug therapy may rarely have symptoms of blood dyscrasias, which can include infection, bleeding, and poor healing.
• Palliative medication may be required for oral side effects.
• Assess salivary flow as a factor in caries, periodontal disease, and candidiasis.
• Consider semisupine chair position for patient comfort if GI side effects occur.
• Avoid elective dental procedures if severe neutropenia (more than 500 cells/mm³) or thrombocytopenia (more than 50,000 cell/mm³) is present.

• Antibiotic prophylaxis is indicated in severely neutropenic patients.
• Patient history should include all medications and herbal or nonherbal remedies taken by the patient.
• Severe side effects may require deferring elective dental procedures until drug therapy is completed.
• Evaluate efficacy of oral hygiene home care; preventive appointments may be necessary.

Consultations:
• Medical consultation may be required to assess disease control.
• In a patient with symptoms of blood dyscrasias, request a medical consultation for blood studies and postpone treatment until normal values are reestablished.
• Liver function tests may be required to determine chronic liver disease.

Teach Patient/Family to:
• Encourage effective oral hygiene to prevent soft tissue inflammation.
• Report oral lesions, soreness, or bleeding to dentist.
• Update medical/drug records if physician makes any changes in evaluation or drug regimens.
• When chronic dry mouth occurs, advise patient to:
  • Avoid mouth rinses with high alcohol content because of drying effects.
  • Use sugarless gum, frequent sips of water, or saliva substitutes.
  • Use daily home fluoride products for anticaries effect.

interferon alfa-2a/2b

in-ter-**fear**′-on **al**′-fa
(Roferon-A)/(Intron-A)

CATEGORY AND SCHEDULE
Pregnancy Risk Category: C

Drug Class: Biologic response modifier

MECHANISM OF ACTION
A biologic response modifier that inhibits viral replication in virus-infected cells.
Therapeutic Effect: Suppresses cell proliferation; increases phagocytic action of macrophages; augments specific lymphocytic cell toxicity.

USES
Treatment of hairy-cell leukemia, malignant melanoma, and AIDS-related Kaposi's sarcoma (KS). They are also used to treat laryngeal papillomatosis (growths in the respiratory tract) in children, genital warts, and some kinds of hepatitis.

PHARMACOKINETICS
Interferon alfa-2a
Well absorbed after IM, subcutaneous administration. Undergoes proteolytic degradation during reabsorption in kidney.
Half-life: IM: 2 hr; Subcutaneous: 3 hr.
Interferon alfa-2b
Well absorbed after IM, subcutaneous administration. Undergoes proteolytic degradation during reabsorption in kidney.
Half-life: 2–3 hr.

INDICATIONS AND DOSAGES
▶ **Hairy-Cell Leukemia**
Interferon alfa-2a
Subcutaneous/IM

Adults. Initially, 3 million units/day for 16–24 wk. Maintenance: 3 million units 3 times a wk. Do not use 36-million-unit vial.
Interferon alfa-2b
Subcutaneous/IM
Adults. 2 million units/m² 3 times a wk. If severe adverse reactions occur, modify dose or temporarily discontinue.

▶ **Chronic Myelocytic Leukemia (CML)**
Interferon alfa-2a
Subcutaneous/IM
Adults. 9 million units daily.

▶ **Condylomata Acuminate**
Interferon alfa-2b
Intralesional
Adults. 1 million units/lesion 3 times a wk for 3 wk. Use only 10-million-unit vial, reconstitute with no more than 1 ml diluent. Use tuberculin (TB) syringe with 25- or 26-gauge needle. Give in evening with acetaminophen, which alleviates side effects.

▶ **Melanoma**
Interferon alfa-2a
Subcutaneous/IM
Adults, Elderly. 12 million units/m² 3 times a wk for 3 mo.
Interferon alfa-2b
IV
Adults. Initially, 20 million units/m² 5 times a wk for 4 wk. Maintenance: 10 million units IM/Subcutaneous for 48 wk.

▶ **AIDS-Related KS**
Interferon alfa-2a
Subcutaneous/IM
Adults. Initially, 36 million units/day for 10–12 wk, may give 3 million units on day 1; 9 million units on day 2; 18 million units on day 3; then begin 36 million units/day for remainder of 10–12 wk.
Maintenance: 36 million units/day 3 times a wk.

Interferon alfa-2b
Subcutaneous/IM
Adults. 30 million units/m² 3 times a wk. Use only 50 million units vials. If severe adverse reactions occur, modify dose or temporarily discontinue.

▶ **Chronic Hepatitis B**
Interferon alfa-2b
Subcutaneous/IM
Adults. 30–35 million units/wk, 5 million units/day or 10 million units 3 times a wk.

▶ **Chronic Hepatitis C**
Interferon alfa-2a
Subcutaneous/IM
Adults. Initially, 6 million units once a day for 3 wk, then 3 million units 3 times a wk for 6 mo.
Interferon alfa-2b
Subcutaneous/IM
Adults. 3 million units 3 times a wk for up to 6 mo, for up to 18–24 mo for chronic hepatitis C.

SIDE EFFECTS/ADVERSE REACTIONS
Frequent
Interferon alfa-2a: Flu-like symptoms, including fever, fatigue, headache, aches, pains, anorexia, chills, nausea, vomiting, coughing, dyspnea, hypotension, edema, chest pain, dizziness, diarrhea, weight loss, taste change, abdominal discomfort, confusion, paresthesia, depression, visual and sleep disturbances, diaphoresis, lethargy
Interferon alfa-2b: Flu-like symptoms, including fever, fatigue, headache, aches, pains, anorexia, and chills, rash with hairy cell leukemia (KS only)
KS: All previously mentioned side effects plus depression, dyspepsia, dry mouth or thirst, alopecia, rigors
Occasional
Interferon alfa-2a: Partial alopecia, rash, dry throat or skin, pruritus,

flatulence, constipation,
hypertension, palpitations, sinusitis
Interferon alfa-2b: Dizziness,
pruritus, dry skin, dermatitis,
alteration in taste
Rare
Interferon alfa-2a: Hot flashes,
hypermotility, Raynaud's syndrome,
bronchospasm, earache, ecchymosis
Interferon alfa-2b: Confusion, leg
cramps, back pain, gingivitis,
flushing, tremors, nervousness, eye
pain

PRECAUTIONS AND CONTRAINDICATIONS

Hypersensitivity to any component
of the formulations
Caution:
Preexisting psoriasis and sarcoidosis,
do not use in patients with platelet
counts less than 50,000/mm^3,
preexisting CV disease, suicidal
tendency, depression, preexisting
psychiatric diseases, depressed bone
marrow; safety and efficacy in
lactation and children younger than
18 yr have not been established

DRUG INTERACTIONS OF CONCERN TO DENTISTRY

• Risk of hepatotoxicity in severe
liver disease: acetaminophen

SERIOUS REACTIONS

! Arrhythmias, stroke, transient
ischemic attacks, CHF, pulmonary
edema, and MI occur rarely with
interferon alfa-2a.
! Hypersensitivity reaction occurs
rarely with interferon alfa-2b.
! Severe adverse reactions of flu-like
symptoms appear dose related with
interferon alfa-2b.

DENTAL CONSIDERATIONS

General:
• Determine why the patient is
taking the drug.

• Monitor vital signs at every
appointment because of
cardiovascular side effects.
• After supine positioning, have
patient sit upright for at least 2 min
to avoid orthostatic hypotension.
• Palliative medication may be
required for oral side effects.
• Assess salivary flow as a factor in
caries, periodontal disease, and
candidiasis.
• Patients on chronic drug therapy
may rarely have symptoms of blood
dyscrasias, which can include
infection, bleeding, and poor
healing.
• Consider semisupine chair position
for patient comfort if GI side effects
occur.
• Avoid elective dental procedures if
severe neutropenia (fewer than 500
cells/mm^3) or thrombocytopenia
(fewer than 50,000 cell/mm^3) is
present.
• Antibiotic prophylaxis is indicated
in severely neutropenic patients.
• Patient history should include all
medications and herbal or nonherbal
remedies taken by the patient.
• Severe side effects may require
deferring elective dental procedures
until drug therapy is completed.
• Evaluate efficacy of oral hygiene
home care; preventive appointments
may be necessary.
Consultations:
• Medical consultation may be
required to assess disease control.
• In a patient with symptoms of
blood dyscrasias, request a medical
consultation for blood studies and
postpone treatment until normal
values are reestablished.
• Liver function tests may be
required to determine chronic liver
disease.
Teach Patient/Family to:
• Encourage effective oral hygiene
to prevent soft tissue inflammation.

- Report oral lesions, soreness, or bleeding to dentist.
- Update medical/drug records if physician makes any changes in evaluation or drug regimens.
- When chronic dry mouth occurs, advise patient to:
  - Avoid mouth rinses with high alcohol content because of drying effects.
  - Use sugarless gum, frequent sips of water, or saliva substitutes.
  - Use daily home fluoride products for anticaries effect.

interferon alfa-2b
in-ter-**fear**'-on **al**'-fa
(Intron-A)
Do not confuse interferon alfa-2b with interferon alfa-2a.

CATEGORY AND SCHEDULE
Pregnancy Risk Category: C

Drug Class: Biologic response modifier

MECHANISM OF ACTION
A biological response modifier that inhibits viral replication in virus-infected cells, suppresses cell proliferation, increases phagocytic action of macrophages, and augments specific cytotoxicity of lymphocytes for target cells.
Therapeutic Effect: Prevents rapid growth of malignant cells; inhibits hepatitis virus.

USES
Treatment of hairy-cell leukemia in patients older than 18 yr, malignant melanoma, chronic hepatitis B, follicular lymphoma, AIDS-related Kaposi's sarcoma (KS), chronic hepatitis C, condylomata acuminata

PHARMACOKINETICS
Well absorbed after IM and subcutaneous administration. Undergoes proteolytic degradation during reabsorption in kidneys.
Half-life: 2–3 hr.

INDICATIONS AND DOSAGES
▸ **Hairy-Cell Leukemia**
IM, Subcutaneous
Adults. 2 million units/m² 3 times a wk. If severe adverse reactions occur, modify dose or temporarily discontinue drug.
▸ **Condyloma Acuminatum**
Intralesional
Adults. 1 million units/lesion 3 times a wk for 3 wk. Use only 10-million-unit vial, and reconstitute with no more than 1 ml diluent.
▸ **AIDS-Related KS**
IM, Subcutaneous
Adults. 30 million units/m² 3 times a wk. Use only 50-million-unit vials. If severe adverse reactions occur, modify dose or temporarily discontinue drug.
▸ **Chronic Hepatitis C**
IM, Subcutaneous
Adults. 3 million units 3 times a wk for up to 6 mo. For patients who tolerate therapy and whose ALT(SGPT) level normalizes within 16 wk, therapy may be extended for up to 18–24 mo.
▸ **Chronic Hepatitis B**
IM, Subcutaneous
Adults. 30–35 million units weekly, either as 5 million units/day or 10 million units 3 times a wk.
▸ **Malignant Melanoma**
IV
Adults. Initially, 20 million units/m² 5 times a wk for 4 wk. Maintenance: 10 million units IM or subcutaneously 3 times a wk for 48 wk.
▸ **Follicular Lymphoma**
Subcutaneous

Adults. 5 million units 3 times a wk for up to 18 mo.

SIDE EFFECTS/ADVERSE REACTIONS

Frequent

Flu-like symptoms, rash (only in patients with hairy-cell leukemia KS)

Patients with KS: All previously mentioned side effects and depression, dyspepsia, dry mouth or thirst, alopecia, rigors

Occasional

Dizziness, pruritus, dry skin, dermatitis, altered taste

Rare

Confusion, leg cramps, back pain, gingivitis, flushing, tremors, nervousness, eye pain

PRECAUTIONS AND CONTRAINDICATIONS

Hypersensitivity

DRUG INTERACTIONS OF CONCERN TO DENTISTRY

• Risk of hepatotoxicity in severe liver disease: acetaminophen

SERIOUS REACTIONS

❗ Hypersensitivity reactions occur rarely.

❗ Severe flu-like symptoms may occur at higher doses.

DENTAL CONSIDERATIONS

General:

• Determine why the patient is taking the drug.

• Monitor vital signs at every appointment because of cardiovascular side effects.

• Palliative medication may be required for oral side effects.

• Assess salivary flow as a factor in caries, periodontal disease, and candidiasis.

• Patients on chronic drug therapy may rarely have symptoms of blood dyscrasias, which can include infection, bleeding, and poor healing.

• Consider semisupine chair position for patient comfort if GI side effects occur.

• Avoid elective dental procedures if severe neutropenia (more than 500 cells/mm^3) or thrombocytopenia (more than 50,000 cell/mm^3) is present.

• Antibiotic prophylaxis is indicated in severely neutropenic patients.

• Patient history should include all medications and herbal or nonherbal remedies taken by the patient.

• Severe side effects may require deferring elective dental procedures until drug therapy is completed.

• Evaluate efficacy of oral hygiene home care; preventive appointments may be necessary.

Consultations:

• Medical consultation may be required to assess disease control.

• In a patient with symptoms of blood dyscrasias, request a medical consultation for blood studies and postpone treatment until normal values are reestablished.

• Liver function tests may be required to determine chronic liver disease.

Teach Patient/Family to:

• Encourage effective oral hygiene to prevent soft tissue inflammation.

• Report oral lesions, soreness, or bleeding to dentist.

• Update medical/drug records if physician makes any changes in evaluation or drug regimens.

• When chronic dry mouth occurs, advise patient to:

  • Avoid mouth rinses with high alcohol content because of drying effects.

• Use sugarless gum, frequent sips of water, or saliva substitutes.
• Use daily home fluoride products for anticaries effect.

interferon alfa-n3
in-ter-**fear'**-on **al'**-fa
(Alferon N)

CATEGORY AND SCHEDULE
Pregnancy Risk Category: C

Drug Class: Biologic response modifier

MECHANISM OF ACTION
A biological response modifier that inhibits viral replication in virus-infected cells, suppresses cell proliferation, increases phagocytic action of macrophages, and augments specific cytotoxicity of lymphocytes for target cells.
Therapeutic Effect: Inhibits viral growth in condylomata acuminatum.

USES
Intralesional treatment of refractory or recurring external condylomata acuminata in patients 18 yr or older

PHARMACOKINETICS
Plasma levels below detectable limits.

INDICATIONS AND DOSAGES
▶ Condyloma Acuminatum
Intralesional
Adults, Children 18 yr and older.
0.05 ml (250,000 international units) per wart twice a wk up to 8 wk. Maximum dose/treatment session: 0.5 ml (2.5 million international units). Do not repeat for 3 mo after initial 8 wk course unless warts enlarge or new warts appear.

SIDE EFFECTS/ADVERSE REACTIONS
Frequent
Flu-like symptoms
Occasional
Dizziness, pruritus, dry skin, dermatitis, altered taste
Rare
Confusion, leg cramps, back pain, gingivitis, flushing, tremor, nervousness, eye pain

PRECAUTIONS AND CONTRAINDICATIONS
Previous history of anaphylactic reaction to egg protein, mouse immunoglobulin, or neomycin
Caution:
CV disease, unstable angina, uncontrolled CHF, severe pulmonary disease, diabetes mellitus with ketoacidosis, coagulation disorders, severe myelosuppression, seizure disorders, risk of transmitting blood-borne infectious disease, lactation, use in children younger than 18 yr has not been established

DRUG INTERACTIONS OF CONCERN TO DENTISTRY
• None reported

SERIOUS REACTIONS
❗ Hypersensitivity reaction occurs rarely.
❗ Severe flu-like symptoms may occur at higher doses.

DENTAL CONSIDERATIONS
General:
• Determine why the patient is taking the drug.
• Following injection, advise patient to take acetaminophen (if there are no contraindications for its use) in PM to ease flu-like symptoms.
• Advise patient if dental drugs prescribed have a potential for photosensitivity.

• Consider semisupine chair position for patient comfort if GI side effects occur.
Consultations:
• Medical consultation may be required to assess disease control.
Teach Patient/Family to:
• Update medical/drug records if physician makes any changes in evaluation or drug regimens.

interferon gamma-1b

in-ter-**fear**'-on **gamm**'-ah
(Actimmune, Imukin[AUS])

CATEGORY AND SCHEDULE
Pregnancy Risk Category: C

Drug Class: Biologic response modifier

MECHANISM OF ACTION
A biological response modifier that induces activation of macrophages in blood monocytes to phagocytes, which is necessary in the body's cellular immune response to intracellular and extracellular pathogens. Enhances phagocytic function and antimicrobial activity of monocytes.
Therapeutic Effect: Decreases signs and symptoms of serious infections in chronic granulomatous disease.

USES
Reduces the severity and frequency of infections associated with chronic granulomatous disease; delays disease progression in patients with severe, malignant osteoporosis

PHARMACOKINETICS
Slowly absorbed after subcutaneous administration.

INDICATIONS AND DOSAGES
▶ Chronic Granulomatous Disease; Severe, Malignant Osteoporosis
Subcutaneous
Adults, Children older than 1 yr.
50 mcg/m² (1.5 million units/m²) in patients with body surface area (BSA) greater than 0.5 m²; 1.5 mcg/kg/dose in patients with BSA 0.5 m² or less. Give 3 times a wk.

SIDE EFFECTS/ADVERSE REACTIONS
Frequent
Fever, headache, rash, chills, fatigue, diarrhea
Occasional
Vomiting, nausea
Rare
Weight loss, myalgia, anorexia

PRECAUTIONS AND CONTRAINDICATIONS
Hypersensitivity to *E. coli*–derived products
Caution:
Cardiac disease, seizure disorders, CNS disorders, myelosuppression, lactation, children younger than 1 yr; monitor hematologic values q3mo

DRUG INTERACTIONS OF CONCERN TO DENTISTRY
• None reported

SERIOUS REACTIONS
! Interferon gamma-1b may exacerbate preexisting CNS disturbances, including decreased mental status, gait disturbance, and dizziness, as well as cardiac disorders.

DENTAL CONSIDERATIONS
General:
• Determine why the patient is taking the drug.

• Patients on chronic drug therapy may rarely have symptoms of blood dyscrasias, which can include infection, bleeding, and poor healing.

• Ask patient about side effects associated with drug use (abnormal hematologic values).

• Consider semisupine chair position for patient comfort if GI side effects occur.

• Place on frequent recall to evaluate healing response.

• Severe side effects may require deferring elective dental procedures until drug therapy is completed.

• Antibiotic prophylaxis is indicated in severely neutropenic patients.

• Avoid elective dental procedures if severe neutropenia (fewer than 500 cells/mm^3) or thrombocytopenia (fewer than 50,000 cell/mm^3) is present.

Consultations:

• In a patient with symptoms of blood dyscrasias, request a medical consultation for blood studies and postpone dental treatment until normal values are reestablished.

• Medical consultation may be required to assess disease control and patient's ability to tolerate stress.

Teach Patient/Family to:

• Encourage effective oral hygiene to prevent soft tissue inflammation.

• Use caution to prevent trauma when using oral hygiene aids.

• Update medical history and drug records if physician makes any changes in evaluation or drug regimens.

ipratropium bromide

eye-pra-**troep**′-ee-um **broh**′-mide
(Apo-Ipravent[CAN],
Aproven[AUS], Atrovent, Atrovent Aerosol[AUS], Atrovent Nasal[AUS], Atrovent NPH, Novo-Ipramide[CAN], Nu-Ipratropium[CAN], PMS-Ipratropium[CAN])

Do not confuse Atrovent with Alupent.

CATEGORY AND SCHEDULE

Pregnancy Risk Category: B

Drug Class: Anticholinergic bronchodilator

MECHANISM OF ACTION

An anticholinergic that blocks the action of acetylcholine at parasympathetic sites in bronchial smooth muscle.

Therapeutic Effect: Causes bronchodilation and inhibits nasal secretions.

USES

Treatment of bronchodilation during bronchospasm in those with COPD, bronchitis, emphysema, asthma; not for rapid bronchodilation, maintenance treatment only; rhinorrhea, rhinorrhea associated with allergic and nonallergic perennial rhinitis in children age 6–11 yr, rhinorrhea associated with common cold

PHARMACOKINETICS

Route	Onset	Peak	Duration
Inhalation	1–3 min	1–2 hr	4–6 hr

Minimal systemic absorption after inhalation. Metabolized in the liver (systemic absorption). Primarily

eliminated in feces. *Half-life:*
1.5–4 hr.

INDICATIONS AND DOSAGES
▸ **Bronchospasm, Acute Treatment**
Inhalation
Adults, Elderly, Children. 4–8 puffs
as needed.
Nebulization
*Adults, Elderly, Children 12 yr and
older.* 500 mcg q30min for 3 doses,
then q2–4h as needed.
Children younger than 12 yr.
250 mcg q20min for 3 doses, then
q2–4h as needed.
▸ **Bronchospasm, Maintenance
Treatment**
Inhalation
*Adults, Elderly, Children 12 yr and
older.* 2–3 puffs q6h.
Children younger than 12 yr. 1–2
puffs q6h.
Nebulization
*Adults, Elderly, Children 12 yr and
older.* 500 mcg q6h.
Children younger than 12 yr.
250–500 mcg q6h.
▸ **Rhinorrhea**
Intranasal
Adults, Children older than 5 yr. 2
sprays of 0.06% solution 3–4 times
a day.
Adults, Children older than 6 yr. 2
sprays of (0.03%) solution 2–3 times
a day.

SIDE EFFECTS/ADVERSE
REACTIONS
Frequent
Inhalation: Cough, dry mouth,
headache, nausea
Nasal: Dry nose and mouth,
headache, nasal irritation
Occasional
Inhalation: Dizziness, transient
increased bronchospasm
Rare
Inhalation: Hypotension, insomnia,
metallic or unpleasant taste,
palpitations, urine retention

Nasal: Diarrhea or constipation, dry
throat, abdominal pain, stuffy nose

PRECAUTIONS AND
CONTRAINDICATIONS
History of hypersensitivity to
atropine
Caution:
Lactation, children younger than
12 yr, narrow-angle glaucoma,
prostatic hypertrophy, bladder neck
obstruction

DRUG INTERACTIONS OF
CONCERN TO DENTISTRY
• Increased effects of anticholinergic
drugs

SERIOUS REACTIONS
! Worsening of angle-closure
glaucoma, acute eye pain, and
hypotension occur rarely.

DENTAL CONSIDERATIONS
General:
• Monitor vital signs at every
appointment because of
cardiovascular and respiratory side
effects.
• Assess salivary flow as a factor in
caries, periodontal disease, and
candidiasis.
• Acute asthmatic episodes may be
precipitated in the dental office.
Sympathomimetic inhalants should
be available for emergency use.
• Consider semisupine chair position
for patients with respiratory disease.
• Place on frequent recall because of
oral side effects.
Consultations:
• Medical consultation may be
required to assess disease control and
patient's ability to tolerate stress.
Teach Patient/Family to:
• Rinse mouth with water after each
inhaled dose to prevent dryness.
• When chronic dry mouth occurs,
advise patient to:

- Avoid mouth rinses with high alcohol content because of drying effects.
- Use sugarless gum, frequent sips of water, or saliva substitutes.
- Use daily home fluoride products for anticaries effect.

irbesartan
erb-ah-**sar′**-tan
(Avapro, Karvea[AUS])

CATEGORY AND SCHEDULE
Pregnancy Risk Category: C (D if used in second or third trimester)

Drug Class: Angiotensin II receptor antagonist, antihypertensive

MECHANISM OF ACTION
An angiotensin II receptor, type AT1, antagonist that blocks the vasoconstrictor and aldosterone-secreting effects of angiotensin II, inhibiting the binding of angiotensin II to the AT1 receptors.
Therapeutic Effect: Causes vasodilation, decreases peripheral resistance, and decreases B/P.

USES
Treatment of hypertension alone or in combination with other antihypertensive drugs; nephropathy in type 2 diabetes

PHARMACOKINETICS
Rapidly and completely absorbed after PO administration. Protein binding: 90%. Undergoes hepatic metabolism to inactive metabolite. Recovered primarily in feces and, to a lesser extent, in urine. Not removed by hemodialysis. *Half-life:* 11–15 hr.

INDICATIONS AND DOSAGES
▶ **Hypertension Alone or in Combination with Other Antihypertensives**
PO
Adults, Elderly, Children 13 yr and older. Initially, 75–150 mg/day. May increase to 300 mg/day.
Children 6–12 yr. Initially, 75 mg/day. May increase to 150 mg/day.
▶ **Nephropathy**
PO
Adults, Elderly. Target dose of 300 mg/day.

SIDE EFFECTS/ADVERSE REACTIONS
Occasional
Upper respiratory tract infection, fatigue, diarrhea, cough
Rare
Heartburn, dizziness, headache, nausea, rash

PRECAUTIONS AND CONTRAINDICATIONS
Bilateral renal artery stenosis, biliary cirrhosis or obstruction, primary hyperaldosteronism, severe hepatic insufficiency
Caution:
Hypersensitivity to other angiotensin II receptor antagonists, volume- or salt-depleted patients, renal impairment, lactation, children

DRUG INTERACTIONS OF CONCERN TO DENTISTRY
- None reported

SERIOUS REACTIONS
! Overdosage may manifest as hypotension and tachycardia. Bradycardia occurs less often.

DENTAL CONSIDERATIONS
General:
- Monitor vital signs at every appointment because of cardiovascular side effects.

• Limit dose or avoid vasoconstrictor.
• Limit use of sodium-containing products, such as saline IV fluids, for those patients with a dietary salt restriction.
• Stress from dental procedures may compromise cardiovascular function; determine patient risk.
• Short appointments and a stress-reduction protocol may be required for anxious patients.
• Use precaution if sedation or general anesthesia is required; risk of hypotensive episode.
• After supine positioning, have patient sit upright for at least 2 min before standing to avoid orthostatic hypotension.
• Consider semisupine chair position for patient comfort if GI side effects occur.
Consultations:
• Consultation with physician may be necessary if sedation or general anesthesia is required.
• Medical consultation may be required to assess disease control and patient's ability to tolerate stress; risk of hypotensive episode.
Teach Patient/Family to:
• Update health and drug history if physician makes any changes in evaluation or drug regimens.

isocarboxazid
eye-soe-kar-**box**′-ah-zid
(Marplan)

CATEGORY AND SCHEDULE
Pregnancy Risk Category: C

Drug Class: Antidepressant-monoamine oxidase inhibitor

MECHANISM OF ACTION
An antidepressant that inhibits the MAO enzyme system at CNS storage sites. The reduced MAO activity causes an increased concentration in epinephrine, norepinephrine, serotonin, and dopamine at neuron receptor sites. **Therapeutic Effect:** Produces antidepressant effect.

USES
Treatment of depression

PHARMACOKINETICS
PO: Good absorption; maximum MAO inhibition 5–10 days, duration up to 2 wk; metabolized by liver; excreted by kidneys.

INDICATIONS AND DOSAGES
▸ **Depression Refractory to Other Antidepressants or Electroconvulsive Therapy**
PO
Adults, Elderly. Initially, 10 mg 3 times a day. May increase to 60 mg/day.

SIDE EFFECTS/ADVERSE REACTIONS
Frequent
Postural hypotension, drowsiness, decreased sexual ability, weakness, trembling, visual disturbances
Occasional
Tachycardia, peripheral edema, nervousness, chills, diarrhea, anorexia, constipation, xerostomia
Rare
Hepatitis, leukopenia, parkinsonian syndrome

PRECAUTIONS AND CONTRAINDICATIONS
Cardiovascular disease (CVD), cerebrovascular disease, liver impairment, pheochromocytoma, liver impairment

Caution:

Suicidal patients, concurrent use with other antidepressants (patients must stop taking MAOI 14 days before initiating therapy with other antidepressants), general anesthesia, severe depression, schizophrenia, diabetes mellitus, lactation, children younger than 16 yr

DRUG INTERACTIONS OF CONCERN TO DENTISTRY

• Increased pressor effects: indirect-acting sympathomimetics (ephedrine)
• Hyperpyretic crisis, convulsions, hypertensive episode: meperidine, possibly other opioids, carbamazepine
• Increased anticholinergic effects: anticholinergics, antihistamines
• Increased effects of alcohol, barbiturates, benzodiazepines, CNS depressants, SSRIs, tricyclic antidepressants, cyclobenzaprine, bupropion, buspirone, dextromethorphan, antihypertensive

SERIOUS REACTIONS

! Hypertensive crisis, marked by severe hypertension, occipital headache radiating frontally, neck stiffness or soreness, nausea, vomiting, sweating, fever or chilliness, clammy skin, dilated pupils, palpitations, tachycardia or bradycardia, and constricting chest pain.

DENTAL CONSIDERATIONS

General:
• Monitor vital signs at every appointment because of cardiovascular side effects.
• After supine positioning, have patient sit upright for at least 2 min to avoid orthostatic hypotension.
• Patients on chronic drug therapy may rarely have symptoms of blood

dyscrasias, which can include infection, bleeding, and poor healing.
• Consider semisupine chair position for patient comfort if GI side effects occur.
• Assess salivary flow as a factor in caries, periodontal disease, and candidiasis.
• Hypertensive episodes are possible even though there are no specific contraindications to vasoconstrictor use in local anesthetics.
• Short appointments and a stress-reduction protocol may be required for anxious patients.

Consultations:
• Medical consultation may be required to assess disease control and patient's ability to tolerate stress.
• In a patient with symptoms of blood dyscrasias, request a medical consultation for blood studies and postpone treatment until normal values are reestablished.

Teach Patient/Family:
• When chronic dry mouth occurs, advise patient to:
  • Avoid mouth rinses with high alcohol content because of drying effects.
  • Use daily home fluoride products for anticaries effect.
  • Use sugarless gum, frequent sips of water, or saliva substitutes.

isoetharine hydrochloride

eye-soe-**eth**´-ah-reen
high-droh-**klor**´-ide
(Beta-2, Bronkometer, Bronkosol, Dey-Lute)

CATEGORY AND SCHEDULE

Pregnancy Risk Category: C

Drug Class: Adrenergic
β_2-agonist

MECHANISM OF ACTION

A sympathomimetic (adrenergic) agonist that stimulates β_2-adrenergic receptors in the lungs, resulting in relaxation of bronchial smooth muscle.
Therapeutic Effect: Relieves bronchospasm, reduces airway resistance.

USES

Treatment of bronchospasm, asthma

PHARMACOKINETICS

Rapidly, well absorbed from the GI tract. Extensive metabolism in GI tract. Unknown extent metabolized in liver and lungs. Excreted in urine.
Half-life: 4 hr.

INDICATIONS AND DOSAGES

▶ **Bronchospasm**
Hand-Bulb Nebulizer
Adults, Elderly. 4 inhalations (range: 3–7 inhalations) undiluted. May be repeated up to 5 times a day.
Metered Dose Inhalation
Adults, Elderly. 1–2 inhalations q4h. Wait 1 min before administering second inhalation.
IPPB, Oxygen Aerolization
Adults, Elderly. 0.5–1 ml of a 0.5% or 0.5 ml of a 1% solution diluted 1:3.

SIDE EFFECTS/ADVERSE REACTIONS

Occasional
Tremor, nausea, nervousness, palpitations, tachycardia, peripheral vasodilation, dryness of mouth, throat, dizziness, vomiting, headache, increased B/P, insomnia

PRECAUTIONS AND CONTRAINDICATIONS

History of hypersensitivity to sympathomimetics

Caution:
Cardiac disorders, hyperthyroidism, diabetes mellitus, prostatic hypertrophy

DRUG INTERACTIONS OF CONCERN TO DENTISTRY

• Increased effects of both drugs: other sympathomimetics
• Increased dysrhythmia: halogenated hydrocarbon anesthetics

SERIOUS REACTIONS

! Excessive sympathomimetic stimulation may produce palpitations, extrasystoles, tachycardia, chest pain, slight increase in B/P followed by a substantial decrease, chills, sweating, and blanching of skin.
! Too frequent or excessive use may lead to loss of bronchodilating effectiveness and severe and paradoxical bronchoconstriction.

DENTAL CONSIDERATIONS

General:
• Assess salivary flow as a factor in caries, periodontal disease, and candidiasis.
• Consider semisupine chair position for patients with respiratory disease.
• Acute asthmatic episodes may be precipitated in the dental office. Sympathomimetic inhalants should be available for emergency use.
Consultations:
• Medical consultation may be required to assess disease control and patient's ability to tolerate stress.
Teach Patient/Family to:
• Rinse mouth with water after each inhaled dose to prevent dryness.
• When chronic dry mouth occurs, advise patient to:
   • Avoid mouth rinses with high alcohol content because of drying effects.

• Use sugarless gum, frequent sips of water, or saliva substitutes.
• Use daily home fluoride products for anticaries effect.

isoniazid
eye-soe-**nye**′-ah-zid
(INH, Isotamine[CAN], Nydrazid, PMS Isoniazid[CAN])

CATEGORY AND SCHEDULE
Pregnancy Risk Category: C

Drug Class: Antitubercular

MECHANISM OF ACTION
An isonicotinic acid derivative that inhibits mycolic acid synthesis and causes disruption of the bacterial cell wall and loss of acid-fast properties in susceptible mycobacteria. Active only during bacterial cell division.
Therapeutic Effect: Bactericidal against actively growing intracellular and extracellular susceptible mycobacteria.

USES
Treatment and prevention of tuberculosis (TB)

PHARMACOKINETICS
Readily absorbed from the GI tract. Protein binding: 10%–15%. Widely distributed (including to CSF). Metabolized in the liver. Primarily excreted in urine. Removed by hemodialysis. *Half-life:* 0.5–5 hr.

INDICATIONS AND DOSAGES
▶ **TB (in Combination with One or More Antituberculars)**
PO, IM
Adults, Elderly. 5 mg/kg/day as a single dose. Maximum 300 mg/day.

Children. 10–15 mg/kg/day as a single dose. Maximum 300 mg/day.
▶ **Prevention of TB**
PO, IM
Adults, Elderly. 300 mg/day as a single dose.
Children. 10 mg/kg/day as a single dose. Maximum 300 mg/day.

SIDE EFFECTS/ADVERSE REACTIONS
Frequent
Nausea, vomiting, diarrhea, abdominal pain
Rare
Pain at injection site, hypersensitivity reaction

PRECAUTIONS AND CONTRAINDICATIONS
Acute hepatic disease, history of hypersensitivity reactions or hepatic injury with previous isoniazid therapy
Caution:
Renal disease; diabetic retinopathy cataracts; ocular defects; hepatic disease; fatal hepatitis, especially in black women and Hispanic women; children younger than 13 yr, monitor liver function

DRUG INTERACTIONS OF CONCERN TO DENTISTRY
• Increased hepatotoxicity: alcohol, acetaminophen, carbamazepine
• Decreased effectiveness: glucocorticoids, especially prednisolone
• Increased plasma concentration: benzodiazepines, alfentanil
• Decreased effect of ketoconazole, miconazole

SERIOUS REACTIONS
! Rare reactions include neurotoxicity (as evidenced by ataxia and paraesthesia), optic neuritis, and hepatotoxicity.

DENTAL CONSIDERATIONS

General:
• Patients on chronic drug therapy may rarely have symptoms of blood dyscrasias, which can include infection, bleeding, and poor healing.
• Patients with active TB should not be treated.
• Medical consultation may be required to assess disease control.
• Examine for evidence of oral signs of disease.
• Do not treat patients with active tuberculosis.

Consultations:
• In a patient with symptoms of blood dyscrasias, request a medical consultation for blood studies and postpone dental treatment until normal values are reestablished.

Teach Patient/Family to:
• Use caution to prevent injury when using oral hygiene aids.

isosorbide

eye-soe-**sor**′-bide
isosorbide dinitrate (Apo-ISDN[CAN], Cedocard[CAN], Dilatrate, Isogen[AUS], Isordil, Sorbidin[AUS]); isosorbide mononitrate (Duride[AUS], Imdur, Imtrate[AUS], ISMO, Monodur Durules[AUS], Monoket)
Do not confuse with Inderal, Isuprel, K-Dur, or Plendil.

CATEGORY AND SCHEDULE
Pregnancy Risk Category: C

Drug Class: Nitrate antianginal

MECHANISM OF ACTION
A nitrate that stimulates intracellular cyclic guanosine monophosphate (GMP).

Therapeutic Effect: Relaxes vascular smooth muscle of both arterial and venous vasculature. Decreases preload and afterload.

USES
Treatment of chronic stable angina pectoris

PHARMACOKINETICS

Route	Onset	Peak	Duration
Sublingual	2–10 min	N/A	1–2 days
Chewable	3 min	N/A	0.5–2 hr
PO	45–60 min	N/A	4–6 hr
Sustained-release	30 min	N/A	6–12 hr

Mononitrate well absorbed after PO administration. Dinitrate poorly absorbed and metabolized in the liver to its active metabolite isosorbide mononitrate. Excreted in urine and feces. *Half-life:* 1–4 hr, dinitrate; 4 hr, mononitrate.

INDICATIONS AND DOSAGES
▶ **Acute Angina, Prophylactic Management in Situations Likely to Provoke Attack**
Sublingual
Adults, Elderly. Initially, 2.5–5 mg. Repeat at 5–10 min intervals. No more than 3 doses in 15–30 min period.
▶ **Acute Prophylactic Management of Angina**
Sublingual
Adults, Elderly. 5–10 mg q2–3h.
▶ **Long-Term Prophylaxis of Angina**
PO
Adults, Elderly. Initially, 5–20 mg 3–4 times a day. Maintenance: 10–40 mg q6h. Consider 2–3 times a day, last dose no later than 7 PM to minimize intolerance.

PO (Mononitrate)
Adults, Elderly. 20 mg 2 times a day,
7 hr apart. First dose upon
awakening in morning.
PO (Extended Release)
Adults, Elderly. Initially, 40 mg.
Maintenance: 40–80 mg 2–3 times a
day. Consider 1–2 times a day, last
dose at 2 PM to minimize intolerance.
PO (Imdur)
Adults, Elderly. 60–120 mg/day as
single dose.
▸ **CHF**
PO (Chewable)
Adults, Elderly. 5–10 mg every
2–3 hr.

SIDE EFFECTS/ADVERSE REACTIONS

Frequent
Burning and tingling at oral point of
dissolution (sublingual), headache
(may be severe) occurs mostly in
early therapy, diminishes rapidly in
intensity, usually disappears during
continued treatment; transient
flushing of face and neck, dizziness
(especially if patient is standing
immobile or is in a warm
environment), weakness, postural
hypotension, nausea, vomiting,
restlessness
Occasional
GI upset, blurred vision, dry mouth

PRECAUTIONS AND CONTRAINDICATIONS

Closed-angle glaucoma, GI
hypermotility or malabsorption
(extended-release tablets), head
trauma, hypersensitivity to nitrates,
increased intracranial pressure,
postural hypotension, severe anemia
(extended-release tablets)
Caution:
Postural hypotension, lactation,
children

DRUG INTERACTIONS OF CONCERN TO DENTISTRY

• Increased effects: alcohol, other
vasodilator-type drugs
• Severe hypotension: sildenafil,
vardenafil, tadalafil

SERIOUS REACTIONS

! Blurred vision or dry mouth may
occur (drug should be discontinued).
! Severe postural hypotension
manifested by fainting,
pulselessness, cold or clammy skin,
and diaphoresis may occur.
! Tolerance may occur with repeated,
prolonged therapy (minor tolerance
with intermittent use of sublingual
tablets). Tolerance may not occur
with extended-release form.
! High dose tends to produce severe
headache.

DENTAL CONSIDERATIONS

General:
• Monitor vital signs at every
appointment because of
cardiovascular side effects.
• After supine positioning, have
patient sit upright for at least 2 min
before standing to avoid orthostatic
hypotension.
• Stress from dental procedures may
compromise cardiovascular function;
determine patient risk.
• Assess salivary flow as a factor in
caries, periodontal disease, and
candidiasis.
• Short appointments and a
stress-reduction protocol may be
required for anxious patients.
• Consider semisupine chair position
for patients with respiratory distress.
• Use vasoconstrictors with caution,
in low doses, and with careful
aspiration. Avoid use of gingival
retraction cord with epinephrine.
• Nitroglycerin should be available
in case of an acute anginal episode.

Consultations:
• Medical consultation may be required to assess disease control and patient's ability to tolerate stress.
Teach Patient/Family:
• When chronic dry mouth occurs, advise patient to:
  • Avoid mouth rinses with high alcohol content because of drying effects.
  • Use sugarless gum, frequent sips of water, or saliva substitutes.
  • Use daily home fluoride products for anticaries effect.

isosorbide dinitrate/ isosorbide mononitrate

ahy-suh-**sawr**′-bayd
dahy-**nahy**′-treyt
isosorbide dinitrate (Apo-ISDN[CAN], Cedocard[CAN], Dilatrate, Isogen[AUS], Isordil, Sorbidin[AUS]); isosorbide mononitrate (Duride[AUS], Imdur, Imdur Durules[AUS], Imtrate[AUS], ISMO, Monodur Durules[AUS], Monoket)
Do not confuse Isordil with Isuprel or Plendil, or Imdur with Inderal or K-Dur.

CATEGORY AND SCHEDULE
Pregnancy Risk Category: C

Drug Class: Nitrate antianginal

MECHANISM OF ACTION
A nitrate that stimulates intracellular cyclic guanosine monophosphate. *Therapeutic Effect:* Relaxes vascular smooth muscle of both arterial and venous vasculature. Decreases preload and afterload.

USES
Treatment of chronic stable angina pectoris

PHARMACOKINETICS

Route	Onset	Peak	Duration
Dinitrate	2–5 min	N/A	1–2 hr
Sublingual oral (chewable)	2–5 min	N/A	1–2 hr
Oral	15–40 min	N/A	4–6 hr
Oral sustained (release)	30 min	N/A	12 hr
Mononitrate oral (extended release)	60 min	N/A	N/A

Dinitrate poorly absorbed and metabolized in the liver to its active metabolite isosorbide mononitrate. Mononitrate well absorbed after PO administration. Excreted in urine and feces. *Half-life:* Dinitrate, 1–4 hr; mononitrate, 4 hr.

INDICATIONS AND DOSAGES
▸ **Angina**
PO (Isosorbide Dinitrate)
Adults, Elderly. 5–40 mg 4 times a day. Sustained-release: 40 mg q8–12h.
PO (Isosorbide Mononitrate)
Adults, Elderly. 5–10 mg twice a day given 7 hr apart. Sustained-release: Initially, 30–60 mg/day in morning as a single dose. May increase dose at 3-day intervals. Maximum: 240 mg/day.

SIDE EFFECTS/ADVERSE REACTIONS
Frequent
Burning and tingling at oral point of dissolution (sublingual), headache (possibly severe) occurs mostly in early therapy, diminishes rapidly in intensity, and usually disappears during continued treatment, transient flushing of face and neck, dizziness (especially if patient is standing immobile or is in a warm

environment), weakness, orthostatic hypotension, nausea, vomiting, restlessness

Occasional

GI upset, blurred vision, dry mouth

PRECAUTIONS AND CONTRAINDICATIONS

Closed-angle glaucoma, GI hypermotility or malabsorption (extended-release tablets), head trauma, hypersensitivity to nitrates, increased intracranial pressure, orthostatic hypotension, severe anemia (extended-release tablets)

DRUG INTERACTIONS OF CONCERN TO DENTISTRY

• Increased effects: alcohol and other drugs that can lower B/P
• Severe hypotension: sildenafil, vardenafil, tadalafil

SERIOUS REACTIONS

! Blurred vision or dry mouth may occur (drug should be discontinued).
! Isosorbide administration may cause severe orthostatic hypotension manifested by fainting, pulselessness, cold or clammy skin, and diaphoresis.
! Tolerance may occur with repeated, prolonged therapy, but may not occur with the extended-release form. Minor tolerance may be seen with intermittent use of sublingual tablets.
! High dosage tends to produce severe headache.

DENTAL CONSIDERATIONS

General:
• Monitor vital signs at every appointment because of cardiovascular side effects.
• After supine positioning, have patient sit upright for at least 2 min before standing to avoid orthostatic hypotension.

• Assess salivary flow as a factor in caries, periodontal disease, and candidiasis.
• Stress from dental procedures may compromise cardiovascular function; determine patient risk.
• Use vasoconstrictors with caution, in low doses, and with careful aspiration. Avoid use of gingival retraction cord with epinephrine.
• Short appointments and a stress-reduction protocol may be required for anxious patients.
• Nitroglycerin should be available in case of acute anginal episode.

Consultations:
• Medical consultation may be required to assess disease control and patient's ability to tolerate stress.

Teach Patient/Family to:
• Encourage effective oral hygiene to prevent soft tissue inflammation.
• When chronic dry mouth occurs, advise patient to:
  • Avoid mouth rinses with high alcohol content because of drying effects.
  • Use sugarless gum, frequent sips of water, or saliva substitutes.
  • Use daily home fluoride products for anticaries effect.

isoxsuprine hydrochloride

eye-**sox**′-soo-preen
high-droh-**klor**′-ide
(Vasodilan)

CATEGORY AND SCHEDULE

Pregnancy Risk Category: C

Drug Class: Peripheral vasodilator

MECHANISM OF ACTION
The mechanism of action of isoxsuprine hydrochloride is not fully understood. Increases muscle blood flow. May have a direct action on vascular smooth muscle. β-adrenergic stimulation of the uterus.
Therapeutic Effect: Relieves symptoms associated with cerebral vascular insufficiency. Inhibits preterm labor.

USES
Treatment of symptoms of cerebrovascular insufficiency; peripheral vascular disease, including arteriosclerosis obliterans, thromboangiitis obliterans, Raynaud's disease

PHARMACOKINETICS
The pharmacokinetics of isoxsuprine hydrochloride is not fully understood. *Half-life:* Unknown.

INDICATIONS AND DOSAGES
▸ Raynaud's Syndrome
IV Infusion
Adults, Elderly. 10–20 mg 3–4 times a day.

SIDE EFFECTS/ADVERSE REACTIONS
Rare
Hypotension, tachyarrhythmia, rash, abdominal discomfort, nausea, dizziness

PRECAUTIONS AND CONTRAINDICATIONS
Arterial bleeding (recent), immediately postpartum
Caution:
Tachycardia

DRUG INTERACTIONS OF CONCERN TO DENTISTRY
• Increased effects: alcohol and drugs that also lower B/P

SERIOUS REACTIONS
! Pulmonary edema occurs rarely.

DENTAL CONSIDERATIONS
General:
• Monitor vital signs at every appointment because of cardiovascular and respiratory side effects.
• After supine positioning, have patient sit upright for at least 2 min before standing to avoid orthostatic hypotension.
• Short appointments and a stress-reduction protocol may be required for anxious patients.
• Drugs used for conscious sedation that lower B/P may potentiate the hypotensive effects.
• Use vasoconstrictors with caution, in low doses, and with careful aspiration. Avoid use of gingival retraction cord with epinephrine.
Consultations:
• Medical consultation may be required to assess disease control and patient's ability to tolerate stress.

isradipine
is-**rad**′-ih-peen
(DynaCirc, DynaCirc CR)
Do not confuse DynaCirc with Dynabac or Dynacin.

CATEGORY AND SCHEDULE
Pregnancy Risk Category: C

Drug Class: Calcium channel blocker

MECHANISM OF ACTION

An antihypertensive that inhibits calcium movement across cardiac and vascular smooth-muscle cell membranes. Potent peripheral vasodilator that does not depress SA or AV nodes.
Therapeutic Effect: Produces relaxation of coronary vascular smooth muscle and coronary vasodilation. Increases myocardial oxygen delivery to those with vasospastic angina.

USES

Treatment of essential hypertension, alone or with a thiazide diuretic; unapproved: angina, Raynaud's disease

PHARMACOKINETICS

Route	Onset	Peak	Duration
PO	2–3 hr	2–4 wk (with multiple doses) 8–16 hr (with single dose)	N/A
PO (controlled-release)	2 hr	8–10 hr	N/A

Well absorbed from the GI tract. Protein binding: 95%. Metabolized in the liver (undergoes first-pass effect). Primarily excreted in urine. Not removed by hemodialysis.
Half-life: 8 hr.

INDICATIONS AND DOSAGES
▶ **Hypertension**
PO
Adults, Elderly. Initially 2.5 mg twice a day. May increase by 2.5 mg at 2- to 4-wk intervals. Range: 5–20 mg/day

SIDE EFFECTS/ADVERSE REACTIONS

Frequent
Peripheral edema, palpitations (higher frequency in females)
Occasional
Facial flushing, cough, gingival enlargement
Rare
Angina, tachycardia, rash, pruritus

PRECAUTIONS AND CONTRAINDICATIONS

Cardiogenic shock, CHF, heart block, hypotension, sinus bradycardia, ventricular tachycardia
Caution:
CHF, hypotension, hepatic disease, lactation, children, renal disease, elderly

DRUG INTERACTIONS OF CONCERN TO DENTISTRY

• Decreased effect: indomethacin, possibly other NSAIDs, phenobarbital
• Increased effect: parenteral and inhalational general anesthetics, other drugs with hypotensive actions, itraconazole
• Increased effects of carbamazepine

SERIOUS REACTIONS

❗ Overdose produces nausea, drowsiness, confusion, and slurred speech.
❗ CHF occurs rarely.

DENTAL CONSIDERATIONS

General:
• Monitor cardiac status; take vital signs at each appointment because of cardiovascular side effects. Consider a stress-reduction protocol to prevent stress-induced angina during the dental appointment.
• After supine positioning, have patient sit upright for at least 2 min

before standing to avoid orthostatic hypotension.
• Place on frequent recall to monitor gingival condition.
• Limit use of sodium-containing products, such as saline IV fluids, for patients with a dietary salt restriction.
• Assess salivary flow as a factor in caries, periodontal disease, and candidiasis.
• Use vasoconstrictors with caution, in low doses, and with careful aspiration. Avoid use of gingival retraction cord with epinephrine.
• Patients on chronic drug therapy may rarely have symptoms of blood dyscrasias, which can include infection, bleeding, and poor healing.

Consultations:
• In a patient with symptoms of blood dyscrasias, request a medical consultation for blood studies and postpone dental treatment until normal values are reestablished.
• Medical consultation may be required to assess disease control and patient's ability to tolerate stress.

Teach Patient/Family to:
• Encourage effective oral hygiene to prevent soft tissue inflammation and minimize gingival enlargement.
• Schedule frequent oral prophylaxis.
• When chronic dry mouth occurs, advise patient to:
  • Avoid mouth rinses with high alcohol content because of drying effects.
  • Use sugarless gum, frequent sips of water, or saliva substitutes.
  • Use daily home fluoride products for anticaries effect.

itraconazole
it-ra-**con**′-ah-zoll
(Sporanox)
Do not confuse Sporanox with Suprax.

CATEGORY AND SCHEDULE
Pregnancy Risk Category: C

Drug Class: Antifungal, systemic (triazole)

MECHANISM OF ACTION
A fungistatic antifungal that inhibits the synthesis of ergosterol, a vital component of fungal cell formation. *Therapeutic Effect:* Damages the fungal cell membrane, altering its function.

USES
Treatment of aspergillosis, blastomycosis, histoplasmosis (pulmonary and extrapulmonary); fungal infections of nails (onychomycosis); *Candida* infections of esophagus or mouth (oral sol only)

PHARMACOKINETICS
Moderately absorbed from the GI tract. Absorption is increased if the drug is taken with food. Protein binding: 99%. Widely distributed, primarily in the fatty tissue, liver, and kidneys. Metabolized in the liver to active metabolite. Primarily excreted in urine. Not removed by hemodialysis. *Half-life:* 21 hr; metabolite, 12 hr.

INDICATIONS AND DOSAGES
▸ **Blastomycosis, Histoplasmosis**
PO
Adults, Elderly. Initially, 200 mg once a day. Maximum: 400 mg/day in 2 divided doses.

IV
Adults, Elderly. 200 mg twice a day for 4 doses, then 200 mg once a day.
▸ **Aspergillosis**
PO
Adults, Elderly. 600 mg/day in 3 divided doses for 3–4 days, then 200–400 mg/day in 2 divided doses.
IV
Adults, Elderly. 200 mg twice a day for 4 doses, then 200 mg once a day.
▸ **Esophageal Candidiasis**
PO
Adults, Elderly. Swish 10 ml in mouth for several seconds, then swallow. Maximum: 200 mg/day.
▸ **Oropharyngeal Candidiasis**
PO
Adults, Elderly. Vigorously swish 10 ml in mouth for several seconds (20 ml total daily dose) once a day.

SIDE EFFECTS/ADVERSE REACTIONS
Frequent
Nausea, rash
Occasional
Vomiting, headache, diarrhea, hypertension, peripheral edema, fatigue, fever
Rare
Abdominal pain, dizziness, anorexia, pruritus

PRECAUTIONS AND CONTRAINDICATIONS
Hypersensitivity to itraconazole, fluconazole, ketoconazole, or miconazole
Caution:
Lactation, liver toxicity, oral anticoagulants (monitor patient), strong inhibitor of CYP3A4 isoenzymes—note drug interactions

DRUG INTERACTIONS OF CONCERN TO DENTISTRY
• Increased risk of rhabdomyolysis: lovastatin, simvastatin
• Increased risk of hypoglycemia: oral antidiabetics
• Increased metabolism: phenobarbital, carbamazepine
• May increase plasma levels of cyclosporine
• Increased CNS depression with triazolam, midazolam (inhibits metabolism of certain benzodiazepines: (e.g., midazolam, triazolam), buspirone, allopurinol (Zyloprim), felodipine)
• Decreased effects: didanosine
• Increased plasma levels: saquinavir, nisoldipine, haloperidol, carbamazepine, erythromycin, clarithromycin
• Avoid itraconazole use with HMG-Co A reductase inhibitors (statins) or lower their dose
• May inhibit warfarin metabolism
• Suspected increase in plasma levels: cola beverages
• Decrease in plasma levels: grapefruit juice
• Decreased effects: didanosine (take 2 hr before didanosine tabs)
• May increase levels and side effects of HMG-Co A reductase inhibitors (statins)
• Increased plasma levels of alfentanil, buspirone, carbamazepine, corticosteroids, zolpidem
• Suspected decrease in oral contractive effectiveness; suggest alternative method of contraception

SERIOUS REACTIONS
! Hepatitis (as evidenced by anorexia, abdominal pain, unusual fatigue or weakness, jaundiced skin or sclera, and dark urine) occurs rarely.

DENTAL CONSIDERATIONS
General:
• Monitor vital signs at every appointment because of cardiovascular side effects.

• Determine why the patient is taking the drug.
• Consider semisupine chair position for patient comfort because of GI effects of drug.
Consultations:
• Medical consultation may be required to assess patient's ability to tolerate stress.

ixabepilone
ix-ab-**ep**′-i-lone
(Ixempra)

CATEGORY AND SCHEDULE
Pregnancy Risk Category: D

Drug Class: Antineoplastic agent, antimicrotubular, epothilone B analog

MECHANISM OF ACTION
Semisynthetic analog of epothilone B. Inhibits microtubules, stops cell division in the G2-M phase and results in subsequent cell death. Suppresses the dynamic instability of beta-tubulin subunits (alpha-beta-II and alpha-beta-III).

USES
Breast cancer, metastatic or locally advanced, as monotherapy in patients whose tumors are resistant or refractory to anthracyclines, taxanes, and capecitabine
Breast cancer, metastatic or locally advanced, in combination with capecitabine in patients who are resistant to treatment with an anthracycline and a taxane, or whose cancer is taxane resistant and for whom further anthracycline therapy is contraindicated

PHARMACOKINETICS
Protein binding: 67% to 77%. Extensively metabolized in liver via CYP450 3A4. At least 30 identified metabolites (inactive). Primarily excreted in feces (65%); urine (21%). *Half-life:* 52 hr.

INDICATIONS AND DOSAGES
Adult. Breast cancer as monotherapy or combination with capecitabine: 40 mg/m^2 IV over 3 hr every 3 wk. Note: All patients must premedicate with an oral H$_1$-antagonist (e.g., diphenhydramine 50 mg) and an oral H$_2$-antagonist (e.g., ranitidine 150–300 mg) 1 hr prior to infusion. Patients with a history of hypersensitivity should premedicate with corticosteroids (e.g., dexamethasone 20 mg) intravenously 30 min prior to infusion or orally 60 min prior to infusion. Body surface area (BSA) is capped at a maximum of 2.2 m^2.
Pediatric. Safety and efficacy have not been established in pediatric patients.

DOSE ADJUSTMENT
Avoid concurrent use of CYP3A4 inhibitors. If concomitant use is necessary, reduce ixabepilone dose to 20 mg/m^2. When a CYP3A4 inhibitor is discontinued, allow a 1-wk washout prior to increasing dose of ixabepilone.
Hepatic impairment (bilirubin greater than 1.5 times upper limit of normal [ULN] and up to 3 times ULN and AST/ALT of up to 10 times ULN), when used as monotherapy: starting dose of 20 mg/m^2; may escalate dose up to 30 mg/m^2 maximum in subsequent cycles.
Febrile neutropenia: reduce dose by 20% when given either as monotherapy or in combination with capecitabine.

SIDE EFFECTS/ADVERSE REACTIONS

Frequent

Alopecia, nail changes, abdominal pain, constipation, diarrhea, nausea, stomatitis, vomiting

Occasional

Edema, hot flush, chest pain, fever, pain, dizziness, insomnia

PRECAUTIONS AND CONTRAINDICATIONS

Contraindicated in combination with capecitabine in patients with AST or ALT greater than 2.5 times ULN or bilirubin greater than 1 time ULN because of increased risk of toxicity and neutropenia-related death
Hypersensitivity reaction to Cremophor El or its derivatives
Contraindicated in patients with neutrophil count less than 1500 cells/mm^3
Contraindicated in patients with platelet count less than 100,000 cells/mm^3
Use with caution in patients with cardiovascular diseases, diabetes (increased risk of severe neuropathy), and in patients taking alcohol-containing products, CYP450 3A4 inhibitors, and inducers. Ixabepilone can cause myelosuppression, peripheral neuropathy (especially during the first 3 cycles of treatment), and cognitive impairment.
Alcohol-containing product (39.8% dehydrated alcohol)

DRUG INTERACTIONS OF CONCERN TO DENTISTRY

• CYP3A4 inhibitors (e.g., erythromycin): May increase levels and adverse effects of ixabepilone

SERIOUS REACTIONS

! Patients with liver impairment may have an increase in the risk of hepatic toxicity and neutropenia-related death.
! Left ventricular dysfunction, myocardial ischemia, myelosuppression, and peripheral neuropathy may occur.

DENTAL CONSIDERATIONS

General:
• If additional analgesia is required for dental pain, consider alternative analgesics (acetaminophen) in patient taking opioids for acute or chronic pain.
• Avoid alcohol-containing products (elixirs, mouth rinses) to assist maintenance of alcohol abstinence.
• Stomatitis, mucositis, and dysgeusia may occur and complicate dental treatment.

Consultations:
• Medical consultation may be required to assess disease control and patient's ability to tolerate stress.

Teach Patient/Family to:
• Encourage effective oral hygiene to prevent soft tissue inflammation.
• Prevent trauma when using oral hygiene aids.
• Avoid mouth rinses with high alcohol content because of drying effect.
• Update health and medication history if physician makes any changes in evaluation or drug regimens; include OTC, herbal, and nonherbal remedies in the update.
• Be alert for the possibility of stomatitis, mucositis, and taste alterations and the need to see dentist immediately if signs of inflammation occur.

kanamycin sulfate
kan-ah-**mye'**-sin **suhl'**-feyt
(Kantrex)

CATEGORY AND SCHEDULE
Pregnancy Risk Category:
Unavailable for irrigating solution

Drug Class: Aminoglycoside;
antibiotic

MECHANISM OF ACTION
An aminoglycoside antibiotic that
irreversibly binds to protein on
bacterial ribosomes.
Therapeutic Effect: Interferes with
protein synthesis of susceptible
microorganisms, bacteriostatic.

USES
Treatment of wound, surgical site
irrigation

INDICATIONS AND DOSAGES
Wound and Surgical Site Irrigation
Adults, Elderly. 0.25% solution to
irrigate pleural space, ventricular or
abscess cavities, wounds, or surgical
sites.

SIDE EFFECTS/ADVERSE REACTIONS
Occasional
Hypersensitivity reactions (fever,
pruritus, rash, urticaria)
Rare
Headache

PRECAUTIONS AND CONTRAINDICATIONS
Hypersensitivity to kanamycin, other
aminoglycosides (cross-sensitivity),
or their components

DRUG INTERACTIONS OF CONCERN TO DENTISTRY
• Increased risk of nephrotoxicity,
ototoxicity and neuromuscular
blockade: concurrent use with other
aminoglycosides
• Risk of inactivation: β-lactam
antiinfectives

SERIOUS REACTIONS
! None known

DENTAL CONSIDERATIONS
General:
• For selected infections in the
hospital setting, provide palliative
emergency dental treatment only.
• Examine for oral manifestation of
opportunistic infection.
• Determine why patient is taking
the drug.
• Caution regarding allergy to
medication.
Consultations:
• Medical consultation may be
required to assess disease control.
Teach Patient/Family to:
• Encourage effective oral hygiene
to prevent soft tissue inflammation.
• Report oral lesions, soreness, or
bleeding to dentist.
• Prevent trauma when using oral
hygiene aids.

ketamine
key'-tah-meen
(Ketalar)

CATEGORY AND SCHEDULE
Pregnancy Risk Category: B

Drug Class: Anesthetic, general

MECHANISM OF ACTION

A rapidly acting general anesthetic that selectively blocks afferent impulses and interacts with CNS transmitter systems.
Therapeutic Effect: Produces an anesthetic state characterized by profound analgesia and normal pharyngeal-laryngeal reflexes.

USES

Production of loss of consciousness before and during surgery

PHARMACOKINETICS

Route	Onset	Peak	Duration
IM (anesthetic)	3–4 min	N/A	12–25 min
IM (analgesic)	30 min	N/A	15–30 min
IV (anesthetic)	30 sec	N/A	5–10 min
IV (analgesic)	10–15 min	N/A	N/A

Rapidly distributed. Metabolized in the liver. Primarily excreted in urine.
Half-life: Distribution: 10–15 min, elimination: 2–3 hr.

INDICATIONS AND DOSAGES

▶ **Sole Anesthetic for Short Diagnostic and Surgical Procedures That Do Not Require Skeletal Muscle Relaxation, Induction of Anesthesia Before Administering Other General Anesthetics, Supplement to Low-Potency Agents**
IV
Adults, Elderly. 1–4.5 mg/kg.
Children. 0.5–2 mg/kg.
IM
Adults, Elderly. 3–8 mg/kg.
Children. 3–7 mg/kg.

SIDE EFFECTS/ADVERSE REACTIONS

Frequent
Increased B/P and pulse rate; emergence reaction (marked by dreamlike state, delirium, hallucinations, and vivid imagery and occasionally accompanied by confusion, excitement, and irrational behavior; lasts from a few hr to 24 hr after ketamine administration)
Occasional
Pain at injection site
Rare
Rash

PRECAUTIONS AND CONTRAINDICATIONS

Aneurysms, angina, CHF, elevated intracranial pressure, hypertension, psychotic disorders, thyrotoxicosis

DRUG INTERACTIONS OF CONCERN TO DENTISTRY

• Increased risk of hypotension and respiratory depression: all CNS depressants

SERIOUS REACTIONS

❗ Continuous or repeated intermittent infusion may result in extreme somnolence and circulatory or respiratory depression.
❗ Too-rapid IV administration of ketamine may produce severe hypotension, respiratory depression, and irregular muscle movements.
❗ Prolonged respiratory depression: nondepolarizing muscle relaxants.

DENTAL CONSIDERATIONS

General:
• Warning: Ketamine should be administered by persons trained in the administration of general anesthesia. Patients must be continually monitored, and facilities for maintenance of a patent airway,

K

ventilatory support, oxygen supplementation, and circulatory resuscitation must be immediately available. Strict aseptic technique must be followed in handling ketamine.

• Monitor for increased B/P and pulse rate; emergence reactions including hallucinations, delirium, dreamlike states, vivid imagery often accompanied by confusion, excitement, and irrational behavior.

• Responsible person must drive the patient home after recovery.

• Use safety measures: side rails, night light, and call bell within reach.

Consultations:

• Consultation with physician may be necessary if sedation or general anesthesia is required.

Teach Patient/Family to:

• Avoid performing tasks that require mental alertness or motor skills for 24 hr after anesthesia has been discontinued.

ketoconazole

kee-toe-**kon**′-ah-zole
(Apo-Ketocomazole[CAN], Nizoral, Nizoral AD, Sebizole[AUS])
Do not confuse Nizoral with Nasarel.

CATEGORY AND SCHEDULE

Pregnancy Risk Category: C
OTC (1% shampoo only)

Drug Class: Imidazole antifungal

MECHANISM OF ACTION

A fungistatic antifungal that inhibits the synthesis of ergosterol, a vital component of fungal cell formation.

Therapeutic Effect: Damages the fungal cell membrane, altering its function.

USES

Treatment of systemic candidiasis, chronic mucocutaneous candidiasis, cutaneous candidiasis, candiduria, coccidioidomycosis, histoplasmosis, chromomycosis, para-coccidioidomycosis, severe recalcitrant cutaneous dermatophyte infections

PHARMACOKINETICS

PO: Peak 1–2 hr. **Half-life:** 2 hr, terminal 8 hr; highly protein bound; metabolized in liver; excreted in bile, feces; requires acid pH for absorption; distributed poorly to CSF.

INDICATIONS AND DOSAGES

▸ **Histoplasmosis, Blastomycosis, Systemic Candidiasis, Chronic Mucocutaneous Candidiasis, Coccidioidomycosis, Paracoccidioidomycosis, Chromomycosis, Seborrheic Dermatitis, Tinea Corporis, Tinea Capitis, Tinea Manus, Tinea Cruris, Tinea Pedis, Tinea Unguium (Onychomycosis), Oral Thrush, Candiduria**
PO
Adults, Elderly. 200–400 mg/day.
Children. 3.3–6.6 mg/kg/day.
Maximum: 800 mg/day in 2 divided doses.
Topical
Adults, Elderly. Apply to affected area 1–2 times a day for 2–4 wk.
Shampoo
Adults, Elderly. Use twice a wk for 4 wk, allowing at least 3 days between shampooing. Use intermittently to maintain control.

SIDE EFFECTS/ADVERSE REACTIONS
Occasional
Nausea, vomiting
Rare
Abdominal pain, diarrhea, headache, dizziness, photophobia, pruritus
Topical: itching, burning, irritation

PRECAUTIONS AND CONTRAINDICATIONS
Hypersensitivity, lactation, fungal meningitis, loratadine, triazolam, dofetilide
Caution:
Renal disease, hepatic disease, drug-induced achlorhydria, potent inhibitor of CYP3A4 isoenzymes

DRUG INTERACTIONS OF CONCERN TO DENTISTRY
• Hepatotoxicity: alcohol, high-dose long-term use, acetaminophen, carbamazepine, sulfonamides
• Decreased absorption: antacids (take 2 hr after ketoconazole), proton pump inhibitors
• Leukocyte disorders: tacrolimus
• Contraindicated with triazolam, lovastatin, dofetilide
• Inhibits the metabolism of benzodiazepines (e.g., midazolam, triazolam)
• May inhibit metabolism of warfarin
• Decreased effects: didanosine (take 2 hr before didanosine tabs)
• May increase plasma levels and side effects of HMG-CoA reductase inhibitors (statins), cyclosporine
• Increased serum levels of indinavir, saquinavir, ritonavir, nisoldipine, haloperidol, carbamazepine, tricyclic antidepressants, buspirone, zolpidem, corticosteroids
• Suspected decrease in oral contraceptive effectiveness; may need to suggest additional contraception

SERIOUS REACTIONS
! Hematologic toxicity (as evidenced by thrombocytopenia, hemolytic anemia, and leukopenia) occurs occasionally.
! Hepatotoxicity may occur within 1 wk to several mo after starting therapy.
! Anaphylaxis occurs rarely.

DENTAL CONSIDERATIONS
General:
• To prevent reinoculation of *Candida* infection, dispose of tooth brush or other contaminated oral hygiene devices used during period of infection.
• Determine if medication controls disease.
• Place on frequent recall to evaluate healing response.
• Assess salivary flow as a factor in caries, periodontal disease, and candidiasis.
Teach Patient/Family to:
• Avoid mouth rinses with high alcohol content because of drying effects.

K

ketoprofen
kee-toe-**proe′**-fen
(Apo-Keto[CAN], Novo-Keto-EC, Orudis[AUS], Orudis KT[CAN], Orudis SR[AUS], Oruvail, Oruvail SR[AUS], Rhodis[CAN])

CATEGORY AND SCHEDULE
Pregnancy Risk Category: B (D if used in third trimester or near delivery)
OTC (tablets)

Drug Class: Nonsteroidal antiinflammatory

MECHANISM OF ACTION
An NSAID that produces analgesic and antiinflammatory effects by inhibiting prostaglandin synthesis. *Therapeutic Effect:* Reduces the inflammatory response and intensity of pain.

USES
Treatment of osteoarthritis, rheumatoid arthritis, dysmenorrhea; OTC: minor aches and pains

PHARMACOKINETICS
PO: Peak 2 hr. *Half-life:* 3–3.5 hr; 99% plasma-protein binding; metabolized in liver; excreted in urine (metabolites), breast milk

INDICATIONS AND DOSAGES
▸ **Acute or Chronic Rheumatoid Arthritis and Osteoarthritis**
PO
Adults. Initially, 75 mg 3 times a day or 50 mg 4 times a day.
Elderly. Initially, 25–50 mg 3–4 times a day. Maintenance: 150–300 mg/day in 3–4 divided doses.
PO (Extended Release)
Adults, Elderly. 100–200 mg once a day.
▸ **Mild-to-Moderate Pain, Dysmenorrhea**
PO
Adults, Elderly. 25–50 mg q6–8h. Maximum: 300 mg/day.
▸ **OTC Dosage**
PO
Adults, Elderly. 12.5 mg q4–6h. Maximum: 6 tabs/day.
▸ **Dosage in Renal Impairment**
Mild. 150 mg/day maximum.
Severe. 100 mg/day maximum.

SIDE EFFECTS/ADVERSE REACTIONS
Frequent
Dyspepsia

Occasional
Nausea, diarrhea or constipation, flatulence, abdominal cramps, headache
Rare
Anorexia, vomiting, visual disturbances, fluid retention

PRECAUTIONS AND CONTRAINDICATIONS
Active peptic ulcer disease, chronic inflammation of the GI tract, GI bleeding or ulceration, history of hypersensitivity to aspirin or NSAIDs
Caution:
Lactation, children, bleeding disorders, GI disorders, cardiac disorders, hypersensitivity to other antiinflammatory agents, elderly, children younger than 16 yr
Potential for increased adverse cardiovascular events in patients at risk for thromboembolism

DRUG INTERACTIONS OF CONCERN TO DENTISTRY
• GI ulceration, bleeding: aspirin, other NSAIDs, alcohol, corticosteroids
• Nephrotoxicity: acetaminophen (prolonged use)
• Possible risk of decreased renal function: cyclosporine
• Increased photosensitizing effect: tetracycline
• SSRIs: NSAIDs increase risk of GI side effects
• When prescribed for dental pain:
  • Risk of increased effects: oral anticoagulants, oral antidiabetics, lithium, methotrexate
  • Decreased effects of diuretics

SERIOUS REACTIONS
! Rare reactions with long-term use include peptic ulcer disease, GI bleeding, gastritis, severe hepatic reactions (cholestasis, jaundice),

nephrotoxicity (dysuria, hematuria, proteinuria, nephrotic syndrome), and severe hypersensitivity reaction (bronchospasm, angioedema).

DENTAL CONSIDERATIONS

General:
• Patients on chronic drug therapy may rarely have symptoms of blood dyscrasias, which can include infection, bleeding, and poor healing.
• Assess salivary flow as a factor in caries, periodontal disease, and candidiasis.
• Avoid prescribing for dental use in pregnancy.
• Avoid prescribing aspirin-containing products or giving to patient taking aspirin.
• Consider semisupine chair position for patients with arthritic disease.
• Severe stomach bleeding may occur in patients who regularly use NSAIDs in recommended doses, when the patient is also taking another NSAID, a blood thinning, or steroid drug, if the patient has GI or peptic ulcer disease, if they are 60 yr or older, or when NSAIDs are taken longer than directed. Warn patients of the potential for severe stomach bleeding.
Consultations:
• In a patient with symptoms of blood dyscrasias, request a medical consultation for blood studies and postpone dental treatment until normal values are reestablished.
• Medical consultation may be required to assess disease control.
Teach Patient/Family to:
• Encourage effective oral hygiene to prevent soft tissue inflammation.
• Use caution to prevent injury when using oral hygiene aids.
 • Warn patient of potential risks of NSAIDs.

• When chronic dry mouth occurs, advise patient to:
 • Avoid mouth rinses with high alcohol content because of drying effects.
 • Use sugarless gum, frequent sips of water, or saliva substitutes.
 • Use daily home fluoride products for anticaries effect.

ketorolac tromethamine
kee-**tor**′-oh-lak
tro-**meth**′-ay-meen
(Acular, Acular LS, Acular PF, Toradol)
Do not confuse Acular with Acthar or Ocular.

K

CATEGORY AND SCHEDULE
Pregnancy Risk Category: C (D if used in third trimester)

Drug Class: Nonsteroidal antiinflammatory

MECHANISM OF ACTION
An NSAID that inhibits prostaglandin synthesis and reduces prostaglandin levels in the aqueous humor.
Therapeutic Effect: Relieves pain stimulus and reduces intraocular inflammation.

USES
Short-term treatment of acute mild-to-moderate pain

PHARMACOKINETICS

Route	Onset	Peak	Duration
PO	30–60 min	1.5–4 hr	4–6 hr
IV/IM	30 min	1–2 hr	4–6 hr

Readily absorbed from the GI tract, after IM administration. Protein binding: 99%. Largely metabolized in the liver. Primarily excreted in urine. Not removed by hemodialysis. *Half-life:* 3.8–6.3 hr (increased with impaired renal function and in the elderly).

INDICATIONS AND DOSAGES
▶ **Short-Term Relief of Mild-to-Moderate Pain (Multiple Doses)**
PO
Adults, Elderly. 10 mg q4–6h. Maximum: 40 mg/24 hr.
IV, IM
Adults younger than 65 yr. 30 mg q6h. Maximum: 120 mg/24 hr.
Adults 65 yr and older, those with renal impairment, those weighing less than 50 kg. 15 mg q6h. Maximum: 60 mg/24 hr.
Children 2–16 yr. 0.5 mg/kg q6h.
▶ **Short-Term Relief of Mild-to-Moderate Pain (Single Dose)**
IV
Adults younger than 65 yr, Children 17 yr and older weighing more than 50 kg. 30 mg.
Adults 65 yr and older, with renal impairment, weighing less than 50 kg. 15 mg.
Children 2–16 yr. 0.5 mg/kg. Maximum: 15 mg.
IM
Adults younger than 65 yr, Children 17 yr and older, weighing more than 50 kg. 60 mg.
Adults 65 yr and older, with renal impairment, weighing less than 50 kg. 30 mg.
Children 2–16 yr. 1 mg/kg. Maximum: 15 kg.
▶ **Allergic Conjunctivitis**
Ophthalmic
Adults, Elderly, Children 3 yr and older. 1 drop 4 times a day.

▶ **Cataract Extraction**
Ophthalmic
Adults, Elderly. 1 drop 4 times a day. Begin 24 hr after surgery and continue for 2 wk.
▶ **Refractive Surgery**
Ophthalmic
Adults, Elderly. 1 drop 4 times a day for 3 days.

SIDE EFFECTS/ADVERSE REACTIONS
Frequent
Headache, nausea, abdominal cramps or pain, dyspepsia, oral lichenoid reaction
Occasional
Diarrhea
Ophthalmic: Transient stinging and burning
Rare
Constipation, vomiting, flatulence, stomatitis, dizziness
Ophthalmic: Ocular irritation, allergic reactions, superficial ocular infection, keratitis

PRECAUTIONS AND CONTRAINDICATIONS
Active peptic ulcer disease, chronic inflammation of GI tract, GI bleeding or ulceration, history of hypersensitivity to aspirin or NSAIDs
Caution:
Children, GI disorders, cardiac disorders, hypersensitivity to other antiinflammatory agents
Increased potential for adverse cardiovascular events in patients at risk for thromboembolism

DRUG INTERACTIONS OF CONCERN TO DENTISTRY
• GI ulceration, bleeding: aspirin, alcohol, corticosteroids
• Contraindicated with probenecid
• Possible risk of decreased renal function: cyclosporine

- SSRIs: NSAIDs increase risk of GI side effects
- When prescribed for dental pain:
  - Risk of increased effects: oral anticoagulants, oral antidiabetics, lithium, methotrexate
  - Decreased antihypertensive effects of diuretics, ß-blockers, ACE inhibitors

SERIOUS REACTIONS

! Rare reactions with long-term use include peptic ulcer disease, GI bleeding, gastritis, severe hepatic reactions (cholestasis, jaundice), nephrotoxicity (glomerular nephritis, interstitial nephritis, nephrotic syndrome), and an acute hypersensitivity reaction (including fever, chills, and joint pain).

DENTAL CONSIDERATIONS

General:
- Assess salivary flow as a factor in caries, periodontal disease, and candidiasis.
- Avoid prescribing in pregnancy.
- Avoid prescribing aspirin or other NSAIDs.
- Avoid long-term use for chronic pain syndromes; combined use of IV or IM and oral doses must not exceed 5 days.
Consultations:
- Medical consultation may be required to assess disease control.
Teach Patient/Family to:
- Avoid mouth rinses with high alcohol content because of drying effects.

▶ Ketorolac Tromethamine (Ocular)
General:
- Determine why patient is taking the drug.
- Avoid dental light in patient's eyes; offer dark glasses for patient comfort.

ketotifen fumarate
kee-toe-tye′-fen fyoo′-mah-rate
(Apo-Ketotifen[CAN], Novo-Ketotifen[CAN], Zaditen[CAN], Zaditor)

CATEGORY AND SCHEDULE
Pregnancy Risk Category: C

Drug Class: Antihistamine

MECHANISM OF ACTION
Selective histamine H_1-antagonist and mast cell stabilizer, suppresses release of mediators from cells involved in hypersensitivity reactions, and decreases chemotaxis and activation of eosinophils.
Therapeutic Effect: Reduces symptoms of allergic conjunctivitis.

USES
Temporary prevention of itching of the eyes caused by allergic conjunctivitis

PHARMACOKINETICS
None reported

INDICATIONS AND DOSAGES
▶ Allergic Conjunctivitis
Ophthalmic
Adults, Elderly, Children 3 yr or older. 1 drop into affected eye q8–12h.

SIDE EFFECTS/ADVERSE REACTIONS
Frequent
Conjunctival infection, headache, rhinitis
Occasional
Allergic reaction, burning, stinging, eyelid disorder, flu-like syndrome, keratitis, mydriasis, ocular discharge or pain, pharyngitis, photophobia, rash

PRECAUTIONS AND CONTRAINDICATIONS

Hypersensitivity to ketotifen or any component of the formulation (the preservative is benzalkonium chloride)

Caution:

Prevent contamination of ophthalmic solution by careful use, do not wear contact lens if eyes are red, delay inserting contacts up to 10 min after drops are placed in eyes; lactation, children younger than 3 yr

DRUG INTERACTIONS OF CONCERN TO DENTISTRY

• None reported

SERIOUS REACTIONS

! No serious signs and symptoms have been seen after ingestion up to 20 mg.

DENTAL CONSIDERATIONS

General:

• Avoid dental light in patient's eyes; offer dark glasses for patient comfort.

K

labetalol hydrochloride
la-**bet**′-ah-lole high-droh-**klor**′-ide
(Normodyne, Presolol[AUS],
Trandate)
Do not confuse Trandate with
tramadol or Trental.

CATEGORY AND SCHEDULE
Pregnancy Risk Category: C (D if
used in second or third trimester)

Drug Class: Nonselective
adrenergic β-blocker and selective
α_1-blocker; antihypertensive

MECHANISM OF ACTION
An antihypertensive that blocks α_1-,
β_1-, and β_2 (large doses)-adrenergic
receptor sites. Large doses increase
airway resistance.
Therapeutic Effect: Slows sinus
heart rate; decreases peripheral
vascular resistance, cardiac output,
and B/P.

USES
Treatment of mild-to-severe
hypertension

PHARMACOKINETICS

Route	Onset	Peak	Duration
PO	0.5–2 hr	2–4 hr	8–12 hr
IV	2.5 min	5–15 min	2–4 hr

Completely absorbed from the GI
tract. Protein binding: 50%.
Undergoes first-pass metabolism.
Metabolized in the liver. Primarily
excreted in urine. Not removed by
hemodialysis. *Half-life:* PO, 6–8 hr;
IV, 5.5 hr.

INDICATIONS AND DOSAGES
▸ **Hypertension**
PO
Adults. Initially, 100 mg twice a day
adjusted in increments of 100 mg
twice a day q2–3 days. Maintenance:
200–400 mg twice a day. Maximum:
2.4 g/day.
Elderly. Initially, 100 mg 1–2 times
a day. May increase as needed.
▸ **Severe Hypertension, Hypertensive
Emergency**
IV
Adults. Initially, 20 mg. Additional
doses of 20–80 mg may be given at
10-min intervals, up to a total dose
of 300 mg.
IV Infusion
Adults. Initially, 2 mg/min up to
total dose of 300 mg.
PO (after IV therapy)
Adults. Initially, 200 mg; then,
200–400 mg in 6–12 hr. Increase
dose at 1-day intervals to desired
level.

SIDE EFFECTS/ADVERSE REACTIONS
Frequent
Drowsiness, difficulty sleeping,
unusual fatigue or weakness,
diminished sexual ability, transient
scalp tingling
Occasional
Dizziness, dyspnea, peripheral
edema, depression, anxiety,
constipation, diarrhea, nasal
congestion, nausea, vomiting,
abdominal discomfort
Rare
Altered taste, dry eyes, increased
urination, paresthesia

PRECAUTIONS AND CONTRAINDICATIONS
Bronchial asthma, cardiogenic
shock, second- or third-degree heart
block, severe bradycardia,
uncontrolled CHF

L

Caution:
Major surgery, lactation, diabetes mellitus, renal disease, thyroid disease, COPD, well-compensated heart failure, CAD, nonallergic bronchospasm

DRUG INTERACTIONS OF CONCERN TO DENTISTRY
• Decreased metabolism: lidocaine
• Decreased effect: sympathomimetics
• Decreased hypotensive effects: indomethacin and other NSAIDs
• Increased hypotension, myocardial depression: hydrocarbon-inhalation anesthetics
• Increased plasma levels: diphenhydramine

SERIOUS REACTIONS
! Labetalol administration may precipitate or aggravate CHF because of decreased myocardial stimulation.
! Abrupt withdrawal may precipitate ischemic heart disease, producing sweating, palpitations, headache, and tremors.
! May mask signs and symptoms of acute hypoglycemia (tachycardia, B/P changes) in patients with diabetes.

DENTAL CONSIDERATIONS

General:
• Monitor vital signs at every appointment because of cardiovascular side effects.
• Patients on chronic drug therapy may rarely have symptoms of blood dyscrasias, which can include infection, bleeding, and poor healing.
• Assess salivary flow as a factor in caries, periodontal disease, and candidiasis.
• Limit dose of vasoconstrictors, or avoid use of vasoconstriction.

• After supine positioning, have patient sit upright for at least 2 min before standing to avoid orthostatic hypotension.
• Limit use of sodium-containing products, such as saline IV fluids, for patients with a dietary salt restriction.
• Stress from dental procedures may compromise cardiovascular function; determine patient risk.
• Short appointments and a stress-reduction protocol may be required for anxious patients.

Consultations:
• Medical consultation may be required to assess disease control and patient's ability to tolerate stress.
• In a patient with symptoms of blood dyscrasias, request a medical consultation for blood studies and postpone dental treatment until normal values are reestablished.

Teach Patient/Family to:
• When chronic dry mouth occurs, advise patient to:
  • Avoid mouth rinses with high alcohol content because of drying effects.
  • Use sugarless gum, frequent sips of water, or saliva substitutes.
  • Use daily home fluoride products for anticaries effect.

lacosamide
(lah-**kose**-a-mide)
(Vimpat)
Do not confuse with lamisil, lanoxin.

CATEGORY AND SCHEDULE
Pregnancy Risk Category: C

Drug Class: Anticonvulsant

MECHANISM OF ACTION

An anticonvulsant and antineuralgic agent whose exact mechanism is unknown but may be related to enhancement of sodium channel inactivation and modulation of collapsing response mediator protein-2 (CRMP-2). Lacosamide decreases the availability of voltage-gated sodium channels.

USES

Adjunctive therapy of partial-onset seizures in patients 17 yr and older

PHARMACOKINETICS

Completely absorbed following oral administration (100%), can be taken with food. Peak plasma concentrations reached in 1–5 hr, widely distributed. Protein binding <15%. Undergoes hepatic metabolism (CYP 2C19). *Half-life:* 13 hr. Excreted primarily by the kidneys.

INDICATIONS AND DOSAGES
▸ **Partial-Onset Seizures**
Adult. PO 50 mg twice daily. May be increased at weekly intervals by 100 mg/day given as 2 divided doses, up to 200–400 mg/day, based on response and tolerability (intravenous form also available when oral administration not feasible).

SIDE EFFECTS/ADVERSE REACTIONS
Frequent
Dizziness, diplopia, blurred vision, headache, nausea
Occasional
Abnormal vision, ataxia, fatigue, nystagmus, somnolence, tremor, vomiting

PRECAUTIONS AND CONTRAINDICATIONS

Hypersensitivity to lacosamide or any of its ingredients, hepatic impairment. Safety in children not established

DRUG INTERACTIONS OF CONCERN TO DENTISTRY
• None reported in dentistry

SERIOUS REACTIONS
! Hypersensitivity

DENTAL CONSIDERATIONS

General:
• Assess salivary flow as a factor in caries, periodontal disease, and candidiasis.
• Morning appointments and stress-reduction protocol may be needed for anxious patients.
• Be prepared to manage seizures and/or nausea.
• After supine positioning, allow patient to sit upright for 2 minutes to avoid occurrence of dizziness.
Consultations:
Consult with physician to determine seizure control and ability to tolerate dental procedures.
Teach Patient/Family to:
• Avoid mouth rinses with high alcohol content because of drying effect.
• Use home fluoride products for anticaries effect.
• Use sugarless/xylitol gum, frequent sips of water, or saliva substitutes if dry mouth occurs.

lamivudine
la-**miv**′-yoo-deen
(Epivir, Epivir-HBV,
Heptovir[CAN], Zeffix[AUS])
Do not confuse lamivudine with
lamotrigine.

CATEGORY AND SCHEDULE
Pregnancy Risk Category: C

Drug Class: Antiviral,
nucleoside analog

MECHANISM OF ACTION
An antiviral that inhibits HIV
reverse transcriptase by viral DNA
chain termination. Also inhibits
RNA- and DNA-dependent DNA
polymerase, an enzyme necessary
for HIV replication.
Therapeutic Effect: Interrupts HIV
replication, slowing the progression
of HIV infection.

USES
Used in combination with
zidovudine for the treatment of HIV
infection and to reduce disease
progression and death in AIDS;
HBV dose form: chronic hepatitis B
associated with evidence of hepatitis
B viral replication and liver
inflammation

PHARMACOKINETICS
Rapidly and completely absorbed
from the GI tract. Protein binding:
less than 36%. Widely distributed
(crosses the blood-brain barrier).
Primarily excreted unchanged in
urine. Not removed by hemodialysis
or peritoneal dialysis. ***Half-life:***
11–15 hr (intracellular), 2–11 hr
(serum, adults), 1.7–2 hr (serum,
children) (increased in impaired
renal function).

INDICATIONS AND DOSAGES
▸ **HIV Infection (in Combination with
Other Antiretrovirals)**
PO
*Adults, Children 12–16 yr, weighing
50 kg (100 lb) or more.* 150 mg
twice a day or 300 mg once a day.
Adults weighing less than 50 kg.
2 mg/kg twice a day.
Children 3 mo–11 yr. 4 mg/kg twice
a day (up to 150 mg/dose).
▸ **Chronic Hepatitis B**
PO
Adults, Children 17 yr and older.
100 mg/day.
Children younger than 17 yr. 3 mg/
kg/day. Maximum: 100 mg/day.
▸ **Dosage in Renal Impairment**
Dosage and frequency are modified
on the basis of creatinine clearance.

Creatinine Clearance	Dosage
50 ml/min or higher	150 mg twice a day
30–49 ml/min	150 mg once a day
15–29 ml/min	150 mg first dose, then 100 mg once a day
5–14 ml/min	150 mg first dose, then 50 mg once a day
Less than 5 ml/min	50 mg first dose, then 25 mg once a day

SIDE EFFECTS/ADVERSE REACTIONS
Frequent
Headache, nausea, malaise and
fatigue, nasal disturbances, diarrhea,
cough, musculoskeletal pain,
neuropathy, insomnia, anorexia,
dizziness, fever or chills
Occasional
Depression, myalgia, abdominal
cramps, dyspepsia, arthralgia

PRECAUTIONS AND CONTRAINDICATIONS
Hypersensitivity, history of
pancreatitis as child

Caution:
Reduce dose in renal disease, lactation

DRUG INTERACTIONS OF CONCERN TO DENTISTRY
• None reported

SERIOUS REACTIONS
! Pancreatitis occurs in 13% of pediatric patients.
! Anemia, neutropenia, and thrombocytopenia occur rarely.

DENTAL CONSIDERATIONS
General:
• Patients on chronic drug therapy may rarely have symptoms of blood dyscrasias, which can include infection, bleeding, and poor healing.
• Examine for oral manifestation of opportunistic infections.
Consultations:
• In a patient with symptoms of blood dyscrasias, request a medical consultation for blood studies and postpone dental treatment until normal values are reestablished.
• Medical consultation may be required to assess disease control and patient's ability to tolerate stress.
Teach Patient/Family to:
• Encourage effective oral hygiene to prevent soft tissue inflammation.
• Use caution to prevent trauma when using oral hygiene aids.
• See dentist immediately if secondary oral infection occurs.

lamotrigine
la-**moe**'-trih-jeen
(Apo-Lamotrigine[CAN], Lamictal, Lamictal CD)
Do not confuse lamotrigine with lamivudine.

CATEGORY AND SCHEDULE
Pregnancy Risk Category: C

Drug Class: Antiepileptic

MECHANISM OF ACTION
An anticonvulsant whose exact mechanism is unknown. May block voltage-gated sodium channels, thus stabilizing neuronal membranes and regulating presynaptic transmitter release of excitatory amino acids.
Therapeutic Effect: Reduces seizure activity.

USES
Adjunctive treatment of refractory partial seizures in adults and adjunctive treatment for Lennox-Gastaut syndrome in pediatric and adult patients; long-term maintenance of bipolar 1 disorder

PHARMACOKINETICS
Rapidly absorbed from the GI tract. Protein binding: 55%. Metabolized primarily by glucuronic acid conjugation. Excreted in the urine.
Half-life: 13–30 hr.

INDICATIONS AND DOSAGES
▸ **Seizure Control in Patients Receiving Enzyme-Inducing Antiepileptic Drug (EIAEDS), But Not Valproic Acid**
PO
Adults, Elderly, Children older than 12 yr. Recommended as add-on therapy: 50 mg once a day for 2 wk, followed by 100 mg/day in 2 divided

doses for 2 wk. Maintenance: Dosage may be increased by 100 mg/day every wk, up to 300–500 mg/day in 2 divided doses.

Children 2–12 yr. 0.6 mg/kg/day in 2 divided doses for 2 wk, then 1.2 mg/kg/day in 2 divided doses for wk 3 and 4. Maintenance: 5–15 mg/kg/day. Maximum: 400 mg/day.

▸ **Seizure Control in Patients Receiving Combination Therapy of EIAEDS and Valproic Acid**

PO

Adults, Elderly, Children older than 12 yr. 25 mg every other day for 2 wk, followed by 25 mg once a day for 2 wk. Maintenance: Dosage may be increased by 25–50 mg/day q1–2wk, up to 150 mg/day in 2 divided doses.

Children 2–12 yr. 0.15 mg/kg/day in 2 divided doses for 2 wk, then 0.3 mg/kg/day in 2 divided doses for wk 3 and 4. Maintenance: 1–5 mg/kg/day in 2 divided doses. Maximum: 200 mg/day.

▸ **Conversion to Monotherapy for Patients Receiving EIAED**

PO

Adults, Elderly, Children 16 yr and older. 500 mg/day in 2 divided doses. Titrate to desired dose while maintaining EIAED at fixed level, then withdraw EIAED by 20% each week over a 4-wk period.

▸ **Conversion to Monotherapy for Patients Receiving Valproic Acid**

PO

Adults, Elderly, Children 16 yr and older. Titrate lamotrigine to 200 mg/day, maintaining valproic acid dose. Maintain lamotrigine dose and decrease valproic acid to 500 mg/day, no greater than 500 mg/day/wk, then maintain 500 mg/day for 1 wk. Increase lamotrigine to 300 mg/day and decrease valproic acid to 250 mg/day. Maintain for 1 wk, then discontinue valproic acid and

increase lamotrigine by 100 mg/day each wk until maintenance dose of 500 mg/day reached.

▸ **Bipolar Disorder in Patients Receiving EIAED**

PO

Adults, Elderly. 50 mg/day for 2 wk, then 100 mg/day for 2 wk, then 200 mg/day for 1 wk, then 300 mg/day for 1 wk, then up to usual maintenance dose 400 mg/day in divided doses.

▸ **Bipolar Disorder in Patients Receiving Valproic Acid**

PO

Adults, Elderly. 25 mg/day every other day for 2 wk, then 25 mg/day for 2 wk, then 50 mg/day for 1 wk, then 100 mg/day. Usual maintenance dose with valproic acid: 100 mg/day.

▸ **Discontinuation Therapy**

Adults, Children older than 12 yr. A dosage reduction of approximately 50% per week over at least 2 wk is recommended.

SIDE EFFECTS/ADVERSE REACTIONS

Frequent

Dizziness, diplopia, headache, ataxia, nausea, blurred vision, somnolence, rhinitis, dry mouth, halitosis

Occasional

Rash, pharyngitis, vomiting, cough, flu-like symptoms, diarrhea, dysmenorrhea, fever, insomnia, dyspepsia

Rare

Constipation, tremors, anxiety, pruritus, vaginitis, hypersensitivity reaction

PRECAUTIONS AND CONTRAINDICATIONS

Hypersensitivity

Caution:

Elderly, children younger than 16 yr, dose adjustment with other anticonvulsants, seizure risk with drug withdrawal, renal or hepatic impairment; can cause Stevens-Johnson syndrome, toxic epidermal necrolysis

DRUG INTERACTIONS OF CONCERN TO DENTISTRY

• Increased excretion: chronic, high-dose acetaminophen (900 mg 3 times a day), but significance is unclear; carbamazepine
• Increased blood levels of carbamazepine

SERIOUS REACTIONS

! Abrupt withdrawal may increase seizure frequency.
! Serious rashes, including Stevens-Johnson syndrome, requiring hospitalization and discontinuation of treatment have been reported.

DENTAL CONSIDERATIONS

General:
• Early-morning appointments and a stress-reduction protocol may be required for anxious patients.
• Determine type of epilepsy, seizure frequency, and quality of seizure control.
• Evaluate respiration characteristics and rate.
• Assess salivary flow as factor in caries, periodontal disease, and candidiasis.
• Patients on chronic drug therapy may rarely have symptoms of blood dyscrasias, which can include infection, bleeding, and poor healing.
• Place on frequent recall because of oral side effects.
Consultations:
• Medical consultation may be required to assess disease control

and the patient's ability to tolerate stress.
• In a patient with symptoms of blood dyscrasias, request a medical consultation for blood studies and postpone dental treatment until normal values are reestablished.
Teach Patient/Family to:
• Encourage effective oral hygiene to prevent soft tissue inflammation.
• Use powered tooth brush if patient has difficulty holding conventional devices.
• When chronic dry mouth occurs, advise patient to:
   • Avoid mouth rinses with high alcohol content because of drying effects.
   • Use daily home fluoride products for anticaries effect.
   • Use sugarless gum, frequent sips of water, or saliva substitutes.

lanreotide
lan-**ree**′-oh-tide
(Somatuline Depot)

CATEGORY AND SCHEDULE
Pregnancy Risk Category: C

Drug Class: Somatostatin

MECHANISM OF ACTION
Octapeptide somatostatin analog that inhibits insulin-like growth factor-1 (IGF-1) and growth hormone. High affinity for somatostatin type 2 (SSTR2) and 5 (SSTR5) receptors in pituitary gland, pancreas, and growth hormone (GH) secreting neoplasms of pituitary gland. Lesser affinity for somatostatin receptors 1, 3, and 4 (SSTR1, SSTR3 and SSTR4).

USES
Acromegaly (long-term therapy in patients who have had inadequate response to surgery and/or radiotherapy; or when surgery and/or radiotherapy is not an option)
For long-term treatment of acromegaly in patients who fail to respond to surgery and radiotherapy.

PHARMACOKINETICS
Protein binding: 79%–83%.
Extensive metabolism in GI tract after biliary excretion.
Bioavailability: 69%–83%. Less than 5% of lanreotide excreted in urine; less than 0.5% recovered unchanged in feces, indicative of some biliary excretion. *Half-life*: 23–36 days.

INDICATIONS AND DOSAGES
SC Injection
Adult. Acromegaly: 90 mg deep SC injection every 4 wk for 3 months. After 3 months adjust dose based on clinical response:
GH >1 to = 2.5 ng/mL, IGF-1 normal and clinical symptoms controlled: maintain dose at 90 mg every 4 wk
GH > 2.5 ng/mL, IGF-1 elevated and/or clinical symptoms uncontrolled, increase dose to 120 mg every 4 wk
GH = 1 ng/mL, IGF-1 normal and clinical symptoms controlled: reduce dose to 60 mg every 4 wk
Dose Adjustments
Renal impairment: 60 mg deep SC injection every 4 wk.
Hepatic impairment: 60 mg deep SC injection every 4 wk.
Geriatric: no dosage adjustment necessary.
Pediatric: Safety and effectiveness in pediatric patients have not been established.

SIDE EFFECTS/ADVERSE REACTIONS
Frequent
Injection site reaction, abdominal pain, diarrhea, nausea, bradycardia, and cholelithiasis

PRECAUTIONS AND CONTRAINDICATIONS
There are no contraindications listed in the manufacturer's labeling.
Use caution in patients with cardiac disease, diabetes mellitus, gallbladder disease, hypothyroidism, renal impairment, and hepatic impairment.

DRUG INTERACTIONS OF CONCERN TO DENTISTRY
• None reported

SERIOUS REACTIONS
! Bradycardia, hypo- and hyperglycemia, gallstones, decreases in thyroid function, renal impairment, and hepatic impairment have occurred.

DENTAL CONSIDERATIONS

General:
• Patient may need assistance in getting into and out of dental chair.
• Adjust chair position for patient comfort.
• Consider semisupine chair position for patient comfort if GI side effects occur.
Consultations:
• Medical consultation may be required to assess disease control and patient's ability to tolerate stress.
• Consultation with physician may be necessary if sedation or general anesthesia is required.

Teach Patient/Family to:
• Update health and medication history if physician makes any changes in evaluation or drug regimens; include OTC, herbal, and nonherbal remedies in the update.
• Use effective oral hygiene to prevent soft tissue inflammation.
• Use caution to prevent injury when using oral hygiene aids.

lansoprazole

lan-**soe**′-pra-zole
(Prevacid, Prevacid IV, Prevacid Solu-Tab, Zoton[AUS])
Do not confuse Prevacid with Pepcid, Pravachol, or Prevpac.

CATEGORY AND SCHEDULE
Pregnancy Risk Category: B

Drug Class: Antisecretory, proton pump inhibitor

MECHANISM OF ACTION
A proton pump inhibitor that selectively inhibits the parietal cell membrane enzyme system (hydrogen-potassium adenosine triphosphatase) or proton pump. *Therapeutic Effect:* Suppresses gastric acid secretion.

USES
Short-term treatment for healing and symptomatic relief of active duodenal ulcer and benign gastric ulcer, erosive esophagitis, and gastroesophageal reflux disease (GERD); maintenance of healing of duodenal ulcers; long-term treatment of pathologic hypersecretory syndromes; NSAID-associated gastric ulcers in patients who continue NSAID use; short-term treatment of symptomatic GERD

PHARMACOKINETICS

Route	Onset	Peak	Duration
PO (15 mg)	2–3 hr	N/A	8–24 hr
PO (30 mg)	1–2 hr	N/A	Longer than 24 hr

Rapid and complete absorption (food may decrease absorption) once drug has left stomach. Protein binding: 97%. Distributed primarily to gastric parietal cells and converted to two active metabolites. Extensively metabolized in the liver. Eliminated in bile and urine. Not removed by hemodialysis.
Half-life: 1.5 hr (increased in the elderly and in those with hepatic impairment).

INDICATIONS AND DOSAGES
▶ **Duodenal Ulcer**
PO
Adults, Elderly. 15 mg/day, before eating, preferably in the morning, for up to 4 wk.
▶ **Erosive Esophagitis**
PO
Adults, Elderly. 30 mg/day, before eating, for up to 8 wk. If healing does not occur within 8 wk (in 5%–10% of cases), may give for additional 8 wk. Maintenance: 15 mg/day.
IV
Adults, Elderly. 30 mg once a day for up to 7 days. Switch to oral lansoprazole therapy as soon as patient can tolerate oral route.
▶ **Gastric Ulcer**
PO
Adults. 30 mg/day for up to 8 wk.
▶ **NSAID Gastric Ulcer**
PO
Adults, Elderly. (Healing): 30 mg/day for up to 8 wk. (Prevention): 15 mg/day for up to 12 wk.

L

▶ **Healed Duodenal Ulcer, GERD**

PO

Adults. 15 mg/day.

▶ **Usual Pediatric Dosage**

Children 3 mo–14 yr, weighing more than 20 kg. 30 mg once daily.

Children 3 mo–14 yr, weighing 10–20 kg. 15 mg once daily.

Children 3 mo–14 yr, weighing less than 10 kg. 7.5 mg once daily.

▶ ***Helicobacter pylori* Infection**

PO

Adults. 30 mg twice a day for 10 days (with amoxicillin and clarithromycin).

▶ **Pathologic Hypersecretory Conditions (Including Zollinger-Ellison Syndrome)**

PO

Adults, Elderly. 60 mg/day. Individualize dosage according to patient needs and for as long as clinically indicated. Administer up to 120 mg/day in divided doses.

SIDE EFFECTS/ADVERSE REACTIONS

Occasional

Diarrhea, abdominal pain, rash, pruritus, altered appetite

Rare

Nausea, headache

PRECAUTIONS AND CONTRAINDICATIONS

Hypersensitivity

Caution:

Children younger than 18 yr, elderly (limit doses to 30 mg/day), severe hepatic disease

DRUG INTERACTIONS OF CONCERN TO DENTISTRY

• Drug interactions not established but potentially can interfere with absorption of amoxicillin, ketoconazole

SERIOUS REACTIONS

❗ Bilirubinemia, eosinophilia, and hyperlipemia occur rarely.

DENTAL CONSIDERATIONS

General:

• Consider semisupine chair position for patient comfort because of GI effects of disease.

• Question the patient about tolerance of NSAIDs or aspirin related to GI problem.

• Patients with GERD may have oral symptoms, including burning mouth, secondary candidiasis, and oral signs of dental erosion.

• Assess salivary flow as factor in caries, periodontal disease, and candidiasis.

Teach Patient/Family to:

• When chronic dry mouth occurs, advise patient to:

• Avoid mouth rinses with high alcohol content because of drying effects.

• Use daily home fluoride products for anticaries effect.

• Use sugarless gum, frequent sips of water, or saliva substitutes.

lanthanum carbonate

lan′-tha-num kar′-boh-nate
(Fosrenol)

CATEGORY AND SCHEDULE

Pregnancy Risk Category: C

Drug Class: Phosphate binder

MECHANISM OF ACTION

A phosphate regulator that dissociates in the acidic environment of the upper GI tract to lanthanum ions, which bind to dietary phosphate released from food during digestion, forming highly insoluble lanthanum phosphate complexes. *Therapeutic Effect:* Reduces phosphate absorption.

USES

Treatment of end-stage renal disease

PHARMACOKINETICS

Phosphate complexes are eliminated in feces.

INDICATIONS AND DOSAGES
▶ **Reduce Serum Phosphate in End-Stage Renal Disease**
PO
Adults, Elderly. 750–1500 mg in divided doses, taken with or immediately after a meal. Dosage may be titrated in 750-mg increments q2–3wk on the basis of serum phosphate levels.

SIDE EFFECTS/ADVERSE REACTIONS
Frequent
Nausea, vomiting, dialysis graft occlusion, abdominal pain

PRECAUTIONS AND CONTRAINDICATIONS
None known

DRUG INTERACTIONS OF CONCERN TO DENTISTRY
• None reported

SERIOUS REACTIONS
! None known

DENTAL CONSIDERATIONS
General:
• Question patient about renal dialysis history and use of other medications.

• Dental drugs known to interact with antacid products should not be taken within 2 hr of lanthanum carbonate.
• Dental procedures must be scheduled to appropriately sequence with dialysis regimen.
• Question patient about coexisting cardiovascular disease, related medications, and any bleeding problems.
• Avoid nephrotoxic drugs; dose adjustment may be required for renal-excreted drugs.
• Oral infections should be eliminated and/or treated aggressively.
• Patient may have AV shunt in place.
• Monitor and record vital signs.
• Consider semisupine chair position for patient comfort if GI side effects occur.
• Question patient about tolerance of NSAIDS or aspirin related to GI disease.
• After supine positioning, have patient sit upright for at least 2 min before standing to avoid orthostatic hypotension.
• Antiinfective prophylaxis may be indicated for patient on dialysis; consult physician.
Consultations:
• Consultation with physician may be necessary if sedation or general anesthesia is required.
• Medical consultation may be required to assess disease control and patient's ability to tolerate stress.
Teach Patient/Family to:
• Encourage effective oral hygiene to prevent soft tissue inflammation.
• Prevent trauma when using oral hygiene aids.
• Update health and medication history if physician makes any changes in evaluation/drug

regimens; include OTC, herbal, and nonherbal drugs in the update.

lapatinib
lah-**pah**′-ti-nib
(Tykerb)

CATEGORY AND SCHEDULE
Pregnancy Risk Category: D

Drug Class: Antineoplastic agent, tyrosine kinase inhibitor; epidermal growth factor receptor (EGFR) inhibitor

MECHANISM OF ACTION
Lapatinib is a 4-anilinoquinazoline kinase inhibitor that inhibits EGFR (ErbB1) and human epidermal receptor type 2 (HER2 [ErbB2]) by reversibly binding to tyrosine kinase, blocking phosphorylation and activation of downstream second messenger (Erk1/2 and Akt), and regulating cellular proliferation and survival in ErbB-expressing tumors.

USES
Combination with capecitabine for patients with advanced or metastatic breast cancer whose tumors overexpress HER2 and for those who have taken an anthracycline, a taxane, and trastuzumab

PHARMACOKINETICS
Incomplete and variable absorption. Protein binding: >99% to albumin and α_1-acid glycoprotein. Metabolized in the liver extensively via CYP3A4 and 3A5 and less extensively via CYP2C19 and 2C8. *Half-life*: about 24 hr. Time to peak in the plasma: 3–6 hr. Excreted unchanged in the feces (27%) and urine (<2%).

INDICATIONS AND DOSAGES
▶ **Breast Cancer**
PO
Adults. 250 mg once daily (in combination with capecitabine). Dosage adjustment for concomitant use with 3A4 inhibitors: 500 mg once daily with careful monitoring. Dosage adjustment for concomitant use with 3A4 inducers: titrate up to 4500 mg/day with careful monitoring.
Dosage in hepatic impairment: 750 mg once daily.
Dosage adjustment for cardiac toxicity: discontinue for decreased left ventricular ejection fraction (LVEF) ≥ grade 2 or LVEF < LLN; consider restarting 1000 mg once daily after 2 wk if normal LVEF and patient experiences no symptoms.
Other toxicities: Discontinue with any toxicity if ≥ grade 2. May restart after if toxicity resolves to = grade 1. 1000 mg once daily for persistent toxicity.

SIDE EFFECTS/ADVERSE REACTIONS
Frequent
Fatigue, palmar-plantar erythrodysesthesia (hand-and-foot syndrome), rash, diarrhea, nausea, vomiting, abdominal pain, mucosal inflammation, stomatitis, dyspepsia, anemia, neutropenia, thrombocytopenia, AST increased, total bilirubin increased, ALT increased, limb pain, back pain, dyspnea
Occasional
Decreased LVEF, insomnia, dry skin

PRECAUTIONS AND CONTRAINDICATIONS
Hypersensitivity to lapatinib or any component of the formulation.

Lapatinib is a hazardous agent. Handle and dispose of with caution. Avoid use in pregnancy and lactation.

Use with caution in patients with a history of use of anthracyclines and chest wall irradiation for the treatment of left ventricular dysfunction.

Use with caution in patients with hepatic impairment. Hepatotoxicity (ALT or AST > 3 times upper limit of normal [ULN] and total bilirubin >1.5 times ULN) has been documented, may be severe and/or fatal.

Caution with CYP 3A4 inhibitors (e.g., erythromycin) and grapefruit; dose adjustments may be needed.

DRUG INTERACTIONS OF CONCERN TO DENTISTRY

• Use with caution when in combination with vasoconstrictors (epinephrine, levonordefrin) in local anesthetic because of the possible risk of QT prolongation (torsade de pointes).

• CYP3A4 inhibitors: Concomitant use with CYP3A4 inhibitors (e.g., erythromycin) may result in increased lapatinib concentrations. Dose reductions are likely.

SERIOUS REACTIONS

! Hepatotoxicity adverse effect (ALT or AST >3 times ULN and total bilirubin >1.5 times ULN) has been documented; may be severe and/or fatal.

! Interstitial lung disease has been reported.

! Decrease in LVEF may occur.

! QTc prolongation may occur.

! Administration during pregnancy or lactation may cause fatal harm.

DENTAL CONSIDERATIONS

General:
• Stomatitis may complicate dental treatment.
• Consider semisupine chair position for patient comfort if GI side effects occur.

Consultations:
• Medical consultation may be required to assess disease control and ability of patient to tolerate dental treatment.

Teach Patient/Family to:
• Use good oral hygiene to prevent soft tissue inflammation.
• Use oral hygiene aids with caution to prevent injury.
• Alert for the possibility of stomatitis and the need to see dentist immediately if signs of inflammation occur.

latanoprost

la-**ta**′-noe-prost
(Xalatan)
Do not confuse with Xanax.

CATEGORY AND SCHEDULE

Pregnancy Risk Category: C

Drug Class: Prostaglandin F_{2a} analogue

MECHANISM OF ACTION

An ophthalmic agent that is a prostanoid selective FP receptor agonist.
Therapeutic Effect: Reduces intraocular pressure (IOP) by reducing aqueous humor production.

USES

Treatment of open-angle glaucoma and ocular hypertension in patients intolerant to other IOP-lowering drugs

PHARMACOKINETICS

Absorbed through the cornea where the isopropyl ester prodrug is hydrolyzed to acid form to become biologically active. Highly lipophilic. The acid of latanoprost can be measured in the aqueous humor during the first 4 hr and in the plasma only during the first hr after local administration. In the cornea, latanoprost is hydrolyzed to the biologically active acid. Metabolized in liver if it reaches systemic circulation. Metabolized to 1,2-dinor metabolite and 1,2,3,4-tetranor metabolite. Primarily eliminated by the kidneys. *Half-life:* 17 min.

INDICATIONS AND DOSAGES
▶ **Glaucoma, Ocular Hypertension**
Ophthalmic
Adults, Elderly. 1 drop (1.5 mcg) in affected eye(s) once daily, in the evening.

SIDE EFFECTS/ADVERSE REACTIONS
Frequent
Blurred vision
Occasional
Eyelash changes, eyelid skin darkening, iris pigmentation
Rare
Macular edema

PRECAUTIONS AND CONTRAINDICATIONS
Hypersensitivity to latanoprost or benzalkonium chloride, or any other component of the formulation
Caution:
Gradual change in eye color, avoid contamination of sterile solution, renal or hepatic impairment, remove contact lens before using, administer at least 5 min apart if other ophthalmic drug is also used, nursing, pediatrics

DRUG INTERACTIONS OF CONCERN TO DENTISTRY
• None reported at this time; avoid use of anticholinergic drugs, atropine-like drugs, propantheline, and diazepam (benzodiazepines) in patient with glaucoma.

SERIOUS REACTIONS
! Pigmentation is expected to increase as long as latanoprost is administered but after discontinuation, pigmentation of the iris is likely to be permanent while pigmentation of the periorbital tissue and eyelash changes has been reported as reversible.
! Inflammation (iritis/uveitis) and macular edema, including cystoid macular edema, have been reported.

DENTAL CONSIDERATIONS

General:
• Check compliance of patient with prescribed drug regimen for glaucoma.
• Avoid dental light in patient's eyes; offer dark glasses for patient comfort.
Consultations:
• Medical consultation may be required to assess disease control.

leflunomide
le-**flu**′-na-mide
(Arava)

CATEGORY AND SCHEDULE
Pregnancy Risk Category: X

Drug Class: Antiarthritic, immunosuppressive

MECHANISM OF ACTION

An immunomodulatory agent that inhibits dihydroorotate dehydrogenase, the enzyme involved in autoimmune process that leads to rheumatoid arthritis.
Therapeutic Effect: Reduces signs and symptoms of rheumatoid arthritis and slows structural damage.

USES

Reduction of signs and symptoms and to retard structural damage in active rheumatoid arthritis as demonstrated by x-ray erosion and joint space narrowing

PHARMACOKINETICS

Well absorbed after PO administration. Protein binding: greater than 99%. Metabolized to active metabolite in the GI wall and liver. Excreted through both renal and biliary systems. Not removed by hemodialysis. *Half-life:* 16 days.

INDICATIONS AND DOSAGES
▸ **Rheumatoid Arthritis**
PO
Adults, Elderly. Initially, 100 mg/day for 3 days, then 10–20 mg/day.

SIDE EFFECTS/ADVERSE REACTIONS
Frequent
Diarrhea, respiratory tract infection, alopecia, rash, nausea

PRECAUTIONS AND CONTRAINDICATIONS
Pregnancy or plans to become pregnant, chronic renal or hepatic insufficiency, rifampin
Caution:
Chronic renal or hepatic insufficiency, rifampin, children younger than 18 yr

DRUG INTERACTIONS OF CONCERN TO DENTISTRY
• None reported

SERIOUS REACTIONS
! Transient thrombocytopenia and leukopenia occur rarely.

DENTAL CONSIDERATIONS
General:
• Monitor vital signs at every appointment because of cardiovascular side effects.
• Consider semisupine chair position for patient comfort if GI side effects occur.
• Examine for oral manifestation of opportunistic infection.
• If acute oral infection occurs, inform physician.
• Assess salivary flow as a factor in caries, periodontal disease, and candidiasis.
Consultations:
• Consult the patient's family if needed.
Teach Patient/Family to:
• Encourage effective oral hygiene to prevent soft tissue inflammation.
• Use powered tooth brush if patient has difficulty holding conventional devices.
• When chronic dry mouth occurs, advise patient to:
   • Avoid mouth rinses with high alcohol content because of drying effects.
• Use daily home fluoride products for anticaries effect.
• Use sugarless gum, frequent sips of water, or saliva substitutes.

L

letrozole
leh'-troe-zoll
(Femara)
Do not confuse Femara with
Femhrt.

CATEGORY AND SCHEDULE
Pregnancy Risk Category: D

Drug Class: Antineoplastic

MECHANISM OF ACTION
Decreases the level of circulating
estrogen by inhibiting aromatase, an
enzyme that catalyzes the final step
in estrogen production.
Therapeutic Effect: Inhibits the
growth of breast cancers that are
stimulated by estrogens.

USES
Treatment of locally advanced or
metastatic breast cancer in
postmenopausal women either
hormone receptor positive or
hormone receptor unknown;
advanced breast cancer in
postmenopausal women with disease
progression following antiestrogen
therapy

PHARMACOKINETICS
Rapidly and completely absorbed.
Metabolized in the liver. Primarily
eliminated by the kidneys. Unknown
if removed by hemodialysis.
Half-life: Approximately 2 days.

INDICATIONS AND DOSAGES
▶ Breast Cancer
PO
Adults, Elderly. 2.5 mg/day.
Continue until tumor progression is
evident.

SIDE EFFECTS/ADVERSE REACTIONS
Frequent
Musculoskeletal pain (back, arm,
leg), nausea, headache
Occasional
Constipation, arthralgia, fatigue,
vomiting, hot flashes, diarrhea,
abdominal pain, cough, rash,
anorexia, hypertension, peripheral
edema
Rare
Asthenia, somnolence, dyspepsia,
weight gain, pruritus

PRECAUTIONS AND CONTRAINDICATIONS
Hypersensitivity
Caution:
Lactation, children (no studies), for
postmenopausal women only,
thrombocytopenia and decreased
lymphocyte counts, liver impairment

DRUG INTERACTIONS OF CONCERN TO DENTISTRY
• None reported

SERIOUS REACTIONS
! None known

DENTAL CONSIDERATIONS

General:
• Patients taking opioids for acute or
chronic pain should be given
alternative analgesics for dental
pain.
• Patients on chronic drug therapy
may rarely have symptoms of blood
dyscrasias, which can include
infection, bleeding, and poor
healing.
• Palliative medication may be
required for management of oral
side effects.
• Examine for oral manifestation of
opportunistic infection.

• Consider semisupine chair position for patient comfort if GI side effects occur.
• Monitor vital signs at every appointment because of cardiovascular and respiratory side effects.

Consultations:
• In a patient with symptoms of blood dyscrasias, request a medical consultation for blood studies and postpone treatment until normal values are reestablished.

Teach Patient/Family to:
• Encourage effective oral hygiene to prevent soft tissue inflammation.
• Be aware of the possibility of secondary oral infection and the need to see dentist immediately if signs of infection occur.

leucovorin calcium (folinic acid, citrovorum factor)

loo-koe-**vor'**-in **kal'**-see-um
(Calcium Leucovorin[AUS], Wellcovorin)
Do not confuse Wellcovorin with Wellbutrin or Wellferon.

CATEGORY AND SCHEDULE
Pregnancy Risk Category: C

Drug Class: Folic acid antagonist antidote, antineoplastic adjunct

MECHANISM OF ACTION
An antidote to folic acid antagonists that may limit methotrexate action on normal cells by competing with methotrexate for the same transport processes into the cells.
Therapeutic Effect: Reverses toxic effects of folic acid antagonists. Reverses folic acid deficiency.

USES
Treatment of megaloblastic or macrocytic anemia caused by folic acid deficiency, overdose of folic acid antagonist, methotrexate toxicity, toxicity caused by pyrimethamine or trimethoprim; used with fluorouracil in colorectal cancer

PHARMACOKINETICS
Readily absorbed from the GI tract. Widely distributed. Primarily concentrated in the liver. Metabolized in the liver and intestinal mucosa to active metabolite. Primarily excreted in urine. *Half-life:* 15 min; metabolite, 30–35 min.

INDICATIONS AND DOSAGES

▸ **Conventional Rescue Dosage in Methotrexate Rescue**
PO, IV, IM
Adults, Elderly, Children. 10 mg/m² IM or IV one time, then PO q6h until serum methotrexate level is less than 0.05 micromolar (µM). If 24-hr serum creatinine level increases by 50% or greater over baseline or methotrexate level exceeds 50 micromolar at 24 hr or 5 micromolar at 48-hr, increase to 100 mg/m² IV q3h until methotrexate level is less than 0.05 micromolar.

▸ **Folic Acid Antagonist Overdose**
PO
Adults, Elderly, Children. 2–15 mg/day for 3 days or 5 mg every 3 days.

▸ **Megaloblastic Anemia**
IM
Adults, Elderly, Children. 3–6 mg/day.

▸ **Megaloblastic Anemia Secondary to Folate Deficiency**
IM
Adults, Elderly, Children. 1 mg/day.

L

▶ **Prevention of Hematologic Toxicity (for Toxoplasmosis), with Sulfadiazine**
PO, IV
Adults, Elderly, Children. 5–10 mg/day, repeat every 3 days.
▶ **Prevention of Hematologic Toxicity with Pyrimethamine, PCP**
PO, IV
Adults, Children. 25 mg once a wk.

SIDE EFFECTS/ADVERSE REACTIONS
Frequent
When combined with chemotherapeutic agents: Diarrhea, stomatitis, nausea, vomiting, lethargy or malaise or fatigue, alopecia, anorexia
Occasional
Urticaria, dermatitis

PRECAUTIONS AND CONTRAINDICATIONS
Pernicious anemia, other megaloblastic anemias secondary to vitamin B$_{12}$ deficiency

DRUG INTERACTIONS OF CONCERN TO DENTISTRY
• None reported

SERIOUS REACTIONS
! Excessive dosage may negate chemotherapeutic effects of folic acid antagonists.
! Anaphylaxis occurs rarely.
! Diarrhea may cause rapid clinical deterioration.

DENTAL CONSIDERATIONS
General:
• Signs of folate deficiency may appear in oral tissues.
• Determine why the patient is taking the drug.
• Patients with severe anemia or cancer or those receiving cancer

chemotherapy may have oral complaints. Palliative therapy may be required.
Consultations:
• Medical consultation may be required to assess disease control.
Teach Patient/Family to:
• Encourage effective oral hygiene to prevent soft tissue inflammation.
• Use caution to prevent trauma when using oral hygiene aids.
• Report oral lesions, soreness, or bleeding to dentist.
• See dentist immediately if secondary oral infection occurs.
• Update medical/drug records if physician makes any changes in evaluation or drug regimens; include OTC, herbal, and nonherbal drugs in the update.

leuprolide acetate
loo´-proe-lide ass´-eh-tayte
(Eligard, Lucrin[AUS], Lucrin Depot Inj[AUS], Lupron, Lupron Depot, Lupron Depot Ped, Viadur)
Do not confuse leuprolide or Lupron with Lopurin or Nuprin.

CATEGORY AND SCHEDULE
Pregnancy Risk Category: X

Drug Class: Antineoplastic hormone; gonadotropin-releasing hormone

MECHANISM OF ACTION
A gonadotropin-releasing hormone analog and antineoplastic agent that stimulates the release of luteinizing hormone (LH) and follicle-stimulating hormone (FSH) from the anterior pituitary gland.
Therapeutic Effect: Produces pharmacologic castration and decreases the growth of abnormal

prostate tissue in males; causes endometrial tissue to become inactive and atrophic in females; and decreases the rate of pubertal development in children with central precocious puberty.

USES
Treatment of metastatic prostate cancer, management of endometriosis, central precocious puberty

PHARMACOKINETICS
Rapidly and well absorbed after subcutaneous administration. Absorbed slowly after IM administration. Protein binding: 43%–49%. *Half-life:* 3–4 hr.

INDICATIONS AND DOSAGES
▸ **Advanced Prostatic Carcinoma**
IM (Lupron Depot)
Adults, Elderly. 7.5 mg every mo or 22.5 mg q3mo or 30 mg q4mo.
Subcutaneous (Eligard)
Adults, Elderly. 7.5 mg every mo or 22.5 mg q3mo or 30 mg q4mo.
Subcutaneous (Lupron)
Adults, Elderly. 1 mg/day.
Subcutaneous (Viadur)
Adults, Elderly. 65 mg implanted q12mo.
▸ **Endometriosis**
IM (Lupron Depot)
Adults, Elderly. 3.75 mg/mo for up to 6 mo or 11.25 mg q3mo for up to 2 doses.
▸ **Uterine Leiomyomata**
IM (with Iron [Lupron Depot])
Adults, Elderly. 3.75 mg/mo for up to 3 mo or 11.25 mg as a single injection.
▸ **Precocious Puberty**
IM (Lupron Depot)
Children. 0.3 mg/kg/dose every 28 days. Minimum: 7.5 mg. If down-regulation is not achieved,

titrate upward in 3.75-mg increments q4wk.
Subcutaneous (Lupron)
Children. 20–45 mcg/kg/day. Titrate upward by 10 mcg/kg/day if down-regulation is not achieved.

SIDE EFFECTS/ADVERSE REACTIONS
Frequent
Hot flashes (ranging from mild flushing to diaphoresis)
Females: Amenorrhea, spotting
Occasional
Arrhythmias; palpitations; blurred vision; dizziness; edema; headache; burning, itching, or swelling at injection site; nausea; insomnia; weight gain
Females: Deepening voice, hirsutism, decreased libido, increased breast tenderness, vaginitis, altered mood
Males: Constipation, decreased testicle size, gynecomastia, impotence, decreased appetite, angina
Rare
Males: Thrombophlebitis

PRECAUTIONS AND CONTRAINDICATIONS
Pernicious anemia, pregnancy

DRUG INTERACTIONS OF CONCERN TO DENTISTRY
• None reported

SERIOUS REACTIONS
! Signs and symptoms of metastatic prostatic carcinoma (such as bone pain, dysuria or hematuria, and weakness or paresthesia of the lower extremities) occasionally worsen 1 to 2 wk after the initial dose but then subside with continued therapy.
! Pulmonary embolism and MI occur rarely.

DENTAL CONSIDERATIONS

General:

• If additional analgesia is required for dental pain, consider alternative analgesics (NSAIDs) in patients taking narcotics for acute or chronic pain.

• Monitor and record vital signs.

• Assess salivary flow as a factor in caries, periodontal disease, and candidiasis.

• This drug may be used in the hospital or on an outpatient basis. Confirm the patient's disease and treatment status.

• Consider semisupine chair position for patient comfort if GI side effects occur.

• Question patient about tolerance of NSAIDS or aspirin related to GI disease.

• Patient on chronic drug therapy may rarely present with symptoms of blood dyscrasias, which can include infection, bleeding, and poor healing. If dyscrasia is present, caution patient to prevent oral tissue trauma when using oral hygiene aids.

• Examine for oral manifestation of opportunistic infection.

Consultations:

• Medical consultation may be required to assess immunologic status during cancer chemotherapy and determine safety risk, if any, posed by the required dental treatment.

• Consider consulting with physician before prescribing drugs that may cause constipation (opioids).

• Medical consultation may be required to assess disease control and patient's ability to tolerate stress.

• In a patient with symptoms of blood dyscrasias, request a medical consultation for blood studies and postpone treatment until normal values are reestablished.

Teach Patient/Family to:

• When chronic dry mouth occurs advise patient to:
  • Avoid mouth rinses with high alcohol content because of drying effects.
  • Use daily home fluoride products for anticaries effect.
  • Use sugarless gum, frequent sips of water, or saliva substitutes.
  • Prevent trauma when using oral hygiene aids.
  • Report oral lesions, soreness, or bleeding to dentist.
  • Update health and medication history if physician makes any changes in evaluation or drug regimens; include OTC, herbal, and nonherbal drugs in the update.

levalbuterol

lee-val-**byoot'**-err-all
(Xopenex)
Do not confuse Xopenex with
Xanax.

CATEGORY AND SCHEDULE
Pregnancy Risk Category: C

Drug Class: Bronchodilator

MECHANISM OF ACTION
A sympathomimetic that stimulates β_2-adrenergic receptors in the lungs resulting in relaxation of bronchial smooth muscle.
Therapeutic Effect: Relieves bronchospasm and reduces airway resistance.

USES

Treatment or prevention of bronchospasm in adults and children older than 6 yr with reversible obstructive airway disease

PHARMACOKINETICS

Route	Onset	Peak	Duration
Inhalation	10–17 min	1.5 hr	5–6 hr

Metabolized in the liver to inactive metabolite. *Half-life:* 3.3–4 hr.

INDICATIONS AND DOSAGES

▶ **Treatment and Prevention of Bronchospasm**
Nebulization
Adults, Elderly, Children 12 yr and older. Initially, 0.63 mg 3 times a day 6–8 hr apart. May increase to 1.25 mg 3 times a day with dose monitoring.
Children 3–11 yr. Initially 0.31 mg 3 times a day. Maximum: 0.63 mg 3 times a day.

SIDE EFFECTS/ADVERSE REACTIONS

Frequent
Tremors, nervousness, headache, throat dryness and irritation
Occasional
Cough, bronchial irritation
Rare
Somnolence, diarrhea, dry mouth, flushing, diaphoresis, anorexia

PRECAUTIONS AND CONTRAINDICATIONS

History of hypersensitivity to sympathomimetics
Caution:
Paradoxic bronchospasm, cardiovascular disorders, seizures, diabetes, hyperthyroidism, coronary insufficiency, cardiac arrhythmias, hypertension, not to exceed recommended dose, β-adrenergic blockers, MAOIs, tricyclic antidepressants, lactation, children younger than 12 yr

DRUG INTERACTIONS OF CONCERN TO DENTISTRY

• Significant reduction of effects: β-adrenergic blockers
• Potentiation of cardiovascular effects: MAOIs, tricyclic antidepressants, methylxanthines
• No specific dental drug interactions reported

SERIOUS REACTIONS

❗ Excessive sympathomimetic stimulation may produce palpitations, extrasystoles, tachycardia, chest pain, a slight increase in B/P followed by a substantial decrease, chills, diaphoresis, and blanching of skin.
❗ Too-frequent or excessive use may lead to decreased bronchodilating effectiveness and severe, paradoxical bronchoconstriction.

DENTAL CONSIDERATIONS

General:
• Monitor vital signs at every appointment because of cardiovascular side effects.
• Assess salivary flow as a factor in caries, periodontal disease, and candidiasis.
• Consider semisupine chair position for patients with respiratory disease.
• Short midday appointments and a stress-reduction protocol may be required for anxious patients.
• Be aware that aspirin or sulfite preservatives in vasoconstrictor-containing products can exacerbate asthma.
• Acute asthmatic episodes may be precipitated in the dental office. Rapid-acting sympathomimetic

inhalants should be available for emergency use. A stress-reduction protocol may be required.
Consultations:
• Medical consultation may be required to assess disease control and patient's ability to tolerate stress.
Teach Patient/Family to:
• Rinse mouth with water after each dose of inhalation dosage forms to prevent dryness.
• When chronic dry mouth occurs, advise patient to:
  • Avoid mouth rinses with high alcohol content because of drying effects.
  • Use daily home fluoride products for anticaries effect.
  • Use sugarless gum, frequent sips of water, or saliva substitutes.

levetiracetam
leva-tir-**ass**'-eh-tam
(Keppra)
Do not confuse Keppra with Kaletra.

CATEGORY AND SCHEDULE
Pregnancy Risk Category: C

Drug Class: Antiepileptic

MECHANISM OF ACTION
An anticonvulsant that inhibits burst firing without affecting normal neuronal excitability.
Therapeutic Effect: Prevents seizure activity.

USES
Adjunctive therapy in adults with partial-onset seizures

PHARMACOKINETICS
PO: Bioavailability 100%, onset 1 hr, peak plasma levels 20 min–2 hr. *Half-life:* 6–8 hr, less than 10% plasma protein bound, limited hepatic metabolism, renal excretion (66%).

INDICATIONS AND DOSAGES
▶ **Partial-Onset Seizures**
PO
Adults, Elderly. Initially, 500 mg q12h. May increase by 1000 mg/day q2wk. Maximum: 3000 mg/day.
Children 4–16 yr. 10–20 mg/kg/day in 2 divided doses. May increase at weekly intervals by 10–20 mg/kg. Maximum: 60 mg/kg.
▶ **Dosage in Renal Impairment**
Dosage is modified on the basis of creatinine clearance.

Creatinine Clearance (ml/min)	Dosage
Higher than 80 ml/min	500–1500 mg q12h
50–80 ml/min	500–1000 mg q12h
30–50 ml/min	250–750 mg q12h
Less than 30 ml/min	250–500 mg q12h
End-stage renal disease using dialysis	500–1000 mg q12h, after dialysis, a 250- to 500-mg supplemental dose is recommended

SIDE EFFECTS/ADVERSE REACTIONS
Frequent
Somnolence, asthenia, headache, infection
Occasional
Dizziness, pharyngitis, pain, depression, nervousness, vertigo, rhinitis, anorexia

Rare

Amnesia, anxiety, emotional lability, cough, sinusitis, anorexia, diplopia

PRECAUTIONS AND CONTRAINDICATIONS

Hypersensitivity reaction
Caution:
Lactation, children, blood dyscrasias

DRUG INTERACTIONS OF CONCERN TO DENTISTRY

• None reported

SERIOUS REACTIONS

! None known

DENTAL CONSIDERATIONS

General:

• Short appointments and a stress-reduction protocol may be required for anxious patients.

• Ask patient about type of epilepsy, seizure frequency, and quality of seizure control.

Consultation:

• Medical consultation may be required to assess disease control and patient's ability to tolerate stress.

• In patients with symptoms of blood dyscrasias, request a medical consultation for blood studies and postpone treatment until normal values are reestablished.

Teach Patient/Family to:

• Update health and drug history if physician makes changes in evaluation or drug regimens; include OTC, herbal, and nonherbal drugs in the update.

levobetaxolol hydrochloride

le-vo-bay-**tax**′-oh-lol
high-droh-**klor**′-ide
(Betaxon)
Do not confuse with levobunolol.

CATEGORY AND SCHEDULE

Pregnancy Risk Category: C

Drug Class: Antiglaucoma agent (ophthalmic)

MECHANISM OF ACTION

An antiglaucoma agent that blocks β_1-adrenergic receptors. Reduces aqueous humor production.
Therapeutic Effect: Reduces intraocular pressure (IOP).

USES

Treatment of certain types of glaucoma

PHARMACOKINETICS

Route	Onset	Peak	Duration
Eye drops	30 min	2 hr	12 hr

INDICATIONS AND DOSAGES

▶ Glaucoma, Ocular Hypertension
Ophthalmic
Adults, Elderly. Instill 1 drop 2 times a day.

SIDE EFFECTS/ADVERSE REACTIONS

Frequent
Ocular discomfort
Occasional
Blurred vision
Rare
Anxiety, dizziness, vertigo, headache

PRECAUTIONS AND CONTRAINDICATIONS

Sinus bradycardia, second- or third-degree atrioventricular (AV) block, cardiogenic shock, overt heart failure, hypersensitivity to betaxolol, levobetaxolol or any component of levobetaxolol formulations

DRUG INTERACTIONS OF CONCERN TO DENTISTRY

• None reported

SERIOUS REACTIONS

❗ Diabetes, hypothyroidism, bradycardia, tachycardia, hypertension, hypotension, heart block, alopecia, dermatitis, psoriasis, arthritis, tendonitis, dyspnea and other respiratory symptoms (e.g., bronchitis, pneumonia, rhinitis, sinusitis, pharyngitis) occur rarely.
❗ Ophthalmic overdosage may produce bradycardia, hypotension, bronchospasm, and acute cardiac failure.

DENTAL CONSIDERATIONS

General:
• Determine why patient is taking the drug.
• Avoid drugs with anticholinergic activity, such as antihistamines, opioids, benzodiazepines, propantheline, atropine, and scopolamine.
• Avoid dental light in patient's eyes; offer dark glasses for patient comfort.
• Question glaucoma patient about compliance with prescribed drug regimen.
Consultations:
• Medical consultation may be required to assess disease control.
Teach Patient/Family to:
• Update health and medication history if physician makes any

changes in evaluation or drug regimens; include OTC, herbal, and nonherbal drugs in the update.

levobunolol hydrochloride

lee-vo-**byoo**′-no-lol high-droh-**klor**′-ide (AK-Beta, Betagan, Novo-Levobunolol[CAN], Optho-Bunolol[CAN], PMS-Levobunolol[CAN])
Do not confuse with levobetaxolol.

CATEGORY AND SCHEDULE

Pregnancy Risk Category: C

Drug Class: Antiglaucoma agent (ophthalmic)

MECHANISM OF ACTION

A nonselective β-blocker that blocks β_1- and β_2-adrenergic receptors.
Therapeutic Effect: Reduces intraocular pressure (IOP). Decreases production of aqueous humor.

USES

Treatment of certain types of glaucoma

PHARMACOKINETICS

Well absorbed after administration. Metabolized in liver. Primarily excreted in urine. *Half-life:* 6.1 hr.

INDICATIONS AND DOSAGES

▸ **Glaucoma, Ocular Hypertension**
Ophthalmic
Adults, Elderly. Instill 1–2 drops in affected eye(s) once daily.

SIDE EFFECTS/ ADVERSE REACTIONS
Frequent
Burning/stinging, eye irritation, visual disturbances
Occasional
Increased light sensitivity, watering of eye
Rare
Dry eye, conjunctivitis, eye pain, diarrhea, dyspepsia

PRECAUTIONS AND CONTRAINDICATIONS
Cardiogenic shock, overt cardiac failure, second- or third-degree heart block, sinus bradycardia, hypersensitivity to levobunolol or any component of the formulation

DRUG INTERACTIONS OF CONCERN TO DENTISTRY
• Patient with glaucoma: avoid use of anticholinergic drugs, atropine-like drugs, propantheline, and diazepam (benzodiazepines)

SERIOUS REACTIONS
! Abrupt withdrawal may result in sweating, headache, and fatigue.
! Ophthalmic overdosage may produce bradycardia, hypotension, bronchospasm, and acute cardiac failure.

DENTAL CONSIDERATIONS
General:
• Check compliance of patient with prescribed drug regimen for glaucoma.
• Avoid dental light in patient's eyes; offer dark glasses for patient comfort.
Consultations:
• Consultation with physician may be necessary if sedation or anesthesia is required.

levocabastine
lev-oh-**kab**'-ah-steen
(Livostin)

CATEGORY AND SCHEDULE
Pregnancy Risk Category: C

Drug Class: Antihistamine, H_1-receptor antagonist

MECHANISM OF ACTION
An antiallergic agent that selectively antagonizes H_1 receptor.
Therapeutic Effect: Blocks histamine-associated symptoms of seasonal allergic conjunctivitis.

USES
Temporary relief of seasonal allergic conjunctivitis

PHARMACOKINETICS
Duration of action is about 2 hr. Minimal systemic absorption.

INDICATIONS AND DOSAGES
▶ Allergic Conjunctivitis
Ophthalmic
Adults, Elderly, Children 12 yr or older. 1 drop 4 times a day, for up to 2 wk.

SIDE EFFECTS/ADVERSE REACTIONS
Frequent
Transient stinging, burning, discomfort, headache
Occasional
Dry mouth, fatigue, eye dryness, lacrimation and discharge, eyelid edema
Rare
Rash, erythema, nausea, dyspnea

PRECAUTIONS AND CONTRAINDICATIONS

Wearing of soft contact lenses (product contains benzalkonium chloride), hypersensitivity to levocabastine or any component of the formulation
Caution:
Lactation, children younger than 12 yr

DRUG INTERACTIONS OF CONCERN TO DENTISTRY

• None reported

SERIOUS REACTIONS

! None reported

DENTAL CONSIDERATIONS

General:
• Question patient about history of allergy to avoid using other potential allergens.
• Avoid dental light in patient's eyes; offer dark glasses for patient comfort.
• Evaluate respiration characteristics and rate.
• Use for less than 2 wk should not present a problem with dry mouth.
Teach Patient/Family to:
• When chronic dry mouth occurs, advise patient to:
  • Avoid mouth rinses with high alcohol content because of drying effects.
  • Use daily home fluoride products for anticaries effect.
  • Use sugarless gum, frequent sips of water, or saliva substitutes.

levocetirizine
(lee-vo-seh-**teer**′-ah-zeen)
(Xyzal [U.S.], Xuzal, Xusal, Xozal, Vozet [intl.])

CATEGORY AND SCHEDULE
Pregnancy Risk Category: B

Drug Class: Nonsedating antihistamine, blocks H_1 receptors

MECHANISM OF ACTION
Active enantiomer of cetirizine, blocks peripheral H_1 histamine receptors, reduces signs and symptoms related to mild allergies.
Therapeutic Effect: Blockade of peripheral actions of histamines results in reduction of bronchial constriction and respiratory and exocrine secretions related to allergy.

USES
Seasonal allergic rhinitis, chronic idiopathic urticaria

PHARMACOKINETICS
Rapidly and extensively absorbed after oral administration, protein binding: 91%. Metabolized in the liver by CYP3A4 (14%) and taurine conjugation; metabolites primarily excreted in urine (85%) and feces (13%). *Half-life:* 8–9 hr.

INDICATIONS AND DOSAGES
▸ **Seasonal Rhinitis**
Adults and Children 12 yr. PO 5 mg (tablet) or 2 tsp (10 ml oral solution) once daily in the evening
Children 6 to 11 yr. PO 2.5 mg (one-half tablet) or 1 tsp (5 ml oral solution) once daily in the evening

SIDE EFFECTS/ADVERSE REACTIONS
Frequent
Somnolence, nasopharyngitis, fatigue, dry mouth, pharyngitis
Occasional
Pyrexia, cough, nosebleed
Rare
Palpitations, fatigue

PRECAUTIONS AND CONTRAINDICATIONS
Activities requiring mental alertness
Nursing
Geriatric patients
Renal impairment
Contraindicated by hypersensitivity to levocetirizine, end-stage renal disease, pediatric patients with impaired renal function

DRUG INTERACTIONS OF CONCERN TO DENTISTRY
• Theoretical potentiation of CNS depressants (e.g., sedatives) in susceptible individuals

SERIOUS REACTIONS
! Hypersensitivity
! Hallucinations, suicidal ideation, orofacial dyskinesia, hypotension
! Cholestasis, glomerulonephritis, still birth

DENTAL CONSIDERATIONS
General:
• Assess salivary flow as a factor in caries, periodontal disease, and candidiasis.
• After supine positioning, allow patient to sit upright for 2 minutes to avoid occurrence of dizziness.
• Consider levocetirizine as an etiologic factor in oral inflammation (pharyngitis).

Consultations:
• Consult with physician to determine disease control and ability to tolerate dental procedures.
Teach Patient/Family to:
• If dry mouth occurs:
  • Avoid mouth rinses with high alcohol content because of drying effect.
  • Use home fluoride products for anticaries effect.
  • Use sugarless/xylitol gum, frequent sips of water, or saliva substitutes.

levodopa
lev-oh-**dope'**-ah
(Dopar, Larodopa)

CATEGORY AND SCHEDULE
Pregnancy Risk Category: C

Drug Class: Antiparkinson agent

MECHANISM OF ACTION
A dopamine prodrug that is converted to dopamine in basal ganglia. Increases dopamine concentrations in the brain, inhibiting hyperactive cholinergic activity.
Therapeutic Effect: Decreases signs and symptoms of Parkinson's disease.

USES
Treatment of Parkinsonism of various causes

PHARMACOKINETICS
About 30% absorbed. May be reduced with high-protein meal. Protein binding: minimal. Crosses blood-brain barrier. Converted to dopamine. Eliminated primarily in urine and to a lesser amount in feces

and expired air. Not removed by hemodialysis. *Half-life:* 0.75–1.5 hr.

INDICATIONS AND DOSAGES
▶ **Parkinsonism**
PO
Adults, Elderly. Initially, 0.5–1 g 2–4 times a day. May increase in increments not exceeding 0.75 g every 3–7 days, up to a maximum of 8 g/day.

SIDE EFFECTS/ADVERSE REACTIONS
Frequent
Uncontrolled body movements of the face, tongue, arms, and upper body; nausea and vomiting; anorexia
Occasional
Depression, anxiety, confusion, nervousness, difficulty urinating, irregular heartbeats, hiccoughs, dizziness, light-headedness, decreased appetite, blurred vision, constipation, dry mouth, flushed skin, headache, insomnia, diarrhea, unusual tiredness, darkening of urine, discolored sweat
Rare
Hypertension, ulcer, hemolytic anemia, marked by tiredness or weakness

PRECAUTIONS AND CONTRAINDICATIONS
Nonselective MAOI therapy, hypersensitivity to levodopa or any component of its formulation
Caution:
Renal disease, cardiac disease, hepatic disease, respiratory disease, MI with dysrhythmia, convulsions, peptic ulcer, asthma, endocrine disease, affective disorders, psychosis, lactation, children younger than 12 yr

DRUG INTERACTIONS OF CONCERN TO DENTISTRY
• Decreased absorption: anticholinergics
• Decreased therapeutic effect: benzodiazepines, pyridoxine (vitamin B_6), tricyclic antidepressants

SERIOUS REACTIONS
❗ High incidence of involuntary dystonic and dyskinetic movements may be noted in patients on long-term therapy.
❗ Mental changes, such as paranoid ideation, psychotic episodes, and depression, may be noted.
❗ Numerous mild-to-severe CNS psychiatric disturbances may include reduced attention span, anxiety, nightmares, daytime somnolence, euphoria, fatigue, paranoia, and hallucinations.

DENTAL CONSIDERATIONS

General:
• Patients on chronic drug therapy may rarely have symptoms of blood dyscrasias, which can include infection, bleeding, and poor healing.
• Assess salivary flow as a factor in caries, periodontal disease, and candidiasis.
• After supine positioning, have patient sit upright for at least 2 min before standing to avoid orthostatic hypotension.
• Avoid dental light in patient's eyes; offer dark glasses for patient comfort.
Consultations:
• In a patient with symptoms of blood dyscrasias, request a medical consultation for blood studies and postpone dental treatment until normal values are reestablished.

- Take precautions if dental surgery is anticipated and anesthesia is required.
- Medical consultation may be required to assess disease control.

Teach Patient/Family to:
- Use powered tooth brush if patient has difficulty holding conventional devices.
- When chronic dry mouth occurs, advise patient to:
  - Avoid mouth rinses with high alcohol content because of drying effects.
  - Use sugarless gum, frequent sips of water, or saliva substitutes.
  - Use daily home fluoride products for anticaries effect.

levofloxacin
lev-oh-**flox**′-ah-sin
(Iquix, Levaquin, Quixin)

CATEGORY AND SCHEDULE
Pregnancy Risk Category: C

Drug Class: Fluoroquinolone antiinfective

MECHANISM OF ACTION
A fluoroquinolone that inhibits the enzyme DNA gyrase in susceptible microorganisms, interfering with bacterial cell replication and repair. *Therapeutic Effect:* Bactericidal.

USES
Treatment of acute infections caused by susceptible bacterial strains causing acute maxillary sinusitis, acute bacterial exacerbation of chronic bronchitis, community-acquired pneumonia, nosocomial pneumonia, complicated and uncomplicated skin and skin-structure infections, uncomplicated UTI, and acute pyelonephritis; nosocomial pneumonia; chronic bacterial prostatitis

PHARMACOKINETICS
Well absorbed after both PO and IV administration. Protein binding: 8%–24%. Penetrates rapidly and extensively into leukocytes, epithelial cells, and macrophages. Lung concentrations are 2–5 times higher than those of plasma. Eliminated unchanged in the urine. Partially removed by hemodialysis. *Half-life:* 8 hr.

INDICATIONS AND DOSAGES
▶ **Bronchitis**
PO, IV
Adults, Elderly. 500 mg q24h for 7 days.
▶ **Community-Acquired Pneumonia**
PO
Adults, Elderly. 750 mg/day for 5 days.
▶ **Pneumonia**
PO, IV
Adults, Elderly. 500 mg q24h for 7–14 days.
▶ **Acute Maxillary Sinusitis**
PO, IV
Adults, Elderly. 500 mg q24h for 10–14 days.
▶ **Skin and Skin-Structure Infections**
PO, IV
Adults, Elderly. 500 mg q24h for 7–10 days.
▶ **UTIs, Acute Pyelonephritis**
PO, IV
Adults, Elderly. 250 mg q24h for 10 days.
▶ **Bacterial Conjunctivitis**
Ophthalmic
Adults, Elderly, Children 1 yr and older. 1–2 drops q2h for 2 days (up to 8 times a day), then 1–2 drops q4h for 5 days.

▸ **Corneal Ulcer**
Ophthalmic
Adults, Elderly, Children older than 5 yr. Days 1–3: Instill 1–2 drops q30min to 2 hr while awake and 4–6 hr after retiring. Days 4 through completion: 1–2 drops q1–4h while awake.

▸ **Dosage in Renal Impairment**
For bronchitis, pneumonia, sinusitis, and skin and skin-structure infections, dosage and frequency are modified on the basis of creatinine clearance.

Creatinine Clearance	Dosage
50–80 ml/min	No change
20–49 ml/min	500 mg initially, then 250 mg q24h
10–19 ml/min	500 mg initially, then 250 mg q48h
Dialysis	500 mg initially, then 250 mg q48h

For UTIs and pyelonephritis, dosage and frequency are modified on the basis of creatinine clearance.

Creatinine Clearance	Dosage
20 ml/min	No change
10–19 ml/min	250 mg initially, then 250 mg q48h

SIDE EFFECTS/ADVERSE REACTIONS

Occasional
Diarrhea, nausea, abdominal pain, dizziness, drowsiness, headache, light-headedness
Ophthalmic: Local burning or discomfort, margin crusting, crystals or scales, foreign body sensation, ocular itching, altered taste
Rare
Flatulence; altered taste; pain; inflammation or swelling in calves, hands, or shoulder; chest pain; difficulty breathing; palpitations; edema; tendon pain; rupture of Achilles tendon
Ophthalmic: Corneal staining, keratitis, allergic reaction, eyelid swelling, tearing, reduced visual acuity

PRECAUTIONS AND CONTRAINDICATIONS

Hypersensitivity to levofloxacin, other fluoroquinolones, or nalidixic acid
Caution:
Children younger than 18 yr; seizure disorders, renal insufficiency, excessive exposure to sunlight, alterations in blood glucose (diabetes), lactation, drink fluids liberally; tendon rupture of shoulder, hand, and Achilles tendon, monitor blood glucose

DRUG INTERACTIONS OF CONCERN TO DENTISTRY

• Interference with absorption: solutions with multivalent cations (e.g., magnesium)
• Increased seizure risk: NSAIDs
• May increase effects of warfarin (monitor bleeding)

SERIOUS REACTIONS

! Antibiotic-associated colitis and other superinfections may occur from altered bacterial balance.
! Hypersensitivity reactions, including photosensitivity (as evidenced by rash, pruritus, blisters, edema, and burning skin), have occurred in patients receiving fluoroquinolones.

DENTAL CONSIDERATIONS

General:
• Determine why patient is taking the drug.

• If dental drugs prescribed, advise patient of potential for photosensitivity.

Consultations:
• Consult with patient's physician if an acute dental infection occurs and another antiinfective is required.

Teach Patient/Family to:
• Minimize exposure to sunlight and wear sunscreen if sun exposure is planned.
• Discontinue treatment and inform dentist immediately if patient experiences pain or inflammation of a tendon, and to rest and refrain from exercise.

levothyroxine

lev-oh-thye-**rox**′-een
(Droxine[AUS], Eltroxin[CAN], Eutroxsig[AUS], Levothroid, Levoxyl, Novothyrox[CAN], Oroxine[AUS], Synthroid, Unithroid)
Do not confuse levothyroxine with liothyronine.

CATEGORY AND SCHEDULE
Pregnancy Risk Category: A

Drug Class: Thyroid hormone

MECHANISM OF ACTION
A synthetic isomer of thyroxine involved in normal metabolism, growth, and development, especially of the CNS in infants. Possesses catabolic and anabolic effects.
Therapeutic Effect: Increases basal metabolic rate, enhances gluconeogenesis, and stimulates protein synthesis.

USES
Treatment of hypothyroidism, myxedema coma, thyroid hormone

replacement, cretinism, chronic thyroiditis, euthyroid goiters, management of thyroid cancer

PHARMACOKINETICS
Variable, incomplete absorption from the GI tract. Protein binding: greater than 99%. Widely distributed. Deiodinated in peripheral tissues, minimal metabolism in the liver. Eliminated by biliary excretion. *Half-life:* 6–7 days.

INDICATIONS AND DOSAGES
▶ **Hypothyroidism**
PO
Adults, Elderly. Initially, 12.5–50 mcg. May increase by 25–50 mcg/day q2-4wk. Maintenance: 100–200 mcg/day.
Children 13 yr and older. 150 mcg/day.
Children 6–12 yr. 100–125 mcg/day.
Children 1–5 yr. 75–100 mcg/day.
Children 7–11 mo. 50–75 mcg/day.
Children 3–6 mo. 25–50 mcg/day.
Children 3 mo and younger. 10–15 mcg/day.
▶ **Thyroid Suppression Therapy**
PO
Adults, Elderly. 2–6 mcg/kg/day for 7–10 days.
▶ **Thyroid-Stimulating Hormone Suppression in Thyroid Cancer, Nodules, Euthyroid Goiters**
PO
Adults, Elderly. 2–6 mcg/kg/day for 7–10 days.
IV
Adults, Elderly, Children. Initial dosage approximately half the previously established oral dosage.

SIDE EFFECTS/ADVERSE REACTIONS
Occasional
Reversible hair loss at the start of therapy (in children)

Rare

Dry skin, GI intolerance, rash, hives, pseudotumor cerebri or severe headache in children

PRECAUTIONS AND CONTRAINDICATIONS

Hypersensitivity to tablet components, such as tartrazine; allergy to aspirin; lactose intolerance; MI and thyrotoxicosis uncomplicated by hypothyroidism; treatment of obesity

Caution

Elderly, angina pectoris, hypertension, ischemia, cardiac disease, lactation

DRUG INTERACTIONS OF CONCERN TO DENTISTRY

• Increased effects of sympathomimetics when thyroid doses are not carefully monitored or in patients with coronary artery disease

SERIOUS REACTIONS

! Excessive dosage produces signs and symptoms of hyperthyroidism, including weight loss, palpitations, increased appetite, tremors, nervousness, tachycardia, hypertension, headache, insomnia, and menstrual irregularities.

! Cardiac arrhythmias occur rarely.

DENTAL CONSIDERATIONS

General:

• Uncontrolled hypothyroid patients may be more responsive to CNS depressants.

• Increased nervousness, excitability, sweating, or tachycardia may indicate a patient with uncontrolled hyperthyroidism or a dose of medication that is too high.

• Uncontrolled patients should be referred for medical treatment.

• Observe appropriate limitations of vasoconstrictor doses.

• Monitor vital signs at every appointment because of CV side effects.

Consultations:

• Medical consultation may be required to assess disease control.

lidocaine hydrochloride

lye′-doe-kane high-droh-**klor′**-ide
(Lidoderm, Lignocaine Gel[AUS], Xylocaine, Xylocaine Aerosol[AUS], Xylocaine Ointment[AUS], Oraqix[US], Xylocaine Viscous Topical Solution[AUS], Xylocard[CAN], Zilactin-L[CAN], Zingo)

CATEGORY AND SCHEDULE

Pregnancy Risk Category: B

Drug Class: Antidysrhythmic (class IB)

MECHANISM OF ACTION

An amide anesthetic that blocks conduction of nerve impulses. **Therapeutic Effect:** Causes temporary loss of feeling and sensation. Also an antiarrhythmic that decreases depolarization, automaticity, excitability of the ventricle during diastole by direct action. Inhibits ventricular arrhythmias.

USES

Ventricular tachycardia, ventricular dysrhythmias during cardiac surgery, MI, digitalis toxicity, cardiac catheterization; for acute management only, local pain control

PHARMACOKINETICS

Route	Onset	Peak	Duration
IV	30–90 sec	N/A	10–20 min
Local Anesthetic	2.5 min	N/A	30–60 min

Completely absorbed after IM administration. Protein binding: 60%–80%. Widely distributed. Metabolized in the liver. Primarily excreted in urine. Minimally removed by hemodialysis. *Half-life:* 1–2 hr.

INDICATIONS AND DOSAGES

▸ **Rapid Control of Acute Ventricular Arrhythmias after an MI, Cardiac Catheterization, Cardiac Surgery, or Digitalis-Induced Ventricular Arrhythmias**

IM
Adults, Elderly. 300 mg (or 4.3 mg/kg). May repeat in 60–90 min.

IV
Adults, Elderly. Initially, 50–100 mg (1 mg/kg) IV bolus at rate of 25–50 mg/min. May repeat in 5 min. Give no more than 200–300 mg in 1 hr. Maintenance: 20–50 mcg/kg/min (1–4 mg/min) as IV Infusion
Children, Infants. Initially, 0.5–1 mg/kg IV bolus; may repeat but total dose not to exceed 3–5 mg/kg. Maintenance: 10–50 mcg/kg/min as IV infusion.

▸ **Dental or Surgical Procedures, Childbirth**

Infiltration or Nerve Block
Adults. Local anesthetic dosage varies with procedure, degree of anesthesia, vascularity, duration. Maximum dose: 4.5 mg/kg. Do not repeat within 2 hr.

▸ **Local Skin Disorders (Minor Burns, Insect Bites, Prickly Heat, Skin Manifestations of Chickenpox, Abrasions), and Mucous Membrane Disorders (Local Anesthesia of Oral, Nasal, and Laryngeal Mucous Membranes; Local Anesthesia of Respiratory, Urinary Tract; Relief of Discomfort of Pruritus Ani, Hemorrhoids, Pruritus Vulvae)**

Topical
Adults, Elderly. Apply to affected areas as needed.

▸ **Treatment of Shingles-Related Skin Pain**

Topical (Dermal Patch)
Adults, Elderly. Apply to intact skin over most painful area (up to 3 applications once for up to 12 hr in a 24-hr period).

SIDE EFFECTS/ADVERSE REACTIONS

CNS effects are generally dose related and of short duration
Occasional
IM: Pain at injection site
Topical: Burning, stinging, tenderness at application site
Rare
Generally with high dose: Drowsiness; dizziness; disorientation; light-headedness; tremors; apprehension; euphoria; sensation of heat, cold, or numbness; blurred or double vision; ringing or roaring in ears (tinnitus); nausea; seizures, post-seizure depression with cardiorespiratory arrest

PRECAUTIONS AND CONTRAINDICATIONS

Adams-Stokes syndrome, hypersensitivity to amide-type local anesthetics, septicemia (spinal anesthesia), supraventricular arrhythmias, Wolff-Parkinson-White syndrome

Caution:
Lactation, children, renal disease,
liver disease, CHF, respiratory
depression, malignant hyperthermia
(questionable), elderly; need to
monitor ECG

DRUG INTERACTIONS OF CONCERN TO DENTISTRY
Patch Form
• None reported
Injectable Form
• Potentiation of other CNS
depressants

SERIOUS REACTIONS
! Although serious adverse reactions
to lidocaine are uncommon, high
dosage by any route may produce
cardiovascular depression,
bradycardia, hypotension,
arrhythmias, heart block,
cardiovascular collapse, and cardiac
arrest.
! CNS toxicity may occur, especially
with regional anesthesia use,
progressing rapidly from mild side
effects to tremors, somnolence,
seizures, vomiting, and respiratory
depression.
! Methemoglobinemia (evidenced by
cyanosis) has occurred following
topical application of lidocaine for
teething discomfort and laryngeal
anesthetic spray.

DENTAL CONSIDERATIONS

▸ **Patch Form**
General:
• Use no more than one patch per
area, remove after 15 min to avoid
toxicity.
Teach Patient/Family to:
• Prevent injury while numbness is
present and to refrain from gum
chewing and eating after dental
treatment.
• Report unresolved oral lesions to
dentist.

lidocaine transoral delivery system
lye′-doe-kane
(DentiPatch)

CATEGORY AND SCHEDULE
Pregnancy Risk Category: B

Drug Class: Amide local
anesthetic

MECHANISM OF ACTION
Inhibits nerve impulses from
sensory nerves, which produces
anesthesia.

USES
Mild topical anesthesia of mucous
membranes of the mouth before
superficial dental procedures

PHARMACOKINETICS
Topical: Onset 2.5 min, duration of
approximately 30 min after removal;
blood levels less than 0.1 ng/ml
limited absorption; hepatic
metabolism, urinary excretion.

INDICATIONS AND DOSAGES
Topical
Adult. Apply one patch to area of
application after drying with gauze;
leave in place until local anesthesia
is produced but no longer than
15 min.

SIDE EFFECTS/ADVERSE REACTIONS
Oral: Taste alteration, stomatitis,
erythema, mucosa irritation
CNS: Headache, excitatory or
depressor actions, dizziness,
nervousness, confusion, tinnitus,
twitching, tremors (associated with
excessive systemic absorption)

CV: Bradycardia, hypotension, cardiovascular collapse (with excessive systemic absorption)
GI: Nausea
Misc: Allergic reactions to this agent or to other ingredients in the formulation (rare)

PRECAUTIONS AND CONTRAINDICATIONS
Hypersensitivity to amide-type local anesthetics
Caution:
Local anesthetic toxicity, no pediatric (children younger than 12 yr) or geriatric studies have been made, liver dysfunction, onset longer for maxilla, lactation, contains phenylalanine (caution phenylketonurics)

DRUG INTERACTIONS OF CONCERN TO DENTISTRY
• None reported

SERIOUS REACTIONS
! CNS excitation and depression, potential respiratory depression (at high blood levels).
! Bradycardia, hypotension, cardiovascular collapse, cardiac arrest (at high blood levels).
! Serious allergic reactions (rare).

DENTAL CONSIDERATIONS
General:
• Use no more than one patch per area, remove after 15 min to avoid toxicity.
Teach Patient/Family to:
• Prevent injury while numbness is present and to refrain from gum chewing and eating after dental treatment.
• Report unresolved oral lesions to dentist.

lincomycin HCl
lin-koe-**my′**-sin
(Bactramycin, Lincocin, Lincomycin)

CATEGORY AND SCHEDULE
Pregnancy Risk Category: B

Drug Class: Antibacterial

MECHANISM OF ACTION
A lincosamide antibiotic that specifically binds on the 50S subunit and affects the process of peptide chain initiation. Bacteriostatic.
Therapeutic Effect: Inhibits protein synthesis of the bacterial cell wall.

USES
Infections caused by group A β-hemolytic streptococci, pneumococci, staphylococci (respiratory tract, skin, soft tissue, UTIs; osteomyelitis; septicemia), and anaerobes

PHARMACOKINETICS
Rapidly absorbed from the GI tract. Protein binding: Unknown. Metabolized in liver. Primarily excreted in urine. Not removed by hemodialysis. *Half-life:* 5.4 hr (prolonged with renal or hepatic impairment).

INDICATIONS AND DOSAGES
▶ **Serious Infection Caused by Susceptible Strains of Streptococci, Pneumococci, and Staphylococci**
PO
Adults. 500 mg 3 times a day (500 mg approximately q8h).
Children older than 1 mo. 30 mg/kg/day (15 mg/lb/day) divided into 3 or 4 equal doses.

> **More Severe Infection Caused by Susceptible Strains of Streptococci, Pneumococci, and Staphylococci**
PO
Adults. 500 mg or more 4 times a day (500 mg or more approximately q6h).
Children older than 1 mo. 60 mg/kg/day (30 mg/lb/day) divided into 3 or 4 equal doses.
> **Serious Infection Caused by Susceptible Strains of Streptococci, Pneumococci, and Staphylococci**
IM
Adults. 600 mg (2 ml) q24h.
Children older than 1 mo. One injection of 10 mg/kg (5 mg/lb) q24h.
> **More Severe Infection Caused by Susceptible Strains of Streptococci, Pneumococci, and Staphylococci**
IM
Adults. 600 mg (2 ml) q12h or more often.
Children older than 1 mo. One injection of 10 mg/kg (5 mg/lb) q12h or more often.
> **Serious Infection Caused by Susceptible Strains of Streptococci, Pneumococci, and Staphylococci**
IV
Adults. 600 mg (2 ml) to 1 g q8–12h.
Children older than 1 mo. One injection of 10 mg/kg (5 mg/lb) q12h or more often. Depending on the severity of the infection, 10–20 mg/kg/day (5–10 mg/lb/day) can be infused in divided doses as described for adults.
> **More Severe Infection Caused by Susceptible Strains of Streptococci, Pneumococci, and Staphylococci**
IV
Adults. 600 mg (2 ml) to 1 g q8–12h. Maximum: 8 g/day.
Intravenous doses are given on the basis of 1 g lincomycin diluted in not less than 100 ml of appropriate

solution and infused over a period of not less than 1 hr.
> **Subconjunctival Injection**
Adults. Inject 0.25 ml (75 mg).
> **Dosage in Renal Impairment**
An appropriate dose is 25%–30% of that recommended for patients with normally functioning kidneys.

SIDE EFFECTS/ADVERSE REACTIONS
Frequent
Abdominal pain, nausea, vomiting, diarrhea
Occasional
Phlebitis, thrombophlebitis with IV administration, pain, induration at IM injection site, allergic reaction, urticaria, pruritus, tinnitus, vertigo
Rare
Dermatitis

PRECAUTIONS AND CONTRAINDICATIONS
History of hypersensitivity to clindamycin or lincomycin
Caution:
Renal disease, liver disease, GI disease, elderly, lactation

DRUG INTERACTIONS OF CONCERN TO DENTISTRY
• Decreased action of erythromycin

SERIOUS REACTIONS
Alert
! Antibiotic-associated colitis, as evidenced by severe abdominal pain and tenderness, fever, and watery and severe diarrhea, may occur during and several weeks after lincomycin therapy.
! Cardiopulmonary arrest and hypotension have been reported.

DENTAL CONSIDERATIONS
General:
• Determine why the patient is taking the drug.
Consultations:
• Medical consultation may be required to assess disease control.
Teach Patient/Family to:
• Encourage effective oral hygiene to prevent soft tissue inflammation.
• Use caution to prevent injury when using oral hygiene aids.
• Notify dentist if diarrhea occurs.
• When used for dental infection, advise patient to:
  • Report sore throat, oral burning sensation, fever, fatigue, any of which could indicate superinfection.
  • Take at prescribed intervals and complete dosage regimen.
  • Immediately notify the dentist if signs or symptoms of infection increase.

linezolid
lin-ez′-oh-lid
(Zyvox, Zyvoxam)
Do not confuse Zyvox with Zovirax.

CATEGORY AND SCHEDULE
Pregnancy Risk Category: C

Drug Class: Antibiotic, oxazolidinone derivative

MECHANISM OF ACTION
An oxalodinone antiinfective that binds to a site on bacterial 23S ribosomal RNA, preventing the formation of a complex that is essential for bacterial translation.

Therapeutic Effect: Bacteriostatic against enterococci and staphylococci; bactericidal against streptococci.

USES
Treatment of vancomycin-resistant *E. faecium* infections; nosocomial pneumonia caused by *S. aureus* (methicillin resistant and susceptible) and *S. pneumoniae* (penicillin susceptible); complicated skin and skin-structure infections caused by *S. aureus* (methicillin resistant and susceptible), *S. pyogenes,* or *S. agalactiae;* uncomplicated skin and skin-structure infections caused by *S. aureus* (methicillin susceptible); community-acquired pneumonia caused by *S. pneumoniae* (penicillin susceptible) or *S. aureus* (methicillin susceptible); and diabetic foot infections without osteomyelitis caused by gram-positive bacteria

PHARMACOKINETICS
Rapidly and extensively absorbed after PO administration. Protein binding: 31%. Metabolized in the liver by oxidation. Excreted in urine.
Half-life: 4–5.4 hr.

INDICATIONS AND DOSAGES
▸ **Vancomycin-Resistant Infections**
PO, IV
Adults, Elderly, Children older than 11 yr. 600 mg q12h for 14–28 days.
▸ **Pneumonia, Complicated Skin, and Skin-Structure Infections**
PO, IV
Adults, Elderly, Children older than 11 yr. 600 mg q12h for 10–14 days.
▸ **Uncomplicated Skin and Skin-Structure Infections**
PO
Adults, Elderly. 400 mg q12h for 10–14 days.

Children older than 11 yr. 600 mg q12h for 10–14 days.
Children 5–11 yr. 10 mg/kg/dose q12h for 10–14 days.
▸ **Usual Neonate Dosage**
PO, IV
Neonates. 10 mg/kg/dose q8–12h.

SIDE EFFECTS/ADVERSE REACTIONS

Occasional
Diarrhea, nausea, headache
Rare
Altered taste, vaginal candidiasis, fungal infection, dizziness, tongue discoloration

PRECAUTIONS AND CONTRAINDICATIONS

Hypersensitivity
Caution:
May promote overgrowth of nonsusceptible bacterial strains, monitor platelet counts in patients at risk for bleeding, lactation, pediatric doses not established, use longer than 28 days, selectively inhibits monoamine oxidase enzymes, potentiation of serotonergic drugs, hepatic disease, hemodialysis patients; risk of myelosuppression, monitor CBC counts, avoid tyramine-containing foods

DRUG INTERACTIONS OF CONCERN TO DENTISTRY

• Potential to increase pressor effects of indirect-action sympathomimetic drugs and vasopressors, such as dopaminergic drugs, phenylephrine, phenylpropanolamine, and pseudoephedrine
• Interactions with vasoconstrictors in local anesthetics has not been studied

SERIOUS REACTIONS

‼ Thrombocytopenia and myelosuppression occur rarely.

‼ Antibiotic-associated colitis and other superinfections may result from altered bacterial balance.

DENTAL CONSIDERATIONS

General:
• Determine why patient is taking the drug.
• Use vasoconstrictor with caution, in low doses, and with careful aspiration. Avoid using gingival retraction cord containing epinephrine.
• Patients on chronic drug therapy may rarely have symptoms of blood dyscrasias, which can include infection, bleeding, and poor healing.
• Examine for oral manifestation of opportunistic infection.
• Consider semisupine chair position for patient comfort if GI side effects occur.
Consultations:
• In a patient with symptoms of blood dyscrasias, request a medical consultation for blood studies and postpone treatment until normal values are reestablished.
• Medical consultation may be required to assess disease control and patient's ability to tolerate stress.
• Physician consultation is advised in the presence of an acute dental infection requiring another antibiotic.
Teach Patient/Family to:
• See dentist immediately if secondary oral infection occurs.
• Report sore throat, oral burning sensation, fever, fatigue, any of which could indicate presence of a superinfection.

liothyronine (T3)
lye-oh-**thye'**-roe-neen
(Cytomel, Tertroxin[AUS],
Triostat)
Do not confuse liothyronine with
levothyroxine.

CATEGORY AND SCHEDULE
Pregnancy Risk Category: A

Drug Class: Thyroid hormone

MECHANISM OF ACTION
A synthetic form of triiodothyronine
(T3), a thyroid hormone involved in
normal metabolism, growth, and
development, especially of the CNS
in infants. Possesses catabolic and
anabolic effects.
Therapeutic Effect: Increases basal
metabolic rate, enhances
gluconeogenesis, and stimulates
protein synthesis.

USES
Treatment of hypothyroidism,
myxedema coma, thyroid hormone
replacement, cretinism, nontoxic
goiter, T3 suppression test;
thyroiditis, euthyroid goiter

PHARMACOKINETICS
PO: Peak 12–48 hr. *Half-life:*
0.6–1.4 days.

INDICATIONS AND DOSAGES
▸ **Hypothyroidism**
PO
Adults, Elderly. Initially, 25 mcg/day.
May increase in increments of
12.5–25 mcg/day q1–2wk.
Maximum 100 mcg/day.
Children. Initially, 5 mcg/day. May
increase by 5 mcg/day q3–4wk.
Maintenance: 100 mcg/day (children
older than 3 yr); 50 mcg/day

(children 1–3 yr); 20 mcg/day
(infants).
▸ **Myxedema**
PO
Adults, Elderly. Initially, 5 mcg/day.
Increase by 5–10 mcg q1–2wk (after
25 mcg/day has been reached, may
increase in 12.5-mcg increments).
Maintenance: 50–100 mcg/day.
▸ **Nontoxic Goiter**
PO
Adults, Elderly. Initially, 5 mcg/day.
Increase by 5–10 mcg/day q1–2wk.
When 25 mcg/day has been reached,
may increase by 12.5–25 mcg/day
q1–2wk. Maintenance: 75 mcg/day.
Children. 5 mcg/day. May increase
by 5 mcg q1–2wk. Maintenance:
15–20 mcg/day.
▸ **Congenital Hypothyroidism**
PO
Children. Initially, 5 mcg/day.
Increase by 5 mcg/day q3–4 days.
Maintenance: Full adult dosage
(children older than 3 yr); 50 mcg/
day (children 1–3 yr); 20 mcg/day
(infants).
▸ **T3 Suppression Test**
PO
Adults, Elderly. 75–100 mcg/day for
7 days; then repeat I131 thyroid
uptake test.
▸ **Myxedema Coma, Precoma**
IV
Adults, Elderly. Initially, 25–50 mcg
(10–20 mcg in patients with
cardiovascular disease). Total dose at
least 65 mcg/day.

SIDE EFFECTS/ADVERSE REACTIONS
Occasional
Reversible hair loss at start of
therapy (in children)
Rare
Dry skin, GI intolerance, rash, hives,
pseudotumor cerebri or severe
headache in children

L

PRECAUTIONS AND CONTRAINDICATIONS

MI and thyrotoxicosis uncomplicated by hypothyroidism; obesity

Caution:

Elderly, angina pectoris, hypertension, ischemia, cardiac disease, lactation

DRUG INTERACTIONS OF CONCERN TO DENTISTRY

- Hypertension, tachycardia: ketamine
- Increased effects of sympathomimetics when thyroid doses are not carefully monitored or in patients with coronary artery disease

SERIOUS REACTIONS

! Excessive dosage produces signs and symptoms of hyperthyroidism, including weight loss, palpitations, increased appetite, tremors, nervousness, tachycardia, hypertension, headache, insomnia, and menstrual irregularities.

! Cardiac arrhythmias occur rarely.

DENTAL CONSIDERATIONS

General:

- Patients with uncontrolled hypothyroidism may be more responsive to CNS depressants.
- Increased nervousness, excitability, sweating, or tachycardia may indicate a patient with uncontrolled hyperthyroidism or a dose of medication that is too high. Uncontrolled patients should be referred for medical treatment.

Consultations:

- Medical consultation may be required to assess disease control.
- Observe appropriate limitations of vasoconstrictor doses.

liotrix
lye'-oh-trix
(Thyrolar, Thyrolar-1, Thyrolar-1/2, Thyrolar-1/4, Thyrolar-2, Thyrolar-3)

CATEGORY AND SCHEDULE
Pregnancy Risk Category: A

Drug Class: Thyroid hormone

MECHANISM OF ACTION

A synthetic form of levothyroxine (T4) and triiodothyronine (T3) involved in normal metabolism, growth, and development, especially the CNS of infants. Possesses catabolic and anabolic effects.
Therapeutic Effect: Increases basal metabolic rate, enhances gluconeogenesis, stimulates protein synthesis.

USES

Treatment of hypothyroidism, thyroid hormone replacement, thyroiditis, euthyroid goiter

PHARMACOKINETICS

T4 is partially absorbed from the GI tract. T3 is almost completely absorbed. Widely distributed. Deiodinated in peripheral tissues, minimal metabolism in the liver.
Half-life: Unknown.

INDICATIONS AND DOSAGES
▸ Hypothyroidism
PO
Adults, Elderly. Initially, 50 mcg (0.05 mg) levothyroxine and 12.5 mcg (0.0125 mg) liothyronine per day, with increments of a like amount at monthly intervals until the desired result is obtained. Maintenance: 50–100 mcg (0.05–0.1 mg) levothyroxine and

12.5–25 mcg (0.0125–0.025 mg) liothyronine per day.

▸ **Congenital Hypothyroidism**
PO
Children older than 12 yr. More than 150 mcg of levothyroxine per day.
Children 6–12 yr. 100–150 mcg of levothyroxine per day.
Children 1–5 yr. 75–100 mcg of levothyroxine per day.
Children 6–12 mo. 50–75 mcg of levothyroxine per day.
Children 0–6 mo. 25–50 mcg of levothyroxine per day.

▸ **Myxedema**
PO
Adults, Elderly. Initially, 12.5 mcg (0.0125 mg) levothyroxine and 3.1 mcg (0.0031 mg) liothyronine per day, with increments of a like amount q2–3wk until the desired result is obtained. Maintenance: 50–100 mcg (0.05–0.1 mg) levothyroxine and 12.5–25 mcg (0.0125–0.025 mg) liothyronine per day.

▸ **Thyroid Cancer**
PO
Adults, Elderly. Larger amounts of thyroid hormone than those used for replacement therapy are required.

▸ **Thyroid Suppression Therapy**
PO
Adults, Elderly. Usual dosage of levothyroxine 2.6 mcg/kg/day for 7–10 days.

SIDE EFFECTS/ADVERSE REACTIONS
Occasional
Reversible hair loss at the start of therapy (in children)
Rare
Dry skin, GI intolerance, rash, hives, pseudotumor cerebri or severe headache in children

PRECAUTIONS AND CONTRAINDICATIONS
Uncorrected adrenal cortical insufficiency, untreated thyrotoxicosis, or hypersensitivity to any of active constituents
Caution:
Elderly, angina pectoris, hypertension, ischemia, cardiac disease, lactation

DRUG INTERACTIONS OF CONCERN TO DENTISTRY
• Hypertension, tachycardia: ketamine
• Increased effects of sympathomimetics when thyroid doses are not carefully monitored or in patients with coronary artery disease

SERIOUS REACTIONS
! Excessive dosage produces signs and symptoms of hyperthyroidism, including weight loss, palpitations, increased appetite, tremors, nervousness, tachycardia, hypertension, headache, insomnia, menstrual irregularities.
! Cardiac arrhythmias occur rarely.

DENTAL CONSIDERATIONS
General:
• Patients with uncontrolled hypothyroidism may be more responsive to CNS depressants.
• Increased nervousness, excitability, sweating, or tachycardia may indicate a patient with uncontrolled hyperthyroidism or a dose of medication that is too high. Uncontrolled patients should be referred for medical treatment.
• Observe appropriate limitations of vasoconstrictor doses.
Consultations:
• Medical consultation may be required to assess disease control.

Teach Patient/Family to:
• Encourage effective oral hygiene to prevent soft tissue inflammation.
• Avoid mouth rinses with high alcohol content because of drying effects.

lisdexamfetamine dimesylate
liz-dex-am-**fet**´-a-meen
(Vyvanase)

CATEGORY AND SCHEDULE
Pregnancy Risk Category: C
Controlled substance: Schedule II

Drug Class: CNS stimulant, amphetamine

MECHANISM OF ACTION
The actual mechanism for attention-deficit/hyperactivity disorder (ADHD) is not known. Prodrug of dextroamphetamine thought to block the neuronal reuptake of norepinephrine and dopamine.

USES
Used for treatment of ADHD.

PHARMACOKINETICS
Rapid absorption. Dextroamphetamine active metabolite. Mean CSF concentrations are 80% those of plasma. **Half-life**: lisdexamfetamine <1 hr and dextroamphetamine 10–13 hr. Metabolized into dextroamphetamine and l-lysine through non–CYP-mediated hepatic or intestinal metabolism. Excreted primarily in the urine (96%), and small amount in feces.

INDICATIONS AND DOSAGES
▸ ADHD
PO
Adults. 30 mg once daily in the morning. May increase in increments of 10 mg or 20 mg/day at weekly intervals until optimal response. Maximum 70 mg/day.
Children (6–12 yr). 30 mg once daily in the morning. May increase in increments of 10 mg or 20 mg/day at weekly intervals until optimal response. Maximum 70 mg/day.

SIDE EFFECTS/ADVERSE REACTIONS
Adult
Frequent
Insomnia, decreased appetite, xerostomia
Occasional
Increase blood pressure, increased heart rate, anxiety, jitteriness, agitation, restlessness, hyperhidrosis, diarrhea, nausea, anorexia, tremor, dyspnea
▸ Children
Frequent
Headache, insomnia, decreased appetite, xerostomia, abdominal pain
Occasional
Irritability, dizziness, affects lability, fever, somnolence, tic, vomiting, weight loss, nausea

PRECAUTIONS AND CONTRAINDICATIONS
Hypersensitivity to lisdexamfetamine, sympathomimetic amines, or its components.
Avoid in patients with pre-existing structural cardiac abnormalities or other heart conditions because serious cardiovascular events including sudden death have been reported.
Avoid in patients with history of ethanol or drug abuse since prolong drug use may lead to dependency.

Avoid in patients with moderate to severe hypertension, arteriosclerosis, hyperthyroidism, or symptomatic cardiovascular diseases.

Use with caution in patients with hypertension and other cardiovascular conditions that might exacerbate increases in blood pressure and/ or heart rate.

Use with caution in patients with history of or pre-existing psychosis, bipolar disorder, aggressive behavior, seizure disorder, and Tourette's syndrome.

Abrupt discontinuation following high doses or for prolonged period may lead to withdrawal syndrome.

DRUG INTERACTIONS OF CONCERN TO DENTISTRY

• Blood pressure should be monitored prior to administering local anesthetic with vasoconstrictors since dextroamphetamine is known to increase blood pressure.

• Tricyclic antidepressants: may potentiate the anticholinergic effects of tricyclic antidepressants.

SERIOUS REACTIONS

! Serious cardiovascular events, including sudden death may, occur in patients with pre-existing structural cardiac abnormalities or other heart conditions.

! Potential for drug dependency may occur with prolonged use.

! Prolonged administration to children with ADHD may produce a temporary suppression of normal weight and height patterns.

DENTAL CONSIDERATIONS

General:

• Monitor vital signs at every appointment because of cardiovascular side effects.

• Observe appropriate limitations of vasoconstrictor doses.

• Assess salivary flow as a factor in caries, periodontal disease, and candidiasis.

• Consider semisupine chair position for patient comfort because of respiratory effects of disease.

Teach Patient/Family to:

• When chronic dry mouth occurs, advise patient to:

   • Avoid mouth rinses with high alcohol content because of drying effects.

   • Use sugarless gum, frequent sips of water, or saliva substitutes.

   • Use daily home fluoride products for anticaries effect.

lisinopril

lye-**sin**'-oh-pril
(Apo-Lisinopril[CAN], Fibsol[AUS], Lisodur[AUS], Prinivil, Zestril)
Do not confuse lisinopril with fosinopril; Prinivil with Desyrel, Plendil, Proventil, or Restoril; Fibsol with Lioresal; or Zestril with Zostrix. Do not confuse lisinopril's combination form Zestoretic with Prilosec.

CATEGORY AND SCHEDULE

Pregnancy Risk Category: C (D if used in second or third trimester)

Drug Class: Angiotensin-converting enzyme (ACE) inhibitor

MECHANISM OF ACTION

This ACE inhibitor suppresses the renin-angiotensin-aldosterone system and prevents conversion of angiotensin I to angiotensin II, a potent vasoconstrictor; may also inhibit angiotensin II at local

vascular and renal sites. Decreases plasma angiotensin II, increases plasma renin activity, and decreases aldosterone secretion.
Therapeutic Effect: Reduces peripheral arterial resistance, B/P, afterload, pulmonary capillary wedge pressure (preload), and pulmonary vascular resistance. In those with heart failure, also decreases heart size, increases cardiac output, and exercise tolerance time.

USES
Treatment of mild-to-moderate hypertension, post-MI if hemodynamically stable, heart failure

PHARMACOKINETICS

Route	Onset	Peak	Duration
PO	1 hr	6 hr	24 hr

Incompletely absorbed from the GI tract. Protein binding: 25%. Primarily excreted unchanged in urine. Removed by hemodialysis.
Half-life: 12 hr (half-life is prolonged in those with impaired renal function).

INDICATIONS AND DOSAGES
▸ **Hypertension (Used Alone)**
PO
Adults. Initially, 10 mg/day. May increase by 5–10 mcg/day at 1- to 2-wk intervals. Maximum: 40 mg/day.
Elderly. Initially, 2.5–5 mg/day. May increase by 2.5–5 mg/day at 1- to 2-wk intervals. Maximum: 40 mg/day.
▸ **Hypertension (Used in Combination with Other Antihypertensives)**

PO
Adults. Initially, 2.5–5 mg/day titrated to patient's needs.
▸ **Adjunctive Therapy for Management of Heart Failure**
PO
Adults, Elderly. Initially, 2.5–5 mg/day. May increase by no more than 10 mg/day at intervals of at least 2 wk. Maintenance: 5–40 mg/day.
▸ **Improve Survival in Patients after an MI**
PO
Adults, Elderly. Initially, 5 mg, then 5 mg after 24 hr, 10 mg after 48 hr, then 10 mg/day for 6 wk. For patients with low systolic B/P, give 2.5 mg/day for 3 days, then 2.5–5 mg/day.
▸ **Dosage in Renal Impairment**
Titrate to patient's needs after giving the following initial dose:

Creatinine Clearance	% Normal Dose
10–50 ml/min	50–75
Less than 10 ml/min	25–50

SIDE EFFECTS/ADVERSE REACTIONS
Frequent
Headache, dizziness, postural hypotension
Occasional
Chest discomfort, fatigue, rash, abdominal pain, nausea, diarrhea, upper respiratory infection
Rare
Palpitations, tachycardia, peripheral edema, insomnia, paresthesia, confusion, constipation, dry mouth, muscle cramps

PRECAUTIONS AND CONTRAINDICATIONS
History of angioedema from previous treatment with ACE inhibitors

Caution:
Lactation, renal disease,
hyperkalemia

DRUG INTERACTIONS OF CONCERN TO DENTISTRY
• Increased hypotension: alcohol, phenothiazines
• Decreased hypotensive effects: indomethacin and possibly other NSAIDs, sympathomimetics
• Suspected reduction in the antihypertensive and vasodilator effects by salicylates; monitor B/P if used concurrently

SERIOUS REACTIONS
❗ Excessive hypotension ("first-dose syncope") may occur in patients with CHF and severe salt and volume depletion.
❗ Angioedema (swelling of face and lips) and hyperkalemia occurs rarely.
❗ Agranulocytosis and neutropenia may be noted in patients with collagen vascular disease, including scleroderma and systemic lupus erythematosus, and impaired renal function.
❗ Nephrotic syndrome may be noted in patients with history of renal disease.

DENTAL CONSIDERATIONS
General:
• Monitor vital signs at every appointment because of cardiovascular and respiratory side effects.
• After supine positioning, have patient sit upright for at least 2 min before standing to avoid orthostatic hypotension.
• Patients on chronic drug therapy may rarely have symptoms of blood dyscrasias, which can include infection, bleeding, and poor healing.

• Assess salivary flow as a factor in caries, periodontal disease, and candidiasis.
• Limit use of sodium-containing products, such as saline IV fluids, for patients with a dietary salt restriction.
• Use vasoconstrictors with caution, in low doses, and with careful aspiration.
• Short appointments and a stress-reduction protocol may be required for anxious patients.
Consultations:
• Medical consultation may be required to assess disease control and patient's ability to tolerate stress.
• In a patient with symptoms of blood dyscrasias, request a medical consultation for blood studies and postpone dental treatment until normal values are reestablished.
• Take precautions if dental surgery is anticipated and sedation or general anesthesia is required; risk of hypotensive episode.
Teach Patient/Family to:
• Encourage effective oral hygiene to prevent soft tissue inflammation.
• Use caution to prevent injury when using oral hygiene aids.
• When chronic dry mouth occurs, advise patient to:
  • Avoid mouth rinses with high alcohol content because of drying effects.
  • Use sugarless gum, frequent sips of water, or saliva substitutes.
  • Use daily home fluoride products for anticaries effect.

lithium carbonate/ lithium citrate

lith′-ee-um
kahr′-buh-neyt/sit′-rayte
lithium carbonate (Duralith[CAN],
Eskalith, Lithi.carb[AUS],
Lithobid, Quilonum SR[AUS]),
lithium citrate (Cibalith-S)
Do not confuse Lithobid with
Levbid, Lithostat, or Lithotabs.

CATEGORY AND SCHEDULE
Pregnancy Risk Category: D

Drug Class: Antimanic,
inorganic salt

MECHANISM OF ACTION
A psychotherapeutic agent that
affects the storage, release, and
reuptake of neurotransmitters.
Antimanic effect may result from
increased norepinephrine reuptake
and serotonin receptor sensitivity.
Therapeutic Effect: Produces
antimanic and antidepressant
effects.

USES
Treatment of manic-depressive
illness (manic phase), prevention of
bipolar manic-depressive psychosis

PHARMACOKINETICS
Rapidly and completely absorbed
from the GI tract. Primarily excreted
unchanged in urine. Removed by
hemodialysis. *Half-life:* 18–24 hr
(increased in elderly).

INDICATIONS AND DOSAGES
Alert
During acute phase, a therapeutic
serum lithium concentration of
1–1.4 mEq/L is required. For
long-term control, the desired level
is 0.5–1.3 mEq/L. Monitor serum

drug concentration and clinical
response.
▶ Prevention or Treatment of Acute
Mania, Manic Phase of Bipolar
Disorder (Manic-Depressive Illness)
PO
Adults. 300 mg 3–4 times a day or
450–900 mg slow-release form
twice a day. Maximum: 2.4 g/day.
Elderly. 300 mg twice a day. May
increase by 300 mg/day q1wk.
Maintenance: 900–1200 mg/day.
Children 12 yr and older. 600–
1800 mg/day in 3–4 divided doses
(2 doses/day for slow-release).
Children younger than 12 yr.
15–60 mg/kg/day in 3–4 divided
doses.

SIDE EFFECTS/ADVERSE REACTIONS
Occasional
Fine hand tremor, polydipsia,
polyuria, mild nausea, dry mouth
Rare
Weight gain, bradycardia or
tachycardia, acne, rash, muscle
twitching, cold and cyanotic
extremities, pseudotumor cerebri
(eye pain, headache, tinnitus, vision
disturbances)

PRECAUTIONS AND CONTRAINDICATIONS
Debilitated patients, severe
cardiovascular disease, severe
dehydration, severe renal disease,
severe sodium depletion
Caution:
Elderly, thyroid disease, seizure
disorders, diabetes mellitus,
systemic infection, urinary retention

DRUG INTERACTIONS OF CONCERN TO DENTISTRY
• Increased toxicity: aspirin,
indomethacin, other NSAIDs,
haloperidol, metronidazole,
carbamazepine

• Increased effects of neuromuscular blocking agents

SERIOUS REACTIONS
! A lithium serum concentration of 1.5–2.0 mEq/L may produce vomiting, diarrhea, drowsiness, confusion, incoordination, coarse hand tremor, muscle twitching, and T-wave depression on ECG.
! A lithium serum concentration of 2.0–2.5 mEq/L may result in ataxia, giddiness, tinnitus, blurred vision, clonic movements, and severe hypotension.
! Acute toxicity may be characterized by seizures, oliguria, circulatory failure, coma, and death.

DENTAL CONSIDERATIONS
General:
• Assess salivary flow as a factor in caries, periodontal disease, and candidiasis.
• After supine positioning, have patient sit upright for at least 2 min before standing to avoid orthostatic hypotension.
Consultations:
• Medical consultation may be required to assess disease control.
Teach Patient/Family to:
• Encourage effective oral hygiene to prevent soft tissue inflammation.
• Use caution to prevent injury when using oral hygiene aids.
• When chronic dry mouth occurs, advise patient to:
  • Avoid mouth rinses with high alcohol content because of drying effects.
  • Use sugarless gum, frequent sips of water, or saliva substitutes.
• Use daily home fluoride products for anticaries effect.

lodoxamide
loe-**dox**′-ah-mide
(Alomide)

CATEGORY AND SCHEDULE
Pregnancy Risk Category: B

Drug Class: Mast cell stabilizer

MECHANISM OF ACTION
A mast cell stabilizer that prevents increase in cutaneous vascular permeability, antigen-stimulated histamine release, and may prevent calcium influx into mast cells. *Therapeutic Effect:* Inhibits sensitivity reaction.

USES
Treatment of vernal keratoconjunctivitis, vernal conjunctivitis, keratitis

PHARMACOKINETICS
Nondetectable absorption. *Half-life:* 8.5 hr.

INDICATIONS AND DOSAGES
▸ **Treatment of Vernal Keratoconjunctivitis, Conjunctivitis, and Keratitis**
Ophthalmic
Adults, Elderly, Children 2 yr or older. 1–2 drops 4 times a day, for up to 3 mo.

SIDE EFFECTS/ADVERSE REACTIONS
Frequent
Transient stinging, burning, instillation discomfort
Occasional
Ocular itching, blurred vision, dry eye, tearing/discharge/foreign body sensation, headache, dry mouth

Rare
Scales on lid/lash, ocular swelling, sticky sensation, dizziness, somnolence, nausea, sneezing, dry nose, rash

PRECAUTIONS AND CONTRAINDICATIONS
Wearing soft contact lenses (product contains benzalkonium chloride), hypersensitivity to lodoxamide tromethamine or any component of the formulation
Caution:
Children younger than 2 yr, lactation

DRUG INTERACTIONS OF CONCERN TO DENTISTRY
• None reported

SERIOUS REACTIONS
! None reported

DENTAL CONSIDERATIONS

General:
• Question patient about history of allergy to avoid use of other potential allergens.
• Avoid dental light in patient's eyes; offer dark glasses for patient comfort.
• Use for less than 2 wk should not present a problem with dry mouth.
Teach Patient/Family to:
• When chronic dry mouth occurs advise patient to:
  • Avoid mouth rinses with high alcohol content because of drying effects.
  • Use daily home fluoride products for anticaries effect.
  • Use sugarless gum, frequent sips of water, or saliva substitutes.

lomefloxacin hydrochloride
low-meh-**flocks**′-ah-sin
high-droh-**klor**′-ide
(Maxaquin)

CATEGORY AND SCHEDULE
Pregnancy Risk Category: C

Drug Class: Fluoroquinolone antiinfective

MECHANISM OF ACTION
A quinolone that inhibits the enzyme DNA gyrase in susceptible microorganisms, interfering with bacterial cell replication and repair. ***Therapeutic Effect:*** Bactericidal.

USES
Treatment of lower respiratory tract infections (pneumonia, bronchitis); GU infections (prostatitis, UTIs); preoperatively to reduce UTIs in transurethral and transrectal surgical procedures caused by susceptible gram-negative organisms

PHARMACOKINETICS
Well absorbed from the GI tract. Protein binding: 10%. Widely distributed. Metabolized in the liver. Primarily excreted in urine. Not removed by hemodialysis. ***Half-life:*** 4–6 hr (increased with impaired renal function and in the elderly).

INDICATIONS AND DOSAGES
▶ **Complicated UTIs**
PO
Adults, Elderly. 400 mg/day for 10–14 days.
▶ **Uncomplicated UTIs**
PO
Adults (Females). 400 mg/day for 3 days.

▸ **Lower Respiratory Tract Infections**
PO
Adults, Elderly. 400 mg/day for 10 days.
▸ **Surgical Prophylaxis**
PO
Adults, Elderly. 400 mg 2–6 hr before surgery.
▸ **Dosage in Renal Impairment**
Dosage and frequency are modified on the basis of creatinine clearance.

Creatinine Clearance	Dosage
41 ml/min and higher	No change
10–40 ml/min	400 mg initially, then 200 mg/day for 10–14 days

SIDE EFFECTS/ADVERSE REACTIONS
Occasional
Nausea, headache, photosensitivity, dizziness
Rare
Diarrhea

PRECAUTIONS AND CONTRAINDICATIONS
Hypersensitivity to quinolones
Caution:
Lactation, children, elderly, renal disease, seizure disorders, excessive sunlight; tendon rupture in shoulder, hand, and Achilles tendons

DRUG INTERACTIONS OF CONCERN TO DENTISTRY
• Decreased effects: antacids
• Increased levels of cyclosporine, caffeine

SERIOUS REACTIONS
! Antibiotic-associated colitis and other superinfections may result from altered bacterial balance.

! Hypersensitivity reactions, including photosensitivity (as evidenced by rash, pruritus, blisters, edema, and burning skin), have occurred in patients receiving fluoroquinolones.
! Arthropathy may occur if the drug is given to children younger than 18 yr.

DENTAL CONSIDERATIONS
General:
• Because of drug interactions, do not use ingestible sodium bicarbonate products, such as the Prophy-Jet air polishing system, until 2 hr after drug use.
• Use caution in prescribing caffeine-containing analgesics.
• Determine why the patient is taking the drug.
• Avoid dental light in patient's eyes; offer dark glasses for patient comfort.
• Ruptures of the shoulder, hand, and Achilles tendons that required surgical repair or resulted in prolonged disability have been reported with this drug.
Consultations:
• Consult with patient's physician if an acute dental infection occurs and another antiinfective is required.
Teach Patient/Family to:
• Use caution to prevent injury when using oral hygiene aids.
• Avoid mouth rinses with high alcohol content because of drying effects.
• Minimize exposure to sunlight and wear sunscreen if sun exposure is planned.
• Discontinue treatment and inform dentist immediately if patient experiences pain or inflammation of a tendon, and to rest and refrain from exercise.

lomustine
low-**mew**'-steen
(CeeNU)

CATEGORY AND SCHEDULE
Pregnancy Risk Category: D

Drug Class: Antineoplastic alkylating agent

MECHANISM OF ACTION
An alkylating agent and nitrosourea that inhibits DNA and RNA protein synthesis by cross-linking with DNA and RNA strands, preventing cell division. Cell cycle–phase nonspecific.
Therapeutic Effect: Interferes with DNA and RNA function.

USES
Treatment of Hodgkin's disease; lymphomas; melanomas; multiple myeloma; brain, lung, bladder, kidney, colon cancer.

PHARMACOKINETICS
PO: Well absorbed. *Half-life:* 16–48 hr; 50% protein bound; metabolized in liver; excreted in urine; crosses blood-brain barrier; excreted in breast milk.

INDICATIONS AND DOSAGES
▶ **Disseminated Hodgkin's Disease, Primary and Metastatic Brain Tumors**
PO
Adults, Elderly. 100–130 mg/m² as single dose. Repeat dose at intervals of at least 6 wk but not until circulating blood elements have returned to acceptable levels. Adjust dose on the basis of hematologic response to previous dose.
Children. 75–150 mg/m² as a single dose every 6 wk.

SIDE EFFECTS/ADVERSE REACTIONS
Frequent
Nausea, vomiting (occurring 45 min–6 hr after dose and lasting 12–24 hr); anorexia (often follows for 2–3 days)
Occasional
Neurotoxicity (confusion, slurred speech), stomatitis, darkening of skin, diarrhea, rash, pruritus, alopecia

PRECAUTIONS AND CONTRAINDICATIONS
Pregnancy
Caution:
Radiation therapy, geriatric patient, lactation

DRUG INTERACTIONS OF CONCERN TO DENTISTRY
• This drug depresses bone marrow function, which may increase risk of bleeding; avoid drugs that can increase bleeding, such as aspirin, NSAIDs

SERIOUS REACTIONS
! Myelosuppression may result in hematologic toxicity, manifested principally as leukopenia, mild anemia, and thrombocytopenia. Leukopenia occurs about 6 wk after a dose, thrombocytopenia about 4 wk after a dose; both persist for 1–2 wk.
! Refractory anemia and thrombocytopenia occur commonly if lomustine therapy continues for more than 1 yr.
! Hepatotoxicity occurs infrequently.
! Large cumulative doses of lomustine may result in renal damage.

DENTAL CONSIDERATIONS

General:

• Patients on chronic drug therapy may rarely have symptoms of blood dyscrasias, which can include infection, bleeding, and poor healing.

• Consider semisupine chair position for patient comfort if GI side effects occur.

• Palliative medication may be required for oral side effects.

• Consider local hemostasis measures to prevent excessive bleeding.

• Prophylactic antibiotics may be indicated to prevent infection if surgery or deep scaling is planned.

• Patients taking opioids for acute or chronic pain should be given alternative analgesics for dental pain.

• Avoid prescribing aspirin-containing products.

Consultations:

• In a patient with symptoms of blood dyscrasias, request a medical consultation for blood studies and postpone dental treatment until normal values are reestablished.

• Patients on cancer chemotherapy should have an adequate WBC count before completing dental procedures that may produce a wound. Consult to determine blood count before appointment.

Teach Patient/Family to:

• Encourage effective oral hygiene to prevent soft tissue inflammation.

• Use caution to prevent trauma when using oral hygiene aids.

• See dentist immediately if secondary oral infection occurs.

• Report oral lesions, soreness, or bleeding to dentist.

• Avoid mouth rinses with high alcohol content because of drying and irritating effects.

• Update medical/drug records if physician makes any changes in evaluation or drug regimens; include OTC, herbal, and nonherbal drugs in the update.

loperamide hydrochloride

loe-**per**′-ah-mide high-droh-**klor**′-ide (Apo-Loperamide[CAN], Gastro-Stop[AUS], Imodium, Imodium A-D, Loperacap[CAN], Novo-Loperamide[CAN])
Do not confuse Imodium with Indocin or Ionamin.

CATEGORY AND SCHEDULE

Pregnancy Risk Category: B
OTC liquid, tablets

Drug Class: Antidiarrheal (opioid)

MECHANISM OF ACTION

An antidiarrheal that directly affects the intestinal wall muscles.
Therapeutic Effect: Slows intestinal motility and prolongs transit time of intestinal contents by reducing fecal volume, diminishing loss of fluid and electrolytes, and increasing viscosity and bulk of stool.

USES

Treatment of diarrhea (cause undetermined), chronic diarrhea, ileostomy discharge

PHARMACOKINETICS

Poorly absorbed from the GI tract. Protein binding: 97%. Metabolized in the liver. Eliminated in feces and excreted in urine. Not removed by hemodialysis. *Half-life:* 9.1–14.4 hr.

INDICATIONS AND DOSAGES
▸ **Acute Diarrhea**
PO (Capsules)
Adults, Elderly. Initially, 4 mg; then 2 mg after each unformed stool. Maximum: 16 mg/day.
Children 9–12 yr, weighing more than 30 kg. Initially, 2 mg 3 times a day for 24 hr.
Children 6–8 yr, weighing 20–30 kg. Initially, 2 mg twice a day for 24 hr.
Children 2–5 yr, weighing 13–20 kg. Initially, 1 mg 3 times a day for 24 hr. Maintenance: 1 mg/10 kg only after loose stool.
▸ **Chronic Diarrhea**
PO
Adults, Elderly. Initially, 4 mg; then 2 mg after each unformed stool until diarrhea is controlled.
Children. 0.08–0.24 mg/kg/day in 2–3 divided doses. Maximum: 2 mg/dose.
▸ **Traveler's Diarrhea**
PO
Adults, Elderly. Initially, 4 mg; then 2 mg after each loose bowel movement (LBM). Maximum: 8 mg/day for 2 days.
Children 9–11 yr. Initially, 2 mg; then 1 mg after each LBM. Maximum: 6 mg/day for 2 days.
Children 6–8 yr. Initially, 1 mg; then 1 mg after each LBM. Maximum: 4 mg/day for 2 days.

SIDE EFFECTS/ADVERSE REACTIONS
Frequent
Dry mouth
Rare
Somnolence, abdominal discomfort, allergic reaction (such as rash and itching)

PRECAUTIONS AND CONTRAINDICATIONS
Acute ulcerative colitis (may produce toxic megacolon), diarrhea associated with pseudomembranous enterocolitis caused by broad-spectrum antibiotics or to organisms that invade intestinal mucosa (such as *Escherichia coli, Shigella,* and *Salmonella*), patients who must avoid constipation
Caution:
Lactation, children younger than 2 yr, liver disease, dehydration, bacterial disease

DRUG INTERACTIONS OF CONCERN TO DENTISTRY
• Increased action: opioid analgesics

SERIOUS REACTIONS
! Toxicity results in constipation, GI irritation, including nausea and vomiting, and CNS depression. Activated charcoal is used to treat loperamide toxicity.

DENTAL CONSIDERATIONS
General:
• Assess salivary flow as a factor in caries, periodontal disease, and candidiasis.
• Evaluate respiration characteristics and rate.
• Consider semisupine chair position for patient comfort because of GI effects of drug.
• This drug product is normally used only for a few doses for acute problems; however, some patients may have to take it for longer time periods as dictated by contributing disease.
Teach Patient/Family to:
• When chronic dry mouth occurs, advise patient to:
  • Avoid mouth rinses with high alcohol content because of drying effects.
  • Use sugarless gum, frequent sips of water, or saliva substitutes.

• Use daily home fluoride products for anticaries effect.

loracarbef
lor-ah-**kar**′-bef
(Lorabid)
Do not confuse loracarbef or Lorabid with Lortab.

CATEGORY AND SCHEDULE
Pregnancy Risk Category: B

Drug Class: Antibiotic, second-generation cephalosporin

MECHANISM OF ACTION
A second-generation cephalosporin that binds to bacterial cell membranes and inhibits cell wall synthesis.
Therapeutic Effect: Bactericidal.

USES
Treatment of gram-negative organisms: *H. influenzae, E. coli, P. mirabilis, Klebsiella*; gram-positive organisms: *S. pneumoniae, S. pyogenes, S. aureus*; upper/lower respiratory tract infection, acute maxillary sinusitis, pharyngitis, tonsillitis; urinary tract and skin infections; otitis media; some in vitro activity against anaerobes

PHARMACOKINETICS
Peak 1 hr. *Half-life:* 1 hr; excreted in urine as unchanged drug.

INDICATIONS AND DOSAGES
▶ **Bronchitis**
PO
Adults, Elderly, Children 12 yr and older. 200–400 mg q12h for 7 days.

▶ **Pharyngitis**
PO
Adults, Elderly, Children 12 yr and older. 200 mg q12h for 10 days.
Children 6 mo–11 yr. 7.5 mg/kg q12h for 10 days.

▶ **Pneumonia**
PO
Adults, Elderly, Children 12 yr and older. 400 mg q12h for 14 days.

▶ **Sinusitis**
PO
Adults, Elderly, Children 12 yr and older. 400 mg q12h for 10 days.
Children 6 mo–11 yr. 15 mg/kg q12h for 10 days.

▶ **Skin and Soft-Tissue Infections**
PO
Adults, Elderly, Children 12 yr and older. 200 mg q12h for 7 days.
Children 6 mo–11 yr. 7.5 mg/kg q12h for 7 days.

▶ **UTIs**
PO
Adults, Elderly, Children 6 mo–12 yr. 200–400 mg q12h for 7–14 days.

▶ **Otitis Media**
PO
Children 6 mo–12 yr. 15 mg/kg q12h for 10 days.

SIDE EFFECTS/ADVERSE REACTIONS
Frequent
Abdominal pain, anorexia, nausea, vomiting, diarrhea
Occasional
Rash, pruritus
Rare
Dizziness, headache, vaginitis

PRECAUTIONS AND CONTRAINDICATIONS
History of anaphylactic reaction to penicillins or hypersensitivity to cephalosporins
Caution:
Lactation, children, renal disease

DRUG INTERACTIONS OF CONCERN TO DENTISTRY
• Decreased effects: tetracyclines, erythromycins, lincomycins

SERIOUS REACTIONS
❗ Antibiotic-associated colitis and other superinfections may result from altered bacterial balance.
❗ Hypersensitivity reactions (ranging from rash, urticaria, and fever to anaphylaxis) occur in less than 5% of patients—most commonly in patients with a history of drug allergies, especially to penicillins.

DENTAL CONSIDERATIONS

General:
• Take precautions regarding allergy to medication.
• Determine why the patient is taking the drug.
• Examine for evidence of oral manifestations of blood dyscrasias (infection, bleeding, poor healing).

Consultations:
• Medical consultation may be required to assess disease control.
• Medical consultation for blood studies (CBC); leukopenic or thrombocytopenic side effects may result in infection, delayed healing, and excessive bleeding. Postpone elective dental treatment until normal values are maintained.

Teach Patient/Family to:
• Encourage effective oral hygiene to prevent soft tissue inflammation.

loratadine
lore-**at**′-ah-deen
(Alavert, Claratyne[AUS], Claritin, Claritin RediTab, Dimetapp, Tavist ND)

CATEGORY AND SCHEDULE
Pregnancy Risk Category: B

Drug Class: Antihistamine, H_1 histamine antagonist

MECHANISM OF ACTION
A long-acting antihistamine that competes with histamine for H_1 receptor sites on effector cells. **Therapeutic Effect:** Prevents allergic responses mediated by histamine, such as rhinitis, urticaria, and pruritus.

USES
Treatment of seasonal allergic rhinitis, idiopathic chronic urticaria

PHARMACOKINETICS

Route	Onset	Peak	Duration
PO	1–3 hr	8–12 hr	Longer than 24 hr

Rapidly and almost completely absorbed from the GI tract. Protein binding: 97%; metabolite, 73%–77%. Distributed mainly to the liver, lungs, GI tract, and bile. Metabolized in the liver to active metabolite; undergoes extensive first-pass metabolism. Eliminated in urine and feces. Not removed by hemodialysis. **Half-life:** 8.4 hr; metabolite, 28 hr (increased in elderly and hepatic impairment).

INDICATIONS AND DOSAGES
▶ **Allergic Rhinitis, Urticaria**
PO
Adults, Elderly, Children 6 yr and older. 10 mg once a day.
Children 2–5 yr. 5 mg once a day.
▶ **Dosage in Hepatic Impairment**
For adults, elderly, and children 6 yr and older dosage is reduced to 10 mg every other day.

SIDE EFFECTS/ADVERSE REACTIONS
Frequent
Headache, fatigue, somnolence
Occasional
Dry mouth, nose, or throat
Rare
Photosensitivity

PRECAUTIONS AND CONTRAINDICATIONS
Hypersensitivity to loratadine or its ingredients
Caution:
Increased intraocular pressure, bronchial asthma, patients at risk for syncope or drowsiness, reduce dose in renal impairment to every other day

DRUG INTERACTIONS OF CONCERN TO DENTISTRY
• Increased CNS depression: all CNS depressants, alcohol
• Increased anticholinergic effect: anticholinergics, antihistamines, antiparkinsonian drugs
• Increased plasma concentration: ketoconazole

SERIOUS REACTIONS
! None known

DENTAL CONSIDERATIONS
General:
• Assess salivary flow as a factor in caries, periodontal disease, and candidiasis.

• Consider semisupine chair position for patients with respiratory disease.
• Conscious sedation drugs may produce synergistic, sedative action.
Teach Patient/Family to:
• Encourage effective oral hygiene to prevent soft tissue inflammation.
• When chronic dry mouth occurs, advise patient to:
  • Avoid mouth rinses with high alcohol content because of drying effects.
  • Use sugarless gum, frequent sips of water, or saliva substitutes.
  • Use daily home fluoride products for anticaries effect.

lorazepam
lor-**ah′**-zeh-pam
(Apo-Lorazepam[CAN], Ativan, Lorazepam Intensol, Novolorazepam[CAN])
Do not confuse lorazepam with Alprazolam.

CATEGORY AND SCHEDULE
Pregnancy Risk Category: D
Controlled Substance Schedule: IV

Drug Class: Benzodiazepine, antianxiety

MECHANISM OF ACTION
A benzodiazepine that enhances the action of the inhibitory neurotransmitter gamma-aminobutyric acid in the CNS, affecting memory, as well as motor, sensory, and cognitive function.
Therapeutic Effect: Produces anxiolytic, anticonvulsant, sedative, muscle relaxant, and antiemetic effects.

USES

Treatment of anxiety, preoperatively in sedation, acute alcohol withdrawal symptoms, muscle spasm

PHARMACOKINETICS

Route	Onset	Peak	Duration
PO	60 min	N/A	8–12 hr
IV	15–30 min	N/A	8–12 hr
IM	30–60 min	N/A	8–12 hr

Well absorbed after PO and IM administration. Protein binding: 85%. Widely distributed. Metabolized in the liver. Primarily excreted in urine. Not removed by hemodialysis. *Half-life:* 10–20 hr.

INDICATIONS AND DOSAGES

▶ **Anxiety**
PO
Adults. 1–10 mg/day in 2–3 divided doses. Average: 2–6 mg/day.
Elderly. Initially, 0.5–1 mg/day. May increase gradually. Range: 0.5–4 mg.
IV
Adults, Elderly. 0.02–0.06 mg/kg q2–6h.
IV Infusion
Adults, Elderly. 0.01–0.1 mg/kg/hr.
PO, IV
Children. 0.05 mg/kg/dose q4–8h. Range: 0.02–0.1 mg/kg. Maximum: 2 mg/dose.

▶ **Insomnia Caused by Anxiety**
PO
Adults. 2–4 mg at bedtime.
Elderly. 0.5–1 mg at bedtime.

▶ **Preoperative Sedation**
IV
Adults, Elderly. 0.044 mg/kg 15–20 min before surgery. Maximum total dose: 2 mg.

IM
Adults, Elderly. 0.05 mg/kg 2 hr before procedure. Maximum total dose: 4 mg.

▶ **Status Epilepticus**
IV
Adults, Elderly. 4 mg over 2–5 min. May repeat in 10–15 min. Maximum: 8 mg in 12-hr period.
Children. 0.1 mg/kg over 2–5 min. May give second dose of 0.05 mg/kg in 15–20 min. Maximum: 4 mg.
Neonates. 0.05 mg/kg. May repeat in 10–15 min.

SIDE EFFECTS/ADVERSE REACTIONS

Frequent
Somnolence (initially in the morning), ataxia, confusion
Occasional
Blurred vision, slurred speech, hypotension, headache
Rare
Paradoxical CNS restlessness or excitement in elderly or debilitated

PRECAUTIONS AND CONTRAINDICATIONS

Angle-closure glaucoma; preexisting CNS depression; severe hypotension; severe uncontrolled pain
Caution:
Elderly, debilitated, hepatic disease, renal disease, myasthenia gravis

DRUG INTERACTIONS OF CONCERN TO DENTISTRY

• Increased effects: alcohol, all CNS depressants, probenecid
• Increased sedation, hallucination: scopolamine
• Possible increase in CNS side effects of kava kava (herb)

SERIOUS REACTIONS

! Abrupt or too-rapid withdrawal may result in pronounced restlessness, irritability, insomnia, hand tremors, abdominal or muscle cramps, diaphoresis, vomiting, and seizures.

! Overdose results in somnolence, confusion, diminished reflexes, and coma.

DENTAL CONSIDERATIONS

General:
• After supine positioning, have patient sit upright for at least 2 min before standing to avoid orthostatic hypotension.
• Elderly persons are more prone to orthostatic hypotension and have increased sensitivity to anticholinergic and sedative effects; use lower dose.
• When administered with opioid analgesic, reduce dose of opioid by one-third.
• Psychologic and physical dependence may occur with chronic administration.
• Have someone drive patient to and from dental office when drug used for conscious sedation.
Consultations:
• Medical consultation may be required to assess disease control.
Teach Patient/Family to:
• Encourage effective oral hygiene to prevent soft tissue inflammation.
• Avoid mouth rinses with high alcohol content because of drying effects.

losartan
lo-**sar**'-tan
(Cozaar)
Do not confuse Cozaar with Zocor.

CATEGORY AND SCHEDULE
Pregnancy Risk Category: C (D if used in second or third trimesters)

Drug Class: Angiotensin II receptor antagonist

MECHANISM OF ACTION
An angiotensin II receptor, type AT1, antagonist that blocks vasoconstrictor and aldosterone-secreting effects of angiotensin II, inhibiting the binding of angiotensin II to the AT1 receptors.
Therapeutic Effect: Causes vasodilation, decreases peripheral resistance, and decreases B/P.

USES
Treatment of hypertension, as a single drug or in combination with other antihypertensives; for reduction of stroke risk in patients with hypertension and left ventricular hypertrophy; nephropathy in Type 2 diabetes mellitus

PHARMACOKINETICS

Route	Onset	Peak	Duration
PO	N/A	6 hr	24 hr

Well absorbed after PO administration. Protein binding: 98%. Undergoes first-pass metabolism in the liver to active metabolites. Excreted in urine and via the biliary system. Not removed by hemodialysis. *Half-life:* 2 hr, metabolite: 6–9 hr.

INDICATIONS AND DOSAGES
▸ **Hypertension**
PO
Adults, Elderly. Initially, 50 mg once a day. Maximum: May be given once or twice a day, with total daily doses ranging from 25–100 mg.
▸ **Nephropathy**
PO
Adults, Elderly. Initially, 50 mg/day. May increase to 100 mg/day based on B/P response.
▸ **Stroke Reduction**
PO
Adults, Elderly. 50 mg/day. Maximum: 100 mg/day.
▸ **Hypertension in Patients with Impaired Hepatic Function**
PO
Adults, Elderly. Initially, 25 mg/day.

SIDE EFFECTS/ADVERSE REACTIONS
Frequent
Upper respiratory tract infection
Occasional
Dizziness, diarrhea, cough
Rare
Insomnia, dyspepsia, heartburn, back and leg pain, muscle cramps, myalgia, nasal congestion, sinusitis

PRECAUTIONS AND CONTRAINDICATIONS
Hypersensitivity, second or third trimester of pregnancy
Caution:
Lactation, children, sodium- and volume-depleted patients, renal impairment.

DRUG INTERACTIONS OF CONCERN TO DENTISTRY
• Potential for increased hypotensive effects with other hypotensive drugs and sedatives
• Suspected increase in antihypertensive effects: fluconazole, ketoconazole; monitor B/P if used concurrently

SERIOUS REACTIONS
! Overdosage may manifest as hypotension and tachycardia. Bradycardia occurs less often.

DENTAL CONSIDERATIONS
General:
• Monitor vital signs at every appointment because of cardiovascular effects.
• Limit use of sodium-containing products, such as saline IV fluids, for patients with a dietary salt restriction.
• Stress from dental procedures may compromise cardiovascular function; determine patient risk.
• Assess salivary flow as a factor in caries, periodontal disease, and candidiasis.
• Short appointments and a stress-reduction protocol may be required for anxious patients.
• Consider semisupine chair position for patient comfort because of respiratory side effects of drug.
• Use precaution if sedation or general anesthesia is required; risk of hypotensive episode.
Consultations:
• Medical consultation may be required to assess disease control and patient's ability to tolerate stress.
Teach Patient/Family to:
• Update health and drug history if physician makes any changes in evaluation or drug regimens; include OTC, herbal, and nonherbal drugs in the update.
• When chronic dry mouth occurs, advise patient to:
  • Avoid mouth rinses with high alcohol content because of drying effects.

- Use daily home fluoride products for anticaries effect.
- Use sugarless gum, frequent sips of water, or saliva substitutes.

loteprednol
loh-teh-**pred'**-nol
(Alrex, Lotemax)

CATEGORY AND SCHEDULE
Pregnancy Risk Category: C

Drug Class: Topical glucocorticoid

MECHANISM OF ACTION
A glucocorticoid that inhibits accumulation of inflammatory cells at inflammation sites, phagocytosis, lysosomal enzyme release and synthesis and/or release of mediators of inflammation.
Therapeutic Effect: Prevents and suppresses cell and tissue immune reactions, inflammatory process.

USES
Treatment of steroid-responsive inflammation of the conjunctiva, cornea, and anterior segments of the globe associated with allergic conjunctivitis, acne rosacea, iritis, superficial punctate keratitis, and so on when topical steroid use is acceptable to reduce inflammation and edema, postoperative inflammation after ocular surgery (Lotemax 0.5%); temporary relief of symptoms of seasonal allergic conjunctivitis (Alrex 0.2%)

PHARMACOKINETICS
Metabolized by enzymes in the eye, minimizing systemic adverse effects.

INDICATIONS AND DOSAGES
▶ **Treatment of Seasonal Allergic Conjunctivitis, Giant Papillary Conjunctivitis, Uritis**
Ophthalmic
Adults, Elderly. Instill 1 drop 4 times a day for 4–6 wk.

SIDE EFFECTS/ADVERSE REACTIONS
Frequent
Blurred vision
Occasional
Decreased vision, watering of eyes, eye pain, nausea, vomiting, burning, stinging, redness of eyes

PRECAUTIONS AND CONTRAINDICATIONS
Acute epithelial herpes simplex keratitis, fungal diseases of ocular structures, vaccinia, varicella, ocular tuberculosis, hypersensitivity, after removal of corneal foreign body, mycobacterial eye infection, acute, purulent, untreated eye infection
Caution:
Prolonged use may result in glaucoma, increased risk of secondary ocular infections, delayed healing after cataract surgery; avoid contamination of sterile container; lactation, safety in children not established

DRUG INTERACTIONS OF CONCERN TO DENTISTRY
- None reported

SERIOUS REACTIONS
! Glaucoma with optic nerve damage, cataract formation, and secondary ocular infection occur rarely.

L

DENTAL CONSIDERATIONS

General:
• Avoid dental light in patient's eyes; offer dark glasses for patient comfort.
• Determine why patient is taking the drug.

loteprednol etabonate; tobramycin

loe-te-**pred**′-nol eh-tah-**bone**′-ayte; toe-bra-**mye**′-sin
(Zylet)

CATEGORY AND SCHEDULE

Pregnancy Risk Category: C

L

Drug Class: Corticosteroid, ophthalmic; antiinflammatory, steroidal, ophthalmic

MECHANISM OF ACTION

A combination ophthalmic product of an aminoglycoside and a glucocorticoid. Loteprednol is a glucocorticoid that inhibits accumulation of inflammatory cells at inflammation sites, phagocytosis, lysosomal enzyme release and synthesis, and/or release of mediators of inflammation. Tobramycin is an antibiotic that irreversibly binds to protein on bacterial ribosomes.
Therapeutic Effect: Prevents and suppresses cell and tissue immune reactions and inflammatory process. Interferes with protein synthesis of susceptible microorganisms.

USES

Treatment of inflammation of the eye, which may occur with certain eye problems or following eye surgery.

PHARMACOKINETICS

Limited systemic absorption.

INDICATIONS AND DOSAGES

▶ **Steroid-Responsive Inflammatory Ocular Conditions for Which a Corticosteroid is Indicated and Where Superficial Bacterial Ocular Infection or a Risk of Bacterial Ocular Infection Exists**
Ophthalmic
Adults, Elderly. Apply 1 or 2 drops into the affected eye(s) q4–6h. During the initial 24–48 hr, the dosing may be increased to every 1–2 hr. Gradually decrease by improvement in clinical signs.

SIDE EFFECTS/ADVERSE REACTIONS

Frequent
Blurred vision
Occasional
Tearing, burning, itching, redness, swelling of eyelid, decreased vision, eye pain
Rare
Nausea, vomiting

PRECAUTIONS AND CONTRAINDICATIONS

Viral diseases of the cornea and conjunctiva including epithelial herpes simplex keratitis (dendritic keratitis), vaccinia, varicella, and mycobacterial infection of the eye and fungal diseases of ocular structures, hypersensitivity to any of loteprednol, tobramycin or any component of the formulation and to other corticosteroids

DRUG INTERACTIONS OF CONCERN TO DENTISTRY

• None reported

SERIOUS REACTIONS

! Glaucoma with optic nerve damage, cataract formation, and

secondary ocular infection occurs rarely.

! Secondary infection, especially fungal infections of the cornea, may occur after use of this medication. These infections are more frequent with long-term applications.

DENTAL CONSIDERATIONS

General:
• Avoid dental light in patient's eyes; offer dark glasses for patient comfort.
• Determine why patient is taking the drug.

lovastatin

lo'-va-sta-tin
(Altoprev, Lotrel, Mevacor)
Do not confuse lovastatin with Leustatin or Livostin, or Mevacor with Mivacron.

CATEGORY AND SCHEDULE
Pregnancy Risk Category: X

Drug Class: Cholesterol-lowering agent

MECHANISM OF ACTION
An antihyperlipidemic that inhibits HMG-CoA reductase, the enzyme that catalyzes the early step in cholesterol synthesis.
Therapeutic Effect: Decreases low-density lipoprotein (LDL) cholesterol, very low-density lipoprotein (VLDL) cholesterol, plasma triglycerides; increases high-density lipoprotein (HDL) cholesterol.

USES
As an adjunct in homozygous familial hypercholesterolemia, mixed hyperlipidemia, elevated serum triglyceride levels, and type IV hyperproteinemia; also reduces total cholesterol LDL-C, apoB, and triglyceride levels; patient should first be placed on cholesterol-lowering diet; primary prevention of CHD and to slow CHD progression

PHARMACOKINETICS

Route	Onset	Peak	Duration
PO	3 days	4–6 wk	N/A

Incompletely absorbed from the GI tract (increased on empty stomach). Protein binding: 95%. Hydrolyzed in the liver to active metabolite. Primarily eliminated in feces. Not removed by hemodialysis. *Half-life:* 1.1–1.7 hr.

INDICATIONS AND DOSAGES
▸ **Hyperlipoproteinemia, Primary Prevention of Coronary Artery Disease**
PO
Adults, Elderly. Initially, 20–40 mg/day with evening meal. Increase at 4-wk intervals up to maximum of 80 mg/day. Maintenance: 20–80 mg/day in single or divided doses.
PO (Extended-Release)
Adults, Elderly. Initially, 20 mg/day. May increase at 4-wk intervals up to 60 mg/day.
Children 10–17 yr. 10–40 mg/day with evening meal.
▸ **Heterozygous Familial Hypercholesterolemia**
PO
Children 10–17 yr. Initially, 10 mg/day. May increase to 20 mg/day after 8 wk and 40 mg/day after 16 wk if needed.

SIDE EFFECTS/ADVERSE REACTIONS

Generally well tolerated. Side effects usually mild and transient.

Frequent

Headache, flatulence, diarrhea, abdominal pain or cramps, rash, and pruritus

Occasional

Nausea, vomiting, constipation, dyspepsia

Rare

Dizziness, heartburn, myalgia, blurred vision, eye irritation

PRECAUTIONS AND CONTRAINDICATIONS

Active liver disease, pregnancy, unexplained elevated liver function tests

Caution:

Past liver disease, alcoholics, severe acute infections, trauma, hypotension, uncontrolled seizure disorders, severe metabolic disorders, electrolyte imbalances

DRUG INTERACTIONS OF CONCERN TO DENTISTRY

• Increased myalgia, rhabdomyolysis: macrolide antibiotics (erythromycin), cyclosporine
• Contraindicated with itraconazole, ketoconazole, erythromycin

SERIOUS REACTIONS

! There is a potential for cataract development.

DENTAL CONSIDERATIONS

General:

• Consider semisupine chair position for patient comfort because of GI side effects.

Teach Patient/Family to:

• Avoid mouth rinses with high alcohol content because of drying effects.

loxapine

lox'-ah-peen

(Apo-Loxapine[CAN], Loxapac[CAN], Loxitane)

CATEGORY AND SCHEDULE

Pregnancy Risk Category: C

Drug Class: Antipsychotic

MECHANISM OF ACTION

A dibenzodiazepine derivative that interferes with the binding of dopamine at postsynaptic receptor sites in brain. Strong anticholinergic effects.

Therapeutic Effect: Suppresses locomotor activity, produces tranquilization.

USES

Treatment of psychotic disorders

PHARMACOKINETICS

Onset of action occurs within 1 hr. Metabolized to active metabolites 8-hydroxyloxapine, 7-hydroxyloxapine, and 8-hydroxyamoxapine. Excreted in urine. **Half-life:** 4 hr.

INDICATIONS AND DOSAGES

▸ **Psychotic Disorders**

PO

Adults. 10 mg 2 times a day. Increase dosage rapidly during first wk to 50 mg, if needed. Usual therapeutic, maintenance range: 60–100 mg daily in 2–4 divided doses. Maximum: 250 mg/day.

SIDE EFFECTS/ADVERSE REACTIONS

Frequent

Blurred vision, confusion, drowsiness, dry mouth, dizziness, light-headedness

Occasional

Allergic reaction (rash, itching), decreased urination, constipation, decreased sexual ability, enlarged breasts, headache, photosensitivity, nausea, vomiting, insomnia, weight gain

PRECAUTIONS AND CONTRAINDICATIONS

Severe CNS depression, comatose states, hypersensitivity to loxapine or any component of the formulation

Caution:

Lactation, seizure disorders, hepatic disease, cardiac disease, prostatic hypertrophy, cardiac conditions, children younger than 16 yr

DRUG INTERACTIONS OF CONCERN TO DENTISTRY

• Increased effects of both drugs: anticholinergics
• Increased CNS depression: alcohol, all CNS depressants
• Decreased effects of sympathomimetics, carbamazepine

SERIOUS REACTIONS

! Extrapyramidal symptoms frequently noted are akathisia (motor restlessness, anxiety). Less frequently noted are akinesia (rigidity, tremors, salivation, mask-like facial expression, reduced voluntary movements). Infrequently noted dystonias: torticollis (neck muscle spasm), opisthotonos (rigidity of back muscles), and oculogyric crisis (rolling back of eyes). Tardive dyskinesia (protrusion of tongue, puffing of cheeks, chewing/puckering of mouth) occurs rarely but may be irreversible. Risk is greater in female elderly patients.

DENTAL CONSIDERATIONS

General:

• Patients on chronic drug therapy may rarely have symptoms of blood dyscrasias, which can include infection, bleeding, and poor healing.
• Assess salivary flow as a factor in caries, periodontal disease, and candidiasis.
• Assess for presence of extrapyramidal motor symptoms, such as tardive dyskinesia and akathisia. Extrapyramidal motor activity may complicate dental treatment.
• After supine positioning, have patient sit upright for at least 2 min before standing to avoid orthostatic hypotension.

Consultations:

• In a patient with symptoms of blood dyscrasias, request a medical consultation for blood studies and postpone dental treatment until normal values are reestablished.
• If signs of tardive dyskinesia or akathisia are present, refer to physician.
• Physician should be informed if significant xerostomic side effects occur (e.g., increased caries, sore tongue, problems eating or swallowing, difficulty wearing prosthesis) so that a medication change can be considered.

Teach Patient/Family to:

• Encourage effective oral hygiene to prevent soft tissue inflammation.

- Use caution to prevent injury when using oral hygiene aids.
- Use powered tooth brush if patient has difficulty holding conventional devices.
- When chronic dry mouth occurs, advise patient to:
  - Avoid mouth rinses with high alcohol content because of drying effects.

- Use sugarless gum, frequent sips of water, or saliva substitutes.
- Use daily home fluoride products for anticaries effect.

L

mafenide
ma′-fe-nide
(Sulfamylon)

CATEGORY AND SCHEDULE
Pregnancy Risk Category: C

Drug Class: Antibacterial, topical; antifungal, topical

MECHANISM OF ACTION
A topical antiinfective that decreases the number of bacteria in avascular tissue of second- and third-degree burns.
Therapeutic Effect: Bacteriostatic. Promotes spontaneous healing of deep partial-thickness burns.

USES
Prevention and treatment of bacterial or fungal infections

PHARMACOKINETICS
Absorbed through devascularized areas into systemic circulation following topical administration. Excreted in the form of its metabolite rhocarboxybenzenes sulfonamide.

INDICATIONS AND DOSAGES
▸ **Burns**
Topical
Adults, Elderly, Children. Apply 1–2 times a day.

SIDE EFFECTS/ADVERSE REACTIONS
Difficult to distinguish side effects and effects of severe burn
Frequent
Pain, burning upon application
Occasional
Allergic reaction (usually 10–14 days after initiation): itching, rash, facial edema, swelling; unexplained syndrome of marked hyperventilation with respiratory alkalosis
Rare
Delay in eschar separation, excoriation of new skin

PRECAUTIONS AND CONTRAINDICATIONS
Hypersensitivity to mafenide or sulfite or any other component of the formulation

DRUG INTERACTIONS OF CONCERN TO DENTISTRY
• None reported

SERIOUS REACTIONS
! Hemolytic anemia, porphyria, bone marrow depression, superinfections (especially with fungi), metabolic acidosis occurs rarely.

M

DENTAL CONSIDERATIONS
General:
• Dental management depends on extent and severity of burns and patient's ability to cooperate; above all use aseptic techniques.
• Provide palliative dental care for dental emergencies only.
• Monitor and record vital signs.
Consultations:
• Medical consultation may be required to assess disease control and patient's ability to tolerate stress.
• Consult patient's physician if an acute dental infection occurs and another antiinfective is required.
Teach Patient/Family to:
• Encourage effective oral hygiene to prevent soft tissue inflammation.
• Prevent trauma when using oral hygiene aids.

magaldrate
mag′-ahl-drate
(Iosopan Plus, Lowsium Plus,
Riopan Plus)

CATEGORY AND SCHEDULE
Pregnancy Risk Category: C

Drug Class: Antacid/aluminum/
magnesium hydroxide

MECHANISM OF ACTION
An antacid that causes fewer
hydrogen ions to be available for
diffusion through the GI mucosa.
Therapeutic Effect: Reduces and
neutralizes gastric acid.

USES
An antacid for hyperacidity

PHARMACOKINETICS
Onset 10–15 min, duration longer
than 3 hr.

INDICATIONS AND DOSAGES
▶ Hyperacidity and Gas
PO
Adults, Elderly. 540–1080 mg
between meals and at bedtime.

SIDE EFFECTS/ADVERSE REACTIONS
Rare
Constipation, diarrhea, fluid
retention, dizziness or light-
headedness, continuing discomfort,
irregular heartbeat, loss of appetite,
mood or mental changes, muscle
weakness, unusual tiredness or
weakness, weight loss, chalky taste

PRECAUTIONS AND CONTRAINDICATIONS
Hypersensitivity to magaldrate,
colostomy or ileostomy, appendicitis,
ulcerative colitis, diverticulitis

Caution:
Elderly, fluid restriction, decreased
GI motility, GI obstruction,
dehydration, renal disease,
sodium-restricted diets, colitis,
gastric outlet obstruction syndrome,
colostomy

DRUG INTERACTIONS OF CONCERN TO DENTISTRY
• Decreased absorption of
anticholinergics, corticosteroids,
sodium fluoride, tetracycline,
ketoconazole, chlordiazepoxide,
ciprofloxacin, metronidazole

SERIOUS REACTIONS
! None known

DENTAL CONSIDERATIONS
General:
• If prescribing oral form of a drug
for which risk of decreased
absorption is reported, advise taking
doses at least 2 hr after or before
antacid use.
• Avoid drugs that could exacerbate
upper GI distress (aspirin and
NSAIDs).
• Consider semisupine chair position
for patient comfort because of GI
effects of disease.

maprotiline
mah-**pro′**-tih-leen
(Ludiomil)

CATEGORY AND SCHEDULE
Pregnancy Risk Category: B

Drug Class: Tetracyclic
antidepressant

MECHANISM OF ACTION
A tetracyclic compound that blocks
reuptake norepinephrine by CNS

presynaptic neuronal membranes, increasing availability at postsynaptic neuronal receptor sites, and enhances synaptic activity. *Therapeutic Effect:* Produces antidepressant effect, with prominent sedative effects and low anticholinergic activity.

USES

Treatment of depression, depression with anxiety, manic depression

PHARMACOKINETICS

Slowly and completely absorbed after PO administration. Protein binding: 88%. Metabolized in liver by hydroxylation and oxidative modification. Excreted in urine. Unknown if removed by hemodialysis. *Half-life:* 27–58 hr.

INDICATIONS AND DOSAGES
▸ **Mild-to-Moderate Depression**
PO
Adults. 75 mg/day to start, in 1–4 divided doses.
Elderly. 50–75 mg/day. In 2 wk, increase dosage gradually in 25 mg increments until therapeutic response is achieved. Reduce to lowest effective maintenance level.
▸ **Severe Depression**
PO
Adults. 100–150 mg/day in 1–4 divided doses. May increase gradually to maximum 225 mg/day.
▸ **Usual Elderly Dosage**
PO
Initially, 25 mg at bedtime. May increase by 25 mg q3–7 days. Maintenance: 50–75 mg/day.

SIDE EFFECTS/ADVERSE REACTIONS
Frequent
Drowsiness, fatigue, dry mouth, blurred vision, constipation, delayed micturition, postural hypotension,

excessive sweating, disturbed concentration, increased appetite, urinary retention
Occasional
GI disturbances (nausea, GI distress, metallic taste sensation), photosensitivity
Rare
Paradoxical reaction (agitation, restlessness, nightmares, insomnia), extrapyramidal symptoms (particularly fine hand tremors)

PRECAUTIONS AND CONTRAINDICATIONS
Acute recovery period following MI, within 14 days of MAOI ingestion, known or suspected seizure disorder, hypersensitivity to maprotiline or any component of the formulation
Caution:
Suicidal patients, severe depression, increased intraocular pressure, narrow-angle glaucoma, urinary retention, cardiac disease, hepatic or renal disease, hypothyroidism, hyperthyroidism, electroshock therapy, elective surgery, elderly, lactation, prostate hypertrophy, schizophrenia, MAOIs

DRUG INTERACTIONS OF CONCERN TO DENTISTRY
• Increased effects of direct-acting sympathomimetics (epinephrine)
• Potential risk of increased CNS depression: alcohol, and all CNS depressants
• Decreased antihypertensive effect: clonidine, guanadrel, guanethidine

SERIOUS REACTIONS
! Higher incidence of seizures than with tricyclic antidepressants, especially in those with no previous history of seizures.
! High dosage may produce cardiovascular effects, such as severe postural hypotension,

M

dizziness, tachycardia, palpitations, and arrhythmias.

! May also result in altered temperature regulation (hyperpyrexia or hypothermia).

! Abrupt withdrawal from prolonged therapy may produce headache, malaise, nausea, vomiting, and vivid dreams.

DENTAL CONSIDERATIONS

General:
• Monitor vital signs at every appointment because of cardiovascular side effects.
• Patients on chronic drug therapy may rarely have symptoms of blood dyscrasias, which can include infection, bleeding, and poor healing.
• Assess salivary flow as a factor in caries, periodontal disease, and candidiasis.
• After supine positioning, have patient sit upright for at least 2 min before standing to avoid orthostatic hypotension.
• Use of epinephrine in gingival retraction cord is contraindicated.
  • Use vasoconstrictors with caution, in low doses, and with careful aspiration.

Consultations:
• In a patient with symptoms of blood dyscrasias, request a medical consultation for blood studies and postpone dental treatment until normal values are reestablished.
• Take precautions if dental surgery is anticipated and anesthesia is required.
• Medical consultation may be required to assess disease control.
• Physician should be informed if significant xerostomic side effects occur (e.g., increased caries, sore tongue, problems eating or swallowing, difficulty wearing

prosthesis) so that a medication change can be considered.

Teach Patient/Family to:
• Encourage effective oral hygiene to prevent soft tissue inflammation.
• Use caution to prevent injury when using oral hygiene aids.
• When chronic dry mouth occurs, advise patient to:
  • Avoid mouth rinses with high alcohol content because of drying effects.
  • Use sugarless gum, frequent sips of water, or saliva substitutes.
  • Use daily home fluoride products for anticaries effect.

mebendazole
meh-**ben**′-dah-zole
(Vermox)

CATEGORY AND SCHEDULE
Pregnancy Risk Category: C

Drug Class: Anthelmintic; carbamate

MECHANISM OF ACTION
A synthetic benzimidazole derivative that degrades parasite cytoplasmic microtubules and irreversibly blocks glucose uptake in helminths and larvae. Vermicidal.
Therapeutic Effect: Depletes glycogen, decreases ATP, causes helminth death.

USES
Treatment of pinworms, roundworms, hookworms, whipworms, thread-worms, pork tapeworms, dwarf tapeworms, beef tapeworms, hydatid cyst

PHARMACOKINETICS
Poorly absorbed from GI tract (absorption increases with food). Metabolized in liver. Primarily eliminated in feces. *Half-life:* 2.5–9 hr (half-life increased with impaired renal function).

INDICATIONS AND DOSAGES
▶ **Trichuriasis, Ascariasis, Hookworm**
PO
Adults, Elderly, Children older than 2 yr. 1 tablet in morning and at bedtime for 3 days.
▶ **Enterobiasis**
PO
Adults, Elderly, Children older than 2 yr. 1 tablet one time.

SIDE EFFECTS/ADVERSE REACTIONS
Occasional
Nausea, vomiting, headache, dizziness, transient abdominal pain, diarrhea with massive infection and expulsion of helminths
Rare
Fever

PRECAUTIONS AND CONTRAINDICATIONS
Hypersensitivity to mebendazole or any component of the formulation

DRUG INTERACTIONS OF CONCERN TO DENTISTRY
• Decreased plasma levels: carbamazepine

SERIOUS REACTIONS
! High dosage may produce reversible myelosuppression (granulocytopenia, leukopenia, neutropenia).

General:
• Determine why patient is taking the drug.
• Patient on chronic drug therapy may rarely present with symptoms of blood dyscrasias, which can include infection, bleeding, and poor healing. If dyscrasia is present, caution patient to prevent oral tissue trauma when using oral hygiene aids.
• Question patient about other drugs he or she is taking.
Consultations:
• In a patient with symptoms of blood dyscrasias, request a medical consultation for blood studies and postpone treatment until normal values are reestablished.

M

mecasermin
mek-ah-**sir**′-men
(Increlex)

CATEGORY AND SCHEDULE
Pregnancy Risk Category: C

Drug Class: Growth hormone

MECHANISM OF ACTION
An insulin-like growth factor-1 (IGF-1) that stimulates the uptake of glucose, fatty acids, and amino acids so that metabolism supports growing tissues.
Therapeutic Effect: Promotes effects of growth hormone.

USES
Treatment for growth failure in children with severe primary IGF-1 deficiency

PHARMACOKINETICS

Absorption has not been determined. Protein binding: greater than 80% bound to IGFBP-3 and acid-labile subunit. Metabolized in liver and kidney. *Half-life:* 5.8 hr.

INDICATIONS AND DOSAGES

▶ **Primary IGF-1 Deficiency (Severe)**
SC
Children. Initially, 0.04–0.08 mg/kg twice a day. Maintenance: May increase by 0.04 mg/kg per dose. Maximum: 0.12 mg/kg twice a day. The drug should be given shortly before or after (20 min) a meal or snack—do not administer when the meal or snack is omitted. Intravenous administration is contraindicated.

SIDE EFFECTS/ADVERSE REACTIONS

Occasional
Hyper/hypoglycemia, headache, snoring, tonsillar hypertrophy, heart murmur, convulsion, dizziness, vomiting, arthralgia, bone pain, extremity pain, muscular atrophy, injection site reactions, papilledema, ear pain, hypoacusis, middle ear fluid, otitis media, serous otitis media, tympanometry abnormal, hematuria, lymphadenopathy, iron-deficiency anemia, ovarian cysts, thymus hypertrophy, thyromegaly, increased liver enzymes
Rare
Hypoglycemic seizure, loss of consciousness secondary to hypoglycemia, intracranial hypertension

PRECAUTIONS AND CONTRAINDICATIONS

Hypersensitivity to mecasermin or its components

Caution:
Avoid in patients with closed epiphyses, active or suspected neoplasia, driving or operating machinery because of hypoglycemic effects

DRUG INTERACTIONS OF CONCERN TO DENTISTRY

• None reported

SERIOUS REACTIONS

! Lymphoid tissue (e.g., tonsillar) hypertrophy associated with complications, such as snoring, sleep apnea, and chronic middle ear effusions have been reported.
! Intracranial hypertension with papilledema, visual changes, headache, nausea and/or vomiting have been reported.
! Local or systemic allergic reactions may occur.

DENTAL CONSIDERATIONS

General:
• Potential acute hypoglycemia

meclizine

mek′-lih-zeen
(Antivert, Bonamine[CAN], Bonine)
Do not confuse Antivert with Axert.

CATEGORY AND SCHEDULE

Pregnancy Risk Category: B

Drug Class: Antihistamine

MECHANISM OF ACTION

An anticholinergic that reduces labyrinthine excitability and diminishes vestibular stimulation of the labyrinth, affecting the chemoreceptor trigger zone.

Therapeutic Effect: Reduces nausea, vomiting, and vertigo.

USES

Treatment of vertigo, motion sickness

PHARMACOKINETICS

Route	Onset	Peak	Duration
PO	30–60 min	N/A	12–24 hr

Well absorbed from the GI tract. Widely distributed. Metabolized in the liver. Primarily excreted in urine. *Half-life:* 6 hr.

INDICATIONS AND DOSAGES
▸ **Motion Sickness**
PO
Adults, Elderly, Children 12 yr and older. 12.5–25 mg 1 hr before travel. May repeat q12–24h. May require a dose of 50 mg.
▸ **Vertigo**
PO
Adults, Elderly, Children 12 yr and older. 25–100 mg/day in divided doses, as needed.

SIDE EFFECTS/ADVERSE REACTIONS
Frequent
Drowsiness
Occasional
Blurred vision; dry mouth, nose, or throat

PRECAUTIONS AND CONTRAINDICATIONS
Hypersensitivity to cyclizines
Caution:
Children, narrow-angle glaucoma, urinary retention, prostatic hypertrophy, elderly, asthma, hypersensitivity to cyclizines

DRUG INTERACTIONS OF CONCERN TO DENTISTRY
• Increased effect of alcohol, other CNS depressants, anticholinergics

SERIOUS REACTIONS
! A hypersensitivity reaction, marked by eczema, pruritus, rash, cardiac disturbances, and photosensitivity, may occur.
! Overdose may produce CNS depression (manifested as sedation, apnea, cardiovascular collapse, or death) or severe paradoxical reactions (such as hallucinations, tremor, and seizures).
! Children may experience paradoxical reactions, including restlessness, insomnia, euphoria, nervousness, and tremors.
! Overdose in children may result in hallucinations, seizures, and death.

DENTAL CONSIDERATIONS
General:
• Assess salivary flow as a factor in caries, periodontal disease, and candidiasis.
Teach Patient/Family to:
• When chronic dry mouth occurs, advise patient to:
  • Avoid mouth rinses with high alcohol content because of drying effects.
  • Use daily home fluoride products for anticaries effect.
  • Use sugarless gum, frequent sips of water, or saliva substitutes.

M

meclofenamate sodium

me-kloe-**fen**′-a-mate **soe**′-dee-um
(Meclomen[CAN])
Do not confuse with meclizine.

CATEGORY AND SCHEDULE

Pregnancy Risk Category: B (D if used in third trimester or near delivery)

Drug Class: Nonsteroidal antiinflammatory

MECHANISM OF ACTION

A nonsteroidal antiinflammatory drug that inhibits prostaglandin synthesis by decreasing activity of the enzyme, cyclooxygenase, which results in decreased formation of prostaglandin precursors.
Therapeutic Effect: Reduces inflammatory response and intensity of pain stimulus reaching sensory nerve endings.

USES

Treatment of mild-to-moderate pain, osteoarthritis, rheumatoid arthritis, dysmenorrhea

PHARMACOKINETICS

PO route, onset 15 min, peak 0.5–1.5 hr, duration 2–4 hr. Completely absorbed from the GI tract. Widely distributed. Protein binding: greater than 99%. Metabolized in liver. Primarily excreted in urine and feces as metabolites. Not removed by hemodialysis. *Half-life:* 2–3.3 hr.

INDICATIONS AND DOSAGES
▸ **Mild-to-Moderate Pain**
PO
Adults, Elderly. 50 mg q4–6h as needed.

▸ **Excessive Menstrual Blood Loss and Primary Dysmenorrhea**
PO
Adults, Elderly. 100 mg 3 times a day for 6 days, starting at the onset of menstrual flow.
▸ **Rheumatoid Arthritis, Osteoarthritis**
PO
Adults, Elderly. 200–400 mg 3–4 times a day.

SIDE EFFECTS/ADVERSE REACTIONS
Frequent
Diarrhea, nausea, abdominal cramping/pain, dyspepsia (heartburn, indigestion, epigastric pain), oral lichenoid reaction
Occasional
Flatulence, rash, dizziness
Rare
Constipation, anorexia, stomatitis, headache, ringing in the ears, rash

PRECAUTIONS AND CONTRAINDICATIONS

Active peptic ulcer disease, chronic inflammation of GI tract, GI bleeding disorders, GI ulceration, history of hypersensitivity to aspirin or NSAIDs
Caution:
Lactation, children younger than 14 yr, bleeding disorders, upper GI disorders, cardiac disorders, hypersensitivity to other antiinflammatory agents

DRUG INTERACTIONS OF CONCERN TO DENTISTRY
• GI ulceration, bleeding: aspirin, alcohol, corticosteroids, bisphosphonates
• Nephrotoxicity: acetaminophen (prolonged use)
• Possible risk of decreased renal function: cyclosporine

- SSRIs: NSAIDs increase risk of GI side effects
- When prescribed for dental pain:
  - Risk of increased effects: oral anticoagulants, oral antidiabetics, lithium, methotrexate
  - Decreased effects of diuretics, β-adrenergic blockers

SERIOUS REACTIONS

! Overdosage may result in headache, seizure, vomiting, and cerebral edema.

! Peptic ulcer disease, GI bleeding, gastritis, severe hepatic reactions, such as jaundice, nephrotoxicity, marked by hematuria, dysuria, proteinuria, and severe hypersensitivity reaction, including bronchospasm, and facial edema occur rarely.

DENTAL CONSIDERATIONS

General:
- Increased potential for adverse cardiovascular events in patients at risk for thromboembolism.
- Patients on chronic drug therapy may rarely have symptoms of blood dyscrasias, which can include infection, bleeding, and poor healing.
- Assess salivary flow as a factor in caries, periodontal disease, and candidiasis.
- Avoid prescribing for dental use in pregnancy.
- Avoid prescribing aspirin-containing products.
- Consider semisupine chair position for patients with rheumatic disease.
- Severe stomach bleeding may occur in patients who regularly use NSAIDs in recommended doses, when the patient is also taking another NSAID, a blood thinning, or steroid drug, if the patient has GI or peptic ulcer disease, if they are 60 yr or older, or when NSAIDs are taken longer than directed. Warn patients of the potential for severe stomach bleeding.

Consultations:
- In a patient with symptoms of blood dyscrasias, request a medical consultation for blood studies and postpone dental treatment until normal values are reestablished.
- Medical consultation may be required to assess disease control.

Teach Patient/Family to:
- Encourage effective oral hygiene to prevent soft tissue inflammation.
- Use caution to prevent injury when using oral hygiene aids.
- Warn patient of potential risks of NSAIDs.
- When chronic dry mouth occurs, advise patient to:
  - Avoid mouth rinses with high alcohol content because of drying effects.
  - Use sugarless gum, frequent sips of water, or saliva substitutes.
  - Use daily home fluoride products for anticaries effect.

M

medroxyprogesterone acetate

me-**drox**′-ee-proe-**jess**′-te-rone **ass**′-ih-tate
(Depo-Provera, Depo-Provera Contraceptive, Novo-Medrone[CAN], Provera, Ralovera[AUS])
Do not confuse medroxyprogesterone with hydroxyprogesterone, methylprednisolone, or methyltestosterone.

CATEGORY AND SCHEDULE
Pregnancy Risk Category: X

Drug Class: Progestogen

MECHANISM OF ACTION

A hormone that transforms endometrium from proliferative to secretory in an estrogen-primed endometrium. Inhibits secretion of pituitary gonadotropins. *Therapeutic Effect:* Prevents follicular maturation and ovulation. Stimulates growth of mammary alveolar tissue and relaxes uterine smooth muscle. Corrects hormonal imbalance.

USES

Treatment of uterine bleeding (abnormal), secondary amenorrhea, endometrial cancer, metastatic renal cancer, contraceptive; with estrogens to reduce incidence of endometrial hyperplasia, cancer

PHARMACOKINETICS

Slowly absorbed after IM administration. Protein binding: 90%. Metabolized in the liver. Primarily excreted in urine. *Half-life:* 30 days.

INDICATIONS AND DOSAGES
▸ **Endometrial Hyperplasia**
PO
Adults. 2.5–10 mg/day for 14 days.
▸ **Secondary Amenorrhea**
PO
Adults. 5–10 mg/day for 5–10 days, beginning at any time during menstrual cycle or 2.5 mg/day.
▸ **Abnormal Uterine Bleeding**
PO
Adults. 5–10 mg/day for 5–10 days, beginning on calculated day 16 or day 21 of menstrual cycle.
▸ **Endometrial, Renal Carcinoma**
IM
Adults, Elderly. Initially, 400–1000 mg; repeat at 1-wk intervals. If improvement occurs and disease is stabilized, begin maintenance with as little as 400 mg/mo.

▸ **Prevention of Pregnancy**
IM
Adults. 150 mg q3mo.

SIDE EFFECTS/ADVERSE REACTIONS
Frequent
Transient menstrual abnormalities (including spotting, change in menstrual flow or cervical secretions, and amenorrhea) at initiation of therapy
Occasional
Edema, weight change, breast tenderness, nervousness, insomnia, fatigue, dizziness
Rare
Alopecia, depression, dermatologic changes, headache, fever, nausea

PRECAUTIONS AND CONTRAINDICATIONS

Carcinoma of breast; estrogen-dependent neoplasm; history of or active thrombotic disorders, such as cerebral apoplexy, thrombophlebitis, or thromboembolic disorders; hypersensitivity to progestins; known or suspected pregnancy; missed abortion; severe hepatic dysfunction; undiagnosed abnormal genital bleeding; use as pregnancy test
Caution:
Lactation, hypertension, asthma, blood dyscrasias, gallbladder disease, CHF, diabetes mellitus, bone disease, depression, migraine headache, convulsive disorders, hepatic disease, renal disease, family history of cancer of breast or reproductive tract

SERIOUS REACTIONS

! Thrombophlebitis, pulmonary or cerebral embolism, and retinal thrombosis occur rarely.

General:
• Place on frequent recall to evaluate inflammatory and healing response.
Teach Patient/Family to:
• Encourage effective oral hygiene to prevent soft tissue inflammation.

---

medrysone
meh'-dri-sone
(HMS Liquifilm)

CATEGORY AND SCHEDULE
Pregnancy Risk Category: C

Drug Class: Antiinflammatory, steroidal, ophthalmic; corticosteroid, ophthalmic

MECHANISM OF ACTION
A topical synthetic corticosteroid that inhibits accumulation of inflammatory cells at inflammation sites.
Therapeutic Effect: Inhibits inflammatory process.

USES
Prevention of permanent damage to the eye, which may occur with certain eye problems. Also provides relief from redness, irritation, and other discomfort.

PHARMACOKINETICS
Absorbed through aqueous humor. Metabolized in liver if absorbed. Excreted in urine and feces.

INDICATIONS AND DOSAGES
▸ **Ophthalmic Disorders**
Ophthalmic
Adults, Elderly, Children 3 yr and older. Instill 1 drop up to every 4 hr.

SIDE EFFECTS/ADVERSE REACTIONS
Frequent
Blurred vision
Occasional
Decreased vision, watering of eyes, eye pain, burning, stinging, redness of eyes, nausea, vomiting

PRECAUTIONS AND CONTRAINDICATIONS
Active superficial herpes simplex, conjunctival or corneal viral disease, fungal diseases of the eye, ocular tuberculosis, hypersensitivity to medrysone or any component of the formulation

DRUG INTERACTIONS OF CONCERN TO DENTISTRY
• None reported

SERIOUS REACTIONS
! Systemic absorption may occur with topical application.
! Cataracts, corneal thinning, corneal ulcers, delayed wound healing, optic nerve damage, and glaucoma have been reported.

General:
• Determine why patient is taking the drug.
• Avoid dental light in patient's eyes; offer dark glasses for patient comfort.

M

mefenamic acid
meh-feh-**nam'**-ik
(Apo-Mefenamic[CAN],
Nu-Mefenamic[CAN], PMS-
Mefenamic Acid[CAN],
Ponstan[CAN], Ponstel)

CATEGORY AND SCHEDULE
Pregnancy Risk Category: C (D if
used in third trimester or near
delivery)

Drug Class: Nonsteroidal
antiinflammatory

MECHANISM OF ACTION
A nonsteroidal antiinflammatory that
produces analgesic and
antiinflammatory effect by inhibiting
prostaglandin synthesis.
Therapeutic Effect: Reduces
inflammatory response and intensity
of pain stimulus reaching sensory
nerve endings.

USES
Treatment of mild-to-moderate
pain, dysmenorrhea, inflammatory
disease

PHARMACOKINETICS
Rapidly absorbed from the GI tract.
Protein binding: high. Metabolized
in liver. Partially excreted in urine
and partially in the feces. Not
removed by hemodialysis. ***Half-life:***
3.5 hr.

INDICATIONS AND DOSAGES
▸ **Mild-to-Moderate Pain, Lower
Back Pain, Dysmenorrhea**
PO
*Adults, Elderly, Children 14 yr and
older.* Initially, 500 mg to start, then
250 mg q4h as needed. Maximum:
1 wk of therapy.

SIDE EFFECTS/ADVERSE REACTIONS
Occasional
Dyspepsia, including heartburn,
indigestion, flatulence, abdominal
cramping, constipation, nausea,
diarrhea, epigastric pain, vomiting,
headache, nervousness, dizziness,
bleeding, elevated liver function
tests, tinnitus, oral lichenoid
reaction
Rare
Fluid retention, arrhythmias,
tachycardia, confusion, drowsiness,
rash, dry eyes, blurred vision, hot
flashes

PRECAUTIONS AND CONTRAINDICATIONS
History of hypersensitivity to aspirin
or NSAIDs, pregnancy
Caution:
Lactation, children, bleeding
disorders, GI disorders, cardiac
disorders, hypersensitivity to other
antiinflammatory agents

DRUG INTERACTIONS OF CONCERN TO DENTISTRY
• GI bleeding, ulceration: aspirin,
alcohol, corticosteroids
• Nephrotoxicity: acetaminophen
(prolonged use and high doses)
• Possible risk of decreased renal
function: cyclosporine
• SSRIs: NSAIDs increase risk of
GI side effects
• When prescribed for dental pain:
  • Risk of increased effects of
  oral anticoagulants, oral
  antidiabetics, lithium,
  methotrexate
  • Decreased effects of diuretics

SERIOUS REACTIONS
! Peptic ulcer, GI bleeding, gastritis,
and severe hepatic reaction, such as
cholestasis and jaundice, occur
rarely.

! Nephrotoxicity, including dysuria, hematuria, proteinuria, and nephrotic syndrome and severe hypersensitivity reaction, marked by bronchospasm, and angioedema occur rarely.

DENTAL CONSIDERATIONS
General:
• Avoid prescribing for dental use in pregnancy.
• Avoid prescribing aspirin-containing products.
• Potential for increased adverse cardiovascular events in patients at risk for thromboembolism.
• Severe stomach bleeding may occur in patients who regularly use NSAIDs in recommended doses, when the patient is also taking another NSAID, a blood thinning, or steroid drug, if the patient has GI or peptic ulcer disease, if they are 60 yr or older, or when NSAIDs are taken longer than directed. Warn patients of the potential for severe stomach bleeding.
Consultations:
• Medical consultation may be required to assess disease control.
Teach Patient/Family to:
• Warn patient of potential risks of NSAIDs.

mefloquine
meh′-flow-quine
(Lariam)
Do not confuse with Librium.

CATEGORY AND SCHEDULE
Pregnancy Risk Category: C

Drug Class: Antimalarial

MECHANISM OF ACTION
A quinolone-methanol compound structurally similar to quinine that destroys the asexual blood forms of malarial pathogens, *Plasmodium falciparum, P. vivax, P. malariae, P. ovale.*
Therapeutic Effect: Inhibits parasite growth.

USES
Prevention or treatment of malaria, a red blood cell infection transmitted by the bite of a mosquito

PHARMACOKINETICS
Well absorbed from the GI tract. Protein binding: 98%. Widely distributed, including CSF. Metabolized in liver. Primarily excreted in urine. *Half-life:* 21–22 days.

INDICATIONS AND DOSAGES
▸ Suppression of Malaria
PO
Adults. 250 mg base weekly starting 1 wk before travel, continuing weekly during travel and for 4 wk after leaving endemic area.
Children more than 45 kg. 250 mg weekly starting 1 wk before travel, continuing weekly during travel and for 4 wk after leaving endemic area.
Children 30–45 kg. 187.5 mg (¾ tablet) weekly starting 1 wk before travel, continuing weekly during travel and for 4 wk after leaving endemic area.
Children 20–30 kg. 125 mg (½ tablet) weekly starting 1 wk before travel, continuing weekly during travel and for 4 wk after leaving endemic area.
Children 10–20 kg. 62.5 mg (¼ tablet) weekly starting 1 wk before travel, continuing weekly during travel and for 4 wk after leaving endemic area.

M

▶ **Treatment of Malaria**
PO
Adults. 1250 mg as a single dose.
Children. 15–25 mg/kg in a single dose. Maximum: 1250 mg.

SIDE EFFECTS/ADVERSE REACTIONS
Occasional
Mild transient headache, difficulty concentrating, insomnia, light-headedness, vertigo, diarrhea, nausea, vomiting, visual disturbances, tinnitus
Rare
Aggressive behavior, anxiety, bradycardia, depression, hallucinations, hypotension, panic attacks, paranoia, psychosis, syncope, tremors

PRECAUTIONS AND CONTRAINDICATIONS
Cardiac abnormalities, severe psychiatric disorders, epilepsy, history of hypersensitivity to mefloquine

DRUG INTERACTIONS OF CONCERN TO DENTISTRY
• None reported

SERIOUS REACTIONS
! Prolonged therapy may result in peripheral neuritis, neuromyopathy, hypotension, ECG changes, agranulocytosis, aplastic anemia, thrombocytopenia, seizures, and psychosis.
! Overdosage may result in headache, vomiting, visual disturbance, drowsiness, and seizures.

DENTAL CONSIDERATIONS
General:
• Consider semisupine chair position for patient comfort if GI side effects occur.

• Question patient about tolerance of NSAIDs or aspirin related to GI disease.
• Determine why patient is taking the drug.
• Be aware of patient's disease, its severity and frequency of NSAIDs or aspirin related to GI disease.
• Monitor and record vital signs.
Consultations:
• Medical consultation may be required to assess disease control and patient's ability to tolerate stress.
Teach Patient/Family to:
• Prevent trauma when using oral hygiene aids.
• Avoid performing tasks that require mental alertness.

megestrol acetate
meh-**jess**′-trole **ass**′-eh-tayte
(Apo-Megestrol[CAN], Megace, Megostat[AUS])

CATEGORY AND SCHEDULE
Pregnancy Risk Category: X (for suspension), D (for tablets)

Drug Class: Progestin

MECHANISM OF ACTION
A hormone and antineoplastic agent that suppresses the release of luteinizing hormone from the anterior pituitary gland by inhibiting pituitary function.
Therapeutic Effect: Shrinks tumors. Also increases appetite by an unknown mechanism.

USES
Treatment of breast, endometrial cancer, renal cell cancer; AIDS wasting syndrome

PHARMACOKINETICS
Well absorbed from the GI tract. Metabolized in the liver; excreted in urine.

INDICATIONS AND DOSAGES
▶ **Palliative Treatment of Advanced Breast Cancer**
PO

Adults, Elderly. 160 mg/day in 4 equally divided doses.
▶ **Palliative Treatment of Advanced Endometrial Carcinoma**
PO

Adults, Elderly. 40–320 mg/day in divided doses. Maximum: 800 mg/day in 1–4 divided doses.
▶ **Anorexia, Cachexia, Weight Loss**
PO

Adults, Elderly. 800 mg (20 ml)/day.

SIDE EFFECTS/ADVERSE REACTIONS
Frequent
Weight gain secondary to increased appetite
Occasional
Nausea, breakthrough bleeding, backache, headache, breast tenderness, carpal tunnel syndrome
Rare
Feelings of coldness

PRECAUTIONS AND CONTRAINDICATIONS
Hypersensitivity

SERIOUS REACTIONS
! Thrombophlebitis and pulmonary embolism occur rarely.

DENTAL CONSIDERATIONS
General:
• Place on frequent recall to evaluate inflammatory and healing response.
• Patients receiving chemotherapy may require palliative treatment for stomatitis.

Teach Patient/Family to:
• Encourage effective oral hygiene to prevent soft tissue inflammation.

meloxicam
mel-**oks**'-ih-kam
(Mobic)

CATEGORY AND SCHEDULE
Pregnancy Risk Category: C (D if used in third trimester or near delivery)

Drug Class: Nonsteroidal antiinflammatory

MECHANISM OF ACTION
An NSAID that produces analgesic and antiinflammatory effects by inhibiting prostaglandin synthesis. *Therapeutic Effect:* Reduces the inflammatory response and intensity of pain.

USES
Relief of signs and symptoms of osteoarthritis

PHARMACOKINETICS

Route	Onset	Peak	Duration
PO (analgesic)	30 min	4–5 hr	N/A

Well absorbed after PO administration. Protein binding: 99%. Metabolized in the liver. Eliminated in urine and feces. Not removed by hemodialysis. *Half-life:* 15–20 hr.

INDICATIONS AND DOSAGES
▶ **Osteoarthritis, Rheumatoid Arthritis**
PO

Adults. Initially, 7.5 mg/day. Maximum: 15 mg/day.

SIDE EFFECTS/ADVERSE REACTIONS

Frequent
Dyspepsia, headache, diarrhea, nausea

Occasional
Dizziness, insomnia, rash, pruritus, flatulence, constipation, vomiting

Rare
Somnolence, urticaria, photosensitivity, tinnitus

PRECAUTIONS AND CONTRAINDICATIONS

Aspirin-induced nasal polyps associated with bronchospasm

Caution:
Preexisting asthma, anaphylactic reactions to NSAIDs, serious GI side effects may occur, GI ulcer or GI bleeding; avoid in late pregnancy, liver dysfunction, dehydration, long-term use, edema, heart failure, hypertension, ACE inhibitors, lactation, elderly

DRUG INTERACTIONS OF CONCERN TO DENTISTRY

- Increased risk of GI side effects: long-duration NSAIDs, aspirin (except low-dose form), oral glucocorticoids, alcoholism, smoking, older age, and generally poor health
- Increased blood levels: lithium
- Reduced natriuretic effect: furosemide and other loop diuretics
- SSRIs: NSAIDs increase risk of GI side effects

SERIOUS REACTIONS

! Rare reactions with long-term use include peptic ulcer disease, GI bleeding, gastritis, severe hepatic reaction (jaundice), nephrotoxicity (hematuria, dysuria, proteinuria), and a severe hypersensitivity reaction (bronchospasm, angioedema).

DENTAL CONSIDERATIONS

General:
- Potential for increased adverse cardiovascular events in patients at risk for thromboembolism.
- Assess salivary flow as a factor in caries, periodontal disease, and candidiasis.
- Avoid prescribing for dental use in pregnancy.
- Patients on chronic drug therapy may rarely have symptoms of blood dyscrasias, which can include infection, bleeding, and poor healing.
- Consider semisupine chair position for patient comfort if GI side effects occur.
- Severe stomach bleeding may occur in patients who regularly use NSAIDs in recommended doses, when the patient is also taking another NSAID, a blood thinning, or steroid drug, if the patient has GI or peptic ulcer disease, if they are 60 yr or older, or when NSAIDs are taken longer than directed. Warn patients of the potential for severe stomach bleeding.

Consultations:
- In a patient with symptoms of blood dyscrasias, request a medical consultation for blood studies and postpone treatment until normal values are reestablished.

Teach Patient/Family to:
- Use powered tooth brush if patient has difficulty holding conventional devices.
- Update health and drug history if physician makes any changes in evaluation or drug regimens; include OTC, herbal, and nonherbal drugs in the update.
- Encourage effective oral hygiene to prevent soft tissue inflammation.

- Prevent trauma when using oral hygiene aids.
- Warn patient of potential risks of NSAIDs.
- When chronic dry mouth occurs, advise patient to:
  - Avoid mouth rinses with high alcohol content because of drying effects.
  - Use daily home fluoride products for anticaries effect.
  - Use sugarless gum, frequent sips of water, or saliva substitutes.

melphalan
mel′-fah-lan
(Alkeran)
Do not confuse Alkeran with Leukeran, or melphalan with Mephyton or Myleran.

CATEGORY AND SCHEDULE
Pregnancy Risk Category: D

Drug Class: Antineoplastic

MECHANISM OF ACTION
An alkylating agent that inhibits protein synthesis primarily by cross-linking with strands of DNA and RNA, producing cell death. Cell cycle–phase nonspecific.
Therapeutic Effect: Disrupts nucleic acid function.

USES
Palliative treatment of multiple myeloma and nonresectable epithelial carcinoma of the ovary

PHARMACOKINETICS
Half-life: 1.5 hr; first-pass hepatic metabolism; plasma levels vary; metabolites excreted in urine.

INDICATIONS AND DOSAGES
▶ **Ovarian Carcinoma**
PO
Adults, Elderly. 0.2 mg/kg/day for 5 successive days. Repeat at 4- to 6-wk intervals.
▶ **Multiple Myeloma**
PO
Adults. Initially, 6 mg once a day, adjusted as indicated; or 0.15 mg/kg/day for 7 days or 0.25 mg/kg/day for 4 days. Repeat at 4- to 6-wk intervals.
IV
Adults. 16 mg/m^2/dose every 2 wk for 4 doses, then repeated monthly according to protocol.
▶ **Dosage in Renal Impairment**
PO, IV
BUN level greater than 30 mg/dl. Decrease melphalan dosage by 50%. Serum creatinine level greater than 1.5 mg/dl. Decrease the melphalan dosage by 50%.

SIDE EFFECTS/ADVERSE REACTIONS
Frequent
Nausea, vomiting (may be severe with large dose)
Occasional
Diarrhea, stomatitis, rash, pruritus, alopecia

PRECAUTIONS AND CONTRAINDICATIONS
Pregnancy, severe myelosuppression
Caution:
Severe bone marrow depression risk, renal impairment

DRUG INTERACTIONS OF CONCERN TO DENTISTRY
- Increased toxicity: antineoplastics, radiation

SERIOUS REACTIONS
! Myelosuppression may cause hematologic toxicity, manifested

principally as leukopenia and thrombocytopenia and, to lesser extent, anemia, pancytopenia, and agranulocytosis. Leukopenia may occur as early as 5 days after drug initiation.

! WBC and platelet counts return to normal levels during the fifth week of therapy, but leukopenia and thrombocytopenia may last more than 6 wk after the drug is discontinued.

! Hyperuricemia, marked by hematuria, crystalluria, and flank pain, may occur.

DENTAL CONSIDERATIONS

General:
• Patients receiving chemotherapy may be taking chronic opioids for pain. Consider NSAIDs for dental pain management.
• Patients receiving chemotherapy may require palliative therapy for stomatitis.
• Patients on chronic drug therapy may rarely have symptoms of blood dyscrasias, which can include infection, bleeding, and poor healing.

Consultations:
• Medical consultation may be required to assess disease control.
• In a patient with symptoms of blood dyscrasias, request a medical consultation for blood studies and postpone dental treatment until normal values are reestablished.

Teach Patient/Family to:
• See dentist immediately if secondary oral infection occurs.
• When chronic dry mouth occurs, advise patient to:
  • Avoid mouth rinses with high alcohol content because of drying effects.

• Use sugarless gum, frequent sips of water, or saliva substitutes.
• Use daily home fluoride products for anticaries effect.

memantine hydrochloride

meh-**man**′-teen
high-droh-**klor**′-ide
(Ebixa[AUS], Namenda)

CATEGORY AND SCHEDULE
Pregnancy Risk Category: B

Drug Class: NMDA receptor antagonist

MECHANISM OF ACTION
A neurotransmitter inhibitor that decreases the effects of glutamate, the principal excitatory neurotransmitter in the brain. Persistent CNS excitation by glutamate is thought to cause the symptoms of Alzheimer's disease.
Therapeutic Effect: May reduce clinical deterioration in moderate to severe Alzheimer's disease.

USES
Treatment of moderate-to-severe dementia of Alzheimer's disease

PHARMACOKINETICS
Rapidly and completely absorbed after PO administration. Protein binding: 45%. Undergoes little metabolism; most of the dose is excreted unchanged in urine.
Half-life: 60–80 hr.

INDICATIONS AND DOSAGES
▸ **Alzheimer's Disease**
PO
Adults, Elderly. Initially, 5 mg once a day. May increase dosage at intervals of at least 1 wk in 5-mg increments to 10 mg/day (5 mg twice a day), then 15 mg/day (5 mg and 10 mg as separate doses), and finally 20 mg/day (10 mg twice a day). Target dose: 20 mg/day.

SIDE EFFECTS/ADVERSE REACTIONS
Occasional
Dizziness, headache, confusion, constipation, hypertension, cough
Rare
Back pain, nausea, fatigue, anxiety, peripheral edema, arthralgia, insomnia

PRECAUTIONS AND CONTRAINDICATIONS
Severe renal impairment
Caution:
Moderate to severe renal impairment, alkaline urine pH, safety and efficacy in nursing mothers and pediatric patients have not been established

DRUG INTERACTIONS OF CONCERN TO DENTISTRY
• None reported

SERIOUS REACTIONS
! None known

DENTAL CONSIDERATIONS
General:
• Monitor vital signs at every appointment because of cardiovascular side effects.
• Patients with Alzheimer's disease may be taking other drugs; get a complete drug history.

• Drug may be used late in disease process; ensure caregiver or responsible person understands informed consent.
• Place on frequent recall to evaluate oral health.
Consultations:
• Consultation with physician may be necessary if sedation or general anesthesia is required.
Teach Patient/Family to:
• Use powered tooth brush if patient has difficulty holding conventional devices.
• Encourage effective oral hygiene to prevent soft tissue inflammation/infection.
• Prevent trauma when using oral hygiene aids.
• Update health and drug history and reporting changes in health status, drug regimen, or disease/treatment status; include OTC, herbal, and nonherbal drugs in the update.

M

meperidine hydrochloride
me-**per**'-ih-deen
high-droh-**klor**'-ide
(Demerol, Pethidine Injection[AUS])
Do not confuse with Demulen or Dymelor.

CATEGORY AND SCHEDULE
Pregnancy Risk Category: B (D if used for prolonged periods or at high dosages at term)
Controlled Substance: Schedule II

Drug Class: Synthetic opioid analgesic

MECHANISM OF ACTION

An opioid agonist that binds to opioid receptors in the CNS. *Therapeutic Effect:* Alters the perception of and emotional response to pain.

USES

Treatment of moderate-to-severe pain, preoperatively in sedation techniques

PHARMACOKINETICS

Route	Onset	Peak	Duration
PO	15 min	60 min	2–4 hr
IV	Less than 5 min	5–7 min	2–3 hr
IM	10–15 min	30–50 min	2–4 hr
SC	10–15 min	30–50 min	2–4 hr

Variably absorbed from the GI tract; well absorbed after IM administration. Protein binding: 60%–80%. Widely distributed. Metabolized in the liver to active metabolite. Primarily excreted in urine. Not removed by hemodialysis. *Half-life:* 2.4–4 hr; metabolite 8–16 hr (increased in hepatic impairment and disease).

INDICATIONS AND DOSAGES

▸ **Analgesia**

PO, IM, Subcutaneous

Adults, Elderly. 50–150 mg q3–4h.

Children. 1.1–1.5 mg/kg q3–4h. Don't exceed single dose of 100 mg.

▸ **Patient-Controlled Analgesia**

IV

Adults. Loading dose: 50–100 mg. Intermittent bolus: 5–30 mg. Lockout interval: 10–20 min. Continuous infusion: 5–40 mg/hr. Maximum (4-hr): 200–300 mg.

▸ **Dosage in Renal Impairment**

Dosage is based on creatinine clearance.

Creatinine Clearance	Dosage
10–50 ml/min	75% of usual dose
Less than 10 ml/min	50% of usual dose

SIDE EFFECTS/ADVERSE REACTIONS

Frequent

Sedation, hypotension (including orthostatic hypotension), diaphoresis, facial flushing, dizziness, nausea, vomiting, constipation

Occasional

Confusion, arrhythmias, tremors, urine retention, abdominal pain, dry mouth, headache, irritation at injection site, euphoria, dysphoria

Rare

Allergic reaction (rash, pruritus), insomnia

PRECAUTIONS AND CONTRAINDICATIONS

Delivery of premature infant, diarrhea because of poisoning, use within 14 days of MAOIs

Caution:

Addictive personality, lactation, increased intracranial pressure, MI (acute), severe heart disease, respiratory depression, hepatic disease, renal disease, children younger than 18 yr

DRUG INTERACTIONS OF CONCERN TO DENTISTRY

• Increased effects with all CNS depressants, neuromuscular blocking agents
• Contraindication: MAOIs, sibutramine
• Increased effects of anticholinergics
• Suspected increase in normeperidine levels: ritonavir
• Increased risk of hypotension: antihypertensive drugs

SERIOUS REACTIONS

! Overdose results in respiratory depression, skeletal muscle flaccidity, cold or clammy skin, cyanosis, and extreme somnolence progressing to seizures, stupor, and coma. The antidote is 0.4 mg naloxone.

! The patient who uses meperidine repeatedly may develop a tolerance to the drug's analgesic effect and physical dependence.

DENTAL CONSIDERATIONS

General:
• Avoid prescribing for dental use in pregnancy.
• After supine positioning, have patient sit upright for at least 2 min before standing to avoid orthostatic hypotension.
• Psychologic and physical dependence may occur with chronic administration.

Teach Patient/Family to:
• Avoid mouth rinses with high alcohol content because of drying effects.

mephentermine sulfate

meh-**fen**′-ter-meen **sull**′-fate
(Wyamine Sulfate)

CATEGORY AND SCHEDULE

Pregnancy Risk Category: C

Drug Class: Sympathomimetic

MECHANISM OF ACTION

A sympathomimetic amine that acts indirectly by releasing norepinephrine and directly by exerting a slight effect on α and β_1 receptors and a moderate effect on β_2 receptors mediating vasodilation. **Therapeutic Effect:** Produces cardiac stimulation.

USES

Treatment of hypotension because of anesthesia, ganglionic blockade, or hemorrhage

PHARMACOKINETICS

Onset of action occurs immediately and persists 15–30 min. Metabolized in liver. Excreted in urine. **Half-life:** 17–18 hr.

INDICATIONS AND DOSAGES

▸ **Hypotension (Secondary to Spinal Anesthesia)**
IM/IV
Adults. 30–45 mg as a single injection.
▸ **Prophylaxis of Hypotension in Spinal Anesthesia**
IM/IV
Adults. 30–45 mg 10–20 min before anesthesia.

SIDE EFFECTS/ADVERSE REACTIONS

Occasional
Anxiety, nervousness, cardiac arrhythmias, increased B/P

PRECAUTIONS AND CONTRAINDICATIONS

Concurrent use or within 14 days of discontinuation of MAOI therapy, hypotension induced by chlorpromazine, hypersensitivity to mephentermine or sympathomimetic amines

DRUG INTERACTIONS OF CONCERN TO DENTISTRY

• Increased risk of arrhythmia: halogenated hydrocarbon anesthetics

SERIOUS REACTIONS

! Mephentermine may produce arrhythmias, including transient extrasystoles, AV block, and hypertension.

M

! CNS effects, including hyperexcitability, prolonged wakefulness, weeping, incoherence, convulsions, flushing, tremors, and hallucinations, may occur with large doses of mephentermine.

DENTAL CONSIDERATIONS

General:
• For use in hospitals or emergency rooms for selected hypotensive episodes.

mephobarbital
me′-foe-**bar**′-bi-tal
(Mebaral)

CATEGORY AND SCHEDULE
Pregnancy Risk Category: D
Controlled substance: Schedule IV

Drug Class: Barbiturate anticonvulsant

MECHANISM OF ACTION
A barbiturate that increases seizure threshold in the motor cortex.
Therapeutic Effect: Depresses monosynaptic and polysynaptic transmission in the CNS.

USES
Treatment of generalized tonic-clonic (grand mal) or absence (petit mal) seizures, sedation

PHARMACOKINETICS
PO route onset 20–60 min, peak N/A, duration 6–8 hr. Well absorbed after PO administration. Widely distributed. Metabolized in liver to active metabolite, a form of phenobarbital. Minimally excreted in urine. Removed by hemodialysis.
Half-life: 34 hr.

INDICATIONS AND DOSAGES
▸ **Epilepsy**
PO
Adults, Elderly. 400–600 mg/day in divided doses or at bedtime.
Children older than 5 yr. 32–64 mg 3 or 4 times a day.
Children younger than 5 yr. 16–32 mg 3 or 4 times a day.
▸ **Sedation**
PO
Adults, Elderly. 32–100 mg/day in 3–4 divided doses.
Children. 16–32 mg in 3–4 divided doses.

SIDE EFFECTS/ADVERSE REACTIONS
Frequent
Dizziness, light-headedness, somnolence
Occasional
Confusion, headache, insomnia, mental depression, nervousness, nightmares, unusual excitement
Rare
Rash, paradoxical CNS hyperactivity or nervousness in children, excitement or restlessness in elderly, generally noted during first 2 wk of therapy, particularly noted in presence of uncontrolled pain

PRECAUTIONS AND CONTRAINDICATIONS
Porphyria, history of hypersensitivity to mephobarbital or other barbiturates
Caution:
Hepatic disease, renal disease, lactation, alcoholism, drug abuse, hyperthyroidism

DRUG INTERACTIONS OF CONCERN TO DENTISTRY
• Increased effects: alcohol, all CNS depressants

• Decreased effects of corticosteroids, doxycycline, carbamazepine

SERIOUS REACTIONS

! Abrupt withdrawal after prolonged therapy may produce effects including markedly increased dreaming, nightmares or insomnia, tremors, sweating, vomiting, to hallucinations, delirium, seizures, and status epilepticus.

! Skin eruptions appear as hypersensitivity reaction.

! Blood dyscrasias, liver disease, and hypocalcemia occur rarely.

! Overdosage produces cold or clammy skin, hypothermia, severe CNS depression, cyanosis, rapid pulse, and Cheyne-Stokes respirations.

! Toxicity may result in severe renal impairment.

DENTAL CONSIDERATIONS

General:

• Determine type of epilepsy, seizure frequency, and quality of seizure control. A stress reduction protocol may be required.

• Avoid use in pregnancy.

• Monitor vital signs at every appointment because of cardiovascular and respiratory side effects.

• Patients on chronic drug therapy may rarely have symptoms of blood dyscrasias, which can include infection, bleeding, and poor healing.

• Barbiturates induce liver microsomal enzymes, which alters the metabolism of other drugs.

• Avoid drugs that may lower seizure threshold (phenothiazines).

• Be sure patient is regularly taking medication.

Consultations:

• In a patient with symptoms of blood dyscrasias, request a medical consultation for blood studies and postpone dental treatment until normal values are reestablished.

• Medical consultation may be required to assess disease control and patient's ability to tolerate stress.

Teach Patient/Family to:

• Encourage effective oral hygiene to prevent soft tissue inflammation.

• Use caution to prevent injury when using oral hygiene aids.

• Avoid mouth rinses with high alcohol content because of drying effects.

---

mepivacaine HCl
me-**piv**′-ah-kane
high-droh-**klor**′-ide
(Carbocaine Caudal 1.5%[AUS], Carbocaine HCl, Polocaine, Polocaine-MPF)

M

CATEGORY AND SCHEDULE
Pregnancy Risk Category: C

Drug Class: Amide local anesthetic

MECHANISM OF ACTION
An amide anesthetic that blocks conduction of nerve impulses. *Therapeutic Effect:* Causes temporary loss of feeling and sensation.

USES
Local dental anesthesia, nerve block, caudal anesthesia, epidural, pain relief, paracervical block, transvaginal block or infiltration

PHARMACOKINETICS

Onset	Peak	Duration
3–20 min	N/A	2–2.5 hr

Protein binding: 75%. Rapidly metabolized in liver. Small amount is excreted in urine. *Half-life:* 1.9–3.2 hr; 8.7–9 hr (neonates).

INDICATIONS AND DOSAGES
▸ Regional Anesthesia
Children younger than 3 yr or weighing less than 30 lb. Maximum dose of mepivacaine should not exceed 4.4 mg/kg.

SIDE EFFECTS/ADVERSE REACTIONS
CNS and cardiovascular effects are generally dose related and of short duration
Occasional
Burning, stinging, tenderness
Rare
Generally with high dose:
Drowsiness, dizziness, disorientation, light-headedness, tremors, apprehension, euphoria, blurred or double vision, ringing or roaring in ears (tinnitus), nausea, sensation of heat, cold, numbness

PRECAUTIONS AND CONTRAINDICATIONS
Hypersensitivity to any local anesthetic agent of the amide-type or to other components of solutions of mepivacaine
Caution:
Elderly, severe drug allergies

DRUG INTERACTIONS OF CONCERN TO DENTISTRY
• CNS depressants: may see increased risk of CNS depression with all CNS depressants, especially in children and when larger doses are used.
• Avoid placing dental cartridges in disinfectant solutions with heavy metals or surface-active agents; may see release of metal ions into local anesthetic solutions with tissue irritation following injection.
• Avoid excessive exposure of dental cartridges to light or heat, which hastens deterioration of vasoconstrictor; observe for color change in local anesthetic solution.
• Risk of cardiovascular side effects: rapid intravascular administration of local anesthetic containing vasoconstrictor, either alone or in patients taking tricyclic antidepressants, MAOIs, digitalis drugs, cocaine, phenothiazines, β-blockers, and in the presence of halogenated-hydrocarbon general anesthetics; use lowest effective vasoconstrictor dose and careful aspiration techniques.
• Avoid use of vasoconstrictors in patients with uncontrolled hyperthyroidism, diabetes, angina, or hypertension; refer these patients for medical treatment before elective dental procedures.

SERIOUS REACTIONS
! CNS toxicity may occur, especially with regional anesthesia use, progressing rapidly from mild side effects to tremors, somnolence, seizures, vomiting, and respiratory depression.
! Allergic reactions, bradyarrhythmia, cardiac arrest, fetal bradycardia, heart block, hypotension, seizure, and ventricular arrhythmia have been reported.
! Allergic reactions occur rarely.

DENTAL CONSIDERATIONS

General:
• Drug is often used with a vasoconstrictor for increased duration of action.
• Monitor vital signs at every appointment because of cardiovascular and respiratory side effects.

Teach Patient/Family to:
• Use care to prevent injury while numbness exists and to refrain from chewing gum and eating following dental anesthesia.
• Report any signs of infection, muscle pain, or fever to dentist when feeling returns.
• Report any unusual soft tissue reactions.

meprobamate
meh-proe-ba′-mate
(Miltown, Novo-Mepro[CAN])

CATEGORY AND SCHEDULE
Pregnancy Risk Category: D
Schedule IV

Drug Class: Sedative-hypnotic, anxiolytic

MECHANISM OF ACTION
A carbamate derivative that affects the thalamus and limbic system. Appears to inhibit multi-neuronal spinal reflexes.
Therapeutic Effect: Relieves pain or muscle spasms.

USES
Treatment of anxiety disorders

PHARMACOKINETICS
Slowly absorbed from the GI tract. Protein binding: 0%–30%.

Metabolized in liver. Excreted in urine and feces. Moderately dialyzable. *Half-life:* 10 hr.

INDICATIONS AND DOSAGES
▶ Anxiety Disorders
PO
Adults, Children 12 yr and older.
400 mg 3–4 times. Maximum: 2400 mg/day.
Children 6–12 yr. 100–200 mg 2–3 times a day.
Elderly. Use lowest effective dose. 200 mg 2–3 times a day.
▶ Dosage in Renal Impairment

Creatinine Clearance	Dosage Interval
10–50 ml/min	Every 9–12 hr
Less than 10 ml/min	Every 12–18 hr

SIDE EFFECTS/ADVERSE REACTIONS
Frequent
Drowsiness, dizziness
Occasional
Tachycardia, palpitations, headache, light-headedness, dermatitis, diarrhea, nausea, vomiting, dyspnea, rash, weakness, blurred vision, wheezing

PRECAUTIONS AND CONTRAINDICATIONS
Acute intermittent porphyria, hypersensitivity to meprobamate or related compounds
Caution:
Suicidal patients, severe depression, renal disease, hepatic disease, elderly

DRUG INTERACTIONS OF CONCERN TO DENTISTRY
• Increased effects: CNS depressants, alcohol

M

SERIOUS REACTIONS

! Agranulocytosis, aplastic anemia, leucopenia, anaphylaxis, cardiac arrhythmias, hypotensive crisis, syncope, Stevens-Johnson syndrome and bullous dermatitis have been reported.

! Overdose may cause CNS depression, ataxia, coma, shock, hypotension, and death.

DENTAL CONSIDERATIONS

General:

• Monitor vital signs at every appointment because of cardiovascular side effects.

• Avoid use in pregnancy.

• Patients on chronic drug therapy may rarely have symptoms of blood dyscrasias, which can include infection, bleeding, and poor healing.

• Assess salivary flow as a factor in caries, periodontal disease, and candidiasis.

• Avoid dental light in patient's eyes; offer dark glasses for patient comfort.

• Determine why the patient is taking the drug.

• Psychologic and physical dependence may occur with chronic administration.

Consultations:

• In a patient with symptoms of blood dyscrasias, request a medical consultation for blood studies and postpone dental treatment until normal values are reestablished.

• Medical consultation may be required to assess disease control.

Teach Patient/Family to:

• Encourage effective oral hygiene to prevent soft tissue inflammation.

• Use caution to prevent injury when using oral hygiene aids.

• When chronic dry mouth occurs, advise patient to:

• Avoid mouth rinses with high alcohol content because of drying effects.

• Use sugarless gum, frequent sips of water, or saliva substitutes.

• Use daily home fluoride products for anticaries effect.

---

mercaptopurine (6-MP)

mur-cap-tow-**pure**′-een

(Purinethol)

CATEGORY AND SCHEDULE

Pregnancy Risk Category: D

Drug Class:

Antineoplastic-antimetabolite

MECHANISM OF ACTION

An antimetabolite that is incorporated into RNA and DNA, blocks purine synthesis, and inhibits DNA and RNA synthesis.

Therapeutic Effect: Causes death of cancer cells.

USES

Treatment of acute lymphatic leukemia (ALL), acute myelogenous leukemia (AML)

PHARMACOKINETICS

Incompletely absorbed when taken orally; metabolized in liver; excreted in urine.

INDICATIONS AND DOSAGES

▸ **ALL**

PO

Adults, Elderly, Children. 2.5–5 mg/kg once a day as induction dose. Maintenance: 1.5–2.5 mg/kg/day.

▶ **Dosage in Renal Impairment**
Creatinine clearance less than
50 ml/min. Administer usual dose
q48h.

SIDE EFFECTS/ADVERSE REACTIONS
Frequent
Myelosuppression (leading to
leukopenia, thrombocytopenia,
anemia), intrahepatic cholestasis,
hepatic necrosis
Occasional
Drug fever, hyperpigmentation, rash,
hyperuricemia, nausea, vomiting,
diarrhea, stomatitis, anorexia,
abdominal pain, mucositis

PRECAUTIONS AND CONTRAINDICATIONS
Pregnancy, severe myelosuppression
or hepatic disease
Caution:
Renal disease

DRUG INTERACTIONS OF CONCERN TO DENTISTRY
• Increased risk of hepatotoxicity:
hepatotoxic drugs

SERIOUS REACTIONS
! Myelosuppression, hepatic
necrosis, and gastroenteritis may
occur.

DENTAL CONSIDERATIONS
General:
• Patients on chronic drug therapy
may rarely have symptoms of blood
dyscrasias, which can include
infection, bleeding, and poor
healing.
• Avoid prescribing aspirin-
containing products.
• Prophylactic antibiotics may be
indicated to prevent infection if
surgery or deep scaling is planned.

• Patients receiving chemotherapy
may require palliative treatment for
stomatitis.
Consultations:
• In a patient with symptoms of
blood dyscrasias, request a medical
consultation for blood studies and
postpone dental treatment until
normal values are reestablished.
Teach Patient/Family to:
• Encourage effective oral hygiene
to prevent soft tissue inflammation.
• Use caution to prevent injury when
using oral hygiene aids.
• Avoid mouth rinses with high
alcohol content.

meropenem
mare-oh-**peh′**-nem
(Merrem IV)

CATEGORY AND SCHEDULE
Pregnancy Risk Category: B

Drug Class: Antiinfective,
miscellaneous; carbapenem

MECHANISM OF ACTION
A carbapenem that binds to
penicillin-binding proteins and
inhibits bacterial cell wall synthesis.
Therapeutic Effect: Produces
bacterial cell death.

USES
Treatment of infections caused by
bacteria

PHARMACOKINETICS
After IV administration, widely
distributed into tissues and body
fluids, including CSF. Protein
binding: 2%. Primarily excreted
unchanged in urine. Removed by
hemodialysis. **Half-life:** 1 hr.

INDICATIONS AND DOSAGES
▶ **Mild-to-Moderate Infections**
IV
Adults, Elderly. 0.5–1 g q8h.
Children 3 mo and older. 20 mg/kg/
dose q8h.
Children younger than 3 mo. 20 mg/
kg/dose q8–12h.
▶ **Meningitis**
IV
*Adults, Elderly, Children weighing
50 kg or more.* 2 g q8h.
*Children 3 mo and older weighing
less than 50 kg.* 40 mg/kg q8h.
Maximum: 2 g/dose.
▶ **Dosage in Renal Impairment**
Dosage and frequency are
modified on the basis of creatinine
clearance.

Creatinine Clearance	Dosage	Interval
26–49 ml/min	Recommended dose (1000 mg)	q12h
10–25 ml/min	½ of recommended dose	q12h
Less than 10 ml/min	½ of recommended dose	q24h

SIDE EFFECTS/ADVERSE REACTIONS
Frequent
Diarrhea, nausea, vomiting,
headache, inflammation at injection
site
Occasional
Oral candidiasis, rash, pruritus
Rare
Constipation, glossitis

PRECAUTIONS AND CONTRAINDICATIONS
None known

DRUG INTERACTIONS OF CONCERN TO DENTISTRY
• Increased or prolonged plasma
levels: probenecid

SERIOUS REACTIONS
❗ Antibiotic-associated colitis
and other superinfections may
occur.
❗ Anaphylactic reactions have been
reported.
❗ Seizures may occur in those with
CNS disorders (including brain
lesions and a history of seizures),
bacterial meningitis, or impaired
renal function.

DENTAL CONSIDERATIONS
General:
• For selected infections in the
hospital setting: provide emergency
dental treatment only.
• Examine for oral manifestation of
opportunistic infection.
• Determine why patient is taking
the drug.
• Caution regarding allergy to
medication.
Consultations:
• Consult patient's physician
if an acute dental infection
occurs and another antiinfective is
required.
• Medical consultation may be
required to assess disease control.
Teach Patient/Family to:
• Encourage effective oral
hygiene to prevent soft tissue
inflammation.
• Report oral lesions, soreness, or
bleeding to dentist.
• Prevent trauma when using oral
hygiene aids.

mesalamine/ 5-aminosalicylic acid (5-ASA)

mez-**al**′-a-meen/ ah-mee-no-sal-i-**sill**′-ik

(Apriso, Asacol, Asacol HD, Canasa, FIV-ASA, Lialda, Mesasal[CAN], Pentasa, Rowasa, Salofalk[CAN])

CATEGORY AND SCHEDULE

Pregnancy Risk Category: B; C (Asacol and Asacol HD)

Drug Class: Gastrointestinals salicylates, antiinflammatory

MECHANISM OF ACTION

A salicylic acid derivative that locally inhibits arachidonic acid metabolite production, thus inhibiting cyclooxygenase, which is increased in patients with chronic inflammatory bowel disease. Interferes with leukotriene synthesis.
Therapeutic Effect: Blocks prostaglandin and leukotriene production and reducing inflammation in the colon.

USES

Ulcerative colitis
Proctosigmoiditis
Proctitis

PHARMACOKINETICS

Poorly absorbed from the colon. Moderately absorbed from the GI tract. Bioavailability: 20%–30% (oral); 10%–35% (rectal). Metabolized in the liver to active metabolite. Unabsorbed portion eliminated in feces; absorbed portion excreted in urine. Unknown if removed by hemodialysis.

Half-life: oral: 0.5–10 hr; metabolite, 2–15 hr; extended release: 9–10 hr; 12–14 hr, metabolite; rectal: 5–7 hr; metabolite, 6–7 hr.

INDICATIONS AND DOSAGES

▶ **Ulcerative Colitis (Induction of Remission), Proctosigmoiditis, Proctitis**

PO (Asacol)
Adults, Elderly. 800 mg 3 times a day (total daily dose of 2.4 g) for 6 wk.

PO (Pentasa)
Adults, Elderly. 1 g (4 Pentasa 250 mg capsules or 2 Pentasa 500 mg capsules) 4 times a day for 8 wk.

PO (Lialda)
Adults. Two to four tablets (1.2 g) once daily with food; total daily dose of 2.4 g or 4.8 g; treatment duration up to 8 wk.

Rectal (Rectal Suspension, Rowasa)
Adults, Elderly. 60 ml (4 g) at bedtime; retain overnight (about 8 hr) for 3–6 wk or if remission is achieved.

Rectal (Suppository, Canasa)
Adults. 1 suppository (1 g), once daily at bedtime. Retain for 1–3 hr or longer to achieve maximum benefit.

▶ **To Maintain Remission in Ulcerative Colitis**

PO (Asacol)
Adults, Elderly. 1.6 g/day in divided doses.

PO (Pentasa)
Adults, Elderly. 1 g 4 times a day

PO (Apriso)
Adults, Elderly. Four capsules (1.5 g/ day) in the morning with or without food.

M

SIDE EFFECTS/ADVERSE REACTIONS

Mesalamine is generally well tolerated, with only mild and transient effects.

Frequent

PO: Abdominal cramps or pain, diarrhea, dizziness, headache, nausea, vomiting, rhinitis, unusual fatigue, flu-like symptoms, nasopharyngitis, sinusitis

Rectal: Abdominal or stomach cramps, flatulence, headache, nausea

Occasional

PO: Hair loss, decreased appetite, back or joint pain, flatulence, acne

Rectal: Hair loss

Rare

PO: Renal impairment, pericarditis, pancreatitis, rectal hemorrhaging, hematologic disorders, hepatitis, hepatotoxicity

Rectal: Anal irritation

PRECAUTIONS AND CONTRAINDICATIONS

Hypersensitivity to mesalamine, any other components of this medication, or salicylates

Rectal suppository: Hypersensitivity to mesalamine (5-aminosalicylic acid) or to the suppository vehicle [saturated vegetable fatty acid esters (hard fat)]; sulfite sensitivity in those using Rowasa

Caution:

Renal disease

Liver disease

Children (safety and efficacy not determined)

DRUG INTERACTIONS OF CONCERN TO DENTISTRY

• Anticoagulants (e.g., low molecular weight heparin, warfarin): May decrease anticoagulant effects
• Varicella virus vaccine: May result in enhanced risk of developing Reye's syndrome

Apriso

• Antacids: May dissolve the coating of the granules of Apriso capsules thereby altering bioavailability

SERIOUS REACTIONS

! Sulfite sensitivity may occur in susceptible patients (with Rowasa), manifested by cramping, headache, diarrhea, fever, rash, hives, itching, and wheezing. Discontinue drug immediately.

! Hepatitis, pancreatitis, pericarditis, and renal impairment occur rarely with oral forms.

DENTAL CONSIDERATIONS

General:

• Determine if the patient has an allergy to sulfa-based products.
• Determine why the patient is using this medication.
• Determine if the patient is pregnant.

Consultations:

• Medical consultation may be required to assess disease control.
• Laboratory tests may be ordered to assess kidney and liver function.

Teach Patient/Family to:

• Report oral lesions, soreness, or bleeding to dentist.
• When chronic dry mouth occurs, advise patient to:
  • Avoid mouth rinses with high alcohol content because of drying effects.
  • Use daily home fluoride products for anticaries effect.
  • Use sugarless gum, frequent sips of water, or saliva substitutes.

M

mesna
mez´-na
(Mesnex, Uromitexan[CAN])

CATEGORY AND SCHEDULE
Pregnancy Risk Category: B

Drug Class: Cytoprotective agent; antineoplastic adjunct, antidote

MECHANISM OF ACTION
An antineoplastic adjunct and cytoprotective agent that binds with and detoxifies urotoxic metabolites of ifosfamide and cyclophosphamide.
Therapeutic Effect: Inhibits ifosfamide- and cyclophosphamide-induced hemorrhagic cystitis.

USES
Detoxifying agent used as a protectant against hemorrhagic cystitis induced by ifosfamide, cyclophosphamide

PHARMACOKINETICS
Rapidly metabolized after IV administration to mesna disulfide, which is reduced to mesna in kidney. Excreted in urine. *Half-life:* 24 min.

INDICATIONS AND DOSAGES
▶ **Prevention of Hemorrhagic Cystitis in Patients Receiving Ifosfamide**
IV
Adults, Elderly. 20% of ifosfamide dose at time of ifosfamide administration and 4 and 8 hr after each dose of ifosfamide. Total dose: 60% of ifosfamide dosage. Range: 60%–160% of the daily ifosfamide dose.

▶ **Prevention of Hemorrhagic Cystitis in Patients Receiving Cyclophosphamide**
PO
Adults, Elderly. 40% of cyclophosphamide dose q4h for 3 doses.
IV
Adults, Elderly. 20% of cyclophosphamide dose at time of cyclophosphamide administration and q3h for 3–4 doses.

SIDE EFFECTS/ADVERSE REACTIONS
Frequent
Bad taste, soft stools
Large doses: Diarrhea, myalgia, headache, fatigue, nausea, hypotension, allergic reaction

PRECAUTIONS AND CONTRAINDICATIONS
None known

DRUG INTERACTIONS OF CONCERN TO DENTISTRY
• None reported

SERIOUS REACTIONS
! Hematuria occurs rarely.

DENTAL CONSIDERATIONS
General:
• Patient will be taking ifosfamide or cyclophosphamide; determine use and disease.
• Question patient about other diseases and medications taken.
• Note side effects and precautions associated with chemotherapeutic drugs.
Consultations:
• Medical consultation should include routine blood counts including platelet counts and bleeding time.

• Consult physician; prophylactic or therapeutic antiinfectives may be indicated if surgery or periodontal treatment is required.
• Medical consultation may be required to assess immunologic status during cancer chemotherapy and determine safety risk, if any, posed by the required dental treatment.
• Medical consultation may be required to assess disease control and patient's ability to tolerate stress.

Teach Patient/Family to:
• Encourage effective oral hygiene to prevent soft tissue inflammation.
• Prevent trauma when using oral hygiene aids.
• Report oral lesions, soreness, or bleeding to dentist.
• Update health and medication history if physician makes any changes in evaluation or drug regimens; include OTC, herbal, and nonherbal drugs in the update.

mesoridazine besylate

mez-oh-**rid**′-ah-zeen **bes**′-il-ayte (Serentil)
Do not confuse Serentil with Proventil, Serevent, or sertraline.

CATEGORY AND SCHEDULE
Pregnancy Risk Category: C

Drug Class: Phenothiazine antipsychotic

MECHANISM OF ACTION
A phenothiazine that blocks dopamine at postsynaptic receptor sites in the brain.

Therapeutic Effect: Diminishes schizophrenic behavior. Also has anticholinergic and sedative effects.

USES
Treatment of psychotic disorders, schizophrenia when inadequate response with other antipsychotic drugs

PHARMACOKINETICS
PO: Onset erratic, peak 2 hr, duration 4–6 hr.
IM: Onset 15–30 min, peak 30 min, duration 6–8 hr. Metabolized by liver, excreted in urine, crosses placenta, excreted in breast milk.

INDICATIONS AND DOSAGES
▶ **Schizophrenia**
PO
Adults, Elderly. 25–50 mg 3 times a day. Maximum: 400 mg/day.
IM
Adults, Elderly. Initially, 25 mg. May repeat in 30–60 min. Range: 25–200 mg.
▶ **Severe Behavioral Problems (Combativeness or Explosive, Hyperexcitable Behavior) Associated with Neurologic Diseases**
PO
Elderly. Initially, 10 mg once or twice a day. May increase at 4–7 day intervals. Maximum: 250 mg.
IM
Adults, Elderly. Initially, 25 mg. May repeat in 30–60 min. Range: 25–200 mg.

SIDE EFFECTS/ADVERSE REACTIONS
Frequent
Orthostatic hypotension, dizziness, syncope (occur frequently after first injection, occasionally after subsequent injections, and rarely with oral form)

Occasional

Somnolence (during early therapy), dry mouth, blurred vision, lethargy, constipation or diarrhea, nasal congestion, peripheral edema, urine retention

Rare

Ocular changes, altered skin pigmentation (in those taking high doses for prolonged periods), darkening of urine

PRECAUTIONS AND CONTRAINDICATIONS

Coma, myelosuppression, severe cardiovascular disease, severe CNS depression, subcortical brain damage

Caution:

Lactation, seizure disorders, hypertension, hepatic disease, cardiac disease, prostatic hypertrophy, intestinal obstruction, respiratory conditions, dose-related prolongation of QTc interval

DRUG INTERACTIONS OF CONCERN TO DENTISTRY

• Increased sedation: other CNS depressants, alcohol, barbiturate anesthetics, opioid analgesics
• Hypotension, tachycardia: epinephrine
• Increased extrapyramidal effects: phenothiazines and related drugs (haloperidol, droperidol), metoclopramide
• Additive photosensitization: tetracyclines
• Increased anticholinergic effects: anticholinergics

SERIOUS REACTIONS

! Abrupt withdrawal after long-term therapy may precipitate nausea, vomiting, gastritis, dizziness, and tremors.

! Blood dyscrasias, particularly agranulocytosis and mild leukopenia, may occur.

! Mesoridazine use may lower the seizure threshold.

DENTAL CONSIDERATIONS

General:

• Monitor vital signs at every appointment because of cardiovascular side effects.
• Patients on chronic drug therapy may rarely have symptoms of blood dyscrasias, which can include infection, bleeding, and poor healing.
• After supine positioning, have patient sit upright for at least 2 min before standing to avoid orthostatic hypotension.
• Assess salivary flow as a factor in caries, periodontal disease, and candidiasis.
• Avoid dental light in patient's eyes; offer dark glasses for patient comfort.
• Assess for presence of extrapyramidal motor symptoms, such as tardive dyskinesia and akathisia. Extrapyramidal motor activity may complicate dental treatment.
• Geriatric patients are more susceptible to drug effects; use lower dose.
• Use vasoconstrictors with caution, in low doses, and with careful aspiration. Avoid use of gingival retraction cord with epinephrine.

Consultations:

• In a patient with symptoms of blood dyscrasias, request a medical consultation for blood studies and postpone dental treatment until normal values are reestablished.
• Take precautions if dental surgery is anticipated and anesthesia is required.
• Refer to physician if signs of tardive dyskinesia or akathisia are present.

M

• Physician should be informed if significant xerostomic side effects occur (e.g., increased caries, sore tongue, problems eating or swallowing, difficulty wearing prosthesis) so that a medication change can be considered.

Teach Patient/Family to:

• Encourage effective oral hygiene to prevent soft tissue inflammation.

• Use caution to prevent injury when using oral hygiene aids.

• Use powered tooth brush if patient has difficulty holding conventional devices.

• When chronic dry mouth occurs, advise patient to:
   • Avoid mouth rinses with high alcohol content because of drying effects.
   • Use sugarless gum, frequent sips of water, or saliva substitutes.
   • Use daily home fluoride products for anticaries effect.

metaproterenol sulfate

met-ah-proe-**ter′**-eh-nole **suhl′**-feyt
(Alupent)
Do not confuse metaproterenol with metipranolol or metoprolol, or Alupent with Atrovent.

CATEGORY AND SCHEDULE
Pregnancy Risk Category: C

Drug Class: Selective β_2-agonist

MECHANISM OF ACTION
A sympathomimetic that stimulates β_2-adrenergic receptors, resulting in relaxation of bronchial smooth muscle.

Therapeutic Effect: Relieves bronchospasm and reduces airway resistance.

USES
Treatment of bronchial asthma, bronchospasm

PHARMACOKINETICS
3% absorbed through lungs after inhalation. Primarily metabolized in the GI tract. Duration 1–5 hr following a single dose (reduced to 1–2.5 hr after repetitive dosing).

INDICATIONS AND DOSAGES
▶ Treatment of Bronchospasm
PO
Adults, Children 10 yr and older. 20 mg 3–4 times a day.
Elderly. 10 mg 3–4 times a day. May increase to 20 mg/dose.
Children 6–9 yr. 10 mg 3–4 times a day.
Children 2–5 yr. 1.3–2.6 mg/kg/day in 3–4 divided doses.
Children younger than 2 yr. 0.4 mg/kg 3–4 times a day.
Inhalation
Adults, Elderly, Children 12 yr and older. 2–3 inhalations q3–4h.
Maximum: 12 inhalations/24 hr.
Nebulization
Adults, Elderly, Children 12 yr and older. 10–15 mg (0.2–0.3 ml) of 5% q4–6h.
Children younger than 12 yr, Infants. 0.5–1 mg/kg (0.01–0.02 ml/kg) of 5% q4–6h.

SIDE EFFECTS/ADVERSE REACTIONS
Frequent
Rigors, tremors, anxiety, nausea, dry mouth
Occasional
Dizziness, vertigo, asthenia, headache, GI distress, vomiting, cough, dry throat

Rare
Somnolence, diarrhea, altered taste

PRECAUTIONS AND CONTRAINDICATIONS
Angle-closure glaucoma, preexisting arrhythmias associated with tachycardia
Caution:
Cardiac disorders, hyperthyroidism, diabetes mellitus, prostatic hypertrophy

DRUG INTERACTIONS OF CONCERN TO DENTISTRY
• Increased effects of both drugs: other sympathomimetics, CNS stimulants
• Increased dysrhythmias: halogenated hydrocarbon anesthetics

SERIOUS REACTIONS
! Excessive sympathomimetic stimulation may cause palpitations, extrasystoles, tachycardia, chest pain, a slight increase in B/P followed by a substantial decrease, chills, diaphoresis, and blanching of skin.
! Too-frequent or excessive use may lead to decreased drug effectiveness and severe, paradoxical bronchoconstriction.

DENTAL CONSIDERATIONS
General:
• Assess salivary flow as a factor in caries, periodontal disease, and candidiasis.
• Consider semisupine chair position for patients with respiratory disease.
• Short appointments and a stress-reduction protocol may be required for anxious patients.
• Be aware that NSAIDs or sulfite preservatives in vasoconstrictor-containing products can exacerbate asthma.

• Acute asthmatic episodes may be precipitated in the dental office. Sympathomimetic inhalants should be available for emergency use.
Consultations:
• Medical consultation may be required to assess disease control and patient's ability to tolerate stress.
Teach Patient/Family to:
• Rinse mouth with water after each inhaled dose to prevent dryness.
• When chronic dry mouth occurs, advise patient to:
  • Avoid mouth rinses with high alcohol content because of drying effects.
  • Use sugarless gum, frequent sips of water, or saliva substitutes.
  • Use daily home fluoride products for anticaries effect.

M

metaraminol
met-ar-**am**′-ih-nol
(Aramine)

CATEGORY AND SCHEDULE
Pregnancy Risk Category: D

Drug Class: Adrenergic agonists

MECHANISM OF ACTION
An α-adrenergic receptor agonist that causes vasoconstriction, reflex bradycardia, inhibits GI smooth muscle and vascular smooth muscle supplying skeletal muscle and increases heart rate and force of heart muscle contraction.
Therapeutic Effect: Increases both systolic and diastolic pressure.

USES
Treatment and prevention of hypotension because of hemorrhage,

spinal anesthesia, and shock associated with brain damage

PHARMACOKINETICS

Route	Onset	Peak	Duration
IM (Pressor Effect)	10 min	N/A	20–60 min
IV	1–2 min	N/A	
SC	5–20 min	N/A	

Metabolized in the liver. Excreted in the urine and the bile.

INDICATIONS AND DOSAGES
▶ **Prevention of Hypotension**
IM/Subcutaneous
Adults, Elderly. 2–10 mg as a single dose.
Children. 0.01 mg/kg as a single dose.
▶ **Adjunctive Treatment of Hypotension**
IV
Adults, Elderly. 15–100 mg IV infusion, administered at a rate to maintain the desired B/P.
▶ **Severe Shock**
IV
Adults, Elderly. 0.5–5 mg direct IV injection followed by 15–100 mg IV infusion in 250–500 ml fluid for control of B/P.

SIDE EFFECTS/ADVERSE REACTIONS
Occasional
Tachycardia, hypertension, cardiac arrhythmias, flushing, palpitations, hypotension, angina, tremors, nervousness, headache, dizziness, weakness, sloughing of skin, nausea, abscess formation, diaphoresis

PRECAUTIONS AND CONTRAINDICATIONS
Cyclopropane or halothane anesthesia, use of MAOIs,

pregnancy, hypersensitivity to metaraminol

DRUG INTERACTIONS OF CONCERN TO DENTISTRY
• Increased risk of arrhythmia: halogenated hydrocarbon anesthetics

SERIOUS REACTIONS
! Overdosage produces hypertension, cerebral hemorrhage, cardiac arrest, and seizures.

DENTAL CONSIDERATIONS

General:
• Acute-use drug for use in hospitals or emergency rooms for selected hypotensive episodes.

metaxalone
me-**tax**′-ah-lone
(Skelaxin)

CATEGORY AND SCHEDULE
Pregnancy Risk Category: C

Drug Class: Muscle relaxant

MECHANISM OF ACTION
A central depressant whose exact mechanism is unknown. Many effects because of its central depressant actions.
Therapeutic Effect: Relieves pain or muscle spasms.

USES
Adjunct to rest, physical therapy, and other measures for relief of discomfort associated with acute, painful musculoskeletal conditions

PHARMACOKINETICS
PO route onset 1 hr, peak 3 hr, duration 4–6 hr. Well absorbed from

the GI tract. Metabolized in liver. Primarily excreted in urine.
Half-life: 9 hr.

INDICATIONS AND DOSAGES
▶ **Muscle Relaxant**
PO
Adults, Elderly, Children older than 12 yr. 800 mg 3–4 times a day.

SIDE EFFECTS/ADVERSE REACTIONS
Occasional
Drowsiness, headache, light-headedness, dermatitis, nausea, vomiting, stomach cramps, dyspnea

PRECAUTIONS AND CONTRAINDICATIONS
Impaired renal or hepatic function, history of drug-induced hemolytic anemias or other anemias, history of hypersensitivity to metaxalone
Caution:
Preexisting hepatic impairment, lactation, children younger than 12 yr, alcohol use

DRUG INTERACTIONS OF CONCERN TO DENTISTRY
• No data reported; however, this drug can cause CNS depression: monitor patients if other CNS depressants are used.

SERIOUS REACTIONS
! Overdose may cause CNS depression, coma, shock, and respiratory depression.

DENTAL CONSIDERATIONS
General:
• Determine why patient is taking the drug.
• Patients on chronic drug therapy may rarely have symptoms of blood dyscrasias, which can include

infection, bleeding, and poor healing.
• Consider semisupine chair position for patient comfort if GI side effects occur.
Consultations:
• In a patient with symptoms of blood dyscrasias, request a medical consultation for blood studies and postpone treatment until normal values are reestablished.
Teach Patient/Family to:
• Update health and drug history if physician makes any changes in evaluation or drug regimens; include OTC, herbal, and nonherbal drugs in the update.

metformin hydrochloride
met-**for**′-min high-droh-**klor**′-ide (Diabex[AUS], Diaformin[AUS], Fortamet, Glucohexal[AUS], Glucomet[AUS], Glucophage, Glucophage XL, Glycon[CAN], Novo-Metformin[CAN], Riomet)

CATEGORY AND SCHEDULE
Pregnancy Risk Category: B

Drug Class: Oral hypoglycemic, biguanide derivative

MECHANISM OF ACTION
An antihyperglycemic that decreases hepatic production of glucose. Decreases absorption of glucose and improves insulin sensitivity.
Therapeutic Effect: Improves glycemic control, stabilizes or decreases body weight, and improves lipid profile.

USES
Treatment of Type 2 diabetes mellitus

PHARMACOKINETICS

Slowly, incompletely absorbed after oral administration. Food delays or decreases the extent of absorption. Protein binding: Negligible. Primarily distributed to intestinal mucosa and salivary glands. Primarily excreted unchanged in urine. Removed by hemodialysis. *Half-life:* 3–6 hr.

INDICATIONS AND DOSAGES

> **Diabetes Mellitus**

PO (500-mg, 1000-mg Tablet)
Adults, Elderly. Initially, 500 mg twice a day, with morning and evening meals. May increase in 500-mg increments every wk, in divided doses. May give twice a day up to 2000 mg/day (e.g., 1000 mg twice a day [with morning and evening meals]). If 2500 mg/day are required, give 3 times a day with meals. Maximum: 2500 mg/day.
Children 10–16 yr. Initially, 500 mg twice a day. May increase by 500 mg/day at weekly intervals. Maximum: 2000 mg/day.
PO (850-mg Tablet)
Adults, Elderly. Initially, 850-mg/day, with morning meal. May increase dosage in 850-mg increments every other week, in divided doses. Maintenance: 850 mg twice a day, with morning and evening meals. Maximum: 2550 mg/day (850 mg 3 times a day).
PO (Extended-Release Tablets)
Adults, Elderly. Initially, 500 mg once a day. May increase by 500 mg/day at weekly intervals. Maximum: 2000 mg once a day.

> **Adjunct to Insulin Therapy**

PO
Adults, Elderly. Initially, 500 mg/day. May increase by 500 mg at 7-day intervals. Maximum: 2500 mg/day (2000 mg/day for extended-release form).

SIDE EFFECTS/ADVERSE REACTIONS

Occasional
GI disturbances (including diarrhea, nausea, vomiting, abdominal bloating, flatulence, and anorexia) that are transient and resolve spontaneously during therapy
Rare
Unpleasant or metallic taste that resolves spontaneously during therapy

PRECAUTIONS AND CONTRAINDICATIONS

Acute CHF, MI, cardiovascular collapse, renal disease or dysfunction, respiratory failure, septicemia
Caution:
Elderly, lactation, children, interferes with vitamin B_{12} absorption; avoid alcohol use

DRUG INTERACTIONS OF CONCERN TO DENTISTRY

• None reported

SERIOUS REACTIONS

! Lactic acidosis occurs rarely but is a fatal complication in 50% of cases. Lactic acidosis is characterized by an increase in blood lactate levels (higher than 5 mmol/L), a decrease in blood pH, and electrolyte disturbances. Signs and symptoms of lactic acidosis include unexplained hyperventilation, myalgia, malaise, and somnolence, which may advance to cardiovascular collapse (shock), acute CHF, acute MI, and prerenal azotemia.

DENTAL CONSIDERATIONS

General:
• Short appointments and a stress-reduction protocol may be required for anxious patients.

- Consider semisupine chair position for patient comfort if GI side effects occur.
- Question patient about self-monitoring of drug's antidiabetic effect, including blood glucose values or finger-stick records.
- Ensure that patient is following prescribed diet and regularly takes medication.
- Diabetics may be more susceptible to infection and have delayed wound healing.
- Place on frequent recall to evaluate healing response.

Consultations:
- Medical consultation may be required to assess disease control and patient's ability to tolerate stress.
- Notify physician immediately if symptoms of lactic acidosis are observed (myalgia, respiratory distress, weakness, diarrhea, malaise, muscle cramps, somnolence).
- Medical consultation may include data from patient's blood glucose monitoring, including glycosylated hemoglobin or HbA$_{1c}$ testing.
- Oral and maxillofacial surgical procedures associated with significantly restricted food intake require a medical consultation and temporary cessation of metformin use.

Teach Patient/Family to:
- Encourage effective oral hygiene to prevent soft-tissue inflammation.
- Understand that alteration of taste may be because of drug side effects.

methadone hydrochloride
meth′-ah-done
high-droh-**klor**′-ide
(Dolophine, Metadol[CAN], Methadone Intensol, Methadose, Physeptone[AUS])

CATEGORY AND SCHEDULE
Pregnancy Risk Category: B (D if used for prolonged periods or at high dosages at term)
Controlled Substance: Schedule II

Drug Class: Synthetic opioid analgesic

MECHANISM OF ACTION
An opioid agonist that binds with opioid receptors in the CNS. *Therapeutic Effect:* Alters the perception of and emotional response to pain; reduces withdrawal symptoms from other opioid drugs.

USES
Treatment of severe pain, opioid withdrawal program

PHARMACOKINETICS

Route	Onset	Peak	Duration
Oral	0.5–1 hr	1.5–2 hr	6–8 hr
IM	10–20 min	N/A	4–5 hr
IV	N/A	15–30 min	3–4 hr

Well absorbed after IM injection. Protein binding: 80%–85%. Metabolized in the liver. Primarily excreted in urine. Not removed by hemodialysis. *Half-life:* 15–25 hr.

INDICATIONS AND DOSAGES
▶ Analgesia
PO
Adults, Elderly. Initially, 5–10 mg q3–4h.

Children. 0.1–0.2 mg/kg q6h as needed. Maximum: 10 mg/dose.
IV, IM, Subcutaneous
Adults, Elderly. Initially, 2.5–10 mg q3–4h.

▸ **Opioid Addiction**
IM, PO
Adults, Elderly. 15–40 mg once daily or as needed. Reduce dose at 1–2 day intervals based on patient response. Maintenance: Individualized.

SIDE EFFECTS/ADVERSE REACTIONS

Frequent
Sedation, decreased B/P (including orthostatic hypotension), diaphoresis, facial flushing, constipation, dizziness, nausea, vomiting
Occasional
Confusion, urine retention, palpitations, abdominal cramps, visual changes, dry mouth, headache, decreased appetite, anxiety, insomnia
Rare
Allergic reaction (rash, pruritus)

PRECAUTIONS AND CONTRAINDICATIONS

Delivery of premature infant, diarrhea because of poisoning, hypersensitivity to narcotics, labor
Caution:
Addictive personality, lactation, increased intracranial pressure, MI (acute), severe heart disease, respiratory depression, hepatic disease, renal disease, children younger than 18 yr

DRUG INTERACTIONS OF CONCERN TO DENTISTRY

• Increased CNS depression: alcohol, narcotics, sedative-hypnotics, skeletal muscle relaxants, benzodiazepines, and other CNS depressants
• Increased effects of anticholinergics

SERIOUS REACTIONS

! Overdose results in respiratory depression, skeletal muscle flaccidity, cold or clammy skin, cyanosis, and extreme somnolence progressing to seizures, stupor, and coma. The antidote is 0.4 mg naloxone.
! The patient who uses methadone long-term may develop a tolerance to the drug's analgesic effect and physical dependence.

DENTAL CONSIDERATIONS

General:
• Assess salivary flow as a factor in caries, periodontal disease, and candidiasis.
• Psychologic and physical dependence may occur with chronic administration.
• Determine why the patient is taking the drug.
• Be aware of the special needs of patients who are in recovery from substance abuse.
• In an opioid-dependent patient, NSAIDs are the drugs of choice for posttreatment pain control.
Consultations:
• Patients in the methadone maintenance program should not receive additional opioids or other controlled substances without a consultation.
Teach Patient/Family:
• When chronic dry mouth occurs, advise patient to:
  • Avoid mouth rinses with high alcohol content because of drying effects.

- Use sugarless gum, frequent sips of water, or saliva substitutes.
- Use daily home fluoride products for anticaries effect.

methamphetamine
meth-am-**fet′**-ah-meen
(Desoxyn, Gradumet)
Do not confuse with Dextran, dextromethorphan, or Excedrin.

CATEGORY AND SCHEDULE
Pregnancy Risk Category: C
Controlled substance: Schedule II

Drug Class: Amphetamine

MECHANISM OF ACTION
A sympathomimetic amine related to amphetamine and ephedrine that enhances CNS stimulant activity. Peripheral actions include elevation of systolic and diastolic B/P and weak bronchodilator and respiratory stimulant action.
Therapeutic Effect: Increases motor activity, mental alertness; decreases drowsiness, fatigue.

USES
Treatment of exogenous obesity, minimal brain dysfunction, attention-deficit/hyperactivity disorder (ADHD)

PHARMACOKINETICS
Rapidly absorbed from the GI tract. Metabolized in liver. Primarily excreted in the urine. Unknown if removed by hemodialysis. *Half-life:* 4–5 hr.

INDICATIONS AND DOSAGES
▶ ADHD
PO
Adults, Children 6 yr and older.
Initially, 2.5–5 mg 1–2 times a day. Increase by 5 mg/day at weekly intervals until therapeutic response achieved.
▶ Appetite Suppressant
PO
Adults, Children 12 yr and older.
5 mg daily, given 30 min before meals. Extended-release 10–15 mg in the morning.

SIDE EFFECTS/ADVERSE REACTIONS
Frequent
Irregular pulse, increased motor activity, talkativeness, nervousness, mild euphoria, insomnia
Occasional
Headache, chills, dry mouth, GI distress, worsening depression in patients who are clinically depressed, tachycardia, palpitations, chest pain

PRECAUTIONS AND CONTRAINDICATIONS
Advanced arteriosclerosis, agitated states, glaucoma, history of drug abuse, history of hypersensitivity to sympathomimetic amines, hyperthyroidism, moderate to severe hypertension, symptomatic cardiovascular disease, within 14 days following discontinuation of an MAOI
Caution:
Gilles de la Tourette's syndrome, lactation, children younger than 6 yr

DRUG INTERACTIONS OF CONCERN TO DENTISTRY
- Increased effect of methamphetamine: CNS stimulants, sympathomimetics

M

• Decreased effects of both drugs: haloperidol, sedative-hypnotics
• Ventricular dysrhythmia: inhalation anesthetics

SERIOUS REACTIONS

! Overdose may produce skin pallor, flushing, arrhythmias, and psychosis.
! Abrupt withdrawal following prolonged administration of high dosage may produce lethargy which may last for weeks.
! Prolonged administration to children with ADHD may produce a temporary suppression of normal weight and height patterns.

DENTAL CONSIDERATIONS

General:
• Monitor vital signs at every appointment due to cardiovascular side effects.
• Assess salivary flow as a factor in caries, periodontal disease, and candidiasis.

Consultations:
• Physician should be informed if significant xerostomic side effects occur (e.g., increased caries, sore tongue, problems eating or swallowing, difficulty wearing prosthesis) so that a medication change can be considered.

Teach Patient/Family to:
• When chronic dry mouth occurs, advise patient to:
  • Avoid mouth rinses with high alcohol content because of drying effects.
  • Use sugarless gum, frequent sips of water, or saliva substitutes.
  • Use daily home fluoride products for anticaries effect.

methazolamide
meth-ah-**zole**′-ah-mide
(Apo-Methazolamide[CAN], GlaucTabs, Neptazane)
Do not confuse with nefazodone.

CATEGORY AND SCHEDULE
Pregnancy Risk Category: C

Drug Class: Carbonic anhydrase inhibitor

MECHANISM OF ACTION
A noncompetitive inhibitor of carbonic anhydrase that inhibits the enzyme at the luminal border of cells of the proximal tubule. Increases urine volume and changes to an alkaline pH with subsequent decreases in the excretion of titratable acid and ammonia.
Therapeutic Effect: Produces a diuretic and antiglaucoma effect.

USES
Treatment of open-angle glaucoma or preoperatively in narrow-angle glaucoma; can be used with miotic, osmotic agents

PHARMACOKINETICS
PO route onset 2–4 hr, peak 6–8 hr, duration 10–18 hr. Well absorbed slowly from the GI tract. Protein binding: 55%. Distributed into the tissues (including CSF). Metabolized slowly from the GI tract. Partially excreted in urine. Not removed by hemodialysis. **Half-life:** 14 hr.

INDICATIONS AND DOSAGES
▶ Glaucoma
PO
Adults, Elderly. 50–100 mg/day 2–3 times a day.

SIDE EFFECTS/ADVERSE REACTIONS
Occasional

Paresthesias, hearing dysfunction or tinnitus, fatigue, malaise, loss of appetite, taste alteration, nausea, vomiting, diarrhea, polyuria, drowsiness, confusion, hypokalemia
Rare

Metabolic acidosis, electrolyte imbalance, transient myopia, urticaria, melena, hematuria, glycosuria, hepatic insufficiency, flaccid paralysis, photosensitivity, convulsions, and rarely, crystalluria, renal calculi

PRECAUTIONS AND CONTRAINDICATIONS

Kidney or liver dysfunction, severe pulmonary obstruction, hypersensitivity to methazolamide or any component of the formulation
Caution:

Hypercalciuria, lactation, children

DRUG INTERACTIONS OF CONCERN TO DENTISTRY

Methazolamide (Neptazane, GlaucTabs)
• Toxicity: salicylates (high doses)
• Hypokalemia: corticosteroids (systemic use)

SERIOUS REACTIONS

! Malaise and complaints of tiredness and myalgia are signs of excessive dosing and acidosis in the elderly.
! Stevens-Johnson syndrome, toxic epidermal necrolysis, fulminant hepatic necrosis, agranulocytosis, aplastic anemia, and other blood dyscrasias have been reported and have caused fatalities.

DENTAL CONSIDERATIONS

General:
• Avoid dental light in patient's eyes; offer dark glasses for patient comfort.
• Avoid prescribing aspirin-containing products.
• Consider semisupine chair position for patient comfort if GI side effects occur.
• Question patient about tolerance of NSAIDs or aspirin related to GI disease.
• Patient on chronic drug therapy may rarely present with symptoms of blood dyscrasias, which can include infection, bleeding, and poor healing.
• Caution patient to prevent oral tissue trauma when using oral hygiene aids.
Consultations:
• In a patient with symptoms of blood dyscrasias, request a medical consultation for blood studies and postpone treatment until normal values are reestablished.
Teach Patient/Family to:
• Encourage effective oral hygiene to prevent soft tissue inflammation.
• Prevent trauma when using oral hygiene aids.
• Update health and medication history if physician makes any changes in evaluation or drug regimens; include OTC, herbal, and nonherbal drugs in the update.

M

methenamine

meh-**theh'**-nah-meen
(Dehydral[CAN], Hiprex,
Hip-Rex[CAN], Mandelamine,
Urasal[CAN], Urex)

CATEGORY AND SCHEDULE

Pregnancy Risk Category: C

Drug Class: Urinary
antiinfective

MECHANISM OF ACTION

A hippuric acid salt that hydrolyzes
to formaldehyde and ammonia in
acidic urine.
Therapeutic Effect: Formaldehyde
has antibacterial action.
Bacteriocidal.

USES

Prophylaxis and treatment of
uncomplicated UTIs

PHARMACOKINETICS

Readily absorbed from the GI tract.
Partially metabolized by hydrolysis
(unless protected by enteric coating)
and partially by the liver. Primarily
excreted in urine. *Half-life:* 3–6 hr.

INDICATIONS AND DOSAGES
▸ **UTI**
PO
Adults, Elderly. 1 g 2 times/day (as
hippurate). 1 g 4 times/day (as
mandelate).
Children 6–12 yr. 25–0 mg/kg/day
q12h (as hippurate). 50–75 mg/kg/
day q6h (as mandelate).

SIDE EFFECTS/ADVERSE
REACTIONS
Occasional
Rash, nausea, dyspepsia, difficulty
urinating

Rare
Bladder irritation, increased liver
enzymes

PRECAUTIONS AND
CONTRAINDICATIONS
Moderate to severe renal
impairment, hepatic impairment
(hippurate salt), tartrazine sensitivity
(Hiprex contains tartrazine),
hypersensitivity to methenamine or
any of its components
Caution:
Renal disease, lactation

DRUG INTERACTIONS OF
CONCERN TO DENTISTRY
• None reported

SERIOUS REACTIONS

! Crystalluria can occur when
methenamine is given in large doses.

DENTAL CONSIDERATIONS

General:
• Determine why the patient is
taking the drug.
• Antibiotics for dental infections
are not contraindicated, but a
physician notification may be
advisable.
• Palliative treatment may be
required for oral side effects.
• Consider semisupine chair position
for patient comfort because of GI
effects of drug.

methimazole

meth-**im'**-ah-zole
(Tapazole)

CATEGORY AND SCHEDULE

Pregnancy Risk Category: D

Drug Class: Thyroid hormone
antagonist

MECHANISM OF ACTION

A thiomidazole derivative that inhibits synthesis of thyroid hormone by interfering with the incorporation of iodine into tyrosyl residues.
Therapeutic Effect: Effectively treats hyperthyroidism by decreasing thyroid hormone levels.

USES

Treatment of hyperthyroidism

PHARMACOKINETICS

PO: Onset 30–40 min, duration 2–4 hr. *Half-life:* 1–2 hr; excreted in urine, bile, breast milk; crosses placenta.

INDICATIONS AND DOSAGES

▸ **Hyperthyroidism**
PO
Adults, Elderly. Initially, 15–60 mg/day in 3 divided doses. Maintenance: 5–15 mg/day.
Children. Initially, 0.4 mg/kg/day in 3 divided doses. Maintenance: $\frac{1}{2}$ the initial dose.

SIDE EFFECTS/ADVERSE REACTIONS

Frequent
Fever, rash, pruritus
Occasional
Dizziness, loss of taste, nausea, vomiting, stomach pain, peripheral neuropathy or numbness in fingers, toes, face
Rare
Swollen lymph nodes or salivary glands

PRECAUTIONS AND CONTRAINDICATIONS

Hypersensitivity, infection, bone marrow depression, hepatic disease, pregnancy (first or second trimester)

Caution:
Infection, bone marrow depression, hepatic disease

DRUG INTERACTIONS OF CONCERN TO DENTISTRY

• Increased cardiovascular side effects in uncontrolled patients: anticholinergics and sympathomimetics
• Patients with uncontrolled hyperthyroidism are at risk when vasoconstrictors are used
• Patients with uncontrolled hypothyroidism may be more responsive to CNS depressants

SERIOUS REACTIONS

❗ Agranulocytosis as long as 4 mo after therapy, pancytopenia, and hepatitis have occurred.

M

DENTAL CONSIDERATIONS

General:
• Monitor vital signs at every appointment because of cardiovascular effects of disease.
• Patients on chronic drug therapy may rarely have symptoms of blood dyscrasias; examine for evidence of oral manifestations of blood dyscrasias (infection, bleeding, poor healing).
• Evaluate for clotting ability during periodontal instrumentation.
• Evaluate for control of hyperthyroidism. Patients with uncontrolled condition should not be treated in the dental office until thyroid values are normalized.
• Patients with uncontrolled condition should be referred for medical evaluation and treatment.
Consultations:
• Medical consultation may be required to assess disease control.
• Medical consultation for blood studies (CBC); leukopenic or

thrombocytopenic side effects may result in infection, delayed healing, and excessive bleeding. Postpone elective dental treatment until normal values are maintained.

Teach Patient/Family to:
• Encourage effective oral hygiene to prevent soft tissue inflammation.
• Use caution in use of oral hygiene aids to prevent injury.

---

methocarbamol
meth-oh-**kar′**-ba-mole
(Carbacot, Robaxin)

CATEGORY AND SCHEDULE
Pregnancy Risk Category: C

Drug Class: Skeletal muscle relaxant

MECHANISM OF ACTION
A carbamate derivative of guaifenesin that causes skeletal muscle relaxation by general CNS depression.
Therapeutic Effect: Relieves muscle spasticity.

USES
Adjunct for relief in painful musculoskeletal conditions

PHARMACOKINETICS
Rapidly and almost completely absorbed from the GI tract. Protein binding: 46%–50%. Metabolized in liver by dealkylation and hydroxylation. Primarily excreted in urine as metabolites. **Half-life:** 1–2 hr.

INDICATIONS AND DOSAGES
▶ **Musculoskeletal Spasm**
IM/IV
Adults, Children 16 yr and older.
1 g q8h for no more than 3 consecutive days. May repeat course of therapy after a drug-free interval of 48 hr.
PO
Adults, Children 16 yr and older.
1.5 g 4 times a day for 2–3 days (up to 8 g/day may be given in severe conditions). Decrease to 4–4.5 g/day in 3–6 divided doses.
Elderly. Initially, 500 mg 4 times a day. May gradually increase dosage.
▶ **Tetanus Spasm**
IV
Adults. 1–3 g q6h until oral dosing is possible. Injection should be used no more than 3 consecutive days.
Children. 15 mg/kg/dose or 500 mg/m^2/dose q6h as needed. Maximum: 1.8 g/m^2/day for 3 days only.

SIDE EFFECTS/ADVERSE REACTIONS
Frequent
Transient drowsiness, weakness, dizziness, light-headedness, nausea, vomiting
Occasional
Headache, constipation, anorexia, hypotension, confusion, blurred vision, vertigo, facial flushing, rash
Rare
Paradoxical CNS excitement and restlessness, slurred speech, tremors, dry mouth, diarrhea, nocturia, impotence, bradycardia, hypotension, syncope

PRECAUTIONS AND CONTRAINDICATIONS
Hypersensitivity to methocarbamol or any component of the

formulation, renal impairment
(injection formulation)
Caution:
Renal disease, hepatic disease,
addictive personalities, myasthenia
gravis, epilepsy

DRUG INTERACTIONS OF CONCERN TO DENTISTRY

• Increased CNS depression:
alcohol, narcotics,
sedative-hypnotics

SERIOUS REACTIONS

! Anaphylactoid reactions,
leukopenia, and seizures
(intravenous form) have been
reported.
! Methocarbamol overdosage
results in cardiac arrhythmias,
nausea, vomiting, drowsiness, and
coma.

DENTAL CONSIDERATIONS

General:
• Determine why the patient is
taking the drug.
• Consider semisupine chair position
for patient comfort if back is
involved.
Teach Patient/Family to:
• Encourage effective oral
hygiene to prevent soft tissue
inflammation.
• Use caution to prevent injury when
using oral hygiene aids.
• Avoid mouth rinses with high
alcohol content because of drying
effects.

methotrexate sodium

meth-oh-**trex**′-ate **soe**′-dee-um
(Apo-Methotrexate[CAN],
Ledertrexate[AUS],
Methoblastin[AUS], Rheumatrex,
Trexall)
Do not confuse Trexall with
Trexan.

CATEGORY AND SCHEDULE

Pregnancy Risk Category: D (X
for patients with psoriasis or
rheumatoid arthritis)

Drug Class: Folic acid
antagonist, antineoplastic

M

MECHANISM OF ACTION

An antimetabolite that competes
with enzymes necessary to reduce
folic acid to tetrahydrofolic acid, a
component essential to DNA, RNA,
and protein synthesis. This action
inhibits DNA, RNA, and protein
synthesis.
Therapeutic Effect: Causes death of
cancer cells.

USES

Treatment of acute lymphocytic
leukemia (ALL), non-Hodgkin's
lymphoma; in combination with
other drugs for breast, lung, head,
neck cancer; lymphosarcoma;
psoriasis; gestational
choriocarcinoma; hydatidiform
mole; rheumatoid arthritis

PHARMACOKINETICS

Variably absorbed from the GI tract.
Completely absorbed after IM
administration. Protein binding:
50%–60%. Widely distributed.
Metabolized intracellularly in the
liver. Primarily excreted in urine.
Removed by hemodialysis but not

by peritoneal dialysis. *Half-life:* 8–12 hr (large doses, 8–15 hr).

INDICATIONS AND DOSAGES

▸ **Trophoblastic Neoplasms**
PO, IM
Adults, Elderly. 15–30 mg/day for 5 days; repeat in 7 days for 3–5 courses.

▸ **Head and Neck Cancer**
PO, IV, IM
Adults, Elderly. 25–50 mg/m^2 once weekly.

▸ **Choriocarcinoma, Chorioadenoma Destruens, Hydatidiform Mole**
PO, IM
Adults, Elderly. 15–30 mg/day for 5 days; repeat 3–5 times with 1–2 wk between courses.

▸ **Breast Cancer**
IV
Adults, Elderly. 30–60 mg/m^2 days 1 and 8 q3–4wk.

▸ **ALL**
PO, IV, IM
Adults, Elderly. Induction: 3.3 mg/m^2/day in combination with other chemotherapeutic agents. Maintenance: 30 mg/m^2/wk PO or IM in divided doses or 2.5 mg/kg IV every 14 days.

▸ **Burkitt's Lymphoma**
PO
Adults. 10–25 mg/day for 4–8 days; repeat with 7- to 10-day rest between courses.

▸ **Lymphosarcoma**
PO
Adults, Elderly. 0.625–2.5 mg/kg/day.

▸ **Mycosis Fungoides**
PO
Adults, Elderly. 2.5–10 mg/day.
IM
Adults, Elderly. 50 mg/wk or 25 mg twice a wk.

▸ **Rheumatoid Arthritis**
PO
Adults, Elderly. 7.5 mg once a wk or 2.5 mg q12h for 3 doses once a wk. Maximum: 20 mg/wk.

▸ **Juvenile Rheumatoid Arthritis**
PO, IM, Subcutaneous
Children. 5–15 mg/m^2/wk as a single dose or in 3 divided doses given q12h.

▸ **Psoriasis**
PO
Adults, Elderly. 10–25 mg once a wk or 2.5–5 mg q12h for 3 doses once a wk.
IM
Adults, Elderly. 10–25 mg once a wk.

▸ **Antineoplastic Dosage for Children**
PO, IM
Children. 7.5–30 mg/m^2/wk or q2wk.
IV
Children. 10–33,000 mg/m^2 bolus or continuous infusion over 6–42 hr.

▸ **Dosage in Renal Impairment**
Creatinine clearance 61–80 ml/min. Reduce dose by 25%.
Creatinine clearance 51–60 ml/min. Reduce dose by 33%.
Creatinine clearance 10–50 ml/min. Reduce dose by 50%–70%.

SIDE EFFECTS/ADVERSE REACTIONS

Frequent
Nausea, vomiting, stomatitis; burning and erythema at psoriatic site (in patients with psoriasis)
Occasional
Diarrhea, rash, dermatitis, pruritus, alopecia, dizziness, anorexia, malaise, headache, drowsiness, blurred vision

PRECAUTIONS AND CONTRAINDICATIONS

Preexisting myelosuppression, severe hepatic or renal impairment
Caution:
Renal disease, lactation, drugs with potential for hepatotoxicity, monitor for hepatic toxicity, methotrexate-induced lung disease

DRUG INTERACTIONS OF CONCERN TO DENTISTRY

· Increased toxicity: aspirin, alcohol, NSAIDs
· Possible fatal interactions: NSAIDs, high-dose IV methotrexate
· Suspected increase in methotrexate toxicity: amoxicillin, tetracycline, doxycycline

SERIOUS REACTIONS

! GI toxicity may produce gingivitis, glossitis, pharyngitis, stomatitis, enteritis, and hematemesis.
! Hepatotoxicity is more likely to occur with frequent small doses than with large intermittent doses.
! Pulmonary toxicity may be characterized by interstitial pneumonitis.
! Hematologic toxicity, which may develop rapidly from marked myelosuppression, may be manifested as leukopenia, thrombocytopenia, anemia, and hemorrhage.
! Dermatologic toxicity may produce a rash, pruritus, urticaria, pigmentation, photosensitivity, petechiae, ecchymosis, and pustules.
! Severe nephrotoxicity may produce azotemia, hematuria, and renal failure.

DENTAL CONSIDERATIONS

General:
· Patients on chronic drug therapy may rarely have symptoms of blood dyscrasias, which can include infection, bleeding, and poor healing.
· Avoid prescribing aspirin- or NSAID-containing products.
· Place on frequent recall because of increased risk for infection and to evaluate healing response.
· Determine why the patient is taking the drug.
· Palliative treatment may be necessary if stomatitis or oral desquamative lesions occur.
Consultations:
· In a patient with symptoms of blood dyscrasias, request a medical consultation for blood studies and postpone dental treatment until normal values are reestablished.
· Medical consultation may be required to assess disease control.
Teach Patient/Family to:
· Encourage effective oral hygiene to prevent soft tissue inflammation.
· Use caution to prevent injury when using oral hygiene aids.
· Use palliative therapy for sore mouth.
· Avoid mouth rinses with high alcohol content because of drying effects.

M

methoxy polyethylene glycol-epoetin beta

meth-**ox**′-ee-pol-ee-**eth**′-il-een-**glye**′-kol-eh-**poe**′-ee-tin-bay-ta
(Mircera)

CATEGORY AND SCHEDULE

Pregnancy Risk Category: C

Drug Class: Anti-anemia agent, continuous erythropoietin receptor activator (CERA)

MECHANISM OF ACTION

Methoxy polyethylene glycol polymer, found in methoxy polyethylene glycol-epoetin beta, attaches to recombinant human erythropoietin in order to remain in the circulation much longer. Methoxy polyethylene glycol-epoetin beta slowly binds to the erythropoietin-receptor and quickly dissociates, which helps prevent internalization and degradation of the molecule. This way it remains biologically active.

USES

Used in treatment of anemia in patients with chronic renal failure (CRF).

PHARMACOKINETICS

Completely absorbed after SC administration. Bioavailability for SC administration is 62%. *Half-life:* 134 ± 65 hr after IV administration and 139 ± 67 hr after SC administration.

INDICATIONS AND DOSAGES
▶ **Patients Not Currently Treated with an Erythropoiesis Stimulating Agent (ESA)**
IV or SC
Adults. Starting 0.6 mcg/kg body weight once every 2 weeks to achieve Hb level >11 g/dl. Dose may be increased by ~25% if Hb increasing rate is <1.0 g/dl over a month. If Hb increase rate is >2 g/dl in a month or if Hb is increasing and approaching 12 g/dl, consider reducing by ~25%. If Hb continues to increase, stop therapy until Hb begins to decrease. If Hb level is >11g/dl, consider maintaining therapy once monthly using the dose equal to twice the previous once every 2-wk dose.

▶ **Patients Currently Treated with an ESA**
IV or SC
Patients currently on an ESA can be directly converted to methoxy polyethylene glycol-epoetin beta once a month. Monthly starting dose is 120 mcg/month, 200 mcg/month, or 360 mcg/month depends on the previous darbepoetin alfa or epoetin (table).

Previous Weekly Starting Dose Darbepoetin Alfa IV or SC Dose (mcg/ week)	Previous Weekly Epoetin Alfa IV or SC Dose (IU/ week)	Monthly Mircera IV or SC Dose (mcg/once monthly)
<40	<8000	120
40–80	8000–16000	200
>80	>16000	360

If a dose adjustment is required to achieve Hb level >11 g/dl, consider increase monthly dose by ~25%.

SIDE EFFECTS/ADVERSE REACTIONS
▶ **Adult**
Frequent
Hypertension
Occasional
Headache, thrombocytopenia, decreased average platelet count, diarrhea, muscle spasm, procedural hypotension, edema, back pain

PRECAUTIONS AND CONTRAINDICATIONS

Hypersensitivity to the active substance or any of the components. Contraindicated in patients with uncontrolled hypertension, hypertensive encephalopathy, and seizures.
Supplemental iron therapy is recommended for all patients with

serum ferritin below 100 mcg/L or transferrin saturation <20%.
Patients with anti-erythropoietin antibodies should not be placed on methoxy polyethylene glycol-epoetin beta because of the risk of pure red cell aplasia.
Methoxy polyethylene glycol-epoetin beta has been studied to have effect on tumor growth and should not be used in patients with any type of malignancy.
Blood pressure should be closely monitored before, during, and after therapy.

DRUG INTERACTIONS OF CONCERN TO DENTISTRY
• None reported

SERIOUS REACTIONS
! Hypertension, hypertensive encephalopathy, and seizures have occurred.

DENTAL CONSIDERATIONS

General:
• Patient's disease, treatment history, and use of other drugs will affect patient evaluation and management.
• Determine why patient is taking the drug.
• Monitor vital signs at every appointment because of cardiovascular side effects.
• Take precautions if dental surgery is anticipated and general anesthesia is required.
• Consider semisupine chair position for patient comfort if GI side effects occur.
Consultations:
• Medical consultation may be required to assess disease control.
• Review patient's medical and drug history.

Teach Patient/Family to:
• Encourage effective oral hygiene to prevent soft tissue inflammation.
• Use caution to prevent injury when using oral hygiene aids.

methsuximide
meth-**sux**′-ih-mide
(Celontin)
Do not confuse with methoxsalen.

CATEGORY AND SCHEDULE
Pregnancy Risk Category: C

Drug Class: Anticonvulsant

MECHANISM OF ACTION
An anticonvulsant agent that increases the seizure threshold, suppresses paroxysmal spike-and-wave pattern in absence seizures, and depresses nerve transmission in the motor cortex.
Therapeutic Effect: Controls absence (petit mal) seizures.

USES
Treatment of refractory absence seizures (petit mal)

PHARMACOKINETICS
Rapidly metabolized in liver to active metabolite, N-desmethylmeth-suximide. Primarily excreted in urine. Unknown if removed by hemodialysis. *Half-life:* 1.4 hr.

INDICATIONS AND DOSAGES
▶ Absence Seizures
PO
Adults, Elderly. Initially, 300 mg/day for the first wk. Increase dosage by 300 mg/day at weekly intervals until response is attained. Maintenance: 1200 mg/day at 2–4 times a day. Do not exceed 1000 mg/day in children

12–15 yr, 1200 mg/day in patients older than 15 yr.
Children. Initially, 10–15 mg/kg/day 3–4 times a day. Increase at weekly intervals. Maximum: 30 mg/kg/day.

SIDE EFFECTS/ADVERSE REACTIONS
Frequent
Drowsiness, dizziness, nausea, vomiting
Occasional
Visual abnormalities, such as spots before eyes, difficulty focusing, blurred vision, dry mouth or pharynx, tongue irritation, nervousness, insomnia, headache, constipation or diarrhea, rash, weight loss, proteinuria, edema

PRECAUTIONS AND CONTRAINDICATIONS
Hypersensitivity to succinimides or any component of the formulation
Caution:
Hepatic disease, renal disease, lactation

DRUG INTERACTIONS OF CONCERN TO DENTISTRY
• Enhanced CNS depression: alcohol, CNS depressants
• Decreased effects: phenothiazines, thioxanthenes, barbiturates
• Changes in seizure pattern, frequency: haloperidol

SERIOUS REACTIONS
❗ Toxic reactions appear as blood dyscrasias, including aplastic anemia, agranulocytosis, thrombocytopenia, leukopenia, leukocytosis, eosinophilia, cardiovascular disturbances, such as CHF, hypotension or hypertension, thrombophlebitis, arrhythmias, and dermatologic effects, such as rash, urticaria, pruritus, photosensitivity.

❗ Abrupt withdrawal may precipitate status epilepticus.

DENTAL CONSIDERATIONS
General:
• Patients on chronic drug therapy may rarely have symptoms of blood dyscrasias, which can include infection, bleeding, and poor healing.
• Avoid dental light in patient's eyes; offer dark glasses for patient comfort.
• Determine type of epilepsy, seizure frequency, and quality of seizure control. A stress-reduction protocol may be required.
• Place on frequent recall to monitor gingival condition.
Consultations:
• In a patient with symptoms of blood dyscrasias, request a medical consultation for blood studies and postpone dental treatment until normal values are reestablished.
• Take precautions if dental surgery is anticipated and anesthesia is required.
• Medical consultation may be required to assess disease control.
Teach Patient/Family to:
• Encourage effective oral hygiene to prevent soft tissue inflammation.
• Use caution to prevent injury when using oral hygiene aids.
• Avoid mouth rinses with high alcohol content if oral side effects occur.

methyldopa/ methyldopate

meth-ill-**doe**′-pa/
meth-ill-**doe**′-payte
(Aldomet, Apo-Methyldopa[CAN],
Hydopa[AUS], Novomedopa[CAN],
Nudopa[AUS])
Do not confuse Aldomet with
Anzemet.

CATEGORY AND SCHEDULE
Pregnancy Risk Category: B

Drug Class: Centrally acting
antihypertensive

MECHANISM OF ACTION
An antihypertensive agent that
stimulates central inhibitory
α-adrenergic receptors, lowers
arterial pressure, and reduces plasma
renin activity.
Therapeutic Effect: Reduces B/P.

USES
Treatment of hypertension

PHARMACOKINETICS
PO: Peak 4–6 hr, duration
12–24 hr.
IV: Peak 2 hr, duration 10–16 hr
Metabolized by liver, excreted in
urine.

INDICATIONS AND DOSAGES
▶ Moderate-to-Severe Hypertension
PO
Adults. Initially, 250 mg 2–3 times a
day for 2 days. Adjust dosage at
intervals of 2 days (minimum).
Elderly. Initially, 125 mg 1–2 times
a day. May increase by 125 mg q2–3
days. Maintenance: 500 mg–2 g/day
in 2–4 divided doses.
Children. Initially, 10 mg/kg/day in
2–4 divided doses. Adjust dosage at
intervals of 2 days (minimum).

Maximum: 65 mg/kg/day or 3 g/day,
whichever is less.
IV
Adults. 250–1000 mg q6–8h.
Maximum: 4 g/day.
Children. Initially, 2–4 mg/kg/dose.
May increase to 5–10 mg/kg/dose in
4–6 hr if no response. Maximum:
65 mg/kg/day or 3 g/day, whichever
is less.

SIDE EFFECTS/ADVERSE REACTIONS
Frequent
Peripheral edema, somnolence,
headache, dry mouth
Occasional
Mental changes (such as anxiety,
depression), decreased sexual
function or libido, diarrhea, swelling
of breasts, nausea, vomiting,
light-headedness, paraesthesia,
rhinitis

PRECAUTIONS AND CONTRAINDICATIONS
Hepatic disease, pheochromocytoma
Caution:
Liver disease, eclampsia, severe
cardiac disease

DRUG INTERACTIONS OF CONCERN TO DENTISTRY
• Decreased effects: indomethacin
and other NSAIDs
• Increased pressor response:
epinephrine and other
sympathomimetics
• Increased sedation: haloperidol,
alcohol, CNS depressants
• Increased hypotensive action of
general anesthetics

SERIOUS REACTIONS
! Hepatotoxicity (abnormal liver
function test results, jaundice,
hepatitis), hemolytic anemia,
unexplained fever and flu-like
symptoms may occur. If these

M

conditions appear, discontinue the medication and contact the physician.

DENTAL CONSIDERATIONS

General:
- Monitor vital signs at every appointment because of cardiovascular side effects.
- Patients on chronic drug therapy may rarely have symptoms of blood dyscrasias, which can include infection, bleeding, and poor healing.
- Assess salivary flow as a factor in caries, periodontal disease, and candidiasis.
- Limit use of sodium-containing products, such as saline IV fluids, for patients with a dietary salt restriction.
- After supine positioning, have patient sit upright for at least 2 min before standing to avoid orthostatic hypotension.
- Stress from dental procedures may compromise cardiovascular function; determine patient risk and consider use of stress-reduction protocol.
Consultations:
- In a patient with symptoms of blood dyscrasias, request a medical consultation for blood studies and postpone dental treatment until normal values are reestablished.
- Medical consultation may be required to assess disease control and patient's ability to tolerate stress.
Teach Patient/Family to:
- Encourage effective oral hygiene to prevent soft tissue inflammation.
- Use caution to prevent injury when using oral hygiene aids.
- When chronic dry mouth occurs, advise patient to:

- Avoid mouth rinses with high alcohol content because of drying effects.
- Use sugarless gum, frequent sips of water, or saliva substitutes.
- Use daily home fluoride products for anticaries effect.

methylergonovine
meth-ill-er-**gon**′-oh-veen
(Methergine)

CATEGORY AND SCHEDULE
Pregnancy Risk Category: C

Drug Class: Oxytocic

MECHANISM OF ACTION
An ergot alkaloid that stimulates α-adrenergic and serotonin receptors, producing arterial vasoconstriction. Causes vasospasm of coronary arteries and directly stimulates uterine muscle.
Therapeutic Effect: Increases strength and frequency of uterine contractions. Decreases uterine bleeding.

USES
Treatment of hemorrhage postpartum or postabortion, uterine contractions

PHARMACOKINETICS

Route	Onset	Peak	Duration
PO	5–10 min	N/A	N/A
IV	Immediate	N/A	3 hr
IM	2–5 min	N/A	N/A

Rapidly absorbed from the GI tract after IM administration. Distributed rapidly to plasma, extracellular fluid, and tissues. Metabolized in the liver

and undergoes first-pass effect. Primarily excreted in urine.
Half-life: IV (alpha phase), 2–3 min or less; IV (beta phase), 20–30 min or longer.

INDICATIONS AND DOSAGES
▶ **Prevention and Treatment of Postpartum and Postabortion Hemorrhage Caused by Atony or Involution**
PO
Adults. 0.2 mg 3–4 times a day. Continue for up to 7 days.
IV, IM
Adults. Initially, 0.2 mg. May repeat q2–4h for no more than a total of 5 doses.

SIDE EFFECTS/ADVERSE REACTIONS
Frequent
Nausea, uterine cramping, vomiting
Occasional
Abdominal pain, diarrhea, dizziness, diaphoresis, tinnitus, bradycardia, chest pain
Rare
Allergic reaction, such as rash and itching; dyspnea; severe or sudden hypertension

PRECAUTIONS AND CONTRAINDICATIONS
Hypertension, pregnancy, toxemia, untreated hypocalcemia

DRUG INTERACTIONS OF CONCERN TO DENTISTRY
• Increased effects: sympathomimetics

SERIOUS REACTIONS
! Severe hypertensive episodes may result in CVA, serious arrhythmias, and seizures.
! Hypertensive effects are more frequent with patient susceptibility, rapid IV administration, and concurrent use of regional anesthesia or vasoconstrictors.
! Peripheral ischemia may lead to gangrene.

DENTAL CONSIDERATIONS
General:
• Acute-use drug normally given in the hospital; provide palliative dental care for dental emergencies only.
Teach Patient/Family to:
• Follow up with definitive dental care at an opportune date.

methylphenidate hydrochloride
meth-ill-**fen′**-ih-date
high-droh-**klor′**-ide
(Attenta[AUS], Concerta, Metadate CD, Metadate ER, Methylin, Methylin ER, PMS-Methylphenidate[CAN], Riphenidate[CAN], Ritalin, Ritalin LA, Ritalin SR)
Do not confuse Ritalin with Rifadin.

CATEGORY AND SCHEDULE
Pregnancy Risk Category: C
Controlled Substance: Schedule II

Drug Class: CNS stimulant, related to amphetamines

MECHANISM OF ACTION
A CNS stimulant that blocks the reuptake of norepinephrine and dopamine into presynaptic neurons.
Therapeutic Effect: Decreases motor restlessness and fatigue; increases motor activity, attention span, and mental alertness; produces mild euphoria.

USES

Treatment of attention-deficit/
hyperactivity disorder (ADHD),
narcolepsy

PHARMACOKINETICS

Onset	Peak	Duration
Immediate release	2 hr	3–5 hr
Sustained release	4–7 hr	3–8 hr
Extended release	N/A	8–12 hr

Slowly and incompletely absorbed
from the GI tract. Protein binding:
15%. Metabolized in the liver.
Eliminated in urine and in feces
by biliary system. Unknown if
removed by hemodialysis. *Half-life:*
2–4 hr.

INDICATIONS AND DOSAGES

▸ **ADHD**
PO
Children 6 yr and older. Immediate
release: Initially, 2.5–5 mg before
breakfast and lunch. May increase
by 5–10 mg/day at weekly intervals.
Maximum: 60 mg/day.
PO (Concerta)
Children 6 yr and older. Initially,
18 mg once a day; may increase by
18 mg/day at weekly intervals.
Maximum: 72 mg/day.
PO (Metadate CD)
Children 6 yr and older. Initially,
20 mg/day. May increase by 20 mg/
day at weekly intervals. Maximum:
60 mg/day.
PO (Ritalin LA)
Children 6 yr and older. Initially,
20 mg/day. May increase by 10 mg/
day at weekly intervals. Maximum:
60 mg/day.
PO (Metadate ER, Methylin ER,
Ritalin SR)
Children 6 yr and older. May
replace regular tablets after daily
dose is titrated and 8-hr dosage

corresponds to sustained-release or
extended-release tablet size.
▸ **Narcolepsy**
PO
Adults, Elderly. 10 mg 2–3 times a
day. Range: 10–60 mg/day.

SIDE EFFECTS/ADVERSE REACTIONS

Frequent
Anxiety, insomnia, anorexia
Occasional
Dizziness, drowsiness, headache,
nausea, abdominal pain, fever, rash,
arthralgia, vomiting
Rare
Blurred vision, Tourette syndrome
(marked by uncontrolled vocal
outbursts, repetitive body
movements, and tics), palpitations

PRECAUTIONS AND CONTRAINDICATIONS

Avoid use within 14 days of
MAOIs
Caution:
Hypertension, depression, seizures,
lactation, drug abuse

DRUG INTERACTIONS OF CONCERN TO DENTISTRY

• Increased effects of CNS
stimulants, tricyclic antidepressants,
SSRIs, sympathomimetics

SERIOUS REACTIONS

❗ Prolonged administration to
children with ADHD may delay
growth.
❗ Overdose may produce
tachycardia, palpitations,
arrhythmias, chest pain,
psychotic episode, seizures, and
coma.
❗ Hypersensitivity reactions and
blood dyscrasias occur rarely.

DENTAL CONSIDERATIONS

General:
• Monitor vital signs at every appointment because of cardiovascular side effects.
• Patients on chronic drug therapy may rarely have symptoms of blood dyscrasias, which can include infection, bleeding, and poor healing.
• Assess salivary flow as a factor in caries, periodontal disease, and candidiasis.
• Use vasoconstrictors with caution, in low doses, and with careful aspiration.
• Determine why the patient is taking the drug.
Consultations:
• In a patient with symptoms of blood dyscrasias, request a medical consultation for blood studies and postpone dental treatment until normal values are reestablished.
• Medical consultation may be required to assess disease control.
Teach Patient/Family to:
• Encourage effective oral hygiene to prevent soft tissue inflammation.
• Use caution to prevent injury when using oral hygiene aids.
• When chronic dry mouth occurs, advise patient to:
  • Avoid mouth rinses with high alcohol content because of drying effects.
  • Use sugarless gum, frequent sips of water, or saliva substitutes.
  • Use daily home fluoride products for anticaries effect.

methylprednisolone

meth-il-pred-**niss′**-oh-lone
methylprednisolone (Medrol)
methylprednisolone acetate (Depo-Medrol, Depo-Nisolone[AUS])
methylprednisolone sodium succinate (A-Methapred, Solu-Medrol)
Do not confuse methylprednisolone with medroxyprogesterone or Medrol with Mebaral.

CATEGORY AND SCHEDULE
Pregnancy Risk Category: C

Drug Class: Glucocorticoid, immediate acting

MECHANISM OF ACTION
An adrenocortical steroid that suppresses migration of polymorphonuclear leukocytes and reverses increased capillary permeability.
Therapeutic Effect: Decreases inflammation.

USES
Treatment of severe inflammation, shock, adrenal insufficiency, collagen disorders

PHARMACOKINETICS

Route	Onset	Peak	Duration
PO	N/A	1–2 hr	30–36 hr
IM	N/A	4–8 days	1–4 wk

Well absorbed from the GI tract after IM administration. Widely distributed. Metabolized in the liver. Excreted in urine. Removed by hemodialysis. *Half-life:* 3.5 hr.

INDICATIONS AND DOSAGES
▶ **Substitution Therapy for Deficiency States: Acute or Chronic Adrenal Insufficiency, Adrenal Insufficiency Secondary to Pituitary Insufficiency, and Congenital Adrenal Hyperplasia; Nonendocrine Disorders: Allergic, Collagen, Hepatic, Intestinal Tract, Ocular, Renal, and Skin Diseases; Arthritis; Bronchial Asthma; Cerebral Edema; Malignancies; and Rheumatic Carditis**

PO
Adults, Elderly. Initially, 4–48 mg/day.

IV (Methylprednisolone Sodium Succinate)
Adults, Elderly. 40–250 mg q4–6h. High dosage: 30 mg/kg over at least 30 min. Repeat q4–6h for 48–72 hr.

▶ **Spinal Cord Injury**

IV Bolus
Adults, Elderly. 30 mg/kg over 15 min. Maintenance dose: 5.4 mg/kg/h over 23 hr, to be given within 45 min of bolus dose.

IM (Methylprednisolone Acetate)
Adults, Elderly. 10–80 mg/day.

Intraarticular, Intralesional
Adults, Elderly. 4–40 mg, up to 80 mg q1–5wk.

▶ **Antiinflammatory/ Immunosuppressant**

PO/IM/IV
Pediatric. 0.5–1.7 mg/kg/day or 5–25 mg/m^2/day in 2–4 divided doses.

SIDE EFFECTS/ADVERSE REACTIONS
Frequent
Insomnia, heartburn, anxiety, abdominal distention, diaphoresis, acne, mood swings, increased appetite, facial flushing, GI distress, delayed wound healing, increased susceptibility to infection, diarrhea or constipation

Occasional
Headache, edema, tachycardia, change in skin color, frequent urination, depression

Rare
Psychosis, increased blood coagulability, hallucinations

PRECAUTIONS AND CONTRAINDICATIONS
Administration of live virus vaccines, systemic fungal infection

Caution:
Diabetes mellitus, glaucoma, osteoporosis, seizure disorders, ulcerative colitis, CHF, myasthenia gravis, renal disease, esophagitis, peptic ulcer, rifampin

DRUG INTERACTIONS OF CONCERN TO DENTISTRY
- Decreased action: barbiturates, rifampin, rifabutin
- Increased GI side effects: alcohol, salicylates, NSAIDs
- Increased action: ketoconazole, macrolide antibiotics
- Hepatotoxicity: acetaminophen (chronic, high doses)

SERIOUS REACTIONS
! Long-term therapy may cause hypocalcemia, hypokalemia, muscle wasting (especially in arms and legs), osteoporosis, spontaneous fractures, amenorrhea, cataracts, glaucoma, peptic ulcer disease, and CHF.
! Abruptly withdrawing the drug after long-term therapy may cause anorexia, nausea, fever, headache, sudden severe myalgia, rebound inflammation, fatigue, weakness, lethargy, dizziness, and orthostatic hypotension.

DENTAL CONSIDERATIONS

General:
• Patients on chronic drug therapy may rarely have symptoms of blood dyscrasias, which can include infection, bleeding, and poor healing.
• Assess salivary flow as a factor in caries, periodontal disease, and candidiasis.
• Symptoms of oral infections may be masked.
• Place on frequent recall to evaluate healing response.
• Prophylactic antibiotics may be indicated to prevent infection if surgery or deep scaling is planned.
• Avoid prescribing NSAID-containing products.
• Determine dose and duration of steroid therapy for each patient to assess risk for stress tolerance and immunosuppression.
• Patients who have been or are currently on chronic steroid therapy (longer than 2 wk) may require supplemental steroids for dental treatment.

Consultations:
• In a patient with symptoms of blood dyscrasias, request a medical consultation for blood studies and postpone dental treatment until normal values are reestablished.
• Medical consultation may be required to assess disease control.
• Consultation may be required to confirm steroid dose and duration of use.

Teach Patient/Family to:
• Encourage effective oral hygiene to prevent soft tissue inflammation.
• Use caution to prevent injury when using oral hygiene aids because of reduced healing response.
• When chronic dry mouth occurs, advise patient to:

• Avoid mouth rinses with high alcohol content because of drying effects.
• Use sugarless gum, frequent sips of water, or saliva substitutes.
• Use daily home fluoride products for anticaries effect.

methyltestosterone

meth-il-tes-**tos**′-te-rone
(Android, Android-10, Android-25, Oreton Methyl, Testred, Virilon)
Do not confuse with methylprednisolone.

CATEGORY AND SCHEDULE
Pregnancy Risk Category: X
Controlled substance: Schedule III

Drug Class: Androgens, hormones/hormone modifiers

M

MECHANISM OF ACTION
A synthetic testosterone derivative with androgen activity that promotes growth and development of male sex organs and maintains secondary sex characteristics in androgen-deficient males.
Therapeutic Effect: Treats hypogonadism and delayed puberty in males.

USES
Replacement of the hormone when the body is unable to produce enough on its own; to stimulate the beginning of puberty in certain boys who are late starting puberty naturally; to treat certain types of breast cancer in females.

PHARMACOKINETICS

Well absorbed from the GI tract.
Protein binding: 98%. Metabolized
in liver. Primarily excreted in urine.
Unknown if removed by
hemodialysis. *Half-life:*
10–100 min.

INDICATIONS AND DOSAGES

▸ **Breast Cancer**
PO
Adults, Elderly. 50–200 mg/day.
▸ **Delayed Puberty**
PO
Adults. 10–50 mg/day.
Adults, Elderly. 50–200 mg/day.
▸ **Hypogonadism**
PO
Adults. 10–50 mg/day.

SIDE EFFECTS/ADVERSE REACTIONS

Frequent
Gynecomastia, acne, amenorrhea or
other menstrual irregularities
Females: Hirsutism, deepening of
voice, clitoral enlargement that may
not be reversible when drug is
discontinued
Occasional
Edema, nausea, insomnia,
oligospermia, priapism, male pattern
of baldness, bladder irritability,
hypercalcemia in immobilized
patients or those with breast cancer,
hypercholesterolemia
Rare
Polycythemia

PRECAUTIONS AND CONTRAINDICATIONS

Pregnancy, prostatic or breast cancer
in males, hypersensitivity to
methyltestosterone or any other
component of its formulation

DRUG INTERACTIONS OF CONCERN TO DENTISTRY

• Edema: ACTH, corticosteroids

SERIOUS REACTIONS

! Cholestatic jaundice,
hepatocellular neoplasms, peliosis
hepatitis, edema with or without
CHF and suppression of clotting
factors II, V, VII, and X have been
reported.

DENTAL CONSIDERATIONS

General:
• Determine why patient is taking
the drug.
• Short appointments and a stress
reduction protocol may be required
for anxious patients.
• Possible risk of bleeding when
used concurrently with oral
anticoagulants and aspirin.
Consultations:
• Medical consultation may be
required to assess disease control.
Teach Patient/Family to:
• Encourage effective oral hygiene
to prevent soft tissue inflammation.
• Update health and medication
history if physician makes any
changes in evaluation or drug
regimens; include OTC, herbal, and
nonherbal drugs in the update.

metipranolol hydrochloride

met-ee-**pran**′-oh-lol
high-droh-**klor**′-ide
(OptiPranolol)
Do not confuse with metoprolol
or propranolol.

CATEGORY AND SCHEDULE

Pregnancy Risk Category: C

Drug Class: Antiglaucoma agent
(ophthalmic)

MECHANISM OF ACTION
An antiglaucoma agent that non-selectively blocks β-adrenergic receptors. Reduces aqueous humor production.
Therapeutic Effect: Reduces intraocular pressure (IOP).

USES
Treatment of certain types of glaucoma

PHARMACOKINETICS

Route	Onset	Peak	Duration
Eye drops	0.5–3 hr	2–7 hr	24 hr or more

Systemic absorption may occur.

INDICATIONS AND DOSAGES
▶ **Glaucoma, Ocular Hypertension**
Ophthalmic
Adults, Elderly. Instill 1 drop 2 times a day.

SIDE EFFECTS/ADVERSE REACTIONS
Frequent
Eye burning/stinging, hyperemia, blurred vision, headache, fatigue
Occasional
Sensitivity to light, dizziness, hypotension
Rare
Dry eye, conjunctivitis, eye pain, rash, muscle pain

PRECAUTIONS AND CONTRAINDICATIONS
Bronchial asthma or chronic obstructive pulmonary disease, cardiogenic shock, overt cardiac failure, second- or third-degree heart AV block, severe sinus bradycardia, hypersensitivity to metipranolol or any component of the formulation

DRUG INTERACTIONS OF CONCERN TO DENTISTRY
• Avoid or use with caution: drugs with anticholinergic effects

SERIOUS REACTIONS
❗ Ophthalmic overdosage may produce bradycardia, hypotension, bronchospasm, and acute cardiac failure.
❗ Arrhythmias and myocardial infarction have been reported.

DENTAL CONSIDERATIONS
General:
• Determine why patient is taking the drug.
• Avoid drugs with anticholinergic activity, such as antihistamines, opioids, benzodiazepines, propantheline, atropine, and scopolamine.
• Avoid dental light in patient's eyes; offer dark glasses for patient comfort.
• Question glaucoma patient about compliance with prescribed drug regimen.
Consultations:
• Medical consultation may be required to assess disease control.
Teach Patient/Family to:
• Update health and medication history if physician makes any changes in evaluation or drug regimens; include OTC, herbal, and nonherbal drugs in the update.

M

metoclopramide

met-oh-kloe-**pra**′-mide
(Apo-Metoclop[CAN],
Maxolon[AUS], Pramin[AUS],
Reglan)
Do not confuse Reglan with
Renagel.

CATEGORY AND SCHEDULE
Pregnancy Risk Category: B

Drug Class: Central dopamine
receptor antagonist

MECHANISM OF ACTION
A dopamine receptor antagonist that
stimulates motility of the upper GI
tract and decreases reflux into the
esophagus. Also raises the threshold
of activity in the chemoreceptor
trigger zone.
Therapeutic Effect: Accelerates
intestinal transit and gastric
emptying; relieves nausea and
vomiting.

USES
Prevention of nausea, vomiting
induced by chemotherapy, radiation,
delayed gastric emptying,
gastroesophageal reflux, diabetic
gastroparesis

PHARMACOKINETICS

Route	Onset	Peak	Duration
PO	30–60 min	N/A	N/A
IV	1–3 min	N/A	N/A
IM	10–15 min	N/A	N/A

Well absorbed from the GI tract.
Metabolized in the liver. Protein
binding: 30%. Primarily excreted in
urine. Not removed by hemodialysis.
Half-life: 4–6 hr.

INDICATIONS AND DOSAGES
▶ **Prevention of Chemotherapy-
Induced Nausea and Vomiting**
IV
Adults, Elderly, Children. 1–2 mg/kg
30 min before chemotherapy; repeat
q2h for 2 doses, then q3h as needed.
▶ **Postoperative Nausea and
Vomiting**
IV
*Adults, Elderly, Children 15 yr and
older.* 10 mg; repeat q6–8h as
needed.
Children 14 yr and younger.
0.1–0.2 mg/kg/dose; repeat q6–8h as
needed.
▶ **Diabetic Gastroparesis**
PO, IV
Adults. 10 mg 30 min before meals
and at bedtime for 2–8 wk.
PO
Elderly. Initially, 5 mg 30 min
before meals and at bedtime. May
increase to 10 mg.
IV
Elderly. 5 mg over 1–2 min. May
increase to 10 mg.
▶ **Symptomatic Gastroesophageal
Reflux**
PO
Adults. 10–15 mg up to 4 times a
day, or single doses up to 20 mg as
needed.
Elderly. Initially, 5 mg 4 times a day.
May increase to 10 mg.
Children. 0.4–0.8 mg/kg/day in 4
divided doses.
▶ **To Facilitate Small Bowel
Intubation (Single Dose)**
IV
Adults, Elderly. 10 mg as a single
dose.
Children 6–14 yr. 2.5–5 mg as a
single dose.
Children younger than 6 yr. 0.1 mg/
kg as a single dose.
▶ **Dosage in Renal Impairment**
Dosage is modified on the basis of
creatinine clearance.

Creatinine Clearance	% of Normal Dose
40–50 ml/min	75
10–40 ml/min	50
Less than 10 ml/min	25–50

SIDE EFFECTS/ADVERSE REACTIONS

Frequent

Somnolence, restlessness, fatigue, lethargy

Occasional

Dizziness, anxiety, headache, insomnia, breast tenderness, altered menstruation, constipation, rash, dry mouth, galactorrhea, gynecomastia

Rare

Hypotension or hypertension, tachycardia

PRECAUTIONS AND CONTRAINDICATIONS

Concurrent use of medications likely to produce extrapyramidal reactions, GI hemorrhage, GI obstruction or perforation, history of seizure disorders, pheochromocytoma

Caution:

Lactation, GI hemorrhage, CHF, asthma, hypertension, renal failure; extrapyramidal diseases, depression, concurrently with or within 14 days of discontinuing MAOIs

DRUG INTERACTIONS OF CONCERN TO DENTISTRY

• Decreased GI action: anticholinergics, opioids
• Increased sedation: alcohol, other CNS depressants
• Increased effects of succinylcholine

SERIOUS REACTIONS

! Extrapyramidal reactions occur most commonly in children and young adults (18–30 yr) receiving large doses (2 mg/kg) during chemotherapy and are usually limited to akathisia (involuntary limb movement and facial grimacing).

DENTAL CONSIDERATIONS

General:

• Assess salivary flow as a factor in caries, periodontal disease, and candidiasis.
• Assess for presence of extrapyramidal motor symptoms, such as tardive dyskinesia and akathisia. Extrapyramidal motor activity may complicate dental treatment.
• Determine why the patient is taking the drug.
• Consider semisupine chair position for patient comfort because of GI effects of disease.

Teach Patient/Family to:

• When chronic dry mouth occurs, advise patient to:
  • Avoid mouth rinses with high alcohol content because of drying effects.
  • Use sugarless gum, frequent sips of water, or saliva substitutes.
  • Use daily home fluoride products for anticaries effect.

M

metolazone

met-**tole**′-ah-zone
(Mykrox, Zaroxolyn)
Do not confuse metolazone with methazolamide or metoprolol, or Zaroxolyn with Zarontin.

CATEGORY AND SCHEDULE

Pregnancy Risk Category: B (D if used in pregnancy-induced hypertension)

Drug Class: Diuretic with thiazide-like effects

MECHANISM OF ACTION

A thiazide-like diuretic and antihypertensive. As a diuretic, blocks reabsorption of sodium, potassium, and chloride at the distal convoluted tubule, increasing renal excretion of sodium and water. As an antihypertensive, reduces plasma and extracellular fluid volume and peripheral vascular resistance. *Therapeutic Effect:* Promotes diuresis and reduces B/P.

USES

Treatment of edema, hypertension, CHF

PHARMACOKINETICS

Route	Onset	Peak	Duration
PO (diuretic)	1 hr	2 hr	12–24 hr

Incompletely absorbed from the GI tract. Protein binding: 95%. Primarily excreted unchanged in urine. Not removed by hemodialysis. *Half-life:* 14 hr.

INDICATIONS AND DOSAGES

▸ **Edema**
PO (Zaroxolyn)
Adults, Elderly. 5–10 mg/day. May increase to 20 mg/day in edema associated with renal disease or heart failure.
Children. 0.2–0.4 mg/kg/day in 1–2 divided doses.
▸ **Hypertension**
PO (Zaroxolyn)
Adults, Elderly. 2.5–5 mg/day.
PO (Mydrox)
Adults, Elderly. Initially, 0.5 mg/day. May increase up to 1 mg/day.

SIDE EFFECTS/ADVERSE REACTIONS

Expected
Increase in urinary frequency and urine volume
Frequent
Dizziness, light-headedness, headache
Occasional
Muscle cramps and spasm, fatigue, lethargy
Rare
Asthenia, palpitations, depression, nausea, vomiting, abdominal bloating, constipation, diarrhea, urticaria

PRECAUTIONS AND CONTRAINDICATIONS

Anuria, hepatic coma or precoma, history of hypersensitivity to sulfonamides or thiazide diuretics, renal decompensation
Caution:
Hypokalemia, renal disease, hepatic disease, gout, COPD, lupus erythematosus, diabetes mellitus

DRUG INTERACTIONS OF CONCERN TO DENTISTRY

• Increased photosensitization: tetracycline
• Decreased hypotensive response: indomethacin and other NSAIDs

SERIOUS REACTIONS

! Vigorous diuresis may lead to profound water and electrolyte depletion, resulting in hypokalemia, hyponatremia, and dehydration.
! Acute hypotensive episodes may occur.
! Hyperglycemia may occur during prolonged therapy.
! Pancreatitis, paresthesia, blood dyscrasias, pulmonary edema, allergic pneumonitis, and dermatologic reactions occur rarely.

! Overdose can lead to lethargy and coma without changes in electrolytes or hydration.

DENTAL CONSIDERATIONS

General:
• Patients on chronic drug therapy may rarely have symptoms of blood dyscrasias, which can include infection, bleeding, and poor healing.
• Assess salivary flow as a factor in caries, periodontal disease, and candidiasis.
• After supine positioning, have patient sit upright for at least 2 min before standing to avoid orthostatic hypotension.
• Short appointments and a stress-reduction protocol may be required for anxious patients.
• Limit use of sodium-containing products, such as saline IV fluids, for patients with a dietary salt restriction.
• Stress from dental procedures may compromise cardiovascular function; determine patient risk.
Consultations:
• In a patient with symptoms of blood dyscrasias, request a medical consultation for blood studies and postpone dental treatment until normal values are reestablished.
• Medical consultation may be required to assess disease control and patient's ability to tolerate stress.
Teach Patient/Family to:
• Encourage effective oral hygiene to prevent soft tissue inflammation.
• Use caution to prevent injury when using oral hygiene aids.
• When chronic dry mouth occurs, advise patient to:
   • Avoid mouth rinses with high alcohol content because of drying effects.

• Use sugarless gum, frequent sips of water, or saliva substitutes.
• Use daily home fluoride products for anticaries effect.

metoprolol tartrate
me-**toe**′-pro-lole **tahr**′-treyt
(Apo-Metoprolol[CAN], Betaloc[CAN], Lopresor[AUS], Lopressor, Metohexal[AUS], Metolol[AUS], Minax[AUS], Nu-Metop[CAN], PMS-Metoprolol[CAN], Toprol XL)
Do not confuse metoprolol with metaproterenol or metolazone.

CATEGORY AND SCHEDULE
Pregnancy Risk Category: C (D if used in second or third trimester)

Drug Class: Antihypertensive, selective β₁-blocker

M

MECHANISM OF ACTION
An antianginal, antihypertensive, and MI adjunct that selectively blocks β₁-adrenergic receptors; high dosages may block β₂-adrenergic receptors. Decreases oxygen requirements. Large doses increase airway resistance.
Therapeutic Effect: Slows sinus node heart rate, decreases cardiac output, and reduces B/P. Also decreases myocardial ischemia severity.

USES
Treatment of mild-to-moderate hypertension, acute MI to reduce risk of cardiovascular mortality, angina pectoris, mild-to-moderate heart failure

PHARMACOKINETICS

Route	Onset	Peak	Duration
PO	10–15 min	N/A	6 hr
PO (extended release)	N/A	6–12 hr	5–8 hr
IV	Immediate	20 min	5–8 hr

Well absorbed from the GI tract. Protein binding: 12%. Widely distributed. Metabolized in the liver (undergoes significant first-pass metabolism). Primarily excreted in urine. Removed by hemodialysis. *Half-life:* 3–7 hr.

INDICATIONS AND DOSAGES
▸ **Mild-to-Moderate Hypertension**
PO
Adults. Initially, 100 mg/day as single or divided dose. Increase at weekly (or longer) intervals. Maintenance: 100–450 mg/day.
Elderly. Initially, 25 mg/day. Range: 25–300 mg/day.
PO (Extended-Release)
Adults. 50–100 mg/day as single dose. May increase at least at weekly intervals until optimal B/P attained. Maximum: 200 mg/ day.
Elderly. Initially, 25–50 mg/day as a single dose. May increase at 1- to 2-wk intervals.
▸ **Chronic, Stable Angina Pectoris**
PO
Adults. Initially, 100 mg/day as single or divided dose. Increase at weekly (or longer) intervals. Maintenance: 100–450 mg/day.
PO (Extended-Release)
Adults. Initially, 100 mg/day as single dose. May increase at least at weekly intervals until optimal clinical response achieved. Maximum: 200 mg/day.

▸ **CHF**
PO (Extended-Release)
Adults. Initially, 25 mg/day. May double dose q2wk. Maximum: 200 mg/day.
▸ **Early Treatment of MI**
IV
Adults. 5 mg q2min for 3 doses, followed by 50 mg orally q6h for 48 hr. Begin oral dose 15 min after last IV dose. Or, in patients who do not tolerate full IV dose, give 25–50 mg orally q6h, 15 min after last IV dose.
▸ **Late Treatment and Maintenance after an MI**
PO
Adults. 100 mg twice a day for at least 3 mo.

SIDE EFFECTS/ADVERSE REACTIONS
Metoprolol is generally well tolerated, with transient and mild side effects
Frequent
Diminished sexual function, drowsiness, insomnia, unusual fatigue or weakness
Occasional
Anxiety, nervousness, diarrhea, constipation, nausea, vomiting, nasal congestion, abdominal discomfort, dizziness, difficulty breathing, cold hands or feet
Rare
Altered taste, dry eyes, nightmares, paraesthesia, allergic reaction (rash, pruritus)

PRECAUTIONS AND CONTRAINDICATIONS
Cardiogenic shock, MI with a heart rate less than 45 beats/min or systolic B/P less than 100 mm Hg, overt heart failure, second- or third-degree heart block, sinus bradycardia

Caution:

Major surgery, lactation, diabetes mellitus, renal disease, thyroid disease, COPD, heart failure, CAD, nonallergic bronchospasm, hepatic disease

DRUG INTERACTIONS OF CONCERN TO DENTISTRY

• Increased hypotension, bradycardia: fentanyl derivatives, inhalation anesthetics
• Decreased antihypertensive effects: NSAIDs, sympathomimetics
• May slow metabolism of lidocaine
• Decreased β-blocking effects (or decreased β-adrenergic effects) of epinephrine, levonordefrin, isoproterenol, and other sympathomimetics
• Increased plasma concentrations: diphenhydramine

SERIOUS REACTIONS

❗ Overdose may produce profound bradycardia, hypotension, and bronchospasm.
❗ Abrupt withdrawal of metoprolol may result in diaphoresis, palpitations, headache, tremulousness, exacerbation of angina, MI, and ventricular arrhythmias.
❗ Metoprolol administration may precipitate CHF and MI in patients with heart disease, thyroid storm in those with thyrotoxicosis, and peripheral ischemia in those with existing peripheral vascular disease.
❗ Hypoglycemia may occur in patients with previously controlled diabetes mellitus.

DENTAL CONSIDERATIONS

General:
• Monitor vital signs at every appointment because of cardiovascular and respiratory side effects.
• After supine positioning, have patient sit upright for at least 2 min before standing to avoid orthostatic hypotension.
• Patients on chronic drug therapy may rarely have symptoms of blood dyscrasias, which can include infection, bleeding, and poor healing.
• Assess salivary flow as a factor in caries, periodontal disease, and candidiasis.
• Stress from dental procedures may compromise cardiovascular function; determine patient risk.
• Short appointments and a stress-reduction protocol may be required for anxious patients.
• Use vasoconstrictors with caution, in low doses, and with careful aspiration. Avoid use of gingival retraction cord with epinephrine.
• Determine why patient is taking the drug.

Consultations:
• In a patient with symptoms of blood dyscrasias, request a medical consultation for blood studies and postpone dental treatment until normal values are reestablished.
• Medical consultation may be required to assess disease control and patient's ability to tolerate stress.
• Take precautions if general anesthesia is required for dental surgery.

Teach Patient/Family to:
• Encourage effective oral hygiene to prevent soft tissue inflammation.
• Use caution to prevent injury when using oral hygiene aids.

M

- When chronic dry mouth occurs, advise patient to:
  - Avoid mouth rinses with high alcohol content because of drying effects.
  - Use sugarless gum, frequent sips of water, or saliva substitutes.
  - Use daily home fluoride products for anticaries effect.

metronidazole hydrochloride

me-troe-**ni**′-da-zole
high-droh-**klor**′-ide
(Apo-Metronidazole[CAN], Flagyl, Flagyl ER, MetroCream, MetroGel, Metrogyl[AUS], MetroLotion, Metronidazole IV[AUS], Metronide[AUS], NidaGel[CAN], Noritate, Novonidazol[CAN], Rozex[AUS])

CATEGORY AND SCHEDULE
Pregnancy Risk Category: B

Drug Class: Trichomonacide, amebicide, antiinfective

MECHANISM OF ACTION
A nitroimidazole derivative that disrupts bacterial and protozoal DNA, inhibiting nucleic acid synthesis.
Therapeutic Effect: Produces bactericidal, antiprotozoal, amebicidal, and trichomonacidal effects. Produces antiinflammatory and immunosuppressive effects when applied topically.

USES
Treatment of intestinal amebiasis, amebic abscess, trichomoniasis, refractory trichomoniasis, bacterial anaerobic infections, giardiasis

PHARMACOKINETICS
Well absorbed from the GI tract; minimally absorbed after topical application. Protein binding: less than 20%. Widely distributed; crosses blood-brain barrier. Metabolized in the liver to active metabolite. Primarily excreted in urine; partially eliminated in feces. Removed by hemodialysis.
Half-life: 8 hr (increased in alcoholic hepatic disease and in neonates).

INDICATIONS AND DOSAGES
▶ **Amebiasis**
PO
Adults, Elderly. 500–750 mg q8h.
Children. 35–50 mg/kg/day in divided doses q8h.
▶ **Trichomoniasis**
PO
Adults, Elderly. 250 mg q8h or 2 g as a single dose.
Children. 15–30 mg/kg/day in divided doses q8h.
▶ **Anaerobic Skin and Skin-Structure, CNS, Lower Respiratory Tract, Bone, Joint, Intraabdominal, and Gynecologic Infections; Endocarditis; Septicemia**
PO, IV
Adults, Elderly, Children. 30 mg/kg/day in divided doses q6h.
Maximum: 4 g/day.
▶ **Antibiotic-Associated Pseudomembranous Colitis**
PO
Adults, Elderly. 250–500 mg 3–4 times a day for 10–14 days.
Children. 30 mg/kg/day in divided doses q6h for 7–10 days.
▶ **Helicobacter Pylori Infections**
PO
Adults, Elderly. 250–500 mg 3 times a day (in combination).
Children. 15–20 mg/kg/day in 2 divided doses.

▸ **Bacterial Vaginosis**
PO
Adults. 750 mg at bedtime for 7 days.
Intravaginal
Adults. One applicatorful twice a day or once a day at bedtime for 5 days.
▸ **Rosacea**
Topical
Adults. Apply thin layer of lotion to affected area twice a day or cream once a day.

SIDE EFFECTS/ADVERSE REACTIONS
Frequent
Systemic: Anorexia, nausea, dry mouth, metallic taste
Vaginal: Symptomatic cervicitis and vaginitis, abdominal cramps, uterine pain
Occasional
Systemic: Diarrhea or constipation, vomiting, dizziness, erythematous rash, urticaria, reddish brown urine
Topical: Transient erythema, mild dryness, burning, irritation, stinging, tearing when applied too close to eyes
Vaginal: Vaginal, perineal, or vulvar itching; vulvar swelling
Rare
Mild, transient leukopenia; thrombophlebitis with IV therapy

PRECAUTIONS AND CONTRAINDICATIONS
Hypersensitivity to metronidazole or other nitroimidazole derivatives (also parabens with topical application)
Caution:
Candida infections; avoid unnecessary use because shown to be carcinogenic in rodents

DRUG INTERACTIONS OF CONCERN TO DENTISTRY
• Disulfiram-like reaction: alcohol, alcohol-containing products
• Decreased action: phenobarbital
• Possible increase in blood levels of tacrolimus
• Enhanced effects of warfarin, carbamazepine

SERIOUS REACTIONS
! Oral therapy may result in furry tongue, glossitis, cystitis, dysuria, pancreatitis, and flattening of T waves on ECG readings.
! Peripheral neuropathy, manifested as numbness and tingling in hands or feet, is usually reversible if treatment is stopped immediately after neurologic symptoms appear.
! Seizures occur occasionally.

DENTAL CONSIDERATIONS

M

General:
• Patients on chronic drug therapy may rarely have symptoms of blood dyscrasias, which can include infection, bleeding, and poor healing.
• Assess salivary flow as a factor in caries, periodontal disease, and candidiasis.
• Determine why the patient is taking the drug.
Consultations:
• In a patient with symptoms of blood dyscrasias, request a medical consultation for blood studies and postpone dental treatment until normal values are reestablished.
• Medical consultation may be required to assess disease control.
Teach Patient/Family to:
• Avoid alcoholic beverages and mouth rinses.
• Report taste alterations.
• Encourage effective oral hygiene to prevent soft tissue inflammation.

• Use caution to prevent injury when using oral hygiene aids.
• When chronic dry mouth occurs, advise patient to:
  • Avoid mouth rinses with high alcohol content because of drying effects.
  • Use sugarless gum, frequent sips of water, or saliva substitutes.
  • Use daily home fluoride products for anticaries effect.

metyrosine
me-tye´-roe-seen
(Demser)

CATEGORY AND SCHEDULE
Pregnancy Risk Category: C

Drug Class: Antihypertensives

MECHANISM OF ACTION
A tyrosine hydroxylase inhibitor that blocks conversion of tyrosine to dihydroxyphenylalanine, the rate-limiting step in the biosynthetic pathway of catecholamines.
Therapeutic Effect: Reduces levels of endogenous catecholamines.

USES
Treatment of high B/P (hypertension) caused by a disease called pheochromocytoma (a noncancerous tumor of the adrenal gland)

PHARMACOKINETICS
Well absorbed from the GI tract. Metabolized in the liver. Excreted primarily in the urine. **Half-life:** 7.2 hr.

INDICATIONS AND DOSAGES
▶ Pheochromocytoma (Preoperative)
PO
Adults, Elderly. Initially, 250 mg 4 times a day. Increase by 250–500 mg/day up to 4 g/day. Maintenance: 2–4 g/day in 4 divided doses for 5–7 days.

SIDE EFFECTS/ADVERSE REACTIONS
Frequent
Drowsiness, extrapyramidal symptoms, diarrhea
Occasional
Galactorrhea, edema of the breasts, nausea, vomiting, dry mouth, impotence, nasal congestion
Rare
Lower extremity edema, urinary problems, urticaria, anemia, depression, disorientation

PRECAUTIONS AND CONTRAINDICATIONS
Hypertension of unknown etiology, hypersensitivity to metyrosine or any component of the formulation

DRUG INTERACTIONS OF CONCERN TO DENTISTRY
• Increased CNS depression with CNS depressants
• NSAIDs may antagonize hypotensive effect

SERIOUS REACTIONS
! Serious or life-threatening allergic reaction characterized by hallucinations, hematuria, hyperstimulation after withdrawal, severe lower extremity edema, and parkinsonism.

DENTAL CONSIDERATIONS

General:
• Medication may be used in anticipation of surgery to remove the adrenal tumor.

• Hypertension may preclude all dental care except for palliative emergency treatment.
• Question patient about compliance with drug therapy.
• Risk of increased CNS depression when other CNS depressants are used.
• Use stress-reduction protocol.
• Trismus may be a symptom of excessive doses of this drug.
• Determine why patient is taking the drug.
• Monitor and record vital signs.
• Use vasoconstrictor with caution, in low doses, and with careful aspiration. Avoid using gingival retraction cord containing epinephrine.
• Assess for presence of extrapyramidal motor symptoms, such as tardive dyskinesia and akathisia; extrapyramidal motor activity may complicate dental treatment. Advise seeing physician if tardive dyskinesia or akathisia is present.
Consultations:
• Medical consultation may be required to assess disease control and patient's ability to tolerate stress.
Teach Patient/Family to:
• Encourage effective oral hygiene to prevent soft tissue inflammation.
• Not drive or perform other tasks requiring mental alertness.

mexiletine hydrochloride
mex-**il′**-eh-teen
high-droh-**klor′**-ide
(Mexitil)

CATEGORY AND SCHEDULE
Pregnancy Risk Category: C

Drug Class: Antidysrhythmic (class IB, lidocaine analog)

MECHANISM OF ACTION
An antiarrhythmic that shortens duration of action potential and decreases effective refractory period in the His-Purkinje system of the myocardium by blocking sodium transport across myocardial cell membranes.
Therapeutic Effect: Suppresses ventricular arrhythmias.

USES
Treatment of documented life-threatening ventricular dysrhythmias

PHARMACOKINETICS
PO: Peak 2–3 hr. *Half-life:* 12 hr; metabolized by liver; excreted unchanged by kidneys (10%); excreted in breast milk.

INDICATIONS AND DOSAGES
▶ Arrhythmia
PO
Adults, Elderly. Initially, 200 mg q8h. Adjust dosage by 50–100 mg at 2- to 3-day intervals. Maximum: 1200 mg/day.

SIDE EFFECTS/ADVERSE REACTIONS
Frequent
GI distress, including nausea, vomiting, and heartburn; dizziness; light-headedness; tremors

Occasional

Nervousness, change in sleep habits, headache, visual disturbances, paresthesia, diarrhea or constipation, palpitations, chest pain, rash, respiratory difficulty, edema

PRECAUTIONS AND CONTRAINDICATIONS

Cardiogenic shock, preexisting second- or third-degree AV block, right bundle-branch block without presence of pacemaker

Caution:

Lactation, children, renal disease, liver disease, CHF, respiratory depression, myasthenia gravis

DRUG INTERACTIONS OF CONCERN TO DENTISTRY

• No specific interactions are reported with dental drugs; however, any drug that could affect the cardiac action of mexiletine should be used in the least effective dose, such as other local anesthetics, vasoconstrictors, and anticholinergics.

SERIOUS REACTIONS

! Mexiletine has the ability to worsen existing arrhythmias or produce new ones.
! CHF may occur, and existing CHF may worsen.

DENTAL CONSIDERATIONS

General:

• Monitor vital signs at every appointment because of cardiovascular side effects.

• Patients on chronic drug therapy may rarely have symptoms of blood dyscrasias, which can include infection, bleeding, and poor healing.

• Assess salivary flow as a factor in caries, periodontal disease, and candidiasis.

• Stress from dental procedures may compromise cardiovascular function; determine patient risk and use stress-reduction protocol.

Consultations:

• In a patient with symptoms of blood dyscrasias, request a medical consultation for blood studies and postpone dental treatment until normal values are reestablished.

• Medical consultation should be made to assess disease control.

• Medical consultation may be required to assess patient's ability to tolerate stress.

Teach Patient/Family to:

• Encourage effective oral hygiene to prevent soft tissue inflammation.

• Use caution to prevent injury when using oral hygiene aids.

• When chronic dry mouth occurs, advise patient to:

  • Avoid mouth rinses with high alcohol content because of drying effects.

  • Use sugarless gum, frequent sips of water, or saliva substitutes.

  • Use daily home fluoride products for anticaries effect.

miconazole

mih-**kon**´-ah-zole
(Femizol-M, Micatin, Micozole[CAN], Monistat[CAN], Monistat-3, Monistat-7, Monistat-Derm)

CATEGORY AND SCHEDULE

Pregnancy Risk Category: C

Drug Class: Antifungal

MECHANISM OF ACTION

An imidazole derivative that inhibits synthesis of ergosterol (vital component of fungal cell formation), damaging cell membrane.
Therapeutic Effect: Fungistatic; may be fungicidal, depending on concentration.

USES

Treatment of tinea pedis, tinea cruris, tinea corporis, tinea versicolor, vaginal or vulval *Candida albicans*

PHARMACOKINETICS

Parenteral: Widely distributed in tissues. Metabolized in liver. Primarily excreted in urine.
Half-life: 24 hr. Topical: No systemic absorption following application to intact skin. Intravaginally: Small amount absorbed systemically.

INDICATIONS AND DOSAGES

▶ **Coccidioidomycosis**
IV
Adults, Elderly. 1.8–3.6 g/day for 3–20 wk or longer.
▶ **Cryptococcosis**
IV
Adults, Elderly. 1.2–2.4 g/day for 3–12 wk or longer.
▶ **Petriellidiosis**
IV
Adults, Elderly. 0.6–3.0 g/day for 5–20 wk or longer.
▶ **Candidiasis**
IV
Adults, Elderly. 0.6–1.8 g/day for 1–20 wk or longer.
▶ **Paracoccidioidomycosis**
IV
Adults, Elderly. 0.2–1.2 g/day for 2–16 wk or longer.

▶ **Usual Dosage for Children**
IV
20–40 mg/kg/day in 3 divided doses. (Do not exceed 15 mg/kg for any 1 infusion.)
▶ **Vulvovaginal Candidiasis**
Intravaginally
Adults, Elderly. One 200 mg suppository at bedtime for 3 days; one 100 mg suppository or one applicatorful at bedtime for 7 days.
▶ **Topical Fungal Infections, Cutaneous Candidiasis**
Topical
Adults, Elderly, Children 2 yr and older. Apply liberally 2 times a day, morning and evening.

SIDE EFFECTS/ADVERSE REACTIONS

Frequent
Phlebitis, fever, chills, rash, itching, nausea, vomiting
Occasional
Dizziness, drowsiness, headache, flushed face, abdominal pain, constipation, diarrhea, decreased appetite
Topical: Itching, burning, stinging, erythema, urticaria
Vaginal: Vulvovaginal burning, itching, irritation, headache, skin rash

PRECAUTIONS AND CONTRAINDICATIONS

Children younger than 1 yr, hypersensitivity to miconazole or any component of the formulation
Topically: Children younger than 2 yr
Caution:
Lactation

DRUG INTERACTIONS OF CONCERN TO DENTISTRY

• Warfarin anticoagulants: potential for increased bleeding

M

• Drugs metabolized by CYP hepatic isoenzyme system: potential increased blood levels of metabolized drugs (e.g., benzodiazepines, phenytoin, anesthetics)

SERIOUS REACTIONS
! Anemia, thrombocytopenia, and liver toxicity occur rarely.

DENTAL CONSIDERATIONS
General:
• Examine oral mucous membranes for signs of fungal infection.
• Broad-spectrum antibiotics may evoke vaginal yeast infections.
Teach Patient/Family to:
• Prevent reinoculation of *Candida* infection by disposing of tooth brush or other contaminated oral hygiene devices used during period of infection.

midazolam hydrochloride
mid-**az**′-zoe-lam
high-droh-**klor**′-ide
(Apo-Midazolam[CAN],
Hypnovel[AUS], Versed)
Do not confuse Versed with
VePesid.

CATEGORY AND SCHEDULE
Pregnancy Risk Category: D
Controlled substance: Schedule
IV

Drug Class: Benzodiazepine,
sedative, anesthesia adjunct

MECHANISM OF ACTION
A benzodiazepine that enhances the action of gamma-aminobutyric acid, one of the major inhibitory neurotransmitters in the brain.

Therapeutic Effect: Produces anxiolytic, hypnotic, anticonvulsant, muscle relaxant, and amnestic effects.

USES
Conscious sedation, general anesthesia induction, sedation for diagnostic endoscopic procedures, intubation, preoperative sedation, amnesia

PHARMACOKINETICS

Route	Onset	Peak	Duration
PO	10–20 min	N/A	N/A
IV	1–5 min	5–7 min	20–30 min
IM	5–15 min	15–60 min	2–6 hr

Well absorbed after IM administration. Protein binding: 97%. Metabolized in the liver to active metabolite. Primarily excreted in urine. Not removed by hemodialysis. *Half-life:* 1–5 hr.

INDICATIONS AND DOSAGES
▸ **Preoperative Sedation**
PO
Children. 0.25–0.5 mg/kg.
Maximum: 20 mg.
IV
Children 6–12 yr. 0.025–0.05 mg/kg.
Children 6 mo–5 yr. 0.05–0.1 mg/kg.
IM
Adults, Elderly. 0.07–0.08 mg/kg 30–60 min before surgery.
Children. 0.1–0.15 mg/kg 30–60 min before surgery. Maximum: 10 mg.
▸ **Conscious Sedation for Diagnostic, Therapeutic, and Endoscopic Procedures**
IV
Adults, Elderly. 1–2.5 mg over 2 min. Titrate as needed. Maximum total dose: 2.5–5 mg.

▸ **Conscious Sedation During Mechanical Ventilation**

IV

Adults, Elderly. 0.01–0.05 mg/kg; may repeat q10–15min until adequately sedated. Then continuous infusion at initial rate of 0.02–0.1 mg/kg/hr (1–7 mg/hr).

Children older than 32 wk. Initially, 1 mcg/kg/min as continuous infusion.

Children 32 wk and younger. Initially, 0.5 mcg/kg/min as continuous infusion.

▸ **Status Epilepticus**

IV

Children older than 2 mo. Loading dose of 0.15 mg/kg followed by continuous infusion of 1 mcg/kg/min. Titrate as needed. Range: 1–18 mcg/kg/min.

SIDE EFFECTS/ADVERSE REACTIONS

Frequent

Decreased respiratory rate, tenderness at IM or IV injection site, pain during injection, oxygen desaturation, hiccups

Occasional

Hypotension, paradoxical CNS reaction

Rare

Nausea, vomiting, headache, coughing

PRECAUTIONS AND CONTRAINDICATIONS

Acute alcohol intoxication, acute angle-closure glaucoma, coma, shock

Caution:

COPD, CHF, chronic renal failure, chills, elderly, debilitated, children younger than 18 yr; to be used only by health care professionals skilled in airway maintenance and ventilation and resuscitation techniques

DRUG INTERACTIONS OF CONCERN TO DENTISTRY

• Prolonged respiratory depression: all CNS depressants, including alcohol, barbiturates, narcotics. All doses of midazolam must be reduced when used in combination with any CNS depressant. Serious respiratory and cardiovascular depression, including death, has occurred when midazolam is used in combination with other CNS depressants or given too rapidly. Medically compromised and elderly patients are at greater risk.

• Increased serum levels and prolonged effect of benzodiazepines: erythromycin, clarithromycin, ketoconazole, itraconazole, fluconazole, miconazole (systemic), diltiazem, fluvoxamine.

• Contraindicated with nelfinavir, ritonavir, indinavir, saquinavir.

• Possible increase in CNS side effects: kava kava (herb).

• Suspected increase in midazolam effects when used in general anesthesia: atorvastatin.

SERIOUS REACTIONS

‼ Inadequate or excessive dosage or improper administration may result in cerebral hypoxia, agitation, involuntary movements, hyperactivity, and combativeness.

‼ A too-rapid IV rate, excessive doses, or a single large dose increases the risk of respiratory depression or arrest.

‼ Respiratory depression or apnea may produce hypoxia and cardiac arrest.

DENTAL CONSIDERATIONS

General:

• Monitor vital signs every 5 min during general anesthesia because of cardiovascular and respiratory side

M

effects. Monitor vital signs at regular intervals during recovery.

• Degree of CNS depression is dose dependent; titrate all doses.

• Drug produces amnesia, especially in the elderly patient.

• Longer recovery period could be observed in an obese patient because half-life may be extended.

• Assist patient with ambulation until drowsy period has passed.

Teach Patient/Family to:

• Avoid driving or potentially hazardous activities until drowsiness or weakness subsides.

• Be aware of anterograde amnesia; events may not be remembered.

• Treat overdose: O_2, vasopressors, flumazenil, resuscitation measures as required.

midodrine

mid′-oh-drin
(Amatine, ProAmatine)
Do not confuse Amatine or
ProAmatine with amantadine or
protamine.

CATEGORY AND SCHEDULE
Pregnancy Risk Category: C

Drug Class: Vasopressor;
orthostatic hypotension adjunct

MECHANISM OF ACTION
A vasopressor that forms the active metabolite desglymidodrine, an α_1-agonist, activating α receptors of the arteriolar and venous vasculature.
Therapeutic Effect: Increases vascular tone and B/P.

USES
Treatment of symptomatic orthostatic; hypotension

PHARMACOKINETICS
Peak 1–2 hr. *Half-life:* 3–4 hr, bioavailability 90%.

INDICATIONS AND DOSAGES
▶ Orthostatic Hypotension
PO
Adults, Elderly. 10 mg 3 times a day. Give during the day when patient is upright, such as upon arising, midday, and late afternoon. Do not give later than 6 PM.
▶ Dosage in Renal Impairment
Adults, Elderly. Give 2.5 mg 3 times a day; increase gradually, as tolerated.

SIDE EFFECTS/ADVERSE REACTIONS
Frequent
Paresthesia, piloerection, pruritus, dysuria, supine hypertension
Occasional
Pain, rash, chills, headache, facial flushing, confusion, dry mouth, anxiety

PRECAUTIONS AND CONTRAINDICATIONS
Acute renal function impairment, persistent hypertension, pheochromocytoma, severe cardiac disease, thyrotoxicosis, urine retention

DRUG INTERACTIONS OF CONCERN TO DENTISTRY
• Risk of increased pressor effects: α-adrenergic agonists

SERIOUS REACTIONS
! None known

DENTAL CONSIDERATIONS

General:
• Carefully review patient's medical and drug history.

- Supine hypotension is a serious side effect; a more upright chair position is highly desirable.
- Determine why patient is taking the drug.
- Monitor and record vital signs at every appointment.
- Use vasoconstrictor with caution, in low doses, and with careful aspiration. Avoid using gingival retraction cord containing epinephrine.
- Examine for oral manifestation of opportunistic infection.
- Assess salivary flow as a factor in caries, periodontal disease, and candidiasis.
- Be aware of patient's disease, its severity, and frequency when known.
- Short appointments and a stress-reduction protocol may be required for anxious patients.
- Precaution if dental surgery is anticipated or general anesthesia is required.

Consultations:
- Medical consultation may be required to assess disease control and patient's ability to tolerate stress.

Teach Patient/Family to:
- Use OTC medications, such as cough, cold, and diet preparations, cautiously because they may affect B/P.
- When chronic dry mouth occurs advise patient to:
  - Avoid mouth rinses with high alcohol content because of drying effects.
  - Use daily home fluoride products for anticaries effect.
  - Use sugarless gum, frequent sips of water, or saliva substitutes.

miglitol
mig′-lee-tall
(Glyset)

CATEGORY AND SCHEDULE
Pregnancy Risk Category: B

Drug Class: Oligosaccharide, glucosidase enzyme inhibitor

MECHANISM OF ACTION
An α-glucosidase inhibitor that delays the digestion of ingested carbohydrates into simple sugars such as glucose.
Therapeutic Effect: Produces smaller rise in blood glucose concentration after meals.

USES
Treatment of type 2 diabetes when diet control is ineffective in controlling blood glucose levels, used as single agent or in combination with other oral hypoglycemics

PHARMACOKINETICS
PO: Peak plasma levels 2–3 hr; negligible plasma protein binding, not metabolized, urinary excretion.

INDICATIONS AND DOSAGES
▸ **Diabetes Mellitus**
PO
Adults, Elderly. Initially, 25 mg 3 times a day with first bite of each main meal. Maintenance: 50 mg 3 times a day. Maximum: 100 mg 3 times a day.

SIDE EFFECTS/ADVERSE REACTIONS
Frequent
Flatulence, loose stools, diarrhea, abdominal pain

M

Occasional
Rash

PRECAUTIONS AND CONTRAINDICATIONS

Colonic ulceration, diabetic ketoacidosis, hypersensitivity to miglitol, inflammatory bowel disease, partial intestinal obstruction
Caution:
Renal impairment, hypoglycemia, lactation, children

DRUG INTERACTIONS OF CONCERN TO DENTISTRY

• None reported

DENTAL CONSIDERATIONS

General:
• Ensure that patient is following prescribed diet and regularly takes medication.
• Type 2 patients may also be using insulin. Should symptomatic hypoglycemia occur while taking this drug, use glucose rather than sucrose because of interference with sucrose metabolism.
• Place on frequent recall to evaluate healing response.
• Short appointments and a stress-reduction protocol may be required for anxious patients.
• Diabetics may be more susceptible to infection and have delayed wound healing.
• Consider semisupine chair position for patient comfort if GI side effects occur.
• Question patient about self-monitoring of drug's antidiabetic effect, including blood glucose values or finger-stick records.
• Examine for oral manifestation of opportunistic infection.
Consultations:
• Medical consultation may be required to assess disease control

and patient's ability to tolerate stress.
• Medical consultation may include data from patient's blood glucose monitoring, including glycosylated hemoglobin or HbA$_{1c}$ testing.
Teach Patient/Family to:
• Update health and drug history if physician makes any changes in evaluation or drug regimens; include OTC, herbal, and nonherbal drugs in update.
• Encourage effective oral hygiene to prevent soft tissue inflammation.

miglustat

mig'-lew-stat
(Zavesca)

CATEGORY AND SCHEDULE

Pregnancy Risk Category: X

Drug Class: Enzyme inhibitor

MECHANISM OF ACTION

A Gaucher's disease agent that inhibits the enzyme, glucosylceramide synthase, reducing the rate of synthesis of most glycosphingolipids. Allows the residual activity of the deficient enzyme, glucocerebrosidase, to be more effective in degrading lysosomal storage within tissues.
Therapeutic Effect: Minimizes conditions associated with Gaucher's disease, such as anemia and bone disease.

USES

Treatment of adult patients with mild to moderate Type 1 Gaucher's disease for whom enzyme replacement therapy is not an option

PHARMACOKINETICS

PO: Maximum plasma levels 2–2.5 hr. *Half-life:* about 6–7 hr; oral bioavailability 97%, no plasma protein binding, excreted unchanged in urine.

INDICATIONS AND DOSAGES

▸ **Gaucher's Disease**

PO

Adults, Elderly. One 100-mg capsule 3 times a day at regular intervals.

▸ **Dosage in Renal Impairment**

Patients with creatinine clearance of 50–70 ml/min. Dosage is reduced to 100 mg twice a day.

Patients with creatinine clearance of 30–49 ml/min. Dosage is 100 mg once a day.

SIDE EFFECTS/ADVERSE REACTIONS

Expected

Diarrhea, weight loss, dry mouth

Frequent

Hand tremors, flatulence, headache, abdominal pain, nausea

Occasional

Paresthesia, anorexia, dyspepsia, leg cramps, vomiting

PRECAUTIONS AND CONTRAINDICATIONS

Women who are or may become pregnant

Caution:

Efficacy and safety not evaluated in patients younger than 18 yr or older than 65 yr, renal impairment, women of reproductive age, provide pretreatment neurologic evaluation, lactation

DRUG INTERACTIONS OF CONCERN TO DENTISTRY

• None reported

SERIOUS REACTIONS

❗ Thrombocytopenia occurs in 7% of patients.

❗ Overdose produces dizziness and neutropenia.

DENTAL CONSIDERATIONS

General:

• Ask patient about disease control.

• Question patient about nosebleeds or other bleeding events.

• Short appointments and a stress-reduction protocol may be required for anxious patients.

• Avoid products that affect platelet function, such as aspirin and NSAIDs.

• Patients on chronic drug therapy may rarely have symptoms of blood dyscrasias, which can include infection, bleeding, and poor healing.

• Assess salivary flow as a factor in caries, periodontal disease, and candidiasis.

• Consider semisupine chair position for patient comfort as needed.

• Place on frequent recall to evaluate healing response.

Consultations:

• Medical consultation may be required to assess disease control and patient's ability to tolerate stress.

• Medical consultation should include routine blood counts, including platelet counts and bleeding time.

• In a patient with symptoms of blood dyscrasias, request a medical consultation for blood studies and postpone treatment until normal values are reestablished.

Teach Patient/Family to:

• Inform dentist of unusual bleeding episodes following dental treatment.

M

• Encourage effective oral hygiene to prevent soft tissue inflammation/ infection.
• Use powered tooth brush if patient has difficulty holding conventional devices.

milnacipran
(mil-nah-**sip**-ran)
(Savella)
Do not confuse with minocycline or Miltown.

CATEGORY AND SCHEDULE
Pregnancy Risk Category: C

Drug Class: Fibromyalgia agent

MECHANISM OF ACTION
Central inhibition of norepinephrine and serotonin reuptake (SNRI). *Therapeutic Effect:* Reduces perception of pain in CNS.

USES
Fibromyalgia pain

PHARMACOKINETICS
Well absorbed orally, 85%–90% bioavailability. Widely distributed, protein binding 13%. Partially metabolized in the liver, *Half-life:* 6–8 hr. Excreted by the kidneys, 55% as unchanged drug.

INDICATIONS AND DOSAGES
▶ Fibromyalgia
PO
Adults, Elderly. 50 mg twice daily, beginning with 12.5 mg total dose on first day of therapy, 12.5 mg twice daily on second and third days of therapy, 25 mg twice daily on days 4 through 7.

SIDE EFFECTS/ADVERSE REACTIONS
Frequent
Anorexia, constipation, dizziness, flushing, headache, hyperhidrosis, hypertension, insomnia, nausea, palpitations, tachycardia, vomiting, dry mouth
Occasional
Blurred vision, chills, disorder of ejaculation, dysuria, migraine, rash, tremors, weight loss
Rare
Abdominal pain and cramps, abnormal liver function tests, delirium, diarrhea, drowsiness, dysgeusia, dyspepsia, dyspnea, ecchymosis, epistaxis, erectile dysfunction, fatigue, fever, hemorrhage, hepatitis, hyperprolactinemia, irritability, leucopenia, changes in libido, pupil dilation, neuroleptic malignant syndrome, night sweats, peripheral edema, muscle pain/rhabdomyolysis, seizures, serotonin syndrome, SIADH syndrome, Stevens-Johnson syndrome, suicidal thoughts, thrombocytopenia, urinary retention

PRECAUTIONS AND CONTRAINDICATIONS
Hypersensitivity milnacipran hydrochloride or its ingredients, children younger than 18 yr, narrow-angle glaucoma, seizure disorder, alcoholism, liver disease, serotonin syndrome, severe renal disease, suicidal patients
Caution:
Children (possible suicide), renal function impairment, pregnancy/ lactation

DRUG INTERACTIONS OF CONCERN TO DENTISTRY
• Increased risk of CNS depression: all CNS depressants, alcohol. May

potentiate mental impairment and somnolence, postural hypotension, avoid alcohol
• Epinephrine: possible hypertension, cardiac dysrhythmias
• MAOIs: increased risk of serotonin syndrome
• Tramadol, tapentadol: increased risk of serotonin syndrome
• Selective serotonin reuptake inhibitors (SSRIs) (e.g., fluoxetine): potentially life-threatening serotonin syndrome

SERIOUS REACTIONS

! Serotonin syndrome (agitation, coma, autonomic instability including tachycardia, neuromuscular abnormalities, diarrhea, nausea, vomiting)
! Increased risk of suicide (children, patients with suicidal tendencies)

DENTAL CONSIDERATIONS

General:
• Avoid postural hypotension.
• Monitor vital signs for possible cardiovascular adverse effects.
• Assess salivary flow as a factor in caries, periodontal disease, and candidiasis.
• Avoid or limit doses of epinephrine in local anesthetic.
• Avoid in patients taking MAOIs or SSRIs.
Teach Patient/Family to:
• Avoid mouth rinses with high alcohol content because of drying effect.
• Use home fluoride products for anticaries effect.
• Use sugarless/xylitol gum, frequent sips of water, or saliva substitutes if dry mouth occurs.

minocycline hydrochloride
mi-noe-sye′-kleen
high-droh-klor′-ide
(Akamin[AUS], Arrestin[US], Dynacin, Minocin, Periostat Minomycin[AUS], Myrac, Novo Minocycline[CAN])
Do not confuse Dynacin with Dynabac or Minocin with Mithracin or niacin.

CATEGORY AND SCHEDULE
Pregnancy Risk Category: D

Drug Class: Tetracycline antiinfective

MECHANISM OF ACTION
A tetracycline antibiotic that inhibits bacterial protein synthesis by binding to ribosomes.
Therapeutic Effect: Bacteriostatic.

USES
Treatment of syphilis, C. trachomatis infection, gonorrhea, lymphogranuloma venereum, rickettsial infections, inflammatory acne, M. marinum, Neisseria meningitidis carriers, actinomycosis, anthrax, acute necrotizing ulcerative gingivitis, AA-induced periodontitis, and other susceptible infections; dental product is an adjunct to scaling and root planing in adult periodontitis

PHARMACOKINETICS
PO: Peak 2–3 hr. Half-life: 11–17 hr; 55%–88% protein bound; excreted in urine, feces, breast milk; crosses placenta.

INDICATIONS AND DOSAGES

▶ **Mild, Moderate, or Severe Prostate, Urinary Tract, and CNS Infections (excluding meningitis); Uncomplicated Gonorrhea; Inflammatory Acne; Brucellosis; Skin Granulomas; Cholera; Trachoma; Nocardiasis; Yaws; and Syphilis When Penicillins Are Contraindicated**

PO

Adults, Elderly. Initially, 100–200 mg, then 100 mg q12h or 50 mg q6h.

IV

Adults, Elderly. Initially, 200 mg, then 100 mg q12h up to 400 mg/day.

PO, IV

Children older than 8 yr. Initially, 4 mg/kg, then 2 mg/kg q12h.

SIDE EFFECTS/ADVERSE REACTIONS

Frequent

Dizziness, light-headedness, diarrhea, nausea, vomiting, abdominal cramps, possibly severe photosensitivity, drowsiness, vertigo

Occasional

Altered pigmentation of skin or mucous membranes, rectal or genital pruritus, stomatitis

PRECAUTIONS AND CONTRAINDICATIONS

Children younger than 8 yr, hypersensitivity to tetracyclines, last half of pregnancy

The use of tetracycline drugs during tooth development (last half of pregnancy, infancy, and childhood up to the age of 8 may cause permanent discoloration of the teeth (yellow-gray-brown). Enamel hypoplasia has also been reported. May also cause retardation of skeletal development and deformations.

Caution:

Hepatic disease, lactation

DRUG INTERACTIONS OF CONCERN TO DENTISTRY

• Decreased effect: antacids, milk, or other calcium- and aluminum-containing products
• Decreased effect of penicillins
• Oral contraceptives: advise patient of a potential risk for decreased contraceptive action, to maintain compliance with oral contraceptive use while using antibiotics, and to consider the use of additional nonhormonal contraception
• Contraindicated with isotretinoin (Accutane)
• Drug interactions of concern to dentistry minocycline HCl (microspheres)

SERIOUS REACTIONS

! Superinfection (especially fungal), anaphylaxis, and benign intracranial hypertension may occur.
! Bulging fontanelles occur rarely in infants.

DENTAL CONSIDERATIONS

General:

• Avoid prescribing during pregnancy.
• This drug is reported to cause intrinsic staining in erupted permanent teeth not associated with the calcification stage.
• The drug readily distributes to gingival crevicular fluid.
• Do not prescribe drug during pregnancy or in patients younger than 8 yr because of tooth discoloration.
• Advise patient if dental drugs prescribed have a potential for photosensitivity.

• Do not use ingestible sodium bicarbonate products, such as the Prophy-Jet air polishing system, at the same time dose is taken; take minocycline 2 hr later.
• Determine why the patient is taking the drug.
• Dental staining or enamel hypoplasia may be associated with exposure to this drug before birth or up to the age of 8. Tetracycline stains may be extremely resistant to ordinary tooth-whitening procedures.
Consultations:
• Medical consultation may be required to assess disease control.
Teach Patient/Family to:
• Encourage effective oral hygiene to prevent soft tissue inflammation.
• Use caution to prevent injury when using oral hygiene aids.
• Avoid mouth rinses with high alcohol content because of drying effects.
• When used for dental infection, advise patient to:
  • Report sore throat, oral burning sensation, fever, fatigue, any of which could indicate superinfection.
  • Take at prescribed intervals and complete dosage regimen.
  • Immediately notify the dentist if signs or symptoms of infection increase.

▸ **Microspheres**
General:
• Follow all general precautions when using tetracyclines.
Teach Patient/Family to:
• Avoid eating hard, crunchy foods for 1 wk.
• Postpone tooth brushing for 12 hr.
• Postpone use of interproximal cleaning devices for 10 days.
• Notify dentist immediately if pain, swelling, or other unexpected symptoms occur.

minoxidil

mih-**nox**′-ih-dill
(Apo-Gain[CAN], Loniten, Milnox[CAN], Regaine[AUS], Rogaine, Rogaine Extra Strength)
Do not confuse Loniten with Lotensin.

CATEGORY AND SCHEDULE
Pregnancy Risk Category: C
OTC (topical solution)

Drug Class: Antihypertensive

MECHANISM OF ACTION
An antihypertensive and hair growth stimulant that has direct action on vascular smooth muscle, producing vasodilation of arterioles.
Therapeutic Effect: Decreases peripheral vascular resistance and B/P; increases cutaneous blood flow; stimulates hair follicle epithelium and hair follicle growth.

USES
Treatment of severe hypertension not responsive to other therapy (used with a diuretic and α-adrenergic antagonist); topically to treat androgenic alopecia

PHARMACOKINETICS

Route	Onset	Peak	Duration
PO	0.5 hr	2–8 hr	2–5 days

Well absorbed from the GI tract; minimal absorption after topical application. Protein binding: None. Widely distributed. Metabolized in the liver to active metabolite. Primarily excreted in urine. Removed by hemodialysis. *Half-life:* 4.2 hr.

INDICATIONS AND DOSAGES

▶ **Severe Symptomatic Hypertension, Hypertension Associated with Organ Damage, Hypertension That Has Failed to Respond to Maximal Therapeutic Dosages of a Diuretic or Two Other Antihypertensives**

PO

Adults. Initially, 5 mg/day. Increase with at least 3-day intervals to 10 mg, then 20 mg, then up to 40 mg/day in 1–2 doses.

Elderly. Initially, 2.5 mg/day. May increase gradually. Maintenance: 10–40 mg/day. Maximum: 100 mg/day.

Children. Initially, 0.1–0.2 mg/kg (5 mg maximum) daily. Gradually increase at a minimum of 3-day intervals. Maintenance: 0.25–1 mg/kg/day in 1–2 doses. Maximum: 50 mg/day.

▶ **Hair Regrowth**

Topical

Adults. 1 ml to affected areas of scalp 2 times a day. Total daily dose not to exceed 2 ml.

SIDE EFFECTS/ADVERSE REACTIONS

Frequent

PO: Edema with concurrent weight gain, hypertrichosis (elongation, thickening, increased pigmentation of fine body hair; develops in 80% of patients within 3–6 wk after beginning therapy)

Occasional

PO: T-wave changes (usually revert to pretreatment state with continued therapy or drug withdrawal)

Topical: Pruritus, rash, dry or flaking skin, erythema

Rare

PO: Breast tenderness, headache, photosensitivity reaction

Topical: Allergic reaction, alopecia, burning sensation at scalp, soreness at hair root, headache, visual disturbances

PRECAUTIONS AND CONTRAINDICATIONS

Pheochromocytoma

Caution:

Lactation, children, renal disease, CAD, CHF

DRUG INTERACTIONS OF CONCERN TO DENTISTRY

• Decreased effects: NSAIDs, indomethacin, sympathomimetics

• Increased hypotension: CNS depressant drug used in conscious sedation technique may also lower B/P

SERIOUS REACTIONS

! Tachycardia and angina pectoris may occur because of increased oxygen demands associated with increased heart rate and cardiac output.

! Fluid and electrolyte imbalance and CHF may occur, especially if a diuretic is not given concurrently with minoxidil.

! Too rapid reduction in B/P may result in syncope, CVA, MI, and ocular or vestibular ischemia.

! Pericardial effusion and tamponade may be seen in patients with impaired renal function who are not on dialysis.

DENTAL CONSIDERATIONS

General:

• Monitor vital signs at every appointment because of cardiovascular side effects.

• Patients on chronic drug therapy may rarely have symptoms of blood dyscrasias, which can include infection, bleeding, and poor healing.

- Limit use of sodium-containing products, such as saline IV fluids, for patients with a dietary salt restriction.
- Short appointments and a stress-reduction protocol may be required for anxious patients.
- After supine positioning, have patient sit upright for at least 2 min before standing to avoid orthostatic hypotension.

Consultations:

- In a patient with symptoms of blood dyscrasias, request a medical consultation for blood studies and postpone dental treatment until normal values are reestablished.
- Medical consultation may be required to assess disease control and patient's ability to tolerate stress.

mirtazapine
mir-**taz**′-ah-peen
(Avanza[AUS], Mirtazon[AUS], Remeron, Remeron Soltab)
Do not confuse Remeron with Premarin.

CATEGORY AND SCHEDULE
Pregnancy Risk Category: C

Drug Class: Tetracyclic antidepressant

MECHANISM OF ACTION
A tetracyclic compound that acts as an antagonist at presynaptic α_2-adrenergic receptors, increasing both norepinephrine and serotonin neurotransmission. Has low anticholinergic activity.
Therapeutic Effect: Relieves depression and produces sedative effects.

USES
Treatment of depression

PHARMACOKINETICS
Rapidly and completely absorbed after PO administration; absorption not affected by food. Protein binding: 85%. Metabolized in the liver. Primarily excreted in urine. Unknown if removed by hemodialysis. **Half-life:** 20–40 hr (longer in males [37 hr] than females [26 hr]).

INDICATIONS AND DOSAGES
▸ **Depression**
PO
Adults. Initially, 15 mg at bedtime. May increase by 15 mg/day q1–2wk. Maximum: 45 mg/day.
Elderly. Initially, 7.5 mg at bedtime. May increase by 7.5–15 mg/day q1–2wk. Maximum: 45 mg/day.

SIDE EFFECTS/ADVERSE REACTIONS
Frequent
Somnolence, dry mouth, increased appetite, constipation, weight gain
Occasional
Asthenia, dizziness, flu-like symptoms, abnormal dreams
Rare
Abdominal discomfort, vasodilation, paresthesia, acne, dry skin, thirst, arthralgia

PRECAUTIONS AND CONTRAINDICATIONS
Use within 14 days of MAOIs
Caution:
Hepatic impairment, renal impairment, elderly, nursing, pediatric, suicidal ideation, cardiovascular or cerebrovascular disease aggravated by hypotension, avoid alcohol use

M

DRUG INTERACTIONS OF CONCERN TO DENTISTRY

• Impairment of cognitive and motor performance with diazepam or other drugs used in conscious sedation
• Use opioid analgesics with caution because of impairment of cognitive or motor performance; NSAIDs may be a more appropriate choice

SERIOUS REACTIONS

! Mirtazapine poses a higher risk of seizures than tricyclic antidepressants, especially in those with no previous history of seizures.
! Overdose may produce cardiovascular effects, such as severe orthostatic hypotension, dizziness, tachycardia, palpitations, and arrhythmias.
! Abrupt discontinuation after prolonged therapy may produce headache, malaise, nausea, vomiting, and vivid dreams.
! Agranulocytosis occurs rarely.

DENTAL CONSIDERATIONS

General:
• Patients on chronic drug therapy may rarely have symptoms of blood dyscrasias, which can include infection, bleeding, and poor healing.
• Assess salivary flow as a factor in caries, periodontal disease, and candidiasis.
• Monitor vital signs at every appointment because of cardiovascular side effects.
• Consider semisupine chair position for patient comfort if GI or MS side effects occur.
• Place on frequent recall if oral side effects are a problem.

Consultations:
• In a patient with symptoms of blood dyscrasias, request a medical consultation for blood studies and postpone dental treatment until normal values are reestablished.
• Take precaution if dental surgery is anticipated and sedation or general anesthesia is required; risk of hypotensive episode.
• Medical consultation may be required to assess disease control.
• Physician should be informed if significant xerostomic side effects occur (e.g., increased caries, sore tongue, problems eating or swallowing, difficulty wearing prosthesis) so that a medication change can be considered.

Teach Patient/Family to:
• Encourage effective oral hygiene to prevent soft tissue inflammation.
• Use caution to prevent soft tissue trauma when using oral hygiene aids.
• Update health history/drug record if physician makes any changes in evaluation or drug regimens; include OTC, herbal, and nonherbal drugs in update.
• Not drive or perform other tasks requiring alertness.
• When chronic dry mouth occurs, advise patient to:
  • Avoid mouth rinses with high alcohol content because of drying effects.
  • Use daily home fluoride products for anticaries effect.
  • Use sugarless gum, frequent sips of water, or saliva substitutes.

misoprostol
mis-oh-**pros'**-toll
(Cytotec)
Do not confuse with Cytomel.

CATEGORY AND SCHEDULE
Pregnancy Risk Category: X

Drug Class: Gastric mucosa
protectant

MECHANISM OF ACTION
A prostaglandin that inhibits basal,
nocturnal gastric acid secretion via
direct action on parietal cells.
Therapeutic Effect: Increases
production of protective gastric
mucus.

USES
Prevention of NSAID-induced
gastric ulcers

PHARMACOKINETICS
Rapidly absorbed from GI tract.
Rapidly converted to active
metabolite. Primarily excreted in
urine. *Half-life:* 20–40 min.

INDICATIONS AND DOSAGES
▶ **Prevention of NSAID-Induced
Gastric Ulcer**
PO
Adults. 200 mcg 4 times a day with
food (last dose at bedtime).
Continue for duration of NSAID
therapy. May reduce dosage to
100 mcg if 200 mcg dose is not
tolerable.
Elderly. 100–200 mcg 4 times a day
with food.

SIDE EFFECTS/ADVERSE
REACTIONS
Frequent
Abdominal pain, diarrhea

Occasional
Nausea, flatulence, dyspepsia,
headache
Rare
Vomiting, constipation

PRECAUTIONS AND
CONTRAINDICATIONS
Pregnancy (produces uterine
contractions), hypersensitivity to
misoprostol or any component of the
formulation
Caution:
Lactation, children, elderly, renal
disease

SERIOUS REACTIONS
! Overdosage may produce sedation,
tremors, convulsions, dyspnea,
palpitations, hypotension, and
bradycardia.

DENTAL CONSIDERATIONS
General:
• Avoid NSAIDs and salicylates in
patients with active upper GI
disease; acetaminophen/opioids are
more appropriate for pain control in
these patients.
Consultations:
• Medical consultation may be
required to assess disease control.

mitotane
my'-tow-tane
(Lysodren)

CATEGORY AND SCHEDULE
Pregnancy Risk Category: C

Drug Class: Antineoplastic

MECHANISM OF ACTION
A hormonal agent that inhibits
activity of the adrenal cortex.

Therapeutic Effect: Suppresses functional and nonfunctional adrenocortical neoplasms by direct cytoxic effect.

USES
Treatment of adrenocortical carcinoma

PHARMACOKINETICS
Adequately absorbed orally (40%). *Half-life:* 18–159 days; hepatic metabolism; excreted in urine, bile.

INDICATIONS AND DOSAGES
▶ **Adrenocortical Carcinomas**
PO
Adults, Elderly. Initially, 2–6 g/day in 3–4 divided doses. Increase by 2–4 g/day every 3–7 days up to 9–10 g/day. Range: 2–16 g/day.

SIDE EFFECTS/ADVERSE REACTIONS
Frequent
Anorexia, nausea, vomiting, diarrhea, lethargy, somnolence, adrenocortical insufficiency, dizziness, vertigo, maculopapular rash, hypouricemia
Occasional
Blurred or double vision, retinopathy, hearing loss, excessive salivation, urine abnormalities (hematuria, cystitis, albuminuria), hypertension, orthostatic hypotension, flushing, wheezing, dyspnea, generalized aching, fever

PRECAUTIONS AND CONTRAINDICATIONS
Known hypersensitivity to mitotane
Caution:
Lactation, hepatic disease, infection; avoid use or discontinue if adrenal cortical suppression occurs

DRUG INTERACTIONS OF CONCERN TO DENTISTRY
• Increased CNS depression: all CNS depressants
• Decreased effects of corticosteroids; if glucocorticoid replacement is necessary, use hydrocortisone

SERIOUS REACTIONS
! Brain damage and functional impairment may occur with long-term, high-dosage therapy.

DENTAL CONSIDERATIONS

General:
• Evaluate respiration characteristics and rate.
• Drug may cause adrenal hypofunction, especially under conditions of stress such as surgery, trauma, or acute illness. Patients should be carefully monitored and given hydrocortisone or mineralocorticoid as needed.
• Consider semisupine chair position for patient comfort if GI side effects occur.
• Patients taking opioids for acute or chronic pain should be given alternative analgesics for dental pain.
Consultations:
• Medical consultation may be required to assess disease control and patient's ability to tolerate stress.
Teach Patient/Family to:
• See dentist immediately if secondary oral infection occurs.
• Report oral lesions, soreness, or bleeding to dentist.
• Update medical/drug records if physician makes any changes in evaluation or drug regimens; include OTC, herbal, and nonherbal drugs in update.

mitoxantrone
my-toe-**zan´**-trone
(Novantrone, Onkotrone[AUS])

CATEGORY AND SCHEDULE
Pregnancy Risk Category: D

Drug Class: Antineoplastic,
antiinfective, immunomodulator;
synthetic anthraquinone

MECHANISM OF ACTION
An anthracenedione that inhibits
B-cell, T-cell, and macrophage
proliferation and DNA and RNA
synthesis. Active throughout the
entire cell cycle.
Therapeutic Effect: Causes cell
death.

PHARMACOKINETICS
Protein binding: 78%. Widely
distributed. Metabolized in the liver.
Primarily eliminated in feces by the
biliary system. Not removed by
hemodialysis. *Half-life:* 2.3–13
days.

USES
Treatment of some kinds of cancer.
It is also used to treat some forms of
multiple sclerosis.

PHARMACOKINETICS
Highly bound to plasma proteins,
metabolized in liver, excreted via
renal, hepatobiliary systems.
Half-life: 24–72 hr.

INDICATIONS AND DOSAGES
▶ **Leukemias**
IV
*Adults, Elderly, Children 2 yr and
older.* 12 mg/m² once a day for 2–3
days.
Children younger than 2 yr. 0.4 mg/
kg once a day for 3–5 days.

▶ **Acute Leukemia in Relapse**
IV
*Adults, Elderly, Children older than
2 yr.* 8–12 mg/m² once a day for 4–5
days.
▶ **Acute Nonlymphocytic Leukemia**
IV
*Adults, Elderly, Children older than
2 yr.* 10 mg/m² once a day for 3–5
days.
▶ **Solid Tumors**
IV
Adults, Elderly. 12–14 mg/m² once
q3–4wk.
Children. 18–20 mg/m² once
q3–4wk.
▶ **Prostate Cancer**
IV
Adults, Elderly. 12–14 mg/m² every
21 days.
▶ **Multiple Sclerosis**
IV
Adults, Elderly. 12 mg/m²/dose
q3mo.

SIDE EFFECTS/ADVERSE REACTIONS
Frequent
Nausea, vomiting, diarrhea, cough,
headache, stomatitis, abdominal
discomfort, fever, alopecia
Occasional
Ecchymosis, fungal infection,
conjunctivitis, UTI
Rare
Arrhythmias

PRECAUTIONS AND CONTRAINDICATIONS
Baseline left ventricular ejection
fraction less than 50%, cumulative
lifetime mitoxantrone dose of
140 mg/m² or more, multiple
sclerosis with hepatic impairment

DRUG INTERACTIONS OF CONCERN TO DENTISTRY
• None reported

SERIOUS REACTIONS

! Myelosuppression may be severe, resulting in GI bleeding, hematologic toxicity, sepsis, and pneumonia.

! Renal failure, seizures, jaundice, and CHF may occur.

! Cardiotoxicity has been reported during therapy.

DENTAL CONSIDERATIONS

General:

• Monitor and record vital signs.

• If additional analgesia is required for dental pain, consider alternative analgesics in patients taking opioids for acute or chronic pain.

• Examine for oral manifestation of opportunistic infection.

• Avoid products that affect platelet function, such as NSAIDs.

• This drug may be used in the hospital or on an outpatient basis. Confirm the patient's disease and treatment status.

• Chlorhexidine mouth rinse prior to and during chemotherapy may reduce severity of mucositis.

• Patient on chronic drug therapy may rarely present with symptoms of blood dyscrasias, which can include infection, bleeding, and poor healing. If dyscrasia is present, caution patient to prevent oral tissue trauma when using oral hygiene aids.

• Palliative medication may be required for management of oral side effects.

• Short appointments and a stress-reduction protocol may be required for anxious patients.

• Provide emergency dental care only during drug use.

• Patients may be at risk of bleeding; check for oral signs.

• Oral infections should be eliminated and treated aggressively.

• Patients may have received other chemotherapy or radiation; confirm medical and drug history.

• Place on frequent recall because of oral side effects.

Consultations:

• Medical consultation should include routine blood counts including platelet counts and bleeding time.

• Consult physician; prophylactic or therapeutic antiinfectives may be indicated if surgery or periodontal treatment is required.

• Medical consultation may be required to assess immunologic status during cancer chemotherapy and determine safety risk, if any, posed by the required dental treatment.

• Medical consultation may be required to assess disease control and patient's ability to tolerate stress.

Teach Patient/Family to:

• See dentist immediately if secondary oral infection occurs.

• Be aware of oral side effects.

• Encourage effective oral hygiene to prevent soft tissue inflammation.

• Report oral lesions, soreness, or bleeding to dentist.

• Prevent trauma when using oral hygiene aids.

• Update health and medication history if physician makes any changes in evaluation or drug regimens; include OTC, herbal, and nonherbal drugs in the update.

modafinil
mode-ah-**feen**′-awl
(Alertec[CAN], Modavigil[AUS],
Provigil)

CATEGORY AND SCHEDULE
Pregnancy Risk Category: C

Drug Class: CNS stimulant

MECHANISM OF ACTION
An α_1-agonist that may bind to
dopamine reuptake carrier sites,
increasing α activity and decreasing
θ and β brain wave activity.
Therapeutic Effect: Reduces the
number of sleep episodes and total
daytime sleep.

USES
Improvement of wakefulness in
narcolepsy, obstructive sleep apnea,
shift work sleep disorder

PHARMACOKINETICS
Well absorbed. Protein binding:
60%. Widely distributed.
Metabolized in the liver. Excreted
by the kidneys. Unknown if
removed by hemodialysis. *Half-life:*
8–10 hr.

INDICATIONS AND DOSAGES
▸ **Narcolepsy, Other Sleep Disorders**
PO
Adults, Elderly. 200–400 mg/day.

SIDE EFFECTS/ADVERSE REACTIONS
Frequent
Anxiety, insomnia, nausea
Occasional
Anorexia, diarrhea, dizziness, dry
mouth or skin, muscle stiffness,
polydipsia, rhinitis, paresthesia,
tremor, headache, vomiting

PRECAUTIONS AND CONTRAINDICATIONS
Hypersensitivity
Caution:
Ischemic heart disease, left
ventricular hypertrophy, mitral valve
prolapse, recent MI, unstable angina,
renal impairment, hepatic
impairment, lactation, children
younger than 16 yr, drug abuse

DRUG INTERACTIONS OF CONCERN TO DENTISTRY
• No documented dental drug
interactions reported; however,
because it induces cytochrome
P-450 isoenzymes, other
P-450 isoenzyme inducers or
inhibitors (antifungal agents,
erythromycin) could result in a drug
interaction.

SERIOUS REACTIONS
❗ Agitation, excitation, hypertension,
and insomnia may occur.

DENTAL CONSIDERATIONS
General:
• Monitor vital signs at every
appointment because of
cardiovascular side effects.
• Assess salivary flow as a factor in
caries, periodontal disease, and
candidiasis.
• Consider semisupine chair position
for patient comfort because of GI
side effects of drug.
• Short appointments and a
stress-reduction protocol may be
required for anxious patients.
Teach Patient/Family to:
• Prevent trauma when using oral
hygiene aids.
• When chronic dry mouth occurs,
advise patient to:
  • Avoid mouth rinses with high
  alcohol content because of
  drying effects.

M

• Use daily home fluoride products for anticaries effect.
• Use sugarless gum, frequent sips of water, or saliva substitutes.

moexipril hydrochloride
moe-**ex**′-ah-pril
high-droh-**klor**′-ide
(Univasc)

CATEGORY AND SCHEDULE
Pregnancy Risk Category: C (D if used in second or third trimesters)

Drug Class: Angiotensin-converting enzyme (ACE) inhibitor

MECHANISM OF ACTION
An ACE inhibitor that suppresses the renin-angiotensin-aldosterone system and prevents conversion of angiotensin I to angiotensin II, a potent vasoconstrictor; may also inhibit angiotensin II at local vascular and renal sites.
Therapeutic Effect: Reduces peripheral arterial resistance and lowers B/P.

USES
Treatment of hypertension as a single drug or in combination with a thiazide diuretic

PHARMACOKINETICS

Route	Onset	Peak	Duration
PO	1 hr	3–6 hr	24 hr

Incompletely absorbed from the GI tract. Food decreases drug absorption. Rapidly converted to active metabolite. Protein binding: 50%. Primarily recovered in feces, partially excreted in urine. Unknown if removed by dialysis. *Half-life:* 1 hr, metabolite 2–9 hr.

INDICATIONS AND DOSAGES
▶ **Hypertension**
PO
Adults, Elderly. For patients not receiving diuretics, initial dose is 7.5 mg once a day 1 hr before meals. Adjust according to B/P effect. Maintenance: 7.5–30 mg a day in 1–2 divided doses 1 hr before meals.
▶ **Hypertension in Patients with Impaired Renal Function**
PO
Adults, Elderly. 3.75 mg once a day in patients with creatinine clearance of 40 ml/min. Maximum: May titrate up to 15 mg/day.

SIDE EFFECTS/ADVERSE REACTIONS
Occasional
Cough, headache, dizziness, fatigue
Rare
Flushing, rash, myalgia, nausea, vomiting

PRECAUTIONS AND CONTRAINDICATIONS
History of angioedema from previous treatment with ACE inhibitors
Caution:
Food retards absorption, renal or hepatic impairment, CHF, SLE, scleroderma, renal artery stenosis, lactation, children

DRUG INTERACTIONS OF CONCERN TO DENTISTRY
• IV fluids containing potassium: risk of hyperkalemia

• Increased hypotension: other hypotensive drugs, alcohol, phenothiazines
• Decreased hypotensive effects: indomethacin, possibly other NSAIDs, sympathomimetics
• Suspected reduction in the antihypertensive and vasodilator effects by salicylates; monitor B/P if used concurrently

SERIOUS REACTIONS

! Excessive hypotension ("first-dose syncope") may occur in patients with CHF and in those who are severely salt or volume depleted.
! Angioedema (swelling of face and lips) and hyperkalemia occur rarely.
! Agranulocytosis and neutropenia may be noted in those with collagen vascular disease, including scleroderma and systemic lupus erythematosus, and impaired renal function.
! Nephrotic syndrome may be noted in those with history of renal disease.

DENTAL CONSIDERATIONS

General:
• Monitor vital signs at every appointment because of cardiovascular side effects.
• After supine positioning, have patient sit upright for at least 2 min before standing to avoid orthostatic hypotension.
• Take precautions if dental surgery is anticipated and general anesthesia is required.
• Patients on chronic drug therapy may rarely have symptoms of blood dyscrasias, which can include infection, bleeding, and poor healing.
• Stress from dental procedures may compromise cardiovascular function; determine patient risk.

• Assess salivary flow as a factor in caries, periodontal disease, and candidiasis.
• Short appointments and a stress-reduction protocol may be required for anxious patients.
Consultations:
• Medical consultation may be required to assess disease control and patient's ability to tolerate stress.
• In a patient with symptoms of blood dyscrasias, request a medical consultation for blood studies and postpone dental treatment until normal values are reestablished.
Teach Patient/Family to:
• Encourage effective oral hygiene to prevent soft tissue inflammation.
• Use caution to prevent trauma when using oral hygiene aids.
• Report oral lesions, soreness, or bleeding to dentist.
• When chronic dry mouth occurs, advise patient to:
  • Avoid mouth rinses with high alcohol content because of drying effects.
  • Use daily home fluoride products for anticaries effect.
  • Use sugarless gum, frequent sips of water, or saliva substitutes.

M

molindone
moe-**lin**′-done
(Moban)
Do not confuse with Mobic.

CATEGORY AND SCHEDULE
Pregnancy Risk Category: C

Drug Class: Antipsychotic

MECHANISM OF ACTION

An indole derivative of dihydroindolone compounds that reduces spontaneous locomotion and aggressiveness.

Therapeutic Effect: Suppresses behavioral response in psychosis.

USES

Treatment of psychotic disorders

PHARMACOKINETICS

Rapidly absorbed from the GI tract. Metabolized in liver. Excreted in feces, and a small amount excreted via lungs as carbon dioxide. Not removed by dialysis. *Half-life:* unknown.

INDICATIONS AND DOSAGES

▶ Schizophrenia

PO

Adults, Children 12 yr and older. Initially, 50–75 mg/day, increased to 100 mg/day in 3–4 days. Maintenance: 5–15 mg 3–4 times a day (mild psychosis). Maintenance: 10–25 mg 3–4 times a day (moderate psychosis). Maintenance: 225 mg/day maximum in divided doses (severe psychosis).

Elderly. Start at a lower dose.

SIDE EFFECTS/ADVERSE REACTIONS

Frequent

Blurred vision, constipation, drowsiness, headache, extrapyramidal symptoms

Occasional

Mental depression

Rare

Skin rash, hot and dry skin, inability to sweat, muscle weakness, confusion, jaundice, convulsions

PRECAUTIONS AND CONTRAINDICATIONS

Severe CNS depression, hypersensitivity to molindone or any component of the formulation

Caution:

Lactation, hypertension, hepatic disease, cardiac disease, Parkinson's disease, brain tumor, glaucoma, urinary retention, diabetes mellitus, respiratory disease, prostatic hypertrophy

DRUG INTERACTIONS OF CONCERN TO DENTISTRY

• Increased sedation: alcohol, other CNS depressants

• Increased anticholinergic effect: anticholinergics, antihistamines

SERIOUS REACTIONS

! Neuroleptic malignant syndrome or tardive dyskinesia has been reported.

DENTAL CONSIDERATIONS

General:

• Patients on chronic drug therapy may rarely have symptoms of blood dyscrasias, which can include infection, bleeding, and poor healing.

• Assess salivary flow as a factor in caries, periodontal disease, and candidiasis.

• After supine positioning, have patient sit upright for at least 2 min before standing to avoid orthostatic hypotension.

• Assess for presence of extrapyramidal motor symptoms, such as tardive dyskinesia and akathisia. Extrapyramidal motor activity may complicate dental treatment.

• Use vasoconstrictors with caution, in low doses, and with careful aspiration.

Consultations:
• In a patient with symptoms of blood dyscrasias, request a medical consultation for blood studies and postpone dental treatment until normal values are reestablished.
• Medical consultation may be required to assess disease control.
Teach Patient/Family to:
• Encourage effective oral hygiene to prevent soft tissue inflammation.
• Use caution to prevent injury when using oral hygiene aids.
• When chronic dry mouth occurs, advise patient to:
  • Avoid mouth rinses with high alcohol content because of drying effects.
  • Use sugarless gum, frequent sips of water, or saliva substitutes.
  • Use daily home fluoride products for anticaries effect.

mometasone furoate monohydrate
mo-**met**′-ah-sone
(Allermax Aqueous[AUS], Asmanex Twisthaler, Elocon Cream[AUS], Elocon Ointment[AUS], Nasonex, Nasonex Nasal Spray[AUS], Novasone Cream[AUS], Novasone Lotion[AUS], Novasone Ointment[AUS])

CATEGORY AND SCHEDULE
Pregnancy Risk Category: C

Drug Class: Synthetic corticosteroid

MECHANISM OF ACTION
An adrenocorticosteroid that inhibits the release of inflammatory cells

into nasal tissue, preventing early activation of the allergic reaction. *Therapeutic Effect:* Decreases response to seasonal and perennial rhinitis.

USES
Treatment of nasal symptoms of seasonal and perennial allergic rhinitis; prophylaxis of nasal symptoms of seasonal allergic rhinitis

PHARMACOKINETICS
Undetectable in plasma. Protein binding: 98%–99%. The swallowed portion undergoes extensive metabolism. Excreted primarily through bile and, to a lesser extent, urine. *Half-life:* 5.8 hr (nasal).

INDICATIONS AND DOSAGES
▸ **Allergic Rhinitis**
Nasal Spray
Adults, Elderly, Children 12 yr and older. 2 sprays in each nostril once a day.
Children 2–11 yr. 1 spray in each nostril once a day.
▸ **Asthma**
Inhalation
Adults, Elderly, Children 12 yr and older. Initially, inhale 220 mcg (1 puff) once a day. Maximum: 880 mcg once a day.
▸ **Skin Disease**
Topical
Adults, Elderly, Children 12 yr and older. Apply cream, lotion, or ointment to affected area once a day.
▸ **Nasal Polyp**
Nasal Spray
Adults, Elderly. 2 sprays in each nostril twice a day.

M

SIDE EFFECTS/ADVERSE REACTIONS

Occasional
Inhalation: Headache, allergic rhinitis, upper respiratory infection, muscle pain, fatigue
Nasal: Nasal irritation, stinging
Topical: Burning
Rare
Inhalation: Abdominal pain, dyspepsia, nausea
Nasal: Nasal or pharyngeal candidiasis
Topical: Pruritus

PRECAUTIONS AND CONTRAINDICATIONS

Hypersensitivity to any corticosteroid, persistently positive sputum cultures for *Candida albicans,* status asthmaticus (inhalation), systemic fungal infections, untreated localized infection involving nasal mucosa
Caution:
Caution in transferring patient from systemic to inhalation steroids; active or quiescent tuberculosis, untreated fungal, bacterial, or viral infections, lactation, safety and efficacy in children younger than 12 yr not established

DRUG INTERACTIONS OF CONCERN TO DENTISTRY

• None reported

SERIOUS REACTIONS

! An acute hypersensitivity reaction, including urticaria, angioedema, and severe bronchospasm, occurs rarely.
! Transfer from systemic to local steroid therapy may unmask previously suppressed bronchial asthma condition.

DENTAL CONSIDERATIONS

General:
• Allergic rhinitis may be a factor in mouth breathing and drying of oral tissues.
• Examine for oral manifestation of opportunistic infection.
Teach Patient/Family to:
• Gargle, rinse mouth with water, and expectorate after each aerosol dose.

---

montelukast
mon-te-**loo**'-kast
(Singulair)

CATEGORY AND SCHEDULE
Pregnancy Risk Category: B

Drug Class: Selective leukotriene receptor antagonist

MECHANISM OF ACTION
An antiasthmatic that binds to cysteinyl leukotriene receptors, inhibiting the effects of leukotrienes on bronchial smooth muscle.
Therapeutic Effect: Decreases bronchoconstriction, vascular permeability, mucosal edema, and mucus production.

USES
Prophylaxis and chronic treatment of asthma, seasonal allergic rhinitis

PHARMACOKINETICS

Route	Onset	Peak	Duration
PO	N/A	N/A	24 hr
PO (chewable)	N/A	N/A	24 hr

Rapidly absorbed from the GI tract. Protein binding: 99%. Extensively metabolized in the liver. Excreted

almost exclusively in feces.
Half-life: 2.7–5.5 hr (slightly longer in the elderly).

INDICATIONS AND DOSAGES
▶ **Bronchial Asthma**
PO
Adults, Elderly, Adolescents older than 14 yr. One 10-mg tablet a day, taken in the evening.
Children 6–14 yr. One 5-mg chewable tablet a day, taken in the evening.
Children 1–5 yr. One 4-mg chewable tablet a day, taken in the evening.

SIDE EFFECTS/ADVERSE REACTIONS
Adults, Adolescents 15 yr and older
Frequent
Headache
Occasional
Influenza
Rare
Abdominal pain, cough, dyspepsia, dizziness, fatigue, dental pain

Children 6–14 yr
Rare
Diarrhea, laryngitis, pharyngitis, nausea, otitis media, sinusitis, viral infection

PRECAUTIONS AND CONTRAINDICATIONS
Hypersensitivity
Caution:
Not for acute asthma attacks, not for treatment of exercise-induced bronchospasm or ASA-induced bronchospasm, chewable tablets contain aspartame, lactation; monitor patients when potent CYP3A4 isoenzyme inducers are used

DRUG INTERACTIONS OF CONCERN TO DENTISTRY
• None reported; however, monitor patients when inhibitors of CYP3A4 or CYP2C9 are prescribed.

SERIOUS REACTIONS
! None known

DENTAL CONSIDERATIONS
General:
• Midday appointments and a stress-reduction protocol may be required for anxious patients.
• Avoid prescribing NSAID-containing products.
• Acute asthmatic episodes may be precipitated in the dental office. Rapid-acting sympathomimetic inhalants should be available for emergency use.
• Be aware that aspirin or sulfite preservatives in vasoconstrictor-containing products can exacerbate asthma.
• Consider semisupine chair position for patients with respiratory disease or if GI side effects occur.
Consultations:
• Medical consultation may be required to assess disease control.
Teach Patient/Family to:
• Update health and drug history if physician makes any changes in evaluation or drug regimens; include OTC, herbal, and nonherbal drugs in the update.

M

moricizine hydrochloride
mor-**iss′**-ih-zeen
high-droh-**klor′**-ide
(Ethmozine)

CATEGORY AND SCHEDULE
Pregnancy Risk Category: B

Drug Class: Antidysrhythmic, type I

MECHANISM OF ACTION
An antiarrhythmic that prevents sodium current across myocardial cell membranes. Has potent local anesthetic activity and membrane stabilizing effects. Slows AV and His-Purkinje conduction and decreases action potential duration and effective refractory period.
Therapeutic Effect: Suppresses ventricular arrhythmias.

USES
Treatment of documented life-threatening dysrhythmias

PHARMACOKINETICS
Peak 0.5–2.2 hr. *Half-life:* 1.5–3.5 hr; protein binding greater than 90%; metabolized by the liver; metabolites excreted in feces, urine.

INDICATIONS AND DOSAGES
▶ **Arrhythmias**
PO
Adults, Elderly. 200–300 mg q8h. May increase by 150 mg/day at no less than 3-day intervals.

SIDE EFFECTS/ADVERSE REACTIONS
Frequent
Dizziness, nausea, headache, fatigue, dyspnea

Occasional
Nervousness, paraesthesia, sleep disturbances, dyspepsia, vomiting, diarrhea, dry mouth

PRECAUTIONS AND CONTRAINDICATIONS
Cardiogenic shock, preexisting second- or third-degree AV block or right bundle-branch block without pacemaker
Caution:
CHF, hypokalemia, hyperkalemia, sick sinus syndrome, lactation, children, impaired hepatic and renal function, cardiac dysfunction

DRUG INTERACTIONS OF CONCERN TO DENTISTRY
• No specific interactions are reported with dental drugs; however, any drug that could affect the cardiac action of moricizine (e.g., other local anesthetics, vasoconstrictors, anticholinergics) should be used in the lowest effective dose.

SERIOUS REACTIONS
! Moricizine may worsen existing arrhythmias or produce new ones.
! Jaundice with hepatitis occurs rarely.
! Overdosage produces vomiting, lethargy, syncope, hypotension, conduction disturbances, exacerbation of CHF, MI, and sinus arrest.

DENTAL CONSIDERATIONS
General:
• Monitor vital signs at every appointment because of cardiovascular side effects.
• Assess salivary flow as a factor in caries, periodontal disease, and candidiasis.

• Stress from dental procedures may compromise cardiovascular function; determine patient risk.
Consultations:
• Medical consultation should be made to assess disease control and patient's ability to tolerate stress.
Teach Patient/Family to:
• Encourage effective oral hygiene to prevent soft tissue inflammation.
• Use caution to prevent injury when using oral hygiene aids.
• When chronic dry mouth occurs, advise patient to:
  • Avoid mouth rinses with high alcohol content because of drying effects.
  • Use sugarless gum, frequent sips of water, or saliva substitutes.
  • Use daily home fluoride products for anticaries effect.

morphine sulfate
mor'-feen sull'-fate
(Anamorph[AUS], Astramorph, Avinza, DepoDur, Duramorph, Infumorph, Kadian, Kapanol[AUS], M-Eslon, Morphine Mixtures[AUS], MS Contin, MSIR, MS Mono[AUS], Oramorph SR, RMS, Roxanol, Statex[CAN])
Do not confuse morphine with hydromorphone, or Roxanol with Roxicet.

CATEGORY AND SCHEDULE
Pregnancy Risk Category: C (D if used for prolonged periods or at high dosages at term)
Controlled Substance: Schedule II

Drug Class: Narcotic opioid

MECHANISM OF ACTION
An opioid agonist that binds with opioid receptors in the CNS. *Therapeutic Effect:* Alters the perception of and emotional response to pain; produces generalized CNS depression.

USES
Treatment of severe pain

PHARMACOKINETICS

Route	Onset	Peak	Duration
Oral solution	N/A	1 hr	3–5 hr
Tablets	N/A	1 hr	3–5 hr
Tablets (ER)	N/A	3–4 hr	8–12 hr
IV	Rapid	0.3 hr	3–5 hr
IM	5–30 min	0.5–1 hr	3–5 hr
Epidural	N/A	1 hr	12–20 hr
Subcutaneous	N/A	1.1–5 hr	3–5 hr
Rectal	N/A	0.5–1 hr	3–7 hr

Variably absorbed from the GI tract. Readily absorbed after IM or subcutaneous administration. Protein binding: 20%–35%. Widely distributed. Metabolized in the liver. Primarily excreted in urine. Removed by hemodialysis. *Half-life:* 2–3 hr (increased in patients with hepatic disease).

INDICATIONS AND DOSAGES
▶ Alert
Dosage should be titrated to desired effect.
▶ Analgesia
PO (Prompt Release)
Adults, Elderly. 10–30 mg q3–4h as needed.
Children. 0.2–0.5 mg/kg q3–4h as needed.
▶ Alert
For the Avinza dosage below, be aware that this drug is to be administered once a day only.

M

> **Alert**

For the Kadian dosage information below, be aware that this drug is to be administered q12h or once a day only.

> **Alert**

Be aware that pediatric dosages of extended-release preparations Kadian and Avinza have not been established.

> **Alert**

For the MSContin and Oramorph SR dosage information below, be aware that the daily dosage is divided and given q8h or q12h.

PO (Extended-Release [Avinza])
Adults, Elderly. Dosage requirement should be established using prompt-release formulations and is based on total daily dose. Avinza is given once a day only.

PO (Extended-Release [Kadian])
Adults, Elderly. Dosage requirement should be established using prompt-release formulations and is based on total daily dose. Dose is given once a day or divided and given q12h.

PO (Extended-Release [MSContin, Oramorph SR])
Adults, Elderly. Dosage requirement should be established using prompt-release formulations and is based on total daily dose. Daily dose is divided and given q8h or q12h.

Children. 0.3–0.6 mg/kg/dose q12h.

IV
Adults, Elderly. 2.5–5 mg q3–4h as needed. Note: Repeated doses (e.g., 1–2 mg) may be given more frequently (e.g., every hour) if needed.
Children. 0.05–0.1 mg/kg q3–4h as needed.

IV Continuous Infusion
Adults, Elderly. 0.8–10 mg/hr. Range: Up to 80 mg/hr.
Children. 10–30 mcg/kg/hr.

IM
Adults, Elderly. 5–10 mg q3–4h as needed.
Children. 0.1 mg/kg q3–4h as needed.

Epidural
Adults, Elderly. Initially, 1–6 mg bolus, infusion rate: 0.1–1 mg/hr. Maximum: 10 mg/24 hr.

Intrathecal
Adults, Elderly. One-tenth of the epidural dose: 0.2–1 mg/dose.

> **PCA**

IV
Adults, Elderly. Loading dose: 5–10 mg. Intermittent bolus: 0.5–3 mg. Lockout interval: 5–12 min. Continuous infusion: 1–10 mg/hr. 4-hr limit: 20–30 mg.

SIDE EFFECTS/ADVERSE REACTIONS

Frequent

Sedation, decreased B/P (including orthostatic hypotension), diaphoresis, facial flushing, constipation, dizziness, somnolence, nausea, vomiting

Occasional

Allergic reaction (rash, pruritus), dyspnea, confusion, palpitations, tremors, urine retention, abdominal cramps, vision changes, dry mouth, headache, decreased appetite, pain or burning at injection site

Rare

Paralytic ileus

PRECAUTIONS AND CONTRAINDICATIONS

Acute or severe asthma, GI obstruction, severe hepatic or renal impairment, severe respiratory depression, asthma, severe liver or renal impairment

Caution:

Addictive personality, lactation, MI (acute), severe heart disease, elderly, respiratory depression, hepatic disease, renal disease, children younger than 18 yr

DRUG INTERACTIONS OF CONCERN TO DENTISTRY

• Increased CNS depression: alcohol, all CNS depressants
• Contraindication: MAOIs
• Increased effects of anticholinergics
• Avoid drugs with opioid antagonist properties (e.g., pentazocine)

SERIOUS REACTIONS

! Overdose results in respiratory depression, skeletal muscle flaccidity, cold or clammy skin, cyanosis, and extreme somnolence progressing to seizures, stupor, and coma.
! The patient who uses morphine repeatedly may develop a tolerance to the drug's analgesic effect and physical dependence.
! The drug may have a prolonged duration of action and cumulative effect in those with hepatic and renal impairment.

DENTAL CONSIDERATIONS

General:
• Monitor vital signs at every appointment because of cardiovascular and respiratory side effects.
• Assess salivary flow as a factor in caries, periodontal disease, and candidiasis.
• After supine positioning, have patient sit upright for at least 2 min before standing to avoid orthostatic hypotension.
• Psychologic and physical dependence may occur with chronic administration.
• Determine why the patient is taking the drug.

• Consider the use of NSAIDs when additional analgesia is required.
Teach Patient/Family to:
• When chronic dry mouth occurs, advise patient to:
  • Use daily home fluoride products for anticaries effect.
  • Avoid mouth rinses with high alcohol content because of drying effects.
  • Use sugarless gum, frequent sips of water, or saliva substitutes.

moxifloxacin hydrochloride

moks-ih-**floks'**-ah-sin
high-dro-**klor'**-ide
(Avelox, Avelox IV, Vigamox)
Do not confuse Avelox with Avonex.

CATEGORY AND SCHEDULE
Pregnancy Risk Category: C

Drug Class: Fluoroquinolone antiinfective

MECHANISM OF ACTION
A fluoroquinolone that inhibits two enzymes, topoisomerase II and IV, in susceptible microorganisms.
Therapeutic Effect: Interferes with bacterial DNA replication. Prevents or delays emergence of resistant organisms. Bactericidal.

USES
Treatment of acute bacterial sinusitis (*S. pneumoniae, H. influenzae,* or *M. catarrhalis*); acute bacterial exacerbation of chronic bronchitis (*S. pneumoniae, H. influenzae, H. parainfluenzae, K. pneumoniae, M. catarrhalis,* or *S. aureus*); community-acquired pneumonia

(*S. pneumoniae, H. influenzae, M. catarrhalis, M. pneumoniae,* or *C. pneumoniae*); bacterial conjunctivitis caused by susceptible bacterial strains including selected aerobic gram-positive species, selected aerobic gram-negative species, and *C. trachomatis*

PHARMACOKINETICS

Well absorbed from the GI tract after PO administration. Protein binding: 50%. Widely distributed throughout body with tissue concentration often exceeding plasma concentration. Metabolized in liver. Primarily excreted in urine with a lesser amount in feces. *Half-life:* 10.7–13.3 hr.

INDICATIONS AND DOSAGES

▸ **Acute Bacterial Sinusitis, Community-Acquired Pneumonia**
PO, IV
Adults, Elderly. 400 mg q24h for 10 days.
▸ **Acute Bacterial Exacerbation of Chronic Bronchitis**
PO, IV
Adults, Elderly. 400 mg q24h for 5 days.
▸ **Skin and Skin–Structure Infection**
PO, IV
Adults, Elderly. 400 mg once a day for 7 days.
▸ **Topical Treatment of Bacterial Conjunctivitis Caused by Susceptible Strains of Bacteria**
Ophthalmic
Adults, Elderly, Children older than 1 yr. 1 drop 3 times a day for 7 days.

SIDE EFFECTS/ADVERSE REACTIONS

Frequent
Nausea, diarrhea

Occasional
Dizziness, headache, abdominal pain, vomiting
Ophthalmic: conjunctival irritation, reduced visual acuity, dry eye, keratitis, eye pain, ocular itching, swelling of tissue around cornea, eye discharge, fever, cough, pharyngitis, rash, rhinitis
Rare
Change in sense of taste, dyspepsia (heartburn, indigestion), photosensitivity; tendon rupture

PRECAUTIONS AND CONTRAINDICATIONS

Hypersensitivity to quinolones
Caution:
Divalent cations, retard absorption, not for use with class 1A and III antiarrhythmics, use in children not studied, cross resistance with other fluoroquinolones, may prolong QT interval in some patients, seizures, use with NSAIDs, children younger than 18 yr, lactation

DRUG INTERACTIONS OF CONCERN TO DENTISTRY

• Increased risk of CNS stimulation and seizures: NSAIDs
• Decreased absorption: divalent and trivalent antacids, iron and zinc salts
• Caution when using erythromycin, tricyclic antidepressants (no data, risk of QT interval)
• Increased risk of life-threatening arrhythmias: procainamide

SERIOUS REACTIONS

! Pseudomembranous colitis as evidenced by fever, severe abdominal cramps or pain, and severe watery diarrhea may occur.
! Superinfection manifested as anal or genital pruritus, moderate to severe diarrhea, and stomatitis may occur.

DENTAL CONSIDERATIONS

General:
• Determine why patient is taking the drug.
• Examine for oral manifestation of opportunistic infection.
• Advise patient if dental drugs prescribed have a potential for photosensitivity.
• Ruptures of the shoulder, hand, and Achilles tendons that required surgical repair or resulted in prolonged disability have been reported with the use of fluoroquinolones. Question patient about history of side effects associated with fluoroquinolone use.
• Monitor vital signs at every appointment because of cardiovascular side effects.
• Patients on chronic drug therapy may rarely have symptoms of blood dyscrasias, which can include infection, bleeding, and poor healing.
• Consider semisupine chair position for patient comfort if GI side effects occur.

Consultations:
• In a patient with symptoms of blood dyscrasias, request a medical consultation for blood studies and postpone treatment until normal values are reestablished.
• Physician consultation is advised in the presence of an acute dental infection requiring another antibiotic.

Teach Patient/Family to:
• If used for dental infection to:
  • Minimize exposure to sunlight and wear sunscreen if sun exposure is planned.
  • Discontinue treatment and inform dentist immediately if patient experiences pain or inflammation of a tendon, and to rest and refrain from exercise.

mupirocin
mew-**peer'**-oh-sin
(Bactroban)
Do not confuse with Bactrim or Bacitracin.

CATEGORY AND SCHEDULE
Pregnancy Risk Category: B

Drug Class: Topical antiinfective, pseudomonic acid A

MECHANISM OF ACTION
An antibacterial agent that inhibits bacterial protein, RNA synthesis. Less effective on DNA synthesis. Nasal: Eradicates nasal colonization of MRSA.
Therapeutic Effect: Prevents bacterial growth and replication. Bacteriostatic.

USES
Treatment of impetigo caused by *S. aureus*, ß-hemolytic streptococci, *S. pyogenes;* nasal membranes: *S. aureus*

PHARMACOKINETICS
Metabolized in skin to inactive metabolite. Transported to skin surface; removed by normal skin desquamation.

INDICATIONS AND DOSAGES
▶ **Impetigo, Infected Traumatic Skin Lesions**
Topical
Adults, Elderly, Children. Apply 3 times a day (may cover with gauze).
▶ **Nasal Colonization of Resistant Staphylococcus Aureus**
Intranasal
Adults, Elderly, Children 12 yr and older. Apply 2 times a day for 5 days.

SIDE EFFECTS/ADVERSE REACTIONS

Frequent
Nasal: Headache, rhinitis, upper respiratory congestion, pharyngitis, altered taste
Occasional
Nasal: Burning, stinging, cough
Topical: Pain, burning, stinging, itching
Rare
Nasal: Pruritus, diarrhea, dry mouth, epistaxis, nausea, rash
Topical: Rash, nausea, dry skin, contact dermatitis

PRECAUTIONS AND CONTRAINDICATIONS

Hypersensitivity to mupirocin or any component of the formulation
Caution:
Lactation

DRUG INTERACTIONS OF CONCERN TO DENTISTRY

- None reported

SERIOUS REACTIONS

! Superinfection may result in bacterial or fungal infections, especially with prolonged or repeated therapy.

DENTAL CONSIDERATIONS

General:
- The dentist may choose to postpone elective dental treatment if the infected site may be affected by dental treatment.

---

mycophenolate mofetil
my-co-**fen′**-oh-late
(CellCept)

CATEGORY AND SCHEDULE
Pregnancy Risk Category: C

Drug Class: Immunosuppressant

MECHANISM OF ACTION

An immunologic agent that suppresses the immunologically mediated inflammatory response by inhibiting inosine monophosphate dehydrogenase, an enzyme that deprives lymphocytes of nucleotides necessary for DNA and RNA synthesis, thus inhibiting the proliferation of T and B lymphocytes.
Therapeutic Effect: Prevents transplant rejection.

USES

Prophylaxis of organ rejection in patients receiving allogenic renal or hepatic transplants, cardiac transplants (in combination with cyclosporine and corticosteroids)

PHARMACOKINETICS

Rapidly and extensively absorbed after PO administration (food decreases drug plasma concentration but doesn't affect absorption). Protein binding: 97%. Completely hydrolyzed to active metabolite mycophenolic acid. Primarily excreted in urine. Not removed by hemodialysis. ***Half-life:*** 17.9 hr.

INDICATIONS AND DOSAGES
▶ **Prevention of Renal Transplant Rejection**
PO, IV
Adults, Elderly. 1 g twice a day.

▶ **Prevention of Heart Transplant Rejection**
PO, IV
Adults, Elderly. 1.5 g twice a day.
▶ **Prevention of Liver Transplant Rejection**
PO
Adults, Elderly. 1.5 g twice a day.
IV
Adults, Elderly. 1 g twice a day.
▶ **Usual Pediatric Dosage**
PO
Children. 600 mg/m²/dose twice a day. Maximum: 2 g/day.

SIDE EFFECTS/ADVERSE REACTIONS

Frequent
UTI, hypertension, peripheral edema, diarrhea, constipation, fever, headache, nausea
Occasional
Dyspepsia; dyspnea; cough; hematuria; asthenia; vomiting; edema; tremors; abdominal, chest, or back pain; oral candidiasis; acne
Rare
Insomnia, respiratory tract infection, rash, dizziness

PRECAUTIONS AND CONTRAINDICATIONS

Hypersensitivity to mycophenolic acid
Caution:
Active GI diseases, lactation, reduce dose in severe chronic renal impairment, increased risk of development of lymphomas or other malignancies and susceptibility to infection

DRUG INTERACTIONS OF CONCERN TO DENTISTRY

• Increased plasma concentration: acyclovir, ganciclovir
• Decreased availability of MPA: drugs that alter the GI flora

SERIOUS REACTIONS

! Significant anemia, leukopenia, thrombocytopenia, neutropenia, and leukocytosis may occur, particularly in those undergoing renal transplant rejection.
! Sepsis and infection occur occasionally.
! GI tract hemorrhage occurs rarely.
! Patients receiving mycophenolate have an increased risk of developing neoplasms.

DENTAL CONSIDERATIONS

General:
• Determine why the patient is taking the drug.
• Short appointments and a stress-reduction protocol may be required for anxious patients.
• Patients who have been or are currently on chronic steroid therapy (longer than 2 wk) may require supplemental steroids for dental treatment.
• Patients on chronic drug therapy may rarely have symptoms of blood dyscrasias, which can include infection, bleeding, and poor healing.
• Place on frequent recall because of oral side effects.
• Determine dose and duration of steroid for patient to assess risk for stress tolerance and immunosuppression.
• Examine for oral manifestations of opportunistic infections.
• Monitor vital signs at every appointment because of cardiovascular and respiratory side effects.
• Consider semisupine chair position for patient comfort if GI side effects occur.
• Antibiotic prophylaxis is usually recommended in patients with organ transplants and immunosuppression.

M

M

• Monitor time since organ/tissue transplant; note duration of transplant and status of renal function.

• Place on frequent recall because of possible blood dyscrasias and oral side effects.

Consultations:

• Medical consultation may be required to assess disease control and patient's ability to tolerate stress.

• In a patient with symptoms of blood dyscrasias, request a medical consultation for blood studies and postpone dental treatment until normal values are reestablished.

• Request baseline B/P in renal transplant patients for patient evaluation before dental treatment.

Teach Patient/Family to:

• See dentist immediately if secondary oral infection occurs.

• Encourage effective oral hygiene to prevent soft tissue inflammation.

• Return to dentist frequently because of possible blood dyscrasias and oral side effects.

• Report oral lesions, soreness, or bleeding to dentist.

nabumetone
na-**byu'**-meh-tone
(Apo-Nabumetone, Relafen)

CATEGORY AND SCHEDULE
Pregnancy Risk Category: C (D if used in third trimester or near delivery)

Drug Class: Nonsteroidal antiinflammatory

MECHANISM OF ACTION
An NSAID that produces analgesic and antiinflammatory effects by inhibiting prostaglandin synthesis. *Therapeutic Effect:* Reduces the inflammatory response and intensity of pain.

USES
Treatment of osteoarthritis, rheumatoid arthritis, acute or chronic treatment

PHARMACOKINETICS
Readily absorbed from the GI tract. Protein binding: 99%. Widely distributed. Metabolized in the liver to active metabolite. Primarily excreted in urine. Not removed by hemodialysis. *Half-life:* 22–30 hr.

INDICATIONS AND DOSAGES
▸ **Acute or Chronic Rheumatoid Arthritis and Osteoarthritis**
PO
Adults, Elderly. Initially, 1000 mg as a single dose or in 2 divided doses. May increase up to 2000 mg/day as a single or in 2 divided doses.

SIDE EFFECTS/ADVERSE REACTIONS
Frequent
Diarrhea, abdominal cramps or pain, dyspepsia, oral lichenoid reaction

Occasional
Nausea, constipation, flatulence, dizziness, headache
Rare
Vomiting, stomatitis, confusion

PRECAUTIONS AND CONTRAINDICATIONS
Active peptic ulcer disease, chronic inflammation of GI tract, GI bleeding or ulceration, history of hypersensitivity to aspirin or NSAIDs, history of significant renal impairment
Caution:
Lactation, children, bleeding disorders, GI disorders, cardiac disorders, renal disorders, hepatic dysfunction, elderly

DRUG INTERACTIONS OF CONCERN TO DENTISTRY
• GI ulceration, bleeding: aspirin, alcohol, corticosteroids
• May decrease effects of nabumetone: salicylates
• Nephrotoxicity: acetaminophen (prolonged use and high doses)
• Possible risk of decreased renal function: cyclosporine
• SSRIs: NSAIDs increase risk of GI side effects

SERIOUS REACTIONS
! Overdose may result in acute hypotension and tachycardia.
! Rare reactions with long-term use include peptic ulcer disease.
! GI bleeding, gastritis, nephrotoxicity (dysuria, cystitis, hematuria, proteinuria, nephrotic syndrome), severe hepatic reactions (cholestasis, jaundice), and severe hypersensitivity reactions (bronchospasm, angioedema).

N

DENTAL CONSIDERATIONS

General:
• Potential increase of adverse cardiovascular events in patients at risk for thromboembolism.
• Patients on chronic drug therapy may rarely have symptoms of blood dyscrasias, which can include infection, bleeding, and poor healing.
• Assess salivary flow as a factor in caries, periodontal disease, and candidiasis.
• Avoid prescribing in pregnancy.
• Avoid prescribing aspirin-containing products.
• Consider semisupine chair position for patients with arthritic disease.
• Severe stomach bleeding may occur in patients who regularly use NSAIDs in recommended doses, when the patient is also taking another NSAID, a blood thinning, or steroid drug, if the patient has GI or peptic ulcer disease, if they are 60 yr or older, or when NSAIDs are taken longer than directed. Warn patients of the potential for severe stomach bleeding.

Consultations:
• In patients with symptoms of blood dyscrasias, request a medical consultation for blood studies and postpone dental treatment until normal values are reestablished.
• Medical consultation may be required to assess disease control.

Teach Patient/Family to:
• Encourage effective oral hygiene to prevent soft tissue inflammation.
• Use caution to prevent injury when using oral hygiene aids.
• Warn patient of potential risks of NSAIDs.
• When chronic dry mouth occurs, advise patient to:

• Avoid mouth rinses with high alcohol content because of drying effects.
• Use daily home fluoride products for anticaries effect.
• Use sugarless gum, frequent sips of water, or saliva substitutes.

nadolol
nay′-doe-lole
(Apo-Nadol[CAN], Corgard, Novo-Nadolol[CAN])

CATEGORY AND SCHEDULE
Pregnancy Risk Category: C (D if used in second or third trimester)

Drug Class: Nonselective β-adrenergic blocker

MECHANISM OF ACTION
A nonselective β-blocker that blocks β_1- and β_2-adrenergic receptors. Large doses increase airway resistance.
Therapeutic Effect: Slows sinus heart rate, decreases cardiac output and B/P. Decreases myocardial ischemia severity by decreasing oxygen requirements.

USES
Treatment of chronic stable angina pectoris, mild-to-moderate hypertension; unapproved: dysrhythmias, MI prophylaxis, vascular headache, mild-to-moderate heart failure

PHARMACOKINETICS
PO: Onset variable, peak 3–4 hr, duration 17–24 hr. *Half-life:* 16–20 hr; not metabolized; excreted in urine (unchanged), bile, breast milk.

INDICATIONS AND DOSAGES
▶ **Mild-to-Moderate Hypertension, Angina**

PO

Adults. Initially, 40 mg/day. May increase by 40–80 mg at 3- to 7-day intervals. Maximum: 240–360 mg/day.

Elderly. Initially, 20 mg/day. May increase gradually. Range: 20–240 mg/day.

▶ **Dosage in Renal Impairment**

Dosage is modified on the basis of creatinine clearance.

Creatinine Clearance	% of Usual Dosage
10–50 ml/min	50
Less than 10 ml/min	25

SIDE EFFECTS/ADVERSE REACTIONS

Nadolol is generally well tolerated, with transient and mild side effects
Frequent
Diminished sexual ability, drowsiness, unusual fatigue, or weakness
Occasional
Bradycardia, difficulty breathing, depression, cold hands or feet, diarrhea, constipation, anxiety, nasal congestion, nausea, vomiting
Rare
Altered taste, dry eyes, itching

PRECAUTIONS AND CONTRAINDICATIONS

Bronchial asthma, cardiogenic shock, CHF secondary to tachyarrhythmias, COPD, patients receiving MAOI therapy, second- or third-degree heart block, sinus bradycardia, uncontrolled cardiac failure
Caution:
Diabetes mellitus, renal disease, lactation, hyperthyroidism, peripheral vascular disease, myasthenia gravis

DRUG INTERACTIONS OF CONCERN TO DENTISTRY

• Sympathomimetics (epinephrine, norepinephrine, isoproterenol): elevated systolic blood pressure, bradycardia or cardiac arrest (limit or avoid vasoconstrictors)
• Slows metabolism of nadolol: lidocaine
• Increased hypotension, myocardial depression: fentanyl derivatives, hydrocarbon inhalation anesthetics
• Decreased hypotensive effect: indomethacin and other NSAIDs

SERIOUS REACTIONS

! Overdose may produce profound bradycardia and hypotension.
! Abrupt withdrawal of nadolol may result in diaphoresis, palpitations, headache, tremors, exacerbation of angina, MI, and ventricular arrhythmias.
! Nadolol administration may precipitate CHF and MI in patients with cardiac disease; thyroid storm in those with thyrotoxicosis; and peripheral ischemia in those with existing peripheral vascular disease.
! Hypoglycemia may occur in patients with previously controlled diabetes.

DENTAL CONSIDERATIONS

General:
• Monitor vital signs at every appointment because of cardiovascular side effects.
• Patients on chronic drug therapy may rarely have symptoms of blood dyscrasias, which can include infection, bleeding, and poor healing.
• After supine positioning, have patient sit upright for at least 2 min

N

before standing to avoid orthostatic hypotension.
• Limit use of sodium-containing products, such as saline IV fluids, for patients with a dietary salt restriction.
• Assess salivary flow as a factor in caries, periodontal disease, and candidiasis.
• Stress from dental procedures may compromise cardiovascular function; determine patient risk. Short appointments and a stress-reduction protocol may be required for anxious patients.
• Consider semisupine chair position for patients with respiratory distress.
Consultations:
• In patients with symptoms of blood dyscrasias, request a medical consultation for blood studies and postpone dental treatment until normal values are reestablished.
• Take precautions if dental surgery is anticipated and anesthesia is required.
• Medical consultation may be required to assess disease control and patient's ability to tolerate stress.
Teach Patient/Family to:
• Encourage effective oral hygiene to prevent soft tissue inflammation.
• Use caution to prevent injury when using oral hygiene aids.
• When chronic dry mouth occurs, advise patient to:
  • Avoid mouth rinses with high alcohol content because of drying effects.
  • Use daily home fluoride products for anticaries effect.
  • Use sugarless gum, frequent sips of water, or saliva substitutes.

nafarelin
naf-**ah**′-rell-in
(Synarel)

CATEGORY AND SCHEDULE
Pregnancy Risk Category: X

Drug Class: Gonadotropin; analog of gonadotropin-releasing hormone

MECHANISM OF ACTION
A gonadotropin inhibitor that initially stimulates the release of the pituitary gonadotropins, luteinizing hormone and follicle-stimulating hormone, then decreases secretion of gonadal steroids.
Therapeutic Effect: Temporarily increases ovarian steroidogenesis, abolishes the stimulatory effect on the pituitary gland, decreases secretion of gonadal steroids.

USES
Treatment of endometriosis, gonadotropin-dependent precocious puberty

PHARMACOKINETICS
Rapidly absorbed after nasal administration. Protein binding: 78%–84%, binds primarily to albumin. Metabolism: unknown. Excreted in urine. *Half-life:* 3 hr.

INDICATIONS AND DOSAGES
▸ Endometriosis
Intranasal
Adults. 400 mcg/day: 200 mcg (1 spray) into 1 nostril in morning, 1 spray into other nostril in evening. For patients with persistent regular menstruation after months of treatment, increase dose to 800 mcg/

day (1 spray into each nostril in morning and evening).

▶ **Central Precocious Puberty**
Intranasal
Children. 1600 mcg/day: 400 mcg (2 sprays into each nostril in morning and evening; total 8 sprays).

SIDE EFFECTS/ADVERSE REACTIONS
Frequent
Hot flashes, muscle pain, decreased breast size, myalgia
Occasional
Nasal irritation, decreased libido, vaginal dryness, headache, emotional lability, acne
Rare
Insomnia, edema, weight gain, seborrhea, depression

PRECAUTIONS AND CONTRAINDICATIONS
Pregnancy, other agonist analogues, undiagnosed abnormal vaginal bleeding, hypersensitivity to nafarelin or any component of the formulation

DRUG INTERACTIONS OF CONCERN TO DENTISTRY
• None reported

SERIOUS REACTIONS
! None reported

DENTAL CONSIDERATIONS
General:
• Determine why patient is taking the drug.

---

naftifine
naf′-ti-feen
(Naftin)
Do not confuse with nafcillin or nafarelin.

CATEGORY AND SCHEDULE
Pregnancy Risk Category: B

Drug Class: Topical antifungal

MECHANISM OF ACTION
An antifungal that selectively inhibits the enzyme squalene epoxidase in a dose-dependent manner, which results in the primary sterol, ergosterol, within the fungal membrane not being synthesized. *Therapeutic Effect:* Results in fungal cell death. Fungistatic and fungicidal.

USES
Treatment of tinea cruris, tinea corporis, tinea pedis

PHARMACOKINETICS
Minimal systemic absorption. Metabolized in the liver. Excreted in the urine, as well as the feces and bile. *Half-life:* 48–72 hr.

INDICATIONS AND DOSAGES
▶ **Tinea Pedis, Tinea Cruris, Tinea Corporis**
Topical
Adults, Elderly, Children 12 yr and older. Apply cream 1 time a day for 4 wk or until signs and symptoms significantly improve. Apply gel 2 times a day for 4 wk or until signs and symptoms significantly improve.

SIDE EFFECTS/ADVERSE REACTIONS
Frequent
Burning, stinging

N

Occasional
Erythema, itching, dryness, irritation

PRECAUTIONS AND CONTRAINDICATIONS

Hypersensitivity to naftifine or any of its components
Caution:
Lactation, children

DRUG INTERACTIONS OF CONCERN TO DENTISTRY

• None reported

SERIOUS REACTIONS

! Excessive irritation may indicate hypersensitivity reaction.

nalbuphine hydrochloride

nal-**byoo′**-feen high-droh-**klor′**-ide
(Nubain)
Do not confuse Nubain with Navane.

CATEGORY AND SCHEDULE

Pregnancy Risk Category: B (D if used for prolonged periods or at high dosages at term)

Drug Class: Opioid agonist, antagonist; opioid analgesic

MECHANISM OF ACTION

A narcotic agonist-antagonist that binds with opioid receptors in the CNS. May displace opioid agonists and competitively inhibit their action; may precipitate withdrawal symptoms.
Therapeutic Effect: Alters the perception of and emotional response to pain.

USES

Relief of moderate-to-severe pain, preoperative sedation, obstetric analgesia, adjunct to anesthesia

PHARMACOKINETICS

Route	Onset	Peak	Duration
IV	2–3 min	30 min	3–6 hr
IM	Less than 15 min	60 min	3–6 hr
Subcutaneous	Less than 15 min	N/A	3–6 hr

Well absorbed after IM or subcutaneous administration. Protein binding: 50%. Metabolized in the liver. Primarily eliminated in feces by biliary secretion. *Half-life:* 3.5–5 hr.

INDICATIONS AND DOSAGES
▶ **Analgesia**
IV, IM, Subcutaneous
Adults, Elderly. 10 mg q3–6h as needed. Don't exceed maximum single dose of 20 mg or daily dose of 160 mg. For patients receiving long-term narcotic analgesics of similar duration of action, give 25% of usual dose.
Children. 0.1–0.15 mg/kg q3–6h as needed.
▶ **Supplement to Anesthesia**
IV
Adults, Elderly. Induction: 0.3–3 mg/kg over 10–15 min. Maintenance: 0.25–0.5 mg/kg as needed.

SIDE EFFECTS/ADVERSE REACTIONS

Frequent
Sedation
Occasional
Diaphoresis, cold and clammy skin, nausea, vomiting, dizziness, vertigo, dry mouth, headache

Rare
Restlessness, emotional lability, paresthesia, flushing, paradoxical reaction

PRECAUTIONS AND CONTRAINDICATIONS
Respiratory rate less than 12 breaths/min

DRUG INTERACTIONS OF CONCERN TO DENTISTRY
• Increased CNS and respiratory depression: all CNS depressants
• Contraindicated with MAOIs
• Avoid use in opioid-dependent persons; risk of withdrawal reactions
• Increased risk of constipation: anticholinergics
• Increased risk of orthostatic hypotension: antihypertensive medications

SERIOUS REACTIONS
! Abrupt withdrawal after prolonged use may produce symptoms of narcotic withdrawal, such as abdominal cramping, rhinorrhea, lacrimation, anxiety, fever, and piloerection (goose bumps).
! Overdose results in severe respiratory depression, skeletal muscle flaccidity, cyanosis, and extreme somnolence progressing to seizures, stupor, and coma.
! Repeated use may result in drug tolerance and physical dependence.

DENTAL CONSIDERATIONS
General:
• Avoid use in an opioid-dependent patient.
• Acute-use drug; question patient about use for pain.
• If additional analgesia is required for dental pain, consider alternative analgesics (NSAIDs) in patients taking opioids for acute or chronic pain.
• Monitor and record vital signs.
• Assess salivary flow as a factor in caries, periodontal disease, and candidiasis.
Consultations:
• Medical consultation may be required to assess disease control.
Teach Patient/Family to:
• Encourage effective oral hygiene to prevent soft tissue inflammation.
• Prevent trauma when using oral hygiene aids.
• Avoid driving or other activities requiring mental alertness.
• Avoid alcohol ingestion or CNS depressants; serious CNS depression may result.
• Avoid OTC preparations that contain CNS depressants (antihistamines, cold remedies).
• When chronic dry mouth occurs advise patient to:
  • Avoid mouth rinses with high alcohol content due to drying effects.
  • Use daily home fluoride products for anticaries effect.
  • Use sugarless gum, frequent sips of water, or saliva substitutes.

nalmefene hydrochloride
nal'-meh-feen high-droh-**klor'**-ide
(Revex)

CATEGORY AND SCHEDULE
Pregnancy Risk Category: B

Drug Class: Opioid antagonist

MECHANISM OF ACTION
Reverses the effects of opioids by competitive antagonism of opioid receptors.

USES
Management of opioid overdose and complete or partial reversal of opioid drug effects, including respiratory depression

PHARMACOKINETICS
IV: Onset 2 min, peak plasma concentration 1.1–2.3 hr; can also be given IM or subcutaneously; hepatic metabolism; excreted in urine.

INDICATIONS AND DOSAGES
▶ **Reversal of Opioid Depression**
IV
Adult. (100 mcg/ml strength) initial dose 0.25 mcg/kg followed by 0.25 mcg/kg, incremental dose at 2–5 min intervals; cumulative doses over 1.0 mcg/kg do not provide additional therapeutic effect; titrate all doses.

Body weight (kg)	ml of 100 mcg/ml Solution
50	0.125
60	0.150
70	0.175
80	0.200
90	0.225
100	0.250

▶ **Known or Suspected Opioid Overdose**
IV
Adult. (1 mg/ml strength) initial 0.5 mg/70 kg; if needed, a second dose of 1.0 mg/70 kg, 2–5 min later; doses over 1.5 mg/70 kg are unlikely to be beneficial.

SIDE EFFECTS/ADVERSE REACTIONS
Oral: Dry mouth

CNS: Dizziness, headache, dysphoria, perception of pain, nervousness
CV: Tachycardia, hypertension, dysrhythmia, hypotension
GI: Nausea, abdominal cramps, vomiting, diarrhea
Resp: Pharyngitis, pulmonary edema
GU: Urinary retention
Integ: Pruritus
MS: Myalgia, joint pain
Misc: Chills

PRECAUTIONS AND CONTRAINDICATIONS
Hypersensitivity
Caution:
Nursing mothers, children, withdrawal symptoms in opioid addicts, renal impairment

DRUG INTERACTIONS OF CONCERN TO DENTISTRY
• None reported

SERIOUS REACTIONS
‼ Precipitation of acute withdrawal syndrome in opioid-dependent individuals.
‼ Tachycardia, hypertension.

DENTAL CONSIDERATIONS

General:
• This drug is intended for acute use only.
• Risk of seizures reported in animal studies; be aware of this potential.
• Serious cardiovascular events have been associated with opioid reversal in postoperative patients; doses should be carefully titrated to reduce these events.
• Buprenorphine depression may not be completely reversed.
• In all cases, the establishment of a patent airway, ventilatory assistance,

oxygen administration, and circulatory access should complement or precede opioid antagonist use.

• Significant opioid depression occurring in the dental office may require relocation of the patient to a medical facility for comprehensive management.

• Patients discharged from the office or emergency facility should be carefully observed for the return of opioid-induced depression.

naloxone hydrochloride
nal-**oks**′-one high-droh-**klor**′-ide
(Narcan)
Do not confuse naltrexone or Narcan with Norcuron.

CATEGORY AND SCHEDULE
Pregnancy Risk Category: B

Drug Class: Narcotic antagonist

MECHANISM OF ACTION
An opioid antagonist that displaces opioids at opioid-occupied receptor sites in the CNS.
Therapeutic Effect: Reverses opioid-induced sleep or sedation, increases respiratory rate, raises B/P to normal range.

USES
Treatment of respiratory depression induced by opioids, to reverse postoperative opioid depression

PHARMACOKINETICS

Route	Onset	Peak	Duration
IV	1–2 min	N/A	20–60 min
IM	2–5 min	N/A	20–60 min
Subcutaneous	2–5 min	N/A	20–60 min

Well absorbed after IM or subcutaneous administration. Metabolized in the liver. Primarily excreted in urine. *Half-life:* 1–1.7hr.

INDICATIONS AND DOSAGES
▸ **Opioid Toxicity**
IV, IM, Subcutaneous
Adults, Elderly. 0.4–2 mg q2–3min as needed. May repeat q20–60min.
Children 5 yr and older and weighing 22 kg or more. 2 mg/dose; if no response, may repeat q2–3min. May need to repeat q20–60min.
Children younger than 5 yr and weighing less than 22 kg. 0.1 mg/kg; if no response, repeat q2–3min. May need to repeat q20–60min.
▸ **Postanesthesia Narcotic Reversal**
IV
Children. 0.01 mg/kg; may repeat q2–3min.
▸ **Neonatal Opioid-Induced Depression**
IV
Neonates. May repeat q2–3min as needed. May need to repeat q1–2h.

SIDE EFFECTS/ADVERSE REACTIONS
None known; little or no pharmacologic effect in absence of narcotics

PRECAUTIONS AND CONTRAINDICATIONS
Respiratory depression due to nonopioid drugs
Caution:
Opioid dependence

N

DRUG INTERACTIONS OF CONCERN TO DENTISTRY

• Antagonizes effects of opioid agonists and mixed agonists/antagonists.

SERIOUS REACTIONS

! Too-rapid reversal of opioid-induced respiratory depression may result in nausea, vomiting, tremors, increased B/P, and tachycardia.
! Excessive dosage in postoperative patients may produce significant excitement, tremors, and reversal of analgesia.
! Patients with cardiovascular disease may experience hypotension or hypertension, ventricular tachycardia and fibrillation, and pulmonary edema.

DENTAL CONSIDERATIONS

General:

• This drug is intended for acute use only, but listed side effects can sometimes be seen.
• Risk of seizures reported in animal studies; be aware of this potential.
• Serious cardiovascular events have been associated with opioid reversal in postoperative patients; doses should be carefully titrated to reduce these events.
• Buprenorphine depression may not be completely reversed.
• In all cases, the establishment of a patent airway, ventilatory assistance, oxygen administration, and circulatory access should complement or precede opioid antagonist use.
• Significant opioid depression occurring in the dental office may require relocation of the patient to a medical facility for comprehensive management.
• Patients discharged from the office/emergency facility should be

carefully observed for the return of opioid-induced depression.

naltrexone hydrochloride

nal-**trex**′-one high-droh-**klor**′-ide
(ReVia)

CATEGORY AND SCHEDULE
Pregnancy Risk Category: C

Drug Class: Narcotic antagonist

MECHANISM OF ACTION

An opioid antagonist that displaces opioids at opioid-occupied receptor sites in the CNS.
Therapeutic Effect: Blocks physical effects of opioid analgesics; decreases craving for alcohol and relapse rate in alcoholism.

USES

Treatment of opioid addiction following detoxification, alcoholism

PHARMACOKINETICS

PO: Onset 15–30 min, peak 1–2 hr, duration is dose dependent.
Half-life: 4 hr; extensive first-pass metabolism; metabolized by liver; excreted by kidneys; crosses placenta; excreted in breast milk.

INDICATIONS AND DOSAGES

▶ **Naloxone Challenge Test to Determine if Patient is Opioid Dependent**

ALERT

Expect to perform the naloxone challenge test if there is any question that the patient is opioid dependent. Do not administer naltrexone until the naloxone challenge test is negative.

IV
Adults, Elderly. Draw 2 ml (0.8 mg) of naloxone into syringe. Inject 0.5 ml (0.2 mg); while needle is still in vein, observe patient for 30 sec for withdrawal signs or symptoms. If no evidence of withdrawal, inject remaining 1.5 ml (0.6 mg); observe patient for additional 20 min for withdrawal signs or symptoms.
Subcutaneous
Adults, Elderly. Inject 2 ml (0.8 mg) of naloxone; observe patient for 45 min for withdrawal signs or symptoms.

▸ **Treatment of Opioid Dependence in Patients Who Have Been Opioid Free for at Least 7–10 Days**
PO
Adults, Elderly. Initially, 25 mg. Observe patient for 1 hr. If no withdrawal signs or symptoms appear, give another 25 mg. May be given as 100 mg every other day or 150 mg every 3 days.

▸ **Adjunctive Treatment of Alcohol Dependence**
PO
Adults, Elderly. 50 mg once a day.

SIDE EFFECTS/ADVERSE REACTIONS
Frequent
Alcoholism: Nausea, headache, depression
Opioid addiction: Insomnia, anxiety, nervousness, headache, low energy, abdominal cramps, nausea, vomiting, arthralgia, myalgia
Occasional
Alcoholism: Dizziness, nervousness, fatigue, insomnia, vomiting, anxiety, suicidal ideation
Narcotic addiction: Irritability, increased energy, dizziness, anorexia, diarrhea or constipation, rash, chills, increased thirst

PRECAUTIONS AND CONTRAINDICATIONS
Acute hepatitis, acute opioid withdrawal, failed naloxone challenge test, hepatic failure, history of hypersensitivity to naltrexone, opioid dependence, positive urine screen for opioids

DRUG INTERACTIONS OF CONCERN TO DENTISTRY
• Decreased effects of opioid narcotics

SERIOUS REACTIONS
! Signs and symptoms of opioid withdrawal include stuffy or runny nose, tearing, yawning, diaphoresis, tremors, vomiting, piloerection, feeling of temperature change, bone pain, arthralgia, myalgia, abdominal cramps, and feeling of skin crawling.
! Accidental naltrexone overdose produces withdrawal symptoms within 5 min of ingestion that may last for up to 48 hr. Symptoms include confusion, visual hallucinations, somnolence, and significant vomiting and diarrhea.
! Hepatocellular injury may occur with large doses.

DENTAL CONSIDERATIONS
General:
• Monitor vital signs at every appointment because of cardiovascular and respiratory side effects.
• Patients on chronic drug therapy may rarely have symptoms of blood dyscrasias, which can include infection, bleeding, and poor healing.
• Patients should not be given opioid analgesics for dental pain management. Substitute with acetaminophen or NSAIDs.

N

• The dental professional must be aware of the patient's disease, and the patient must be active in treatment for chemical dependency.

Consultations:

• In patients with symptoms of blood dyscrasias, request a medical consultation for blood studies and postpone dental treatment until normal values are reestablished.

• Medical consultation may be required to assess disease control.

• Inform aftercare provider or counselor if sedative medications are required for proper management.

Teach Patient/Family to:

• Encourage effective oral hygiene to prevent soft tissue inflammation.

• Use caution to prevent injury when using oral hygiene aids.

naphazoline

naf-**az**′-oh-leen
(AK-Con, Albalon Liquifilm[AUS],
Clear Eyes[AUS], Naphcon,
Naphcon Forte[AUS], Privine,
Vasocon)

CATEGORY AND SCHEDULE
Pregnancy Risk Category: C

Drug Class: Ophthalmic vasoconstrictor

MECHANISM OF ACTION
A sympathomimetic that directly acts on α-adrenergic receptors in conjunctival arterioles and nasal blood vessels.
Therapeutic Effect: Causes vasoconstriction, resulting in decreased congestion.

USES
Relief of hyperemia, irritation in superficial corneal vascularity

PHARMACOKINETICS
Instillation: Duration 2–3 hr.

INDICATIONS AND DOSAGES
▶ **Nasal Congestion Resulting from Acute or Chronic Rhinitis, Common Cold, Hay Fever, or Other Allergies**
Intranasal
Adults, Elderly, Children older than 12 yr. 1–2 drops or sprays in each nostril q3–6h.
Children 6–12 yr. 1 spray or drop in each nostril q6h as needed.
▶ **Control of Hyperemia in Patients with Superficial Corneal Vascularity; Relief of Congestion and Inflammation; for Use During Ocular Diagnostic Procedures**
Ophthalmic
Adults, Elderly, Children older than 6 yr. 1–2 drops in affected eye q3–4h for 3–4 days.

SIDE EFFECTS/ADVERSE REACTIONS
Occasional
Nasal: Burning, stinging, or drying of nasal mucosa; sneezing; rebound congestion
Ophthalmic: Blurred vision, dilated pupils, increased eye irritation

PRECAUTIONS AND CONTRAINDICATIONS
Angle-closure glaucoma, before peripheral iridectomy, patients with a narrow angle who do not have glaucoma
Caution:
Hypertension, hyperthyroidism, elderly, severe arteriosclerosis, cardiac disease

DRUG INTERACTIONS OF CONCERN TO DENTISTRY
• Increased pressor effects: tricyclic antidepressants

SERIOUS REACTIONS

! If naphazoline is systemically absorbed, the patient may experience tachycardia, palpitations, headache, insomnia, light-headedness, nausea, nervousness, and tremors.

! Large doses may produce tachycardia, palpitations, light-headedness, nausea, and vomiting.

! Overdose in patients older than 60 yr may produce hallucinations, CNS depression, and seizures.

DENTAL CONSIDERATIONS

General:

• Monitor vital signs at every appointment because of cardiovascular side effects.

• Avoid dental light in patient's eyes; offer dark glasses for patient comfort.

naproxen/naproxen sodium

na-**prox**'-en **soe**'-dee-um
naproxen: (Crysanal[AUS],
EC-Naprosyn, Inza[AUS],
Naprelan, Naprosyn) naproxen
sodium: (Aleve, Anaprox,
Anaprox DS, Apo-
Naprosyn[CAN], Naprogesic[AUS],
Novo-Naprox[CAN],
Nu-Naprox[CAN], Pamprin)
Do not confuse Aleve with Alesse
or Anaprox with Anaspaz.

CATEGORY AND SCHEDULE

Pregnancy Risk Category: B (D if used in third trimester or near delivery)
OTC (220 mg gelcaps, 220 mg tablets)

Drug Class: Nonsteroidal antiinflammatory

MECHANISM OF ACTION

An NSAID that produces analgesic and antiinflammatory effects by inhibiting prostaglandin synthesis. *Therapeutic Effect:* Reduces the inflammatory response and intensity of pain.

USES

Treatment of mild-to-moderate pain, osteoarthritis, rheumatoid, juvenile, gouty arthritis, ankylosing spondylitis, primary dysmenorrhea; unapproved: migraine, PMS, fever

PHARMACOKINETICS

Route	Onset	Peak	Duration
PO (analgesic)	Less than 1 hr	N/A	7 hr or less
PO (anti-rheumatic)	Less than 14 days	2–4 wk	N/A

Completely absorbed from the GI tract. Protein binding: 99%. Metabolized in the liver. Primarily excreted in urine. Not removed by hemodialysis. *Half-life:* 13 hr.

INDICATIONS AND DOSAGES
▶ **Rheumatoid Arthritis, Osteoarthritis, Ankylosing Spondylitis**
PO
Adults, Elderly. 250–500 mg naproxen (275–550 mg naproxen sodium) twice a day or 250 mg naproxen (275 mg naproxen sodium) in morning and 500 mg naproxen (550 mg naproxen sodium) in evening. Naprelan: 750–1000 mg once a day.
▶ **Acute Gouty Arthritis**
PO
Adults, Elderly. Initially, 750 mg naproxen (825 mg naproxen sodium), then 250 mg naproxen (275 mg naproxen sodium) q8h until

N

attack subsides. Naprelan: Initially,
1000–1500 mg, then 1000 mg once
a day until attack subsides.

▶ **Mild-to-Moderate Pain,
Dysmenorrhea, Bursitis, Tendinitis**
PO
Adults, Elderly. Initially, 500 mg
naproxen (550 mg naproxen
sodium), then 250 mg naproxen
(275 mg naproxen sodium) q6–8h as
needed. Maximum: 1.25 g/day
naproxen (1.375 g/day naproxen
sodium). Naprelan: 1000 mg once a
day.

▶ **Juvenile Rheumatoid Arthritis**
PO (Naproxen Only)
Children. 10–15 mg/kg/day in 2
divided doses. Maximum: 1000 mg/
day.

SIDE EFFECTS/ADVERSE
REACTIONS

Frequent
Nausea, constipation, abdominal
cramps or pain, heartburn, dizziness,
headache, somnolence, oral
lichenoid reaction
Occasional
Stomatitis, diarrhea, indigestion
Rare
Vomiting, confusion

PRECAUTIONS AND
CONTRAINDICATIONS

Hypersensitivity to aspirin,
naproxen, or other NSAIDs
Caution:
Lactation, children, bleeding
disorders, GI disorders, cardiac
disorders, hypersensitivity to other
antiinflammatory agents, elderly,
more than 2 alcohol drinks daily

DRUG INTERACTIONS OF
CONCERN TO DENTISTRY

• GI ulceration, bleeding: aspirin,
alcohol, corticosteroids
  • Nephrotoxicity: acetaminophen
(chronic use and high doses)

• Possible risk of decreased renal
function: cyclosporine
• Increased photosensitization:
tetracycline
• Increased plasma levels:
probenecid
• SSRIs: NSAIDs increase risk of
GI side effects
• When prescribed for dental pain:
  • Risk of increased effects: oral
anticoagulants, oral antidiabetics,
trium, methotrexate
  • Decreased antihypertensive
effects of diuretics, β-adrenergic
blockers, and ACE inhibitors

SERIOUS REACTIONS

! Rare reactions with long-term use
include peptic ulcer disease.
! GI bleeding, gastritis, severe
hepatic reactions (cholestasis,
jaundice), nephrotoxicity (dysuria,
hematuria, proteinuria, nephrotic
syndrome), and a severe
hypersensitivity reaction (fever,
chills, bronchospasm).

DENTAL CONSIDERATIONS

General:
• Possible increased adverse
cardiovascular events in patients at
risk for thromboembolism.
• Patients on chronic drug therapy
may rarely have symptoms of blood
dyscrasias, which can include
infection, bleeding, and poor
healing.
• Assess salivary flow as a factor in
caries, periodontal disease, and
candidiasis.
• Avoid prescribing for dental use in
pregnancy.
• Avoid prescribing aspirin-
containing products.
• Consider semisupine chair position
for patients with arthritic disease.
• Severe stomach bleeding may
occur in patients who regularly use

NSAIDs in recommended doses, when the patient is also taking another NSAID, a blood thinning, or steroid drug, if the patient has GI or peptic ulcer disease, if they are 60 yr or older, or when NSAIDs are taken longer than directed. Warn patients of the potential for severe stomach bleeding.

Consultations:

• In patients with symptoms of blood dyscrasias, request a medical consultation for blood studies and postpone dental treatment until normal values are reestablished.

• Medical consultation may be required to assess disease control.

Teach Patient/Family to:

• Encourage effective oral hygiene to prevent soft tissue inflammation.

• Use caution to prevent injury when using oral hygiene aids.

• Warn patient of potential risks of NSAIDs.

• When chronic dry mouth occurs, advise patient to:

  • Avoid mouth rinses with high alcohol content because of drying effects.

  • Use daily home fluoride products for anticaries effect.

  • Use sugarless gum, frequent sips of water, or saliva substitutes.

naratriptan

nare-ah-**trip**′-tan
(Amerge, Naramig[AUS])
Do not confuse Amerge with Amaryl.

CATEGORY AND SCHEDULE
Pregnancy Risk Category: C

Drug Class: Serotonin agonist

MECHANISM OF ACTION

A serotonin receptor agonist that binds selectively to vascular receptors, producing a vasoconstrictive effect on cranial blood vessels.
Therapeutic Effect: Relieves migraine headache.

USES

Acute treatment of migraine attacks with or without aura in adults

PHARMACOKINETICS

Well absorbed after PO administration. Protein binding: 28%–31%. Metabolized by the liver to inactive metabolite. Eliminated primarily in urine and, to a lesser extent, in feces. *Half-life:* 6 hr (increased in hepatic or renal impairment).

INDICATIONS AND DOSAGES
▶ **Acute Migraine Attack**
PO
Adults. 1 mg or 2.5 mg. If headache improves but then returns, dose may be repeated after 4 hr. Maximum: 5 mg/24 hr.
▶ **Dosage in Mild-to-Moderate Hepatic or Renal Impairment**
A lower starting dose is recommended. Do not exceed 2.5 mg/24 hr.

SIDE EFFECTS/ADVERSE REACTIONS
Occasional
Nausea
Rare
Paresthesia; dizziness; fatigue; somnolence; jaw, neck, or throat pressure

PRECAUTIONS AND CONTRAINDICATIONS

Basilar or hemiplegic migraine, cerebrovascular or peripheral

N

vascular disease, coronary artery disease, ischemic heart disease (including angina pectoris, history of MI, silent ischemia, and Prinzmetal's angina), severe hepatic impairment (Child-Pugh grade C), severe renal impairment (serum creatinine less than 15 ml/min), uncontrolled hypertension, use within 24 hr of ergotamine-containing preparations or another serotonin receptor agonist, use within 14 days of MAOIs

Caution:
Risk of serious cardiovascular events, including ischemia and MI; renal/hepatic dysfunction, SSRI antidepressants, lactation, use in children not established, not recommended in elderly

DRUG INTERACTIONS OF CONCERN TO DENTISTRY

• No specific interactions with dental drugs reported.
• Should not be used within 24 hr of another 5-HT1 agonist.

SERIOUS REACTIONS

! Corneal opacities and other ocular defects may occur.
! Cardiac reactions (including ischemia, coronary artery vasospasm, and MI) and noncardiac vasospasm-related reactions (such as hemorrhage and CVA), occur rarely, particularly in patients with hypertension, diabetes, or a strong family history of coronary artery disease; obese patients; smokers; males older than 40 yr; and postmenopausal women.

DENTAL CONSIDERATIONS

General:
• This is an acute-use drug; it is doubtful that patients will come to

the office if acute migraine is present.
• Be aware of patient's disease, its severity, and its frequency when known.

Consultations:
• If treating chronic orofacial pain, consult with physician of record.
• Medical consultation may be required to assess disease control and patient's ability to tolerate stress.

Teach Patient/Family to:
• Update health and drug history if physician makes any changes in evaluation or drug regimens; include OTC, herbal, and nonherbal drugs in update.
• Avoid mouth rinses with high alcohol content because of additional drying effects.

nateglinide
na-**teg**′-lin-ide
(Starlix)

CATEGORY AND SCHEDULE
Pregnancy Risk Category: C

Drug Class: Oral antidiabetic, meglitinide class

MECHANISM OF ACTION
An antihyperglycemic that stimulates release of insulin from β cells of the pancreas by depolarizing β cells, leading to an opening of calcium channels. Resulting calcium influx induces insulin secretion.
Therapeutic Effect: Lowers blood glucose concentration.

USES
Treatment of Type 2 diabetes mellitus when hyperglycemia cannot be controlled by diet and exercise,

can be used in combination with metformin, not for patients who have been chronically treated with other antidiabetic drugs

PHARMACOKINETICS
PO: Rapid absorption, peak plasma levels 1 hr, bioavailability 73%, plasma protein binding 98%, hepatic metabolism (CYP450 2C9 isoenzyme [70%] and CYP450 3A4 isoenzyme [30%]); excretion renal (83%), feces (10%).

INDICATIONS AND DOSAGES
▶ Diabetes Mellitus
PO
Adult, Elderly. 120 mg 3 times a day before meals. Initially, 60 mg may be given.

SIDE EFFECTS/ADVERSE REACTIONS
Frequent
Upper respiratory tract infection
Occasional
Back pain, flu symptoms, dizziness, arthropathy, diarrhea
Rare
Bronchitis, cough

PRECAUTIONS AND CONTRAINDICATIONS
Diabetic ketoacidosis, type 1
Diabetes mellitus
Caution:
Hypoglycemia (geriatric, malnourished, adrenal insufficiency or pituitary insufficiency more susceptible to hypoglycemia), β-blocker may mask hypoglycemia, administer before meals, infection, hepatic dysfunction, lactation, children

DRUG INTERACTIONS OF CONCERN TO DENTISTRY
• Most drug interactions not clearly identified; may act as an inhibitor of

CYP450 2C9 enzymes but not CYP450 3A4. Does not appear to interact with highly protein-bound drugs
• Potentiation of hypoglycemic effects: NSAIDs, salicylates, nonselective β-blockers

SERIOUS REACTIONS
! Hypoglycemia occurs in less than 2% of patients.

DENTAL CONSIDERATIONS
General:
• If dentist prescribes any of the drugs listed in the drug interaction section, monitor patient's blood sugar levels.
• Consider semisupine chair position for patient comfort if GI side effects occur.
• Ensure that patient is following prescribed diet and regularly takes medication.
• Place on frequent recall to evaluate healing response.
• Short appointments and a stress-reduction protocol may be required.
• Diabetics may be more susceptible to infection and have delayed wound healing.
Consultations:
• Medical consultation may include data from patient's blood glucose monitoring, including glycosylated hemoglobin or HbA$_{1c}$ testing.
• Medical consultation may be required to assess disease control and patient's ability to tolerate stress.
Teach Patient/Family to:
• Prevent trauma when using oral hygiene aids.
• Update health and drug history if physician makes any changes in evaluation or drug regimens.

nebivolol
ne-**biv**-oh-lole
(Bystolic)

CATEGORY AND SCHEDULE
Pregnancy Risk Category: C

Drug Class: Antihypertensive,
β-adrenergic blocker (selective)

MECHANISM OF ACTION
An antihypertensive that possesses
selective β_1 blocking activity, but
loses selectivity at higher doses.
Causes vasodilation through nitric
oxide (NO)-production, potentiating
its actions, and reducing total
peripheral vascular resistance.
Therapeutic Effect: Decreases B/P,
heart rate, and myocardial
contractility; suppresses renin
activity.

USES
Hypertension

PHARMACOKINETICS
Rapidly absorbed. Bioavailability of
approximately 12% (extensive
metabolizers) to 96% (poor
metabolizers). Protein binding: 98%,
mostly albumin. Extensively
metabolized in the liver to active
metabolites by glucuronidation and
CYP450 2D6. Excreted in urine
(38% in extensive metabolizers;
67% in poor metabolizers) and in
feces (44% in extensive
metabolizers; 13% in poor
metabolizers). **Half-life:** 12–19 hr;
10–12 hr in extensive metabolizers
and 19–32 hr in poor metabolizers.

INDICATIONS AND DOSAGES
▶ **Hypertension**
PO
Adults, Elderly. 5–40 mg/day.
Initially, 5 mg/day. May increase at
2-wk intervals. Maximum: 40 mg/
day.
▶ **Dosage in Renal Impairment**
*Adults (creatinine clearance less
than 30 ml/min).* Initially, 2.5 mg/
day.
Increase with caution.
▶ **Dosage in Hepatic Impairment
(Moderate)**
Adults. 2.5 mg/day.
Increase with caution.
Not recommended in patients with
severe hepatic impairment

SIDE EFFECTS/ADVERSE
REACTIONS
Adults
Frequent
Fatigue, dizziness, headache
Occasional
Nausea, diarrhea, somnolence, pain,
peripheral edema
Rare
Bradycardia, dyspnea, chest pain,
rash, acute renal failure, erectile
dysfunction, Raynaud's
phenomenon, syncope,
bronchospasm, acute pulmonary
edema

PRECAUTIONS AND
CONTRAINDICATIONS
Hypersensitivity to nebivolol or any
component of the formulation
Severe bradycardia
Heart block >first degree
Cardiogenic shock
Decompensated HF
Bronchospastic disease
Caution:
Sick sinus syndrome (unless a
permanent pacemaker is in place)
Severe hepatic impairment (Child
Pugh >B)

Abrupt cessation of therapy
Cardiac failure, angina, acute MI
Diabetes (hypoglycemia)
Thyrotoxicosis
Peripheral vascular disease
Concurrent use with CYP2D6 inhibitors
Impaired renal or hepatic function
Anesthesia/surgery
Concomitant use with other β-blockers
Pheochromocytoma

DRUG INTERACTIONS OF CONCERN TO DENTISTRY

• Diuretics, other antihypertensives: May increase hypotensive effect of nebivolol.
• Sympathomimetics, xanthines: Increased systolic BP, bradycardia. May antagonize the effects and reduce bronchodilation.
• CYP450 2D6 inhibitors: May increase concentrations of nebivolol.
• Oral hypoglycemics and insulin: May mask symptoms of hypoglycemia and prolong hypoglycemic effect of insulin and oral hypoglycemics.
• NSAIDs: May reduce the antihypertensive effect of nebivolol.
• Digoxin: May cause serious bradycardia.
• Calcium channel blockers (verapamil, diltiazem): May cause hypotension and bradycardia.

SERIOUS REACTIONS

! Second- and third-degree atrioventricular block has been reported.
! Abrupt withdrawal may result in rebound or withdrawal hypertension, severe exacerbation of angina, myocardial infarction, and ventricular arrhythmia.
! Nebivolol administration may precipitate CHF and MI in patients with heart disease, thyroid storm in those with thyrotoxicosis, and peripheral ischemia in those with existing peripheral vascular disease.
! Hypoglycemia may occur in patients with previously controlled diabetes.

DENTAL CONSIDERATIONS

General:
• Monitor vital signs at every appointment because of cardiovascular side effects.
• Avoid vasoconstrictors or limit doses.
• After supine positioning, have patient sit upright for at least 2 min before standing to avoid orthostatic hypotension.
• Assess salivary flow as a factor in caries, periodontal disease, and candidiasis.
• Limit use of sodium-containing products, such as saline IV fluids, for those patients with dietary salt restriction.
• Stress from dental procedures may compromise cardiovascular function; determine patient risk.
Consultations:
• Medical consultation may be required to assess disease control.
Teach Patient/Family to:
• Report oral lesions, soreness, or bleeding to dentist.
• When chronic dry mouth occurs, advise patient to:
  • Avoid mouth rinses with high alcohol content because of drying effects.
  • Use daily home fluoride products for anticaries effect.
  • Use sugarless gum, frequent sips of water, or saliva substitutes.

N

nedocromil sodium

ned-oh-**crow**′-mil **soe**′-dee-um
(Alocril, Mireze[CAN], Tilade,
Tilade CFC Free[AUS])

CATEGORY AND SCHEDULE
Pregnancy Risk Category: B

Drug Class: Antiasthmatic, mast
cell stabilizer

MECHANISM OF ACTION
A mast cell stabilizer that prevents
the activation and release of
inflammatory mediators, such as
histamine, leukotrienes, mast cells,
eosinophils, and monocytes.
Therapeutic Effect: Prevents both
early and late asthmatic responses.

USES
Maintenance therapy in mild-to-
moderate asthma; ophthalmic
solution for allergic conjunctivitis

PHARMACOKINETICS
Inhalation: Peak 15 min, duration
4–6 hr. *Half-life:* 80 min; excreted
unchanged in feces.

INDICATIONS AND DOSAGES
▸ **Mild-to-Moderate Asthma**
Oral Inhalation
*Adults, Elderly, Children 6 yr and
older.* 2 inhalations 4 times a day.
May decrease to 3 times a day then
twice a day as asthma becomes
controlled.
▸ **Allergic Conjunctivitis**
Ophthalmic
*Adults, Elderly, Children 3 yr and
older.* 1–2 drops in each eye twice a
day.

SIDE EFFECTS/ADVERSE REACTIONS
Frequent
Cough, pharyngitis, bronchospasm,
headache, altered taste
Occasional
Rhinitis, upper respiratory tract
infection, abdominal pain, fatigue
Rare
Diarrhea, dizziness

PRECAUTIONS AND CONTRAINDICATIONS
Hypersensitivity to this drug or
lactose, status asthmaticus
Caution:
Lactation, renal disease, hepatic
disease, safety and efficacy of
inhalation in children younger than
6 yr or ophthalmic solution in
children younger than 3 yr not
established

DRUG INTERACTIONS OF CONCERN TO DENTISTRY
• None reported

SERIOUS REACTIONS
! None known

DENTAL CONSIDERATIONS

Nedocromil Sodium (Alocril)
General:
• Determine why patient is taking
the drug.
• Avoid dental light in patient's eyes;
offer dark glasses for patient
comfort.
• Users may report unpleasant taste
while using this product.
Nedocromil Sodium
General:
• Assess salivary flow as a factor in
caries, periodontal disease, and
candidiasis.
• Consider semisupine chair position
for patients with respiratory disease.

• Short appointments and a stress-reduction protocol may be required for anxious patients.
• Be aware that aspirin or sulfite preservatives in vasoconstrictor-containing products can exacerbate asthma.
Consultations:
• Medical consultation may be required to assess disease control.
Teach Patient/Family to:
• Avoid mouth rinses with high alcohol content because of drying effects.
• Rinse mouth with water after each inhaled dose to prevent dryness.

nefazodone hydrochloride
neh-**faz**′-oh-doan
high-droh-**klor**′-ide
(Serzone)

CATEGORY AND SCHEDULE
Pregnancy Risk Category: C

Drug Class: Antidepressant

MECHANISM OF ACTION
Exact mechanism is unknown. Appears to inhibit neuronal uptake of serotonin and norepinephrine and to antagonize α_1-adrenergic receptors.
Therapeutic Effect: Relieves depression.

USES
Treatment of major depressive disorders

PHARMACOKINETICS
Rapidly and completely absorbed from the GI tract; food delays absorption. Protein binding: 99%. Widely distributed in body tissues, including CNS. Extensively metabolized to active metabolites. Excreted in urine and eliminated in feces. Unknown if removed by hemodialysis. *Half-life:* 2–4 hr.

INDICATIONS AND DOSAGES
▶ **Depression, Prevention of Relapse of Acute Depressive Episode**
PO
Adults. Initially, 200 mg/day in 2 divided doses. Gradually increase by 100–200 mg/day at intervals of at least 1 wk. Range: 300–600 mg/day.
Elderly. Initially, 100 mg/day in 2 divided doses. Subsequent dosage titration based on clinical response. Range: 200–400 mg/day.
Children. 300–400 mg/day.

SIDE EFFECTS/ADVERSE REACTIONS
Frequent
Headache, dry mouth, somnolence, nausea, dizziness, constipation, insomnia, asthenia, light-headedness
Occasional
Dyspepsia, blurred vision, diarrhea, infection, confusion, abnormal vision, pharyngitis, increased appetite, orthostatic hypotension, flushing, feeling of warmth, peripheral edema, cough, flu-like symptoms

PRECAUTIONS AND CONTRAINDICATIONS
Use within 14 days of MAOIs
Caution:
Mania, hypomania, suicidal tendencies, seizures, history of MI or unstable heart conditions, hepatic impairment, lactation, children younger than 18 yr, elderly (requires dose adjustment), priapism history, alcohol use; risk in operating auto or hazardous machinery

N

DRUG INTERACTIONS OF CONCERN TO DENTISTRY

• Must not be used concurrently with or within 14 days of discontinuing MAOI
• Risk of significant adverse drug interaction with triazolam, alprazolam, alcohol-containing products
• Increased sedation: St. John's wort (herb)
• Acts as an inhibitor of CYP3A4 isoenzymes: risk of interaction with drugs metabolized by CYP3A4

SERIOUS REACTIONS

! Serious reactions, such as hyperthermia, rigidity, myoclonus, extreme agitation, delirium, and coma, will occur if the patient takes an MAOI concurrently or fails to let enough time elapse when switching from an MAOI to nefazodone or vice versa.

DENTAL CONSIDERATIONS

General:
• Assess salivary flow as a factor in caries, periodontal disease, and candidiasis.
• Take vital signs at every appointment because of cardiovascular side effects.
• After supine positioning, have patient sit upright for at least 2 min before standing to avoid postural hypotension.
• There is no information concerning the use of vasoconstrictors in patients taking this drug.
• Advise patient if dental drugs prescribed have a potential for photosensitivity.

Consultations:
• Medical consultation may be required to assess disease control.

• Physician should be informed if significant xerostomic side effects occur (e.g., increased caries, sore tongue, problems eating or swallowing, difficulty wearing prosthesis) so that a medication change can be considered.
• Because there is no experience with the use of conscious sedation or general anesthesia in patients taking this drug, a medical consultation is recommended for risk evaluation.
• Patients showing anorexia, jaundice, GI complaints, or malaise should be referred for medical evaluation before treatment.

Teach Patient/Family to:
• When chronic dry mouth occurs, advise patient to:
    • Avoid mouth rinses with high alcohol content because of drying effects.
    • Use daily home fluoride products for anticaries effect.
    • Use sugarless gum, frequent sips of water, or saliva substitutes.

nelarabine

nel-**ay**′-reh-been
(Arranon)

CATEGORY AND SCHEDULE

Pregnancy Risk Category: D

Drug Class: Antineoplastic

MECHANISM OF ACTION

A prodrug of deoxyguanosine analogue 9-β-D-arabinofuranosylguanine (ara-G) that disrupts DNA synthesis.
Therapeutic Effect: Induces cellular apoptosis.

USES
Treatment of relapsed or refractory T-cell acute lymphoblastic leukemia (ALL) and T-cell lymphoblastic lymphoma

PHARMACOKINETICS
Protein binding: less than 25%. Metabolized in liver to ara-G (active); also hydrolyzed to methyl guanine. Excreted in urine.
Half-life: 30 min (nelarabine); 3 hr (ara-G).

INDICATIONS AND DOSAGES
▸ **T-cell ALL (Relapsed or Refractory)**
IV
Adults. 1500 mg/m^2 delivered as a 2-hr infusion on days 1, 3, and 5 of a 21-day treatment cycle. Treatment cycles should be repeated until evidence of disease progression is observed.
Children. 650 mg/m^2 delivered as a 1-hr infusion daily for days 1–5 of a 21-day treatment cycle. Treatment cycles should be repeated until evidence of disease progression is observed.
▸ **T-cell Lymphoblastic Lymphoma (Relapsed or Refractory)**
IV
Adults. 1500 mg/m^2 delivered as a 2-hr infusion on days 1, 3, and 5 of a 21-day treatment cycle. Treatment cycles should be repeated until evidence of disease progression is observed.
Children. 650 mg/m^2 delivered as a 1-hr infusion daily for days 1–5 of a 21-day treatment cycle. Treatment cycles should be repeated until evidence of disease progression is observed.

SIDE EFFECTS/ADVERSE REACTIONS
Frequent
Anemia, neutropenia, thrombocytopenia, fatigue, nausea, leukopenia, cough, fever, diarrhea, vomiting, somnolence, dizziness, constipation, peripheral neuropathy, dyspnea, headache, hypoesthesia, weakness, peripheral edema, febrile neutropenia, hypokalemia, petechiae, edema, pain, albumin decreased, bilirubin increased, pleural effusion
Occasional
Abdominal pain, anorexia, arthralgia, infection, ataxia, back pain, muscle weakness, rigors, stomatitis, hypotension, tachycardia, hypocalcemia, confusion, epistaxis, pneumonia, sinusitis, insomnia, dehydration, limb pain, abnormal gait, depressed level of consciousness, hypomagnesemia, depression, seizure, hyper-/hypoglycemia, abdominal distension, AST increased, creatinine increased, noncardiac chest pain, wheezing, chest pain, tremor, blurred vision, motor dysfunction, taste perversion, amnesia, balance disorder, nerve paralysis, sensory loss
Rare
Aphasia, cerebral hemorrhage, coma, encephalopathy, hemiparesis, hydrocephalus, lethargy, leukoencephalopathy, loss of consciousness, mental impairment, neuropathic pain, nerve palsy, nystagmus, paralysis, sciatica, sensory disturbance, speech disorder, demyelination, ascending peripheral neuropathy, dysarthria, hyporeflexia, hypertonia, incoordination, sinus headache (1%)

PRECAUTIONS AND CONTRAINDICATIONS
Hypersensitivity to nelarabine or its components

Caution:
Do not breast-feed, compromised bone marrow reserve, chickenpox, herpes zoster, history of gout, infection

DRUG INTERACTIONS OF CONCERN TO DENTISTRY
• None reported

SERIOUS REACTIONS
! Severe neurologic events have been reported with the use of nelarabine including altered mental states, severe somnolence, convulsions, peripheral neuropathy ranging from numbness and paresthesias to motor weakness and paralysis.
! Demyelination and ascending peripheral neuropathies similar in appearance to Guillain-Barré syndrome have been reported.
! Leukopenia, anemia, neutropenia, and thrombocytopenia have been associated with nelarabine therapy.

DENTAL CONSIDERATIONS
General:
• Monitor vital signs at every appointment because of cardiovascular and respiratory adverse effects.
• Avoid aspirin and NSAIDs to prevent gastrointestinal irritation and excessive bleeding.
• Examine patient carefully for oral manifestations of opportunistic infections, blood dyscrasias, and stomatitis and mucositis.
• Confirm patient's disease status and treatment regimen.
• Chlorhexidine mouthrinse prior to and during chemotherapy may reduce severity of mucositis.
• Palliative medication may be required for management of oral adverse effects of drug.

• Patient may be taking prophylactic antiinfective drug.
• Place patient on frequent recall due to adverse oral effects of drug.
Consultations:
• Consult physician to determine control of disease and ability of patient to tolerate dental procedures.
• Consult physician to determine need for prophylactic or therapeutic antiinfective medications if oral surgery or periodontal treatment is required.
• Consult physician to assess patient's immunologic and coagulation status and determine safety risk, if any, posed by the required dental treatment.
Teach Patient/Family to:
• Be aware of oral adverse effects of drug.
• Use atraumatic, effective oral hygiene measures to prevent or minimize soft tissue inflammation.
• Report oral lesions, soreness, or bleeding to dentist.
• Update health and medication history if physician makes any changes in evaluation or drug regimen; include OTC, herbal, and nonherbal drug in update.

nelfinavir
nel-**fin**′-eh-veer
(Viracept)

CATEGORY AND SCHEDULE
Pregnancy Risk Category: B

Drug Class: Antiviral

MECHANISM OF ACTION
Inhibits the activity of HIV-1 protease, the enzyme necessary for the formation of infectious HIV.

Therapeutic Effect: Formation of immature noninfectious viral particles rather than HIV replication.

USES

Treatment of HIV infection when indicated by surrogate marker changes in patients receiving nelfinavir in combination with nucleoside analogues or alone for up to 24 wk

PHARMACOKINETICS

Well absorbed after PO administration (absorption increased with food). Protein binding: 98%. Metabolized in the liver. Highly bound to plasma proteins. Eliminated primarily in feces. Unknown if removed by hemodialysis. *Half-life:* 3.5–5 hr.

INDICATIONS AND DOSAGES
▶ HIV Infection
PO
Adults. 750 mg (three 250-mg tablets) 3 times a day or 1250 mg twice a day in combination with nucleoside analogs (enhances antiviral activity).
Children 2–13 yr. 0–30 mg/kg/dose 3 times a day. Maximum: 750 mg q8h.

SIDE EFFECTS/ADVERSE REACTIONS
Frequent
Diarrhea
Occasional
Nausea, rash
Rare
Flatulence, asthenia

PRECAUTIONS AND CONTRAINDICATIONS
Concurrent administration with midazolam, rifampin, or triazolam

Caution:
Pediatric use, phenylketonuria (powder contains phenylalanine), diabetes mellitus, hyperglycemia, hepatic impairment, development of resistance, hemophilia, lactation, children younger than 2 yr, an inhibitor of CYP3A4 isoenzymes; use with caution with drugs that are inducers of CYP3A4 or CYP2C19 isoenzymes

DRUG INTERACTIONS OF CONCERN TO DENTISTRY
• Contraindicated with triazolam, midazolam, and other drugs dependent on CYP3A4 for metabolism
• Increased plasma levels: azithromycin, ketoconazole
• Increased plasma concentrations of fentanyl

SERIOUS REACTIONS
• None known

DENTAL CONSIDERATIONS

General:
• Examine for oral manifestation of opportunistic infection.
• Patients on chronic drug therapy may rarely have symptoms of blood dyscrasias, which can include infection, bleeding, and poor healing.
• Palliative medication may be required for management of oral side effects.
Consultations:
• In a patient with symptoms of blood dyscrasias, request a medical consultation for blood studies and postpone treatment until normal values are reestablished.
• Medical consultation may be required to assess disease control.

N

Teach Patient/Family to:
• Encourage effective oral hygiene to prevent soft tissue inflammation.
• Use caution to prevent trauma when using oral hygiene aids.
• Update health and drug history if physician makes any changes in evaluation or drug regimens; include OTC, herbal, and nonherbal drugs in the update.
• See dentist immediately if secondary oral infection occurs.

neostigmine
nee-oh-**stig**′-meen
(Prostigmin)
Do not confuse neostigmine with physostigmine.

CATEGORY AND SCHEDULE
Pregnancy Risk Category: C

Drug Class: Cholinesterase inhibitor

MECHANISM OF ACTION
A cholinergic that prevents destruction of acetylcholine by inhibiting the enzyme acetylcholinesterase, thus enhancing impulse transmission across the myoneural junction.
Therapeutic Effect: Improves intestinal and skeletal muscle tone; stimulates salivary and sweat gland secretions.

USES
Myasthenia gravis, nondepolarizing neuromuscular blocker, antagonist, bladder distention, postoperative ileus

PHARMACOKINETICS
PO: Onset 45–75 min, duration 2.5–4 hr.
IM/Subcutaneous: Onset 10–30 min, duration 2.5–4 hr.
IV: Onset 4–8 min, duration 2–4 hr
Metabolized in liver, excreted in urine.

INDICATIONS AND DOSAGES
▸ **Myasthenia Gravis**
PO
Adults, Elderly. Initially, 15–30 mg 3–4 times a day. Increase as necessary. Maintenance: 150 mg/day (range of 15–375 mg).
Children. 2 mg/kg/day or 60 mg/m²/day divided q3–4h.
IV, IM, Subcutaneous
Adults. 0.5–2.5 mg as needed.
Children. 0.01–0.04 mg/kg q2–4h.
▸ **Diagnosis of Myasthenia Gravis**
IM
Adults, Elderly. 0.022 mg/kg. If cholinergic reaction occurs, discontinue tests and administer 0.4–0.6 mg or more atropine sulfate IV.
Children. 0.025–0.04 mg/kg preceded by atropine sulfate 0.011 mg/kg subcutaneously.
▸ **Prevention of Postoperative Urinary Retention**
IM, Subcutaneous
Adults, Elderly. 0.25 mg q4–6h for 2–3 days.
▸ **Postoperative Abdominal Distention and Urine Retention**
IM, Subcutaneous
Adults, Elderly. 0.5–1 mg.
Catheterize patient if voiding does not occur within 1 hr. After voiding, administer 0.5 mg q3h for 5 injections.
▸ **Reversal of Neuromuscular Blockade**
IV
Adults, Elderly. 0.5–2.5 mg given slowly.
Children. 0.025–0.08 mg/kg/dose.
Infants. 0.025–0.1 mg/kg/dose.

SIDE EFFECTS/ADVERSE REACTIONS

Frequent

Muscarinic effects (diarrhea, diaphoresis, increased salivation, nausea, vomiting, abdominal cramps or pain)

Occasional

Muscarinic effects (urinary urgency or frequency, increased bronchial secretions, miosis, lacrimation)

PRECAUTIONS AND CONTRAINDICATIONS

GI or GU obstruction, peritonitis

Caution:

Bradycardia, hypotension, seizure disorders, bronchial asthma, coronary occlusion, hyperthyroidism, dysrhythmias, peptic ulcer, megacolon, poor GI motility, lactation, children

DRUG INTERACTIONS OF CONCERN TO DENTISTRY

• Decreased action: hydrocarbon inhalation anesthetics, corticosteroids
• Decreased action of anticholinergics (may be contraindicated)
• Increased action of succinylcholine
• Increased toxicity of ester-type local anesthetics

SERIOUS REACTIONS

! Overdose produces a cholinergic crisis manifested as abdominal discomfort or cramps, nausea, vomiting, diarrhea, flushing, facial warmth, excessive salivation, diaphoresis, lacrimation, pallor, bradycardia or tachycardia, hypotension, bronchospasm, urinary urgency, blurred vision, miosis, and fasciculation (involuntary muscular contractions visible under the skin).

DENTAL CONSIDERATIONS

General:

• Monitor vital signs at every appointment because of cardiovascular and respiratory side effects.
• Early-morning and brief appointments are preferred because of effects of disease on oral musculature.

Consultations:

• Take precautions if dental surgery is anticipated and anesthesia is required.
• Medical consultation may be required to assess disease control and patient's tolerance for stress.

nevirapine

neh-**veer**'-ah-peen

(Viramune)

CATEGORY AND SCHEDULE

Pregnancy Risk Category: C

Drug Class: Antiviral

MECHANISM OF ACTION

A nonnucleoside reverse transcriptase inhibitor that binds directly to HIV-1 reverse transcriptase, thus changing the shape of this enzyme and blocking RNA- and DNA-dependent polymerase activity.

Therapeutic Effect: Interferes with HIV replication, slowing the progression of HIV infection.

USES

Treatment in combination with nucleoside analogs for HIV-1 infection in adults who have demonstrated clinical or immunologic deterioration

PHARMACOKINETICS

Readily absorbed after PO administration. Protein binding: 60%. Widely distributed. Extensively metabolized in the liver. Excreted primarily in urine. *Half-life:* 45 hr (single dose), 25–30 hr (multiple doses).

INDICATIONS AND DOSAGES
▸ **HIV Infection**
PO
Adults. 200 mg once a day for 14 days (to reduce the risk of rash). Maintenance: 200 mg twice a day in combination with nucleoside analogs.
Children older than 8 yr. 4 mg/kg once a day for 14 days; then 4 mg/kg twice a day. Maximum: 400 mg/day.
Children 2 mo–8 yr. 4 mg/kg once a day for 14 days; then 7 mg/kg twice a day.

SIDE EFFECTS/ADVERSE REACTIONS
Frequent
Rash, fever, headache, nausea, granulocytopenia (more common in children)
Occasional
Stomatitis (burning, erythema, or ulceration of the oral mucosa; dysphagia)
Rare
Paresthesia, myalgia, abdominal pain

PRECAUTIONS AND CONTRAINDICATIONS
Hypersensitivity, protease inhibitors
Caution:
Severe life-threatening skin reactions (Stevens-Johnson syndrome), fatal

hepatotoxicity has occurred, renal dysfunction, lactation, children

DRUG INTERACTIONS OF CONCERN TO DENTISTRY
• Should not be given with ketoconazole; monitor patients when other CYP3A4 isoenzyme inhibitors are used.

SERIOUS REACTIONS
! Hepatitis and rash may become severe and life threatening.

DENTAL CONSIDERATIONS

General:
• Determine why patient is taking the drug.
• Examine for oral manifestation of opportunistic infection.
Consultations:
• Medical consultation may be required to assess disease control.
Teach Patient/Family to:
• Encourage effective oral hygiene to prevent soft tissue inflammation.
• Report oral lesions, soreness, or bleeding to dentist.
• Update health history/drug record if physician makes any changes in evaluation or drug regimens; include OTC, herbal, and nonherbal drugs in the update.
• See dentist immediately if secondary oral infection occurs.

niacin, nicotinic acid

nye′-ah-sin, nih-**koh**′-tin-ik **ass**′-id
(Niacor, Niaspan, Nicotinex, Slo-Niacin)

Do not confuse niacin, Niacor, or Niaspan with Minocin or nitro-bid.

CATEGORY AND SCHEDULE

Pregnancy Risk Category: A (C if used at dosages above the recommended daily allowance)

OTC

Drug Class: Vitamin B₃

MECHANISM OF ACTION

An antihyperlipidemic, water-soluble vitamin that is a component of 2 coenzymes needed for tissue respiration, lipid metabolism, and glycogenolysis. Inhibits synthesis of very low-density lipoproteins (VLDLs).
Therapeutic Effect: Reduces total, low-density lipoprotein (LDL), and VLDL cholesterol levels and triglyceride levels; increases high-density lipoprotein (HDL) cholesterol concentration.

USES

Treatment of pellagra, hyperlipidemias (niacin), peripheral vascular disease (niacin)

PHARMACOKINETICS

Readily absorbed from the GI tract. Widely distributed. Metabolized in the liver. Primarily excreted in urine.
Half-life: 45 min.

INDICATIONS AND DOSAGES

▶ **Hyperlipidemia**
PO (Immediate-Release)

Adults, Elderly. Initially, 50–100 mg twice a day for 7 days. Increase gradually by doubling dose every wk up to 1–1.5 g/day in 2–3 doses. Maximum: 3 g/day.
Children. Initially, 100–250 mg/day (maximum: 10 mg/kg/day) in 3 divided doses. May increase by 100 mg/wk or 250 mg q2–3wk. Maximum: 2250 mg/day.
PO (Timed-Release)
Adults, Elderly. Initially, 500 mg/day in 2 divided doses for 1 wk; then increase to 500 mg twice a day. Maintenance: 2 g/day.
▶ **Nutritional Supplement**
PO
Adults, Elderly. 10–20 mg/day. Maximum: 100 mg/day.
▶ **Pellagra**
PO
Adults, Elderly. 50–100 mg 3–4 times a day. Maximum: 500 mg/day.
Children. 50–100 mg 3 times a day.

SIDE EFFECTS/ADVERSE REACTIONS

Frequent
Flushing (especially of the face and neck) occurring within 20 min of drug administration and lasting for up to 30–60 min, GI upset, pruritus
Occasional
Dizziness, hypotension, headache, blurred vision, burning or tingling of skin, flatulence, nausea, vomiting, diarrhea
Rare
Hyperglycemia, glycosuria, rash, hyperpigmentation, dry skin

PRECAUTIONS AND CONTRAINDICATIONS

Active peptic ulcer disease, arterial hemorrhaging, hepatic dysfunction, hypersensitivity to niacin or tartrazine (frequently seen in

patients sensitive to aspirin), severe hypotension.
Caution:
Glaucoma, cardiovascular disease, CAD, diabetes mellitus, gout, schizophrenia

DRUG INTERACTIONS OF CONCERN TO DENTISTRY

• None reported

SERIOUS REACTIONS

! Arrhythmias occur rarely.

DENTAL CONSIDERATIONS

General:
• Take vital signs at every appointment because of cardiovascular side effects.
• After supine positioning, have patient sit upright for at least 2 min before standing to avoid postural hypotension.
• Assess salivary flow as a factor in caries, periodontal disease, and candidiasis.
Teach Patient/Family to:
• When chronic dry mouth occurs, advise patient to:
  • Avoid mouth rinses with high alcohol content because of drying effects.
  • Use daily home fluoride products for anticaries effect.
  • Use sugarless gum, frequent sips of water, or saliva substitutes.

nicardipine hydrochloride

nye-**card**′-ih-peen
high-droh-**klor**′-ide
(Cardene, Cardene IV, Cardene SR)
Do not confuse nicardipine with nifedipine, Cardene with codeine, or Cardene SR with Cardizem SR or codeine.

CATEGORY AND SCHEDULE

Pregnancy Risk Category: C

Drug Class: Calcium channel blocker

MECHANISM OF ACTION

An antianginal and antihypertensive agent that inhibits calcium ion movement across cell membranes, depressing contraction of cardiac and vascular smooth muscle.
Therapeutic Effect: Increases heart rate and cardiac output. Decreases systemic vascular resistance and B/P.

USES

Treatment of chronic stable angina pectoris, hypertension

PHARMACOKINETICS

Route	Onset	Peak	Duration
PO	N/A	1–2 hr	8 hr

Rapidly, completely absorbed from the GI tract. Protein binding: 95%. Undergoes first-pass metabolism in the liver. Primarily excreted in urine. Not removed by hemodialysis.
Half-life: 2–4 hr.

INDICATIONS AND DOSAGES
▸ **Chronic Stable (Effort-Associated) Angina**
PO
Adults, Elderly. Initially, 20 mg 3 times a day. Range: 20–40 mg 3 times a day.
▸ **Essential Hypertension**
PO
Adults, Elderly. Initially, 20 mg 3 times a day. Range: 20–40 mg 3 times a day.
PO (Sustained-Release)
Adults, Elderly. Initially, 30 mg twice a day. Range: 30–60 mg twice a day.
▸ **Short-Term Treatment of Hypertension When Oral Therapy Is Not Feasible or Desirable (Substitute for Oral Nicardipine)**
IV
Adults, Elderly. 0.5 mg/hr (for patient receiving 20 mg PO q8h); 1.2 mg/hr (for patient receiving 30 mg PO q8h); 2.2 mg/hr (for patient receiving 40 mg PO q8h).
▸ **Patients Not Already Receiving Nicardipine**
IV
Adults, Elderly (gradual B/P decrease). Initially, 5 mg/hr. May increase by 2.5 mg/hr q15min. After B/P goal is achieved, decrease rate to 3 mg/hr.
Adults, Elderly (rapid B/P decrease). Initially, 5 mg/hr. May increase by 2.5 mg/hr q5min. Maximum: 15 mg/hr until desired B/P attained. After B/P goal achieved, decrease rate to 3 mg/hr.
▸ **Changing From IV to Oral Antihypertensive Therapy**
Adults, Elderly. Begin antihypertensives other than nicardipine when IV has been discontinued; for nicardipine, give first dose 1 hr before discontinuing IV.

▸ **Dosage in Hepatic Impairment**
Adults, Elderly. Initially give 20 mg twice a day; then titrate.
▸ **Dosage in Renal Impairment**
Adults, Elderly. Initially give 20 mg q8h (30 mg twice a day [sustained-release capsules]); then titrate.

SIDE EFFECTS/ADVERSE REACTIONS
Frequent
Headache, facial flushing, peripheral edema, light-headedness, dizziness
Occasional
Asthenia (loss of strength, energy), palpitations, angina, tachycardia
Rare
Nausea, abdominal cramps, dyspepsia, dry mouth, rash

PRECAUTIONS AND CONTRAINDICATIONS
Atrial fibrillation or flutter associated with accessory conduction pathways, cardiogenic shock, CHF, second- or third-degree heart block, severe hypotension, sinus bradycardia, ventricular tachycardia, within several hr of IV β-blocker therapy
Caution:
CHF, hypotension, hepatic injury, lactation, children, renal disease, elderly

DRUG INTERACTIONS OF CONCERN TO DENTISTRY
• Decreased effect: indomethacin, possibly other NSAIDs, phenobarbital, St. John's wort (herb)
• Increased effect: parenteral and inhalational general anesthetics or other drugs with hypotensive actions
• Possible risk of increased plasma level, monitor patient: erythromycin, ketoconazole, other CYP3A4 inhibitors

N

• Increased effects of nondepolarizing muscle relaxants
• Increased effects of carbamazepine

SERIOUS REACTIONS

! Overdose produces confusion, slurred speech, somnolence, marked hypotension, and bradycardia.

DENTAL CONSIDERATIONS

General:
• Monitor cardiac status; take vital signs at each appointment because of CV side effects. Consider a stress-reduction protocol to prevent stress-induced angina during the dental appointment.
• After supine positioning, have patient sit upright for at least 2 min before standing to avoid orthostatic hypotension.
• Place on frequent recall to monitor possible gingival enlargement.
• Limit use of sodium-containing products, such as saline IV fluids, for patients with a dietary salt restriction.
• Assess salivary flow as a factor in caries, periodontal disease, and candidiasis.
• Use vasoconstrictors with caution, in low doses, and with careful aspiration. Avoid use of gingival retraction cord with epinephrine.
Consultations:
• Medical consultation may be required to assess disease control and tolerance for stress.
Teach Patient/Family to:
• Encourage effective oral hygiene to prevent soft tissue inflammation and minimize gingival enlargement.
• Schedule frequent oral prophylaxis if hyperplasia occurs.
• When chronic dry mouth occurs, advise patient to:

• Avoid mouth rinses with high alcohol content because of drying effects.
• Use daily home fluoride products for anticaries effect.
• Use sugarless gum, frequent sips of water, or saliva substitutes.

nicotine

nik'-oh-teen
(Commit, Habitrol[CAN], Nicabate[AUS], Nicabate CQ Clear[AUS], Nicabate CQ Lozenges[AUS], NicoDerm[CAN], NicoDerm CQ, Nicorette, Nicorette Plus[CAN], Nicotinell[AUS], Nicotrol, Nicotrol NS, Nicotrol Patch[CAN])
Do not confuse NicoDerm with Nitroderm.

CATEGORY AND SCHEDULE

Pregnancy Risk Category: D (transdermal)
OTC (NicoDerm transdermal patch, Nicotrol transdermal patch, Nicorette chewing gum)

Drug Class: Smoking deterrent

MECHANISM OF ACTION

A cholinergic-receptor agonist binds to acetylcholine receptors, producing both stimulating and depressant effects on the peripheral and central nervous systems.
Therapeutic Effect: Provides a source of nicotine during nicotine withdrawal and reduces withdrawal symptoms.

USES

Adjunct to cigarette smoking cessation program

PHARMACOKINETICS

Absorbed slowly after transdermal administration. Protein binding: 5%. Metabolized in the liver. Excreted primarily in urine. *Half-life:* 4 hr.

INDICATIONS AND DOSAGES
▶ **Smoking Cessation Aid to Relieve Nicotine Withdrawal Symptoms**
PO (Chewing Gum)
Adults, Elderly. Usually, 10–12 pieces/day. Maximum: 30 pieces/day.
PO (Lozenge)
Adults, Elderly. One 4-mg or 2-mg lozenge q1–2h for the first 6 wk; 1 lozenge q2–4h for wk 7–9; and 1 lozenge q4–8h for wk 10–12. Maximum: 1 lozenge at a time, 5 lozenges/6 hr, 20 lozenges/day.
Transdermal
Adults, Elderly who smoke 10 cigarettes or more per day. Follow the guidelines below.
  Step 1: 21 mg/day for 4–6 wk.
  Step 2: 14 mg/day for 2 wk.
  Step 3: 7 mg/day for 2 wk.
Adults, Elderly who smoke fewer than 10 cigarettes per day. Follow the guidelines below.
  Step 1: 14 mg/day for 6 wk.
  Step 2: 7 mg/day for 2 wk.
Patients weighing less than 100 lb, patients with a history of cardiovascular disease. Initially, 14 mg/day for 4–6 wk, then 7 mg/day for 2–4 wk.
Transdermal (Nicotrol)
Adults, Elderly. 1 patch a day for 6 wk.
Nasal
Adults, Elderly. 1–2 doses/hr (1 dose = 2 sprays [1 in each nostril] = 1 mg). Maximum: 5 doses (5 mg)/hr; 40 doses (40 mg)/day.
Inhaler (Nicotrol)
Adults, Elderly. Puff on nicotine cartridge mouthpiece for about 20 min as needed.

SIDE EFFECTS/ADVERSE REACTIONS
Frequent
All forms: Hiccups, nausea
Gum: Mouth or throat soreness, nausea, hiccups
Transdermal: Erythema, pruritus, or burning at application site
Occasional
All forms: Eructation, GI upset, dry mouth, insomnia, diaphoresis, irritability
Gum: Hiccups, hoarseness
Inhaler: Mouth or throat irritation, cough
Rare
All forms: Dizziness, myalgia, arthralgia

PRECAUTIONS AND CONTRAINDICATIONS
Immediate post-MI period, life-threatening arrhythmias, severe or worsening angina
Caution:
Skin disease, angina pectoris, MI, renal or hepatic insufficiency, peptic ulcer, serious cardiac dysrhythmias, hyperthyroidism, pheochromocytoma, insulin-dependent diabetes, elderly

DRUG INTERACTIONS OF CONCERN TO DENTISTRY
• Decreased dose at cessation of smoking: acetaminophen, caffeine, oxazepam, pentazocine
• Decreased metabolism of propoxyphene (increased blood levels)

SERIOUS REACTIONS
! Overdose produces palpitations, tachyarrhythmias, seizures, depression, confusion, diaphoresis, hypotension, rapid or weak pulse, and dyspnea. Lethal dose for adults is 40–60 mg. Death results from respiratory paralysis.

N

DENTAL CONSIDERATIONS

General:
• Assess salivary flow as a factor in caries, periodontal disease, and candidiasis.

Teach Patient/Family to:
• When chronic dry mouth occurs, advise patient to:
  • Avoid mouth rinses with high alcohol content because of drying effects.
  • Use daily home fluoride products to prevent caries.
  • Use sugarless gum, frequent sips of water, or saliva substitutes.
• When used in conjunction with a smoking cessation program in the dental office, teach:
  • All aspects of product drug; give package insert to patient and explain:
  • That patch is to be used only to deter smoking.
  • Not to use during pregnancy; birth defects may occur.
  • To keep used and unused system out of reach of children and pets; potentially toxic if chewed or swallowed.
  • To apply once per day to a non-hairy, clean, dry area of skin on upper body or upper outer arm.
  • To stop smoking immediately when beginning treatment with patch.
  • To apply promptly after removing from protective covering; system may lose strength.

Nicotine Polacrilex

General:
• Take vital signs at every appointment because of cardiovascular side effects.

• Temporomandibular joint (TMJ) disorder may be aggravated by chewing because of heavier viscosity of gum.

Teach Patient/Family to:
• Encourage effective oral hygiene to prevent periodontal inflammation.
• When chronic dry mouth occurs, advise patient to:
  • Avoid mouth rinses with high alcohol content because of drying effects.
  • Use daily home fluoride products for anticaries effect.
  • Use sugarless gum, frequent sips of water, or saliva substitutes.
• When used in conjunction with a smoking cessation program in the dental office, teach:
  • All aspects of product use; give package insert to patient and explain:
  • That gum is to be used only to deter smoking.
  • To avoid use in pregnancy; birth defects may occur.
  • To stop smoking when beginning treatment with gum.
  • To dispose of gum carefully because nicotine will still be present; to protect from children and pets.

nifedipine

nye-fed'-ih-peen
(Adalat 5[AUS], Adalat 10[AUS],
Adalat 20[AUS], Adalat CC,
Adalat Oros[AUS], Apo-
Nifed[CAN], Nifecard[AUS],
Nifedicol XL, Nifehexal[AUS],
Novo-Nifedin[CAN], Nyefax[AUS],
Procardia, Procardia XL)
Do not confuse nifedipine with
nicardipine or nimodipine.

CATEGORY AND SCHEDULE

Pregnancy Risk Category: C

Drug Class: Calcium channel
blocker

MECHANISM OF ACTION

An antianginal and antihypertensive
agent that inhibits calcium ion
movement across cell membranes,
depressing contraction of cardiac
and vascular smooth muscle.
Therapeutic Effect: Increases heart
rate and cardiac output. Decreases
systemic vascular resistance and B/P.

USES

Treatment of chronic stable angina
pectoris, vasospastic angina,
hypertension (sustained release only)

PHARMACOKINETICS

Route	Onset	Peak	Duration
Sublingual	1–5 min	N/A	N/A
PO	20–30 min	N/A	4–8 hr
PO (extended release)	2 hr	N/A	24 hr

Rapidly, completely absorbed from
the GI tract. Protein binding:
92%–98%. Undergoes first-pass
metabolism in the liver. Primarily

excreted in urine. Not removed by
hemodialysis. **Half-life:** 2–5 hr.

INDICATIONS AND DOSAGES

▶ **Prinzmetal's Variant Angina,
Chronic Stable (Effort-Associated)
Angina**
PO
Adults, Elderly. Initially, 10 mg 3
times a day. Increase at 7- to 14-day
intervals. Maintenance: 10 mg 3
times a day up to 30 mg 4 times a
day.
PO (Extended-Release)
Adults, Elderly. Initially, 30–60 mg/
day. Maintenance: Up to 120 mg/
day.
▶ **Essential Hypertension**
PO (Extended-Release)
Adults, Elderly. Initially, 30–60 mg/
day. Maintenance: Up to 120 mg/
day.

SIDE EFFECTS/ADVERSE REACTIONS

Frequent
Peripheral edema, headache, flushed
skin, dizziness
Occasional
Nausea, shakiness, muscle cramps
and pain, somnolence, palpitations,
nasal congestion, cough, dyspnea,
wheezing, oral gingival enlargement
Rare
Hypotension, rash, pruritus,
urticaria, constipation, abdominal
discomfort, flatulence, sexual
difficulties

PRECAUTIONS AND CONTRAINDICATIONS

Advanced aortic stenosis, severe
hypotension
Caution:
CHF, hypotension, sick sinus
syndrome, second- or third-degree
heart block, hypotension less than
90 mm Hg systolic, hepatic injury,
lactation, children, renal disease

N

DRUG INTERACTIONS OF CONCERN TO DENTISTRY

• Decreased effect: indomethacin, possibly other NSAIDs, phenobarbital
• Increased effect: parenteral and inhalational general anesthetics or other drugs with hypotensive actions
• Possible increase in effects, monitor patients: inhibitors of CYP3A4 isoenzyme
• Increased effects of nondepolarizing muscle relaxants
• Increased effects of carbamazepine

SERIOUS REACTIONS

! Nifedipine may precipitate CHF and MI in patients with cardiac disease and peripheral ischemia.
! Overdose produces nausea, somnolence, confusion, and slurred speech.

DENTAL CONSIDERATIONS

General:
• Monitor cardiac status; take vital signs at each appointment because of cardiovascular side effects. Consider a stress-reduction protocol to prevent stress-induced angina during the dental appointment.
• After supine positioning, have patient sit upright for at least 2 min before standing to avoid orthostatic hypotension at dismissal.
• Place on frequent recall to monitor possible gingival enlargement.
• Limit use of sodium-containing products, such as saline IV fluids, for patients with a dietary salt restriction.
• Assess salivary flow as a factor in caries, periodontal disease, and candidiasis.
• Use vasoconstrictors with caution, in low doses, and with careful aspiration. Avoid use of gingival retraction cord with epinephrine.

Consultations:
• Medical consultation may be required to assess disease control and stress tolerance.
Teach Patient/Family to:
• Encourage effective oral hygiene to prevent soft tissue inflammation and minimize gingival overgrowth.
• Schedule frequent oral prophylaxis if gingival enlargement occurs.
• When chronic dry mouth occurs, advise patient to:
    • Avoid mouth rinses with high alcohol content because of drying effects.
    • Use daily home fluoride products for anticaries effect.
    • Use sugarless gum, frequent sips of water, or saliva substitutes.

nilotinib
nye-**loe**′-ti-nib
(Tasigna)

CATEGORY AND SCHEDULE
Pregnancy Risk Category: D

Drug Class: Antineoplastic agent, tyrosine kinase inhibitor

MECHANISM OF ACTION
Selectively inhibits Bcr-Abl kinase. Binds to and stabilizes the inactive conformation of the kinase domain of Abl protein. Also exhibits activity in imatinib-resistant Bcr-Abl kinase mutations.

USES
Treatment of chronic phase and accelerated phase of Philadelphia chromosome-positive chronic myelogenous leukemia (CML) in patients resistant or intolerant to prior imatinib therapy

PHARMACOKINETICS

98% protein binding. Metabolized hepatically via oxidation and hydroxylation by CYP3A4 into inactive metabolites. Bioavailability is increased by 82% when administered 30 min after a high-fat meal. *Half-life:* 15–17 hr. Excreted in the feces (93%; 69% as parent drug).

INDICATIONS AND DOSAGES

Treatment of chronic phase and accelerated phase Philadelphia chromosome-positive CML in patients resistant or intolerant to prior imatinib therapy
PO
Adults. 400 mg twice daily (every 12 hr).
Dosage adjustment for concomitant use with CYP3A4 inhibitors: avoid concomitant use. If required, consider reducing nilotinib by 50% to 400 mg once daily with careful monitoring.
Dosage adjustment for concomitant use with CYP3A4 inducers: avoid concomitant use. If required, consider increasing dose of nilotinib with careful monitoring.
Dosage adjustment for hepatotoxicity: If bilirubin >3 times upper limit of normal (ULN) (= grade 3): withhold nilotinib, monitor bilirubin, resume at 400 mg once daily when bilirubin returns to = 1.5 times ULN (= grade 1). If ALT or AST >5 times ULN (= grade 3): withhold nilotinib, monitor transaminases, resume at 400 mg once daily when ALT or AST returns to = 2.5 times ULN (= grade 1).
Dosage adjustment for hematologic toxicity (neutropenia and thrombocytopenia): absolute neutrophil count (ANC) <1000/mm^3 and/or platelets <50,000/mm^3: stop nilotinib, monitor blood counts. ANC >1000/mm^3 and platelets >50,000/mm^3 within 2 wk: continue at 400 mg twice daily.
ANC <1000/mm^3 and/or platelets <50,000/mm^3 for >2 wk: reduce dose to 400 mg once daily.
Dosage adjustment for QT prolongation:
QTc >480 msec: stop nilotinib, monitor and correct potassium and magnesium levels. QTcF returns to <450 msec and to within 20 msec of baseline within 2 wk: continue at 400 mg twice daily.
QTcF returns to 450–480 msec within 2 wk: reduce dose to 400 mg once daily. QTcF >480 msec after dosage reduction to 400 mg once daily, discontinue therapy.

SIDE EFFECTS/ADVERSE REACTIONS
Adult
Frequent
Peripheral edema, headache, fatigue, fever, rash, pruritus, hyperglycemia, nausea, diarrhea, constipation, vomiting, increased lipase, abdominal pain, neutropenia, thrombocytopenia, anemia, arthralgia, limb pain, myalgia, weakness, muscle spasm, bone pain, back pain, cough, nasopharyngitis, dyspnea
Occasional
Flushing, hypertension, palpitation, prolonged QT interval, dizziness, dysphonia, insomnia, vertigo, alopecia, dry skin, eczema, erythema, hyperhidrosis, urticaria, hypophosphatemia (10%), hypokalemia (5%), hyperkalemia (4%), hypocalcemia (4%), hyponatremia (3%), decreased albumin (1%), abdominal discomfort, dyspepsia, pancreatitis (<1%), pleural effusion (<1%), hyperbilirubinemia (10%), increased

N

ALT (4%), increased phosphatase (3%), increased AST (1%)

PRECAUTIONS AND CONTRAINDICATIONS

Hypokalemia
Hypomagnesemia
Long QT syndrome
Avoid comitant use with
QT-prolonging agents and CYP3A4 inhibitors/inducers
Use with caution in patients with bone marrow suppression, electrolyte imbalances, pancreatitis, and hepatic impairment
Administer nilotinib on an empty stomach, at least 1 hr before and 2 hr after food

DRUG INTERACTIONS OF CONCERN TO DENTISTRY

• CYP3A4 inhibitors (e.g., erythromycin): May increase the blood levels and adverse effects of nilotinib.

SERIOUS REACTIONS

! QT prolongation, which can lead to sudden death, has been reported.
! Fetal damage can occur when used in pregnant women.

DENTAL CONSIDERATIONS

General:
• Stomatitis and mouth ulceration may complicate dental treatment and oral hygiene.
• Consider semisupine chair position for patient comfort if GI side effects occur.
• Use with caution when in combination with vasoconstrictors (epinephrine, levonordefrin) in the local anesthetic regimen due to the possible risk of QT prolongation (torsade de pointes).
Consultations:
• Medical consultation may be required to assess disease control

and ability of patient to tolerate dental treatment.
Teach Patient/Family to:
• Encourage effective oral hygiene to prevent soft tissue inflammation.
• Use caution to prevent injury when using oral hygiene aids.
• Be alert for the possibility of stomatitis and mouth ulcerations and the need to see dentist immediately if signs of inflammation and ulceration occur.

nilutamide
nih-**lute′**-ah-myd
(Anandron[CAN], Nilandron)

CATEGORY AND SCHEDULE
Pregnancy Risk Category: C

Drug Class: Hormone; antineoplastic

MECHANISM OF ACTION

An antiandrogen hormone and antineoplastic agent that competitively inhibits androgen action by binding to androgen receptors in target tissue.
Therapeutic Effect: Decreases growth of abnormal prostate tissue.

USES

Treatment of cancer of the prostate gland

PHARMACOKINETICS

Rapidly and completed absorbed; excreted in urine and feces as metabolites.

INDICATIONS AND DOSAGES
▸ Prostatic Carcinoma
PO
Adults, Elderly. 300 mg once a day for 30 days, then 150 mg once a

day. Begin on day of, or day after, surgical castration.

SIDE EFFECTS/ADVERSE REACTIONS

Frequent

Hot flashes, delay in recovering vision after bright illumination (such as sun, television, bright lights), decreased libido, diminished sexual function, mild nausea, gynecomastia, alcohol intolerance

Occasional

Constipation, hypertension, dizziness, dyspnea, UTIs

PRECAUTIONS AND CONTRAINDICATIONS

Severe hepatic impairment, severe respiratory insufficiency

DRUG INTERACTIONS OF CONCERN TO DENTISTRY

• Avoid drugs that may aggravate urinary retention when symptoms are present.
• This is an inhibitor of CYP3A4 isoenzymes; no specific studies have been done, but use caution when prescribing drugs metabolized by this enzyme.

SERIOUS REACTIONS

! Interstitial pneumonitis occurs rarely.

DENTAL CONSIDERATIONS

General:
• Monitor and record vital signs.
• If additional analgesia is required for dental pain, consider alternative analgesics (NSAIDs) in patients taking narcotics for acute or chronic pain.
• Avoid dental light in patient's eyes; offer dark glasses for patient comfort.

• This drug may be used in the hospital or on an outpatient basis. Confirm the patient's disease and treatment status.
• Short appointments and a stress-reduction protocol may be required for anxious patients.
Consultations:
• Medical consultation may be required to assess immunologic status during cancer chemotherapy and determine safety risk, if any, posed by the required dental treatment.
• Medical consultation may be required to assess disease control and patient's ability to tolerate stress.
Teach Patient/Family to:
• Encourage effective oral hygiene to prevent soft tissue inflammation.
• Prevent trauma when using oral hygiene aids.
• Report oral lesions, soreness, or bleeding to dentist.
• Update health and medication history if physician makes any changes in evaluation or drug regimens; include OTC, herbal, and nonherbal in the update.

N

nimodipine

nye-**mode′**-ih-peen
(Nimotop)
Do not confuse nimodipine with nifedipine.

CATEGORY AND SCHEDULE

Pregnancy Risk Category: C

Drug Class: Calcium channel blockers

MECHANISM OF ACTION

A cerebral vasospasm agent that inhibits movement of calcium ions

across vascular smooth-muscle cell membranes.
Therapeutic Effect: Produces favorable effect on severity of neurologic deficits due to cerebral vasospasm. Exerts greatest effect on cerebral arteries; may prevent cerebral spasm.

USES

Relief of and control of angina pectoris (chest pain)

PHARMACOKINETICS

Rapidly absorbed from the GI tract. Protein binding: 95%. Metabolized in the liver. Excreted in urine; eliminated in feces. Not removed by hemodialysis. *Half-life:* terminal, 3 hr.

INDICATIONS AND DOSAGES
▸ **Improvement in Neurologic Deficits after Subarachnoid Hemorrhage from Ruptured Congenital Aneurysms**
PO
Adults, Elderly. 60 mg q4h for 21 days. Begin within 96 hr of subarachnoid hemorrhage.

SIDE EFFECTS/ADVERSE REACTIONS
Occasional
Hypotension, peripheral edema, diarrhea, headache
Rare
Allergic reaction (rash, hives), tachycardia, flushing of skin

PRECAUTIONS AND CONTRAINDICATIONS

Atrial fibrillation or flutter, cardiogenic shock, CHF, heart block, sinus bradycardia, ventricular tachycardia, within several hr of IV β-blocker therapy

DRUG INTERACTIONS OF CONCERN TO DENTISTRY
• Hypotension: anesthetics, other antihypertensive medications
• Antagonism of antihypertensive effect: indomethacin and possibly other NSAIDs
• Possible reduction in antihypertensive effects: sympathomimetics

SERIOUS REACTIONS
! Overdose produces nausea, weakness, dizziness, somnolence, confusion, and slurred speech.

DENTAL CONSIDERATIONS

General:
• Patients may have significant neurologic deficit; dental care may not be practical.
• Avoid vasoconstrictors or limit doses appropriately.
• Caution: potential for interactions with drugs used in dentistry.
• Determine why patient is taking the drug.
• Monitor for possible gingival enlargement.
• Monitor and record vital signs.
• After supine positioning, have patient sit upright for at least 2 min before standing to avoid orthostatic hypotension.
Consultations:
• This drug may be used in the hospital or on an outpatient basis. Confirm the patient's disease and treatment status.
• Medical consultation may be required to assess disease control and patient's ability to tolerate stress.
Teach Patient/Family to:
• Encourage effective oral hygiene to prevent soft tissue inflammation.
• Update health and medication history if physician makes any

changes in evaluation or drug regimens; include OTC, herbal, and nonherbal drugs in the update.

nipradilol
ni-**pra**-dih-lole
(Hypadil [JAPAN])

CATEGORY AND SCHEDULE

Drug Class: β-adrenergic blocker (non-selective)

MECHANISM OF ACTION
Non-selective β blocker with α-1 blocking activity. Nitroglycerin-like vasodilator properties.
Therapeutic Effect: Reduces B/P, improved myocardial ischemia, reduces heart rate. Reduces intraocular pressure. Decreases peripheral vascular resistance.

USES
Essential hypertension
Angina pectoris
Open-angle glaucoma
Ocular hypertension
Cardiomyopathy
Parkinsonian tremor

PHARMACOKINETICS
Bioavailability: 29%–47%. Protein binding: less than 30%. Extensively distributed in tissues. Ophthalmic: rapidly reaches ocular tissue.
Half-life: 2 hr.

INDICATIONS AND DOSAGES
▶ **Hypertension, Essential**
PO
Adults. 3–9 mg twice day.
▶ **Angina**
PO
Adults. 3–6 mg twice a day.
▶ **Cardiomyopathy**
PO
Adults. 1.5–9 mg/day.
▶ **Parkinsonian Tremor**
PO
Adults. 3 mg twice a day.
▶ **Glaucoma**
Ophthalmic
Adults. Apply 0.25% twice/day.
▶ **Ocular Hypertension**
Ophthalmic
Adults. 0.25% twice/day.

SIDE EFFECTS/ADVERSE REACTIONS
Frequency not defined
Oral: Bradycardia, circulatory disturbances, shortness of breath, dizziness, headache, drowsiness, insomnia, GI symptoms, weakness, sweating, tinnitus, hypersensitivity, orthostatic hypotension, arrhythmias, hypoglycemia, nausea, anorexia, thrombocytosis, vertigo
Ophthalmic: Blepharitis, eyelid pruritus, punctate keratitis, corneal erosion, eyelid contact eczema, eye irritation and redness

PRECAUTIONS AND CONTRAINDICATIONS
Hypersensitivity to nipradilol or any component of the formulation
Bronchial asthma or related bronchospastic conditions
Cardiogenic shock
Pulmonary edema
Second- or third-degree AV block
Severe bradycardia
Diabetic ketoacidosis
Metabolic acidosis
Left ventricular dysfunction
Caution:
Anesthesia/surgery
Abrupt withdrawal
Bronchial asthma or related bronchospastic conditions
Cerebrovascular insufficiency

CHF
Diabetes mellitus
Hyperthyroidism/thyrotoxicosis
Myasthenic conditions
Peripheral vascular disease
Hepatic dysfunction
Renal dysfunction

DRUG INTERACTIONS OF CONCERN TO DENTISTRY

• Diuretics, other antihypertensives: May increase hypotensive effect of nipradilol.
• Sympathomimetics, xanthines: Possible increased systolic BP, bradycardia. May antagonize the effects and reduce bronchodilation.
• Oral hypoglycemics and insulin: May mask symptoms of hypoglycemia and prolong hypoglycemic effect of insulin and oral hypoglycemics.
• NSAIDs: May reduce the antihypertensive effect of nipradilol.
• Digoxin: May cause serious bradycardia.
• Calcium channel blockers (verapamil, diltiazem): May cause hypotension and bradycardia.
• Latanoprost: Additive effects.

SERIOUS REACTIONS

! Ophthalmic overdose may produce bradycardia, hypotension, bronchospasm, and acute cardiac failure.

DENTAL CONSIDERATIONS

General:
• Monitor vital signs at every appointment because of cardiovascular side effects.
• Assess salivary flow as a factor in caries, periodontal disease, and candidiasis.
• Limit use of sodium-containing products, such as saline IV fluids, for those patients with dietary salt restriction.

Consultations:
• Medical consultation may be required to assess disease control.
Teach Patient/Family to:
• Report oral lesions, soreness, or bleeding to dentist.
• When chronic dry mouth occurs, advise patient to:
 • Avoid mouth rinses with high alcohol content because of drying effects.
 • Use daily home fluoride products for anticaries effect.
 • Use sugarless gum, frequent sips of water, or saliva substitutes.

nisoldipine
nye-**soul**′-dih-peen
(Sular)
Do not confuse with nicardipine.

CATEGORY AND SCHEDULE
Pregnancy Risk Category: C

Drug Class: Calcium channel antagonist (dihydropyridine group)

MECHANISM OF ACTION
A calcium channel blocker that inhibits calcium ion movement across cell membrane, depressing contraction of cardiac and vascular smooth muscle.
Therapeutic Effect: Increases heart rate and cardiac output. Decreases systemic vascular resistance and B/P.

USES
Hypertension as a single agent or in combination with other antihypertensive medications

PHARMACOKINETICS
Poor absorption from the GI tract. Food increases bioavailability.

Protein binding: more than 99%. Metabolism occurs in the gut wall. Primarily excreted in urine. Not removed by hemodialysis. *Half-life:* 7–12 hr.

INDICATIONS AND DOSAGES
▶ **Hypertension**
PO
Adults. Initially, 20 mg once daily, then increase by 10 mg/wk, or longer intervals until therapeutic B/P response is attained.
Initially, 10 mg once daily. Increase by 10 mg/wk to therapeutic response. Maintenance: 20–40 mg once daily. Maximum: 60 mg once daily.

SIDE EFFECTS/ADVERSE REACTIONS
Frequent
Giddiness, dizziness, light-headedness, peripheral edema, headache, flushing, weakness, nausea, oral gingival enlargement
Occasional
Transient hypotension, heartburn, muscle cramps, nasal congestion, cough, wheezing, sore throat, palpitations, nervousness, mood changes
Rare
Increase in frequency, intensity, duration of anginal attack during initial therapy

PRECAUTIONS AND CONTRAINDICATIONS
Sick-sinus syndrome or second- or third-degree AV block (except in presence of pacemaker), hypersensitivity to nisoldipine or any component of the formulation
Caution:
Avoid high-fat meals, severe coronary artery disease, monitor B/P, CHF, severe hepatic

impairment, do not break or crush tablets, lactation, geriatric patients

SERIOUS REACTIONS
May precipitate CHF and MI in patients with cardiac disease and peripheral ischemia.
Overdose produces nausea, drowsiness, confusion, and slurred speech.

DENTAL CONSIDERATIONS
General:
• Stress from dental procedures may compromise cardiovascular function; determine patient risk.
• Avoid vasoconstrictors or limit doses appropriately.
• Monitor vital signs at every appointment because of cardiovascular side effects.
• Short appointments and a stress-reduction protocol may be required for anxious patients.
• Grapefruit juice may increase plasma levels.
• Monitor for possible gingival enlargement.
• Limit use of sodium-containing products, such as saline IV fluids, for patients with a dietary salt restriction.
• After supine positioning, have patient sit upright for at least 2 min before standing to avoid orthostatic hypotension.
• Assess salivary flow as a factor in caries, periodontal disease, and candidiasis.
Consultations:
• Medical consultation may be required to assess disease control and patient's ability to tolerate stress.
Teach Patient/Family to:
• Schedule frequent oral prophylaxis if gingival enlargement occurs.
• When chronic dry mouth occurs, advise patient to:

N

• Avoid mouth rinses with high alcohol content because of drying effects.
• Use daily home fluoride products for anticaries effect.
• Use sugarless gum, frequent sips of water, or saliva substitutes.

nitazoxanide
nigh-taz-**oks**'-ah-nide
(Alinia)

CATEGORY AND SCHEDULE
Pregnancy Risk Category: B

Drug Class: Antiprotozoals

MECHANISM OF ACTION
An antiparasitic that interferes with the body's reaction to pyruvate ferredoxin oxidoreductase, an enzyme essential for anaerobic energy metabolism.
Therapeutic Effect: Produces antiprotozoal activity, reducing or terminating diarrheal episodes.

USES
Treatment of diarrhea that is caused by certain types of protozoa (tiny, 1-celled animals)

PHARMACOKINETICS
Rapidly hydrolyzed to an active metabolite. Protein binding: 99%. Excreted in the urine, bile, and feces. *Half-life:* 2–4 hr.

INDICATIONS AND DOSAGES
▸ **Diarrhea**
PO
Children 12 yr and older. 200 mg q12h.

Children 4–11 yr. 200 mg (10 ml) q12h for 3 days.
Children 12–47 mo. 100 mg (5 ml) q12h for 3 days.

SIDE EFFECTS/ADVERSE REACTIONS
Occasional
Abdominal pain
Rare
Diarrhea, vomiting, headache

PRECAUTIONS AND CONTRAINDICATIONS
History of sensitivity to aspirin and salicylates

DRUG INTERACTIONS OF CONCERN TO DENTISTRY
• None reported

SERIOUS REACTIONS
! None known

DENTAL CONSIDERATIONS

General:
• This is an acute-use drug; patients highly unlikely to present for dental care.
• Ensure patients are well hydrated and electrolytes reestablished following recovery if they present for dental treatment.
Consultations:
• Medical consultation may be required to assess disease control.
Teach Patient/Family to:
• Maintain or reestablish oral hygiene care.

nitrofurantoin sodium

nye-troe-**fyoor**'-an-toyn
soe'-dee-um

(Apo-Nitrofurantoin[CAN],
Furadantin, Macrobid,
Macrodantin, Novo-Furan[CAN],
Ralodantin[AUS])

CATEGORY AND SCHEDULE

Pregnancy Risk Category: B

Drug Class: Urinary tract
antiinfective

MECHANISM OF ACTION

An antibacterial UTI agent that
inhibits the synthesis of bacterial
DNA, RNA, proteins, and cell walls
by altering or inactivating ribosomal
proteins.
Therapeutic Effect: Bacteriostatic
(bactericidal at high concentrations).

USES

Treatment of UTIs caused by
*E. coli, Klebsiella, Pseudomonas,
P. vulgaris, P. morganii, Serratia,
Citrobacter, S. aureus*

PHARMACOKINETICS

Microcrystalline form rapidly and
completely absorbed;
macrocrystalline form more slowly
absorbed. Food increases absorption.
Protein binding: 40%. Primarily
concentrated in urine and kidneys.
Metabolized in most body tissues.
Primarily excreted in urine.
Removed by hemodialysis. *Half-life:*
20–60 min.

INDICATIONS AND DOSAGES

▶ UTIs

PO (Furadantin, Macrodantin)
Adults, Elderly. 50–100 mg q6h.
Maximum: 400 mg/day.

Children. 5–7 mg/kg/day in divided
doses q6h. Maximum: 400 mg/day.
PO (Macrobid)
Adults, Elderly. 100 mg twice a day.
Maximum: 400 mg/day.
▶ **Long-Term Prevention of UTIs**
PO
Adults, Elderly. 50–100 mg at
bedtime.
Children. 1–2 mg/kg/day as a single
dose. Maximum: 100 mg/day.

SIDE EFFECTS/ADVERSE REACTIONS

Frequent
Anorexia, nausea, vomiting, dark
urine
Occasional
Abdominal pain, diarrhea, rash,
pruritus, urticaria, hypertension,
headache, dizziness, drowsiness
Rare
Photosensitivity, transient alopecia,
asthmatic exacerbation in those with
history of asthma

PRECAUTIONS AND CONTRAINDICATIONS

Anuria, oliguria, substantial renal
impairment (creatinine clearance
less than 40 ml/min); infants
younger than 1 mo because of the
risk of hemolytic anemia
Caution:
Lactation

DRUG INTERACTIONS OF CONCERN TO DENTISTRY

• Increased effects: anticholinergic
drugs

SERIOUS REACTIONS

! Superinfection, hepatotoxicity,
peripheral neuropathy (may be
irreversible), Stevens-Johnson
syndrome, permanent pulmonary
function impairment, and
anaphylaxis occur rarely.

DENTAL CONSIDERATIONS

General:
• Determine why the patient is taking the drug.
Consultations:
• Medical consultation may be required to assess disease control and to select an antiinfective if a dental infection is diagnosed.

nitrofurazone

nye-troe-**fyoor**′-ah-zone
(Furacin)
Do not confuse with nitrofurantoin.

CATEGORY AND SCHEDULE
Pregnancy Risk Category: C
OTC (ointment)

Drug Class: Antibacterial, topical

MECHANISM OF ACTION
A synthetic nitrofuran that inhibits bacterial enzymes involved in carbohydrate metabolism.
Therapeutic Effect: Inhibits a variety of enzymes. Bactericidal.

USES
Surface skin infections, including
*S. aureus, streptococci, E. coli,
C. perfringens, E. aerogens, Proteus*
spp.

PHARMACOKINETICS
Not known

INDICATIONS AND DOSAGES
▶ Burns, Catheter-Related UTI, Skin Grafts
Topical
Adults. Apply directly on lesion with spatula or place on a piece of gauze first. Use of a bandage is optional.

Preparation should remain on lesion for at least 24 hr. Dressing may be changed several times daily or left on the lesion for a longer period.

SIDE EFFECTS/ADVERSE REACTIONS
Occasional
Itching, rash, swelling

PRECAUTIONS AND CONTRAINDICATIONS
Hypersensitivity to nitrofurazone or any of its components

DRUG INTERACTIONS OF CONCERN TO DENTISTRY
• None reported

SERIOUS REACTIONS
! Use of nitrofurazone may result in bacterial or fungal overgrowth of nonsusceptible pathogens, which may lead to secondary infection.

DENTAL CONSIDERATIONS

General:
• Dental management depends on extent and severity of burns and patient's ability to cooperate; use aseptic techniques.
• Provide palliative dental care for dental emergencies only.
• Monitor and record vital signs.
Consultations:
• Medical consultation may be required to assess disease control and patient's ability to tolerate stress.
• Consult patient's physician if an acute dental infection occurs and another antiinfective is required.
Teach Patient/Family to:
• Encourage effective oral hygiene to prevent soft tissue inflammation.
• Prevent trauma when using oral hygiene aids.

N

nitroglycerin
nye-troe-**gli**′-ser-in
(Anginine[AUS], Minitran,
Nitradisc[AUS], Nitrek, Nitro-Bid,
Nitro-Dur, Nitrogard,
Nitroject[CAN], Nitrolingual,
Nitrolingual Spray[AUS],
Nitrong-SR, NitroQuick,
Nitrostat, Nitro-Tab,
Rectogesic[AUS], Transiderm
Nitro[AUS], Trinipatch[CAN])
Do not confuse nitroglycerin with
nitroprusside; Nitro-Bid with
Nicobid; Nitro-Dur with
NicoDerm; Nitrostat with
Hyperstat, Nilstat, or Nystatin; or
Nitrong-SR with Nizoral.

CATEGORY AND SCHEDULE
Pregnancy Risk Category: B

Drug Class: Inorganic nitrate,
vasodilator

MECHANISM OF ACTION
A nitrate that decreases myocardial
oxygen demand. Reduces left
ventricular preload and afterload.
Therapeutic Effect: Dilates
coronary arteries and improves
collateral blood flow to ischemic
areas within myocardium.
IV form produces peripheral
vasodilation.

USES
Treatment of chronic stable angina
pectoris, prophylaxis of angina pain,
CHF associated with acute MI,
controlled hypotension in surgical
procedures

PHARMACOKINETICS

Route	Onset	Peak	Duration
Sublingual	1–3 min	4–8 min	30–60 min
Translingual spray	2 min	4–10 min	30–60 min
Buccal tablet	2–5 min	4–10 min	2 hr
PO (extended release)	20–45 min	45–120 min	4–8 hr
Topical	15–60 min	30–120 min	2–12 hr
Transdermal patch	40–60 min	60–180 min	18–24 hr
IV	1–2 min	Immediate	3–5 min

Well absorbed after PO, sublingual,
and topical administration.
Undergoes extensive first-pass
metabolism. Metabolized in the liver
and by enzymes in the bloodstream.
Primarily excreted in urine. Not
removed by hemodialysis. *Half-life:*
1–4 min.

INDICATIONS AND DOSAGES
▸ **Acute Relief of Angina Pectoris,
Acute Prophylaxis**
Lingual Spray
Adults, Elderly. 1 spray onto or
under tongue q3–5min until relief is
noted (no more than 3 sprays in
15-min period).
Sublingual
Adults, Elderly. 0.4 mg q5min until
relief is noted (no more than 3 doses
in 15-min period). Use
prophylactically 5–10 min before
activities that may cause an acute
attack.
▸ **Long-Term Prophylaxis of Angina**
PO (Extended-Release)
Adults, Elderly. 2.5–9 mg
q8–12h.
Topical
Adults, Elderly. Initially, 1/2 inch
q8h. Increase by 1/2 inch with each

N

application. Range: 1–2 inches q8h up to 4–5 inches q4h.

Transdermal Patch

Adults, Elderly. Initially, 0.2–0.4 mg/hr. Maintenance: 0.4–0.8 mg/hr. Consider patch on for 12–14 hr, patch off for 10–12 hr (prevents tolerance).

▶ **CHF Associated with Acute MI**

IV

Adults, Elderly. Initially, 5 mcg/min via infusion pump. Increase in 5-mcg/min increments at 3- to 5-min intervals until B/P response is noted or until dosage reaches 20 mcg/min; then increase as needed by 10 mcg/min. Dosage may be further titrated according to clinical, therapeutic response up to 200 mcg/min.

Children. Initially, 0.25–0.5 mcg/kg/min; titrate by 0.5–1 mcg/kg/min up to 20 mcg/kg/min.

SIDE EFFECTS/ADVERSE REACTIONS

Frequent

Headache (possibly severe; occurs mostly in early therapy, diminishes rapidly in intensity, and usually disappears during continued treatment), transient flushing of face and neck, dizziness (especially if patient is standing immobile or is in a warm environment), weakness, orthostatic hypotension

Sublingual: Burning, tingling sensation at oral point of dissolution

Ointment: Erythema, pruritus

Occasional

GI upset

Transdermal: Contact dermatitis

PRECAUTIONS AND CONTRAINDICATIONS

Allergy to adhesives (transdermal), closed-angle glaucoma, constrictive pericarditis (IV), early MI (sublingual), GI hypermotility or malabsorption (extended-release),

head trauma, hypotension (IV), inadequate cerebral circulation (IV), increased intracranial pressure, nitrates, orthostatic hypotension, pericardial tamponade (IV), severe anemia, uncorrected hypovolemia (IV)

Caution:

Postural hypotension, lactation

DRUG INTERACTIONS OF CONCERN TO DENTISTRY

• Increased hypotensive effects: alcohol, opioids, benzodiazepines, phenothiazines, and other drugs used in conscious sedation techniques

SERIOUS REACTIONS

❗ Nitroglycerin should be discontinued if blurred vision or dry mouth occurs.

❗ Severe orthostatic hypotension may occur, manifested by fainting, pulselessness, cold or clammy skin, and diaphoresis.

❗ Tolerance may occur with repeated, prolonged therapy; minor tolerance may occur with intermittent use of sublingual tablets.

❗ High doses of nitroglycerin tend to produce severe headache.

DENTAL CONSIDERATIONS

General:

• Take vital signs at every appointment because of cardiovascular side effects.

• After supine positioning, have patient sit upright for at least 2 min before standing to avoid orthostatic hypotension.

• Assess salivary flow as a factor in caries, periodontal disease, and candidiasis.

• Ensure that patient's drug is easily available if angina occurs.

- A benzodiazepine or nitrous oxide/oxygen may be prescribed to allay anxiety.
- Check expiration date on prescription to ensure drug activity. If bottle has been opened, the shelf life is 3 mo.
- Stress from dental procedures may compromise cardiovascular function; determine patient risk.
- Talk with patient about disease control (frequency of angina episodes).
- Use vasoconstrictors with caution, in low doses, and with careful aspiration. Avoid gingival retraction cord with epinephrine.
- Short appointments and a stress-reduction protocol may be required for anxious patients.
- Consider semisupine chair position for patients with cardiovascular disease.

Consultations:
- Medical consultation may be required to assess disease control and patient's ability to tolerate stress.

Teach Patient/Family to:
- Encourage effective oral hygiene to prevent soft tissue inflammation.
- Use caution to prevent injury when using oral hygiene aids.
- When chronic dry mouth occurs, advise patient to:
  - Avoid mouth rinses with high alcohol content because of drying effects.
  - Use daily home fluoride products for anticaries effect.
  - Use sugarless gum, frequent sips of water, or saliva substitutes.

nizatidine
ni-**za**′-ti-deen
(Apo-Nizatidine[CAN], Axid, Axid AR, Tazac[AUS])
Do not confuse Axid with Ansaid.

CATEGORY AND SCHEDULE
Pregnancy Risk Category: B
OTC (75 mg capsules)

Drug Class: Histamine H$_2$-receptor antagonist

MECHANISM OF ACTION
An antiulcer agent and gastric acid secretion inhibitor that inhibits histamine action at H$_2$ receptors of parietal cells.
Therapeutic Effect: Inhibits basal and nocturnal gastric acid secretion.

USES
Treatment of duodenal ulcer, Zollinger-Ellison syndrome, gastric ulcers, hypersecretory conditions, gastroesophageal reflux disease (GERD), stress ulcers; unapproved: GI symptoms associated with NSAID use in rheumatoid arthritis

PHARMACOKINETICS
Rapidly well absorbed from the GI tract. Protein binding: 35%. Metabolized in the liver. Primarily excreted in urine. Not removed by hemodialysis. *Half-life:* 1–2 hr (increased with impaired renal function).

INDICATIONS AND DOSAGES
▶ **Active Duodenal Ulcer**
PO
Adults, Elderly. 300 mg at bedtime or 150 mg twice a day.

▶ **Prevention of Duodenal Ulcer Recurrence**
PO
Adults, Elderly. 150 mg at bedtime.
▶ **GERD**
PO
Adults, Elderly. 150 mg twice a day.
▶ **Active Benign Gastric Ulcer**
PO
Adults, Elderly. 150 mg twice a day or 300 mg at bedtime.
PO, Oral Solution
Children 12 yr and older. 2 tsp twice a day.
▶ **Dyspepsia**
PO
Adults, Elderly. 75 mg 30–60 min before meals; no more than 2 tablets a day.
▶ **Dosage in Renal Impairment**
Dosage adjustment is based on creatinine clearance.

Creatinine Clearance	Active Ulcer	Maintenance Therapy
20–50 ml/min	150 mg every bedtime	150 mg every other day
Less than 20 ml/min	150 mg every bedtime	150 mg q3days

SIDE EFFECTS/ADVERSE REACTIONS
Occasional
Somnolence, fatigue
Rare
Diaphoresis, rash

PRECAUTIONS AND CONTRAINDICATIONS
Hypersensitivity to other H$_2$-antagonists
Caution:
Hepatic disease, renal disease, lactation, children younger than 16 yr

DRUG INTERACTIONS OF CONCERN TO DENTISTRY
• Increased serum salicylate when administered with high doses of aspirin
• Decreased absorption of ketoconazole (take doses 2 hr apart)

SERIOUS REACTIONS
! Asymptomatic ventricular tachycardia, hyperuricemia not associated with gout, and nephrolithiasis occur rarely.

DENTAL CONSIDERATIONS
General:
• Avoid prescribing aspirin-containing products in patients with active GI disease.
Teach Patient/Family to:
• Avoid mouth rinses with high alcohol content because of drying effects.

norethindrone
nor-**eth′**-in-drone
(Aygestin, Camila, Errin, Jolivette, Micronor, Nora-BE, Nor-QD, Norlutate[CAN])

CATEGORY AND SCHEDULE
Pregnancy Risk Category: X

Drug Class: Progesterone derivative

MECHANISM OF ACTION
A synthetic progestin that is used as a single agent or in combination with estrogens for the treatment of gynecological disorders. It inhibits secretion of pituitary gonadotropin (LH), which prevents follicular maturation and ovulation.
Therapeutic Effect: Transforms endometrium from proliferative to

secretory in an estrogen-primed endometrium, promotes mammary gland development, relaxes uterine smooth muscle.

USES
Treatment of uterine bleeding (abnormal), amenorrhea, endometriosis

PHARMACOKINETICS
Rapidly absorbed from the GI tract. Widely distributed. Protein binding: 61%. Metabolized in liver. Excreted in urine and feces. *Half-life:* 4–13 hr.

INDICATIONS AND DOSAGES
▸ **Contraception**
PO
Adults. 1 tablet/day.
▸ **Amenorrhea and Abnormal Uterine Bleeding**
PO
Adults. 5–20 mg/day cyclically (21 days on; 7 days off or continuously) or for acetate salt formulation, 2.5–10 mg cyclically.
▸ **Endometriosis**
PO
Adults. 10 mg/day for 2 wk increase at increments of 5 mg/day every 2 wk until 30 mg/day; continue for 6–9 mo or until breakthrough bleeding demands temporary termination. For acetate salt formulation, 5 mg/day for 14 days increase at increments of 2.5 mg/day every 2 wk up to 15 mg/day; continue for 6–9 mo or until breakthrough bleeding demands temporary termination.

SIDE EFFECTS/ADVERSE REACTIONS
Occasional
Breast tenderness, dizziness, headache, breakthrough bleeding,

amenorrhea, menstrual irregularity, nausea, weakness
Rare
Mental depression, fever, insomnia, rash, acne, increased breast tenderness, weight gain/loss, changes in cervical erosion and secretions, cholestatic jaundice

PRECAUTIONS AND CONTRAINDICATIONS
Acute liver disease, benign or malignant liver tumors, hypersensitivity to norethindrone and any component of the formulation, known or suspected carcinoma of the breast, known or suspected pregnancy, undiagnosed abnormal genital bleeding
Caution:
Lactation, hypertension, asthma, blood dyscrasias, gallbladder disease, CHF, diabetes mellitus, bone disease, depression, migraine headache, convulsive disorders, hepatic disease, renal disease, family history of breast or reproductive tract cancer

DRUG INTERACTIONS OF CONCERN TO DENTISTRY
• Decreased effectiveness of oral contraceptives (low risk), antibiotics, barbiturates

SERIOUS REACTIONS
! Thrombophlebitis, cerebrovascular disorders, retinal thrombosis, cholestatic jaundice, and pulmonary embolism occur rarely.

DENTAL CONSIDERATIONS
General:
• Place on frequent recall to evaluate gingival inflammation, if present.
• Increased incidence of dry socket has been reported after extraction.

• Monitor vital signs at each appointment.
Teach Patient/Family to:
• Encourage effective oral hygiene to prevent periodontal inflammation.
• Use additional method of birth control while undergoing antibiotic therapy.

norfloxacin

nor-**flox**′-ah-sin
(Apo-Norflox[CAN], Insensye[AUS], Norfloxacine[CAN], Noroxin, Novo-Norfloxacin[CAN], PMS-Norfloxacin[CAN], Roxin[AUS])

CATEGORY AND SCHEDULE
Pregnancy Risk Category: C

Drug Class: Fluoroquinolone antiinfective

MECHANISM OF ACTION
A quinolone that inhibits DNA gyrase in susceptible microorganisms, interfering with bacterial cell replication and repair.
Therapeutic Effect: Bactericidal.

USES
Treatment of adult UTIs (including complicated) caused by *E. coli, E. cloacae, P. mirabilis, K. pneumoniae,* group D strep, indole-positive *Proteus, C. freundii, S. aureus;* sexually transmitted disease caused by *N. gonorrhoeae;* prostatitis caused by *E. coli*

PHARMACOKINETICS
PO: Peak 1 hr, steady state 2 days.
Half-life: 3–4 hr; excreted in urine as active drug, metabolites.

INDICATIONS AND DOSAGES
▸ UTIs
PO
Adults, Elderly. 400 mg twice a day for 7–21 days.
▸ Prostatitis
PO
Adults. 400 mg twice a day for 28 days.
▸ Uncomplicated Gonococcal Infections
PO
Adults. 800 mg as a single dose.
▸ Dosage in Renal Impairment
Dosage and frequency are modified on the basis of creatinine clearance.

Creatinine Clearance	Dosage
30 ml/min or higher	400 mg twice a day
Less than 30 ml/min	400 mg once a day

SIDE EFFECTS/ADVERSE REACTIONS
Frequent
Nausea, headache, dizziness
Rare
Vomiting, diarrhea, dry mouth, bitter taste, nervousness, drowsiness, insomnia, photosensitivity, tinnitus, crystalluria, rash, fever, seizures

PRECAUTIONS AND CONTRAINDICATIONS
Children younger than 18 yr because of risk of arthropathy; hypersensitivity to norfloxacin, other quinolones, or their components
Caution:
Children, renal disease, seizure disorders, tendon rupture in shoulder, hand, and Achilles tendons

DRUG INTERACTIONS OF CONCERN TO DENTISTRY
• Decreased absorption: sodium bicarbonate

SERIOUS REACTIONS

! Superinfection, anaphylaxis, Stevens-Johnson syndrome, and arthropathy occur rarely.

! Hypersensitivity reactions, including photosensitivity (as evidenced by rash, pruritus, blisters, edema, and burning skin), have occurred in patients receiving fluoroquinolones.

DENTAL CONSIDERATIONS

General:
• Assess salivary flow as a factor in caries, periodontal disease, and candidiasis.
• Determine why the patient is taking the drug.
• Because of drug interaction, do not use ingestible sodium bicarbonate products, such as the Prophy-Jet air polishing system, until 2 hr after drug use.
• Avoid dental light in patient's eyes; offer dark glasses for patient comfort.
• Ruptures of the shoulder, hand, and Achilles tendons that required surgical repair or resulted in prolonged disability have been reported.

Consultations:
• Consult with patient's physician if an acute dental infection occurs and another antiinfective is required.

Teach Patient/Family to:
• Avoid mouth rinses with high alcohol content because of drying effects.
• Discontinue treatment and inform dentist immediately if patient experiences pain or inflammation of a tendon, and to rest and refrain from exercise.

norgestrel

nor-**jes**′-trel
(Ovrette)

CATEGORY AND SCHEDULE

Pregnancy Risk Category: X

Drug Class: Progesterone derivative

MECHANISM OF ACTION

A progestin that inhibits secretion of pituitary gonadotropin (LH), which prevents follicular maturation and ovulation.

Therapeutic Effect: Transforms endometrium from proliferative to secretory in an estrogen-primed endometrium, promotes mammary gland development, relaxes uterine smooth muscle.

USES

Oral contraception

PHARMACOKINETICS

Well absorbed from the GI tract. Widely distributed. Protein binding: 97%. Metabolized in liver via reduction and conjugation. Primarily excreted in urine.
Half-life: 20 hr.

INDICATIONS AND DOSAGES

▸ **Contraception, Female**
PO
Adults. 0.075 mg/day.

SIDE EFFECTS/ADVERSE REACTIONS

Frequent
Breakthrough bleeding or spotting at beginning of therapy, amenorrhea, change in menstrual flow, breast tenderness

Occasional

Edema, weight gain or loss, rash, pruritus, photosensitivity, skin pigmentation

Rare

Pain or swelling at injection site, acne, mental depression, alopecia, hirsutism

PRECAUTIONS AND CONTRAINDICATIONS

Hypersensitivity to norgestrel or any component of the formulation, hypersensitivity to tartrazine, thromboembolic disorders, severe hepatic disease; breast cancer; undiagnosed vaginal bleeding, pregnancy

Caution:

Lactation, hypertension, asthma, blood dyscrasias, gallbladder disease, CHF, diabetes mellitus, bone disease, depression, migraine headache, convulsive disorders, hepatic disease, renal disease, family history of breast or reproductive tract cancer

DRUG INTERACTIONS OF CONCERN TO DENTISTRY

• Decreased effectiveness of oral contraceptives: antibiotics, barbiturates

SERIOUS REACTIONS

! Thrombophlebitis, cerebrovascular disorders, retinal thrombosis, and pulmonary embolism occur rarely.

DENTAL CONSIDERATIONS

General:

• Place on frequent recall to evaluate gingival inflammation, if present.
• Increased incidence of dry socket has been reported after extraction.
• Monitor vital signs at each appointment.

Teach Patient/Family to:

• Encourage effective oral hygiene to prevent periodontal inflammation.
• Quit smoking because it decreases risk of serious and adverse cardiovascular side effects.
• Use an additional method of birth control while undergoing antibiotic therapy.

nortriptyline hydrochloride

nor-**trip**′-ti-leen
high-droh-**klor**′-ide
(Allegron[AUS], Apo-Nortriptyline[CAN], Aventyl, Norventyl, Novo-Nortriptyline [CAN], Pamelor)
Do not confuse nortriptyline with amitriptyline, or Aventyl with Ambenyl or Bentyl.

CATEGORY AND SCHEDULE

Pregnancy Risk Category: D

Drug Class:

Antidepressant-tricyclic

MECHANISM OF ACTION

A tricyclic antidepressant that blocks reuptake of the neurotransmitters norepinephrine and serotonin at neuronal presynaptic membranes, increasing their availability at postsynaptic receptor sites.
Therapeutic Effect: Relieves depression.

USES

Treatment of major depression

PHARMACOKINETICS

Well absorbed from the GI tract. Protein binding: 86%–95%. Metabolized in the liver. Primarily excreted in urine. *Half-life:* 17.6 hr.

INDICATIONS AND DOSAGES
▶ **Depression**
PO
Adults. 75–100 mg/day in 1–4 divided doses until therapeutic response is achieved. Reduce dosage gradually to effective maintenance level.
Elderly. Initially, 10–25 mg at bedtime. May increase by 25 mg every 3–7 days. Maximum: 150 mg/day.
Children 12 yr and older. 30–50 mg/day in 3–4 divided doses. Maximum: 150 mg/day.
Children 6–11 yr. 10–20 mg/day in 3–4 divided doses.
▶ **Enuresis**
PO
Children 12 yr and older. 25–35 mg/day.
Children 8–11 yr. 10–20 mg/day.
Children 6–7 yr. 10 mg/day.

SIDE EFFECTS/ADVERSE REACTIONS
Frequent
Somnolence, fatigue, dry mouth, blurred vision, constipation, delayed micturition, orthostatic hypotension, diaphoresis, impaired concentration, increased appetite, urine retention
Occasional
GI disturbances (nausea, GI distress, metallic taste), photosensitivity
Rare
Paradoxic reactions (agitation, restlessness, nightmares, insomnia), extrapyramidal symptoms (particularly fine hand tremors)

PRECAUTIONS AND CONTRAINDICATIONS
Acute recovery period after MI; use within 14 days of MAOIs
Caution:
Suicidal patients, severe depression, increased intraocular pressure, narrow-angle glaucoma, urinary retention, cardiac disease, hepatic disease, hyperthyroidism, electroshock therapy, elective surgery, MAOIs

DRUG INTERACTIONS OF CONCERN TO DENTISTRY
• Increased anticholinergic effects: muscarinic blockers, antihistamines, phenothiazines
• Increased effects of direct-acting sympathomimetics (epinephrine, levonordefrin)
• Potential risk of increased CNS depression: alcohol, barbiturates, benzodiazepines, and other CNS depressants
• Decreased antihypertensive effect: clonidine, guanadrel, guanethidine
• Avoid concurrent use with St. John's wort (herb)

SERIOUS REACTIONS
! Overdose may produce seizures; cardiovascular effects, such as severe orthostatic hypotension, dizziness, tachycardia, palpitations, and arrhythmias; and altered temperature regulation, such as hyperpyrexia or hypothermia.
! Abrupt discontinuation after prolonged therapy may produce headache, malaise, nausea, vomiting, and vivid dreams.

DENTAL CONSIDERATIONS
General:
• Take vital signs at every appointment because of cardiovascular side effects.
• Assess salivary flow as a factor in caries, periodontal disease, and candidiasis.
• Patients on chronic drug therapy may rarely have symptoms of blood dyscrasias, which can include infection, bleeding, and poor healing.

N

• After supine positioning, have patient sit upright for at least 2 min before standing to avoid orthostatic hypotension.
• Use vasoconstrictors with caution, in low doses, and with careful aspiration. Avoid use of gingival retraction cord with epinephrine.
• Place on frequent recall because of oral side effects.

Consultations:
• In patients with symptoms of blood dyscrasias, request a medical consultation for blood studies and postpone dental treatment until normal values are reestablished.
• Medical consultation may be required to assess disease control.
• Physician should be informed if significant xerostomic side effects occur (e.g., increased caries, sore tongue, problems eating or swallowing, difficulty wearing prosthesis) so that a medication change can be considered.

Teach Patient/Family to:
• Encourage effective oral hygiene to prevent soft tissue inflammation.
• Use caution to prevent injury when using oral hygiene aids.
• When chronic dry mouth occurs, advise patient to:
   • Avoid mouth rinses with high alcohol content because of drying effects.
   • Use daily home fluoride products for anticaries effect.
   • Use sugarless gum, frequent sips of water, or saliva substitutes.

nystatin
nye-**stat**'-in
(Mycostatin, Nilstat[CAN], Nyaderm, Nystop)
Do not confuse nystatin or Mycostatin with Nitrostat.

CATEGORY AND SCHEDULE
Pregnancy Risk Category: C

Drug Class: Antifungal

MECHANISM OF ACTION
A fungistatic antifungal that binds to sterols in the fungal cell membrane. *Therapeutic Effect:* Increases fungal cell-membrane permeability, allowing loss of potassium and other cellular components.

USES
Treatment of *Candida* species causing oral, vaginal, intestinal infections

PHARMACOKINETICS
PO: Poorly absorbed from the GI tract. Eliminated unchanged in feces. Topical: Not absorbed systemically from intact skin.

INDICATIONS AND DOSAGES
▶ **Intestinal Infections**
PO
Adults, Elderly. 500,000–1,000,000 units q8h.
▶ **Oral Candidiasis**
PO
Adults, Elderly, Children. 400,000–600,000 units 4 times a day.
Infants. 200,000 units 4 times a day.
▶ **Vaginal Infections**
Vaginal
Adults, Elderly, Adolescents. 1 tablet/day at bedtime for 14 days.

▸ **Cutaneous Candidal Infections**
Topical
Adults, Elderly, Children. Apply 2–4
times a day.

SIDE EFFECTS/ADVERSE REACTIONS
Occasional
PO: None known
Topical: Skin irritation
Vaginal: Vaginal irritation

PRECAUTIONS AND CONTRAINDICATIONS
Hypersensitivity

SERIOUS REACTIONS
! High dosages of oral form may
produce nausea, vomiting, diarrhea,
and GI distress.

DENTAL CONSIDERATIONS

General:
• Determine why the patient is
taking the drug.
• Broad-spectrum antibiotic may
contribute to oral *Candida*
infections.

Teach Patient/Family to:
• Complete entire course of
medication.
• Not use commercial mouthwashes
for mouth infection unless
prescribed by dentist.
• Soak full or partial dentures in a
suitable antifungal solution nightly.
• Prevent reinoculation of *Candida*
infection by disposing of tooth brush
or other contaminated oral hygiene
devices used during period of
infection.

N

octreotide acetate
ok-**tree**′-oh-tide **ass**′-ih-tate
(Sandostatin, Sandostatin LAR)
Do not confuse octreotide with
OctreoScan, or Sandostatin with
Sandimmune or Sandoglobulin.

CATEGORY AND SCHEDULE
Pregnancy Risk Category: B

Drug Class: Secretory inhibitor,
growth hormone suppressant

MECHANISM OF ACTION
An antidiarrheal and growth
hormone suppressant that suppresses
the secretion of serotonin and
gastroenteropancreatic peptides and
enhances fluid and electrolyte
absorption from the GI tract.
Therapeutic Effect: Prolongs
intestinal transit time.

USES
Treatment of severe diarrhea and
other symptoms that occur with
certain intestinal tumors

PHARMACOKINETICS

Route	Onset	Peak	Duration
Subcutaneous	N/A	N/A	Up to 12 hr

Rapidly and completely absorbed
from injection site. Excreted in
urine. Removed by hemodialysis.
Half-life: 1.5 hr.

INDICATIONS AND DOSAGES
▸ **Diarrhea**
IV (Sandostatin)
Adults, Elderly. Initially, 50–
100 mcg q8h. May increase by
100 mcg/dose q48h. Maximum:
500 mcg q8h.

Subcutaneous (Sandostatin)
Adults, Elderly. 50 mcg 1–2 times a
day.
IV, Subcutaneous (Sandostatin)
Children. 1–10 mcg/kg q12h.
▸ **Carcinoid Tumors**
IV, Subcutaneous (Sandostatin)
Adults, Elderly. 100–600 mcg/day in
2–4 divided doses.
IM (Sandostatin LAR)
Adults, Elderly. 20 mg q4wk.
▸ **VIPomas**
IV, Subcutaneous (Sandostatin)
Adults, Elderly. 200–300 mcg/day in
2–4 divided doses.
IM (Sandostatin LAR)
Adults, Elderly. 20 mg q4wk.
▸ **Esophageal Varices**
IV (Sandostatin)
Adults, Elderly. Bolus of 25–50 mcg
followed by IV infusion of
25–50 mcg/hr.
▸ **Acromegaly**
IV, Subcutaneous (Sandostatin)
Adults, Elderly. 50 mcg 3 times a
day. Increase as needed. Maximum:
500 mcg 3 times a day.
IM (Sandostatin LAR)
Adults, Elderly. 20 mg q4wk for
3 mo. Maximum: 40 mg q4wk.

SIDE EFFECTS/ADVERSE REACTIONS
Frequent
Diarrhea, nausea, abdominal
discomfort, headache, injection site
pain
Occasional
Vomiting, flatulence, constipation,
alopecia, facial flushing, pruritus,
dizziness, fatigue, arrhythmias,
ecchymosis, blurred vision
Rare
Depression, diminished libido,
vertigo, palpitations, dyspnea

PRECAUTIONS AND CONTRAINDICATIONS
None known

DRUG INTERACTIONS OF CONCERN TO DENTISTRY

• May cause decrease in vitamin B$_{12}$ levels.

SERIOUS REACTIONS

! Patients using octreotide may develop cholelithiasis or, with prolonged high dosages, hypothyroidism.

! GI bleeding, hepatitis, and seizures occur rarely.

DENTAL CONSIDERATIONS

General:

• This drug is administered in several disease states; determine patient's medical and drug history and exact use to accurately plan patient management.

• Monitor and record vital signs.

• Consider semisupine chair position for patient comfort if GI side effects occur.

• Question patient about tolerance of NSAIDs or aspirin related to GI disease.

• This drug may be used in the hospital or on an outpatient basis. Confirm the patient's disease and treatment status.

• Patient may need assistance in getting into and out of dental chair. Adjust chair position for patient comfort.

• Examine for oral manifestation of opportunistic infection.

Consultations:

• Medical consultation may be required to assess disease control and patient's ability to tolerate stress.

Teach Patient/Family to:

• Encourage effective oral hygiene to prevent soft tissue inflammation.

• Prevent trauma when using oral hygiene aids.

• Use powered tooth brush if patient has difficulty holding conventional devices.

• Update health and medication history if physician makes any changes in evaluation or drug regimens; include OTC, herbal, and nonherbal drugs in the update.

ofloxacin

o-**flox**′-ah-sin

(Apo-Oflox[CAN], Floxin, Floxin Otic, Ocuflox)

Do not confuse Floxin with Flexeril or Flexon, or Ocuflox with Ocufen.

CATEGORY AND SCHEDULE

Pregnancy Risk Category: C

Drug Class: Fluoroquinolone antiinfective

MECHANISM OF ACTION

A fluoroquinolone antibiotic that inhibits DNA gyrase in susceptible microorganisms, interfering with bacterial cell replication and repair. ***Therapeutic Effect:*** Bactericidal.

USES

Treatment of lower respiratory tract infections (pneumonia, bronchitis), genitourinary infections (prostatitis, UTIs) caused by *E. coli, K. pneumoniae, C. trachomatis, N. gonorrhoeae;* skin and skin-structure infections

PHARMACOKINETICS

Rapidly and well absorbed from the GI tract. Protein binding: 20%–25%. Widely distributed (including to CSF). Metabolized in the liver. Primarily excreted in urine. Removed by hemodialysis.

Half-life: 4.7–7 hr (increased in impaired renal function, cirrhosis, and the elderly).

INDICATIONS AND DOSAGES
▸ **UTIs**
PO, IV
Adults. 200 mg q12h.
▸ **Pelvic Inflammatory Disease (PID)**
PO
Adults. 400 mg q12h for 10–14 days.
▸ **Lower Respiratory Tract, Skin and Skin-Structure Infections**
PO, IV
Adults. 400 mg q12h for 10 days.
▸ **Prostatitis, Sexually Transmitted Diseases (Cervicitis, Urethritis)**
PO
Adults. 300 mg q12h.
▸ **Prostatitis**
IV
Adults. 300 mg q12h.
▸ **Sexually Transmitted Diseases**
IV
Adults. 400 mg as a single dose.
▸ **Acute, Uncomplicated Gonorrhea**
PO
Adults. 400 mg 1 time.
▸ **Usual Elderly Dosage**
PO
Elderly. 200–400 mg q12–24h for 7 days up to 6 wk.
▸ **Bacterial Conjunctivitis**
Ophthalmic
Adults, Elderly. 1–2 drops q2–4h for 2 days, then 4 times a day for 5 days.
▸ **Corneal Ulcers**
Ophthalmic
Adults. 1–2 drops q30min while awake for 2 days, then q60min while awake for 5–7 days, then 4 times a day.
▸ **Acute Otitis Media**
Otic
Children 1–12 yr. 5 drops into the affected ear 2 times a day for 10 days.

▸ **Otitis Externa**
Otic
Adults, Elderly, Children 12 yr and older. 10 drops into the affected ear once a day for 7 days.
Children 6 mo–11 yr. 5 drops into the affected ear once a day for 7 days.
▸ **Dosage in Renal Impairment**
After a normal initial dose, dosage and frequency are based on creatinine clearance.

Creatinine Clearance	Adjusted Dose	Dosage Interval
Greater than 50 ml/min	None	q12h
10–50 ml/min	None	q24h
Less than 10 ml/min	1/2	q24h

SIDE EFFECTS/ADVERSE REACTIONS
Frequent
Nausea, headache, insomnia
Occasional
Abdominal pain, diarrhea, vomiting, dry mouth, flatulence, dizziness, fatigue, drowsiness, rash, pruritus, fever
Rare
Constipation, paraesthesia

PRECAUTIONS AND CONTRAINDICATIONS
Hypersensitivity to any quinolones
Caution:
Lactation, children younger than 18 yr, elderly, renal disease, seizure disorders, excessive sunlight, tendon rupture in shoulder, hand, and Achilles tendons

DRUG INTERACTIONS OF CONCERN TO DENTISTRY
• Decreased effects: antacids
• Possible increased risk of life-threatening dysrhythmias: procainamide

SERIOUS REACTIONS

! Antibiotic-associated colitis and other superinfections may occur from altered bacterial balance.

! Hypersensitivity reactions, including photosensitivity (as evidenced by rash, pruritus, blisters, edema, and burning skin), have occurred in patients receiving fluoroquinolones.

! Arthropathy (swelling, pain, and clubbing of fingers and toes, degeneration of stress-bearing portion of a joint) may occur if the drug is given to children.

DENTAL CONSIDERATIONS

General:

• Because of drug interaction, do not use ingestible sodium bicarbonate products, such as the Prophy-Jet air polishing system, until 2 hr after drug use.

• Examine for oral manifestation of opportunistic infections.

• Avoid dental light in patient's eyes; offer dark glasses for patient comfort.

• Minimize exposure to sunlight and wear sunscreen if sun exposure is planned.

• Ruptures of the shoulder, hand, and Achilles tendons that required surgical repair or resulted in prolonged disability have been reported with this drug.

Consultations:

• Consult with patient's physician if an acute dental infection occurs and another antiinfective is required.

Teach Patient/Family to:

• Encourage effective oral hygiene to prevent soft tissue inflammation.

• Avoid mouth rinses with high alcohol content because of drying effects.

• Discontinue treatment and inform dentist immediately if patient experiences pain or inflammation of a tendon, and to rest and refrain from exercise.

Ofloxacin (Optic)

General:

• Avoid dental light in patient's eyes; offer dark glasses for patient comfort and safety protection during dental treatment.

Ofloxacin Otic Solution

General:

• Determine why the patient is taking the drug.

• Severity or discomfort of infection may require postponement of elective dental treatment.

Consultations:

• Consult with patient's physician if an acute dental infection occurs and another antiinfective is required.

• Medical consultation may be required to assess disease control in the patient.

Teach Patient/Family to:

• When chronic dry mouth occurs, advise patient to:

  • Avoid mouth rinses with high alcohol content because of drying effects.

  • Use daily home fluoride products for anticaries effect.

  • Use sugarless gum, frequent sips of water, or saliva substitutes.

olanzapine

oh-**lan´**-za-peen

(Zyprexa, Zyprexa Intramuscular, Zyprexa Zydis)

Do not confuse olanzapine with olsalazine, or Zyprexa with Zyrtec.

CATEGORY AND SCHEDULE

Pregnancy Risk Category: C

Drug Class: Antipsychotic

MECHANISM OF ACTION
A dibenzepin derivative that antagonizes α_1-adrenergic, dopamine, histamine, muscarinic, and serotonin receptors. Produces anticholinergic, histaminic, and CNS depressant effects.
Therapeutic Effect: Diminishes manifestations of psychotic symptoms.

USES
Treatment of psychotic disorders, schizophrenia, bipolar disorder; acute manic episode in bipolar 1 disorder in combination with lithium or valproate

PHARMACOKINETICS
Well absorbed after PO administration. Protein binding: 93%. Extensively distributed throughout the body. Undergoes extensive first-pass metabolism in the liver. Excreted primarily in urine and, to a lesser extent, in feces. Not removed by dialysis. *Half-life:* 21–54 hr.

INDICATIONS AND DOSAGES
▶ **Schizophrenia**
PO
Adults. Initially, 5–10 mg once daily. May increase by 10 mg/day at 5–7 day intervals. If further adjustments are indicated, may increase by 5–10 mg/day at 7-day intervals. Range: 10–30 mg/day.
Elderly. Initially, 2.5 mg/day. May increase as indicated. Range: 2.5–10 mg/day.
Children. Initially, 2.5 mg/day. Titrate as needed up to 20 mg/day.
▶ **Bipolar Mania**
PO
Adults. Initially, 10–15 mg/day. May increase by 5 mg/day at intervals of at least 24 hr. Maximum: 20 mg/day.

Children. Initially, 2.5 mg/day. Titrate as needed up to 20 mg/day.
▶ **Dosage for Elderly or Debilitated Patients and Those Predisposed to Hypotensive Reactions**
The initial dosage for these patients is 5 mg/day.
▶ **Control Agitation in Schizophrenic or Bipolar Patients**
IM
Adults, Elderly. 2.5–10 mg. May repeat 2 hr after first dose and 4 hr after second dose. Maximum: 30 mg/day.

SIDE EFFECTS/ADVERSE REACTIONS
Frequent
Somnolence, agitation, insomnia, headache, nervousness, hostility, dizziness, rhinitis
Occasional
Anxiety, constipation, nonaggressive atypical behavior, dry mouth, weight gain, orthostatic hypotension, fever, arthralgia, restlessness, cough, pharyngitis, visual changes (dim vision)
Rare
Tachycardia; back, chest, abdominal, or extremity pain; tremors

PRECAUTIONS AND CONTRAINDICATIONS
Hypersensitivity
Caution:
Lactation, paralytic ileus, elderly; combination of age, smoking, and gender (female) may increase clearance rate; neuroleptic malignant syndrome, cardiovascular disease, cerebrovascular disease, seizures, orthostatic hypotension, Alzheimer's dementia, prostate hypertrophy, glaucoma; patients should be monitored for signs and symptoms of diabetes mellitus

DRUG INTERACTIONS OF CONCERN TO DENTISTRY
• Potentiation of orthostatic hypotension: diazepam, alcohol, other CNS depressants
• Increased anticholinergic effects: anticholinergic drugs
• Suspected reduction of plasma levels: carbamazepine

SERIOUS REACTIONS
! Rare reactions include seizures and neuroleptic malignant syndrome, a potentially fatal syndrome characterized by hyperpyrexia, muscle rigidity, irregular pulse or B/P, tachycardia, diaphoresis, and cardiac arrhythmias.
! Extrapyramidal symptoms and dysphagia may also occur.
! Overdose produces drowsiness and slurred speech.

DENTAL CONSIDERATIONS

General:
• Consider semisupine chair position for patient comfort because of GI effects of drug.
• Assess salivary flow as factor in caries, periodontal disease, and candidiasis.
• Monitor vital signs at every appointment because of cardiovascular side effects.
• After supine positioning, have patient sit upright for at least 2 min before standing to avoid orthostatic hypotension.
• Patients on chronic drug therapy may rarely have symptoms of blood dyscrasias, which can include infection, bleeding, and poor healing.
• Assess for presence of extrapyramidal motor symptoms, such as tardive dyskinesia and akathisia. Extrapyramidal motor activity may complicate dental treatment.

Consultations:
• In a patient with symptoms of blood dyscrasias, request a medical consultation for blood studies and postpone dental treatment until normal values are reestablished.
• Medical consultation may be required to assess disease control.
• Physician should be informed if significant xerostomic side effects occur (e.g., increased caries, sore tongue, problems eating or swallowing, difficulty wearing prosthesis) so that a medication change can be considered.
Teach Patient/Family to:
• Encourage effective oral hygiene to prevent soft tissue inflammation.
• Use powered tooth brush if patient has difficulty holding conventional devices.
• Use caution when driving or performing other tasks requiring alertness.
• When chronic dry mouth occurs, advise patient to:
  • Avoid mouth rinses with high alcohol content because of drying effects.
  • Use daily home fluoride products for anticaries effect.
  • Use sugarless gum, frequent sips of water, or saliva substitutes.

olmesartan
ol-meh-**sar′**-tan
(Benicar)

CATEGORY AND SCHEDULE
Pregnancy Risk Category: C (1st trimester) and D (2nd and 3rd trimesters).

Drug Class: Antihypertensive, angiotensin (AT) II receptor blocker.

MECHANISM OF ACTION

Blocks the vasoconstrictor effects of angiotensin II by blocking the binding of angiotensin II to the AT 1 receptor in smooth muscle. Olmesartan increases urinary flow rate.

USES

Treatment of hypertension as monotherapy or in combination with other antihypertensive agents

PHARMACOKINETICS

Rapidly, completely absorbed after PO administration. Protein binding: 99%. Olmesartan medoxomil is an inactive drug. It is hydrolyzed in the gastrointestinal tract to active olmesartan which is absorbed. Bioavailability: 26%. Food does not affect the bioavailability of olmesartan. Dose not cross blood-brain barrier. Primarily excreted in feces and to a lesser extent in urine. *Half-life:* 13 hr.

INDICATIONS AND DOSAGES
▸ **Hypertension (with or without Other Antihypertensive Agents)**
PO
Adults. Initially, 20 mg once daily. May be increased to 40 mg once daily after 2 wk. Lower starting dose in patients receiving volume depleting drugs (e.g., diuretics). *Elderly.* May start at 5–10 mg/day. Dosage in Hepatic Impairment: no adjustment necessary. Dosage in Renal Impairment: no adjustment necessary.

SIDE EFFECTS/ADVERSE REACTIONS
Adults
Frequent
Dizziness, headache, diarrhea

Occasional
Abdominal pain, chest pain, insomnia, tachycardia, cough, hyperglycemia

Children
Safety and efficacy have not been established in children

PRECAUTIONS AND CONTRAINDICATIONS

Hypertensive to olmesartan or its components
Use caution in patients with aortic/ mitral stenosis, hypovolemia, renal artery stenosis, and renal impairment.
Hyperkalemia may occur.
Pregnancy: [U.S. Boxed Warning]: "Based on human data, drugs that act on the angiotensin system can cause injury and death to the developing fetus when used in the second and third trimesters. Angiotensin receptor blockers should be discontinued as soon as possible once pregnancy is detected."

DRUG INTERACTIONS OF CONCERN TO DENTISTRY

• NSAIDs: May reduce efficacy of olmesartan.

SERIOUS REACTIONS

! Allergic reactions are reported rarely with angiotensin receptor antagonists.
! Bradycardia may occur.
! Rhabdomyolysis has been reported.

DENTAL CONSIDERATIONS

General:
• Monitor vital signs at every appointment because of cardiovascular side effects.
• Avoid or limit dose of vasoconstrictor.

- After supine positioning, have patient sit upright for at least 2 min to avoid dizziness.
- Stress from dental procedure may compromise cardiovascular function; determine patient risk.

Consultations:
- Medical consultation may be required to assess disease control and to determine ability of patient to tolerate dental treatment.

Teach Patient/Family to:
- Prevent injury when using oral hygiene aids.
- Encourage effective oral hygiene to prevent soft tissue inflammation.

olmesartan medoxomil
ol-meh-**sar**′-tan
(Benicar)

CATEGORY AND SCHEDULE
Pregnancy Risk Category: C (D if used in second or third trimester)

Drug Class: Angiotensin II (ATI) receptor antagonist

MECHANISM OF ACTION
An angiotensin II receptor, type ATI, antagonist that blocks the vasoconstrictor and aldosterone-secreting effects of angiotensin II, inhibiting the binding of angiotensin II to the ATI receptors.
Therapeutic Effect: Causes vasodilation, decreases peripheral resistance, and decreases B/P.

USES
Treatment of hypertension, as a single drug or in combination with other antihypertensives

PHARMACOKINETICS
Rapidly and completely absorbed after PO administration. Metabolized in the liver. Recovered primarily in feces and, to a lesser extent, in urine. Not removed by hemodialysis. *Half-life:* 13 hr.

INDICATIONS AND DOSAGES
▶ **Hypertension**
PO
Adults, Elderly, Patients with mildly impaired hepatic or renal function. 20 mg once a day in patients who are not volume depleted. After 2 wk of therapy, if further reduction in B/P is necessary, may increase dosage to 40 mg/day.

SIDE EFFECTS/ADVERSE REACTIONS
Occasional
Dizziness
Rare
Headache, diarrhea, upper respiratory tract infection

PRECAUTIONS AND CONTRAINDICATIONS
Bilateral renal artery stenosis
Caution:
Discontinue drug if pregnancy occurs, use in volume- or salt-depleted patients, or in nursing mothers or pediatric patients has not been established, impaired renal function, CHF, renal artery stenosis

DRUG INTERACTIONS OF CONCERN TO DENTISTRY
- No significant drug interactions have been reported, but increased hypotensive effects always are possible when used with other antihypertensives or sedatives.

O

SERIOUS REACTIONS

❗ Overdosage may manifest as hypotension and tachycardia. Bradycardia occurs less often.

DENTAL CONSIDERATIONS

General:

• Monitor vital signs at every appointment because of cardiovascular side effects.

• Avoid or limit dose of vasoconstrictor.

• Consider semisupine chair position for patient comfort if GI side effects occur.

• Limit use of sodium-containing products, such as saline IV fluids, for patients with a dietary salt restriction.

• Stress from dental procedures may compromise cardiovascular function; determine patient risk.

• Patients with hypertensive disease may be taking more than one drug to control B/P; although not specifically noted for this drug, postural hypotension is always a possibility.

• After supine positioning, have patient sit upright for at least 2 min before standing to avoid orthostatic hypotension.

• Short appointments and a stress-reduction protocol may be required for anxious patients.

• Use precaution if sedation or general anesthesia is required; risk of hypotensive episode.

Consultations:

• Medical consultation may be required to assess disease control and patient's ability to tolerate stress.

Teach Patient/Family to:

• Update health and drug history if physician makes any changes in evaluation or drug regimens; include OTC, herbal, and nonherbal drugs in the update.

olopatadine
(oh-loh-**pat**′-ah-deen)
(Patanase [U.S.], Pataday, Patanol, Patanol S, Opatanol [INTL.])

CATEGORY AND SCHEDULE
Pregnancy Risk Category: C

Drug Class: Ophthalmic and nasal antihistamine

MECHANISM OF ACTION
Blocks release of histamine from mast cells and blocks effect of histamine on H_1 receptors in tissues of eye.
Therapeutic Effect: Reduces effects of ophthalmic (allergic conjunctivitis) and nasal allergic reactions.

USES
Allergic conjunctivitis and rhinitis

PHARMACOKINETICS
Low systemic exposure after topical administration. *Half-life:* 3 hr. Excreted primarily (60%–70%) as parent drug in urine

INDICATIONS AND DOSAGES
▸ **Allergic Conjunctivitis**
Topical, Ophthalmic/Intranasal
Adult. One drop two times per day q6–8h.

SIDE EFFECTS/ADVERSE REACTIONS
Frequent
Headache
Occasional
Asthenia, blurred vision, burning or stinging, cold syndrome, dry eye, foreign body sensation, hyperemia, hypersensitivity, keratitis, lid edema, nausea, pharyngitis, rhinitis, pruritus, sinusitis, dysgeusia

PRECAUTIONS AND CONTRAINDICATIONS
Hypersensitivity
Nursing
Contraindicated by hypersensitivity to olopatadine or any of its ingredients

DRUG INTERACTIONS OF CONCERN TO DENTISTRY
• None reported

SERIOUS REACTIONS
! None reported

DENTAL CONSIDERATIONS
General:
• Consider drug as etiologic factor in dysgeusia.
Consultations:
• Consult with physician to determine disease control and ability to tolerate dental procedures.
Teach Patient/Family to:
• Report changes in taste sensation or other oral adverse effects.

olsalazine sodium
ohl-**sal**'-ah-zeen **soe**'-dee-um
(Dipentum)
Do not confuse olsalazine with olanzapine.

CATEGORY AND SCHEDULE
Pregnancy Risk Category: C

Drug Class: Antiinflammatory, salicylate derivative

MECHANISM OF ACTION
A salicylic acid derivative that is converted to mesalamine in the colon by bacterial action.
Blocks prostaglandin production in bowel mucosa.

Therapeutic Effect: Reduces colonic inflammation in inflammatory bowel disease.

USES
Maintenance of remission of ulcerative colitis in patients intolerant to sulfasalazine

PHARMACOKINETICS
PO: Partially absorbed, peak 1.5 hr.
Half-life: 5–10 hr; excreted in urine as 5-aminosalicylic acid and metabolites; crosses placenta.

INDICATIONS AND DOSAGES
▶ **Maintenance of Controlled Ulcerative Colitis**
PO
Adults, Elderly. 1 g/day in 2 divided doses, preferably q12h.

SIDE EFFECTS/ADVERSE REACTIONS
Frequent
Headache, diarrhea, abdominal pain or cramps, nausea
Occasional
Depression, fatigue, dyspepsia, upper respiratory tract infection, decreased appetite, rash, itching, arthralgia
Rare
Dizziness, vomiting, stomatitis

PRECAUTIONS AND CONTRAINDICATIONS
History of hypersensitivity to salicylates
Caution:
Lactation, impaired hepatic function, severe allergy, bronchial asthma, renal disease

SERIOUS REACTIONS
! Sulfite sensitivity may occur in susceptible patients, manifested by cramping, headache, diarrhea, fever,

rash, hives, itching, and wheezing. Discontinue drug immediately.
! Excessive diarrhea associated with extreme fatigue is noted rarely.

DENTAL CONSIDERATIONS

General:
• Consider semisupine chair position for patient comfort because of GI effects of disease.
Consultations:
• Avoid drugs that could aggravate an inflammatory colon disease; consultation is recommended before selection of an antibiotic.
Teach Patient/Family to:
• Encourage effective oral hygiene to prevent soft tissue inflammation.
• Use caution to prevent injury when using oral hygiene aids.
• Avoid mouth rinses with high alcohol content because of drying effects.

omalizumab
oh-mah-**liz**'-uw-mab
(Xolair)

CATEGORY AND SCHEDULE
Pregnancy Risk Category: B

Drug Class: Anti-IgE monoclonal antibody

MECHANISM OF ACTION
A monoclonal antibody that selectively binds to human immunoglobulin E (IgE), preventing it from binding to the surface of mast cells and basophils.
Therapeutic Effect: Prevents or reduces the number of asthmatic attacks.

USES
Reduction of asthma exacerbation in patients with moderate to severe asthma who have a positive skin test or in vitro reactivity to a perennial aeroallergen not adequately controlled by inhaled glucocorticoids

PHARMACOKINETICS
Absorbed slowly after subcutaneous administration, with peak concentration in 7–8 days. Excreted in the liver, reticuloendothelial system, and endothelial cells.
Half-life: 26 days.

INDICATIONS AND DOSAGES
▶ **Moderate-to-Severe Persistent Asthma in Patients Who Are Reactive to a Perennial Allergen and Whose Asthma Symptoms Have Been Inadequately Controlled with Inhaled Corticosteroids**
Subcutaneous
Adults, Elderly, Children 12 yr and older. 150–375 mg every 2 or 4 wk; dose and dosing frequency are individualized on the basis of weight and pretreatment IgE level (as shown below).
4-wk Dosing Table

Pretreatment Serum IgE Levels (units/ml)	Weight 30–60 kg	Weight 61–70 kg	Weight 71–90 kg	Weight 91–150 kg
30–100	150 mg	150 mg	150 mg	300 mg
101–200	300 mg	300 mg	300 mg	See next table
201–300	300 mg	See next table	See next table	See next table

2-wk Dosing Table

Pretreatment Serum IgE (units/ml)	Weight 30–60 kg	Weight 61–70 kg	Weight 71–90 kg	Weight 91–150 kg
101–200	See preceding table	See preceding table	See preceding table	225 mg
201–300	See preceding table	225 mg	225 mg	300 mg
301–400	225 mg	225 mg	300 mg	Do not dose
401–500	300 mg	300 mg	375 mg	Do not dose
501–600	300 mg	375 mg	Do not dose	Do not dose
601–700	375 mg	Do not dose	Do not dose	Do not dose

SIDE EFFECTS/ADVERSE REACTIONS

Frequent

Injection site ecchymosis, redness, warmth, stinging, and urticaria; viral infections; sinusitis; headache; pharyngitis

Occasional

Arthralgia, leg pain, fatigue, dizziness

Rare

Arm pain, earache, dermatitis, pruritus

PRECAUTIONS AND CONTRAINDICATIONS

Hypersensitivity

Caution:

Possible risk of malignancy, anaphylactic reactions, not for acute asthma or status asthmaticus, do not abruptly discontinue glucocorticoid therapy, use in nursing mothers or children younger than 12 yr has not been established

DRUG INTERACTIONS OF CONCERN TO DENTISTRY

• None reported

SERIOUS REACTIONS

! Anaphylaxis occurs within 2 hr of the first dose or subsequent doses in 0.1% of patients.
! Malignant neoplasms occur in 0.5% of patients.

DENTAL CONSIDERATIONS

General:

• Determine why patient is taking the drug.
• Be aware of patient's disease, its severity, and its frequency, when known.
• Question patient about other medications used for asthma or to prevent bronchoconstriction.
• Avoid drugs that may aggravate asthma.
• Short appointments and a stress reduction protocol may be required for anxious patients.
• Have patient bring personal short-acting bronchodilator to appointment for use in emergency.
• Acute asthmatic episodes may be precipitated in the dental office. Rapid-acting sympathomimetic inhalants should be available for emergency use. A stress-reduction protocol may be required.

Consultations:

• Consultation with physician may be necessary if sedation or general anesthesia is required.
• Medical consultation may be required to assess disease control and patient's ability to tolerate stress.

Teach Patient/Family to:

• Encourage effective oral hygiene to prevent soft tissue inflammation/infection.
• Update health and drug history and report changes in health status, drug regimen, or disease/treatment status.

omega-3 fatty acids
(Lovaza)

CATEGORY AND SCHEDULE
Pregnancy Risk Category: C

Drug Class: Antihyperlipidemic agent

MECHANISM OF ACTION
A combination of ethyl esters of omega 3 fatty acids, principally eicosapentaenoic acid (EPA) and docosahexaenoic acid (DHA) but the mechanism of action is not well understood. May inhibit acyl-CoA:1,2-diacylglycerol acyltransferase, increase mitochondrial and peroxisomal β-oxidation in the liver, decrease lipogenesis in the liver, and increase plasma lipoprotein lipase activity. *Therapeutic Effect:* Lowers serum triglyceride level.

USES
Hypertriglyceridemia, severe (≥500 mg/dl), adjunct to diet

PHARMACOKINETICS
Absorbed when administered as ethyl esters following PO administration.

INDICATIONS AND DOSAGES
▶ **Hypertriglyceridemia, Severe (≥500 mg/dl), Adjunct to Diet**
PO

Adults. 4-g dose (4 capsules) or as two 2-g doses (2 capsules twice daily).

SIDE EFFECTS/ADVERSE REACTIONS
Frequent
Eructation, infection

Occasional
Flu syndrome, dyspepsia, back pain, pain (general), angina, rash, dysgeusia
Rare
Elevated LDL cholesterol levels

PRECAUTIONS AND CONTRAINDICATIONS
Hypersensitivity to omega-3 fatty acids or any component of the formulation
Caution:
Hepatic impairment
Fish allergy
Pregnancy
Nursing mothers
Elevated LDL cholesterol levels
Prolongation of bleeding time

DRUG INTERACTIONS OF CONCERN TO DENTISTRY
• Anticoagulants, antiplatelets: May increase the risk of bleeding.

SERIOUS REACTIONS
! ALT and AST should be monitored periodically in patients with hepatic impairment.
! Lipid profile should be monitored.

DENTAL CONSIDERATIONS

General:
• Monitor vital signs at every appointment because of cardiovascular side effects.
• After supine positioning, have patient sit upright for at least 2 min before standing to avoid orthostatic hypotension.
• Assess salivary flow as a factor in caries, periodontal disease, and candidiasis.
• Stress from dental procedures may compromise cardiovascular function; determine patient risk.

Consultations:
• Medical consultation may be required to assess disease control.
Teach Patient/Family to:
• Report oral lesions, soreness, or bleeding to dentist.
• When chronic dry mouth occurs, advise patient to:
  • Avoid mouth rinses with high alcohol content because of drying effects.
  • Use daily home fluoride products for anticaries effect.
  • Use sugarless gum, frequent sips of water, or saliva substitutes.

omeprazole
oh-**mep'**-rah-zole
(Losec[CAN], Maxor[AUS], Prilosec, Prilosec OTC, Probitor[AUS], Zegerid)
Do not confuse Prilosec with prilocaine, Prinivil, or Prozac.

CATEGORY AND SCHEDULE
Pregnancy Risk Category: C

Drug Class: Antisecretory, proton pump inhibitor

MECHANISM OF ACTION
A benzimidazole that is converted to active metabolites that irreversibly bind to and inhibit hydrogen-potassium adenosine triphosphatase, an enzyme on the surface of gastric parietal cells. Inhibits hydrogen ion transport into gastric lumen.
Therapeutic Effect: Increases gastric pH, reduces gastric acid production.

USES
Treatment of gastroesophageal reflux disease (GERD), severe erosive esophagitis, poorly responsive systemic GERD, pathologic hypersecretory conditions (Zollinger-Ellison syndrome, systemic mastocytosis, multiple endocrine adenomas), with clarithromycin, short-term treatment of gastric ulcers; not approved for long-term ulcer maintenance therapy

PHARMACOKINETICS

Route	Onset	Peak	Duration
PO	1 hr	2 hr	72 hr

Rapidly absorbed from the GI tract. Protein binding: 99%. Primarily distributed into gastric parietal cells. Metabolized extensively in the liver. Primarily excreted in urine. Unknown if removed by hemodialysis. *Half-life:* 0.5–1 hr (increased in patients with hepatic impairment).

INDICATIONS AND DOSAGES
▸ **Erosive Esophagitis, Poorly Responsive GERD, Active Duodenal Ulcer, Prevention and Treatment of NSAID-Induced Ulcers**
PO
Adults, Elderly. 20 mg/day.
▸ **To Maintain Healing of Erosive Esophagitis**
PO
Adults, Elderly. 20 mg/day.
▸ **Pathologic Hypersecretory Conditions**
PO
Adults, Elderly. Initially, 60 mg/day up to 120 mg 3 times a day.
▸ **Duodenal Ulcer Caused by *H. pylori***
PO
Adults, Elderly. 20 mg twice a day for 10 days.

O

▸ **Active Benign Gastric Ulcer**
PO
Adults, Elderly. 40 mg/day for
4–8 wk.
▸ **Usual Pediatric Dosage**
*Children older than 2 yr, weighing
20 kg and more.* 20 mg/day.
*Children older than 2 yr, weighing
less than 20 kg.* 10 mg/day.

SIDE EFFECTS/ADVERSE REACTIONS
Frequent
Headache
Occasional
Diarrhea, abdominal pain, nausea
Rare
Dizziness, asthenia or loss of
strength, vomiting, constipation,
upper respiratory tract infection,
back pain, rash, cough

PRECAUTIONS AND CONTRAINDICATIONS
Hypersensitivity
Caution:
Lactation, children

DRUG INTERACTIONS OF CONCERN TO DENTISTRY
• Increased serum levels: diazepam

SERIOUS REACTIONS
! None known

DENTAL CONSIDERATIONS

General:
• Question the patient about
tolerance of NSAIDs or aspirin
related to GI problem.
• Consider semisupine chair position
for patient comfort because of GI
effects of disease.
• Assess salivary flow as a factor in
caries, periodontal disease, and
candidiasis.

Teach Patient/Family to:
• Use caution to prevent injury when
using oral hygiene aids.
• When chronic dry mouth occurs,
advise patient to:
  • Avoid mouth rinses with high
  alcohol content because of
  drying effects.
  • Use daily home fluoride
  products to prevent caries.
  • Use sugarless gum, frequent
  sips of water, or saliva
  substitutes.

oprelvekin (interleukin-2, IL-2)
oh-**prel′**-vee-kinn
(Neumega)
Do not confuse Neumega with
Neupogen.

CATEGORY AND SCHEDULE
Schedule IV
Pregnancy Risk Category: C

Drug Class: Hematopoietic;
platelet growth factor

MECHANISM OF ACTION
A hematopoietic that stimulates
production of blood platelets,
essential to the blood-clotting
process.
Therapeutic Effect: Increases
platelet production.

USES
Prevention of low platelet counts
caused by treatment with some
cancer medicines

PHARMACOKINETICS
Peak 3.2 hr following single
subcutaneous dose. *Half-life:* 6.9 hr.
Rapidly excreted by the kidneys.

INDICATIONS AND DOSAGES
▸ **Prevention of Thrombocytopenia**
Subcutaneous
Adults. 50 mcg/kg once a day.
Children. 75–100 mcg/kg once a
day. Continue for 14–28 days or
until platelet count reaches 50,000
cells/mcl after its nadir.

SIDE EFFECTS/ADVERSE REACTIONS
Frequent
Nausea or vomiting, fluid retention,
neutropenic fever, diarrhea, rhinitis,
headache, dizziness, fever, insomnia,
cough, rash, pharyngitis,
tachycardia, vasodilation

PRECAUTIONS AND CONTRAINDICATIONS
None known

DRUG INTERACTIONS OF CONCERN TO DENTISTRY
• No data available

SERIOUS REACTIONS
! Transient atrial fibrillation or
flutter occurs in 10% of patients and
may be caused by increased plasma
volume; oprelvekin is not directly
dysrhythmogenic. Dysrhythmias are
usually brief in duration and convert
spontaneously to normal sinus
rhythm.
! Papilledema may occur in
children.

DENTAL CONSIDERATIONS

General:
• If bleeding problem has not been
diagnosed, refer for evaluation prior
to any dental treatment.
• Question patient about medical
and drug history in relationship to
bleeding problems.
• Provide dental treatment in
conjunction with hematologist.

• Patients may present with
localized gingival bleeding with
incomplete clotting.
• Avoid elective dental procedures if
severe neutropenia (more than 500
cells/mm³) or thrombocytopenia
(fewer than 50,000 cells/mm³) is
present.
• Avoid products that affect platelet
function, such as aspirin and
NSAIDs.
• Monitor and record vital signs.
• Consider local hemostasis
measures to prevent excessive
bleeding.
• Short appointments and a
stress-reduction protocol may be
required for anxious patients.
• Place on frequent recall to evaluate
healing response.
Consultations:
• Consultation with hematologist or
physician of record required.
• Medical consultation should
include routine blood counts,
including platelet counts and
bleeding time.
• Consultation with physician may
be necessary if sedation or general
anesthesia is required.
• In a patient with symptoms of
blood dyscrasias, request a medical
consultation for blood studies and
postpone treatment until normal
values are reestablished.
• Medical consultation should
include PPT or INR.
Teach Patient/Family to:
• Use soft tooth brush to prevent
trauma to oral tissues and risk of
bleeding.
• Encourage effective oral
hygiene to prevent soft tissue
inflammation.
• Report oral lesions, soreness, or
bleeding to dentist.
• Update health and medication
history if physician makes any
changes in evaluation or drug

regimens; include OTC, herbal, and nonherbal drugs in the update.
• Prevent trauma when using oral hygiene aids.

orlistat
ohr′-lih-stat
(Xenical)
Do not confuse Xenical with Xeloda.

CATEGORY AND SCHEDULE
Pregnancy Risk Category: B

Drug Class: Antiobesity

MECHANISM OF ACTION
A gastric and pancreatic lipase inhibitor that inhibits absorption of dietary fats by inactivating gastric and pancreatic enzymes.
Therapeutic Effect: Resulting caloric deficit may positively affect weight control.

USES
Obesity management, including weight loss and maintenance in conjunction with a reduced-calorie diet; used in patients with a defined body mass index with other risk factors for cardiovascular disease

PHARMACOKINETICS
Minimal absorption after administration. Protein binding: 99%. Primarily eliminated unchanged in feces. Unknown if removed by hemodialysis. *Half-life:* 1–2 hr.

INDICATIONS AND DOSAGES
▶ **Weight Reduction**
PO
Adults, Elderly, Children 12–16 yr.
120 mg 3 times a day.

SIDE EFFECTS/ADVERSE REACTIONS
Frequent
Headache, abdominal discomfort, flatulence, fecal urgency, fatty or oily stool
Occasional
Back pain, menstrual irregularity, nausea, fatigue, diarrhea, dizziness
Rare
Anxiety, rash, myalgia, dry skin, vomiting

PRECAUTIONS AND CONTRAINDICATIONS
Cholestasis, chronic malabsorption syndrome
Caution:
Adherence to dietary guidelines, supplemental fat-soluble vitamins may be required, along with beta-carotene, nephrolithiasis, use in children not established

DRUG INTERACTIONS OF CONCERN TO DENTISTRY
• None reported

SERIOUS REACTIONS
! None known

DENTAL CONSIDERATIONS
General:
• Although no dental drug interactions are reported, observe expected outcomes of systemically administered drugs.
• Severely obese patients may have Type 2 diabetes or cardiovascular diseases.
• Consider semisupine chair position for patient comfort if GI side effects occur.
• Ensure that patient is following prescribed diet and regularly takes medication.

Consultations:
• Medical consultation may be required to assess disease control.
Teach Patient/Family to:
• Update health and drug history if physician makes any changes in evaluation or drug regimens; include OTC, herbal, and nonherbal drugs in the update.

orphenadrine
or-**fen**′-ah-dreen
(Norflex, Orphenace[CAN], Rhoxal-orphenadrine[CAN])

CATEGORY AND SCHEDULE
Pregnancy Risk Category: C

Drug Class: Skeletal muscle relaxant

MECHANISM OF ACTION
A skeletal muscle relaxant that is structurally related to diphenhydramine and is thought to indirectly affect skeletal muscle by central atropine-like effects.
Therapeutic Effect: Relieves musculoskeletal pain.

USES
Treatment of pain in musculoskeletal conditions

PHARMACOKINETICS
Well absorbed after PO and IM absorption. Protein binding: low. Metabolized in liver. Primarily excreted in urine and feces.
Half-life: 14 hr.

INDICATIONS AND DOSAGES
▶ Musculoskeletal Pain
IM/IV
Adults, Elderly. 60 mg 2 times a day. Switch to oral form for maintenance.

PO
Adults, Elderly. 100 mg 2 times a day.

SIDE EFFECTS/ADVERSE REACTIONS
Frequent
Drowsiness, dizziness, muscular weakness, hypotension, dry mouth, nose, throat, and lips, urinary retention, thickening of bronchial secretions
Elderly. Sedation, dizziness, hypotension
Occasional
Elderly. Flushing, visual or hearing disturbances, paresthesia, diaphoresis, chill

PRECAUTIONS AND CONTRAINDICATIONS
Angle-closure glaucoma, myasthenia gravis, pyloric or duodenal obstruction, stenosing peptic ulcer, prostatic hypertrophy, obstruction of the bladder neck, achalasia, cardiospasm (megaesophagus), hypersensitivity to orphenadrine or any component of the formulation
Caution:
Children, cardiac disease, tachycardia, caution in lactation

DRUG INTERACTIONS OF CONCERN TO DENTISTRY
• Increased CNS effects: CNS depressants, alcohol
• Increased anticholinergic effect: other anticholinergics

SERIOUS REACTIONS
! Hypersensitivity reaction, such as eczema, pruritus, rash, cardiac disturbances, and photosensitivity, may occur.
! Overdosage may vary from CNS depression, including sedation, apnea, hypotension, cardiovascular

O

collapse, or death, to severe paradoxical reaction, such as hallucinations, tremors, and seizures.

DENTAL CONSIDERATIONS

General:
• Consider semisupine chair position for patients with back pain.
• Patients on chronic drug therapy may rarely have symptoms of blood dyscrasias, which can include infection, bleeding, and poor healing.
• Assess salivary flow as a factor in caries, periodontal disease, and candidiasis.

Consultations:
• In a patient with symptoms of blood dyscrasias, request a medical consultation for blood studies and postpone dental treatment until normal values are reestablished.
• Medical consultation may be required to assess disease control.

Teach Patient/Family to:
• Encourage effective oral hygiene to prevent soft tissue inflammation.
• Use caution to prevent injury when using oral hygiene aids.
• Use caution when driving or operating equipment because of risk of dizziness.
• When chronic dry mouth occurs, advise patient to:
  • Avoid mouth rinses with high alcohol content because of drying effects.
  • Use daily home fluoride products to prevent caries.
  • Use sugarless gum, frequent sips of water, or saliva substitutes.

oseltamivir
oh-sell-**tam**′-ah-veer
(Tamiflu)

CATEGORY AND SCHEDULE
Pregnancy Risk Category: C

Drug Class: Antiviral

MECHANISM OF ACTION
A selective inhibitor of influenza virus neuraminidase, an enzyme essential for viral replication. Acts against both influenza A and B viruses.
Therapeutic Effect: Suppresses the spread of infection within the respiratory system and reduces the duration of clinical symptoms.

USES
Treatment of uncomplicated acute illness caused by influenza infection in adults who have been symptomatic for no more than 2 days; more effective against influenza type A virus; prophylaxis for adults and children older than 13 yr

PHARMACOKINETICS
Readily absorbed. Protein binding: 3%. Extensively converted to active drug in the liver. Primarily excreted in urine. **Half-life:** 6–10 hr.

INDICATIONS AND DOSAGES
▸ **Influenza**
PO
Adults, Elderly. 75 mg 2 times a day for 5 days.
Children weighing more than 40 kg. 75 mg twice a day.
Children weighing 24–40 kg. 60 mg twice a day.
Children weighing 15–23 kg. 45 mg twice a day.

Children weighing less than 15 kg.
30 mg twice a day.
▸ **Prevention of Influenza**
PO
Adults, Elderly. 75 mg once a day.
▸ **Dosage in Renal Impairment**
PO
Adults, Elderly. Dosage is decreased
to 75 mg once a day for at least 7
days and possibly up to 6 wk.

SIDE EFFECTS/ADVERSE REACTIONS
Frequent
Nausea, vomiting, diarrhea
Occasional
Abdominal pain, bronchitis,
dizziness, headache, cough,
insomnia, fatigue, vertigo

PRECAUTIONS AND CONTRAINDICATIONS
Hypersensitivity
Caution:
Renal impairment, lactation

DRUG INTERACTIONS OF CONCERN TO DENTISTRY
• None reported

SERIOUS REACTIONS
! Colitis, pneumonia, and pyrexia
occur rarely.

DENTAL CONSIDERATIONS
General:
• Acute influenza patients are
unlikely to be seen in the dental
office except for dental
emergencies.
• Consider semisupine chair position
for patient comfort because of
respiratory effects of disease.

oxacillin
ox-ah-**sill**´-in

CATEGORY AND SCHEDULE
Pregnancy Risk Category: B

Drug Class: Broad-spectrum
antiinfective; beta lactamase-
resistant penicillin

MECHANISM OF ACTION
A penicillin that binds to bacterial
membranes.
Therapeutic Effect: Bactericidal.

USES
Treatment of infections caused by
beta lactamase-producing bacteria

PHARMACOKINETICS
PO/IM: Peak 30–60 min, duration
4–6 hr **IV:** Peak 5 min, duration
4–6 hr. *Half-life:* 30–60 min.
Metabolized in the liver; excreted in
urine, bile, breast milk, crosses
placenta.

INDICATIONS AND DOSAGES
▸ **Upper Respiratory Tract, Skin, and Skin-Structure Infections**
IV, IM
*Adults, Elderly, Children weighing
40 kg or more.* 250–500 mg
q4–6h.
Children weighing less than 40 kg.
50 mg/kg/day in divided doses q6h.
Maximum: 12 g/day.
▸ **Lower Respiratory Tract and Other Serious Infections**
IV, IM
*Adults, Elderly, Children weighing
40 kg or more.* 1 g q4–6h.
Maximum: 12 g/day.
Children weighing less than 40 kg.
100 mg/kg/day in divided doses
q4–6h.

SIDE EFFECTS/ADVERSE REACTIONS

Frequent

Mild hypersensitivity reaction (fever, rash, pruritus), GI effects (nausea, vomiting, diarrhea)

Occasional

Phlebitis, thrombophlebitis (more common in elderly), hepatotoxicity (with high IV dosage)

PRECAUTIONS AND CONTRAINDICATIONS

Hypersensitivity to any penicillin

DRUG INTERACTIONS OF CONCERN TO DENTISTRY

• Increased or prolonged plasma levels: probenecid
• Aminoglycosides: injections must be separated by 1 hr
• Possible decrease in antimicrobial effectiveness: tetracyclines, erythromycins, lincomycins
• Suspected increase in methotrexate toxicity

SERIOUS REACTIONS

! Antibiotic-associated colitis and other superinfections may result from altered bacterial balance.
! A mild to severe hypersensitivity reaction may occur in those allergic to penicillins.

DENTAL CONSIDERATIONS

General:
• Determine why patient is taking the drug.
• Caution regarding allergy to medication.

Consultations:
• Consult patient's physician if an acute dental infection occurs and another antiinfective is required.
• Medical consultation may be required to assess disease control.

Teach Patient/Family to:
• Encourage effective oral hygiene to prevent soft tissue inflammation.
• Prevent trauma when using oral hygiene aids.
• When antibiotics are used for dental infection:
    • Report sore throat, oral burning sensation, fever, or fatigue, any of which could indicate presence of a superinfection.

oxaliplatin

ahks-al-eh-**plah**′-tin
(Eloxatin)

CATEGORY AND SCHEDULE

Pregnancy Risk Category: D

Drug Class: Antineoplastic; platinum coordination complex

MECHANISM OF ACTION

A platinum-containing complex that cross-links with DNA strands, preventing cell division. Cell cycle-phase nonspecific.
Therapeutic Effect: Inhibits DNA replication.

USES

Treatment of metastatic carcinoma of the colon or rectum in combination with 5-FU/leucovorin

PHARMACOKINETICS

Rapidly distributed. Protein binding: 90%. Undergoes rapid, extensive nonenzymatic biotransformation. Excreted in urine. *Half-life:* 70 hr.

INDICATIONS AND DOSAGES
▶ **Metastatic Colon or Rectal Cancer in Patients Whose Disease Has Recurred or Progressed During or Within 6 Mo of Completing First-Line Therapy with Bolus 5-Fluorouracil (5-FU), Leucovorin, and Irinotecan**
IV
Adults. Day 1: Oxaliplatin 85 mg/m^2 in 250–500 ml D5W and leucovorin 200 mg/m^2, both given simultaneously over more than 2 hr in separate bags using a Y-line, followed by 5-FU 400 mg/m^2 IV bolus given over 2–4 min, followed by 5-FU 600 mg/m^2 in 500 ml D5W as a 22-hr continuous IV infusion. Day 2: Leucovorin 200 mg/m^2 IV infusion given over more than 2 hr, followed by 5-FU 400 mg/m^2 IV bolus given over 2–4 min, followed by 5-FU 600 mg/m^2 in 500 ml D5W as a 22-hr continuous IV infusion.
▶ **Ovarian Cancer**
IV
Adults. Cisplatin 100 mg/m^2 and oxaliplatin 130 mg/m^2 every 3 wk.

SIDE EFFECTS/ADVERSE REACTIONS
Frequent
Peripheral or sensory neuropathy (usually occurs in hands, feet, perioral area, and throat but may present as jaw spasm, abnormal tongue sensation, eye pain, chest pressure, or difficulty walking, swallowing, or writing), nausea, fatigue, diarrhea, vomiting, constipation, abdominal pain, fever, anorexia
Occasional
Stomatitis, earache, insomnia, cough, difficulty breathing, backache, edema

Rare
Dyspepsia, dizziness, rhinitis, flushing, alopecia

PRECAUTIONS AND CONTRAINDICATIONS
History of allergy to platinum compounds

DRUG INTERACTIONS OF CONCERN TO DENTISTRY
• None reported

SERIOUS REACTIONS
! Peripheral or sensory neuropathy can occur, sometimes precipitated or exacerbated by drinking or holding a glass of cold liquid during the IV infusion.
! Pulmonary fibrosis, characterized by a nonproductive cough, dyspnea, crackles, and radiologic pulmonary infiltrates, may require drug discontinuation.
! Hypersensitivity reaction (rash, urticaria, pruritus) occurs rarely.

DENTAL CONSIDERATIONS
General:
• If additional analgesia is required for dental pain, consider alternative analgesics (NSAIDs) in patients taking opioids for acute or chronic pain.
• Examine for oral manifestation of opportunistic infection.
• Avoid products that affect platelet function, such as aspirin and NSAIDs.
• This drug may be used in the hospital or on an outpatient basis. Confirm the patient's disease and treatment status.
• Chlorhexidine mouth rinse prior to and during chemotherapy may reduce severity of mucositis.
• Patient on chronic drug therapy may rarely present with symptoms

of blood dyscrasias, which can include infection, bleeding, and poor healing. If dyscrasia is present, caution patient to prevent oral tissue trauma when using oral hygiene aids.
• Palliative medication may be required for management of oral side effects.
• Short appointments and a stress-reduction protocol may be required for anxious patients.
• Provide palliative emergency dental care during drug use.
• Patients may be at risk of bleeding; check for oral signs.
• Oral infections should be eliminated and treated aggressively.
• Monitor vital signs.
Consultations:
• Medical consultation should include routine blood counts, including platelet counts and bleeding time.
• Consult physician; prophylactic or therapeutic antiinfectives may be indicated if surgery or periodontal treatment is required.
• Medical consultation may be required to assess immunologic status during cancer chemotherapy and determine safety risk, if any, posed by the required dental treatment.
• Medical consultation may be required to assess disease control and patient's ability to tolerate stress.
Teach Patient/Family to:
• See dentist immediately if secondary oral infection occurs.
• Be aware of oral side effects.
• Encourage effective oral hygiene to prevent soft tissue inflammation.
• Report oral lesions, soreness, or bleeding to dentist.
• Prevent trauma when using oral hygiene aids.

• Update health and medication history if physician makes any changes in evaluation or drug regimens; include OTC, herbal, and nonherbal drugs in the update.
• Avoid ice water rinses and exposure to cold to prevent exacerbation of neuropathy symptoms.

oxandrolone
ox-**an**′-droe-lone
(Lonavar[AUS], Oxandrin)
Do not confuse with testolactone.

CATEGORY AND SCHEDULE
Pregnancy Risk Category: X
Controlled substance: Schedule III

Drug Class: Androgenic anabolic steroid

MECHANISM OF ACTION
A synthetic testosterone derivative that promotes growth and development of male sex organs, maintains secondary sex characteristics in androgen-deficient males.
Therapeutic Effect: Androgenic and anabolic actions.

USES
Promotion of weight gain in catabolic or tissue wasting processes, such as extensive surgery, burns, infection, or trauma; HIV wasting syndrome; Turner's syndrome

PHARMACOKINETICS
Well absorbed from the GI tract. Protein binding: 94%–97%. Metabolized in liver. Primarily excreted in urine. Unknown if

removed by hemodialysis. *Half-life:* 5–13 hr.

INDICATIONS AND DOSAGES
▸ **Weight Gain**
Adults, Elderly. 2.5–20 mg in divided doses 2–4 times a day usually for 2–4 wk. Course of therapy is based on individual response. Repeat intermittently as needed.
Children. Total daily dose is 0.1 mg/kg. Repeat intermittently as needed.

SIDE EFFECTS/ADVERSE REACTIONS
Frequent
Gynecomastia, acne, amenorrhea, other menstrual irregularities
Females: Hirsutism, deepening of voice, clitoral enlargement that may not be reversible when drug is discontinued
Occasional
Edema, nausea, insomnia, oligospermia, priapism, male pattern of baldness, bladder irritability, hypercalcemia in immobilized patients or those with breast cancer, hypercholesterolemia
Rare
Polycythemia with high dosage

PRECAUTIONS AND CONTRAINDICATIONS
Nephrosis, carcinoma of breast or prostate hypercalcemia, pregnancy, hypersensitivity to oxandrolone or any component of the formulation
Caution:
Diabetes mellitus, cardiovascular disease, MI, increased risk of prostatic hypertrophy, prostatic carcinoma, virilization (women), increased PT

DRUG INTERACTIONS OF CONCERN TO DENTISTRY
• Increased risk of bleeding: aspirin
• Edema: adrenocorticotropic hormone (ACTH), adrenal steroids

SERIOUS REACTIONS
! Peliotic hepatitis of the liver, spleen replaced with blood-filled cysts, hepatic neoplasms and hepatocellular carcinoma have been associated with prolonged high-dosage, anaphylactic reactions.

DENTAL CONSIDERATIONS

General:
• Monitor vital signs at every appointment because of cardiovascular side effects.
• Determine why the patient is taking the drug.
• Consider local hemostasis measures to prevent excessive bleeding.
• Short appointments and a stress-reduction protocol may be required for anxious patients.
• Avoid prescribing aspirin-containing products.
Consultations:
• If signs of anemia are observed in oral tissues, physician consultation may be required.
• Medical consultation may be required to assess disease control and patient's ability to tolerate stress.
• Medical consultation should include INR.
Teach Patient/Family to:
• Encourage effective oral hygiene to prevent soft tissue inflammation.
• See dentist immediately if secondary oral infection occurs.

oxaprozin
ox-ah-**pro**′-zin
(Daypro)
Do not confuse oxaprozin with
oxazepam.

CATEGORY AND SCHEDULE
Pregnancy Risk Category: C (D if
used in third trimester or near
delivery)

Drug Class: Nonsteroidal
antiinflammatory

MECHANISM OF ACTION
An NSAID that produces analgesic
and antiinflammatory effects by
inhibiting prostaglandin synthesis.
Therapeutic Effect: Reduces the
inflammatory response and intensity
of pain.

USES
Treatment of rheumatoid arthritis,
osteoarthritis, and ankylosing
spondylitis

PHARMACOKINETICS
Well absorbed from the GI tract.
Protein binding: 99%. Widely
distributed. Metabolized in the liver.
Primarily excreted in urine; partially
eliminated in feces. Not removed by
hemodialysis. *Half-life:* 42–50 hr.

INDICATIONS AND DOSAGES
▸ **Osteoarthritis**
PO
Adults, Elderly. 1200 mg once a day
(600 mg in patients with low body
weight or mild disease). Maximum:
1800 mg/day.
▸ **Rheumatoid Arthritis**
PO
Adults, Elderly. 1200 mg once a day.
Range: 600–1800 mg/day.

▸ **Juvenile Rheumatoid Arthritis**
Children weighing more than 54 kg.
1200 mg/day.
Children weighing 32–54 kg.
900 mg/day.
Children weighing 22–31 kg.
600 mg/day.
▸ **Dosage in Renal Impairment**
For adults and elderly patients with
renal impairment, the recommended
initial dose is 600 mg/day; may be
increased up to 1200 mg/day.

SIDE EFFECTS/ADVERSE REACTIONS
Occasional
Nausea, diarrhea, constipation,
dyspepsia, edema
Rare
Vomiting, abdominal cramps or
pain, flatulence, anorexia, confusion,
tinnitus, insomnia, somnolence

PRECAUTIONS AND CONTRAINDICATIONS
Active peptic ulcer disease, chronic
inflammation of GI tract, GI
bleeding or ulceration, history of
hypersensitivity to aspirin or
NSAIDs
Caution:
• Lactation, children, bleeding
disorders, GI disorders, cardiac
disorders, hypersensitivity to other
antiinflammatory agents, diabetes

DRUG INTERACTIONS OF CONCERN TO DENTISTRY
• GI ulceration, bleeding: aspirin,
alcohol, corticosteroids
• Decreased action: salicylates
• Nephrotoxicity: acetaminophen
(prolonged use and high doses)
• Possible risk of decreased renal
function: cyclosporine
• SSRIs: increased risk of GI side
effects
• When prescribed for dental pain:

• Risk of increased effects: oral anticoagulants, oral antidiabetics, lithium, methotrexate
• Decreased antihypertensive effects of diuretics, β-adrenergic blockers, and ACE inhibitors

SERIOUS REACTIONS

! Hypertension, acute renal failure, respiratory depression, GI bleeding, and coma occur rarely.

DENTAL CONSIDERATIONS

General:
• Patients on chronic drug therapy may rarely have symptoms of blood dyscrasias, which can include infection, bleeding, and poor healing.
• Assess salivary flow as a factor in caries, periodontal disease, and candidiasis.
• Avoid prescribing for dental use in pregnancy.
• Consider semisupine chair position for patients with arthritic disease.
• Severe stomach bleeding may occur in patients who regularly use NSAIDs in recommended doses, when the patient is also taking another NSAID, an anticoagulent/ antiplatelet drug, or steroid drug, if the patient has GI or peptic ulcer disease, if they are 60 yr or older, or when NSAIDs are taken longer than directed. Warn patients of the potential for severe stomach bleeding.
Consultations:
• Medical consultation may be required to assess disease control.
• In a patient with symptoms of blood dyscrasias, request a medical consultation for blood studies and postpone dental treatment until normal values are reestablished.

Teach Patient/Family to:
• Encourage effective oral hygiene to prevent soft tissue inflammation.
• Use caution to prevent injury when using oral hygiene aids.
• Warn patient of potential risks of NSAIDs.
• When chronic dry mouth occurs, advise patient to:
  • Avoid mouth rinses with high alcohol content because of drying effects.
  • Use daily home fluoride products to prevent caries.
  • Use sugarless gum, frequent sips of water, or saliva substitutes.

oxazepam

ox-a′-ze-pam
(Alepam[AUS], Apo-Oxazepam[CAN], Murelax[AUS], Serax, Serepax[AUS])
Do not confuse oxazepam with oxaprozin, or Serax with Eurax or Xerac.

CATEGORY AND SCHEDULE

Pregnancy Risk Category: D
Controlled Substance Schedule IV

Drug Class: Benzodiazepine

MECHANISM OF ACTION

A benzodiazepine that potentiates the effects of gamma-aminobutyric acid and other inhibitory neurotransmitters by binding to specific receptors in the CNS.
Therapeutic Effect: Produces anxiolytic effect and skeletal muscle relaxation.

USES
Treatment of anxiety, alcohol withdrawal

PHARMACOKINETICS
Well absorbed from the GI tract. Protein binding: 97%. Metabolized in the liver. Primarily excreted in urine. Not removed by hemodialysis. *Half-life:* 5–20 hr.

INDICATIONS AND DOSAGES
▸ **Mild-to-Moderate Anxiety**
PO
Adults. 10–15 mg 3–4 times a day.
▸ **Severe Anxiety**
PO
Adults. 15–30 mg 3–4 times a day.
▸ **Alcohol Withdrawal**
PO
Adults. 15–30 mg 3–4 times a day.
Elderly. Initially, 10–20 mg 3 times a day. May gradually increase up to 30–45 mg/day.

SIDE EFFECTS/ADVERSE REACTIONS
Frequent
Mild, transient somnolence at beginning of therapy
Occasional
Dizziness, headache
Rare
Paradoxic CNS reactions, such as hyperactivity or nervousness in children and excitement or restlessness in the elderly or debilitated (generally noted during the first 2 wk of therapy)

PRECAUTIONS AND CONTRAINDICATIONS
Angle-closure glaucoma; preexisting CNS depression; severe, uncontrolled pain
Caution:
Elderly, debilitated, hepatic disease, renal disease

DRUG INTERACTIONS OF CONCERN TO DENTISTRY
• Increased effects: CNS depressants, alcohol, and anticonvulsant medications
• Possible increase in CNS side effects of kava kava (herb)

SERIOUS REACTIONS
! Abrupt or too-rapid withdrawal may result in pronounced restlessness, irritability, insomnia, hand tremors, abdominal or muscle cramps, diaphoresis, vomiting, and seizures.
! Overdose results in somnolence, confusion, diminished reflexes, and coma.

DENTAL CONSIDERATIONS
General:
• Monitor vital signs at every appointment because of cardiovascular side effects.
• Avoid use in pregnancy.
• Psychologic and physical dependence may occur with chronic administration.
• Geriatric patients are more susceptible to drug effects; use lower dose.
• Assess salivary flow as a factor in caries, periodontal disease, and candidiasis.
Consultations:
• Medical consultation may be required to assess disease control.
Teach Patient/Family to:
• Avoid mouth rinses with high alcohol content because of drying effects.

oxcarbazepine
oks-kar-**bays**'-uh-peen
(Trileptal)

CATEGORY AND SCHEDULE
Pregnancy Risk Category: C

Drug Class: Anticonvulsant

MECHANISM OF ACTION
An anticonvulsant that blocks sodium channels, resulting in stabilization of hyperexcited neural membranes, inhibition of repetitive neuronal firing, and diminishing synaptic impulses.
Therapeutic Effect: Prevents seizures.

USES
Monotherapy or adjunctive therapy of partial seizures in adults with epilepsy; monotherapy or adjunctive therapy for partial seizures in children (4–16 yr) with epilepsy

PHARMACOKINETICS
Completely absorbed from GI tract and extensively metabolized in the liver to active metabolite. Protein binding: 40%. Primarily excreted in urine. *Half-life:* 2 hr; metabolite, 6–10 hr.

INDICATIONS AND DOSAGES
▶ **Adjunctive Treatment of Seizures**
PO
Adults, Elderly. Initially, 600 mg/day in 2 divided doses. May increase by up to 600 mg/day at weekly intervals. Maximum: 2400 mg/day.
Children 4–16 yr. 8–10 mg/kg. Maximum: 600 mg/day.
Maintenance (based on weight): 1800 mg/day for children weighing more than 39 kg; 1200 mg/day for children weighing 29.1–39 kg; and 900 mg/day for children weighing 20–29 kg.
▶ **Conversion to Monotherapy**
PO
Adults, Elderly. 600 mg/day in 2 divided doses (while decreasing concomitant anticonvulsant over 3–6 wk). May increase by 600 mg/day at weekly intervals up to 2400 mg/day.
Children. Initially, 8–10 mg/kg/day in 2 divided doses with simultaneous initial reduction of dose of concomitant antiepileptic.
▶ **Initiation of Monotherapy**
PO
Adults, Elderly. 600 mg/day in 2 divided doses. May increase by 300 mg/day every 3 days up to 1200 mg/day.
Children. Initially, 8–10 mg/kg/day in 2 divided doses. Increase at 3 day intervals by 5 mg/kg/day to achieve maintenance dose by weight;
(70 kg): 1500–2100 mg/day;
(60–69 kg): 1200–2100 mg/day;
(50–59 kg): 1200–1800 mg/day;
(41–49 kg): 1200–1500 mg/day;
(35–40 kg): 900–1500 mg/day;
(25–34 kg): 900–1200 mg/day;
(20–24 kg): 600–900 mg/day.
▶ **Dosage in Renal Impairment**
For patients with creatinine clearance less than 30 ml/min, give 50% of normal starting dose, then titrate slowly to desired dose.

SIDE EFFECTS/ADVERSE REACTIONS
Frequent
Dizziness, nausea, headache
Occasional
Vomiting, diarrhea, ataxia, nervousness, heartburn, indigestion, epigastric pain, constipation
Rare
Tremors, rash, back pain, epistaxis, sinusitis, diplopia

O

PRECAUTIONS AND CONTRAINDICATIONS

Hypersensitivity to this drug or carbamazepine

Caution:

Development of hyponatremia, withdraw drug slowly to avoid seizures, cognitive CNS adverse effects, decreases effect of oral contraceptives, caution when used with other anticonvulsants, renal impairment, lactation

DRUG INTERACTIONS OF CONCERN TO DENTISTRY

• No dental drug interactions reported; CYP450 3A4/5 enzyme inducers may decrease plasma levels
• Possible increase in CNS depression: all CNS depressants, alcohol

SERIOUS REACTIONS

! Clinically significant hyponatremia may occur.

DENTAL CONSIDERATIONS

General:

• Monitor vital signs at every appointment because of cardiovascular side effects.
• Patients on chronic drug therapy may rarely have symptoms of blood dyscrasias, which can include infection, bleeding, and poor healing.
• Assess salivary flow as a factor in caries, periodontal disease, and candidiasis.
• Consider semisupine chair position for patient comfort if GI side effects occur.
• Short appointments and a stress-reduction protocol may be required for anxious patients.
• Determine type of epilepsy, seizure frequency, and quality of seizure control.

Consultations:

• In a patient with symptoms of blood dyscrasias, request a medical consultation for blood studies and postpone treatment until normal values are reestablished.
• Medical consultation may be required to assess disease control and patient's ability to tolerate stress.

Teach Patient/Family to:

• Encourage effective oral hygiene to prevent soft tissue inflammation.
• Prevent trauma when using oral hygiene aids.
• When chronic dry mouth occurs, advise patient to:
  • Avoid mouth rinses with high alcohol content because of drying effects.
  • Use daily home fluoride products for anticaries effect.
  • Use sugarless gum, frequent sips of water, or saliva substitutes.

oxiconazole

ox-i-**con**′-a-zole
(Oxistat, Oxizole[CAN])
Do not confuse with Nitrostat.

CATEGORY AND SCHEDULE

Pregnancy Risk Category: B

Drug Class: Antifungals, topical, dermatologics

MECHANISM OF ACTION

An antifungal agent that inhibits ergosterol synthesis.
Therapeutic Effect: Destroys cytoplasmic membrane integrity of fungi. Fungicidal.

USES

Treatment of infections caused by a fungus

PHARMACOKINETICS

Low systemic absorption. Absorbed and distributed in each layer of the dermis. Excreted in the urine.

INDICATIONS AND DOSAGES

▶ **Tinea pedis**

Topical

Adults, Elderly, Children 12 yr and older. Apply 1–2 times a day for 1 mo or until signs and symptoms significantly improve.

▶ **Tinea cruris, Tinea corporis**

Topical

Adults, Elderly, Children 12 yr and older. Apply 1–2 times a day for 2 wk or until signs and symptoms significantly improve.

SIDE EFFECTS/ADVERSE REACTIONS

Occasional

Itching, local irritation, stinging, dryness

PRECAUTIONS AND CONTRAINDICATIONS

Not for ophthalmic use, hypersensitivity to oxiconazole or any other azole fungals

DRUG INTERACTIONS OF CONCERN TO DENTISTRY

• None reported

SERIOUS REACTIONS

! Hypersensitivity reactions characterized by rash, swelling, pruritus, maceration, and a sensation of warmth may occur.

DENTAL CONSIDERATIONS

General:

• Determine why the patient is using this medication.

---

oxidized cellulose
oks′-ih-dye-zed **cell**′-you-lose
(Interceed, Surgicel)

CATEGORY AND SCHEDULE
Pregnancy Risk Category: Not reported

Drug Class: Cellulose hemostatic

MECHANISM OF ACTION

Oxidized cellulose is saturated with blood at the bleeding site and swells into a gelatinous mass that aids in clot formation. When used in small amounts, it is absorbed from the sites of implantation with minimal tissue reaction.
Therapeutic Effect: Reduces bleeding.

USES

Hemostasis in surgery, oral surgery, exodontia

PHARMACOKINETICS

Absorption occurs in 7–14 days.
Half-life: Unknown.

INDICATIONS AND DOSAGES

▶ **Surgical Procedures to Assist in the Control of Capillary, Venous, and Small Arterial Hemorrhage When Ligation or Other Conventional Methods of Control Are Impractical or Ineffective**

Topical

Adults. Minimal amounts of an appropriate size are laid on the bleeding site or held firmly against the tissues until hemostasis is obtained.

SIDE EFFECTS/ADVERSE REACTIONS

Frequency Not Defined
Headache, nasal burning or stinging, sneezing, encapsulation of fluid

PRECAUTIONS AND CONTRAINDICATIONS

Use for packing or implantation in fractures or laminectomies, hemorrhage from large arteries, and nonhemorrhagic oozing surfaces; use as a wrap; use around the optic nerve and chiasm; applied as wadding or packing as a hemostatic agent; hypersensitivity to oxidized cellulose or any component of the formulation
Caution:
Do not autoclave; inactivation of topical thrombin

SERIOUS REACTIONS

! Pain, numbness, and paralysis have been reported.

0

DENTAL CONSIDERATIONS

General:
• Apply dry; use only amount needed to control bleeding.
• Place loosely and avoid packing; remove excess before closure in surgery; irrigate first, then remove using sterile technique.
• Ensure therapeutic response: decreased bleeding in surgery.
• Can be left in situ when necessary but should be removed once bleeding is controlled.
• Application of topical thrombin solution to the cellulose gauze will inactivate thrombin because of acidity.

oxybutynin

ox-ih-**byoo**′-ti-nin
(Ditropan, Ditropan XL, Oxytrol)
Do not confuse oxybutynin with OxyContin, or Ditropan with diazepam.

CATEGORY AND SCHEDULE

Pregnancy Risk Category: B

Drug Class: Antispasmodic

MECHANISM OF ACTION

An anticholinergic that exerts antispasmodic (papaverine-like) and antimuscarinic (atropine-like) action on the detrusor smooth muscle of the bladder.
Therapeutic Effect: Increases bladder capacity and delays desire to void.

USES

Antispasmodic for neurogenic bladder, overactive bladder

PHARMACOKINETICS

Route	Onset	Peak	Duration
PO	0.5–1 hr	3–6 hr	6–10 hr

Rapidly absorbed from the GI tract. Metabolized in the liver. Primarily excreted in urine. Unknown if removed by hemodialysis. *Half-life:* 1–2.3 hr.

INDICATIONS AND DOSAGES
▸ **Neurogenic Bladder**
PO
Adults. 5 mg 2–3 times a day up to 5 mg 4 times a day.
Elderly. 2.5–5 mg twice a day. May increase by 2.5 mg/day every 1–2 days.

Children 5 yr and older. 5 mg twice a day up to 5 mg 4 times a day.
Children 1–4 yr. 0.2 mg/kg/dose 2–4 times a day.
PO (Extended-Release)
Adults. 5–10 mg/day up to 30 mg/ day.
Transdermal
Adults. 3.9 mg applied twice a week. Apply every 3–4 days.

SIDE EFFECTS/ADVERSE REACTIONS

Frequent
Constipation, dry mouth, somnolence, decreased perspiration
Occasional
Decreased lacrimation or salivation, impotence, urinary hesitancy and retention, suppressed lactation, blurred vision, mydriasis, nausea or vomiting, insomnia

PRECAUTIONS AND CONTRAINDICATIONS

GI or GU obstruction, glaucoma, myasthenia gravis, toxic megacolon, ulcerative colitis
Caution:
Lactation, suspected glaucoma, children younger than 12 yr, hiatal hernia, esophageal reflux, coronary heart disease, CHF, hypertension

DRUG INTERACTIONS OF CONCERN TO DENTISTRY

• Increased anticholinergic effect: anticholinergic drugs
• Increased depressant effect of both drugs: CNS depressants, alcohol

SERIOUS REACTIONS

! Overdose produces CNS excitation (including nervousness, restlessness, hallucinations, and irritability), hypotension or hypertension, confusion, tachycardia, facial flushing, and respiratory depression.

DENTAL CONSIDERATIONS

General:
• Assess salivary flow as a factor in caries, periodontal disease, and candidiasis.
• Monitor vital signs at every appointment because of cardiovascular side effects.
• Avoid dental light in patient's eyes; offer dark glasses for patient comfort.
• Consider semisupine chair position for patient comfort if GI side effects occur.
Consultations:
• Physician should be informed if significant xerostomic side effects occur (e.g., increased caries, sore tongue, problems eating or swallowing, difficulty wearing prosthesis) so that a medication change can be considered.
Teach Patient/Family to:
• Encourage effective oral hygiene to prevent soft tissue inflammation.
• When chronic dry mouth occurs, advise patient to:
  • Avoid mouth rinses with high alcohol content because of drying effects.
  • Use daily home fluoride products to prevent caries.
  • Use sugarless gum, frequent sips of water, or saliva substitutes.

O

oxycodone
ox-ee-**koe**'-done
(Endone[AUS], OxyContin,
Oxydose, OxyFast, OxyIR,
Oxynorm[AUS], Roxicodone,
Roxicodone Intensol)
Do not confuse oxycodone with
oxybutynin.

CATEGORY AND SCHEDULE
Pregnancy Risk Category: B (D if
used for prolonged periods or at
high dosages at term)
Controlled Substance: Schedule II

Drug Class: Synthetic opioid
analgesic

MECHANISM OF ACTION
An opioid analgesic that binds with
opioid receptors in the CNS.
Therapeutic Effect: Alters the
perception of and emotional
response to pain.

USES
Treatment of moderate-to-severe
pain, normally used in combination
with aspirin or acetaminophen;
combination products

PHARMACOKINETICS

Route	Onset	Peak	Duration
PO, immediate release	N/A	N/A	4–5 hr
PO, controlled release	N/A	N/A	12 hr

Moderately absorbed from the GI
tract. Protein binding: 38%–45%.
Widely distributed. Metabolized in
the liver. Excreted in urine.
Unknown if removed by
hemodialysis. *Half-life:* 2–3 hr
(3.2 hr controlled-release).

INDICATIONS AND DOSAGES
▸ **Analgesia**
PO (Controlled-Release)
Adults, Elderly. Initially, 10 mg
q12h. May increase every 1–2 days
by 25%–50%. Usual: 40 mg/day
(100 mg/day for cancer pain).
PO (Immediate-Release)
Adults, Elderly. Initially, 5 mg q6h
as needed. May increase up to
30 mg q4h. Usual: 10–30 mg q4h as
needed.
Children. 0.05–0.15 mg/kg/dose
q4–6h.

SIDE EFFECTS/ADVERSE REACTIONS
Frequent
Somnolence, dizziness, hypotension
(including orthostatic hypotension),
anorexia
Occasional
Confusion, diaphoresis, facial
flushing, urine retention,
constipation, dry mouth, nausea,
vomiting, headache
Rare
Allergic reaction, depression,
paradoxic CNS hyperactivity or
nervousness in children, paradoxic
excitement and restlessness in
elderly or debilitated patients

PRECAUTIONS AND CONTRAINDICATIONS
Hypersensitivity, addiction (narcotic)
Caution:
Addictive personality, lactation,
increased intracranial pressure, MI
(acute), severe heart disease,
respiratory depression, hepatic
disease, renal disease, children
younger than 18 yr, physical
dependence

DRUG INTERACTIONS OF CONCERN TO DENTISTRY

• Increased effects with other CNS depressants: alcohol, other narcotics, sedative-hypnotics, skeletal muscle relaxants, phenothiazines, benzodiazepines
• Contraindication: MAOIs
• Increased effects of anticholinergics
• Partial antagonists (e.g., pentazocine) may precipitate withdrawal

SERIOUS REACTIONS

! Overdose results in respiratory depression, skeletal muscle flaccidity, cold or clammy skin, cyanosis, and extreme somnolence progressing to seizures, stupor, and coma.
! Hepatotoxicity may occur with overdose of the acetaminophen component of fixed-combination products.
! The patient who uses oxycodone repeatedly may develop a tolerance to the drug's analgesic effect and physical dependence.

DENTAL CONSIDERATIONS

General:
• Monitor vital signs at every appointment because of cardiovascular and respiratory side effects.
• Assess salivary flow as a factor in caries, periodontal disease, and candidiasis.
• Psychologic and physical dependence may occur with chronic administration.
• Determine why the patient is taking the drug.
Teach Patient/Family to:
• Avoid mouth rinses with high alcohol content because of drying effects.

oxymetazoline

ox-ee-met-**az**′-oh-leen
(Afrin, Afrin 12-Hour, Afrin Children's Strength Nose Drops, OcuClear, Sinex 12 Hour Long-Acting)

CATEGORY AND SCHEDULE

Pregnancy Risk Category: C
OTC

Drug Class: Nasal decongestant, sympathomimetic amine

MECHANISM OF ACTION

A direct-acting sympathomimetic amine that acts on α-adrenergic receptors in arterioles of the nasal mucosa to produce constriction. *Therapeutic Effect:* Causes vasoconstriction resulting in decreased blood flow and decreased nasal congestion.

USES

Treatment of nasal congestion

PHARMACOKINETICS

Onset of action is about 10 min, and duration of action is 7 hr or more. Absorption occurs from the nasal mucosa and can produce systemic effects, primarily following overdose or excessive use. Excreted mostly in the urine, as well as the feces. *Half-life:* 5–8 hr.

INDICATIONS AND DOSAGES
▶ Rhinitis
Intranasal
Adults, Elderly, Children older than 6 yr. 2–3 drops/sprays (0.05% nasal solution) in each nostril q12h.
Children 2–5 yr. 2–4 drops or sprays (0.025% nasal solution) in each nostril q12h for up to 3 days.

▸ **Conjunctivitis**
Ophthalmic
Adults, Elderly, Children older than 6 yr. 1–2 drops (0.025% ophthalmic solution) q6h for 3–4 days.

SIDE EFFECTS/ADVERSE REACTIONS
Occasional
Burning, stinging, drying nasal mucosa, sneezing, rebound congestion, insomnia, nervousness

PRECAUTIONS AND CONTRAINDICATIONS
Narrow-angle glaucoma or hypersensitivity to oxymetazoline or other adrenergic agents
Caution:
Children younger than 6 yr, elderly, diabetes, cardiovascular disease, hypertension, hyperthyroidism, increased intracranial pressure, prostatic hypertrophy, glaucoma

DRUG INTERACTIONS OF CONCERN TO DENTISTRY
• Increased risk of hypertension: tricyclic antidepressants, but it requires adequate systemic absorption of oxymetazoline

SERIOUS REACTIONS
! Large doses may produce tachycardia, hypertension, arrhythmias, palpitations, light-headedness, nausea, and vomiting.

DENTAL CONSIDERATIONS

General:
• Excessive use can lead to rebound congestion and cardiovascular side effects; follow recommended dosing intervals.
• Extensive nasal swelling and congestion may interfere with optimal use of nitrous oxide/oxygen sedation.

oxymetholone
ox-ee-**meth**′-oh-lone
(Anadrol, Anapolon[CAN])
Do not confuse with oxycodone.

CATEGORY AND SCHEDULE
Pregnancy Risk Category: X
Controlled substance: Schedule III

Drug Class: Androgenic anabolic steroid

MECHANISM OF ACTION
An androgenic-anabolic steroid that is a synthetic derivative of testosterone synthesized to accentuate anabolic as opposed to androgenic effects.
Therapeutic Effect: Improves nitrogen balance in conditions of unfavorable protein metabolism with adequate caloric and protein intake, stimulates erythropoiesis, suppresses gonadotropic functions of pituitary, and may exert a direct effect upon the testes.

USES
Anemia associated with bone marrow failure and red cell production deficiencies; aplastic anemia, myelofibrosis, and anemia caused by myelotoxic drugs

PHARMACOKINETICS
The pharmacokinetics of oxymetholone has been studied. Metabolized in the liver via reduction and oxidation. Unchanged oxymetholone and its metabolites are excreted in urine. *Half-life:* Unknown.

INDICATIONS AND DOSAGES
▶ **Anemia, Chronic Renal Failure, Acquired Aplastic Anemia, Chemotherapy-Induced Myelosuppression, Fanconi's Anemia, Red Cell Aplasia**
PO
Adults, Elderly, Children. 1–5 mg/kg/day. Response is not immediate, and a minimum of 3–6 mo should be given.

SIDE EFFECTS/ADVERSE REACTIONS
Frequent
Gynecomastia, acne, amenorrhea, menstrual irregularities
Females: Hirsutism, deepening of voice, clitoral enlargement that may not be reversible when drug is discontinued
Occasional
Edema, nausea, insomnia, oligospermia, priapism, male pattern of baldness, bladder irritability, hypercalcemia in immobilized patients or those with breast cancer, hypercholesterolemia, inflammation and pain at IM injection site
Transdermal: Itching, erythema, skin irritation
Rare
Liver damage, hypersensitivity

PRECAUTIONS AND CONTRAINDICATIONS
Cardiac impairment, hypercalcemia, pregnancy/lactation, prostatic or breast cancer in males, metastatic breast cancer in women with active hypercalcemia, nephrosis or nephritic phase nephritis, severe liver disease, hypersensitivity to oxymetholone or any of its components
Caution:
Diabetes mellitus, cardiovascular disease, MI, increased risk of prostatic hypertrophy, prostatic

carcinoma, virilization (women), increased PT

DRUG INTERACTIONS OF CONCERN TO DENTISTRY
• Increased risk of bleeding: aspirin
• Edema: ACTH, adrenal steroids

SERIOUS REACTIONS
! Cholestatic jaundice, hepatic necrosis and death occur rarely but have been reported in association with long-term androgenic-anabolic steroid use.

DENTAL CONSIDERATIONS
General:
• Monitor vital signs at every appointment because of cardiovascular side effects.
• Determine why the patient is taking the drug.
• Consider local hemostasis measures to prevent excessive bleeding.
• Short appointments and a stress-reduction protocol may be required for anxious patients.
• Avoid prescribing aspirin-containing products.
Consultations:
• Physician consultation may be required if signs of anemia are observed in oral tissues.
• Medical consultation may be required to assess disease control and patient's ability to tolerate stress.
• Medical consultation should include INR.
Teach Patient/Family to:
• Encourage effective oral hygiene to prevent soft tissue inflammation.
• See dentist immediately if secondary oral infection occurs.

paclitaxel

pak-leh-**tax'**-ell
(Abraxane, Anzatax[AUS], Onxol, Taxol)
Do not confuse paclitaxel with Paxil, or Taxol with Taxotere.

CATEGORY AND SCHEDULE
Pregnancy Risk Category: D

Drug Class: Antineoplastic

MECHANISM OF ACTION
An antimitotic agent in the taxoids family that disrupts the microtubular cell network, which is essential for cellular function. Blocks cells in the late G2 phase and M phase of the cell cycle.
Therapeutic Effect: Inhibits cellular mitosis and replication.

USES
Treatment of metastatic ovarian cancer, non–small-cell lung cancer; second-line treatment for AIDS-related Kaposi's sarcoma (KS); adjuvant treatment of node-positive breast cancer sequential to a course of standard doxorubicin-containing combination chemotherapy

PHARMACOKINETICS
Does not readily cross the blood-brain barrier. Protein binding: 89%–98%. Metabolized in the liver to active metabolites; eliminated by bile. Not removed by hemodialysis.
Half-life: 1.3–8.6 hr.

INDICATIONS AND DOSAGES
▸ **Ovarian Cancer**
IV
Adults. 135–175 mg/m^2/dose over 1–24 hr q3wk.

▸ **Breast Carcinoma**
IV (Onxol, Taxol)
Adults, Elderly. 175 mg/m^2 over 3 hr q3wk.
PO (Abraxane)
Adults, Elderly. 260 mg/m^2 over 30 min q3wk.

▸ **Non–Small-Cell Lung Carcinoma**
IV
Adults, Elderly. 135 mg/m^2 over 24 hr, followed by cisplatin 75 mg/m^2 q3wk.

▸ **KS**
IV
Adults, Elderly. 135 mg/m^2/dose over 3 hr q3wk or 100 mg/m^2/dose over 3 hr q2wk.

▸ **Dosage in Hepatic Impairment**

Total Bilirubin	Total Dose
More than 3 mg/dl	Less than 50 mg/m^2
1.6–3 mg/dl	Less than 75 mg/m^2
1.5 mg/dl or less	Less than 135 mg/m^2

SIDE EFFECTS/ADVERSE REACTIONS
Expected
Diarrhea, alopecia, nausea, vomiting
Frequent
Myalgia or arthralgia, peripheral neuropathy
Occasional
Mucositis, hypotension during infusion, pain or redness at injection site
Rare
Bradycardia

PRECAUTIONS AND CONTRAINDICATIONS
Baseline neutropenia (neutrophil count 1500 cells/mm^3), hypersensitivity to drugs developed with Cremophor EL (polyoxyethylated castor oil)
Caution:
Bone marrow depression, AV block, hepatic impairment, lactation,

children, recent MI, angina pectoris, CHF history, current use of drug with effect on cardiac conduction system

DRUG INTERACTIONS OF CONCERN TO DENTISTRY

• Possible (not demonstrated) increase in action by strong inhibitors of CYP2C8 and CYP3A4 isoenzymes: diazepam, ketoconazole, midazolam (monitor patient if prescribed)

SERIOUS REACTIONS

! Neutropenic nadir occurs at approximately day 11 of paclitaxel therapy.
! Anemia and leukopenia are common reactions.
! Thrombocytopenia occurs occasionally.
! A severe hypersensitivity reaction, including dyspnea, severe hypotension, angioedema, and generalized urticaria, occurs rarely.

DENTAL CONSIDERATIONS

General:
• Consider semisupine chair position for patient comfort if GI side effects occur.
• Patients receiving chemotherapy may require palliative therapy for stomatitis.
• Patients on chronic drug therapy may rarely have symptoms of blood dyscrasias, which can include infection, bleeding, and poor healing.
Consultations:
• Medical consultation may be required to assess disease control.
Teach Patient/Family to:
• Encourage effective oral hygiene to prevent soft tissue inflammation.
• Use caution to prevent trauma when using oral hygiene aids.

paliperidone
pal-ee-**per'**-i-done
(Invega, Invega Sustenna)

CATEGORY AND SCHEDULE
Pregnancy Risk Category: C

Drug Class: Antipsychotic

MECHANISM OF ACTION
The active metabolite of risperidone that may antagonize dopamine and serotonin receptors. Exhibits α-adrenergic and H_1 receptor antagonistic activity.
Therapeutic Effect: Suppresses psychotic behavior; decreases both positive and negative symptoms of schizophrenia.

USES
Schizophrenia

PHARMACOKINETICS
Paliperidone ER uses the osmotic drug-release technology that delivers the drug at a controlled rate. Oral bioavailability of paliperidone ER is 28%. Protein binding: 74%. Paliperidone dissolves slowly following IM injection. Not extensively metabolized in the liver. Extensively excreted in the kidney unchanged; minimal in feces.
Half-life: 23 hr (PO); 25–49 days (IM).

INDICATIONS AND DOSAGES
▸ Schizophrenia
PO (Extended-Release)
Adults. 6 mg a day, administered in the morning. Maximum: 12 mg a day. Titration should not occur more frequently than 5 days.

▶ **Renal Impairment**
PO (Extended-Release)
Creatinine clearance 50 to 80 ml/min. Initially, 3 mg/day. Maximum dose is 6 mg/day.
Creatinine clearance 10 to 50 ml/min. Initially, 1.5 mg/day. Maximum dose is 3 mg/day.

SIDE EFFECTS/ADVERSE REACTIONS
Frequent
Tachycardia, headache, somnolence, parkinsonism, insomnia, tremor
Occasional
Anxiety, extrapyramidal side effects, akathisia, dizziness, constipation, dyspepsia, nausea, weight gain, nasopharyngitis, appetite changes, sleep disturbances, back pain
Rare
Arrhythmia, fatigue, asthenia, orthostatic hypotension, abdominal pain, cough, myalgia, hyperprolactinemia, xerostomia

PRECAUTIONS AND CONTRAINDICATIONS
Hypersensitivity to paliperidone, risperidone, or its components
Caution:
Elderly with dementia-related psychosis (increased mortality)—black box warning
Renal impairment
Hepatic impairment
Neuroleptic malignant syndrome
Tardive dyskinesia
Seizures
Leukopenia, neutropenia, agranulocytosis
Patients at risk for suicide
Cognitive and motor impairment
Hyperglycemia, diabetes, patients should be monitored for signs and symptoms of hyperglycemia
QT prolongation; electrolyte disturbances; serum potassium and magnesium should be monitored as hypokalemia and hypomagnesemia may increase the risk of QT prolongation

DRUG INTERACTIONS OF CONCERN TO DENTISTRY
• CNS depressants, alcohol: Additive CNS depressant effects
• Antihypertensive agents: May enhance the hypotensive effects
• Dopamine agonists, levodopa: May block the effects of dopamine agonists and levodopa
• QT-interval prolonging drugs: May cause additive effects
• Carbamazepine: May decrease the levels of paliperidone

SERIOUS REACTIONS
! Prolongation of QT interval may produce torsades de pointes. Patients with bradycardia, hypokalemia, hypomagnesemia are at increased risk.
! Orthostatic hypotension including dizziness, tachycardia, and syncope with standing may occur.
! Agranulocytosis, leucopenia, and neutropenia may occur.

DENTAL CONSIDERATIONS
General:
• Monitor vital signs at every appointment because of cardiovascular side effects.
• After supine positioning, have patient sit upright for at least 2 min before standing to avoid orthostatic hypotension.
• Assess salivary flow as a factor in caries, periodontal disease, and candidiasis.
• Assess for presence of extrapyramidal motor symptoms such as tardive dyskinesia and akathisia. Extrapyramidal motor

activity may complicate dental treatment.

• Consider semisupine chair position for patient comfort if GI side effects occur.

Consultations:

• In a patient with symptoms of blood dyscrasias, request a medical consultation for blood studies and postpone treatment until normal values are reestablished.

• Medical consultation may be required to assess disease control.

• Physician should be informed if significant xerostomic side effects occur (e.g., increased caries, sore tongue, problems eating or swallowing, difficulty wearing prosthesis) so that medication change can be considered.

• Consultation with physician may be necessary if sedation or general anesthesia is required.

Teach Patient/Family to:

• Encourage effective oral hygiene to prevent soft tissue inflammation.

• Prevent trauma when using oral hygiene aids.

• When chronic dry mouth occurs, advise patient to:

  • Avoid mouth rinses with high alcohol content because of drying effects.

  • Use daily home fluoride products for anticaries effect.

  • Use sugarless gum, frequent sips of water, or saliva substitutes.

palonosetron hydrochloride
pal-oh-**noe**′-seh-tron
high-droh-**klor**′-ide
(Aloxi)

CATEGORY AND SCHEDULE
Pregnancy Risk Category: B

Drug Class: Antiemetics/ antivertigo, serotonin receptor antagonists

MECHANISM OF ACTION
A 5-HT$_3$ receptor antagonist that acts centrally in the chemoreceptor trigger zone and peripherally at vagal nerve endings.

USES
Prevention of nausea and vomiting associated with chemotherapy

PHARMACOKINETICS
Protein binding: 52%. Eliminated in urine. *Half-life:* 40 hr.

INDICATIONS AND DOSAGES
▸ Chemotherapy-Induced Nausea and Vomiting
IV
Adults, Elderly. 0.25 mg as a single dose 30 min before starting chemotherapy.

SIDE EFFECTS/ADVERSE REACTIONS
Occasional
Headache, constipation
Rare
Diarrhea, dizziness, fatigue, abdominal pain, insomnia

PRECAUTIONS AND CONTRAINDICATIONS
None known

P

DRUG INTERACTIONS OF CONCERN TO DENTISTRY
• None reported

SERIOUS REACTIONS
! Overdose may produce a combination of CNS stimulant and depressant effects.

DENTAL CONSIDERATIONS

General:
• For acute use in hospitals or cancer treatment centers.
Teach Patient/Family to:
• Be aware of possible oral side effects from concurrent chemotherapy.

pamidronate disodium
pam-id'-row-nate die-soe'-dee-um (Aredia, Pamisol[AUS])
Do not confuse Aredia with Adriamycin.

CATEGORY AND SCHEDULE
Pregnancy Risk Category: D

Drug Class: Bone-resorption inhibitor, electrolyte modifier

MECHANISM OF ACTION
A bisphosphate that binds to bone and inhibits osteoclast-mediated calcium resorption.
Therapeutic Effect: Lowers serum calcium concentrations.

USES
Treatment of moderate-to-severe Paget's disease, mild-to-moderate hypercalcemia associated with malignancy with or without bone metastases, osteolytic bone metastases in breast cancer, multiple myeloma patients

PHARMACOKINETICS

Route	Onset	Peak	Duration
IV	24–48 hr	5–7 days	N/A

After IV administration, rapidly absorbed by bone. Slowly excreted unchanged in urine. Unknown if removed by hemodialysis. *Half-life:* bone, 300 days; unmetabolized, 2.5 hr.

INDICATIONS AND DOSAGES
▶ Hypercalcemia
IV Infusion
Adults, Elderly. Moderate hypercalcemia (corrected serum calcium level 12–13.5 mg/dl): 60–90 mg. Severe hypercalcemia (corrected serum calcium level greater than 13.5 mg/dl): 90 mg.
▶ Paget's Disease
IV Infusion
Adults, Elderly. 30 mg/day for 3 days.
▶ Osteolytic Bone Lesion
90 mg over 4 hr once monthly.

SIDE EFFECTS/ADVERSE REACTIONS
Frequent
Temperature elevation (at least 1°C) 24–48 hr after administration; redness, swelling, induration, pain at catheter site in patients receiving 90 mg; anorexia, nausea, fatigue
Occasional
Constipation, rhinitis

PRECAUTIONS AND CONTRAINDICATIONS
Hypersensitivity to other bisphosphonates, such as etidronate, tiludronate, risedronate, and alendronate. Dental implants are contraindicated for patients taking this drug.

DRUG INTERACTIONS OF CONCERN TO DENTISTRY

• None reported

SERIOUS REACTIONS

! Hypophosphatemia, hypokalemia, hypomagnesemia, and hypocalcemia occur more frequently with higher dosages.

! Anemia, hypertension, tachycardia, atrial fibrillation, and somnolence occur more frequently with 90-mg doses.

! GI hemorrhage occurs rarely.

! Osteonecrosis of the jaw.

DENTAL CONSIDERATIONS

General:

• Evaluate patient for signs and symptoms of osteonecrosis of the jaw.

• Determine why patient is taking the drug.

• This drug may be used in the hospital or on an outpatient basis. Confirm the patient's disease and treatment status.

• Examine for oral manifestation of opportunistic infection.

• Monitor and record vital signs.

• Consider semisupine chair position for patient comfort if GI side effects occur.

• Question patient about tolerance of NSAIDs or aspirin related to GI disease.

• Be aware of the oral manifestations of Paget's disease (macrognathia, alveolar pain).

• Patients may have received other chemotherapy or radiation; confirm medical and drug history.

Consultations:

• Medical consultation may be required to assess disease control and patient's ability to tolerate stress.

Teach Patient/Family to:

• Observe regular recall schedule and practice effective oral hygiene to minimize risk of osteonecrosis of the jaw.

• Avoid drugs containing calcium, vitamin D, and antacids; possible antagonism of pamidronate.

pancreatin/ pancrelipase

pan-kree-**ah**′-tin/
pan-kree-**lie**′-pace
(pancreatin: Ku-Zyme, Pancreatin;
pancrelipase: Cotazym-S[AUS],
Cotazym-S Forte[AUS], Creon,
Pancrease[CAN], Pancrease MT,
Ultrase, Viokase)

CATEGORY AND SCHEDULE

Pregnancy Risk Category: B
(Pancrease, Pancrease MT); C
(Creon, Kutrase, Lipram,
Pancrelipase, Panokase, Plaretase,
Ultrase, Ultrase MT, Viokase)

Drug Class: Digestive enzyme, oral

P

MECHANISM OF ACTION

A pancreatic digestive enzyme combination (protease, lipase, amylase) that hydrolyzes fats to glycerol and fatty acids, converts proteins into peptides and amino acids, and converts starch into dextrins and maltose.

USES

Enzyme replacement therapy for pancreatic insufficiency, such as in cystic fibrosis, chronic pancreatitis, post-pancreatectomy, ductal obstructions causes by pancreatic or bile duct tumors, steatorrhea of malabsorption, and post-gastrectomy.

PHARMACOKINETICS

Locally inactivated in the GI tract by anti-enzymes, excreted by the intestinal mucosa, or by the action of protease enzymes. Digested enzyme fragments may be absorbed by blood and are excreted in urine, or excreted in feces.

INDICATIONS AND DOSAGES
▶ **Pancreatic Insufficiency**
Adult. PO 4000 to 20,000 units as capsules or tablets with meals or snacks and with sufficient liquids.
Children 7 to 12 yr. PO 4000 to 12,000 units with each meal and snacks.
Children 1-6 yr. PO 4000 to 8000 units with each meal and snacks.
Dosages vary from product to product and preparations are not interchangeable due to variations in bioequivalence.

SIDE EFFECTS/ADVERS REACTIONS
Frequent
Gastrointestinal upset
Occasional
Diarrhea, abdominal pain, vomiting, intestinal obstruction or stenosis, constipation, dermatitis, flatulence, nausea, melena, weight loss, pain, bloating, cramping
Rare
Allergic reactions

PRECAUTIONS AND CONTRAINDICATIONS
Fibrotic strictures, primarily in cystic fibrosis patients. GI obstructions; hyperuricosuria and hyperuricemia (high doses)

DRUG INTERACTIONS OF CONCERN TO DENTISTRY
• None reported in dentistry

SERIOUS REACTIONS
! Hypersensitivity, hyperuricosuria, hyperuricemia, fibrotic strictures

DENTAL CONSIDERATIONS

General:
• Know why patient is taking drug.
• Plan dental care to avoid disruptions of patient's diet.
Consultations:
• Consult with physician to determine severity of systemic disease and ability to tolerate dental procedures.
Teach Patient/Family to:
• Report changes in medical status and update medical history of prescription drugs.

panitumumab
pan-ih-**tu**′-mue-mab
(Vectibix)

CATEGORY AND SCHEDULE
Pregnancy Risk Category: C

Drug Class: Antineoplastic, monoclonal antibody

MECHANISM OF ACTION
An antineoplastic agent that binds specifically to epidermal growth factor (EGFR) on normal and tumor cells, and competitively inhibits the binding of ligands for EGFR. Blocks phosphorylation and activation of intracellular tyrosine kinases, resulting in inhibition of cell survival, growth, proliferation, and transformation.
Therapeutic Effect: Inhibits growth and survival of selected human tumor cell lines expressing EGFR.

USES
Treatment of EGFR-positive metastatic colorectal cancer

PHARMACOKINETICS
Half-life: 4–11 days. Other pharmacokinetic parameters have not been clearly established.

INDICATIONS AND DOSAGES
▶ **EGFR-Positive Metastatic Colorectal Cancer**
IV Infusion
Adults. 6 mg/kg administered over 60 min every 14 days. Doses higher than 1000 mg should be administered over 90 min.
▶ **Dosing Adjustments**
Infusion Reactions
Infusion reactions, mild-to-moderate (grade 1 or 2). Reduce the infusion rate by 50% for the duration of infusion. Infusion reactions, severe (grade 3 or 4). Immediately and permanently discontinue.
▶ **Dermatologic Toxicity**
Dermatologic toxicity (grade 3 or 4). Withhold panitumumab if skin toxicity does not improve to grade 2 or lower within 1 mo, permanently discontinue.
Dermatologic toxicity (grade 2 or lower), and the patient is symptomatically improved after withholding no more than 2 doses of panitumumab. Treatment may be resumed at 50% of the original dose. If toxicities recur, permanently discontinue drug. If toxicities do not recur, subsequent doses may be increased in increments of 25% of the original dose until the recommended dose of 6 mg/kg is obtained.
Safety and efficacy have not been established in children.

SIDE EFFECTS/ADVERSE REACTIONS
Frequent
Dermatologic toxicity, erythema, acneiform rash, pruritus, hypomagnesemia, fatigue, exfoliation, abdominal pain, paronychia, nausea, rash, diarrhea, constipation, fissures, vomiting, cough, acne, peripheral edema, dry skin
Occasional
Nail disorder, stomatitis, mucositis, eyelash growth, conjunctivitis, ocular hyperemia, lacrimation increased
Rare
Infusion reactions, eye/eyelid irritation

PRECAUTIONS AND CONTRAINDICATIONS
Hypersensitivity to panitumumab or its components; sunlight may exacerbate skin reactions

DRUG INTERACTIONS OF CONCERN TO DENTISTRY
• None reported

SERIOUS REACTIONS
! Dermatologic toxicities have been reported.
! Severe infusion-related reactions have been reported.
! Pulmonary fibrosis has been reported.

DENTAL CONSIDERATIONS
General:
• Examine patient for signs of adverse drug effects, including stomatitis and mucositis.
• Be prepared to manage nausea and vomiting related to drug use.
• Avoid aspirin and NSAIDs to reduce GI irritation.

Consultations:
• Consult physician to determine degree of disease control and ability of patient to tolerate dental procedures.

Teach Patient/Family to:
• Be aware of oral side effects of drug.
• Report oral lesions, soreness or bleeding to dentist.
• Use effective, atraumatic oral hygiene to minimize soft tissue inflammation.
• Update health and medication history if physician makes any changes in evaluation or drug regimen; include OTC, herbal, and nonherbal drugs in the update.

pantoprazole

pan-**toe**´-pra-zole
(Protonix, Pantoloc, Somac[AUS])
Do not confuse Protonix with Lotronex.

CATEGORY AND SCHEDULE
Pregnancy Risk Category: B

Drug Class: Gastrointestinal, proton pump inhibitor

MECHANISM OF ACTION
A benzimidazole that is converted to active metabolites that irreversibly bind to and inhibit hydrogen-potassium adenosine triphosphate, an enzyme on the surface of gastric parietal cells. Inhibits hydrogen ion transport into gastric lumen.
Therapeutic Effect: Increases gastric pH and reduces gastric acid production.

USES
Short-term treatment of esophageal erosion and ulceration associated with gastroesophageal reflux disease (GERD)

PHARMACOKINETICS

Route	Onset	Peak	Duration
PO	N/A	N/A	24 hr

Rapidly absorbed from the GI tract. Protein binding: 98%. Primarily distributed into gastric parietal cells. Metabolized extensively in the liver. Primarily excreted in urine. Not removed by hemodialysis. **Half-life:** 1 hr.

INDICATIONS AND DOSAGES
▸ **Erosive Esophagitis**
PO
Adults, Elderly. 40 mg/day for up to 8 wk. If not healed after 8 wk, may continue an additional 8 wk.
IV
Adults, Elderly. 40 mg/day for 7–10 days.
▸ **Hypersecretory Conditions**
PO
Adults, Elderly. Initially, 40 mg twice a day. May increase to 240 mg/day.
IV
Adults, Elderly. 80 mg twice a day. May increase to 80 mg q8hr.

SIDE EFFECTS/ADVERSE REACTIONS
Rare
Diarrhea, headache, dizziness, pruritus, rash

PRECAUTIONS AND CONTRAINDICATIONS
Caution is warranted with a chronic or current hepatic disease. It is unknown if pantoprazole crosses the placenta or is distributed in breast milk. Safety and efficacy of pantoprazole have not been

established in children. No age-related precautions have been noted in the elderly. Serum chemistry laboratory values, including serum creatinine and cholesterol levels, should be obtained before therapy.

DRUG INTERACTIONS OF CONCERN TO DENTISTRY
• None reported

SERIOUS REACTIONS
! None known

DENTAL CONSIDERATIONS

General:
• Avoid aspirin and NSAIDs for pain control if GI disease requires.
• Consider semisupine chair position for patient comfort because of possible regurgitation of stomach contents.
• Patients with gastroesophageal reflux may have oral symptoms, including burning mouth, secondary candidiasis, and dental erosion

Consultations:
• Consultation is only required if GI disease is severe or associated with other systemic conditions.

Teach Patient/Family to:
• Report symptoms of oral adverse effects of GI disease.

papaverine hydrochloride
pa-**pav′**-er-een
(Papacon, Para-Time SR, Pavabid Plateau, Pavacot, Pavagen)

CATEGORY AND SCHEDULE
Pregnancy Risk Category: C

Drug Class: Peripheral vasodilator

MECHANISM OF ACTION
A vasodilating agent that acts directly on the heart muscle to depress conduction and prolong the refractory period.
Therapeutic Effect: Relaxes smooth muscle.

USES
Treatment of arterial spasm resulting in cerebral and peripheral ischemia; myocardial ischemia associated with vascular spasm or dysrhythmias; angina pectoris; peripheral pulmonary embolism; visceral spasm as in ureteral, biliary, and GI colic PVD; unapproved: with phentolamine or alprostadil for intracavernous injection for impotence

PHARMACOKINETICS
Protein binding: 90%. Primarily excreted in urine as inactive metabolites. **Half-life:** Unknown.

INDICATIONS AND DOSAGES
▶ Vascular Spasm
IV/IM
Adults, Elderly. Inject 1–4 ml slowly and repeat q3h as indicated.
PO
Adults, Elderly. One capsule q12h. In difficult cases, administration may be increased to one capsule q8h or 2 capsules q12h.

SIDE EFFECTS/ADVERSE REACTIONS
Frequency Not Defined
Capsules: Nausea, abdominal distress, anorexia, constipation, malaise, drowsiness, vertigo, perspiration, headache, diarrhea, skin rash
Injection: General discomfort, nausea, abdominal discomfort, anorexia, constipation, diarrhea, skin rash, malaise, vertigo, headache,

intensive flushing of the face, perspiration, increased depth of respiration, increased heart rate, slight rise in B/P, excessive sedation

PRECAUTIONS AND CONTRAINDICATIONS

Complete atrioventricular heart block, impotence by intracorporeal injection, hypersensitivity to papaverine or any component of the formulation

Caution:
Cardiac dysrhythmias, glaucoma, pregnancy category C, lactation, drug dependency, children, hepatic hypersensitivity, Parkinson's disease

DRUG INTERACTIONS OF CONCERN TO DENTISTRY

• Increased hypotension: alcohol, other drugs that may also lower B/P

SERIOUS REACTIONS

! Hepatotoxicity has been reported.
! Priapism has been reported.

DENTAL CONSIDERATIONS

General:
• Monitor vital signs at every appointment because of cardiovascular and respiratory side effects.
• Short appointments and a stress-reduction protocol may be required for anxious patients.
Consultations:
• Stress from dental procedures may compromise cardiovascular function; determine patient risk.
• Medical consultation may be required to assess disease control.
Teach Patient/Family to:
• Avoid mouth rinses with high alcohol content.
• Encourage effective oral hygiene to prevent soft tissue inflammation.

paregoric

par-eh-**gor**'-ik
Do not confuse with opium tincture.

CATEGORY AND SCHEDULE

Pregnancy Risk Category: B (D if used for prolonged periods, high dosages at term)
Controlled substance: Schedule III

Drug Class: Antidiarrheal

MECHANISM OF ACTION

An opioid agonist that contains many opioid alkaloids, including morphine. It inhibits gastric motility due to its morphine content.
Therapeutic Effect: Decreases digestive secretions, increases GI muscle tone, and reduces GI propulsion.

USES

Treatment of diarrhea

PHARMACOKINETICS

Variably absorbed from the GI tract. Protein binding: low. Metabolized in liver. Primarily excreted in urine primarily as morphine glucuronide conjugates and unchanged drug—morphine, codeine, papaverine, etc. Unknown if removed by hemodialysis. *Half-life:* 2–3 hr.

INDICATIONS AND DOSAGES

▸ Antidiarrheal
PO
Adults, Elderly. 5–10 ml 1–4 times a day.
Children. 0.25–0.5 ml/kg/dose 1–4 times a day.

SIDE EFFECTS/ADVERSE REACTIONS

Frequent
Constipation, drowsiness, nausea, vomiting
Occasional
Paradoxical excitement, confusion, pounding heartbeat, facial flushing, decreased urination, blurred vision, dizziness, dry mouth, headache, hypotension, decreased appetite, redness, burning, pain at injection site
Rare
Hallucinations, depression, stomach pain, insomnia

PRECAUTIONS AND CONTRAINDICATIONS

Diarrhea caused by poisoning until the toxic material is removed, hypersensitivity to morphine sulfate or any component of the formulation, pregnancy (prolonged use or high dosages near term)
Caution:
Liver disease, addiction-prone individuals, prostatic hypertrophy (severe), caution in lactation, safety and efficacy in pediatric patients not established

DRUG INTERACTIONS OF CONCERN TO DENTISTRY

• Increased action of both drugs: alcohol, all other CNS depressants
• Decreased peristalsis: anticholinergic drugs

SERIOUS REACTIONS

! Overdosage results in cold or clammy skin, confusion, convulsions, decreased B/P, restlessness, pinpoint pupils, bradycardia, respiratory depression, decreased level of consciousness, and severe weakness.

! Tolerance to analgesic effect and physical dependence may occur with repeated use.

DENTAL CONSIDERATIONS

General:
• Psychologic and physical dependence may occur with chronic administration.
• Determine why the patient is taking the drug.
Teach Patient/Family to:
• Avoid mouth rinses with high alcohol content because of drying effects.

pargyline
par-gi-leen
(Eutonyl)

CATEGORY AND SCHEDULE

Pregnancy Risk Category: NA

Drug Class: Monoamine oxidase inhibitor; antihypertensive

P

MECHANISM OF ACTION

A monoamine oxidase inhibitor that inhibits the metabolism of catecholamines and tyramine.
Therapeutic Effect: Decreases blood pressure.

USES

Hypertension, moderate to severe

PHARMACOKINETICS

Not available

INDICATIONS AND DOSAGES
▶ **Hypertension**
PO
Adults. Initially, 25 mg daily. May be titrated by weekly intervals. Maintenance: 5–75 mg daily.

SIDE EFFECTS/ADVERSE REACTIONS

Side effects based on other monoamine oxidase inhibitors

Frequent

Orthostatic hypotension, restlessness, GI upset, insomnia, dizziness, lethargy, weakness, dry mouth, peripheral edema, fainting, palpitations

Occasional

Flushing, diaphoresis, rash, urinary frequency, increased appetite, transient impotence

Rare

Visual disturbances, impotence

PRECAUTIONS AND CONTRAINDICATIONS

Hypersensitivity to pargyline or any component of the formulation

Pheochromocytoma

Malignant hypertension

Advanced renal failure

Schizophrenia

Hyperthyroidism

Caution:

Cardiac arrhythmias

Hypertension

Suicidal tendencies

Pregnancy

Children

DRUG INTERACTIONS OF CONCERN TO DENTISTRY

• Tyramine-containing foods: May increase the risk of hypertensive crisis.

SERIOUS REACTIONS

! Manic psychosis has been reported.

DENTAL CONSIDERATIONS

General:

• Monitor vital signs at every appointment because of cardiovascular side effects.

• After supine positioning, have patient sit upright for at least 2 min before standing to avoid orthostatic hypotension.

• Assess salivary flow as a factor in caries, periodontal disease, and candidiasis.

• Stress from dental procedures may compromise cardiovascular function; determine patient risk.

Consultations:

• Medical consultation may be required to assess disease control.

Teach Patient/Family to:

• Report oral lesions, soreness, or bleeding to dentist.

• When chronic dry mouth occurs, advise patient to:

• Avoid mouth rinses with high alcohol content because of drying effects.

• Use daily home fluoride products for anticaries effect.

• Use sugarless gum, frequent sips of water, or saliva substitutes.

paromomycin

par-oh-moe-**mye′**-sin
(Humatin)
Do not confuse with Humira.

CATEGORY AND SCHEDULE

Pregnancy Risk Category: C

Drug Class: Amebicide antibiotic

MECHANISM OF ACTION

An antibacterial agent that acts directly on amoebas and against normal and pathogenic organisms in the GI tract. Interferes with bacterial protein synthesis by binding to 30S ribosomal subunits.

Therapeutic Effect: Produces amoebicidal effects.

USES

Treatment of intestinal amebiasis, adjunct in hepatic coma

PHARMACOKINETICS

Poorly absorbed from the GI tract and most of the dose is eliminated unchanged in feces.

INDICATIONS AND DOSAGES

▶ **Intestinal Amebiasis**
PO
Adults, Elderly, Children. 25–35 mg/kg/day q8h for 5–10 days.
▶ **Hepatic Coma**
PO
Adults, Elderly. 4 g/day q6–12h for 5–6 days.

SIDE EFFECTS/ADVERSE REACTIONS

Occasional
Diarrhea, abdominal cramps, nausea, vomiting, heartburn
Rare
Rash, pruritus, vertigo

PRECAUTIONS AND CONTRAINDICATIONS

Intestinal obstruction, renal failure, hypersensitivity to paromomycin or any of its components

DRUG INTERACTIONS OF CONCERN TO DENTISTRY

• Possible degradation by penicillins and cephalosporins

SERIOUS REACTIONS

! Overdosage may result in nausea, vomiting, and diarrhea.

DENTAL CONSIDERATIONS

General:
• Determine why patient is taking the drug.

• Consider semisupine chair position for patient comfort due to GI effects of disease.
• Question patient about tolerance of NSAIDs or aspirin related to GI disease.
• Postpone elective dental treatment until symptoms are controlled.
Consultations:
• Medical consultation may be required to assess disease control.
Teach Patient/Family to:
• Update health and medication history if physician makes any changes in evaluation or drug regimens; include OTC, herbal, and nonherbal drugs in the update.
• Report sore throat, oral burning sensation, fever, or fatigue, any of which could indicate presence of a superinfection.

---

paroxetine hydrochloride

par-**ox**′-eh-teen
high-droh-**klor**′-ide
(Aropax 20[AUS], Paxeva, Paxil, Paxil CR, Paxtine[AUS])
Do not confuse paroxetine with pyridoxine, or Paxil with Doxil or Taxol.

P

CATEGORY AND SCHEDULE

Pregnancy Risk Category: C

Drug Class: Antidepressant

MECHANISM OF ACTION

An antidepressant, anxiolytic, and antiobsessional agent that selectively blocks uptake of the neurotransmitter serotonin at neuronal presynaptic membranes, thereby increasing its availability at postsynaptic receptor sites.

Therapeutic Effect: Relieves depression, reduces obsessive-compulsive behavior, decreases anxiety.

USES

Treatment of depression, panic disorder, obsessive-compulsive disorder, social anxiety disorder; generalized anxiety disorder, posttraumatic stress disorder; premenstrual dysphoric disorder

PHARMACOKINETICS

Well absorbed from the GI tract. Protein binding: 95%. Widely distributed. Metabolized in the liver. Excreted in urine. Not removed by hemodialysis. ***Half-life:*** 24 hr.

INDICATIONS AND DOSAGES

▸ **Depression**

PO

Adults. Initially, 20 mg/day. May increase by 10 mg/day at intervals of more than 1 wk. Maximum: 50 mg/day.

PO (Controlled-Release)

Adults. Initially, 25 mg/day. May increase by 12.5 mg/day at intervals of more than 1 wk. Maximum: 62.5 mg/day.

▸ **Generalized Anxiety Disorder**

PO

Adults. Initially, 20 mg/day. May increase by 10 mg/day at intervals of more than 1 wk. Range: 20–50 mg/day.

▸ **Obsessive-Compulsive Disorder**

PO

Adults. Initially, 20 mg/day. May increase by 10 mg/day at intervals of more than 1 wk. Range: 20–60 mg/day.

▸ **Panic Disorder**

PO

Adults. Initially, 10–20 mg/day. May increase by 10 mg/day at intervals of more than 1 wk. Range: 10–60 mg/day.

▸ **Social Anxiety Disorder**

PO

Adults. Initially, 20 mg/day. Range: 20–60 mg/day.

▸ **Posttraumatic Stress Disorder**

PO

Adults. Initially, 20 mg/day. May increase by 10 mg/day at intervals of more than 1 wk. Range: 20–50 mg/day.

▸ **Premenstrual Dysphoric Disorder**

PO (Paxil CR)

Adults. Initially, 12.5 mg/day. May increase by 12.5 mg at weekly intervals to a maximum of 25 mg/day.

▸ **Usual Elderly Dosage**

PO

Initially, 10 mg/day. May increase by 10 mg/day at intervals of more than 1 wk. Maximum: 40 mg/day.

PO (Controlled-Release)

Initially, 12.5 mg/day. May increase by 12.5 mg/day at intervals of more than 1 wk. Maximum: 50 mg/day.

SIDE EFFECTS/ADVERSE REACTIONS

Frequent

Nausea, somnolence, headache, dry mouth, asthenia, constipation, dizziness, insomnia, diarrhea, diaphoresis, tremor

Occasional

Decreased appetite, respiratory disturbance (such as increased cough), anxiety, nervousness, flatulence, paresthesia, yawning, decreased libido, sexual dysfunction, abdominal discomfort

Rare

Palpitations, vomiting, blurred vision, altered taste, confusion

PRECAUTIONS AND CONTRAINDICATIONS

Use within 14 days of MAOIs

Caution:
Lactation, elderly, oral anticoagulants, renal or hepatic impairment, children with suspected higher risk of suicide ideation, other serotonergic drugs

DRUG INTERACTIONS OF CONCERN TO DENTISTRY
• Possible increased side effects: highly protein-bound drugs (aspirin), other antidepressants, alcohol
• Possible inhibition of fluoxetine metabolism: erythromycin, clarithromycin
• Increased half-life of diazepam
• NSAIDs: increased risk of GI side effects

SERIOUS REACTIONS
! Abnormal bleeding, hyponatremia, seizures, hypomania, and suicidal thoughts have been reported.

DENTAL CONSIDERATIONS

General:
• After supine positioning, have patient sit upright for at least 2 min before standing to avoid orthostatic hypotension.
• Assess salivary flow as a factor in caries, periodontal disease, and candidiasis.
• Avoid dental light in patient's eyes; offer dark glasses for patient comfort.
Consultations:
• Medical consultation may be required to assess disease control and patient's ability to tolerate stress.
• Physician should be informed if significant xerostomic side effects occur (e.g., increased caries, sore tongue, problems eating or swallowing, difficulty wearing prosthesis) so that a medication change can be considered.

Teach Patient/Family to:
• When chronic dry mouth occurs, advise patient to:
  • Avoid mouth rinses with high alcohol content because of drying effects.
  • Use daily home fluoride products to prevent caries.
  • Use sugarless gum, frequent sips of water, or saliva substitutes.

pazopanib
paz-**oh**′-pa-nib
(Votrient)

CATEGORY AND SCHEDULE
Pregnancy Risk Category: D

Drug Class: Antineoplastic (tyrosine kinase inhibitor), vascular endothelial growth factor inhibitor

MECHANISM OF ACTION
A multi-tyrosine kinase inhibitor of angiogenesis. Inhibits vascular endothelial growth factor receptor (VEGFR)–1, VEGFR-2, VEGFR-3, platelet-derived growth factor receptor (PDGFR)–alpha and PDGFR-beta, fibroblast growth factor receptor (FGFR)–1 and FGFR-3, cytokine receptor, interleukin-2 receptor inducible T-cell kinase, leukocyte-specific protein tyrosine kinase, and transmembrane glycoprotein receptor tyrosine kinase.
Therapeutic Effect: Inhibits tumor growth by inhibiting angiogenesis, decreases growth and spread of renal cell carcinoma.

USES
Advanced renal cell carcinoma

P

PHARMACOKINETICS

Well absorbed following PO administration. Food increases absorption. Protein binding: 99%. Primarily metabolized in liver by CYP3A4, minor metabolism by CYP1A2 and 2C8. Primarily eliminated in the feces; minimal excretion in urine. *Half-life:* 30.9 hr.

INDICATIONS AND DOSAGES
▶ Advanced Renal Cell Carcinoma (RCC)
PO
Adults. 800 mg a day, without food (at least 1 hr before or 2 hr after a meal).
Adults, taking strong CYP3A4 inhibitor. 400 mg a day, without food.
▶ Dosage in Hepatic Impairment
Moderate impairment. 200 mg a day. No adjustment necessary for renal impairment.

SIDE EFFECTS/ADVERSE REACTIONS
Frequent
Hypertension, fatigue, asthenia, headache, diarrhea, nausea, anorexia, vomiting, abdominal pain, hair color changes, hemorrhage, leucopenia, neutropenia, thrombocytopenia, lymphocytopenia, elevated LFTs, elevated/reduced glucose, elevated TSH, elevated lipase, decreased phosphorus, sodium, and magnesium
Occasional
MI/ischemia, QT prolongation, rash, alopecia, skin depigmentation, dysgeusia, dyspepsia, proteinuria, hematuria, hypothyroidism, hemoptysis, weight loss, palmar-plantar erythrodysesthesia, chest pain
Rare
TIA, CVA, torsades de pointes, rectal hemorrhage, facial edema, fatal hemorrhage, GI perforation or fistula

PRECAUTIONS AND CONTRAINDICATIONS
Hypersensitivity to pazopanib or its components
Severe hepatic impairment—black box warning
History of hemoptysis, cerebral or GI bleeding in preceding 6 months
Risk/history of arterial thrombotic events, including MI, angina or ischemic stroke within preceding 6 months
Pregnancy
Lactation
Caution:
Prolonged QTc interval, drugs that prolong QTc
Electrolyte abnormalities
Gastrointestinal perforation/fistula
Surgery (pazopanib should be stopped 7 days prior to surgery and restarted if clinical judgment indicates adequate wound healing)
Hypertension
Hypothyroidism (may worsen condition)
Moderate hepatic impairment (reduce dose)
Concurrent use of strong CYP3A4 inhibitors (reduce dose of pazopanib)
Concurrent use of strong CYP3A4 inducers (may decrease effectiveness)
Concurrent use with CYP3A4, CYP2D6, or CYP2C8 substrates

DRUG INTERACTIONS OF CONCERN TO DENTISTRY
• CYP3A4, CYP2C8, CYP2D6 substrates: May increase drug levels (e.g., triazolam)
• CYP3A4 inducers: May reduce pazopanib concentrations
• CYP3A4 inhibitors: May increase pazopanib concentrations

- QT prolonging agents: May increase the risk of QT prolongation, including torsades de pointes
- Grapefruit juice: May increase pazopanib concentrations
- Lapatinib: May increase pazopanib concentrations; may increase risk of QT prolongation
- Midazolam: May increase midazolam concentrations
- Paclitaxel: May increase paclitaxel concentrations

SERIOUS REACTIONS

! Severe and fatal hepatotoxicity has been reported; liver function tests should be performed when treatment is initiated and at least once every 4 wk for the first 4 months of therapy, monitor periodically thereafter.

DENTAL CONSIDERATIONS

General:
- Patient on chronic drug therapy may rarely have symptoms of blood dyscrasias, which include infection, bleeding, and poor healing.
- Avoid dental light in patient's eyes; offer dark glasses for patient comfort.
- Place on frequent recall because of oral side effects.
- Consider semisupine chair position for patient comfort if GI side effects occur.
Consultations:
- In a patient with symptoms of blood dyscrasias, request a medical consultation for blood studies and postpone treatment until normal values are reestablished.
- Medical consultation may be required to assess disease control.
Teach Patient/Family to:
- Encourage effective oral hygiene to prevent soft tissue inflammation.

- Prevent trauma when using oral hygiene aids.
- Be alert for the possibility of secondary oral infection and the need to see dentist immediately if signs of infection occur.

pegfilgrastim
peg-fil-**gras'**-tim
(Neulasta)
Do not confuse Neulasta with Neumega.

CATEGORY AND SCHEDULE
Pregnancy Risk Category: C

Drug Class: Hematopoietic agent

MECHANISM OF ACTION

A colony-stimulating factor that regulates production of neutrophils within bone marrow. Also a glycoprotein that primarily affects neutrophil progenitor proliferation, differentiation, and selected end-cell functional activation.
Therapeutic Effect: Increases phagocytic ability and antibody-dependent destruction; decreases incidence of infection.

USES

To decrease infection in patients receiving antineoplastics that are myelosuppressive; to increase WBC in patients with drug-induced neutropenia

PHARMACOKINETICS

Readily absorbed after subcutaneous administration. *Half-life:* 15–80 hr.

INDICATIONS AND DOSAGES
▶ **Myelosuppression**
Subcutaneous
Adults, Elderly. Give as a single
6-mg injection once per
chemotherapy cycle.

SIDE EFFECTS/ADVERSE REACTIONS
Frequent

Bone pain, nausea, fatigue, alopecia,
diarrhea, vomiting, constipation,
anorexia, abdominal pain, arthralgia,
generalized weakness, peripheral
edema, dizziness, stomatitis,
mucositis, neutropenic fever

PRECAUTIONS AND CONTRAINDICATIONS
Hypersensitivity to *Escherichia
coli*–derived proteins, within 14 days
before and 24 hr after cytotoxic
chemotherapy

DRUG INTERACTIONS OF CONCERN TO DENTISTRY
• None reported

SERIOUS REACTIONS
! Allergic reactions, such as
anaphylaxis, rash, and urticaria,
occur rarely.
! Cytopenia resulting from an
antibody response to growth factors
occurs rarely.
! Splenomegaly occurs rarely; assess
for left upper abdominal or shoulder
pain.
! Adult respiratory distress
syndrome (ARDS) may occur in
patients with sepsis.

DENTAL CONSIDERATIONS

General:
• Patients may have a history of
chemotherapy or radiation; confirm
medical and drug history.

• Determine type of
chemotherapeutic agents used and
related oral side effects.
• Monitor and record vital signs.
• Examine for oral manifestation of
opportunistic infection.
Consultations:
• Medical consultation may be
required to assess disease control
and patient's ability to tolerate
stress.
Teach Patient/Family to:
• Encourage effective oral hygiene
to prevent soft tissue inflammation.
• Prevent trauma when using oral
hygiene aids.
• Report oral lesions, soreness, or
bleeding to dentist.

peginterferon alfa-2a
peg-inn-ter-**fear**'-on **al**'-fah
(Pegasys)

CATEGORY AND SCHEDULE
Pregnancy Risk Category: C

Drug Class: Biologic response
modifier

MECHANISM OF ACTION
An immunomodulator that binds to
specific membrane receptors on the
cell surface, inhibiting viral
replication in virus-infected cells,
suppressing cell proliferation, and
producing reversible decreases in
leukocyte and platelet counts.
Therapeutic Effect: Inhibits
hepatitis C virus.

USES
Treatment of adults with chronic
hepatitis C with compensated liver
disease who have not been

previously treated with interferon-alfa.

PHARMACOKINETICS

Subcutaneous: Peak serum levels 72–96 hr; cleared from the body at 94 ml/hr; no data in children. Readily absorbed after subcutaneous administration. Excreted by the kidneys. *Half-life:* 80 hr.

INDICATIONS AND DOSAGES
▸ **Hepatitis C**
Subcutaneous
Adults 18 yr and older, Elderly.
180 mcg (1 ml) injected in abdomen or thigh once weekly for 48 wk.
▸ **Dosage in Renal Impairment**
For patients who require hemodialysis, dosage is 135 mg injected in abdomen or thigh once weekly for 48 wk.
▸ **Dosage in Hepatic Impairment**
For patients with progressive ALT (SGPT) increases above baseline values, dosage is 90 mcg injected in abdomen or thigh once weekly for 48 wk.

SIDE EFFECTS/ADVERSE REACTIONS
Frequent
Headache
Occasional
Alopecia, nausea, insomnia, anorexia, dizziness, diarrhea, abdominal pain, flu-like symptoms, psychiatric reactions (depression, irritability, anxiety), injection site reaction, impaired concentration, diaphoresis, dry mouth, nausea, vomiting

PRECAUTIONS AND CONTRAINDICATIONS
Autoimmune hepatitis, decompensated hepatic disease, infants, neonates

Caution:
Preexisting cardiac disease, may aggravate hypothyroidism, hyperthyroidism, hyperglycemia, hypoglycemia, diabetes, ophthalmologic disorders, lactation, children; closely monitor patients, severe life-threatening neuropsychiatric, autoimmune, ischemic, or infectious disorders may cause or aggravate these conditions

DRUG INTERACTIONS OF CONCERN TO DENTISTRY
• Risk of hepatotoxicity in severe liver disease: acetaminophen

SERIOUS REACTIONS
! Serious, acute hypersensitivity reactions, such as urticaria, angioedema, bronchoconstriction, and anaphylaxis, may occur. Other rare reactions include pancreatitis, colitis, endocrine disorders (e.g., diabetes mellitus), hyperthyroidism or hypothyroidism, ophthalmologic disorders, and pulmonary disorders.

P

DENTAL CONSIDERATIONS
General:
• Determine why patient is taking the drug.
• Assess salivary flow as a factor in caries, periodontal disease, and candidiasis.
• Consider semisupine chair position for patient comfort if GI side effects occur.
• Question patient about tolerance of NSAIDs or aspirin related to GI disease.
• Patients on chronic drug therapy may rarely have symptoms of blood dyscrasias, which can include infection, bleeding, and poor healing.

• Avoid elective dental procedures if severe neutropenia (fewer than 500 cells/mm³) or thrombocytopenia (fewer than 50,000 cell/mm³) is present.

• Severe side effects may require postponing elective dental procedures until drug therapy is completed.

Consultations:

• Medical consultation may be required to assess disease control in the patient.

• In a patient with symptoms of blood dyscrasias, request a medical consultation for blood studies and postpone treatment until normal values are reestablished.

• Liver function tests may be required to determine chronic liver disease.

Teach Patient/Family to:

• Encourage effective oral hygiene to prevent soft tissue inflammation/infection.

• Evaluate efficacy of oral hygiene home care; preventive appointments may be necessary.

• Prevent trauma when using oral hygiene aids.

• When chronic dry mouth occurs, advise patient to:
  • Avoid mouth rinses with high alcohol content because of drying effects.
  • Use daily home fluoride products for anticaries effect.
  • Use sugarless gum, frequent sips of water, or saliva substitutes.

peginterferon alfa-2b
peg-inn-ter-**fear**′-on **al**′-fah (PEG-Intron)

CATEGORY AND SCHEDULE
Pregnancy Risk Category: C

Drug Class: Biologic response modifier

MECHANISM OF ACTION
An immunomodulator that inhibits viral replication in virus-infected cells, suppresses cell proliferation, increases phagocytic action of macrophages, and augments specific cytotoxicity of lymphocytes for target cells.
Therapeutic Effect: Inhibits hepatitis C virus.

USES
Treatment of adults with chronic hepatitis C with compensated liver disease who have not been previously treated with interferon-alfa; peginterferon alfa-2b can be used with ribavirin.

PHARMACOKINETICS
Subcutaneous: Peak serum levels 72–96 hr; cleared from the body at 94 ml/hr; no data in children, pharmacokinetic data are limited.

INDICATIONS AND DOSAGES
▶ **Chronic Hepatitis C, Monotherapy**
Subcutaneous
Adults 18 yr and older, Elderly.
Administer appropriate dosage (see chart below) once weekly for 1 yr on the same day each week.

Vial Strength	Weight (kg)	mcg*	ml*
100 mcg/ml	37–45	40	0.4
	46–56	50	0.5
160 mcg/ml	57–72	64	0.4
	73–88	80	0.5
240 mcg/ml	89–106	96	0.4
	107–136	120	0.5
300 mcg/ml	137–160	150	0.5

*Of peginterferon alpha-2b to administer

▶ **Chronic Hepatitis C**
Subcutaneous combination therapy with ribavirin (400 mg twice a day). Initially, 1.5 mcg/kg/wk.

SIDE EFFECTS/ADVERSE REACTIONS
Frequent
Flu-like symptoms; inflammation, bruising, pruritus, and irritation at injection site
Occasional
Psychiatric reactions (depression, anxiety, emotional lability, irritability), insomnia, alopecia, diarrhea
Rare
Rash, diaphoresis, dry skin, dizziness, flushing, vomiting, dyspepsia

PRECAUTIONS AND CONTRAINDICATIONS
Autoimmune hepatitis, decompensated hepatic disease, history of psychiatric disorders
Caution:
Preexisting cardiac disease, may aggravate hypothyroidism, hyperthyroidism, hyperglycemia, hypoglycemia, diabetes, ophthalmologic disorders, lactation, children; closely monitor patients, severe life-threatening neuropsychiatric, autoimmune, ischemic, or infectious disorders may cause or aggravate these conditions

DRUG INTERACTIONS OF CONCERN TO DENTISTRY
• Risk of hepatotoxicity in severe liver disease: acetaminophen

SERIOUS REACTIONS
❗ Serious, acute hypersensitivity reactions (such as urticaria, angioedema, bronchoconstriction, and anaphylaxis), pulmonary disorders, endocrine disorders (e.g., diabetes mellitus), hypothyroidism, hyperthyroidism, and pancreatitis occur rarely.
❗ Ulcerative colitis may occur within 12 wk of starting treatment.

DENTAL CONSIDERATIONS
General:
• Determine why patient is taking the drug.
• Assess salivary flow as a factor in caries, periodontal disease, and candidiasis.
• Consider semisupine chair position for patient comfort if GI side effects occur.
• Question patient about tolerance of NSAIDs or aspirin related to GI disease.
• Patients on chronic drug therapy may rarely have symptoms of blood dyscrasias, which can include infection, bleeding, and poor healing.
• Avoid elective dental procedures if severe neutropenia (fewer than 500 cells/mm^3) or thrombocytopenia (fewer than 50,000 cell/mm^3) is present.
• Severe side effects may require postponing elective dental procedures until drug therapy is completed.
Consultations:
• Medical consultation may be required to assess disease control in the patient.

P

• In a patient with symptoms of blood dyscrasias, request a medical consultation for blood studies and postpone treatment until normal values are reestablished.
• Liver function tests may be required to determine chronic liver disease.

Teach Patient/Family to:
• Encourage effective oral hygiene to prevent soft tissue inflammation/infection.
• Evaluate efficacy of oral hygiene home care; preventive appointments may be necessary.
• Prevent trauma when using oral hygiene aids.
• When chronic dry mouth occurs, advise patient to:
  • Avoid mouth rinses with high alcohol content because of drying effects.
  • Use daily home fluoride products for anticaries effect.
  • Use sugarless gum, frequent sips of water, or saliva substitutes.

pegvisomant

peg-**vis**′-oh-mant
(Somavert)
Do not confuse Somavert with somatrem or somatropin.

CATEGORY AND SCHEDULE
Pregnancy Risk Category: B

Drug Class: Acromegaly agent

MECHANISM OF ACTION
A protein that selectively binds to growth hormone (GH) receptors on cell surfaces, blocking the binding of endogenous GHs and interfering with GH signal transduction.

Therapeutic Effect: Decreases serum concentrations of insulin-like growth factor 1 (IGF-1) and other GH-responsive serum proteins.

USES
Treatment of acromegaly in those patients who have an inadequate response to other treatment

PHARMACOKINETICS
Not distributed extensively into tissues after subcutaneous administration. Less than 1% excreted in urine. *Half-life:* 6 days.

INDICATIONS AND DOSAGES
▸ **Acromegaly**
Subcutaneous
Adults, Elderly. Initially, 40 mg as a loading dose, then 10 mg daily. After 4–6 wk, adjust dosage in 5-mg increments if serum IGF-1 level is still elevated, or in 5-mg decrements if IGF-1 level has decreased below the normal range. Maximum: 30 mg daily.

SIDE EFFECTS/ADVERSE REACTIONS
Frequent
Infection (cold symptoms, upper respiratory tract infection, blister, ear infection)
Occasional
Back pain, dizziness, injection site reaction, peripheral edema, sinusitis, nausea
Rare
Diarrhea, paresthesia

PRECAUTIONS AND CONTRAINDICATIONS
Latex allergy (stopper on vial contains latex)

DRUG INTERACTIONS OF CONCERN TO DENTISTRY
• Opioids: decreased serum levels

SERIOUS REACTIONS

! Pegvisomant use may markedly elevate liver function test results, including serum transaminase levels.
! Substantial weight gain occurs rarely.

DENTAL CONSIDERATIONS

General:
• Confirm history of previous medical, surgical, or radiation treatment for this disease.
• Monitor vital signs.
• Patient may complain of temporomandibular dysfunction (TMD) due to disease.
• Place on frequent recall to evaluate healing response.
Consultations:
• Physician consultation should include liver function tests.
Teach Patient/Family to:
• Encourage effective oral hygiene to prevent soft tissue inflammation.
• Prevent trauma when using oral hygiene aids.
• Update health and medication history if physician makes any changes in evaluation or drug regimens; include OTC, herbal, and nonherbal drugs in the update.

pemirolast potassium
peh-**meer**'-oh-last
poe-**tass**'-ee-um
(Alamast)

CATEGORY AND SCHEDULE
Pregnancy Risk Category: C

Drug Class: Ophthalmic

MECHANISM OF ACTION

An antiallergic agent that prevents activation and release of mediators of inflammation (e.g., mast cells). *Therapeutic Effect:* Reduces symptoms of allergic conjunctivitis.

USES
Relief of allergic conjunctivitis

PHARMACOKINETICS
Detected in plasma. Excreted in urine. *Half-life:* 4.5 hr.

INDICATIONS AND DOSAGES
▸ **Allergic Conjunctivitis**
Ophthalmic
Adults, Elderly, Children 3 yr and older. 1–2 drops in affected eye(s) 4 times a day.

SIDE EFFECTS/ADVERSE REACTIONS
Frequent
Headache, rhinitis, cold and flu symptoms
Occasional
Transient ocular stinging, burning, itching, dry eye, foreign body sensation, tearing
Rare
Sinusitis, sneezing/nasal congestion

PRECAUTIONS AND CONTRAINDICATIONS
Hypersensitivity to pemirolast potassium or any other component of the formulation
Caution:
Lactation, children, do not wear contact lens if eyes are red, may affect soft contact lens, if no red eyes wait 10 min after using to place soft contacts

DRUG INTERACTIONS OF CONCERN TO DENTISTRY
• None reported

P

SERIOUS REACTIONS
! None reported

DENTAL CONSIDERATIONS

General:
• Question patient about history of allergies to avoid using other potential allergens.
• Avoid dental light in patient's eyes; offer dark glasses for patient comfort.

pemoline
pem'-oh-leen
(Cylert, PemADD, PemADD CT)

CATEGORY AND SCHEDULE
Pregnancy Risk Category: B
Controlled Substance: Schedule IV

Drug Class: CNS stimulant

MECHANISM OF ACTION
A CNS stimulant that blocks the reuptake mechanism present in dopaminergic neurons in the cerebral cortex and subcortical structures.
Therapeutic Effect: Reduces motor restlessness and fatigue, increases alertness, elevates mood.

USES
Treatment of attention-deficit/hyperactivity disorder (ADHD)

PHARMACOKINETICS
PO: Peak 2–4 hr, duration 8 hr.
Half-life: 12 hr; metabolized (50%) by liver; excreted (40%) by kidneys.

INDICATIONS AND DOSAGES
▸ ADHD
PO
Children 6 yr and older. Initially, 37.5 mg/day as a single dose in morning. May increase by 18.75 mg at weekly intervals until therapeutic response is achieved. Range: 56.25–75 mg/day. Maximum: 112.5 mg/day.

SIDE EFFECTS/ADVERSE REACTIONS
Frequent
Anorexia, insomnia
Occasional
Nausea, abdominal discomfort, diarrhea, headache, dizziness, somnolence

PRECAUTIONS AND CONTRAINDICATIONS
Family history of Tourette syndrome, hepatic impairment, motor tics
Caution:
Renal disease, lactation, drug abuse, children younger than 6 yr; liver function monitoring recommended

DRUG INTERACTIONS OF CONCERN TO DENTISTRY
• Increased irritability, stimulation: caffeine-containing products and food

SERIOUS REACTIONS
! Visual disturbances, rash, and dyskinetic movements of the tongue, lips, face, and extremities have occurred.
! Large doses of pemoline may produce extreme nervousness and tachycardia.
! Hepatic effects, such as hepatitis and jaundice, appear to be reversible when the drug is discontinued.
! Prolonged administration to children with ADHD may temporarily delay growth.

DENTAL CONSIDERATIONS

General:
• Keep dental appointments short because of effects of disease.
Teach Patient/Family to:
• Use powered tooth brush for effective plaque control.

penbutolol
pen-**beaut´**-oh-lol
(Levatol)
Do not confuse with pindolol.

CATEGORY AND SCHEDULE
Pregnancy Risk Category: C (D if used in the second or third trimester)

Drug Class: Nonselective β-adrenergic blocker

MECHANISM OF ACTION
An antihypertensive that possesses nonselective β-blocking. Has moderate intrinsic sympathomimetic activity.
Therapeutic Effect: Reduces cardiac output, decreases B/P, increases airway resistance, and decreases myocardial ischemia severity.

USES
Treatment of hypertension alone or with other antihypertensive drugs, mild-to-moderate heart failure

PHARMACOKINETICS
Rapidly and extensively absorbed from the GI tract. Protein binding: 80%–90%. Metabolized in liver. Excreted primarily via urine.
Half-life: 17–26 hr.

INDICATIONS AND DOSAGES
▶ **Hypertension**
PO
Adults. Initially, 20 mg/day as a single dose. May increase to 40–80 mg/day.
Elderly. Initially, 10 mg/day.

SIDE EFFECTS/ADVERSE REACTIONS
Frequent
Decreased sexual ability, drowsiness, trouble sleeping, unusual tiredness/ weakness
Occasional
Diarrhea, bradycardia, depression, cold hands/feet, constipation, anxiety, nasal congestion, nausea, vomiting
Rare
Altered taste, dry eyes, itching, numbness of fingers, toes, scalp

PRECAUTIONS AND CONTRAINDICATIONS
Bronchial asthma or related bronchospastic conditions, cardiogenic shock, pulmonary edema, second- or third-degree AV block, severe bradycardia, overt cardiac failure, hypersensitivity to penbutolol or any component of the formulation
Caution:
Diabetes mellitus, renal disease, lactation, hyperthyroidism, COPD, hepatic disease, children, myasthenia gravis, peripheral vascular disease, hypotension

DRUG INTERACTIONS OF CONCERN TO DENTISTRY
• Decreased hypotensive effect: indomethacin, NSAIDs
• Increased hypotension, myocardial depression: hydrocarbon inhalation anesthetics

P

- Hypertension, bradycardia: sympathomimetics (epinephrine, ephedrine)
- Slow metabolism of lidocaine

SERIOUS REACTIONS

! Abrupt withdrawal may result in sweating, palpitations, headache, and tremulousness.

! Hypoglycemia may occur in patients with previously controlled diabetes.

DENTAL CONSIDERATIONS

General:
- Monitor vital signs at every appointment because of cardiovascular side effects.
- Patients on chronic drug therapy may rarely have symptoms of blood dyscrasias, which can include infection, bleeding, and poor healing.
- Limit use of sodium-containing products, such as saline IV fluids, for patients with a dietary salt restriction.
- Assess salivary flow as a factor in caries, periodontal disease, and candidiasis.
- After supine positioning, have patient sit upright for at least 2 min before standing to avoid orthostatic hypotension.
- Stress from dental procedures may compromise cardiovascular function; determine patient risk.
- Short appointments and a stress-reduction protocol may be required for anxious patients.
- Use vasoconstrictor with caution, in low doses, and with careful aspiration.
- Avoid using gingival retraction cord containing epinephrine.
Consultations:
- In a patient with symptoms of blood dyscrasias, request a medical consultation for blood studies and postpone dental treatment until normal values are reestablished.
- Medical consultation may be required to assess disease control and patient's ability to tolerate stress.

Teach Patient/Family to:
- Use caution to prevent injury when using oral hygiene aids.
- Encourage effective oral hygiene to prevent soft tissue inflammation.
- If taste alterations occur, consider drug as potential cause.
- When chronic dry mouth occurs, advise patient to:
  - Avoid mouth rinses with high alcohol content because of drying effects.
  - Use daily home fluoride products to prevent caries.
  - Use sugarless gum, frequent sips of water, or saliva substitutes.

penciclovir

pen-sye′-kloe-veer
(Denavir, Vectavir[South Africa, Costa Rica, Dominican Republic, El Salvador, Germany, Guatemala, Honduras, Israel, Nicaragua, Panama])
Do not confuse with acyclovir.

CATEGORY AND SCHEDULE
Pregnancy Risk Category: B

Drug Class: Antiviral

MECHANISM OF ACTION
Penciclovir triphosphate inhibits HSV polymerase competitively with deoxyguanosine triphosphate. Consequently, herpes viral DNA synthesis and, therefore, replication are selectively inhibited.

Therapeutic Effect: An antiviral compound that has inhibitory activity against human herpes virus types 1 and 2.

USES
Treatment of recurrent herpes labialis (cold sores)

PHARMACOKINETICS
Measurable penciclovir concentrations were not detected in plasma or urine. The systemic absorption of penciclovir following topical administration has not been evaluated.

INDICATIONS AND DOSAGES
▶ **Herpes Labialis (Cold Sores)**
Topical
Adolescents, Adults. Penciclovir should be applied every 2 hr during waking hours for a period of 4 days. Treatment should be started as early as possible (i.e., during the prodrome or when lesions appear).

SIDE EFFECTS/ADVERSE REACTIONS
Frequent
Headache
Occasional
Dysgeusia; decreased sensitivity of skin, particularly to touch; redness of the skin; skin rash (maculopapular, erythematous), local edema, skin discoloration; pruritus; hypoesthesia; paresthesias; parosmia; urticaria; oral/pharyngeal edema
Rare
Mild pain, burning, or stinging

PRECAUTIONS AND CONTRAINDICATIONS
Hypersensitivity to penciclovir or any of its components

Caution:
Acyclovir-resistant herpes viruses, patients younger than 18 yr, use on mucous membranes not recommended, avoid applications near the eye, lactation

DRUG INTERACTIONS OF CONCERN TO DENTISTRY
• None reported

SERIOUS REACTIONS
! None reported

DENTAL CONSIDERATIONS
General:
• Use in immunocompromised patients not established.
• Postpone dental treatment when oral herpetic lesions are present.
Teach Patient/Family to:
• Dispose of tooth brush or other contaminated oral hygiene devices used during period of infection to prevent reinoculation of herpetic infection.
• Apply with a finger cot or latex glove to prevent herpes infection on fingers.

P

penicillin G benzathine
pen-ih-**sil′**-lin G **benz′**-ah-thene
(Bicillin LA, Permapen)
Do not confuse penicillin G benzathine with penicillin G potassium or penicillin G procaine.

CATEGORY AND SCHEDULE
Pregnancy Risk Category: B

Drug Class: Benzathine salt of natural penicillin G

MECHANISM OF ACTION

A penicillin that inhibits bacterial cell wall synthesis by binding to one or more of the penicillin-binding proteins of bacteria.
Therapeutic Effect: Bactericidal.

USES

Treatment of respiratory infections, scarlet fever, erysipelas, otitis media, pneumonia, skin and soft tissue infections, bejel, pinta, yaws; effective for gram-positive cocci (*Staphylococcus, S. pyogenes, S. viridans, S. faecalis, S. bovis, S. pneumoniae*), gram-negative cocci (*N. gonorrhoeae*), gram-positive bacilli (*B. anthracis, C. perfringens, C. tetani, C. diphtheriae, L. monocytogenes*), gram-negative bacilli (*E. coli, P. mirabilis, Salmonella, Shigella, Enterobacter, S. moniliformis*), spirochetes (*T. pallidum*), Actinomyces

PHARMACOKINETICS

IM: Very slow absorption, hydrolyzed to penicillin G, duration 21–28 days. *Half-life:* 30–60 min; excreted in urine, breast milk; crosses placenta.

INDICATIONS AND DOSAGES
▶ **Group A Streptococcal Infections**
IM
Adults, Elderly. 1.2 million units as a single dose.
Children. 25,000–50,000 units/kg as a single dose.
▶ **Prevention of Rheumatic Fever**
IM
Adults, Elderly. 1.2 million units every 3–4 wk or 600,000 units twice monthly.
Children. 25,000–50,000 units/kg every 3–4 wk.

▶ **Early Syphilis**
IM
Adults, Elderly. 2.4 million units divided and administered in 2 separate injection sites.
▶ **Congenital Syphilis**
IM
Children. 50,000 units/kg weekly for 3 wk.
▶ **Syphilis of More Than 1 Yr Duration**
IM
Adults, Elderly. 2.4 million units divided and administered in 2 separate injection sites weekly for 3 wk.
Children. 50,000 units/kg weekly for 3 wk.

SIDE EFFECTS/ADVERSE REACTIONS

Occasional
Lethargy, fever, dizziness, rash, pain at injection site
Rare
Seizures, interstitial nephritis

PRECAUTIONS AND CONTRAINDICATIONS

Hypersensitivity to any penicillin
Caution:
Hypersensitivity to cephalosporins

DRUG INTERACTIONS OF CONCERN TO DENTISTRY

• Decreased antimicrobial effect of penicillin: tetracyclines, erythromycins, lincomycins
• Increased penicillin concentrations: aspirin, probenecid
• Suspected increased risk of methotrexate toxicity

SERIOUS REACTIONS

! Hypersensitivity reactions, ranging from chills, fever, and rash to anaphylaxis, may occur.

DENTAL CONSIDERATIONS

General:
- Take precautions regarding allergy to medication.
- Determine why the patient is taking the drug.
- Place on frequent recall to evaluate healing response.

Consultations:
- Medical consultation may be required to assess disease control.

Teach Patient/Family to:
- When used for dental infection, advise patient to:
  - Report sore throat, oral burning sensation, fever, fatigue, any of which could indicate superinfection.
  - Take at prescribed intervals and complete dosage regimen.
  - Immediately notify the dentist if signs or symptoms of infection increase.

penicillin G potassium

pen-ih-**sil**'-lin G poe-**tass**'-ee-um
(Megacillin[CAN], Novepen-G[CAN], Pfizerpen)
Do not confuse penicillin G potassium with penicillin G benzathine or penicillin G procaine.

CATEGORY AND SCHEDULE

Pregnancy Risk Category: B

Drug Class: Antibiotics, penicillins

MECHANISM OF ACTION

A penicillin that inhibits bacterial cell wall synthesis by binding to one or more of the penicillin-binding proteins of bacteria.
Therapeutic Effect: Bactericidal.

USES

Treatment of sepsis, meningitis, pericarditis, endocarditis, pneumonia due to susceptible gram-positive organisms (not *Staphylococcus aureus*), and some gram-negative organisms

PHARMACOKINETICS

Completely absorbed from intramuscular injection sites. Peak blood levels reached rapidly after intravenous infusion. Bound primarily to albumin. Widely distributed, but has limited penetration into cerebrospinal fluid. 60% excreted within 5 hr by kidney.

INDICATIONS AND DOSAGES

▶ **Sepsis, Meningitis, Pericarditis, Endocarditis, Pneumonia Caused by Susceptible Gram-Positive Organisms (Not Staphylococcus aureus) and Some Gram-Negative Organisms**
IV, IM
Adults, Elderly. 2–24 million units/kg/day in divided doses q4–6h.
Children. 100,000–400,000 units/kg/day in divided doses q4–6h.
▶ **Dosage in Renal Impairment**
Dosage interval is modified on the basis of creatinine clearance.

Creatinine Clearance	Dosage Interval
10–30 ml/min	Usual dose q8–12h
Less than 10 ml/min	Usual dose q12–18h

SIDE EFFECTS/ADVERSE REACTIONS

Occasional
Lethargy, fever, dizziness, rash, electrolyte imbalance, diarrhea, thrombophlebitis
Rare
Seizures, interstitial nephritis

PRECAUTIONS AND CONTRAINDICATIONS
Hypersensitivity to any penicillin

DRUG INTERACTIONS OF CONCERN TO DENTISTRY
• Increased or prolonged plasma levels: probenecid
• Possible decrease in antimicrobial effectiveness: tetracyclines, erythromycins, lincomycins

SERIOUS REACTIONS
! Hypersensitivity reactions ranging from rash, fever, and chills to anaphylaxis occur.

DENTAL CONSIDERATIONS

General:
• Determine why patient is taking the drug.
• Caution regarding allergy to medication.
• Use with caution in patients with a history of antibiotic-associated colitis.

Consultations:
• Consult patient's physician if an acute dental infection occurs and another antiinfective is required.
• Medical consultation may be required to assess disease control.

Teach Patient/Family to:
• Encourage effective oral hygiene to prevent soft tissue inflammation.
• Prevent trauma when using oral hygiene aids.
• Report sore throat, oral burning sensation, fever, or fatigue, any of which could indicate presence of a superinfection.

penicillin V potassium
pen-ih-**sil**′-in V poe-**tass**′-ee-um
(Abbocillin VK[AUS], Apo-Pen-VK[CAN], Cilicaine VK[AUS], L.P.V.[AUS], Novo-Pen-VK[CAN], Veetids)

CATEGORY AND SCHEDULE
Pregnancy Risk Category: B

Drug Class: Semisynthetic penicillin

MECHANISM OF ACTION
A penicillin that inhibits cell wall synthesis by binding to bacterial cell membranes.
Therapeutic Effect: Bactericidal.

USES
Effective for treatment of gram-positive cocci (*S. aureus, S. viridans, S. faecalis, S. bovis, S. pneumoniae*), gram-negative cocci (*N. gonorrhoeae, N. meningitidis*), gram-positive bacilli (*B. anthracis, C. perfringens, C. tetani, C. diphtheriae*), gram-negative bacilli (*S. moniliformis*), spirochetes (*T. pallidum*), *Actinomyces, Peptococcus,* and *Peptostreptococcus* species

PHARMACOKINETICS
Moderately absorbed from the GI tract. Protein binding: 80%. Widely distributed. Metabolized in the liver. Primarily excreted in urine.
Half-life: 1 hr (increased in impaired renal function).

INDICATIONS AND DOSAGES

▶ **Mild-to-Moderate Respiratory Tract or Skin or Skin-Structure Infections, Otitis Media, Necrotizing Ulcerative Gingivitis**

PO

Adults, Elderly, Children 12 yr and older. 125–500 mg q6–8h.

Children younger than 12 yr. 25–50 mg/kg/day in divided doses q6–8h. Maximum: 3 g/day.

▶ **Primary Prevention of Rheumatic Fever**

PO

Adults, Elderly. 500 mg 2–3 times a day for 10 days.

Children. 250 mg 2–3 times a day for 10 days.

SIDE EFFECTS/ADVERSE REACTIONS

Frequent

Mild hypersensitivity reaction (chills, fever, rash), nausea, vomiting, diarrhea

Rare

Bleeding

PRECAUTIONS AND CONTRAINDICATIONS

Hypersensitivity to any penicillin

Caution:

Hypersensitivity to cephalosporins, lactation

DRUG INTERACTIONS OF CONCERN TO DENTISTRY

• Decreased antimicrobial effectiveness of penicillin: tetracyclines, erythromycins, lincomycins

• Increased penicillin concentrations: probenecid

• Food: reduced absorption and effectiveness

SERIOUS REACTIONS

! Severe hypersensitivity reactions, including anaphylaxis, may occur.

! Nephrotoxicity, antibiotic-associated colitis, and other superinfections may result from high dosages or prolonged therapy.

DENTAL CONSIDERATIONS

General:

• Take precautions regarding allergy to medication.

• Determine why the patient is taking the drug.

• If used for dental infection, place on frequent recall to evaluate healing response.

Consultations:

• Medical consultation may be required to assess disease control.

Teach Patient/Family:

• When used for dental infection, advise patient to:

• Report sore throat, oral burning sensation, fever, fatigue, any of which could indicate superinfection.

• Take at prescribed intervals and complete dosage regimen.

• Immediately notify the dentist if signs or symptoms of infection or allergy occur.

P

pentamidine isethionate

pen-**tam′**-ih-deen
ice-eth-**eyé**-oh-nate
(NebuPent, Pentacarinat[CAN], Pentam-300)

CATEGORY AND SCHEDULE

Pregnancy Risk Category: C

Drug Class: Antiprotozoal

MECHANISM OF ACTION
An antiinfective that interferes with nuclear metabolism and incorporation of nucleotides, inhibiting DNA, RNA, phospholipid, and protein synthesis.
Therapeutic Effect: Produces antibacterial and antiprotozoal effects.

USES
Treatment of *Pneumocystis carinii* infections in immunocompromised patients (injection); prevention in high-risk HIV-infected patients (INH)

PHARMACOKINETICS
Well absorbed after IM administration; minimally absorbed after inhalation. Widely distributed. Primarily excreted in urine. Minimally removed by hemodialysis. *Half-life:* 6.5 hr (increased in impaired renal function). Powder for Nebulization (NebuPent): 300 mg.

INDICATIONS AND DOSAGES
▶ *Pneumocystis carinii* Pneumonia (PCP)
IV, IM
Adults, Elderly. 4 mg/kg/day once a day for 14–21 days.
Children. 4 mg/kg/day once a day for 10–14 days.
▶ Prevention of PCP
Inhalation
Adults, Elderly. 300 mg once q4wk.
Children 5 yr and older. 300 mg q3–4wk.
Children younger than 5 yr. 8 mg/kg/dose once q3–4wk.

SIDE EFFECTS/ADVERSE REACTIONS
Frequent
Injection: Abscess, pain at injection site

Inhalation: Fatigue, metallic taste, shortness of breath, decreased appetite, dizziness, rash, cough, nausea, vomiting, chills
Occasional
Injection: Nausea, decreased appetite, hypotension, fever, rash, altered taste, confusion
Inhalation: Diarrhea, headache, anemia, muscle pain
Rare
Injection: Neuralgia, thrombocytopenia, phlebitis, dizziness

PRECAUTIONS AND CONTRAINDICATIONS
Concurrent use with didanosine
Caution:
Blood dyscrasias, hepatic disease, renal disease, diabetes mellitus, cardiac disease, hypocalcemia

DRUG INTERACTIONS OF CONCERN TO DENTISTRY
• None reported

SERIOUS REACTIONS
! Rare reactions include life-threatening or fatal hypotension, arrhythmias, hypoglycemia, leukopenia, nephrotoxicity or renal failure, anaphylactic shock, Stevens-Johnson syndrome, and toxic epidural necrolysis.
! Hyperglycemia and insulin-dependent diabetes mellitus (often permanent) may occur even months after therapy has stopped.

DENTAL CONSIDERATIONS
General:
• Monitor vital signs at every appointment because of cardiovascular side effects.
• Patients on chronic drug therapy may rarely have symptoms of blood dyscrasias, which can include

infection, bleeding, and poor healing.

• Place on frequent recall to evaluate healing response.

• Assess salivary flow as a factor in caries, periodontal disease, and candidiasis.

• Consider semisupine chair position for patients with respiratory disease.

• For inhalation dosage forms, rinse mouth with water after each dose to prevent dryness.

• Place on frequent recall because of oral side effects.

Consultations:

• In a patient with symptoms of blood dyscrasias, request a medical consultation for blood studies and postpone dental treatment until normal values are reestablished.

• Medical consultation may be required to assess disease control.

Teach Patient/Family to:

• See dentist immediately if secondary oral infection occurs.

• Encourage effective oral hygiene to prevent soft tissue inflammation.

• Use caution to prevent injury when using oral hygiene aids.

• Use dietary suggestions to maintain oral and systemic health.

• When chronic dry mouth occurs, advise patient to:

  • Avoid mouth rinses with high alcohol content because of drying effects.

  • Use daily home fluoride products to prevent caries.

  • Use sugarless gum, frequent sips of water, or saliva substitutes.

pentazocine hydrochloride; naloxone hydrochloride

pen-**taz**′oh-seen high-droh-**klor**′-ide; nah-**lok**′-sohn high-droh-**klor**′-ide

(Talwin Nx)

CATEGORY AND SCHEDULE

Pregnancy Risk Category: C
Controlled Substance: Schedule IV

Drug Class: Synthetic opioid/ mixed agonist/antagonist

MECHANISM OF ACTION

Pentazocine is both an opioid agonist and antagonist that induces analgesia by stimulating the kappa and sigma opioid receptors. Naloxone is an opioid antagonist that displaces opiates at opiate-occupied receptor sites in the CNS.

Therapeutic Effect: Pentazocine: induces analgesia. Naloxone: blocks opioid effects if injected; reverses opiate-induced sleep or sedation; increases respiratory rate, returns B/P to normal.

USES

Treatment of moderate-to-severe pain alone or in combination with aspirin or acetaminophen

PHARMACOKINETICS

Well absorbed. Metabolized in liver. Primarily excreted in urine. Minimal excretion in bile and feces.
Half-life: 2–3 hr.

P

INDICATIONS AND DOSAGES

▶ **Pain, Moderate-to-Severe**

PO

Adults, Elderly, Children 12 yr and older. 1 tablet every 3–4 hr. May be increased to 2 tablets when needed. Maximum: 12 tablets/day.

SIDE EFFECTS/ADVERSE REACTIONS

Occasional

Confusion, dizziness, fatigue, light-headedness, drowsiness, mood changes, headache, GI upset, vomiting, constipation, stomach pain, rash, difficulty urinating

PRECAUTIONS AND CONTRAINDICATIONS

Hypersensitivity to pentazocine or naloxone or any component on the formulation

Caution:

Addictive personality, lactation, increased intracranial pressure, head injury, MI (acute), severe heart disease, respiratory depression, hepatic disease, renal disease, children 12 yr, acute abdominal conditions, Addison's disease, prostatic hypertrophy, patients taking other narcotics

DRUG INTERACTIONS OF CONCERN TO DENTISTRY

• Increased effects: all CNS depressants, alcohol
• Contraindication: MAOIs
• Do not mix in solutions or syringe with barbiturates
• Additive side effects of opioid agonists
• Increased effects of anticholinergics

• Decreased effects of opioid agonists, precipitation of withdrawal

SERIOUS REACTIONS

❗ Respiratory depression and serious skin reactions, such as Stevens-Johnson syndrome, have been reported but occur rarely.

DENTAL CONSIDERATIONS

General:

• Monitor vital signs at every appointment because of cardiovascular and respiratory side effects.
• Assess salivary flow as a factor in caries, periodontal disease, and candidiasis.
• Consider semisupine chair position for patient comfort if GI side effects occur.
• Psychologic and physical dependence may occur with chronic administration.

Teach Patient/Family:

• When chronic dry mouth occurs, advise patient to:
  • Avoid mouth rinses with high alcohol content because of drying effects.
  • Use daily home fluoride products to prevent caries.
  • Use sugarless gum, frequent sips of water, or saliva substitutes.

pentazocine
pen-**tah**'-zoe-seen
(Talwin)

COMBINATION PRODUCTS
With naloxone, an opioid antagonist (oral) (Talwin NX); with aspirin (oral) (Talwin Compound); w/acetaminophen (oral) (Talacen)

CATEGORY AND SCHEDULE
Pregnancy Risk Category: C
Controlled substance: Schedule IV

Drug Class: Opioid analgesics

MECHANISM OF ACTION
An opioid antagonist that binds with opioid receptors within CNS.
Therapeutic Effect: Alters processes affecting pain perception, emotional response to pain.

USES
Relief of moderate-to-severe pain associated with surgical procedures

PHARMACOKINETICS
Well absorbed after administration. Widely distributed including in CSF. Metabolized in liver via oxidative and glucuronide conjugation pathways, extensive first-pass effect. Excreted in small amounts as unchanged drug. *Half-life:* 2–3 hr, prolonged with hepatic impairment.

INDICATIONS AND DOSAGES
▶ **Analgesia**
PO (with Naloxone)
Adults. 50 mg q3–4h. May increase to 100 mg q3–4h, if needed. Maximum: 600 mg/day.
Elderly. 50 mg q4h.

▶ **Subcutaneous/IM/IV (without Naloxone)**
Adults. 30 mg q3–4h. Do not exceed 30 mg IV or 60 mg subcutaneous/IM per dose. Maximum: 360 mg/day.
IM
Elderly. 25 mg q4h.
▶ **Obstetric Labor (without Naloxone)**
IM
Adults. 30 mg as a single dose.
IV
Adults. 20 mg when contractions are regular. May repeat 2–3 times q2–3h.

SIDE EFFECTS/ADVERSE REACTIONS
Frequent
Drowsiness, euphoria, nausea, vomiting
Occasional
Allergic reaction, histamine reaction (decreased B/P, increased sweating, flushing, wheezing), decreased urination, altered vision, constipation, dizziness, dry mouth, headache, hypotension, pain/burning at injection site

PRECAUTIONS AND CONTRAINDICATIONS
Hypersensitivity to pentazocine or any component of the formulation

DRUG INTERACTIONS OF CONCERN TO DENTISTRY
• Increased effects: all CNS depressants, alcohol
• Contraindication: MAOIs
• Do not mix with barbiturates in solutions or syringe
• Additive side effects of opioid agonists
• Increased effects of anticholinergics
• Decreased effects of opioid agonists, precipitation of withdrawal

P

SERIOUS REACTIONS

❗ Overdosage results in severe respiratory depression, skeletal muscle flaccidity, cyanosis, extreme somnolence progressing to convulsions, stupor, and coma.
❗ Abrupt withdrawal after prolonged use may produce symptoms of narcotic withdrawal (abdominal cramps, rhinorrhea, lacrimation, nausea, vomiting, restlessness, anxiety, increased temperature, piloerection).

DENTAL CONSIDERATIONS

General:
• Monitor vital signs at every appointment because of cardiovascular and respiratory side effects.
• Assess salivary flow as a factor in caries, periodontal disease, and candidiasis.
• Consider semisupine chair position for patient comfort if GI side effects occur.
• Psychologic and physical dependence may occur with chronic administration.
Teach Patient/Family:
• When chronic dry mouth occurs, advise patient to:
  • Avoid mouth rinses with high alcohol content because of drying effects.
  • Use daily home fluoride products to prevent caries.
  • Use sugarless gum, frequent sips of water, or saliva substitutes.

pentobarbital

pen-toe-**bar**'-bi-tal
(Nembutal, Phenobarbitone[AUS])
Do not confuse with phenobarbital.

CATEGORY AND SCHEDULE

Pregnancy Risk Category: D
Controlled substance: Schedule II (capsules, injection), Schedule III (suppositories)

Drug Class: Sedative-hypnotic barbiturate

MECHANISM OF ACTION

A barbiturate that binds at the gamma-aminobutyric acid (GABA) receptor complex, enhancing GABA activity.
Therapeutic Effect: Depresses CNS activity and reticular activating system.

USES

Treatment of insomnia, sedation, preoperative medication, increased intracranial pressure (ICP), dental anesthetic

PHARMACOKINETICS

Well absorbed after PO, parenteral administration. Protein binding: 35%–55%. Rapidly, widely distributed. Metabolized in liver. Primarily excreted in urine. Removed by hemodialysis. **Half-life:** 15–48 hr.

INDICATIONS AND DOSAGES

▸ **Preanesthetic**
PO
Adults, Elderly. 100 mg.
Children. 2–6 mg/kg. Maximum: 100 mg/dose.
IM
Adults, Elderly. 150–200 mg.

Children. 2–6 mg/kg. Maximum: 100 mg/dose.

Rectal

Children 12–14 yr. 60 or 120 mg.
Children 5–12 yr. 60 mg.
Children 1–4 yr. 30–60 mg.
Children 2 mo–1 yr. 30 mg.

▶ **Hypnotic**

PO

Adults, Elderly. 100 mg at bedtime.

IM

Adults, Elderly. 150–200 mg at bedtime.
Children. 2–6 mg/kg. Maximum: 100 mg/dose at bedtime.

IV

Adults, Elderly. 100 mg initially then, after 1 min, may give additional small doses at 1-min intervals, up to 500 mg total.
Children. 50 mg initially then, after 1 min, may give additional small doses at 1-min intervals, up to desired effect.

Rectal

Adults, Elderly. 120–200 mg at bedtime.
Children 12–14 yr. 60 or 120 mg at bedtime.
Children 5–12 yr. 60 mg at bedtime.
Children 1–4 yr. 30–60 mg at bedtime.
Children 2 mo–1 yr. 30 mg at bedtime.

▶ **Anticonvulsant**

IV

Adults, Elderly. 2–15 mg/kg loading dose given slowly over 1–2 hr. Maintenance infusion: 0.5–5 mg/kg/hr.
Children. 5–15 mg/kg loading dose given slowly over 1–2 hr. Maintenance infusion: 0.5–3 mg/kg/hr.

SIDE EFFECTS/ADVERSE REACTIONS

Occasional

Agitation, confusion, dizziness, somnolence

Rare

Confusion, paradoxic CNS hyperactivity or nervousness in children, excitement or restlessness in elderly

PRECAUTIONS AND CONTRAINDICATIONS

Porphyria, hypersensitivity to barbiturates

Caution:

Anemia, lactation, hepatic disease, renal disease, hypertension, elderly, acute/chronic pain

DRUG INTERACTIONS OF CONCERN TO DENTISTRY

• Hepatotoxicity: halogenated-hydrocarbon anesthetics
• Increased CNS depression: alcohol, all other CNS depressants
• Increased metabolism of carbamazepine, tricyclic antidepressants, corticosteroids
• Decreased half-life of doxycycline

SERIOUS REACTIONS

! Agranulocytosis, megaloblastic anemia, apnea, hypoventilation, bradycardia, hypotension, syncope, hepatic damage, and Stevens-Johnson syndrome occur rarely.
! Abrupt withdrawal after prolonged therapy may produce effects ranging from markedly increased dreaming, nightmares or insomnia, tremor, sweating and vomiting, to hallucinations, delirium, seizures, and status epilepticus.
! Skin eruptions appear as hypersensitivity reactions.
! Overdosage produces cold or clammy skin, hypothermia, severe

CNS depression, cyanosis, and rapid pulse.

DENTAL CONSIDERATIONS

General:
• Determine why the patient is taking the drug.
• Monitor vital signs at every appointment because of cardiovascular side effects. Evaluate respiration characteristics and rate.
• Patients on chronic drug therapy may rarely have symptoms of blood dyscrasias, which can include infection, bleeding, and poor healing.
• When used for sedation in dentistry:
  • Assess vital signs before use and q30min after use as sedative.
  • Observe respiratory dysfunction: respiratory depression, character, rate, rhythm; hold drug if respirations are fewer than 10/min or if pupils are dilated.
  • After supine positioning, have patient sit upright for at least 2 min before standing to avoid orthostatic hypotension.
  • Have someone escort patient to and from dental office when drug is used for conscious sedation.
  • Barbiturates induce liver microsomal enzymes, which alter the metabolism of other drugs.
  • Geriatric patients are more susceptible to drug effects; use lower dose.
Consultations:
• In a patient with symptoms of blood dyscrasias, request a medical consultation for blood studies and postpone dental treatment until normal values are reestablished.

Teach Patient/Family to:
• Avoid driving or other activities requiring alertness.
• Avoid alcohol ingestion or CNS depressants; serious CNS depression may result.
• Avoid OTC preparations (antihistamines, cold remedies) that contain CNS depressants.

pentosan polysulfate
pen′-toe-san poll-ee-**sull**′-fate
(Elmiron)
Do not confuse with pentostatin.

CATEGORY AND SCHEDULE
Pregnancy Risk Category: B

Drug Class: Anticoagulant

MECHANISM OF ACTION
A negatively-charged synthetic sulfated polysaccharide with heparin-like properties that appear to adhere to bladder wall mucosal membrane, may act as a buffering agent to control cell permeability, preventing irritating solutes in the urine. Has anticoagulant/fibrinolytic effects.
Therapeutic Effect: Relieves bladder pain.

USES
Relief of interstitial cystitis symptoms

PHARMACOKINETICS
Poorly and erratically absorbed from the gastrointestinal tract. Distributed in uroepithelium of GU tract with lesser amount found in the liver, spleen, lung, skin, periosteum, and bone marrow. Metabolized in liver and kidney (secondary). Eliminated in the urine. *Half-life:* 4.8 hr.

INDICATIONS AND DOSAGES
▸ **Interstitial Cystitis**
PO
Adults, Elderly. 100 mg 3 times a day.

SIDE EFFECTS/ADVERSE REACTIONS
Frequent
Alopecia areata (a single area on the scalp), diarrhea, nausea, headache, rash, abdominal pain, dyspepsia
Occasional
Dizziness, depression, increased liver function tests

PRECAUTIONS AND CONTRAINDICATIONS
Hypersensitivity to pentosan polysulfate sodium or structurally related compounds

DRUG INTERACTIONS OF CONCERN TO DENTISTRY
• Potential risk of bleeding: high-dose aspirin

SERIOUS REACTIONS
! Ecchymosis, epistaxis, gum hemorrhage have been reported (drug produces weak anticoagulant effect).
! Overdose may produce liver function abnormalities.

DENTAL CONSIDERATIONS
General:
• Possesses weak anticoagulant activity; question patient about bleeding or bruising.
• Consider semisupine chair position for patient comfort if GI side effects occur.
• Question patient about tolerance of NSAIDs or aspirin related to GI disease.

• Avoid products that affect platelet function, such as aspirin and NSAIDs.
• Consider local hemostasis measures to prevent excessive bleeding.
Consultations:
• Confer with physician if bleeding is a problem; epistaxis, spontaneous gingival bleeding.
• Medical consultation should include routine blood counts, including platelet counts and bleeding time.
Teach Patient/Family to:
• Encourage effective oral hygiene to prevent soft tissue inflammation.
• Prevent trauma when using oral hygiene aids.
• Report oral lesions, soreness, or bleeding to dentist.
• Importance of updating health and medication history if physician makes any changes in evaluation or drug regimens; include OTC, herbal, and nonherbal drugs in the update.

P

pentostatin
pen-toe-**stat**′-in
(Nipent)
Do not confuse with pravastatin.

CATEGORY AND SCHEDULE
Pregnancy Risk Category: D

Drug Class: Antineoplastic, enzyme inhibitor

MECHANISM OF ACTION
An antimetabolite that inhibits the enzyme adenosine deaminase (ADA) (increases intracellular levels of adenine deoxynucleotide). Greatest activity in T cells of lymphoid system. Inhibits ADA and RNA synthesis. Produces DNA damage.

Therapeutic Effect: Leads to death of tumor cells.

USES
Treatment of α-interferon–refractory hairy cell leukemia

PHARMACOKINETICS
After IV administration, rapidly distributed to body tissues (poorly distributed to cerebrospinal fluid). Protein binding: 4%. Excreted primarily in urine unchanged or as active metabolite. *Half-life:* 5.7 hr (2.6–10 hr).

INDICATIONS AND DOSAGES
▶ **Hairy Cell Leukemia**
IV
Adults, Elderly. 4 mg/m² q2wk until complete response attained (without any major toxicity). Discontinue if no response in 6 mo; partial response in 12 mo.
▶ **Dosage in Renal Impairment**
Only when benefits justify risks, give 2–3 mg/m² in patients with creatinine clearance 50–60 ml/min.

SIDE EFFECTS/ADVERSE REACTIONS
Frequent
Nausea, vomiting, fever, fatigue, rash, pain, cough, upper respiratory tract infection, anorexia, diarrhea
Occasional
Headache, pharyngitis, sinusitis, myalgia, chills, arthralgia, peripheral edema, anorexia, blurred vision, conjunctivitis, skin discoloration, sweating, anxiety, depression, dizziness, confusion

PRECAUTIONS AND CONTRAINDICATIONS
Hypersensitivity to pentostatin

SERIOUS REACTIONS
❗ Bone marrow depression is manifested as hematologic toxicity (principally leukopenia, anemia, thrombocytopenia).
❗ Doses higher than recommended (20–50 mg/m² in divided doses for more than 5 days) may produce severe renal, hepatic, pulmonary, or CNS toxicity.

DENTAL CONSIDERATIONS
• Increased susceptibility to infections.
• Increased bleeding.
• Anemia.
• Oral ulcerations, mucositis (use palliative measures for relief).
• Increased nausea, vomiting.
• Consult physician to determine disease control and ability of patient to tolerate dental procedures.

pentoxifylline
pen-tox-**if**′-ih-lin
(Albert[CAN], Apo-Pentoxifylline SR[CAN], Pentoxifylline[CAN], Pentoxyl, Trental)
Do not confuse Trental with Tegretol or Trandate.

CATEGORY AND SCHEDULE
Pregnancy Risk Category: C

Drug Class: Hemorheologic agent

MECHANISM OF ACTION
A blood viscosity-reducing agent that alters the flexibility of RBCs; inhibits production of tumor necrosis factor, neutrophil activation, and platelet aggregation.
Therapeutic Effect: Reduces blood viscosity and improves blood flow.

USES

Treatment of intermittent claudication related to chronic occlusive arterial disease of the limbs

PHARMACOKINETICS

Well absorbed after oral administration. Undergoes first-pass metabolism in the liver. Primarily excreted in urine. Unknown if removed by hemodialysis.
Half-life: 24–48 min; metabolite, 60–90 min.

INDICATIONS AND DOSAGES

▶ **Intermittent Claudication**
PO
Adults, Elderly. 400 mg 3 times a day. Decrease to 400 mg twice a day if GI or CNS adverse effects occur. Continue for at least 8 wk.

SIDE EFFECTS/ADVERSE REACTIONS

Occasional
Dizziness, nausea, altered taste, dyspepsia, marked by heartburn, epigastric pain, and indigestion
Rare
Rash, pruritus, anorexia, constipation, dry mouth, blurred vision, edema, nasal congestion, anxiety

PRECAUTIONS AND CONTRAINDICATIONS

History of intolerance to xanthine derivatives, such as caffeine, theophylline, or theobromine; recent cerebral or retinal hemorrhage
Caution:
Angina pectoris, cardiac disease, lactation, children, impaired renal function

DRUG INTERACTIONS OF CONCERN TO DENTISTRY

• Increased bleeding: ASA, NSAIDs

SERIOUS REACTIONS

❗ Angina and chest pain occur rarely and may be accompanied by palpitations, tachycardia, and arrhythmias.
❗ Signs and symptoms of overdose, such as flushing, hypotension, nervousness, agitation, hand tremor, fever, and somnolence, appear 4–5 hr after ingestion and last for 12 hr.

DENTAL CONSIDERATIONS

General:
• Monitor vital signs at every appointment because of cardiovascular side effects.
• Assess salivary flow as a factor in caries, periodontal disease, and candidiasis.
• Stress from dental procedures may compromise cardiovascular function; determine patient risk.
• Short appointments and a stress-reduction protocol may be required for anxious patients.
• Talk with patient about potential systemic diseases (e.g., diabetes, cardiovascular disease) that may be associated with claudication.
Consultations:
• Medical consultation may be required to assess disease control and patient's ability to tolerate stress.
Teach Patient/Family to:
• Encourage effective oral hygiene to prevent soft tissue inflammation.
• Prevent injury when using oral hygiene aids.
• When chronic dry mouth occurs, advise patient to:
  • Avoid mouth rinses with high alcohol content because of drying effects.
  • Use home fluoride products to prevent caries.

P

• Use sugarless gum, frequent sips of water, or saliva substitutes.

perindopril
per-**in**′-doh-pril
(Aceon)

CATEGORY AND SCHEDULE
Pregnancy Risk Category: C (D if used in second or third trimester)

Drug Class: Angiotensin-converting enzyme (ACE) inhibitor

MECHANISM OF ACTION
An ACE inhibitor that suppresses the renin-angiotensin-aldosterone system and prevents conversion of angiotensin I to angiotensin II, a potent vasoconstrictor; may also inhibit angiotensin II at local vascular and renal sites.
Therapeutic Effect: Reduces peripheral arterial resistance and B/P.

USES
Treatment of essential hypertension as monotherapy or in combination with other antihypertensive medication

PHARMACOKINETICS
PO: Absolute bioavailability 20%–30%, metabolized to active metabolite, perindoprilat, peak plasma levels 1 hr, active metabolite 3–4 hr; protein binding 10%–20%, hepatic metabolism, excreted mostly in urine (75%)

INDICATIONS AND DOSAGES
▶ **Hypertension**
PO
Adults, Elderly. 2–8 mg/day as single dose or in 2 divided doses. Maximum: 16 mg/day.

SIDE EFFECTS/ADVERSE REACTIONS
Occasional
Cough, back pain, sinusitis, upper extremity pain, dyspepsia, fever, palpitations, hypotension, dizziness, fatigue, syncope

PRECAUTIONS AND CONTRAINDICATIONS
History of angioedema from previous treatment with ACE inhibitors
Caution:
Renal insufficiency, hypertension with CHF, severe CHF, renal artery stenosis, autoimmune disease, collagen vascular disease, pregnancy category C (first trimester); pregnancy category D (second and third trimesters), lactation

DRUG INTERACTIONS OF CONCERN TO DENTISTRY
• Decreased hypotensive effects: NSAIDs, aspirin
• Increased hypotension: caution in use of other drugs that have hypotensive effects
• Suspected reduction in the antihypertensive and vasodilator effects by salicylates; monitor B/P if used concurrently

SERIOUS REACTIONS
! Excessive hypotension ("first-dose syncope") may occur in patients with CHF and in those who are severely salt or volume depleted.
! Angioedema (swelling of face and lips) and hyperkalemia occur rarely.

! Agranulocytosis and neutropenia may be noted in those with collagen vascular disease, including scleroderma and systemic lupus erythematosus, and impaired renal function.

! Nephrotic syndrome may be noted in those with history of renal disease.

DENTAL CONSIDERATIONS

General:
• Monitor vital signs at every appointment because of cardiovascular side effects.
• Limit use of sodium-containing products, such as saline IV fluids, for patients with a dietary salt restriction.
• Stress from dental procedures may compromise cardiovascular function; determine patient risk.
• Short appointments and a stress-reduction protocol may be required for anxious patients.
• After supine positioning, have patient sit upright for at least 2 min before standing to avoid orthostatic hypotension.
• Use precaution if sedation or general anesthesia is required; risk of hypotensive episode.
• Assess salivary flow as a factor in caries, periodontal disease, and candidiasis.
• Consider semisupine chair position for patient comfort if GI or respiratory side effects occur.
• Patients on chronic drug therapy may rarely have symptoms of blood dyscrasias, which can include infection, bleeding, and poor healing.
Consultations:
• In a patient with symptoms of blood dyscrasias, request a medical consultation for blood studies and

postpone treatment until normal values are reestablished.
• Medical consultation may be required to assess disease control and patient's ability to tolerate stress.
Teach Patient/Family to:
• Update health and drug history if physician makes any changes in evaluation or drug regimens; include OTC, herbal, and nonherbal drugs in the update.
• Encourage effective oral hygiene to prevent soft tissue inflammation.
• Prevent trauma when using oral hygiene aids.
• When chronic dry mouth occurs, advise patient to:
  • Avoid mouth rinses with high alcohol content because of drying effects.
  • Use daily home fluoride products for anticaries effect.
  • Use sugarless gum, frequent sips of water, or saliva substitutes.

P

perphenazine
per-**fen**′-ah-zeen
(Trilafon)
Do not confuse perphenazine with promazine.

CATEGORY AND SCHEDULE
Pregnancy Risk Category: C

Drug Class: Phenothiazine antipsychotic

MECHANISM OF ACTION
An antipsychotic agent and antiemetic that blocks postsynaptic dopamine receptor sites in the brain. *Therapeutic Effect:* Suppresses behavioral response in psychosis, and relieves nausea and vomiting.

USES
Treatment of psychotic disorders, schizophrenia, alcoholism, nausea, vomiting

PHARMACOKINETICS
PO: Onset erratic, peak 2–4 hr IM: Onset 10 min, peak 1–2 hr, duration 6 hr, occasionally 12–24 hr Metabolized by liver, excreted in urine, crosses placenta, excreted in breast milk.

INDICATIONS AND DOSAGES
▶ **Severe Schizophrenia**
PO
Adults. 4–16 mg 2–4 times a day. Maximum: 64 mg/day.
Elderly. Initially, 2–4 mg/day. May increase at 4–7 day intervals by 2–4 mg/day up to 32 mg/day.
▶ **Severe Nausea and Vomiting**
PO
Adults. 8–16 mg/day in divided doses up to 24 mg/day.

SIDE EFFECTS/ADVERSE REACTIONS
Occasional
Marked photosensitivity, somnolence, dry mouth, blurred vision, lethargy, constipation or diarrhea, nasal congestion, peripheral edema, urine retention
Rare
Ocular changes, altered skin pigmentation, hypotension, dizziness, syncope

PRECAUTIONS AND CONTRAINDICATIONS
Coma, myelosuppression, severe cardiovascular disease, severe CNS depression, subcortical brain damage
Caution:
Lactation, seizure disorders, hypertension, hepatic disease, cardiac disease

DRUG INTERACTIONS OF CONCERN TO DENTISTRY
• Increased sedation: other CNS depressants, alcohol, barbiturate anesthetics, opioid analgesics
• Hypotension, tachycardia: epinephrine
• Increased extrapyramidal effects: phenothiazines and related drugs (haloperidol, droperidol), metoclopramide
• Additive photosensitization: tetracyclines, fluoroquinolones
• Increased anticholinergic effects: anticholinergics

SERIOUS REACTIONS
❗ Extrapyramidal symptoms appear to be dose-related and are divided into three categories: akathisia (characterized by inability to sit still, tapping of feet), parkinsonian symptoms (including mask-like face, tremors, shuffling gait, hypersalivation), and acute dystonias (such as torticollis, opisthotonos, and oculogyric crisis).
❗ Tardive dyskinesia occurs rarely.
❗ Abrupt withdrawal after long-term therapy may precipitate nausea, vomiting, gastritis, dizziness, and tremors.

DENTAL CONSIDERATIONS

General:
• Monitor vital signs at every appointment because of cardiovascular side effects.
• Patients on chronic drug therapy may rarely have symptoms of blood dyscrasias, which can include infection, bleeding, and poor healing.
• After supine positioning, have patient sit upright for at least 2 min before standing to avoid orthostatic hypotension.

• Assess salivary flow as a factor in caries, periodontal disease, and candidiasis.
• Avoid dental light in patient's eyes; offer dark glasses for patient comfort.
• Assess for presence of extrapyramidal motor symptoms, such as tardive dyskinesia and akathisia. Extrapyramidal motor activity may complicate dental treatment.
• Geriatric patients are more susceptible to drug effects; use lower dose.
• Use vasoconstrictors with caution, in low doses, and with careful aspiration. Avoid use of gingival retraction cord with epinephrine.

Consultations:
• In a patient with symptoms of blood dyscrasias, request a medical consultation for blood studies and postpone dental treatment until normal values are reestablished.
• Take precautions if dental surgery is anticipated and anesthesia is required.
• If signs of tardive dyskinesia or akathisia are present, refer to physician.
• Physician should be informed if significant xerostomic side effects occur (e.g., increased caries, sore tongue, problems eating or swallowing, difficulty wearing prosthesis) so that a medication change can be considered.

Teach Patient/Family to:
• Encourage effective oral hygiene to prevent soft tissue inflammation.
• Use caution to prevent injury when using oral hygiene aids.
• Use powered tooth brush if patient has difficulty holding conventional devices.
• When chronic dry mouth occurs, advise patient to:

• Avoid mouth rinses with high alcohol content because of drying effects.
• Use daily home fluoride products to prevent caries.
• Use sugarless gum, frequent sips of water, or saliva substitutes.

---

phenazopyridine hydrochloride

fen-az-oh-**peer**′-ih-deen high-droh-**klor**′-ide
(Azo-Gesic, Azo-Standard, Phenazo[CAN], Prodium, Pyridium, Uristat)
Do not confuse phenazopyridine with pyridoxine, or Prodium with Perdiem.

CATEGORY AND SCHEDULE
Pregnancy Risk Category: B

Drug Class: Urinary tract analgesic

MECHANISM OF ACTION
An interstitial cystitis agent that exerts topical analgesic effect on urinary tract mucosa.
Therapeutic Effect: Relieves urinary pain, burning, urgency, and frequency.

USES
Treatment of urinary tract irritation/infection

PHARMACOKINETICS
Well absorbed from the GI tract. Partially metabolized in the liver. Primarily excreted in urine.

P

INDICATIONS AND DOSAGES
▶ **Urinary Analgesic**
PO
Adults. 100–200 mg 3–4 times a day.
Children 6 yr and older. 12 mg/kg/ day in 3 divided doses for 2 days.
▶ **Dosage in Renal Impairment**
Dosage interval is modified on the basis of creatinine clearance.

Creatinine Clearance	Interval
50–80 ml/min	Usual dose q8–16h
Less than 50 ml/min	Avoid use

SIDE EFFECTS/ADVERSE REACTIONS
Occasional
Headache, GI disturbance, rash, pruritus

PRECAUTIONS AND CONTRAINDICATIONS
Hepatic or renal insufficiency
Caution:
Renal disease

DRUG INTERACTIONS OF CONCERN TO DENTISTRY
• None reported

SERIOUS REACTIONS
! Overdose may lead to hemolytic anemia, nephrotoxicity, or hepatotoxicity. Patients with renal impairment or severe hypersensitivity to the drug may also develop these reactions.
! A massive and acute overdose may result in methemoglobinemia.

DENTAL CONSIDERATIONS

General:
• Consider semisupine chair position for patient comfort if GI side effects occur.

• Patients on chronic drug therapy may rarely have symptoms of blood dyscrasias, which can include infection, bleeding, and poor healing.
• Be aware that patient might have UTI; question if antiinfectives are also being used.

phendimetrazine
fen-dye-**me**′-tra-zeen
(Adipost, Bontril PDM, Bontril Slow-Release, Melfiat, Obezine, Phendiet, Phendiet-105, Plegine, Prelu-2)

CATEGORY AND SCHEDULE
Pregnancy Risk Category: C
Controlled Substance: Schedule III

Drug Class: Anorexiant, amphetamine-like

MECHANISM OF ACTION
A phenylalkylamine sympathomimetic with activity similar to amphetamines that stimulates the CNS and elevates B/P most likely mediated via norepinephrine and dopamine metabolism. Causes stimulation of the hypothalamus.
Therapeutic Effect: Decreases appetite.

USES
Treatment of exogenous obesity

PHARMACOKINETICS
The pharmacokinetics of phendimetrazine tartrate has not been well established. Metabolized to active metabolite, phendimetrazine. Excreted in urine.
Half-life: 2–4 hr.

INDICATIONS AND DOSAGES
▶ **Obesity**
PO
Adults, Elderly. 105 mg/day in the morning or before the morning meal (sustained release); 35 mg 2–3 times a day (immediate release). Maximum: 70 mg 3 times a day.

SIDE EFFECTS/ADVERSE REACTIONS
Occasional
Constipation, nausea, diarrhea, dry mouth, dysuria, libido changes, flushing, hypertension, insomnia, nervousness, headache, dizziness, irritability, agitation, restlessness, palpitations, increased heart rate, sweating, tremor, urticaria

PRECAUTIONS AND CONTRAINDICATIONS
Advanced arteriosclerosis, agitated states, glaucoma, history of drug abuse, history of hypersensitivity to sympathomimetic amines, hyperthyroidism, moderate-to-severe hypertension, symptomatic cardiovascular disease, use within 14 days of discontinuation MAOI, hypersensitivity to phendimetrazine or sympathomimetics
Caution:
Drug abuse, anxiety, lactation

DRUG INTERACTIONS OF CONCERN TO DENTISTRY
• Hypertensive crisis: MAOIs or within 14 days of MAOIs
• Increased risk of dysrhythmia: hydrocarbon inhalation, general anesthetics, epinephrine
• Decreased effect: tricyclic antidepressants, ascorbic acid, phenothiazines
• Caffeine or caffeine-containing products: may increase risk of insomnia and dry mouth

SERIOUS REACTIONS
! Multivalvular heart disease, primary pulmonary hypertension, and arrhythmias occur rarely.
! Overdose may produce flushing, arrhythmias, and psychosis.
! Abrupt withdrawal following prolonged administration of high doses may produce extreme fatigue and depression.

DENTAL CONSIDERATIONS
General:
• Monitor vital signs at every appointment because of cardiovascular side effects.
• Avoid or limit dose of vasoconstrictor.
• Assess salivary flow as a factor in caries, periodontal disease, and candidiasis.
• Determine why the patient is taking the drug.
• Psychologic and physical dependence may occur with chronic administration.
• Patients on chronic drug therapy may rarely have symptoms of blood dyscrasias, which can include infection, bleeding, and poor healing.
Consultations:
• In a patient with symptoms of blood dyscrasias, request a medical consultation for blood studies and postpone dental treatment until normal values are reestablished.
Teach Patient/Family to:
• Encourage effective oral hygiene to prevent soft tissue inflammation.
• Report oral lesions, soreness, or bleeding to dentist.
• Use caution to prevent injury when using oral hygiene aids.
• When chronic dry mouth occurs, advise patient to:
  • Avoid mouth rinses with high alcohol content because of drying effects.

• Use daily home fluoride products to prevent caries.
• Use sugarless gum, frequent sips of water, or saliva substitutes.

phenelzine sulfate
fen´-el-zeen **sull**´-fate
(Nardil)

CATEGORY AND SCHEDULE
Pregnancy Risk Category: C

Drug Class: Antidepressant, monoamine oxidase inhibitor (MAOI)

MECHANISM OF ACTION
An MAOI that inhibits the activity of the enzyme monoamine oxidase at CNS storage sites, leading to increased levels of the neurotransmitters epinephrine, norepinephrine, serotonin, and dopamine at neuronal receptor sites. *Therapeutic Effect:* Relieves depression.

USES
Treatment of depression when uncontrolled by other means

PHARMACOKINETICS
Well absorbed from GI tract. Metabolized in the liver. Primarily excreted in urine. *Half-life:* 1.2 hr.

INDICATIONS AND DOSAGES
▸ **Depression Refractory to Other Antidepressants or Electroconvulsive Therapy**
PO
Adults. 5 mg 3 times a day. May increase to 60–90 mg/day.
Elderly. Initially, 7.5 mg/day. May increase by 7.5–15 mg/day q3–4wk up to 60 mg/day in divided doses.

SIDE EFFECTS/ADVERSE REACTIONS
Frequent
Orthostatic hypotension, restlessness, GI upset, insomnia, dizziness, headache, lethargy, asthenia, dry mouth, peripheral edema
Occasional
Flushing, diaphoresis, rash, urinary frequency, increased appetite, transient impotence
Rare
Visual disturbances

PRECAUTIONS AND CONTRAINDICATIONS
Cardiovascular or cerebrovascular disease, hepatic or renal impairment, pheochromocytoma
Caution:
Suicidal patients, convulsive disorders, severe depression, schizophrenia, hyperactivity, diabetes mellitus

DRUG INTERACTIONS OF CONCERN TO DENTISTRY
• Increased anticholinergic effect: anticholinergics, haloperidol, phenothiazines, antihistamines
• Hyperpyretic crisis, convulsions, hypertensive episode: meperidine, carbamazepine, cyclobenzaprine
• Cardiac dysrhythmia: caffeine-containing medications
• Increased risk of serotonin syndrome: tricyclic antidepressants, other serotonin reuptake inhibitors
• Increased sedative effects of alcohol, barbiturates, benzodiazepines, CNS depressants
• Increased pressor effects: indirect-acting sympathomimetics, such as ephedrine, amphetamine

SERIOUS REACTIONS
❗ Hypertensive crisis occurs rarely and is marked by severe

hypertension, occipital headache radiating frontally, neck stiffness or soreness, nausea, vomiting, diaphoresis, fever or chilliness, clammy skin, dilated pupils, palpitations, tachycardia or bradycardia, and constricting chest pain.

! Intracranial bleeding has been reported in association with severe hypertension.

DENTAL CONSIDERATIONS

General:
• Monitor vital signs at every appointment because of cardiovascular side effects.
• Assess salivary flow as a factor in caries, periodontal disease, and candidiasis.
• After supine positioning, have patient sit upright for at least 2 min before standing to avoid orthostatic hypotension.
• Hypertensive episodes are possible even though there are no specific contraindications to vasoconstrictor use in local anesthetics.
• Avoid prescribing caffeine-containing products.
• Take precautions if dental surgery is anticipated and general anesthesia is required.

Consultations:
• Medical consultation may be required to assess disease control and patient's ability to tolerate stress.

Teach Patient/Family to:
• Use powered tooth brush if patient has difficulty holding conventional devices.
• When chronic dry mouth occurs, advise patient to:
  • Avoid mouth rinses with high alcohol content because of drying effects.

• Use daily home fluoride products to prevent caries.
• Use sugarless gum, frequent sips of water, or saliva substitutes.

phenobarbital
fee-noe-**bar**′-bi-tal
(Luminal, Phenobarbitone[AUS])
Do not confuse phenobarbital with pentobarbital, or Luminal with Tuinal.

CATEGORY AND SCHEDULE
Pregnancy Risk Category: D
Controlled Substance: Schedule IV

Drug Class: Barbiturate anticonvulsant

MECHANISM OF ACTION
A barbiturate that enhances the activity of gamma-aminobutyric acid (GABA) by binding to the GABA receptor complex.
Therapeutic Effect: Depresses CNS activity.

USES
Treatment of all forms of epilepsy, status epilepticus, febrile seizures in children, sedation, insomnia; unapproved: hyperbilirubinemia, chronic cholestasis

PHARMACOKINETICS

Route	Onset	Peak	Duration
PO	20–60 min	N/A	6–10 hr
IV	5 min	30 min	4–10 hr

Well absorbed after PO or parenteral administration. Protein binding: 35%–50%. Rapidly and widely

P

distributed. Metabolized in the liver. Primarily excreted in urine. Removed by hemodialysis. *Half-life:* 53–118 hr.

INDICATIONS AND DOSAGES
▸ **Status Epilepticus**
IV
Adults, Elderly, Children, Neonates. Loading dose of 15–20 mg/kg as a single dose or in divided doses.
▸ **Seizure Control**
PO, IV
Adults, Elderly, Children older than 12 yr. 1–3 mg/kg/day.
Children 6–12 yr. 4–6 mg/kg/day.
Children 1–5 yr. 6–8 mg/kg/day.
Children younger than 1 yr. 5–6 mg/ kg/day.
Neonates. 3–4 mg/kg/day.
▸ **Sedation**
PO, IM
Adults, Elderly. 30–120 mg/day in 2–3 divided doses.
Children. 2 mg/kg 3 times a day.
▸ **Hypnotic**
PO, IV, IM, Subcutaneous
Adults, Elderly. 100–320 mg at bedtime.
Children. 3–5 mg/kg at bedtime.

SIDE EFFECTS/ADVERSE REACTIONS
Occasional
Somnolence
Rare
Confusion; paradoxic CNS reactions, such as hyperactivity or nervousness in children and excitement or restlessness in the elderly (generally noted during first 2 wk of therapy, particularly in presence of uncontrolled pain)

PRECAUTIONS AND CONTRAINDICATIONS
Porphyria, preexisting CNS depression, severe pain, severe respiratory disease

Caution:
Anemia

DRUG INTERACTIONS OF CONCERN TO DENTISTRY
• Increased effects: alcohol, all CNS depressants, saquinavir
• Decreased effects of corticosteroids, doxycycline, carbamazepine

SERIOUS REACTIONS
! Abrupt withdrawal after prolonged therapy may produce increased dreaming, nightmares, insomnia, tremor, diaphoresis, vomiting, hallucinations, delirium, seizures, and status epilepticus.
! Skin eruptions may be a sign of a hypersensitivity reaction.
! Blood dyscrasias, hepatic disease, and hypocalcemia occur rarely.
! Overdose produces cold or clammy skin, hypothermia, severe CNS depression, cyanosis, tachycardia, and Cheyne-Stokes respirations.
! Toxicity may result in severe renal impairment.

DENTAL CONSIDERATIONS
General:
• Determine why the patient is taking the drug.
• Monitor vital signs at every appointment because of cardiovascular side effects. Evaluate respiration characteristics and rate.
• Patients on chronic drug therapy may rarely have symptoms of blood dyscrasias, which can include infection, bleeding, and poor healing.
• When used for sedation in dentistry:
    • Assess vital signs before and during use and after use as sedative.

• Observe respiratory dysfunction: respiratory depression, character, rate, rhythm; hold drug if respirations are less frequent than 10/min or if pupils are dilated.
• After supine positioning, have patient sit upright for at least 2 min before standing to avoid orthostatic hypotension.
• Have someone escort patient to and from dental office when drug used for conscious sedation.
• Barbiturates induce liver microsomal enzymes, which alter the metabolism of other drugs.
• Geriatric patients are more susceptible to drug effects; use lower dose.
Consultations:
• In a patient with symptoms of blood dyscrasias, request a medical consultation for blood studies and postpone dental treatment until normal values are reestablished.
Teach Patient/Family to:
• Avoid driving or other activities requiring alertness.
• Avoid alcohol ingestion or CNS depressants; serious CNS depression may result.
• Use OTC preparations with caution because they may contain other CNS depressants (e.g., antihistamines, cold remedies).

phenoxybenzamine
fen-ox-ee-**ben**′-za-meen
(Dibenzyline)

CATEGORY AND SCHEDULE
Pregnancy Risk Category: C

Drug Class: Antihypertensive, pheochromocytoma

MECHANISM OF ACTION
An antihypertensive that produces long-lasting, noncompetitive α-adrenergic blockade of postganglionic synapses in exocrine glands and smooth muscles. Relaxes urethra and increases opening of the bladder.
Therapeutic Effect: Controls hypertension.

USES
Treatment of hypertension caused by pheochromocytoma

PHARMACOKINETICS
Well absorbed from the GI tract. Distributed into fatty tissue. Metabolized in liver. Eliminated in urine and feces. Not removed by hemodialysis. ***Half-life:*** 24 hr.

INDICATIONS AND DOSAGES
▸ **Pheochromocytoma**
PO
Adults. Initially, 10 mg twice daily. May increase dose every other day to 20–40 mg 2–3 times/day.
Children. 1–2 mg/kg/day in divided doses.

SIDE EFFECTS/ADVERSE REACTIONS
Frequent
Headache, lethargy, confusion, fatigue
Occasional
Nausea, postural hypotension, syncope, dry mouth
Rare
Palpitations, diarrhea, constipation, inhibition of ejaculation, weakness, altered vision, dizziness

PRECAUTIONS AND CONTRAINDICATIONS
Any condition compromised by hypotension, hypersensitivity to

P

phenoxybenzamine or any component of the formulation

DRUG INTERACTIONS OF CONCERN TO DENTISTRY
• Exaggerated hypotension, tachycardia: epinephrine, other α-adrenergic agonists

SERIOUS REACTIONS
! Overdosage produces severe hypotension, irritability, lethargy, tachycardia, dizziness, and shock.

DENTAL CONSIDERATIONS

General:
• Medication may be used in anticipation of surgery to remove the adrenal tumor.
• Hypertension may preclude all dental care except for palliative emergency treatment.
• Question patient about compliance with drug therapy.
• Risk of increased CNS depression when other CNS depressants are used.
• Determine why patient is taking the drug.
• Monitor and record vital signs.
• Use vasoconstrictor with caution, in low doses, and with careful aspiration. Avoid using gingival retraction cord containing epinephrine.
• After supine positioning, have patient sit upright for at least 2 min before standing to avoid orthostatic hypotension.
Consultations:
• Medical consultation may be required to assess disease control and patient's ability to tolerate stress.
Teach Patient/Family to:
• Encourage effective oral hygiene to prevent soft tissue inflammation.

• Not drive or perform other tasks requiring mental alertness.

phentermine
fen′-ter-meen
(Adipex-P, Fastin, Ionamin, Oby-Cap, Phentercot, Pro-Fast HS, Pro-Fast SA, Pro-Fast SR, T-Diet, Teramine, Zantryl)

CATEGORY AND SCHEDULE
Pregnancy Risk Category: B
Controlled Substance: Schedule IV

Drug Class: Sympathomimetic, anorexiant

MECHANISM OF ACTION
A sympathomimetic amine structurally similar to dextroamphetamine and is most likely mediated via norepinephrine and dopamine metabolism. Causes stimulation of the hypothalamus. *Therapeutic Effect:* Decreased appetite.

USES
Treatment of exogenous obesity

PHARMACOKINETICS
Well absorbed from the GI tract; resin absorbed slower. Excreted unchanged in urine. *Half-life:* 20 hr.

INDICATIONS AND DOSAGES
▸ Obesity
PO
Adults, Children older than 16 yr.
Adipex-P: 37.5 mg as a single daily dose or in divided doses.
Ionamin: 15–37.5 mg/day before breakfast or 1–2 hr after breakfast.
Fastin: 30 mg/day taken in the morning.

SIDE EFFECTS/ADVERSE REACTIONS

Occasional

Restlessness, insomnia, tremor, palpitations, tachycardia, elevation in B/P, headache, dizziness, dry mouth, unpleasant taste, diarrhea or constipation, changes in libido

PRECAUTIONS AND CONTRAINDICATIONS

Advanced arteriosclerosis, agitated states, cardiovascular disease, concurrent use or within 14 days of discontinuation of MAOI therapy, glaucoma, history of drug abuse, hypertension (moderate to severe), hyperthyroidism, hypersensitivity to phentermine or sympathomimetic amines

Caution:

Lactation, drug abuse, anxiety, tolerance

DRUG INTERACTIONS OF CONCERN TO DENTISTRY

• Hypertensive crisis: MAOIs or within 14 days of MAOIs
• Increased risk of dysrhythmia: hydrocarbon inhalation general anesthetics
• Decreased effect: tricyclic antidepressants, ascorbic acid, phenothiazines
• Caffeine or caffeine-containing products may increase risk of insomnia

SERIOUS REACTIONS

❗ Primary pulmonary hypertension (PPH), psychotic episodes, and valvular heart disease rarely occur.
❗ Anorectic agents have been associated with regurgitant multivalvular heart disease involving mitral, aortic, and/or tricuspid valves.
❗ Prolonged use may cause physical or psychological dependence.

DENTAL CONSIDERATIONS

General:

• Monitor vital signs at every appointment because of cardiovascular side effects.
• Assess salivary flow as a factor in caries, periodontal disease, and candidiasis.
• Determine why the patient is taking the drug.
• Psychologic and physical dependence may occur with chronic administration.
• Patients on chronic drug therapy may rarely have symptoms of blood dyscrasias, which can include infection, bleeding, and poor healing.

Consultations:

• In a patient with symptoms of blood dyscrasias, request a medical consultation for blood studies and postpone dental treatment until normal values are reestablished.
• Determine need for possible antibiotic prophylaxis.

Teach Patient/Family to:

• Encourage effective oral hygiene to prevent soft tissue inflammation.
• Prevent injury when using oral hygiene aids.
• Report oral lesions, soreness, or bleeding to dentist.
• When chronic dry mouth occurs, advise patient to:
  • Avoid mouth rinses with high alcohol content because of drying effects.
  • Use daily home fluoride products to prevent caries.
  • Use sugarless gum, frequent sips of water, or saliva substitutes.

P

phentolamine
fen-**tole**′-ah-meen
(Regitine, Oraverse)

CATEGORY AND SCHEDULE
Pregnancy Risk Category: C

Drug Class: Antihypertensive

MECHANISM OF ACTION
Blocks α-adrenergic receptors.
Therapeutic Effect: Produces
relaxation of vascular smooth
muscle, vasodilation and increased
blood flow, systemically reducing
blood pressure and locally increasing
the rate of vascular uptake of dental
local anesthetics containing a
vasoconstrictor.

USES
Treatment of hypertension, diagnosis
of pheochromocytoma, control of
acute hypertension, prevention and
treatment of dermal necrosis
following extravasation of
norepinephrine or dopamine
(unapproved with papaverine for
intracavernous injection for
impotence) (Regitine); reversal of
dental local anesthetic-related
soft-tissue anesthesia and associated
functional deficits (Oraverse)

PHARMACOKINETICS
Poorly absorbed from the GI tract;
rapidly absorbed after parenteral
administration. Protein binding 72%.
Metabolized primarily in the liver;
metabolites excreted in urine and
feces. ***Half-life***: 2–3 hr.

INDICATIONS AND DOSAGES
▸ **Extravasation of Norepinephrine**
Subcutaneous
Adults, Elderly. Infiltrate area with a
small amount (1 ml) of solution

made by diluting 5–10 mg in 10 ml
of normal saline within 12 hr of
extravasation. Do not exceed
0.1–0.2 mg/kg or 5 mg total. If dose
is effective, normal skin color
should return to the blanched area
within 1 hr.
Children. Infiltrate area with small
amount (1 ml) of solution made by
diluting 5–10 mg in 10 ml of normal
saline within 12 hr of extravasation.
Do not exceed 0.1–0.2 mg/kg or
5 mg total.
▸ **Diagnosis of Pheochromocytoma**
IM/IV
Adults, Elderly. 5 mg as a single
dose.
Children. 0.05–0.1 mg/kg/dose,
maximum single dose 5 mg.
▸ **Surgery for Pheochromocytoma**
Hypertension
IM/IV
Adults, Elderly. 5 mg given 1–2 hr
before procedure and repeated as
needed every 2–4 hr.
Children. 0.05–0.1 mg/kg/dose given
1–2 hr before procedure. Repeat as
needed every 2–4 hr until
hypertension is controlled.
Maximum single dose: 5 mg
▸ **Hypertensive Crisis**
IV
Adults, Elderly. 5–20 mg as a single
dose.
▸ **Reversal of Soft-Tissue Anesthesia**
Related to Dental Local Anesthetics
0.2 to 0.8 mg (0.25–2 1.7-ml dental
cartridges), using the same
location(s) and technique(s)
employed for the administration of
the vasoconstrictor-containing local
anesthetic (infiltration or block
technique).

SIDE EFFECTS/ADVERSE
REACTIONS
Occasional
Hypotension, tachycardia,
bradycardia, flushing, orthostatic

hypotension, weakness, dizziness, nausea, vomiting, diarrhea, nasal congestion, pulmonary hypertension, injection site pain
Rare
Acute, prolonged hypotension, cardiac dysrhythmias
Contraindications
Hypersensitivity

PRECAUTIONS AND CONTRAINDICATIONS
Myocardial infarction, cerebrovascular spasm and cerebrovascular occlusion have been reported following parenteral administration of phentolamine, in association with hypotension producing shock-like states. Contraindicated in patients with hypersensitivity to phentolamine.

DRUG INTERACTIONS OF CONCERN TO DENTISTRY
• None reported

SERIOUS REACTIONS
! Symptoms of overdosage include tachycardia, shock, vomiting, and dizziness.
! Mixed-acting (e.g., epinephrine) agents may result in greater hypotension.

DENTAL CONSIDERATIONS
General:
• When used for reversal of soft-tissue anesthesia associated with dental local anesthetic, use to reverse soft-tissue effects of vasoconstrictor-containing local anesthetics and explain use and effects of drug to patient.
• This is an acute-use drug for hypertension and pheochromocytoma, which are the principal immediate, systemic concerns.

• Assess vital signs at each appointment because of nature of disease.
• Patients with untreated pheochromocytoma or with extreme, uncontrolled hypertension are not candidates for elective dental treatment.
• Stress from dental procedures may compromise cardiovascular function; determine patient risk.
• Short appointments and stress-reduction protocol may be required for anxious patients.
• Use vasoconstrictors with caution, in low doses and with careful aspiration.
Consultations:
• Consult with physician to determine disease control and ability to tolerate dental procedures.
Teach Patient/Family to:
• Update medical history based on most recent medical evaluation.

phenylephrine hydrochloride
fen-ill-**eh′**-frin high-droh-**klor′**-ide
(AD-Nephrin, AK-Dilate, Isopto Frin[AUS], Mydfrin, Neo-Synephrine, Neo-Synephrine Ophthalmic Viscous 10%[AUS], Prefrin)

CATEGORY AND SCHEDULE
Pregnancy Risk Category: C
OTC (nasal solution, nasal spray, ophthalmic solution)

Drug Class: Nasal decongestant, sympathomimetic

MECHANISM OF ACTION
A sympathomimetic, α receptor stimulant that acts on the α-adrenergic receptors of vascular

smooth muscle. Causes vasoconstriction of arterioles of nasal mucosa or conjunctiva, activates dilator muscle of the pupil to cause contraction, produces systemic arterial vasoconstriction. *Therapeutic Effect:* Decreases mucosal blood flow and relieves congestion and increases systolic B/P.

USES
Treatment of nasal congestion (temporary relief)

PHARMACOKINETICS

Route	Onset	Peak	Duration
IV	Immediate	N/A	15–20 min
IM	10–15 min	N/A	0.5–2 hr
Subcuta-neous	10–15 min	N/A	1 hr

Minimal absorption after intranasal and ophthalmic administration. Metabolized in the liver and GI tract. Primarily excreted in urine. *Half-life:* 2.5 hr.

INDICATIONS AND DOSAGES
▶ **Nasal Decongestant**
Nasal Spray, Nasal Solution
Adults, Elderly, Children 12 yr and older. 2–3 drops or 1–2 sprays of 0.25%–0.5% solution into each nostril.
Children 6–11 yr. 2–3 drops or 1–2 sprays of 0.25% solution into each nostril.
Children younger than 6 yr. 2–3 drops of 0.125% solution (dilute 0.5% solution with 0.9% NaCl to achieve 0.125%) in each nostril. Repeat q4h as needed. Do not use for more than 3 days.

▶ **Conjunctival Congestion, Itching, and Minor Irritation; Whitening of Sclera**
Ophthalmic
Adults, Elderly, Children 12 yr and older. 1–2 drops of 0.12% solution q3–4h.
▶ **Hypotension, Shock**
IM, Subcutaneous
Adults, Elderly. 2–5 mg/dose q1–2h.
Children. 0.1 mg/kg/dose q1–2h.
IV Bolus
Adults, Elderly. 0.1–0.5 mg/dose q10–15min as needed.
Children. 5–20 mcg/kg/dose q10–15min.
IV Infusion
Adults, Elderly. 100–180 mcg/min.
Children. 0.1–0.5 mcg/kg/min.
Titrate to desired effect.

SIDE EFFECTS/ADVERSE REACTIONS
Frequent
Nasal: Rebound nasal congestion caused by overuse, especially when used longer than 3 days
Occasional
Mild CNS stimulation (restlessness, nervousness, tremors, headache, insomnia, particularly in those hypersensitive to sympathomimetics, such as elderly patients)
Nasal: Stinging, burning, drying of nasal mucosa
Ophthalmic: Transient burning or stinging, brow ache, blurred vision

PRECAUTIONS AND CONTRAINDICATIONS
Acute pancreatitis, heart disease, hepatitis, narrow-angle glaucoma, pheochromocytoma, severe hypertension, thrombosis, ventricular tachycardia
Caution:
Children younger than 6 yr, elderly, diabetes, cardiovascular disease, hypertension, hyperthyroidism,

increased intraocular pressure, prostatic hypertrophy, glaucoma, ischemic heart disease, excessive use

DRUG INTERACTIONS OF CONCERN TO DENTISTRY
• None reported with normal topical use

SERIOUS REACTIONS
! Large doses may produce tachycardia and palpitations (particularly in those with cardiac disease), light-headedness, nausea, and vomiting.
! Overdose in those older than 60 yr may result in hallucinations, CNS depression, and seizures.
! Prolonged nasal use may produce chronic swelling of nasal mucosa and rhinitis.

DENTAL CONSIDERATIONS

General:
• Consider semisupine chair position for patient comfort because of respiratory effects of disease.
• Assess salivary flow as a factor in caries, periodontal disease, and candidiasis.
• Patients with significant nasal congestion may complicate nasal administration of nitrous oxide/oxygen sedation.
Teach Patient/Family:
• That this product is not indicated for prolonged use because of congestion rebound.

phenylephrine hydrochloride; sulfacetamide sodium
fen-ill-**eh′**-frin high-droh-**klor′**-ide; sul-fa-**see′**-ta-mide **soe′**-dee-um
(Vasosulf)

CATEGORY AND SCHEDULE
Pregnancy Risk Category: C

Drug Class: Antibacterial, sympathomimetic, ophthalmic

MECHANISM OF ACTION
Phenylephrine is a sympathomimetic that acts on α-adrenergic receptors of vascular smooth muscle. Sulfacetamide is a sulfonamide that interferes with synthesis of folic acid that bacteria require for growth.
Therapeutic Effect: Increases systolic/diastolic B/P, produces constriction of blood vessels, conjunctival arterioles, nasal arterioles. Prevents bacterial growth.

USES
Treatment of generalized tonic-clonic (grand mal) seizures, status epilepticus, nonepileptic seizures, trigeminal neuralgia, cardiac dysrhythmias (class Ib) caused by digitalis-type drugs

PHARMACOKINETICS
Minimal absorption following ophthalmic administration.

P

INDICATIONS AND DOSAGES
▶ Topical Application to Conjunctiva That Relieves Congestion, Itching, Minor Irritation; Whitens Sclera of Eye
Ophthalmic
Adults, Elderly, Children 12 yr and older. Instill 1–2 drops q3–4h.

SIDE EFFECTS/ADVERSE REACTIONS
Occasional
Transient burning/stinging, brow ache, blurred vision

PRECAUTIONS AND CONTRAINDICATIONS
Angle-closure glaucoma, those with soft contact lenses, hypersensitivity to phenylephrine, sulfacetamide, or any component of the formulation

DRUG INTERACTIONS OF CONCERN TO DENTISTRY
• None reported with normal topical use

SERIOUS REACTIONS
! None reported

DENTAL CONSIDERATIONS
General:
• Consider semisupine chair position for patient comfort because of respiratory effects of disease.
• Assess salivary flow as a factor in caries, periodontal disease, and candidiasis.
• Patients with significant nasal congestion may complicate nasal administration of nitrous oxide/oxygen sedation.
Teach Patient/Family:
• That this product is not indicated for prolonged use because of congestion rebound.

phenytoin
fen'-ih-toyn
(Dilantin)

CATEGORY AND SCHEDULE
Pregnancy Risk Category: D

Drug Class: Anticonvulsant, hydantoin; antiarrhythmic agent, class Ib

MECHANISM OF ACTION
Phenytoin is an anticonvulsant drug that can stabilize neuronal membranes and decreases seizure activity by increasing efflux or decreasing influx of sodium ions across cell membranes from neurons of the motor cortex.
Acts as an antiarrhythmic by suppressing abnormal ventricular automaticity of cardiac tissue and shortening refractory period and QT interval.

USES
Status epilepticus, other seizure disorders
Prevention and treatment of seizures following head trauma/neurosurgery
Cardiac dysrhythmia

PHARMACOKINETICS
Slowly absorbed after oral administration. Highly protein bound: neonates greater or equal to 80%, infants greater or equal to 85%, and adults between 90%–95%. *Half-life:* 7–42 hr. Renal excretion (<5% as unchanged drug) and its metabolites occur partly with glomerular filtration but more importantly by tubular secretion.

INDICATIONS AND DOSAGES
IV
Adults, Elderly. Status epilepticus:
Loading dose: 10–15 mg/kg;
Maintenance dose: 300 mg/day or
4–6 mg/kg/day in 2–3 divided doses.
Cardiac dysrhythmia: 1.25 mg/kg
every 5 min as needed. May repeat
to a max dose of 15 mg/kg.
IM
Seizure, during and following
neurosurgery; treatment and
prophylaxis: 100–200 mg IM every
4 hr during surgery and continued
during the postoperative period.
PO
Adults, Elderly. Seizure control:
Loading dose: 15–20 mg/kg in 3
divided doses 2–4 hr apart.
Maintenance dose: 300 mg/day or
4–6 mg/kg/day in 2–3 divided doses.
▸ **Status Epilepticus**
IV
Children 10–16 yr. 6–7 mg/kg/day.
Children 7–9 yr. 7–8 mg/kg/day.
Children 4–6 yr. 7.5–9 mg/kg/day.
Children 6 mo–3 yr. 8–10 mg/kg/
day.
Neonates. Loading dose: 15–20 mg/
kg; Maintenance dose: 5–8 mg/kg/
day.
PO
Seizure control: Loading dose:
15–20 mg/kg in 3 divided doses
2–4 hr apart. Maintenance dose:
300 mg/day or 4–6 mg/kg/day in
2–3 divided doses.
Dosage adjustments
Dosage adjustments may be required
in the elderly: Initially, 3 mg/kg/day,
in divided doses, the dosage being
adjusted according to serum
hydantoin concentrations and patient
response.
Obese patients: the IV loading dose
should be calculated on the basis of
ideal body weight plus 1.33 times
the excess weight over ideal weight,
because phenytoin preferentially
distributes into fat.
Pregnancy: phenytoin requirements
are greater during pregnancy,
requiring increases in doses in some
patients. After delivery, the dose
should be decreased to avoid
toxicity.
Liver disease: there may be an
increase in unbound phenytoin
concentrations in patients with
hepatic insufficiency, recommended
to measuring unbound phenytoin
concentrations level.
Renal impairment: there may be an
increase in unbound phenytoin
concentrations in patients with renal
impairment, recommended to
measuring unbound phenytoin
concentrations level.

SIDE EFFECTS/ADVERSE REACTIONS
▸ **Dose-Related**
Frequent
Headache, blurred vision, sleepy,
nausea and vomiting,
constipation
Occasional
Confusion, rash, feeling nervous,
hypokalemia
Frequent
Headache, blurred vision, sleepy,
nausea and vomiting, constipation
Occasional
Confusion, rash, feeling nervous,
hypokalemia

PRECAUTIONS AND CONTRAINDICATIONS
Contraindications
Hypersensitivity to phenytoin,
fosphenytoin, or hydantoins
Sinus bradycardia, SA block, second
and third-degree AV block and
Adams-Stokes syndrome
(intravenous phenytoin only)

P

Seizures Caused by Hypoglycemia
Use caution in patients with respiratory depression, CHF, MI, or damaged myocardium (IV route only).

Use with caution in patients with preexisting diseases such as liver impairment, diabetes mellitus (hyperglycemia has occurred in diabetics), history of renal disease, and alcohol use (acute use: increases levels; chronic use: decrease levels); hypotension.

Do not abruptly withdraw this medicine because of precipitate status epilepticus.

It is important to discontinue if skin rash occurs (do not resume if rash is exfoliative, purpuric, or bullous, or if lupus erythematosus or Stevens-Johnson syndrome is suspected).

DRUG INTERACTIONS OF CONCERN TO DENTISTRY

• Alcohol, other CNS depressants: May increase CNS depression.
• Fluconazole, ketoconazole, miconazole: May increase phenytoin blood concentration.
• Glucocorticoids: Phenytoin may decrease the effects of glucocorticoids.
• Lidocaine, propranolol: Phenytoin may increase cardiac depressant effects.

SERIOUS REACTIONS

! Increased risk of suicidal behavior has been observed.
! Phenytoin should be discontinued if a skin rash appears.
! Hyperglycemia, resulting from the drug's inhibitory effects on insulin release, has been reported.
! Osteomalacia has been associated with phenytoin therapy and is considered to be due to phenytoin's interference with vitamin D metabolism.

DENTAL CONSIDERATIONS

General:
• Gingival enlargement is a common problem observed primarily during the first 6 months of phenytoin therapy appearing with gingivitis.
• To minimize severity and growth rate of gingival tissue, begin a program of professional cleaning and patient plaque control within 10 days of starting anticonvulsant therapy.
• Consider semisupine chair position for patient comfort because of GI side effects.
• Monitor vital signs every appointment because of cardiovascular side effects.
• Avoid or limit dose of vasoconstrictor in patients with dysrhythmias.
• Avoid any agents that contain alcohol (propylene glycol and ethanol) due to increased risk of hypotension, bradycardia, and arrhythmias.

Consultations:
• Medical consultation may be required to assess disease control and patient's ability to tolerate stress.

Teach Patient/Family to:
• Update health and drug history, reporting changes in health status, drug regimen changes.
• Avoid mouth rinses with high alcohol content because of drying effects.
• When chronic dry mouth occurs advise patient to:
    • Suggest xylitol gum/products to stimulate saliva and for anticaries effect.

physostigmine
fih-zoe-**stig'**-meen
(Antilirium)
Do not confuse physostigmine
with Prostigmin or
pyridostigmine.

CATEGORY AND SCHEDULE
Pregnancy Risk Category: C

Drug Class:
Parasympathomimetic
(cholinergic)

MECHANISM OF ACTION
A cholinergic that inhibits
destruction of acetylcholine by
enzyme acetylcholinesterase, thus
enhancing impulse transmission
across the myoneural junction.
Therapeutic Effect: Improves
skeletal muscle tone, stimulates
salivary and sweat gland
secretions.

USES
Antidote for reversal of toxic CNS
effects due to anticholinergic drugs,
tricyclic antidepressants

INDICATIONS AND DOSAGES
▶ To Reverse CNS Effects of
Anticholinergic Drugs and Tricyclic
Antidepressants
IV, IM
Adults, Elderly. Initially, 0.5–2 mg.
If no response, repeat q20min until
response or adverse cholinergic
effects occur. If initial response
occurs, may give additional doses of
1–4 mg q30–60 min as life-
threatening signs, such as
arrhythmias, seizures, and deep
coma, recur.
Children. 0.01–0.03 mg/kg. May
give additional doses q5–10 min
until response or adverse cholinergic

effects occur or total dose of 2 mg
given.

SIDE EFFECTS/ADVERSE
REACTIONS
Expected
Miosis, increased GI and skeletal
muscle tone, bradycardia, sweating,
excessive salivation
Occasional
Marked drop in B/P (hypertensive
patients)
Rare
Allergic reaction

PRECAUTIONS AND
CONTRAINDICATIONS
Active uveal inflammation,
angle-closure glaucoma before
iridectomy, asthma, cardiovascular
disease, concurrent use of
ganglionic-blocking agents, diabetes,
gangrene, glaucoma associated with
iridocyclitis, hypersensitivity to
cholinesterase inhibitors or their
components, mechanical obstruction
of intestinal or urogenital tract,
vagotonic state

DRUG INTERACTIONS OF
CONCERN TO DENTISTRY
• Contraindicated: succinylcholine

SERIOUS REACTIONS
! Parenteral overdose produces a
cholinergic crisis manifested as
abdominal discomfort or cramps,
nausea, vomiting, diarrhea, flushing,
facial warmth, excessive salivation,
diaphoresis, urinary urgency, and
blurred vision. If overdose occurs,
stop all anticholinergic drugs and
immediately administer 0.6–1.2 mg
atropine sulfate IM or IV for adults,
or 0.01 mg/kg for infants and
children younger than 12 yr.

P

DENTAL CONSIDERATIONS

General:
• For acute use in hospitals and emergency rooms.
Teach Patient/Family to:
• Avoid driving at night or participating in activities requiring visual acuity in the presence of dim lighting.

phytonadione
(vitamin K₁)
fye-toe-na-**dye**′-own
(Aqua Mephyton, Mephyton)

CATEGORY AND SCHEDULE
Pregnancy Risk Category: C

Drug Class: Vitamin K₁, fat-soluble vitamin

MECHANISM OF ACTION
Needed for adequate blood clotting (factors II, VII, IX, X)

USES
Treatment of vitamin K malabsorption, hypoprothrombinemia, prevention of hypoprothrombinemia caused by oral anticoagulants

PHARMACOKINETICS
PO/Injection: Readily absorbed from duodenum and requires bile salts, rapid hepatic metabolism, onset of action 6–12 hr, normal PT in 12–24 hr, crosses placenta, renal and biliary excretion; because of severe side effects, restrict IV route when other administration routes are not available.

INDICATIONS AND DOSAGES
▶ Hypoprothrombinemia Caused by Vitamin K Malabsorption
PO/IM
Adult. 2–25 mg; may repeat or increase to 50 mg.
Child. 5–10 mg.
Infants. 2 mg.
▶ Prevention of Hemorrhagic Disease of the Newborn
Subcutaneous/IM
Neonate. 0.5–1 mg after birth; repeat in 6–8 hr if required.
▶ Hypoprothrombinemia Caused by Oral Anticoagulants
PO/Subcutaneous/IM
Adult. 2.5–10 mg; may repeat 12–48 hr after PO dose or 6–8 hr after subcutaneous/IM dose, based on PT.

SIDE EFFECTS/ADVERSE REACTIONS
Occasional
Dysgeusia, headache, cardiac irregularities (tachycardia), nausea, vomiting, hemoglobinuria, rash, urticaria, flushing, erythema, sweating, bronchospasms, dyspnea, cramplike pain
Rare
Hyperbilirubinemia

PRECAUTIONS AND CONTRAINDICATIONS
Hypersensitivity, severe hepatic disease, last few weeks of pregnancy

DRUG INTERACTIONS OF CONCERN TO DENTISTRY
• Decreased action: broad-spectrum antibiotics, salicylates (high doses)
• Antagonist to oral anticoagulants

SERIOUS REACTIONS
! Severe hypersensitivity reactions

DENTAL CONSIDERATIONS

General:
• Determine why the patient is taking this drug. Medical consultation should be made before dental treatment.
• Patients on chronic drug therapy may rarely have symptoms of blood dyscrasias, which can include infection, bleeding, and poor healing.
Consultations:
• Medical consultation to determine coagulation stability.

pilocarpine hydrochloride

pye-loe-**kar**′-peen
high-droh-**klor**′-ide
(Isopto Carpin[AUS], Ocusert Pilo-20[AUS], Ocusert Pilo-40[AUS], Pilopt Eye Drops[AUS], P.V. Carpine Liquifilm Ophthalmic Solution[AUS], Salagen)

CATEGORY AND SCHEDULE
Pregnancy Risk Category: C

Drug Class: Miotic, cholinergic agonist

MECHANISM OF ACTION
A cholinergic that increases exocrine gland secretions by stimulating cholinergic receptors.
Therapeutic Effect: Improves symptoms of dry mouth in patients with salivary gland hypofunction.

USES
Treatment of primary glaucoma, early stages of wide-angle glaucoma (less useful in advanced stages), chronic open-angle glaucoma, acute narrow-angle glaucoma before emergency surgery; also used to neutralize mydriatics used during eye exam; may be used alternately with mydriatics to break adhesions between iris and lens

PHARMACOKINETICS

Route	Onset	Peak	Duration
PO	20 min	1 hr	3–5 hr

Absorption decreased if taken with a high-fat meal. Inactivation of pilocarpine thought to occur at neuronal synapses and probably in plasma. Excreted in urine. *Half-life:* 4–12 hr.

INDICATIONS AND DOSAGES
▸ **Dry Mouth Associated with Radiation Treatment for Head and Neck Cancer**
PO
Adults, Elderly. 5 mg 3 times a day. Range: 15–30 mg/day. Maximum: 2 tablets/dose.
▸ **Dry Mouth Associated with Sjögren's Syndrome**
PO
Adults, Elderly. 5 mg 4 times a day. Range: 20–40 mg/day.
▸ **Dosage in Hepatic Impairment**
Dosage decreased to 5 mg twice a day for adults and elderly with hepatic impairment.

SIDE EFFECTS/ADVERSE REACTIONS
Frequent
Diaphoresis, excessive salivation
Occasional
Headache, dizziness, urinary frequency, flushing, dyspepsia, nausea, asthenia, lacrimation, visual disturbances
Rare
Diarrhea, abdominal pain, peripheral edema, chills

P

PRECAUTIONS AND CONTRAINDICATIONS

Conditions in which miosis is undesirable, such as acute iritis and angle-closure glaucoma; uncontrolled asthma
Caution:
Bronchial asthma, hypertension

DRUG INTERACTIONS OF CONCERN TO DENTISTRY

• Anticholinergic drugs, which reduce salivation antagonize therapeutic action

SERIOUS REACTIONS

! Patients with diaphoresis who don't drink enough fluids may develop dehydration.

DENTAL CONSIDERATIONS

General:
• Avoid drugs with anticholinergic activity, such as antihistamines, opioids, benzodiazepines, propantheline, atropine, and scopolamine.
• Avoid dental light in patient's eyes; offer dark glasses for patient comfort.
• Monitor vital signs at every appointment because of cardiovascular and respiratory side effects.
Consultations:
• Medical consultation may be required to assess disease control.
▸ **Pilocarpine HCl (Oral)**
General:
• Patients receiving chemotherapy may require palliative treatment for stomatitis.
• Assess salivary flow as a factor in caries, periodontal disease, and candidiasis.
• Monitor vital signs at every appointment because of cardiovascular side effects.

• Place on frequent recall because of oral effects of head and neck radiation.
Consultations:
• Medical consultation may be required to assess disease control.
• Medical consultation may be necessary before prescribing for patients with cardiovascular, retinal, or respiratory disease.
Teach Patient/Family to:
• Use caution when driving at night or performing hazardous activities in reduced lighting (visual blurring).
• Take plenty of fluids, observe for dehydration, or discontinue drug.

pimecrolimus
pim-eh-crow-**lee**′-mus
(Elidel)

CATEGORY AND SCHEDULE
Pregnancy Risk Category: C

Drug Class: Topical antiinflammatory

MECHANISM OF ACTION
An immunomodulator that inhibits release of cytokine, an enzyme that produces an inflammatory reaction.
Therapeutic Effect: Produces antiinflammatory activity.

USES
Short-term and intermittent long-term treatment of mild to moderate atopic dermatitis in non-immunocompromised patients age 2 yr and older in whom conventional therapies cannot be used because of potential risks; in patients with an inadequate response; or in patients who are not responsive to conventional therapies

PHARMACOKINETICS

Minimal systemic absorption with topical application. Metabolized in liver. Excreted in feces.

INDICATIONS AND DOSAGES

▶ **Atopic Dermatitis (Eczema)**
Topical
Adults, Elderly, Children 2–17 yr.
Apply to affected area twice daily for up to 3 wk (up to 6 wk in adolescents, children 2–17 yr). Rub in gently and completely.

SIDE EFFECTS/ADVERSE REACTIONS

Rare

Transient application-site sensation of burning or feeling of heat

PRECAUTIONS AND CONTRAINDICATIONS

Hypersensitivity to pimecrolimus or any component of the formulation, Netherton's syndrome (potential for increased systemic absorption), application to active cutaneous viral infections

Caution:

Do not use for active cutaneous viral infections, infected dermatitis, natural or artificial sunlight exposure, no data on excretion in human milk, children younger than 2 yr

DRUG INTERACTIONS OF CONCERN TO DENTISTRY

• Drug interactions have not been evaluated. Low blood levels were measured in some patients. Use drugs that inhibit CYP3A4 isoenzymes with caution in patients with widespread and erythrodermic disease.

SERIOUS REACTIONS

! Lymphadenopathy and phototoxicity occur rarely.

General:

• Determine why the patient is taking this drug.

pimozide

pim′-oh-zide
(Orap)

CATEGORY AND SCHEDULE

Pregnancy Risk Category: C

Drug Class: Antipsychotic, antidyskinetic

MECHANISM OF ACTION

A diphenylbutylpiperidine that blocks dopamine at postsynaptic receptor sites in the brain.
Therapeutic Effect: Suppresses behavioral response in psychosis.

USES

Treatment of motor and phonic tics in Gilles de la Tourette's syndrome; unapproved: psychotic disorders

PHARMACOKINETICS

PO: Onset erratic, peak 6–8 hr.
Half-life: 50–55 hr; metabolized by liver; excreted in urine, feces.

INDICATIONS AND DOSAGES

▶ **Tourette's Disorder**
PO
Adults, Elderly. 1–2 mg/day in divided doses 3 times a day. Maximum: 10 mg/day.
Children older than 12 yr. Initially, 0.5 mg/kg/day. Maximum: 10 mg/day.

P

SIDE EFFECTS/ADVERSE REACTIONS

Occasional

Akathisia, dystonic extrapyramidal effects, parkinsonian extrapyramidal effects, tardive dyskinesia, blurred vision, ocular changes, constipation, decreased sweating, dry mouth, nasal congestion, dizziness, drowsiness, orthostatic hypotension, urinary retention, somnolence

Rare

Rash, cholestatic jaundice, priapism

PRECAUTIONS AND CONTRAINDICATIONS

Aggressive schizophrenics when sedation is required; concurrent administration of pemoline; methylphenidate or amphetamines; concurrent administration with dofetilide, sotalol, quinidine, other Class IA and III anti-arrhythmics, mesoridazine, thioridazine, chlorpromazine, droperidol, sparfloxacin, gatifloxacin, moxifloxacin, halofantrine, mefloquine, pentamidine, arsenic trioxide, levomethadyl acetate, dolasetron mesylate, probucol, tacrolimus, ziprasidone, sertraline, macrolide antibiotics, drugs that cause QT prolongation, and less potent inhibitors of CYP3A; congenital or drug-induced long QT syndrome; doses greater than 10 mg daily; history of cardiac arrhythmias, Parkinson's disease; patients with known hypokalemia or hypomagnesemia; severe central nervous system depression; simple tics or tics not associated with Tourette's syndrome; hypersensitivity to pimozide or any of its components

Caution:

Children younger than 12 yr, lactation, hypertension, hepatic disease, cardiac disease, renal disease, breast cancer, hypokalemia

DRUG INTERACTIONS OF CONCERN TO DENTISTRY

• Increased CNS depression: alcohol, CNS depressants
• Increased effects of both drugs: phenothiazines
• Increased effects of anticholinergic drugs
• Prolonged QT interval, fatal cardiac arrhythmia; contraindicated: clarithromycin, erythromycin, azithromycin, dirithromycin, itraconazole

SERIOUS REACTIONS

❗ Serious reactions such as blood dyscrasias, agranulocytosis, leukocytopenia, thrombocytopenia, cholestatic jaundice, neuroleptic malignant syndrome (NMS), constipation or paralytic ileus, priapism, QT prolongation and torsades de pointes, seizure, systemic lupus erythematosus-like syndrome, and temperature regulation dysfunction (heatstroke or hypothermia) occur rarely.
❗ Abrupt withdrawal following long-term therapy may precipitate nausea, vomiting, gastritis, dizziness, and tremors.

DENTAL CONSIDERATIONS

General:

• Assess salivary flow as a factor in caries, periodontal disease, and candidiasis.
• Monitor vital signs at every appointment because of cardiovascular side effects.
• Assess for presence of extrapyramidal motor symptoms, such as tardive dyskinesia and akathisia. Extrapyramidal motor activity may complicate dental treatment.

• After supine positioning, have patient sit upright for at least 2 min before standing to avoid orthostatic hypotension.
• Consider action of drug in assessment of dysgeusia.
Consultations:
• Medical consultation may be required to assess disease control.
• If signs of tardive dyskinesia or akathisia are present, refer to physician.
Teach Patient/Family to:
• Encourage effective oral hygiene to prevent soft tissue inflammation.
• Use caution to prevent injury when using oral hygiene aids.
• When chronic dry mouth occurs, advise patient to:
    • Avoid mouth rinses with high alcohol content because of drying effects.
    • Use daily home fluoride products to prevent caries.
    • Use sugarless gum, frequent sips of water, or saliva substitutes.

pindolol
pin´-doe-loll
(Apo-Pindol[CAN], Visken)

CATEGORY AND SCHEDULE
Pregnancy Risk Category: B (D if used in second or third trimester)

Drug Class: Nonselective β-adrenergic blocker

MECHANISM OF ACTION
A nonselective beta blocker that blocks β_1- and β_2-adrenergic receptors.
Therapeutic Effect: Slows heart rate, decreases cardiac output, decreases B/P, and exhibits antiarrhythmic activity. Decreases myocardial ischemia severity by decreasing oxygen requirements.

USES
Treatment of mild-to-moderate hypertension, mild-to-moderate heart failure

PHARMACOKINETICS
Completely absorbed from GI tract. Metabolized in liver. Primarily excreted in urine. *Half-life:* 3–4 hr (half-life increased with impaired renal function, elderly).

INDICATIONS AND DOSAGES
▸ **Mild-to-Moderate Hypertension**
PO
Adults. Initially, 5 mg 2 times a day. Gradually increase dose by 10 mg/day at 2- to 4-wk intervals. Maintenance: 10–30 mg/day in 2–3 divided doses. Maximum: 60 mg/day.
▸ **Usual Elderly Dosage**
PO
Initially, 5 mg/day. May increase by 5 mg q3–4wk.

SIDE EFFECTS/ADVERSE REACTIONS
Frequent
Decreased sexual ability, drowsiness, trouble sleeping, unusual tiredness or weakness
Occasional
Bradycardia, depression, cold hands/feet, diarrhea, constipation, anxiety, nasal congestion, nausea, vomiting
Rare
Altered taste, dry eyes, itching, numbness of fingers, toes, and scalp

P

PRECAUTIONS AND CONTRAINDICATIONS

Bronchial asthma, COPD, uncontrolled cardiac failure, sinus bradycardia, heart block greater than first degree, cardiogenic shock, CHF, unless secondary to tachyarrhythmias

Caution:

Major surgery, diabetes mellitus, renal disease, thyroid disease, COPD, well-compensated heart failure, CAD, nonallergic bronchospasm, impaired hepatic function, children

DRUG INTERACTIONS OF CONCERN TO DENTISTRY

• Increased hypotension, bradycardia: anticholinergics, hydrocarbon inhalation anesthetics, fentanyl derivatives
• Decreased antihypertensive effects: indomethacin, sympathomimetics
• Increased effect of both drugs: phenothiazines, xanthines
• Decreased bronchodilation: theophyllines
• Hypertension, bradycardia: epinephrine, ephedrine
• Slow metabolism of drug: lidocaine

SERIOUS REACTIONS

❗ Overdosage may produce profound bradycardia and hypotension.
❗ Abrupt withdrawal may result in sweating, palpitations, headache, and tremulousness.
❗ May precipitate CHF or MI in patients with heart disease; thyroid storm in those with thyrotoxicosis; or peripheral ischemia in those with existing peripheral vascular disease.
❗ Hypoglycemia may occur in previously controlled diabetics.

❗ Signs of thrombocytopenia, such as unusual bleeding or bruising, occur rarely.

DENTAL CONSIDERATIONS

General:
• Monitor vital signs at every appointment because of cardiovascular side effects.
• Patients on chronic drug therapy may rarely have symptoms of blood dyscrasias, which can include infection, bleeding, and poor healing.
• Stress from dental procedures may compromise cardiovascular function; determine patient risk; use stress-reduction protocol.
• Use vasoconstrictors with caution, in low doses, and with careful aspiration. Avoid use of gingival retraction cord with epinephrine.
• Consider semisupine chair position for patient comfort if GI side effects occur.
• Assess salivary flow as a factor in caries, periodontal disease, and candidiasis.
• Consider drug effects if taste alteration occurs.

Consultations:
• In a patient with symptoms of blood dyscrasias, request a medical consultation for blood studies and postpone dental treatment until normal values are reestablished.
• Medical consultation may be required to assess disease control and patient's ability to tolerate stress.

Teach Patient/Family to:
• Encourage effective oral hygiene to prevent soft tissue inflammation.
• Use caution to prevent injury when using oral hygiene aids.
• When chronic dry mouth occurs, advise patient to:

- Avoid mouth rinses with high alcohol content because of drying effects.
- Use daily home fluoride products to prevent caries.
- Use sugarless gum, frequent sips of water, or saliva substitutes.

pioglitazone
pye-oh-**gli**′-ta-zone
(Actos)

CATEGORY AND SCHEDULE
Pregnancy Risk Category: C

Drug Class: Antidiabetic, oral

MECHANISM OF ACTION
An antidiabetic that improves target-cell response to insulin without increasing pancreatic insulin secretion. Decreases hepatic glucose output and increases insulin-dependent glucose utilization in skeletal muscle.
Therapeutic Effect: Lowers blood glucose concentration.

USES
Monotherapy, as an adjunct to diet and exercise in patients with Type 2 diabetes mellitus; may also be used with metformin when metformin, diet, and exercise are not adequate for control

PHARMACOKINETICS
Rapidly absorbed. Highly protein bound (99%), primarily to albumin. Metabolized in the liver. Excreted in urine. Unknown if removed by hemodialysis. **Half-life:** 16–24 hr.

INDICATIONS AND DOSAGES
▶ **Diabetes Mellitus, Combination Therapy**
PO
Adult, Elderly. With insulin: Initially, 15–30 mg once a day. Initially continue current insulin dosage; then decrease insulin dosage by 10%–25% if hypoglycemia occurs or plasma glucose level decreases to less than 100 mg/dl. Maximum: 45 mg/day. With sulfonylureas: Initially, 15–30 mg/day. Decrease sulfonylurea dosage if hypoglycemia occurs. With metformin: Initially, 15–30 mg/day. As monotherapy: Monotherapy is not to be used if patient is well controlled with diet and exercise alone. Initially, 15–30 mg/day. May increase dosage in increments until 45 mg/day is reached.

SIDE EFFECTS/ADVERSE REACTIONS
Frequent
Headache, upper respiratory tract infection
Occasional
Sinusitis, myalgia, pharyngitis, aggravated diabetes mellitus

PRECAUTIONS AND CONTRAINDICATIONS
Active hepatic disease; diabetic ketoacidosis; increased serum transaminase levels, including ALT (SGPT) greater than 2.5 times normal serum level
Caution:
Hepatic dysfunction (reduce dose), renal impairment, lactation, children younger than 18 yr

DRUG INTERACTIONS OF CONCERN TO DENTISTRY
- None reported

SERIOUS REACTIONS
! None known

DENTAL CONSIDERATIONS

General:
• Ensure that patient is following prescribed diet and regularly takes medication.
• Place on frequent recall to evaluate healing response.
• Short appointments and a stress-reduction protocol may be required for anxious patients.
• Diabetics may be more susceptible to infection and have delayed wound healing.
• Question patient about self-monitoring of drug's antidiabetic effect, including blood glucose values or finger-stick records.
• Consider semisupine chair position for patient comfort if GI side effects occur.

Consultations:
• Medical consultation may be required to assess disease control and patient's ability to tolerate stress.
• Medical consultation may include data from patient's blood glucose monitoring, including glycosylated hemoglobin or HbA$_{1c}$ testing.

Teach Patient/Family to:
• Prevent trauma when using oral hygiene aids.
• Update health and drug history if physician makes any changes in evaluation or drug regimens; include OTC, herbal, and nonherbal drugs in the update.
• Encourage effective oral hygiene to prevent soft tissue inflammation.

pirbuterol
peer-**beut'**-er-all
(Maxair, Maxair Autohaler)

CATEGORY AND SCHEDULE
Pregnancy Risk Category: C

Drug Class: Bronchodilator

MECHANISM OF ACTION
A sympathomimetic, adrenergic agonist, that stimulates β_2-adrenergic receptors in the lungs, resulting in relaxation of bronchial smooth muscle.
Therapeutic Effect: Relieves bronchospasm, reduces airway resistance.

USES
Treatment of reversible bronchospasm (prevention, treatment), including asthma; may be given with theophylline or steroids

PHARMACOKINETICS
Absorbed from bronchi following inhalation. Metabolized in liver. Primarily excreted in urine. Unknown if removed by hemodialysis. **Half-life:** 2–3 hr.

INDICATIONS AND DOSAGES
▸ **Prevention of Bronchospasm**
Inhalation
Adults, Elderly, Children 12 yr and older. 2 inhalations q4–6h.
Maximum: 12 inhalations daily.
▸ **Treatment of Bronchospasm**
Inhalation
Adults, Elderly, Children 12 yr and older. 2 inhalations separated by at least 1–3 min, followed by a third inhalation. Maximum: 12 inhalations daily.

SIDE EFFECTS/ADVERSE REACTIONS

Occasional

Nervousness, tremor, headache, palpitations, nausea, dizziness, tachycardia, cough

PRECAUTIONS AND CONTRAINDICATIONS

History of hypersensitivity to pirbuterol, albuterol, or any of its components

Caution:

Lactation, cardiac disorders, hyperthyroidism, diabetes mellitus, prostatic hypertrophy

DRUG INTERACTIONS OF CONCERN TO DENTISTRY

• None reported

SERIOUS REACTIONS

! Excessive sympathomimetic stimulation may produce palpitations, extrasystoles, tachycardia, chest pain, slight increases in B/P followed by a substantial decrease, chills, sweating and blanching of skin.

! Too-frequent or excessive use may lead to loss of bronchodilating effectiveness and severe, paradoxical bronchoconstriction.

DENTAL CONSIDERATIONS

General:

• Acute asthmatic episodes may be precipitated in the dental office. Sympathomimetic inhalants should be available for emergency use.

• Be aware that aspirin or sulfite preservatives in vasoconstrictor-containing products can exacerbate asthma.

• Monitor vital signs at every appointment because of cardiovascular and respiratory side effects.

• Assess salivary flow as a factor in caries, periodontal disease, and candidiasis.

• Consider semisupine chair position for patients with respiratory disease.

• Short appointments and a stress-reduction protocol may be required for anxious patients.

Consultations:

• Medical consultation may be required to assess disease control and patient's ability to tolerate stress.

Teach Patient/Family to:

• Rinse mouth with water after each dose to prevent dryness (for inhalation dosage forms).

• When chronic dry mouth occurs, advise patient to:

  • Avoid mouth rinses with high alcohol content because of drying effects.

  • Use daily home fluoride products to prevent caries.

  • Use sugarless gum, frequent sips of water, or saliva substitutes.

P

piroxicam

peer-**ox**′-ih-kam

(Apo-Piroxicam[CAN], Candyl-D[AUS], Feldene, Fexicam[CAN], Mobilis[AUS], Novo-Pirocam[CAN], Pyrahexyl-D [AUS], Rosig[AUS], Rosig-D[AUS])

Do not confuse Feldene with Seldane.

CATEGORY AND SCHEDULE

Pregnancy Risk Category: C (D if used in third trimester or near delivery)

Drug Class: Nonsteroidal antiinflammatory

MECHANISM OF ACTION

An NSAID that produces analgesic and antiinflammatory effects by inhibiting prostaglandin synthesis. *Therapeutic Effect:* Reduces inflammatory response and intensity of pain.

USES

Treatment of osteoarthritis, rheumatoid arthritis; unapproved: gouty arthritis

PHARMACOKINETICS

PO: Peak 2 hr. *Half-life:* 3–3.5 hr; 99% protein binding; metabolized in liver; excreted in urine (metabolites), breast milk.

INDICATIONS AND DOSAGES
▸ **Acute or Chronic Rheumatoid Arthritis and Osteoarthritis**
PO
Adults, Elderly. Initially, 10–20 mg/day as a single dose or in divided doses. Some patients may require up to 30–40 mg/day.
Children. 0.2–0.3 mg/kg/day. Maximum: 15 mg/day.

SIDE EFFECTS/ADVERSE REACTIONS

Frequent
Dyspepsia, nausea, dizziness
Occasional
Diarrhea, constipation, abdominal cramps or pain, flatulence, stomatitis
Rare
Hypertension, urticaria, dysuria, ecchymosis, blurred vision, insomnia, phototoxicity

PRECAUTIONS AND CONTRAINDICATIONS

Active peptic ulcer disease, chronic inflammation of the GI tract, GI bleeding or ulceration, history of hypersensitivity to aspirin or NSAIDs

Caution:
Lactation, children, bleeding disorders, GI disorders, cardiac disorders, hypersensitivity to other antiinflammatory agents, hypertension

DRUG INTERACTIONS OF CONCERN TO DENTISTRY

• GI ulceration, bleeding: aspirin, alcohol, corticosteroids
• Nephrotoxicity: acetaminophen (prolonged use and high doses)
• Possible risk of decreased renal function: cyclosporine
• Decreased action: salicylates
• SSRIs: increased risk of GI side effects
• When prescribed for dental pain:
  • Risk of increased effects of oral anticoagulants, oral antidiabetics, lithium, methotrexate
  • Decreased antihypertensive effects of diuretics, α-adrenergic blockers, ACE inhibitors

SERIOUS REACTIONS

! Rare reactions with long-term use include peptic ulcer disease, GI bleeding, gastritis, severe hepatic reaction (cholestasis, jaundice), nephrotoxicity (dysuria, hematuria, proteinuria, nephrotic syndrome), hematologic sensitivity (anemia, leukopenia, eosinophilia, thrombocytopenia), and a severe hypersensitivity reaction (fever, chills, bronchospasm).

DENTAL CONSIDERATIONS

General:
• Patients on chronic drug therapy may rarely have symptoms of blood dyscrasias, which can include infection, bleeding, and poor healing.

• Assess salivary flow as a factor in caries, periodontal disease, and candidiasis.
• Avoid prescribing during pregnancy.
• Minimize use of aspirin-containing products.
• Consider semisupine chair position for patients with arthritic disease or if GI side effects occur.
Consultations:
• In a patient with symptoms of blood dyscrasias, request a medical consultation for blood studies and postpone dental treatment until normal values are reestablished.
• Medical consultation may be required to assess disease control.
Teach Patient/Family to:
• Encourage effective oral hygiene to prevent soft tissue inflammation.
• Use caution to prevent injury when using oral hygiene aids.
• Report oral lesions, soreness, or bleeding to dentist.
• When chronic dry mouth occurs, advise patient to:
  • Avoid mouth rinses with high alcohol content because of drying effects.
  • Use daily home fluoride products to prevent caries.
  • Use sugarless gum, frequent sips of water, or saliva substitutes.

pitavastatin
pit´-a-vah´-stah-tin
(Livalo)
Do not confuse with Levatol.

CATEGORY AND SCHEDULE
Pregnancy Risk Category: X

Drug Class: Antihyperlipidemics, HMG CoA reductase inhibitors

MECHANISM OF ACTION
An antihyperlipidemic that inhibits HMG-CoA reductase, the enzyme that catalyzes the early step in cholesterol synthesis.
Therapeutic Effect: Increases the amount of LDL receptors on hepatocyte membranes thereby decreasing LDL and VLDL cholesterol as well as plasma triglyceride levels; also increases HDL cholesterol.

USES
Hypercholesterolemia
Mixed dyslipidemia

PHARMACOKINETICS
Rapidly and well absorbed after PO administration. Bioavailability: 51%. Protein binding: >99%. Distributed primarily to the liver. Major metabolite is a lactone, formed by glucuronidation. Metabolized in the liver, via UGT1A3 and UGT2B7; mildly by CYP2C9 and 2C8. Primarily excreted in feces; minimally in urine. **Half-life:** 9–12 hr.

INDICATIONS AND DOSAGES
▸ **Hypercholesterolemia, Mixed Dyslipidemia**
PO
Adults. Initially, 2 mg a day. May increase after 4 wk. Range: 1–4 mg/day. Maximum: 4 mg/day.
Concomitant use with erythromycin: Maximum: 1 mg/day.
Concomitant use with rifampin: Maximum: 2 mg/day.
▸ **Dosage in Renal Impairment**
Mild to moderate impairment (CrCl 30 to less than 60 ml/min or ESRD on hemodialysis). 1 mg a day (Maximum: 2 mg/day).
Moderate to severe impairment (CrCl less than 30 ml/min and not

P

on hemodialysis). Not recommended.

SIDE EFFECTS/ADVERSE REACTIONS

Pitavastatin is generally well tolerated. Side effects are usually mild and transient.

Occasional

Constipation, diarrhea, back pain, myalgia, arthralgia, pain in extremities, headache, rash or pruritus, allergy, influenza, nasopharyngitis, headache, increased CPK, increased alkaline phosphatase and bilirubin

Rare

Rhabdomyolysis

PRECAUTIONS AND CONTRAINDICATIONS

Hypersensitivity to pitavastatin or its components
Active liver disease
Lactation
Pregnancy
Unexplained elevated hepatic function test results
Concomitant use with cyclosporine or lopinavir/ritonavir
Severe renal impairment (CrCl <30 ml/min without dialysis)
Cholestasis or jaundice
Hepatitis
Hepatic encephalopathy

Caution:

Mild to moderate renal impairment
Alcohol consumption
Seizure disorder
Major surgery or trauma

DRUG INTERACTIONS OF CONCERN TO DENTISTRY

• Cyclosporine, lopinavir/ritonavir: May potentiate the effects of pitavastatin
• CYP450 inducers: May decrease pitavastatin levels
• CYP450 inhibitors: May increase pitavastatin levels (e.g., macrolide antibiotics)
• Fibric acids, niacin: May cause additive effects; increase risk of myopathy

SERIOUS REACTIONS

! Cases of rhabdomyolysis have been reported with pitavastatin.
! Discontinue pitavastatin if myopathy or elevated CK levels occur.
! Elevated liver transaminases have been reported. Liver function should be assessed before therapy, at 4 wk after starting or when increasing dose, then periodically. Reduce dose if serum transaminases are 3 times ULN.

DENTAL CONSIDERATIONS

General:

• Consider semisupine chair position for patient comfort if GI side effects occur.

Consultations:

• Medical consultation may be required to assess disease control.

Teach Patient/Family to:

• Encourage effective oral hygiene to prevent soft tissue inflammation.
• Prevent trauma when using oral hygiene aids.
• Be alert for the possibility of secondary oral infection and the need to see dentist immediately if signs of infection occur.

podofilox
poe-doe-**fil**′-ox
(Condyline[CAN], Condyline
Paint[AUS], Condylox)

CATEGORY AND SCHEDULE
Pregnancy Risk Category: C

Drug Class: Antimitotic agent

MECHANISM OF ACTION
An active component of podophyllin
resin that binds to tubulin to prevent
formation of microtubules resulting
in mitotic arrest. Exercises many
biological effects, such as damages
endothelium of small blood vessels,
attenuates nucleoside transport,
suppresses immune responses,
inhibits macrophage metabolism,
induces interleukin-1 and
interleukin-2, decreases
lymphocytes' response to mitogens,
and enhances macrophage growth.
Therapeutic Effect: Removes
genital warts.

USES
Removal of certain types of warts
on the outside skin of the genital
areas (penis or vulva)

PHARMACOKINETICS
Time to peak occurs in 1–2 hr.
Some degree of absorption.
Half-life: 1–4.5 hr.

INDICATIONS AND DOSAGES
▶ **Anogenital Warts**
Topical
Adults. Apply 0.5% gel for 3 days,
then withhold for 4 days. Repeat
cycle up to 4 times.

▶ **Genital Warts (Condylomata
Acuminate)**
Topical
Adults. Apply 0.5% solution or gel
q12h in the morning and evening for
3 days, then withhold for 4 days.
Repeat cycle up to 4 times.

SIDE EFFECTS/ADVERSE
REACTIONS
Occasional
Erosion, inflammation, itching, pain,
burning
Rare
Nausea, vomiting

PRECAUTIONS AND
CONTRAINDICATIONS
Bleeding warts, moles, birthmarks
or unusual warts with hair, diabetes,
poor blood circulation, pregnancy,
steroid use, hypersensitivity to
podofilox or any component of its
formulation

DRUG INTERACTIONS OF
CONCERN TO DENTISTRY
• None reported

P

SERIOUS REACTIONS
! Nausea and vomiting occur rarely
and usually after cumulative doses.

DENTAL CONSIDERATIONS
General:
• Determine why patient is taking
the drug.
• Examine oral mucous membranes
for lesions; overuse may be
associated with oral ulcers.
• Tactful questions related to STD
may be appropriate.
• Explore medical and drug history.
• Not for use on mucous
membranes.
Consultations:
• Medical consultation may be
required to assess disease control.

Teach Patient/Family to:
• Encourage effective oral hygiene to prevent soft tissue inflammation.
• Prevent trauma when using oral hygiene aids.
• Update health and medication history if physician makes any changes in evaluation or drug regimens; include OTC, herbal, and nonherbal drugs in the update.

podophyllum resin
po-**dof**′-fil-um rez-in
(Podocon-25, Pododerm)

CATEGORY AND SCHEDULE
Pregnancy Risk Category: X

Drug Class: Cytotoxic, topical

MECHANISM OF ACTION
A cytotoxic agent that directly affects epithelial cell metabolism by arresting mitosis through binding to a protein subunit of spindle microtubules.
Therapeutic Effect: Removes soft genital warts.

USES
Removal of benign growths

PHARMACOKINETICS
Topical podophyllum is systemically absorbed. Absorption may be increased if applied to bleeding, friable, or recently biopsied warts.

INDICATIONS AND DOSAGES
▶ Genital Warts (Condylomata Acuminate)
Topical
Adults, Elderly, Children. Apply 10%–25% solution in compound benzoin tincture to dry surface. Use 1 drop at a time allowing drying

between drops until area is covered. Total volume should be limited to less than 0.5 ml per treatment session.

SIDE EFFECTS/ADVERSE REACTIONS
Occasional
Pruritus, nausea, vomiting, abdominal pain, diarrhea

PRECAUTIONS AND CONTRAINDICATIONS
Diabetes mellitus, concomitant steroid therapy, circulation disorders, bleeding warts, moles, birthmarks or unusual warts with hair growing from them, pregnancy, hypersensitivity to podophyllum resin preparations

DRUG INTERACTIONS OF CONCERN TO DENTISTRY
• None reported

SERIOUS REACTIONS
! Paresthesia, polyneuritis, paralytic ileus, pyrexia, leukopenia, thrombocytopenia, coma, and death have been reported with podophyllum resin use.

DENTAL CONSIDERATIONS
General:
• Determine why patient is taking the drug.
• This medication is applied in physician's office.
• Questions related to sexually transmitted diseases may be appropriate.
Consultations:
• Medical consultation may be required to assess disease control.
Teach Patient/Family to:
• Encourage effective oral hygiene to prevent soft tissue inflammation.

• Prevent trauma when using oral hygiene aids.
• Update health and medication history if physician makes any changes in evaluation or drug regimens; include OTC, herbal, and nonherbal drugs in the update.

polymyxin B
polly-**mix**'-in
(Aerosporin)

CATEGORY AND SCHEDULE
Pregnancy Risk Category: B

Drug Class: Antibiotics, polymyxins

MECHANISM OF ACTION
An antibiotic that alters cell membrane permeability in susceptible microorganisms. *Therapeutic Effect:* Bactericidal.

USES
Treatment of superficial external infections

PHARMACOKINETICS
Negligible absorption. Protein binding: low. Excreted in urine. Poor removal in hemodialysis. *Half-life:* 6 hr.

INDICATIONS AND DOSAGES
▸ **Mild-to-Moderate Infections**
IV
Adults, Elderly, Children 2 yr and older. 15,000–25,000 units/kg/day in divided doses q12h.
Infants. Up to 40,000 units/kg/day.
IM
Adults, Elderly, Children 2 yr and older. 25,000–30,000 units/kg/day in divided doses q4–6h.
Infants. Up to 40,000 units/kg/day.

▸ **Usual Irrigation Dosage**
Continuous Bladder Irrigation
Adults, Elderly. 1 ml urogenital concentrate (contains 200,000 units polymyxin B, 57 mg neomycin) added to 1000 ml 0.9% NaCl. Give each 1000 ml >24 hr for up to 10 days (may increase to 2000 ml/day when urine output is greater than 2 L/day).
▸ **Usual Ophthalmic Dosage**
Ophthalmic
Adults, Elderly, Children. 1 drop q3–4h.

SIDE EFFECTS/ADVERSE REACTIONS
Frequent
Severe pain, irritation at IM injection sites, phlebitis, thrombophlebitis with IV administration
Occasional
Fever, urticaria

PRECAUTIONS AND CONTRAINDICATIONS
Hypersensitivity to polymyxin B or any component of the formulation
Caution:
Hypokalemia, renal disease, hepatic disease, gout, COPD, lupus erythematosus, diabetes mellitus

SERIOUS REACTIONS
! Nephrotoxicity, especially with concurrent/sequential use of other nephrotoxic drugs, renal impairment, concurrent/sequential use of muscle relaxants.
! Superinfection, especially with fungi, may occur.

DENTAL CONSIDERATIONS
General:
• Avoid dental light in patient's eyes; offer dark glasses for patient

P

comfort and safety during dental treatment.

polymyxin B sulfate; trimethoprim sulfate

pol-ee-**mix**'-in bee **sul**'-fate;
trye-**meth**'-oh-prim **sul**'-fate
(Polytrim)

CATEGORY AND SCHEDULE
Pregnancy Risk Category: C

Drug Class: Antiinfective, ophthalmic

MECHANISM OF ACTION
Polymyxin B damages bacterial cytoplasmic membrane that causes leakage of intracellular components. Trimethoprim is a folate antagonist that blocks bacterial biosynthesis of nucleic acids and proteins by interfering with metabolism of folinic acid.
Therapeutic Effect: Prevents inflammatory process. Interferes with bacterial protein synthesis. Produces antibacterial activity.

USES
Treatment of superficial external ocular infections

PHARMACOKINETICS
Absorption through intact skin and mucous membranes is insignificant.

INDICATIONS AND DOSAGES
▸ **Treatment of Surface Ocular Bacterial Conjunctivitis and Blepharoconjunctivitis**
Ophthalmic
Adults, Elderly, Children. Instill 1–2 drops in eye(s) every 3 hr for 7–10 days. Maximum: 6 doses/day.

SIDE EFFECTS/ADVERSE REACTIONS
Occasional
Local irritation, redness, burning, stinging, itching

PRECAUTIONS AND CONTRAINDICATIONS
Hypersensitivity to polymyxin B, trimethoprim sulfate, or any component of the formulation

DRUG INTERACTIONS OF CONCERN TO DENTISTRY
• None reported

SERIOUS REACTIONS
! Prolonged use may result in overgrowth of nonsusceptible organisms, including superinfection.
! Hypersensitivity reactions consisting of lid edema, itching, increased redness, tearing, and/or circumocular rash have been reported.
! Photosensitivity has been reported in patients taking oral trimethoprim.

DENTAL CONSIDERATIONS

General:
• Avoid dental light in patient's eyes; offer dark glasses for patient comfort and safety during dental treatment.

posaconazole

poe-sah-**kone**'-ah-zole
(Noxafil)

CATEGORY AND SCHEDULE
Pregnancy Risk Category: C

Drug Class: Antifungal

MECHANISM OF ACTION

A triazole antifungal that blocks the synthesis of ergosterol, a key component of fungal cell membrane, through the inhibition of the enzyme lanosterol 14a-α-demethylase and accumulation of methylated sterol precursors. *Therapeutic Effect:* Inhibits fungal cell membrane formation.

USES

Prophylaxis of invasive *Aspergillus* and *Candida* infections in patients who are severely immunocompromised

PHARMACOKINETICS

Food increases absorption. Protein binding: greater than 98%. Not significantly metabolized; undergoes glucuronidation into metabolites. Primarily eliminated in feces (71%, 66% unchanged); partial excretion in urine (13%, less than 0.2% unchanged). *Half-life:* 35 hr.

INDICATIONS AND DOSAGES
▶ **Prophylaxis of Invasive Fungal Infections**
PO
Adults, Children 13 yr and older. 200 mg (5 ml) three times a day.
▶ **Oropharyngeal Candidiasis**
PO
Adults, Children 13 yr and older. Initially, 100 mg (2.5 ml) twice a day on the first day. Maintenance: 100 mg (2.5 ml) once a day for 13 days.
▶ **Oropharyngeal Candidiasis, Refractory to Itraconazole and/or Fluconazole**
PO
Adults, Children 13 yr and older. 400 mg (10 ml) twice a day.

SIDE EFFECTS/ADVERSE REACTIONS
Adult
Frequent
Diarrhea
Occasional
Nausea, neutropenia, headache, vomiting, abdominal pain, flatulence, QTc prolongation, rash, hypokalemia, anemia, fever, bilirubin increased, ALT increased, AST increased, GGT increased, dizziness, weakness, anorexia, fatigue, insomnia, mucositis, thrombocytopenia, alkaline phosphatase increased, serum creatinine increased, myalgia, pruritus, dyspepsia, xerostomia
Rare
Hypertension, blurred vision, tremor, hepatocellular damage, taste perversion, constipation, somnolence

PRECAUTIONS AND CONTRAINDICATIONS

Hypersensitivity to azole antifungals, posaconazole or its components; avoid coadministration with ergot alkaloids
Caution:
Do not breast-feed, hepatic impairment, patients with an increased risk of arrhythmia, electrolyte abnormalities

DRUG INTERACTIONS OF CONCERN TO DENTISTRY

• Calcium channel blockers: may increase the levels and effects of calcium channel blockers
• Cimetidine: may decrease the levels and effects of posaconazole; avoid concurrent use
• Cyclosporine: may increase the levels and effects of cyclosporine
• CYP3A4 substrates: may increase the levels and effects of CYP3A4

P

substrates (e.g., midazolam, triazolam)
• Ergot alkaloids: may increase the levels and effects of ergot alkaloids
• HMG-CoA reductase inhibitors: may increase the levels and effects of HMG-CoA reductase inhibitors
• Phenytoin: may increase the levels and effects of phenytoin; avoid concurrent use
• QT-prolonging agents: increased risk of arrhythmia (torsade de pointes)
• Rifabutin: may increase the levels and effects of rifabutin; avoid concurrent use
• Sirolimus: may increase the levels and effects of sirolimus
• Tacrolimus: may increase the levels and effects of tacrolimus
• Vinca alkaloids: may increase the levels and effects of vinca alkaloids

SERIOUS REACTIONS

! Hepatic dysfunction may occur.
! Arrhythmia (torsade de pointes) has been reported.

DENTAL CONSIDERATIONS

General:
• Monitor vital signs at every appointment due to possible adverse cardiovascular effects.
• Determine why patient is taking the drug.
• Consider semisupine chair position for patient comfort due to adverse GI effects of drug.
• To prevent reinoculation of candidal infection, dispose of tooth brush and other contaminated oral hygiene devices used during period of infection.
• Assess salivary flow as a factor in caries, periodontal disease, and candidiasis.

• Disinfect or remake removable prostheses that may harbor residual candidal organisms.
• Consider drug effect in evaluating taste changes versus restorative materials.
Consultations:
• Medical consult may be necessary to determine patient's ability to tolerate dental procedures.
Teach Patient/Family to:
• Avoid mouth rinses with high alcohol content because of drying effects.

potassium chloride

poe-**tass'**-ee-um **klor'**-ide
(Apo-K[CAN], Cena K; Ed K10, KCare; K-10, K-8, Kaochlor, Kaochlor S-F, Kaon-CI, Kaon-CL 10, Kaon-CL 20%, Kato, Kay Ciel, KCl-20, KCl-40, K-Dur 10, K-Dur 20, K-Lor; Klor-Con, Klor-Con/25, Klor-Con 10, Klor-Con 8, Klor-Con M10, Klor-Con M15, Klor-Con M20, Klotrix, K-Lyte CI, K-Norm, K-Sol, K-Tab, Micro-K, Micro-K 10, Rum-K)
Do not confuse with Cardura or Slow-FE.

CATEGORY AND SCHEDULE

Pregnancy Risk Category: C

Drug Class: Potassium electrolyte

MECHANISM OF ACTION

An electrolyte that is necessary for multiple cellular metabolic processes. Primary action is intracellular.
Therapeutic Effect: Necessary for nerve impulse conduction,

contraction of cardiac, skeletal, and smooth muscle; maintains normal renal function and acid-base balance.

USES
Prevention and treatment of hypokalemia

PHARMACOKINETICS
Well absorbed from the GI tract. Enters cells via active transport from extracellular fluid. Primarily excreted in urine.

INDICATIONS AND DOSAGES
▶ **Prevention of Hypokalemia (on Diuretic Therapy)**
PO
Adults, Elderly. 20–40 mEq/day in 1–2 divided doses.
Children. 1–2 mEq/kg in 1–2 divided doses.
▶ **Treatment of Hypokalemia**
IV
Adults, Elderly. 5–10 mEq/hr. Maximum: 400 mEq/day.
Children. 1 mEq/kg over 1–2 hr.
PO
Adults, Elderly. 40–80 mEq/day, further doses based on laboratory values.
Children. 1–2 mEq/day, further doses based on laboratory values.

SIDE EFFECTS/ADVERSE REACTIONS
Occasional
Nausea, vomiting, diarrhea, flatulence, abdominal discomfort with distention, phlebitis with IV administration (particularly when potassium concentration of greater than 40 mEq/L is infused)
Rare
Rash

PRECAUTIONS AND CONTRAINDICATIONS
Digitalis toxicity, heat cramps, hyperkalemia, patients receiving potassium-sparing diuretics, postoperative oliguria, severe burns, severe renal impairment, shock with dehydration or hemolytic reaction, untreated Addison's disease, hypersensitivity to any component of the formulation
Caution:
Cardiac disease, potassium-sparing diuretic therapy, systemic acidosis, pregnancy category A, renal impairment

DRUG INTERACTIONS OF CONCERN TO DENTISTRY
• Decreased potassium requirement: corticosteroids
• Increased GI side effects: anticholinergic drugs, NSAIDs
• Increased serum potassium: NSAIDs, cyclosporine

SERIOUS REACTIONS
! Hyperkalemia (observed particularly in elderly or in patients with impaired renal function) manifested as paresthesia of extremities, heaviness of legs, cold skin, grayish pallor, hypotension, mental confusion, irritability, flaccid paralysis, and cardiac arrhythmias.

DENTAL CONSIDERATIONS
General:
• Patients taking potassium supplements will normally be taking a diuretic. Compliance with potassium supplements can be a problem. Verify serum potassium levels as required.
• Consider semisupine chair position for patient comfort if GI side effects occur.

P

potassium acetate/ potassium bicarbonate-citrate/ potassium chloride/ potassium gluconate

poe-**tah**′-see-um **ass**′-eh-tayte
(potassium bicarbonate-citrate:
K-Lyte, Klor-Con EF, Effer K,
K-Lyte DS; potassium chloride:
Apo-K[CAN], Kaochlor, K-Dur,
K-Lor, K-Lor-Con M 15,
Kaon-Cl, KSR[AUS], KSR-
600[AUS], Micro-K, Slow-K[AUS],
Span-K[AUS]; potassium
gluconate: Kaon)
Do not confuse K-dur with
Cardura.

CATEGORY AND SCHEDULE
Pregnancy Risk Category: C (A
for potassium chloride)

Drug Class: Potassium
electrolyte

MECHANISM OF ACTION
An electrolyte that is necessary for
multiple cellular metabolic
processes. Primary action is
intracellular.
Therapeutic Effect: Is necessary for
nerve impulse conduction and
contraction of cardiac, skeletal, and
smooth muscle; maintains normal
renal function and acid-base
balance.

USES
Prevention and treatment of
hypokalemia

PHARMACOKINETICS
Well absorbed from the GI tract.
Enters cells by active transport from
extracellular fluid. Primarily
excreted in urine.

INDICATIONS AND DOSAGES
▸ **Prevention of Hypokalemia (in Patients on Diuretic Therapy)**
PO
Adults, Elderly. 20–40 mEq/day in
1–2 divided doses.
Children. 1–2 mEq/kg/day in 1–2
divided doses.
▸ **Treatment of Hypokalemia**
PO
Adults, Elderly. 40–80 mEq/day;
further doses based on laboratory
values.
Children. 2–5 mEq/day; further
doses based on laboratory values.
IV
Adults, Elderly. 5–10 mEq/hr.
Maximum: 400 mEq/day.
Children. 1 mEq/kg over 1–2 hr.

SIDE EFFECTS/ADVERSE REACTIONS
Occasional
Nausea, vomiting, diarrhea,
flatulence, abdominal discomfort
with distention, phlebitis with IV
administration (particularly when
higher concentrations are infused
IV)
Rare
Rash

PRECAUTIONS AND CONTRAINDICATIONS
Concurrent use of potassium-sparing
diuretics, digitalis toxicity, heat
cramps, hyperkalemia, postoperative
oliguria, severe burns, severe renal
impairment, shock with dehydration
or hemolytic reaction, untreated
Addison's disease
Caution:
Cardiac disease, potassium-sparing
diuretic therapy, systemic acidosis,
renal impairment

DRUG INTERACTIONS OF CONCERN TO DENTISTRY
• Decreased potassium requirement: corticosteroids
• Increased GI side effects: anticholinergic drugs, NSAIDs
• Increased serum potassium: NSAIDs, cyclosporine

SERIOUS REACTIONS
❗ Hyperkalemia (more common in elderly patients and those with impaired renal function) may be manifested as paresthesia, feeling of heaviness in the lower extremities, cold skin, grayish pallor, hypotension, confusion, irritability, flaccid paralysis, and cardiac arrhythmias.

DENTAL CONSIDERATIONS
General:
• Patients taking potassium supplements will normally be taking a diuretic. Compliance with potassium supplements can be a problem. Verify serum potassium levels as required.
• Consider semisupine chair position for patient comfort if GI side effects occur.

povidone iodine
poe′-vi-done
(ACU-dyne, Aerodine, Betadine, Betagen, Biodyne, Efodine, Iodex-P, Mallisol, Minidyne, Operand, Polydine Proviodine)

CATEGORY AND SCHEDULE
Pregnancy Risk Category: D (vaginal antiseptic)

Drug Class: Iodophor disinfectant

MECHANISM OF ACTION
Destroys a wide variety of microorganisms by local irritation, germicidal action.

USES
Cleansing wounds, disinfection, preoperative skin preparation removal

INDICATIONS AND DOSAGES
Topical
Adults, Children. Use as needed on infected body surface.

SIDE EFFECTS/ADVERSE REACTIONS
Frequent
Skin irritation

PRECAUTIONS AND CONTRAINDICATIONS
Hypersensitivity to iodine
Caution:
Extensive burns

DRUG INTERACTIONS OF CONCERN TO DENTISTRY
• Do not use with alcohol or hydrogen peroxide

SERIOUS REACTIONS
❗ Severe allergic reactions

DENTAL CONSIDERATIONS
General:
• Assess for allergies to seafood; if present, drug should not be used.
• Store in tight, light-resistant container.
• Evaluate area of the body involved for irritation, rash, breaks, dryness, and scales.
Teach Patient/Family to:
• Discontinue use if rash, irritation, or redness occurs.

pramipexole
pram-eh-**pex**′-ol
(Mirapex)
Do not confuse Mirapex with
Mifeprex or MiraLAX.

CATEGORY AND SCHEDULE
Pregnancy Risk Category: C

Drug Class: Antiparkinson agent

MECHANISM OF ACTION
An antiparkinson agent that
stimulates dopamine receptors in the
striatum.
Therapeutic Effect: Relieves signs
and symptoms of Parkinson's
disease.

USES
Treatment of idiopathic Parkinson's
disease

PHARMACOKINETICS
Rapidly and extensively absorbed
after PO administration. Protein
binding: 15%. Widely distributed.
Steady-state concentrations achieved
within 2 days. Primarily eliminated
in urine. Not removed by
hemodialysis. *Half-life:* 8 hr (12 hr
in patients older than 65 yr).

INDICATIONS AND DOSAGES
▸ **Parkinson's Disease**
PO
Adults, Elderly. Initially, 0.375 mg/
day in 3 divided doses. Do not
increase dosage more frequently
than every 5–7 days. Maintenance:
1.5–4.5 mg/day in 3 equally divided
doses.
▸ **Dosage in Renal Impairment**
Dosage and frequency are modified
on the basis of creatinine clearance.

Creatinine Clearance	Initial Dose	Maximum Dose
Greater than 60 ml/min	0.125 mg 3 times a day	1.5 mg 3 times a day
35–59 ml/min	0.125 mg twice a day	1.5 mg twice a day
15–34 ml/min	0.125 mg once a day	1.5 mg once a day

SIDE EFFECTS/ADVERSE REACTIONS
Frequent
Early Parkinson's disease: Nausea,
asthenia, dizziness, somnolence,
insomnia, constipation
Advanced Parkinson's disease:
Orthostatic hypotension,
extrapyramidal reactions, insomnia,
dizziness, hallucinations
Occasional
Early Parkinson's disease: Edema,
malaise, confusion, amnesia,
akathisia, anorexia, dysphagia,
peripheral edema, vision changes,
impotence
Advanced Parkinson's disease:
Asthenia, somnolence, confusion,
constipation, abnormal gait, dry
mouth
Rare
Advanced Parkinson's disease:
General edema, malaise, chest pain,
amnesia, tremor, urinary frequency
or incontinence, dyspnea, rhinitis,
vision changes

PRECAUTIONS AND CONTRAINDICATIONS
History of hypersensitivity to
pramipexole
Caution:
Orthostatic hypotension,
hallucination risk higher than 65 yr,
renal insufficiency, caution in
driving a car (somnolence), risk of
falling asleep while performing daily

P

activities, lactation, use not
established in children

DRUG INTERACTIONS OF CONCERN TO DENTISTRY
• Increased CNS depression: all
CNS depressants
• Possible decreased effects:
dopamine antagonists
(phenothiazines, butyrophenones, or
thioxanthenes) and metoclopramide

SERIOUS REACTIONS
! None known

DENTAL CONSIDERATIONS
General:
• Monitor vital signs at every
appointment because of
cardiovascular side effects.
• Assess salivary flow as factor in
caries, periodontal disease, and
candidiasis.
• Consider semisupine chair position
for patient comfort if GI side effects
occur.
• After supine positioning, have
patient sit upright for at least 2 min
before standing to avoid orthostatic
hypotension.
Consultations:
• Medical consultation may be
required to assess disease control
and patient's ability to tolerate
stress.
Teach Patient/Family to:
• Encourage effective oral hygiene
to prevent soft tissue inflammation.
• Use caution to prevent trauma
when using oral hygiene aids.
• Use powered tooth brush if patient
has difficulty holding conventional
devices.
• Update health and drug history if
physician makes any changes in
evaluation or drug regimens; include
OTC, herbal, and nonherbal drugs in
the update.

• When chronic dry mouth occurs,
advise patient to:
  • Avoid mouth rinses with high
  alcohol content because of
  drying effects.
  • Use daily home fluoride
  products for anticaries effect.
  • Use sugarless gum, frequent
  sips of water, or saliva
  substitutes.

---

prasugrel
pra-soo-grel
(Effient)
Do not confuse with prazosin.

CATEGORY AND SCHEDULE
Pregnancy Risk Category: C

Drug Class: Platelet aggregation
inhibitor

MECHANISN OF ACTION
Binds selectively and irreversibly to
platelet P2Y12 receptors and inhibits
ADP-induced platelet activation and
aggregation.

USES
Reduction of adverse thrombotic
cardiovascular events, including
stent thrombosis, in patients with
acute coronary syndrome, with
unstable angina or non-ST-elevation
myocardial infarction and those with
ST-elevation myocardial infarction
managed with primary or delayed
percutaneous coronary intervention
(PCI)

PHARMACOKINETICS
Rapidly hydrolyzed in the intestine
to a thiolactone metabolite, which is
then absorbed. Metabolized in the
liver primarily by CYP 3A4 and
2B6, with numerous metabolites.

Half-life: 7 hr. 70% excreted by the kidneys, 25% in the feces. Metabolism and excretion not significantly affected by mild-to-moderate hepatic or renal impairment.

INDICATIONS AND DOSAGES
▶ **Antiplatelet Therapy**
PO
Adult, Elderly (under the age of 75). 60-mg loading dose, then 10 mg once daily, in combination with low-dose aspirin (75–325 mg).

SIDE EFFECTS/ADVERSE REACTIONS
Frequent
Bleeding, hypertension, hypercholesterolemia, hyperlipidemia, headache, back pain, dyspnea, nausea, dizziness, cough, hypotension, fatigue, non-cardiac chest pain
Occasional
Anemia
Rare
Thrombocytopenia, abnormal hepatic function, allergic reactions, angioedema

PRECAUTIONS AND CONTRAINDICATIONS
Severe bleeding, especially elderly over the age of 75 and less than 60 kg body weight

DRUG INTERACTIONS OF CONCERN TO DENTISTRY
• Increased risk of serious bleeding: NSAIDs
• Epinephrine: coexisting cardiovascular disease
• CYP Inhibitors: increased bleeding (erythromycin, clarithromycin, azole antifungal drugs, benzodiazepines)

SERIOUS REACTIONS
! Excessive bleeding, hypersensitivity

DENTAL CONSIDERATIONS
General:
• Avoid discontinuation for dental procedures because of increased risk of thromboembolism.
• Use careful surgical technique and local hemostatic measures to prevent excessive bleeding.
• Question patient about concurrent use of aspirin, other NSAIDs.
• Avoid or limit doses of epinephrine in local anesthetic due to cardiovascular disease status.
• Monitor vital signs at every appointment due to cardiovascular disease status.
Consultations:
• Medical consultation may be required to assess disease control and patient's ability to tolerate stress.
• Consultation should include data on bleeding time.
• In a patient with signs or symptoms of blood dyscrasias, request a medical consultation for blood studies and postpone treatment until normal values are reestablished.
Teach Patient/Family to:
• Update health and drug history if physician makes any changes in evaluation or drug regimens.
• Use caution to prevent trauma when using oral hygiene aids.
• Report any unusual or prolonged bleeding episodes after dental treatment.

pravastatin
prav-ih-**sta´**-tin
(Pravachol)
Do not confuse pravastatin with
Prevacid, or Pravachol with
propranolol.

CATEGORY AND SCHEDULE
Pregnancy Risk Category: X

Drug Class: Antihyperlipidemic

MECHANISM OF ACTION
An HMG-CoA reductase inhibitor
that interferes with cholesterol
biosynthesis by preventing the
conversion of HMG-CoA reductase
to mevalonate, a precursor to
cholesterol.
Therapeutic Effect: Lowers serum
low-density lipoproteins (LDLs) and
very low-density lipoproteins
(VLDLs), cholesterol, and plasma
triglyceride levels; increases serum
high-density lipoprotein (HDL)
concentration.

USES
As an adjunct in homozygous or
heterozygous familial
hypercholesterolemia, mixed
hyperlipidemia, elevated serum
triglyceride levels, and type IV
hyperproteinemia; also reduces total
cholesterol LDL-C, apo B, and
triglyceride levels; patient should
first be placed on cholesterol-
lowering diet; primary prevention of
coronary events, secondary
prevention of cardiovascular events

PHARMACOKINETICS
Poorly absorbed from the GI tract.
Protein binding: 50%. Metabolized
in the liver (minimal active
metabolites). Primarily excreted in
feces via the biliary system. Not

removed by hemodialysis. **Half-life:**
2.7 hr.

INDICATIONS AND DOSAGES
▸ **Hyperlipidemia, Primary and
Secondary Prevention of
Cardiovascular Events in Patients
with Elevated Cholesterol Levels**
PO
Adults, Elderly. Initially, 40 mg/day.
Titrate to desired response. Range:
10–80 mg/day.
Children 14–18 yr. 40 mg/day.
Children 8–13 yr. 20 mg/day.
▸ **Dosage in Hepatic and Renal
Impairment**
For adults, give 10 mg/day initially.
Titrate to desired response.

SIDE EFFECTS/ADVERSE REACTIONS
Pravastatin is generally well
tolerated. Side effects are usually
mild and transient.
Occasional
Nausea, vomiting, diarrhea,
constipation, abdominal pain,
headache, rhinitis, rash, pruritus
Rare
Heartburn, myalgia, dizziness,
cough, fatigue, flu-like symptoms

PRECAUTIONS AND CONTRAINDICATIONS
Active hepatic disease or
unexplained, persistent elevations of
liver function test results
Caution:
Past liver disease, alcoholics, severe
acute infections, trauma,
hypotension, uncontrolled seizure
disorders, severe metabolic
disorders, electrolyte imbalances

DRUG INTERACTIONS OF CONCERN TO DENTISTRY
• Increased risk of myopathy or
rhabdomyolysis: erythromycin,
itraconazole

P

SERIOUS REACTIONS
! Malignancy and cataracts may occur.
! Hypersensitivity occurs rarely.

DENTAL CONSIDERATIONS

General:
• Monitor vital signs at every appointment because of possible cardiovascular disease.
• Consider semisupine chair position for patient comfort if GI side effects occur.

prazosin hydrochloride
pra'-zoe-sin high-droh-**klor'**-ide
(Minipress, Prasig[AUS], Pratisol[AUS], Pressin[AUS])

CATEGORY AND SCHEDULE
Pregnancy Risk Category: C

Drug Class: Antihypertensive, α-adrenergic antagonist

MECHANISM OF ACTION
An antidote, antihypertensive, and vasodilator that selectively blocks α_1-adrenergic receptors, decreasing peripheral vascular resistance.
Therapeutic Effect: Produces vasodilation of veins and arterioles, decreases total peripheral resistance, and relaxes smooth muscle in bladder neck and prostate.

USES
Treatment of hypertension; unapproved: CHF, urinary retention in prostatic hypertrophy, pheochromocytoma

PHARMACOKINETICS
PO: Onset 2 hr, peak 1–3 hr, duration 6–12 hr. *Half-life:* 2–4 hr; metabolized in liver; excreted via bile, feces (greater than 90%), in urine (less than 10%).

INDICATIONS AND DOSAGES
▶ Mild-to-Moderate Hypertension
PO
Adults, Elderly. Initially, 1 mg 2–3 times a day. Maintenance: 3–15 mg/day in divided doses. Maximum: 20 mg/day.
Children. 5 mcg/kg/dose q6h. Gradually increase up to 25 mcg/kg/dose.

SIDE EFFECTS/ADVERSE REACTIONS
Frequent
Dizziness, somnolence, headache, asthenia (loss of strength, energy)
Occasional
Palpitations, nausea, dry mouth, nervousness
Rare
Angina, urinary urgency

PRECAUTIONS AND CONTRAINDICATIONS
Hypersensitivity, severe CHF
Caution:
Children

DRUG INTERACTIONS OF CONCERN TO DENTISTRY
• Increased effects: epinephrine
• Decreased effect: indomethacin, NSAIDs

SERIOUS REACTIONS
! First-dose syncope (hypotension with sudden loss of consciousness) may occur 30–90 min following initial dose of more than 2 mg, a too-rapid increase in dosage, or addition of another antihypertensive agent to therapy. First-dose syncope may be preceded by tachycardia (pulse rate of 120–160 beats/min).

DENTAL CONSIDERATIONS

General:
• Monitor vital signs at every appointment because of cardiovascular side effects.
• Avoid or limit dose of vasoconstrictor.
• After supine positioning, have patient sit upright for at least 2 min before standing to avoid orthostatic hypotension.
• Assess salivary flow as a factor in caries, periodontal disease, and candidiasis.
• Limit use of sodium-containing products, such as saline IV fluids, for patients with a dietary salt restriction.
• Stress from dental procedures may compromise cardiovascular function; determine patient risk.
• Short appointments and a stress-reduction protocol may be required.

Consultations:
• Medical consultation may be required to assess disease control.

Teach Patient/Family to:
• When chronic dry mouth occurs, advise patient to:
  • Avoid mouth rinses with high alcohol content because of drying effects.
  • Use daily home fluoride products to prevent caries.
  • Use sugarless gum, frequent sips of water, or saliva substitutes.

prednisolone
pred-**niss'**-oh-lone
(AK-Pred, AK-Tate[CAN], Inflamase Forte, Inflamase Mild, Minims-Prednisolone[CAN], Novo-Prednisolone[CAN], Orapred, Pediapred, Pred Forte, Pred Mild, Prelone, Solone[AUS])
Do not confuse prednisolone with prednisone or primidone.

CATEGORY AND SCHEDULE
Pregnancy Risk Category: C (D if used in first trimester)

Drug Class: Glucocorticoid, immediate acting

MECHANISM OF ACTION
An adrenocortical steroid that inhibits accumulation of inflammatory cells at inflammation sites, phagocytosis, lysosomal enzyme release and synthesis, and release of mediators of inflammation.
Therapeutic Effect: Prevents or suppresses cell-mediated immune reactions. Decreases or prevents tissue response to inflammatory process.

USES
Treatment of severe inflammation, immunosuppression, neoplasms, adrenal insufficiency, acute exacerbation of multiple sclerosis

PHARMACOKINETICS
PO: Peak 1–2 hr, duration 2 days.
IM: Peak 3–45 hr.

INDICATIONS AND DOSAGES

▶ **Substitution Therapy for Deficiency States: Acute or Chronic Adrenal Insufficiency, Congenital Adrenal Hyperplasia, and Adrenal Insufficiency Secondary to Pituitary Insufficiency; Nonendocrine Disorders: Arthritis; Rheumatic Carditis; Allergic, Collagen, Intestinal Tract, Liver, Ocular, Renal, Skin Diseases; Bronchial Asthma; Cerebral Edema; Malignancies**

PO

Adults, Elderly. 5–60 mg/day in divided doses.
Children. 0.1–2 mg/kg/day in 1–4 divided doses.

▶ **Treatment of Conjunctivitis and Corneal Injury**

Ophthalmic

Adults, Elderly. 1–2 drops every hr during day and q2h during night. After response, decrease dosage to 1 drop q4h, then 1 drop 3–4 times a day.

SIDE EFFECTS/ADVERSE REACTIONS

Frequent

Insomnia, heartburn, nervousness, abdominal distention, increased sweating, acne, mood swings, increased appetite, facial flushing, delayed wound healing, increased susceptibility to infection, diarrhea or constipation

Occasional

Headache, edema, change in skin color, frequent urination

Rare

Tachycardia, allergic reaction (such as rash and hives), psychological changes, hallucinations, depression
Ophthalmic: stinging or burning, posterior subcapsular cataracts

PRECAUTIONS AND CONTRAINDICATIONS

Acute superficial herpes simplex keratitis, systemic fungal infections, varicella

Caution:

Diabetes mellitus, glaucoma, osteoporosis, seizure disorders, ulcerative colitis, CHF, myasthenia gravis, ulcerative GI disease, rifampin

DRUG INTERACTIONS OF CONCERN TO DENTISTRY

• Decreased action: barbiturates, rifampin, rifabutin
• Increased side effects: alcohol, salicylates, NSAIDs
• Increased action: ketoconazole, macrolide antibiotics (erythromycin, clarithromycin, azithromycin)
• Hepatotoxicity: acetaminophen (chronic use, high doses)

SERIOUS REACTIONS

! Long-term therapy may cause hypocalcemia, hypokalemia, muscle wasting (especially in the arms and legs), osteoporosis, spontaneous fractures, amenorrhea, cataracts, glaucoma, peptic ulcer disease, and CHF.
! Abruptly withdrawing the drug after long-term therapy may cause anorexia, nausea, fever, headache, severe or sudden joint pain, rebound inflammation, fatigue, weakness, lethargy, dizziness, and orthostatic hypotension.
! Suddenly discontinuing prednisolone may be fatal.

DENTAL CONSIDERATIONS

General:

• Monitor vital signs at every appointment because of cardiovascular side effects.

• Patients on chronic drug therapy may rarely have symptoms of blood dyscrasias, which can include infection, bleeding, and poor healing.

• Assess salivary flow as a factor in caries, periodontal disease, and candidiasis.

• Avoid prescribing aspirin-containing products.

• Place on frequent recall to evaluate healing response.

• Prophylactic antibiotics may be indicated to prevent infection if surgery or deep scaling is planned.

• Symptoms of oral infections may be masked.

• Determine dose and duration of steroid therapy for each patient to assess risk for stress tolerance and immunosuppression.

• Patients who have been or are currently on chronic steroid therapy longer than 2 wk may require supplemental steroids for stressful dental treatment.

• Determine why the patient is taking the drug.

Consultations:

• In a patient with symptoms of blood dyscrasias, request a medical consultation for blood studies and postpone dental treatment until normal values are reestablished.

• Medical consultation may be required to assess disease control.

• Consultation may be required to confirm steroid dose and duration of use.

Teach Patient/Family to:

• Encourage effective oral hygiene to prevent soft tissue inflammation.

• Use caution to prevent injury when using oral hygiene aids.

• When chronic dry mouth occurs, advise patient to:

  • Avoid mouth rinses with high alcohol content because of drying effects.

• Use daily home fluoride products to prevent caries.

• Use sugarless gum, frequent sips of water, or saliva substitutes.

---

prednisolone acetate
pred-**niss**′-oh-lone **as**′-ih-tate
(AK-Pred, Econopred Plus, Inflamase Forte, Inflamase Mild, Ocu-Pred, Ocu-Pred-A, Ocu-Pred Forte, Pred Forte, Pred Mild, Prednisol)

CATEGORY AND SCHEDULE
Pregnancy Risk Category: C

Drug Class: Glucocorticoid, immediate acting

MECHANISM OF ACTION
An adrenal corticosteroid that inhibits accumulation of inflammatory cells at inflammation sites, phagocytosis, lysosomal enzyme release and synthesis, and release of mediators of inflammation.

Therapeutic Effect: Prevents or suppresses cell-mediated immune reactions. Decreases or prevents tissue response to inflammatory process.

USES
Treatment of severe inflammation, immunosuppression, neoplasms, adrenal insufficiency, acute exacerbation of multiple sclerosis

PHARMACOKINETICS
Absorbed into aqueous humor, cornea, iris, choroids, ciliary body, and retina. Systemic absorption may occur, but significant only at high dosages.

P

INDICATIONS AND DOSAGES
▶ **Conjunctivitis**
Ophthalmic
Adults, Elderly, Children. 1–2 drops
2–4 times a day.

SIDE EFFECTS/ADVERSE REACTIONS
Occasional
Stinging or burning

PRECAUTIONS AND CONTRAINDICATIONS
Fungal, mycobacterial, or viral
infections of the eye,
hypersensitivity to prednisolone
acetate or any component of the
formulation
Caution:
Diabetes mellitus, glaucoma,
osteoporosis, seizure disorders,
ulcerative colitis, CHF, myasthenia
gravis, ulcerative GI disease,
rifampin

DRUG INTERACTIONS OF CONCERN TO DENTISTRY
• Decreased action: barbiturates,
rifampin, rifabutin
• Increased side effects: alcohol,
salicylates, NSAIDs
• Increased action: ketoconazole,
macrolide antibiotics (erythromycin,
clarithromycin, azithromycin)
• Hepatotoxicity: acetaminophen
(chronic use, high doses)

SERIOUS REACTIONS
❗ Prolonged use of corticosteroids
may result in glaucoma with damage
to the optic nerve, defects in visual
acuity and fields of vision, posterior
subcapsular cataract formation, and
delayed wound healing.
❗ Long-term use may cause corneal
and scleral thinning.
❗ Systemic effects are uncommon,
but systemic hypercorticoidism has
been reported.

❗ Acute anterior uveitis and
perforation of the globe, keratitis,
conjunctivitis, corneal ulcers,
mydriasis, conjunctival hyperemia,
loss of accommodation, and ptosis
have occasionally been reported.
❗ The development of secondary
ocular infection has occurred.
Fungal and viral infections of the
cornea may develop with long-term
applications of steroid.

DENTAL CONSIDERATIONS

General:
• Monitor vital signs at every
appointment because of
cardiovascular side effects.
• Patients on chronic drug therapy
may rarely have symptoms of blood
dyscrasias, which can include
infection, bleeding, and poor
healing.
• Assess salivary flow as a factor in
caries, periodontal disease, and
candidiasis.
• Avoid prescribing aspirin-
containing products.
• Place on frequent recall to evaluate
healing response.
• Prophylactic antibiotics may be
indicated to prevent infection if
surgery or deep scaling is planned.
• Symptoms of oral infections may
be masked.
• Determine dose and duration of
steroid therapy for each patient to
assess risk for stress tolerance and
immunosuppression.
• Patients who have been or are
currently on chronic steroid therapy
longer than 2 wk may require
supplemental steroids for stressful
dental treatment.
• Determine why the patient is
taking the drug.
Consultations:
• In a patient with symptoms of
blood dyscrasias, request a medical

consultation for blood studies and postpone dental treatment until normal values are reestablished.
• Medical consultation may be required to assess disease control.
• Consultation may be required to confirm steroid dose and duration of use.

Teach Patient/Family to:
• Encourage effective oral hygiene to prevent soft tissue inflammation.
• Use caution to prevent injury when using oral hygiene aids.
• When chronic dry mouth occurs, advise patient to:
  • Avoid mouth rinses with high alcohol content because of drying effects.
  • Use daily home fluoride products to prevent caries.
  • Use sugarless gum, frequent sips of water, or saliva substitutes.

prednisolone acetate; sulfacetamide sodium

pred-**niss**′-oh-lone **ass**′-eh-tate; sul-fa-**see**′-ta-mide **soe**′-dee-um (AK-Cide; Blephamide; Blephamide S.O.P.; Medasulf; Metimyd; Ocu-Lone C; Vasocidin)

CATEGORY AND SCHEDULE
Pregnancy Risk Category: C

Drug Class: Glucocorticoid, immediate acting

MECHANISM OF ACTION
Prednisolone is an adrenal corticosteroid that inhibits accumulation of inflammatory cells at inflammation sites, phagocytosis, lysosomal enzyme release and synthesis, and release of mediators of inflammation. Sulfacetamide is a sulfonamide that interferes with synthesis of folic acid that bacteria require for growth.
Therapeutic Effect: Prevents or suppresses cell-mediated immune reactions. Decreases or prevents tissue response to inflammatory process. Prevents further bacterial growth; bacteriostatic.

USES
Treatment of severe inflammation, immunosuppression, neoplasms, adrenal insufficiency, acute exacerbation of multiple sclerosis

PHARMACOKINETICS
None reported

INDICATIONS AND DOSAGES
▸ **Steroid-Responsive Inflammatory Ocular Conditions for Which a Corticosteroid is Indicated and Where Superficial Bacterial Ocular Infection or a Risk of Bacterial Ocular Infection Exists**
Ophthalmic Ointment
Adults, Elderly, Children. Apply 3 or 4 times a day and once at bedtime.
Ophthalmic Suspension
Adults, Elderly, Children. Instill 2–3 drops every 1–2 hr while awake.

SIDE EFFECTS/ADVERSE REACTIONS
Occasional
Local irritation
Rare
Elevation of intraocular pressure

PRECAUTIONS AND CONTRAINDICATIONS
Epithelial herpes simplex keratitis (dendritic keratitis), vaccinia, varicella, and other viral diseases of the cornea or conjunctiva, mycobacterial infection of the eye,

P

and fungal diseases of ocular structure, known or suspected hypersensitivity to other sulfonamides or other corticosteroids or any component of the formulation

DRUG INTERACTIONS OF CONCERN TO DENTISTRY

• Decreased action: barbiturates, rifampin, rifabutin
• Increased side effects: alcohol, salicylates, NSAIDs
• Increased action: ketoconazole, macrolide antibiotics (erythromycin, clarithromycin, azithromycin)
• Hepatotoxicity: acetaminophen (chronic use, high doses)

SERIOUS REACTIONS

! Prolonged use of corticosteroids may result in glaucoma with damage to the optic nerve, defects in visual acuity and fields of vision, posterior subcapsular cataract formation, and delayed wound healing.
! Long-term use may cause corneal and scleral thinning.
! Systemic effects are uncommon, but systemic hypercorticoidism has been reported.
! Acute anterior uveitis and perforation of the globe, keratitis, conjunctivitis, corneal ulcers, mydriasis, conjunctival hyperemia, loss of accommodation, and ptosis have occasionally been reported.
! The development of secondary ocular infection has occurred. Fungal and viral infections of the cornea may develop with long-term applications of steroid.
! Fatalities caused by reactions to sulfonamides including Stevens-Johnson syndrome, toxic epidermal necrolysis, fulminant hepatic necrosis, agranulocytosis, aplastic anemia, and other blood dyscrasias have occurred.

DENTAL CONSIDERATIONS

General:
• Monitor vital signs at every appointment because of cardiovascular side effects.
• Patients on chronic drug therapy may rarely have symptoms of blood dyscrasias, which can include infection, bleeding, and poor healing.
• Assess salivary flow as a factor in caries, periodontal disease, and candidiasis.
• Avoid prescribing aspirin-containing products.
• Place on frequent recall to evaluate healing response.
• Prophylactic antibiotics may be indicated to prevent infection if surgery or deep scaling is planned.
• Symptoms of oral infections may be masked.
• Determine dose and duration of steroid therapy for each patient to assess risk for stress tolerance and immunosuppression.
• Patients who have been or are currently on chronic steroid therapy longer than 2 wk may require supplemental steroids for stressful dental treatment.
• Determine why the patient is taking the drug.
Consultations:
• In a patient with symptoms of blood dyscrasias, request a medical consultation for blood studies and postpone dental treatment until normal values are reestablished.
• Medical consultation may be required to assess disease control.
• Consultation may be required to confirm steroid dose and duration of use.
Teach Patient/Family to:
• Encourage effective oral hygiene to prevent soft tissue inflammation.

- Use caution to prevent injury when using oral hygiene aids.
- When chronic dry mouth occurs, advise patient to:
  - Avoid mouth rinses with high alcohol content because of drying effects.
  - Use daily home fluoride products to prevent caries.
  - Use sugarless gum, frequent sips of water, or saliva substitutes.

prednisolone sodium phosphate
pred-**nis**′-oh-lone **soe**′-dee-um **foss**′-fate
(AK-Pred, Inflamase Forte, Inflamase Mild, Orapred, Pediapred)

CATEGORY AND SCHEDULE
Pregnancy Risk Category: C

Drug Class: Glucocorticoid, antiinflammatory

MECHANISM OF ACTION
An adrenal corticosteroid that inhibits accumulation of inflammatory cells at inflammation sites, phagocytosis, lysosomal enzyme release and synthesis, and release of mediators of inflammation.
Therapeutic Effect: Prevents or suppresses cell-mediated immune reactions. Decreases or prevents tissue response to inflammatory process.

USES
Primary or secondary adrenocortical insufficiency; adjunctive therapy of rheumatoid arthritis; collagen diseases; skin inflammatory disorders; allergy; respiratory diseases; hematologic disorders; neoplastic diseases; multiple sclerosis

PHARMACOKINETICS
Rapidly and well absorbed from the GI tract following oral administration. Protein binding: 90%–95%. Widely distributed. Metabolized in the liver. Excreted in the urine as sulfate and glucuronide conjugates. *Half-life:* 2–4 hr. Absorbed into aqueous humor, cornea, iris, choroid, ciliary body, and retina following ocular administration. Systemic absorption occurs but may be significant only at higher dosages or in extended pediatric therapy.

INDICATIONS AND DOSAGES
▶ **Asthma**
PO
Children. 1–2 mg/kg/day in single or divided doses for 3–10 days.
▶ **Endocrine Disorders, Hematologic and Neoplastic Disorders, Inflammatory Conditions**
PO
Adults, Elderly. 5–60 mg/day.
Children. 0.14–2 mg/kg/day divided into 3 or 4 doses.
▶ **Multiple Sclerosis Exacerbations**
PO
Adults, Elderly. 200 mg/day for 1 wk, followed by 80 mg every other day for 1 mo.
▶ **Nephrotic Syndrome**
PO
Children. 60 mg/m² daily. Maximum: 80 mg/day divided 3 times a day for 4 wk, then 40 mg/m² every other day for 4 wk.
▶ **Ophthalmic Disorders**
Ophthalmic Suspension
Adults, Elderly, Children. Instill 1 or 2 drops up to 6 times a day.

SIDE EFFECTS/ADVERSE REACTIONS

Frequent

Insomnia, heartburn, nervousness, abdominal distention, increased sweating, acne, mood swings, increased appetite, facial flushing, delayed wound healing, increased susceptibility to infection, diarrhea or constipation

Occasional

Headache, edema, change in skin color, frequent urination

Rare

Tachycardia, allergic reaction, such as rash and hives, psychic changes, hallucinations, depression

Ophthalmic: stinging or burning, posterior subcapsular cataracts

PRECAUTIONS AND CONTRAINDICATIONS

Systemic fungal infections, live or live attenuated vaccines, hypersensitivity to prednisolone sodium phosphate or any component of the formulation

DRUG INTERACTIONS OF CONCERN TO DENTISTRY

• Decreased action: barbiturates, rifampin, rifabutin
• Increased side effects: alcohol, salicylates, NSAIDs
• Increased action: ketoconazole, macrolide antibiotics (erythromycin, clarithromycin, azithromycin)
• Hepatotoxicity: acetaminophen (chronic use, high doses)

SERIOUS REACTIONS

! Prolonged use of corticosteroids may result in glaucoma with damage to the optic nerve, defects in visual acuity and fields of vision, posterior subcapsular cataract formation, and delayed wound healing.
! Long-term use may cause corneal and scleral thinning.

! Systemic effects are uncommon, but systemic hypercorticoidism has been reported.
! Acute anterior uveitis and perforation of the globe, keratitis, conjunctivitis, corneal ulcers, mydriasis, conjunctival hyperemia, loss of accommodation and ptosis have occasionally been reported.
! The development of secondary ocular infection has occurred. Fungal and viral infections of the cornea may develop with long-term applications of steroid.

DENTAL CONSIDERATIONS

General:

• Monitor vital signs at every appointment because of cardiovascular side effects.
• Patients on chronic drug therapy may rarely have symptoms of blood dyscrasias, which can include infection, bleeding, and poor healing.
• Assess salivary flow as a factor in caries, periodontal disease, and candidiasis.
• Avoid prescribing aspirin-containing products.
• Place on frequent recall to evaluate healing response.
• Prophylactic antibiotics may be indicated to prevent infection if surgery or deep scaling is planned.
• Symptoms of oral infections may be masked.
• Determine dose and duration of steroid therapy for each patient to assess risk for stress tolerance and immunosuppression.
• Patients who have been or are currently on chronic steroid therapy longer than 2 wk may require supplemental steroids for stressful dental treatment.
• Determine why the patient is taking the drug.

Consultations:
• In a patient with symptoms of blood dyscrasias, request a medical consultation for blood studies and postpone dental treatment until normal values are reestablished.
• Medical consultation may be required to assess disease control.
• Consultation may be required to confirm steroid dose and duration of use.

Teach Patient/Family to:
• Encourage effective oral hygiene to prevent soft tissue inflammation.
• Use caution to prevent injury when using oral hygiene aids.
• When chronic dry mouth occurs, advise patient to:
  • Avoid mouth rinses with high alcohol content because of drying effects.
  • Use daily home fluoride products to prevent caries.
  • Use sugarless gum, frequent sips of water, or saliva substitutes.

prednisone

pred′-ni-sone
(Apo-Prednisone[CAN], Deltasone, Panafcort[AUS], Prednisone Intensol, Sone[AUS], Sterapred, Sterapred DS, Winpred[CAN])
Do not confuse prednisone with prednisolone or primidone.

CATEGORY AND SCHEDULE
Pregnancy Risk Category: C (D if used in first trimester)

Drug Class: Glucocorticoid, intermediate acting

MECHANISM OF ACTION
An adrenocortical steroid that inhibits accumulation of inflammatory cells at inflammation sites, phagocytosis, lysosomal enzyme release and synthesis, and release of mediators of inflammation.
Therapeutic Effect: Prevents or suppresses cell-mediated immune reactions. Decreases or prevents tissue response to inflammatory process.

USES
Treatment of severe inflammation, immunosuppression, neoplasms, multiple sclerosis, collagen disorders, dermatologic disorders, acute exacerbation of multiple sclerosis

PHARMACOKINETICS
Well absorbed from the GI tract. Protein binding: 70%–90%. Widely distributed. Metabolized in the liver and converted to prednisolone. Primarily excreted in urine. Not removed by hemodialysis. *Half-life:* 3.4–3.8 hr.

INDICATIONS AND DOSAGES
▸ **Substitution Therapy in Deficiency States: Acute or Chronic Adrenal Insufficiency, Congenital Adrenal Hyperplasia, and Adrenal Insufficiency Secondary to Pituitary Insufficiency; Nonendocrine Disorders: Arthritis; Rheumatic Carditis; Allergic, Collagen, Intestinal Tract, Liver, Ocular, Renal, Skin Diseases; Bronchial Asthma; Cerebral Edema; Malignancies**
PO
Adults, Elderly. 5–60 mg/day in divided doses.
Children. 0.05–2 mg/kg/day in 1–4 divided doses.

SIDE EFFECTS/ADVERSE REACTIONS

Frequent
Insomnia, heartburn, nervousness, abdominal distention, increased sweating, acne, mood swings, increased appetite, facial flushing, delayed wound healing, increased susceptibility to infection, diarrhea or constipation

Occasional
Headache, edema, change in skin color, frequent urination

Rare
Tachycardia, allergic reaction (including rash and hives), psychological changes, hallucinations, depression

PRECAUTIONS AND CONTRAINDICATIONS

Acute superficial herpes simplex keratitis, systemic fungal infections, varicella

Caution:
Diabetes mellitus, glaucoma, osteoporosis, seizure disorders, ulcerative colitis, CHF, myasthenia gravis, renal disease, esophagitis, peptic ulcer, rifampin

DRUG INTERACTIONS OF CONCERN TO DENTISTRY

• Decreased action: barbiturates, rifampin, rifabutin
• Increased side effects: alcohol, salicylates, NSAIDs
• Increased action: ketoconazole, macrolide antibiotics
• Hepatotoxicity: acetaminophen (chronic, high doses)

SERIOUS REACTIONS

! Long-term therapy may cause muscle wasting in the arms and legs, osteoporosis, spontaneous fractures, amenorrhea, cataracts, glaucoma, peptic ulcer disease, and CHF.

! Abruptly withdrawing the drug following long-term therapy may cause anorexia, nausea, fever, headache, sudden or severe joint pain, rebound inflammation, fatigue, weakness, lethargy, dizziness, and orthostatic hypotension.
! Suddenly discontinuing prednisone may be fatal.

DENTAL CONSIDERATIONS

General:
• Monitor vital signs at every appointment because of cardiovascular side effects.
• Patients on chronic drug therapy may rarely have symptoms of blood dyscrasias, which can include infection, bleeding, and poor healing.
• Avoid aspirin-containing products.
• Assess salivary flow as a factor in caries, periodontal disease, and candidiasis.
• Symptoms of oral infections may be masked.
• Place on frequent recall to evaluate healing response.
• Prophylactic antibiotics may be indicated to prevent infection if surgery or deep scaling is planned.
• Determine dose and duration of steroid therapy for each patient to assess risk for stress tolerance and immunosuppression.
• Patients who have been or are currently on chronic steroid therapy longer than 2 wk may require supplemental steroids for stressful dental treatment.
• Determine why the patient is taking the drug.

Consultations:
• In a patient with symptoms of blood dyscrasias, request a medical consultation for blood studies and postpone dental treatment until normal values are reestablished.

• Medical consultation may be required to assess disease control.
• Consultation may be required to confirm steroid dose and duration of use.

Teach Patient/Family to:
• Encourage effective oral hygiene to prevent soft tissue inflammation.
• Use caution to prevent injury when using oral hygiene aids.
• When chronic dry mouth occurs, advise patient to:
  • Avoid mouth rinses with high alcohol content because of drying effects.
  • Use daily home fluoride products to prevent caries.
  • Use sugarless gum, frequent sips of water, or saliva substitutes.

pregabalin
pre-**gab**-a-lin
(Lyrica)
Do not confuse with Premarin.

CATEGORY AND SCHEDULE
Pregnancy Risk Category: C

Drug Class: Anticonvulsant, analgesic

MECHANISM OF ACTION
An anticonvulsant and antineuralgic agent whose exact mechanism is unknown but may be related to binding to and modulation of calcium channels with a resulting decrease in the calcium-dependent release of neurotransmitters.

USES
Partial-onset seizures, post-herpetic neuralgia, neuropathic pain associated with diabetic neuropathy

PHARMACOKINETICS
Well absorbed following oral administration (90%), can be taken with food. Peak plasma concentrations reached in 0.7–1.5 hr, widely distributed, not protein-bound. Does not undergo hepatic metabolism. *Half-life:* 4.6–6.8 hr. 98% excreted unchanged by the kidneys.

INDICATIONS AND DOSAGES
▸ **Partial-Onset Seizures**
PO
Adults. 150–600 mg per day, beginning at 150 mg/day (75 mg bid or 50 mg tid). May be increased to a maximum dose of 600 mg/day based on efficacy and tolerability.
▸ **Neuropathic Pain Associated with Diabetic Neuropathy**
PO
Adults. 50 mg tid initially; increased to 300 mg per day within 1 wk based on efficacy and tolerability.
▸ **Post-Herpetic Neuralgia**
PO
Adults. 75–100 mg bid or 50–100 mg tid, beginning at 75 mg bid or 50 mg tid. May be increased to 300 mg/day within 1 wk based on efficacy and tolerability.

SIDE EFFECTS/ADVERSE REACTIONS
Frequent
Dizziness, somnolence, peripheral edema, dry mouth, constipation, accidental injury, asthenia, weight gain, blurred vision, abnormal thought
Occasional
Amnesia, speech impairment, abnormal gait, twitching, confusion, myoclonus, constipation, diplopia, ecchymosis, arthralgia, leg cramps, myalgia, myasthenia

P

PRECAUTIONS AND CONTRAINDICATIONS

Hypersensitivity to pregabalin or any of its ingredients, weight gain, peripheral edema, creatine kinase elevations (associated with myopathy), thrombocytopenia, mild PR prolongation, may cause dizziness, somnolence and mental impairment. Can cause blurring or other changes in vision. Abrupt discontinuation can result in recurrence of seizures and insomnia, nausea, headache, and diarrhea. Safety in children not established.

DRUG INTERACTIONS OF CONCERN TO DENTISTRY

Increased risk of CNS depression: all CNS depressants, alcohol. May potentiate mental impairment and somnolence.

SERIOUS REACTIONS

! Increased risk of congestive circulatory failure in patients at-risk for peripheral edema

DENTAL CONSIDERATIONS

General:
• Assess salivary flow as a factor in caries, periodontal disease, and candidiasis.
• Early-morning appointments and stress-reduction protocol may be needed for anxious patients.
• Be prepared to manage seizures.
• After supine positioning, allow patient to sit upright for 2 min to avoid occurrence of dizziness.
Consultations:
• Consult with physician to determine seizure control and ability to tolerate dental procedures.
Teach Patient/Family to:
• Avoid mouth rinses with high alcohol content because of drying effect.

• Use home fluoride products for anticaries effect.
• Use sugarless/xylitol gum, frequent sips of water, or saliva substitutes if dry mouth occurs.

prilocaine hydrochloride (local)
pry′-lo-kane high-droh-klor′-ide
(Citanest)
With vasoconstrictor:
(Citanest Forte with epinephrine)

CATEGORY AND SCHEDULE
Pregnancy Risk Category: B

Drug Class: Amide local anesthetic

MECHANISM OF ACTION

Inhibits ion fluxes across membranes; decreases rise of depolarization phase of action potential; blocks nerve action potential.

USES

Local dental anesthesia

PHARMACOKINETICS

Injection: Onset 2–10 min, duration 2–4 hr; metabolized in liver; excreted in urine.

INDICATIONS AND DOSAGES
▶ Dental Injection: Infiltration or Conduction Block

Prilocaine 4% without vasoconstrictor: Maximum dose of 400 mg over a 2-hr period per dental appointment for healthy adult patient*; doses must be adjusted for medically compromised, debilitated, or elderly and for each individual patient. Doses in excess of 400 mg have caused methemoglobinemia.

Always use the lowest effective dose, a slow injection rate, and a careful aspiration technique. In considering the dose of local anesthesia with vasoconstrictor, the dose of epinephrine must also be considered. The recommended dose of epinephrine in a local anesthetic solution is 3 mcg/kg, not to exceed a total dose of 0.2 mg per appointment for a healthy adult. For adult patients with clinically significant cardiovascular disease, the dose limit of epinephrine is 0.04 mg per appointment. The dose limits of epinephrine will affect the amount of local anesthetic allowable in a given appointment.

▸ **Example Calculations Illustrating Amount of Drug Administered per Dental Cartridge(s):**

No. of Dental Cartridges (1.8 ml)	mg of Prilocaine (4%)
1	72
2	144
3	216
4	288

Prilocaine 4% with epinephrine 1:200,000: Recommended doses are the same; adjust doses for each individual as previously indicated. Also available in 1.7-ml cartridges.

*Maximum dose cited from Malamed SF: *Handbook of local anesthesia,* ed 6, 2011, Mosby, as well as manufacturer's package insert. Doses may differ in other published reference resources.

▸ **Example Calculations Illustrating Amount of Drug Administered per Dental Cartridge(s):**

No. of Dental Cartridges (1.8 ml)	mg of Prilocaine (4%)	mg (mcg) Vasoconstrictor (1:200,000)
1	72	0.009 (9)
2	144	0.018 (18)
4	288	0.036 (36)

Available forms include: 4% solution, 4% solution with epinephrine 1:200,000.

SIDE EFFECTS/ADVERSE REACTIONS
Occasional

Numbness, tingling, trismus, convulsions, loss of consciousness, drowsiness, disorientation, tremors, shivering, anxiety, restlessness, myocardial depression, cardiac arrest, dysrhythmias, bradycardia, hypotension, hypertension, nausea, vomiting, methemoglobinemia, rash, urticaria, allergic reactions
Rare

Status asthmaticus, respiratory arrest, anaphylaxis

PRECAUTIONS AND CONTRAINDICATIONS
Hypersensitivity, cross-sensitivity among amides (rare), severe liver disease
Caution:

Elderly, large doses of local anesthetic in myasthenia gravis, risk of methemoglobinemia

DRUG INTERACTIONS OF CONCERN TO DENTISTRY
• CNS depressants: increased risk of CNS depression with all CNS depressants, especially in children and when larger doses are used
• Avoid placing dental cartridges in disinfection solutions with heavy metals or surface-active agents; may see release of ions into local

P

anesthetic solutions with tissue irritation following injection
• Avoid excessive exposure of dental cartridges to light or heat; hastens deterioration of vasoconstrictor; observe for color change in local anesthetic solution
• Risk of cardiovascular side effects; rapid intravascular administration of local anesthetic containing vasoconstrictor, either alone or in patients taking tricyclic antidepressants, MAOIs, digitalis drugs, cocaine, phenothiazines, β-blockers, and in the presence of halogenated-hydrocarbon general anesthetics; use smallest effective vasoconstrictor dose and careful aspiration technique
• Avoid use of vasoconstrictors in patients with uncontrolled hyperthyroidism, diabetes, angina, or hypertension; refer these patients for medical treatment before elective dental treatment

SERIOUS REACTIONS
! Methemoglobinemia (at higher doses)

DENTAL CONSIDERATIONS
General:
• Monitor vital signs at every appointment because of cardiovascular side effects.
• Often used with vasoconstrictor for increased duration of action.
• Lubricate dry lips before injection or dental treatment as required.
Teach Patient/Family to:
• Use care to prevent injury while numbness exists and to refrain from chewing gum and eating following dental anesthesia.
• Report any signs of infection, muscle pain, or fever to dentist when feeling returns.

• Report any unusual soft tissue reactions (e.g., paresthesia).

primaquine
prim'-ah-kween
(Primacin[AUS])
Do not confuse with primidone.

CATEGORY AND SCHEDULE
Pregnancy Risk Category: C

Drug Class: Antiprotozoal

MECHANISM OF ACTION
An antimalarial and antirheumatic that eliminates tissue exoerythrocytic forms of *Plasmodium falciparum.* Disrupts mitochondria and binds to DNA.
Therapeutic Effect: Inhibits parasite growth.

USES
Treatment of malaria caused by *P. vivax;* unapproved: with clindamycin in the treatment of *P. carinii* in AIDS

PHARMACOKINETICS
Well absorbed. Metabolized in the liver to the active metabolite, carboxyprimaquine. Excreted in the urine in small amounts as unchanged drug. *Half-life:* 4–6 hr.

INDICATIONS AND DOSAGES
▸ Treatment of Malaria
PO
Adults, Elderly. 15-mg base daily for 14 days.
Children. 0.3-mg base/kg/wk once daily for 14 days.
▸ Malaria Prophylaxis
PO
Adults, Elderly. 30 mg base daily. Begin 1 day before departure and

continue for 7 days after leaving malarious area.

SIDE EFFECTS/ADVERSE REACTIONS
Frequent
Abdominal pain, nausea, vomiting
Rare
Leukopenia, hemolytic anemia, methemoglobinemia

PRECAUTIONS AND CONTRAINDICATIONS
Concomitant medications that cause bone marrow suppression, rheumatoid arthritis, lupus erythematosus, glucose-6-phosphate dehydrogenase deficiency, pregnancy, hypersensitivity to primaquine or any of its components

DRUG INTERACTIONS OF CONCERN TO DENTISTRY
• None reported

SERIOUS REACTIONS
! Leukopenia, hemolytic anemia, methemoglobinemia occur rarely.
! Overdosage include symptoms of abdominal cramps, vomiting, burning epigastric distress, central nervous system and cardiovascular disturbances, cyanosis, methemoglobinemia, moderate leukocytosis or leukopenia, and anemia.
! Acute hemolysis occurs, but patients recover completely if the dosage is discontinued.

DENTAL CONSIDERATIONS
General:
• Patients on chronic drug therapy may rarely have symptoms of blood dyscrasias, which can include infection, bleeding, and poor healing.

• Avoid dental light in patient's eyes; offer dark glasses for patient comfort.
Consultations:
• In a patient with symptoms of blood dyscrasias, request a medical consultation for blood studies and postpone dental treatment until normal values are reestablished.
Teach Patient/Family to:
• Encourage effective oral hygiene to prevent soft tissue inflammation.
• Use caution to prevent injury when using oral hygiene aids.

primidone
prih'-mih-done
(Apo-Primidone[CAN], Mysoline)
Do not confuse primidone with prednisone.

CATEGORY AND SCHEDULE
Pregnancy Risk Category: D
Controlled Substance: Schedule IV

Drug Class: Anticonvulsant, barbiturate derivative

P

MECHANISM OF ACTION
A barbiturate that decreases motor activity from electrical and chemical stimulation and stabilizes the seizure threshold against hyperexcitability.
Therapeutic Effect: Reduces seizure activity.

USES
Treatment of generalized tonic-clonic (grand mal), complex-partial psychomotor seizures

PHARMACOKINETICS
PO: Peak 4 hr. *Half-life:* 3–24 hr; excreted by kidneys, in breast milk.

INDICATIONS AND DOSAGES
▸ **Seizure Control**
PO
Adults, Elderly, Children 8 yr and older. 125–150 mg/day at bedtime. May increase by 125–250 mg/day every 3–7 days. Maximum: 2 g/day.
Children younger than 8 yr. Initially, 50–125 mg/day at bedtime. May increase by 50–125 mg/day every 3–7 days. Usual dose: 10–25 mg/kg/day in divided doses.
Neonates. 12–20 mg/kg/day in divided doses.

SIDE EFFECTS/ADVERSE REACTIONS
Frequent
Ataxia, dizziness
Occasional
Anorexia, drowsiness, mental changes, nausea, vomiting, paradoxical excitement
Rare
Rash

PRECAUTIONS AND CONTRAINDICATIONS
History of bronchopneumonia, porphyria
Caution:
COPD, hepatic disease, renal disease, abrupt withdrawal, lactation, hyperactive children

DRUG INTERACTIONS OF CONCERN TO DENTISTRY
• Increased CNS depression: alcohol, other CNS depressants
• Increased metabolism/hepatotoxicity: halothane, halogenated-hydrocarbon inhalation anesthetics
• Increased seizure threshold: haloperidol, phenothiazines
• Decreased effects of acetaminophen, corticosteroids, doxycycline, fenoprofen

• Lower blood concentrations: carbamazepine

SERIOUS REACTIONS
! Abrupt withdrawal after prolonged therapy may produce effects ranging from increased dreaming, nightmares, insomnia, tremor, diaphoresis, and vomiting to hallucinations, delirium, seizures, and status epilepticus.
! Skin eruptions may be a sign of a hypersensitivity reaction.
! Blood dyscrasias, hepatic disease, and hypocalcemia occur rarely.
! Overdose produces cold or clammy skin, hypothermia, and severe CNS depression, followed by high fever and coma.

DENTAL CONSIDERATIONS

General:
• Ask about type of epilepsy, seizure frequency, and quality of seizure control.
• After supine positioning, have patient sit upright for at least 2 min before standing to avoid orthostatic hypotension.
• Patients on chronic drug therapy may rarely have symptoms of blood dyscrasias, which can include infection, bleeding, and poor healing.
• Short appointments and a stress-reduction protocol may be required for anxious patients.
Consultations:
• Medical consultation may be required to assess disease control and patient's ability to tolerate stress.
• In a patient with symptoms of blood dyscrasias, request a medical consultation for blood studies and postpone dental treatment until normal values are reestablished.

Teach Patient/Family to:
• Encourage effective oral hygiene to prevent soft tissue inflammation.
• Use caution to prevent injury when using oral hygiene aids.
• Avoid mouth rinses with high alcohol content because of drying effects.

probenecid
proe-**ben**′-eh-sid
(Benuryl[CAN], Pro-Cid[AUS])
Do not confuse probenecid with procainamide.

CATEGORY AND SCHEDULE
Pregnancy Risk Category: C

Drug Class: Uricosuric

MECHANISM OF ACTION
A uricosuric that competitively inhibits reabsorption of uric acid at the proximal convoluted tubule. Also, inhibits renal tubular secretion of weak organic acids, such as penicillins.
Therapeutic Effect: Promotes uric acid excretion, reduces serum uric acid level, and increases plasma levels of penicillins and cephalosporins.

USES
Treatment of hyperuricemia in gout, gouty arthritis, adjunct to cephalosporin or penicillin treatment by reducing excretion and maintaining high blood levels

PHARMACOKINETICS
Hyperuricemia in gout, gouty arthritis, adjunct to cephalosporin or penicillin treatment by reducing excretion and maintaining high blood levels.

INDICATIONS AND DOSAGES
▸ **Gout**
PO
Adults, Elderly. Initially, 250 mg twice a day for 1 wk; then 500 mg twice a day. May increase by 500 mg q4wk. Maximum: 2–3 g/day. Maintenance: Dosage that maintains normal uric acid level.
▸ **As Adjunct to Penicillin or Cephalosporin Therapy to Prolong Antibiotic Plasma Levels**
PO
Adults, Elderly. 2 g/day in divided doses.
Children weighing more than 50 kg. Receive adult dosage.
Children 2–14 yr. Initially, 25 mg/kg. Maintenance: 40 mg/kg/day in 4 divided doses.
▸ **Gonorrhea**
PO
Adults, Elderly. 1 g 30 min before penicillin, ampicillin, or amoxicillin.

SIDE EFFECTS/ADVERSE REACTIONS
Frequent
Headache, anorexia, nausea, vomiting
Occasional
Lower back or side pain, rash, hives, itching, dizziness, flushed face, frequent urge to urinate, gingivitis

PRECAUTIONS AND CONTRAINDICATIONS
Blood dyscrasias, children younger than 2 yr, concurrent high-dose aspirin therapy, severe renal impairment, uric acid calculi
Caution:
Severe respiratory disease, lactation, cardiac edema

P

DRUG INTERACTIONS OF CONCERN TO DENTISTRY

- Increased toxicity: dapsone, indomethacin, other NSAIDs, acyclovir
- Increased sedation: benzodiazepines
- Decreased action: alcohol, salicylates
- Increased duration of action: penicillins, cephalosporins

SERIOUS REACTIONS

! Severe hypersensitivity reactions, including anaphylaxis, occur rarely and usually within a few hr after administration following previous use. If severe hypersensitivity reactions develop, discontinue the drug immediately and contact the physician.
! Pruritic maculopapular rash, possibly accompanied by malaise, fever, chills, arthralgia, nausea, vomiting, leukopenia, and aplastic anemias should be considered a toxic reaction.

DENTAL CONSIDERATIONS

General:
- Avoid prescribing aspirin-containing products.

Teach Patient/Family to:
- Encourage effective oral hygiene to prevent soft tissue inflammation.
- Use caution to prevent injury when using oral hygiene aids.
- Avoid mouth rinses with high alcohol content because of drying effects.

procaine
proe′-kane
(Novocain, Mericaine)

CATEGORY AND SCHEDULE
Pregnancy Risk Category: C

Drug Class: Anesthetics, local

MECHANISM OF ACTION
Procaine causes a reversible blockade of nerve conduction by decreasing nerve membrane permeability to sodium.
Therapeutic Effect: Local anesthesia.

USES
Treatment of pain by local infiltration, nerve block, spinal

PHARMACOKINETICS
Highly plasma protein-bound and distributed to all body tissues. Excreted in the urine (80%).
Half-life: 40 ± 9 sec in adults, 84 ± 30 sec in neonates.

INDICATIONS AND DOSAGES
▶ **Spinal Anesthesia**
Intrathecal
Adults. 0.5–1 ml of a 10% solution (50–100 mg) mixed with an equal volume of diluent injected into the third or fourth lumbar interspace (perineum and lower extremities). 2 ml of a 10% solution (200 mg) mixed with 1 ml of diluent injected into the second, third, or fourth interspace.
▶ **Infiltration Anesthesia, Dental Anesthesia, Control of Severe Pain (Postherpetic Neuralgia, Cancer Pain, or Burns)**
Topical
Adults. A single dose of 350–600 mg using a 0.25 or 0.5%

solution. Use 0.9% sodium chloride for dilution.

Children. 15 mg/kg of a 0.5% solution is the maximum recommended dose.

▸ **Peripheral or Sympathetic Nerve Block (Regional Anesthesia)**
Topical
Adults. Up to 200 ml of a 0.5% solution (1 g), 100 ml of a 1% solution (1 g), or 50 ml of a 2% solution (1 g). The 2% solution should only be used when a small volume of anesthetic is required.

SIDE EFFECTS/ADVERSE REACTIONS
Frequent
Numbness or tingling of the face or mouth, pain at the injection site, dizziness, drowsiness, light-headedness, nausea, vomiting, back pain, headache
Rare
Anxiety, restlessness, difficulty breathing, shortness of breath, seizures (convulsions), skin rash, itching (hives), slow, irregular heartbeat (palpitations), swelling of the face or mouth, tremors, QT prolongation, PR prolongation, atrial fibrillation, sinus bradycardia, hypotension, angina, cardiovascular collapse, fecal or urinary incontinence, loss of perineal sensation and sexual function, persistent motor, sensory, and/or autonomic (sphincter control) deficit

PRECAUTIONS AND CONTRAINDICATIONS
Hypersensitivity to ester local anesthetics, sulfites, PABA, patients on anticoagulant therapy, and in patients with coagulopathy, infection, thrombocytopenia. Should not be given by the intraarterial, intrathecal, or intravenous routes.

DRUG INTERACTIONS OF CONCERN TO DENTISTRY
• Possible prolonged effects of succinylcholine
• Increased CNS depression with all CNS depressants, especially in children and when larger doses are used
• Risk of cardiovascular side effects: rapid intravascular injection
• Suspected interference with antimicrobial activity of sulfonamides

SERIOUS REACTIONS
❗ Procaine-induced CNS toxicity usually presents with symptoms of stimulation, such as anxiety, apprehension, restlessness, nervousness, disorientation, confusion, dizziness, blurred vision, tremor, nausea/vomiting, shivering, or seizures. Subsequently, depressive symptoms can occur including drowsiness, unconsciousness, and respiratory arrest.
❗ If higher concentrations are introduced into the bloodstream, depression of cardiac excitability and contractility may cause AV block, ventricular arrhythmias, or cardiac arrest. CNS toxicity including dizziness, tongue numbness, visual impairment and disturbances, and muscular twitching appear to occur before cardiotoxic effects.
Alert
❗ Procaine should be used with caution in patients that have asthma because there is the increased risk of anaphylactoid reactions including bronchospasm and status asthmaticus.
Alert
❗ Local anesthetics can cause varying degrees of maternal, fetal, and neonatal toxicities during labor and obstetric delivery. Fetal heart

rate should be monitored, as well as the presence of symptoms indicating fetal bradycardia, fetal acidosis, and maternal hypotension. Epidural procaine may cause decreased uterine contractility or maternal expulsion efforts and alter the forces of parturition.

Alert

! Unintentional fetal intracranial injection of procaine occurring during pudendal or paracervical block has been shown to lead to neonatal depression at birth and can lead to seizures within 6 hr as a result of high serum concentrations.

DENTAL CONSIDERATIONS

General:
• Not available for use in dental local anesthetic cartridges.

procarbazine hydrochloride

pro-**car**′-bah-zeen
high-droh-**klor**′-ide
(Matulane, Natulan[CAN])
Do not confuse procarbazine with dacarbazine.

CATEGORY AND SCHEDULE

Pregnancy Risk Category: D

Drug Class: Antineoplastic, miscellaneous

MECHANISM OF ACTION

A methylhydrazine derivative that inhibits DNA, RNA, and protein synthesis. May also directly damage DNA. Cell cycle-phase specific for S phase of cell division.
Therapeutic Effect: Causes cell death.

USES

Treatment of lymphoma, Hodgkin's disease, cancers resistant to other therapy

PHARMACOKINETICS

PO: Peak levels 1 hr; concentrates in liver, kidney, skin; metabolized in liver, excreted in urine.

INDICATIONS AND DOSAGES
▶ Advanced Hodgkin's Disease
PO
Adults, Elderly. Initially, 2–4 mg/kg/day as a single dose or in divided doses for 1 wk, then 4–6 mg/kg/day. Maintenance: 1–2 mg/kg/day.
Children. 50–100 mg/m^2/day for 10–14 days of a 28-day cycle. Continue until maximum response occurs, leukocyte count falls below 4000/mm^3, or platelet count falls below 100,000/mm^3. Maintenance: 50 mg/m^2/day.

SIDE EFFECTS/ADVERSE REACTIONS

Frequent

Severe nausea, vomiting, respiratory disorders (cough, effusion), myalgia, arthralgia, drowsiness, nervousness, insomnia, nightmares, diaphoresis, hallucinations, seizures

Occasional

Hoarseness, tachycardia, nystagmus, retinal hemorrhage, photophobia, photosensitivity, urinary frequency, nocturia, hypotension, diarrhea, stomatitis, paraesthesia, unsteadiness, confusion, decreased reflexes, footdrop

Rare

Hypersensitivity reaction (dermatitis, pruritus, rash, urticaria), hyperpigmentation, alopecia

PRECAUTIONS AND CONTRAINDICATIONS

Myelosuppression, hypersensitivity, thrombocytopenia, bone marrow depression

Caution:
Renal disease, hepatic disease, radiation therapy

DRUG INTERACTIONS OF CONCERN TO DENTISTRY

• Increased CNS depression: barbiturates, antihistamines, narcotics
• Disulfiram-like reaction: ethyl alcohol
• Hypertension: indirect-acting sympathomimetics
• Increased anticholinergic effect: anticholinergic drugs, antihistamines
• Increased risk of severe toxic reactions: tricyclic antidepressants, meperidine and other opioids, tyramine-containing foods and other MAOIs; may include cyclobenzaprine and carbamazepine

SERIOUS REACTIONS

! Major toxic effects are myelosuppression manifested as hematologic toxicity (mainly leukopenia, thrombocytopenia, and anemia) and hepatotoxicity manifested as jaundice and ascites.
! UTIs may occur secondary to leukopenia.

DENTAL CONSIDERATIONS

General:
• Patients on chronic drug therapy may rarely have symptoms of blood dyscrasias, which can include infection, bleeding, and poor healing.
• Monitor vital signs at every appointment because of cardiovascular side effects.

• Consider semisupine chair position for patient comfort if GI side effects occur.
• Assess salivary flow as a factor in caries, periodontal disease, and candidiasis.
• After supine positioning, have patient sit upright for at least 2 min before standing to avoid orthostatic hypotension.
• Avoid dental light in patient's eyes; offer dark glasses for patient comfort.
• Avoid aspirin-containing products because of bleeding risk.
• Avoid use of gingival retraction cord with epinephrine.
• Patients receiving chemotherapy may require palliative treatment for stomatitis.

Consultations:
• In a patient with symptoms of blood dyscrasias, request a medical consultation for blood studies and postpone dental treatment until normal values are reestablished.
• Take precautions if dental surgery is anticipated and sedation or general anesthesia is required (risk of hypotension).

Teach Patient/Family to:
• Encourage effective oral hygiene to prevent soft tissue inflammation.
• Use caution to prevent injury when using oral hygiene aids.
• Report oral lesions, soreness, or bleeding to dentist.
• When chronic dry mouth occurs, advise patient to:
  • Avoid mouth rinses with high alcohol content because of drying effects.
  • Use daily home fluoride products to prevent caries.
  • Use sugarless gum, frequent sips of water, or saliva substitutes.

P

prochlorperazine
proe-klor-**per**′-ah-zeen
(Compazine, Stemetil[CAN], Stemzine[AUS])
Do not confuse prochlorperazine with chlorpromazine, or Compazine with Copaxone.

CATEGORY AND SCHEDULE
Pregnancy Risk Category: C

Drug Class: Antipsychotic

MECHANISM OF ACTION
A phenothiazine that acts centrally to inhibit or block dopamine receptors in the chemoreceptor trigger zone and peripherally to block the vagus nerve in the GI tract.
Therapeutic Effect: Relieves nausea and vomiting and improves psychotic conditions.

PHARMACOKINETICS

Route	Onset*	Peak	Duration
Tablets, oral solution	30–40 min	N/A	3–4 hr
Capsules (extended release)	30–40 min	N/A	10–12 hr
Rectal	60 min	N/A	3–4 hr

*As an antiemetic.

Variably absorbed after PO administration. Widely distributed. Metabolized in the liver and GI mucosa. Primarily excreted in urine. Unknown if removed by hemodialysis. **Half-life:** 23 hr.

INDICATIONS AND DOSAGES
▸ **Nausea and Vomiting**
PO
Adults, Elderly. 5–10 mg 3–4 times a day.

Children. 0.4 mg/kg/day in 3–4 divided doses.
PO (Extended-Release)
Adults, Elderly. 10 mg twice a day or 15 mg once a day.
IV
Adults, Elderly. 2.5–10 mg. May repeat q3–4h.
Children. 0.1–0.15 mg/kg/dose q8–12h. Maximum: 40 mg/day.
IM
Adults, Elderly. 5–10 mg q3–4h.
Children. 0.1–0.15 mg/kg/dose q8–12h. Maximum: 40 mg/day.
Rectal
Adults, Elderly. 25 mg twice a day.
Children. 0.4 mg/kg/day in 3–4 divided doses.
▸ **Psychosis**
PO
Adults, Elderly. 5–10 mg 3–4 times a day. Maximum: 150 mg/day.
Children. 2.5 mg 2–3 times a day. Maximum: 25 mg for children 6–12 yr; 20 mg for children 2–5 yr.
IM
Adults, Elderly. 10–20 mg q4h.
Children. 0.13 mg/kg/dose.

SIDE EFFECTS/ADVERSE REACTIONS
Frequent
Somnolence, hypotension, dizziness, fainting (commonly occurring after first dose, occasionally after subsequent doses, and rarely with oral form)
Occasional
Dry mouth, blurred vision, lethargy, constipation, diarrhea, myalgia, nasal congestion, peripheral edema, urine retention

PRECAUTIONS AND CONTRAINDICATIONS
Angle-closure glaucoma, CNS depression, coma, myelosuppression, severe cardiac or hepatic

P

impairment, severe hypotension or hypertension

Caution:
Children younger than 2 yr, elderly

DRUG INTERACTIONS OF CONCERN TO DENTISTRY

• Increased sedation: other CNS depressants, alcohol, barbiturate anesthetics, opioid analgesics
• Hypotension, tachycardia: epinephrine
• Increased extrapyramidal effects: phenothiazines and related drugs (haloperidol, droperidol), metoclopramide
• Additive photosensitization: tetracyclines
• Increased anticholinergic effects: anticholinergics

SERIOUS REACTIONS

! Extrapyramidal symptoms appear to be dose-related and are divided into three categories: akathisia (marked by inability to sit still, tapping of feet), parkinsonian symptoms (including mask-like face, tremors, shuffling gait, hypersalivation), and acute dystonias (such as torticollis, opisthotonos, and oculogyric crisis). A dystonic reaction may also produce diaphoresis or pallor.
! Tardive dyskinesia, manifested as tongue protrusion, puffing of the cheeks, and puckering of the mouth, is a rare reaction that may be irreversible.
! Abrupt withdrawal after long-term therapy may precipitate nausea, vomiting, gastritis, dizziness, and tremors.
! Blood dyscrasias, particularly agranulocytosis and mild leukopenia, may occur.
! Prochlorperazine use may lower the seizure threshold.

DENTAL CONSIDERATIONS

General:
• Monitor vital signs at every appointment because of cardiovascular side effects.
• Patients on chronic drug therapy may rarely have symptoms of blood dyscrasias, which can include infection, bleeding, and poor healing.
• After supine positioning, have patient sit upright for at least 2 min before standing to avoid orthostatic hypotension.
• Assess salivary flow as a factor in caries, periodontal disease, and candidiasis.
• Avoid dental light in patient's eyes; offer dark glasses for patient comfort.
• Assess for presence of extrapyramidal motor symptoms, such as tardive dyskinesia and akathisia. Extrapyramidal motor activity may complicate dental treatment.
• Geriatric patients are more susceptible to drug effects; use lower dose.
• Use vasoconstrictors with caution, in low doses, and with careful aspiration.

Consultations:
• In a patient with symptoms of blood dyscrasias, request a medical consultation for blood studies and postpone dental treatment until normal values are reestablished.
• Take precautions if dental surgery is anticipated and anesthesia is required.
• If signs of tardive dyskinesia or akathisia are present, refer to physician.

Teach Patient/Family to:
• Encourage effective oral hygiene to prevent soft tissue inflammation.

P

• Use caution to prevent injury when using oral hygiene aids.
• Use powered tooth brush if patient has difficulty holding conventional devices.
• When chronic dry mouth occurs, advise patient to:
  • Avoid mouth rinses with high alcohol content because of drying effects.
  • Use daily home fluoride products to prevent caries.
  • Use sugarless gum, frequent sips of water, or saliva substitutes.

procyclidine
proe-**sye**′-kli-deen
(Kemadrin)

CATEGORY AND SCHEDULE
Pregnancy Risk Category: C

Drug Class: Anticholinergic, antidyskinetic

MECHANISM OF ACTION
An anticholinergic agent that exerts an atropine-like action and produces an antispasmodic effect on smooth muscle, is a potent mydriatic, and inhibits salivation.
Therapeutic Effect: Relieves symptoms of Parkinson's disease and drug-induced extrapyramidal symptoms.

USES
Treatment of Parkinson symptoms, extrapyramidal symptoms associated with neuroleptic drugs

PHARMACOKINETICS
Well absorbed from the GI tract. Protein binding: extensive. Metabolized in liver, undergoes extensive first-pass effect. Primarily excreted in urine. Unknown if removed by hemodialysis. **Half-life:** 7.7–16.1 hr.

INDICATIONS AND DOSAGES
▶ **Drug-Induced Extrapyramidal Reactions**
PO
Adults, Elderly. Initially, 2.5 mg 3 times a day. May increase by 2.5 mg/day as needed. Maintenance: 10–20 mg/day in divided doses 3 times a day.
▶ **Parkinson's Disease**
PO
Adults, Elderly. Initially, 2.5 mg 3 times a day after meals.
Maintenance: 2.5–5 mg mg/day in divided doses 3 times a day after meals.
▶ **Hepatic Function Impairment**
PO
Adults, Elderly. 2.5–5 mg mg/day in divided doses twice a day after meals.

SIDE EFFECTS/ADVERSE REACTIONS
Frequent
Blurred vision, mydriasis, disorientation, light-headedness, nausea, vomiting, dry mouth, nose, throat, and lips

PRECAUTIONS AND CONTRAINDICATIONS
Angle-closure glaucoma
Elderly, lactation, tachycardia, prostatic hypertrophy, children, kidney or liver disease, drug abuse, hypotension, hypertension, psychiatric patients

DRUG INTERACTIONS OF CONCERN TO DENTISTRY
• Increased anticholinergic effect: antihistamines, anticholinergics, meperidine

• Increased CNS depression: alcohol, CNS depressants

SERIOUS REACTIONS

! Overdosage may vary from severe anticholinergic effects, such as unsteadiness, severe drowsiness, severe dryness of mouth, nose, or throat, tachycardia, shortness of breath, and skin flushing.

! Also produces severe paradoxical reaction, marked by hallucinations, tremor, seizures, and toxic psychosis.

DENTAL CONSIDERATIONS

General:

• Monitor vital signs at every appointment because of cardiovascular side effects.

• Assess salivary flow as a factor in caries, periodontal disease, and candidiasis.

• After supine positioning, have patient sit upright for at least 2 min before standing to avoid orthostatic hypotension.

• Avoid dental light in patient's eyes; offer dark glasses for patient comfort.

• Do not ingest sodium bicarbonate products, such as the Prophy-Jet air polishing system, until 1 hr after drug use.

• Place on frequent recall because of oral side effects.

Consultations:

• Medical consultation may be required to assess disease control.

• Medical consultation may be required to assess patient's ability to tolerate stress.

Teach Patient/Family to:

• Use powered tooth brush if patient has difficulty holding conventional devices.

• Encourage effective oral hygiene to prevent soft tissue inflammation.

• Use caution to prevent injury when using oral hygiene aids.

• When chronic dry mouth occurs, advise patient to:

• Avoid mouth rinses with high alcohol content because of drying effects.

• Use daily home fluoride products for anticaries effect.

• Use sugarless gum, frequent sips of water, or saliva substitutes.

progesterone
proe-**jess'**-ter-one
(Crinone, Prochieve, Prometrium)

CATEGORY AND SCHEDULE
Pregnancy Risk Category: D

Drug Class: Contraceptives, hormones/hormone modifiers, progestins

MECHANISM OF ACTION
A natural steroid hormone that promotes mammary gland development and relaxes uterine smooth muscle.
Therapeutic Effect: Decreases abnormal uterine bleeding; transforms endometrium from proliferative to secretory in an estrogen-primed endometrium.

USES
Prevention of endometrial hyperplasia, secondary amenorrhea, abnormal uterine bleeding, treatment of infertility

PHARMACOKINETICS
IM, Rectal, Vaginal: Duration 24 hr, excreted in urine, feces; metabolized in liver.

P

INDICATIONS AND DOSAGES
▶ **Amenorrhea**
PO
Adults. 400 mg daily in evening for 10 days.
IM
Adults. 5–10 mg for 6–8 days. Withdrawal bleeding expected in 48–72 hr if ovarian activity produced proliferative endometrium.
Vaginal
Adults. Apply 45 mg (4% gel) every other day for 6 or fewer doses.
▶ **Abnormal Uterine Bleeding**
IM
Adults. 5–10 mg for 6 days. When estrogen given concomitantly, begin progesterone after 2 wk of estrogen therapy; discontinue when menstrual flow begins.
▶ **Prevention of Endometrial Hyperplasia**
PO
Adults. 200 mg in evening for 12 days per 28-day cycle in combination with daily conjugated estrogen.
▶ **Infertility**
Vaginal
Adults. 90 mg (8% gel) once a day (twice a day in women with partial or complete ovarian failure).

SIDE EFFECTS/ADVERSE REACTIONS
Frequent
Breakthrough bleeding or spotting at beginning of therapy, amenorrhea, change in menstrual flow, breast tenderness
Gel: drowsiness
Occasional
Edema, weight gain or loss, rash, pruritus, photosensitivity, skin pigmentation
Rare
Pain or swelling at injection site, acne, depression, alopecia, hirsutism

PRECAUTIONS AND CONTRAINDICATIONS
Breast cancer; history of active cerebral apoplexy; thromboembolic disorders or thrombophlebitis; missed abortion; severe hepatic dysfunction; undiagnosed vaginal bleeding; use as a pregnancy test

DRUG INTERACTIONS OF CONCERN TO DENTISTRY
• None reported

SERIOUS REACTIONS
! Thrombophlebitis, cerebrovascular disorders, retinal thrombosis, and pulmonary embolism occur rarely.

DENTAL CONSIDERATIONS

General:
• Determine why patient is taking the drug.
• Advise patient if dental drugs prescribed have a potential for photosensitivity.
• Monitor vital signs.
• Some patients may experience drowsiness; inquire before using CNS depressants.
Teach Patient/Family to:
• Not drive or perform other tasks requiring mental alertness.
• Encourage effective oral hygiene to prevent soft tissue inflammation.
• Prevent trauma when using oral hygiene aids.
• Update health and medication history if physician makes any changes in evaluation or drug regimen; include OTC, herbal, and nonherbal drugs in the update.

promethazine hydrochloride

proe-**meth**'-ah-zeen
high-droh-**klor**'-ide
(Insomn-Eze[AUS], Phenadoz,
Phenergan)
Do not confuse promethazine
with promazine.

CATEGORY AND SCHEDULE
Pregnancy Risk Category: C

Drug Class: Antihistamine,
H₁-receptor antagonist

MECHANISM OF ACTION
A phenothiazine that acts as an
antihistamine, antiemetic, and
sedative-hypnotic. As an
antihistamine, inhibits histamine at
histamine receptor sites. As an
antiemetic, diminishes vestibular
stimulation, depresses labyrinthine
function, and acts on the
chemoreceptor trigger zone. As a
sedative-hypnotic, produces CNS
depression by decreasing stimulation
of the brainstem reticular formation.
Therapeutic Effect: Prevents
allergic responses mediated by
histamine, such as rhinitis, urticaria,
and pruritus. Prevents and relieves
nausea and vomiting.

USES
Motion sickness, rhinitis, allergy
symptoms, sedation, nausea,
preoperative or postoperative
sedation

PHARMACOKINETICS

Route	Onset	Peak	Duration
PO	20 min	N/A	2–8 hr
IV	3–5 min	N/A	2–8 hr
IM	20 min	N/A	2–8 hr
Rectal	20 min	N/A	2–8 hr

Well absorbed from the GI tract
after IM administration. Widely
distributed. Metabolized in the liver.
Primarily excreted in urine. Not
removed by hemodialysis. *Half-life:*
16–19 hr.

INDICATIONS AND DOSAGES
▶ **Allergic Symptoms**
PO
Adults, Elderly. 6.25–12.5 mg 3
times a day plus 25 mg at bedtime.
Children. 0.1 mg/kg/dose
(maximum: 12.5 mg) 3 times a day
plus 0.5 mg/kg/dose (maximum:
25 mg) at bedtime.
IV, IM
Adults, Elderly. 25 mg. May repeat
in 2 hr.
▶ **Motion Sickness**
PO
Adults, Elderly. 25 mg 30–60 min
before departure; may repeat in
8–12 hr, then every morning on
rising and before evening meal.
Children. 0.5 mg/kg 30–60 min
before departure; may repeat in
8–12 hr, then every morning on
rising and before evening meal.
▶ **Prevention of Nausea and
Vomiting**
PO, IV, IM, Rectal
Adults, Elderly. 12.5–25 mg q4–6h
as needed.
Children. 0.25–1 mg/kg q4–6h as
needed.
▶ **Preoperative and Postoperative
Sedation; Adjunct to Analgesics**
IV, IM
Adults, Elderly. 25–50 mg.
Children. 12.5–25 mg.
▶ **Sedative**
PO, IV, IM, Rectal
Adults, Elderly. 25–50 mg/dose.
May repeat q4–6h as needed.
Children. 0.5–1 mg/kg/dose q6h as
needed. Maximum: 50 mg/dose.

P

SIDE EFFECTS/ADVERSE REACTIONS

Expected

Somnolence, disorientation; in elderly, hypotension, confusion, syncope

Frequent

Dry mouth, nose, or throat; urine retention; thickening of bronchial secretions

Occasional

Epigastric distress, flushing, visual disturbances, hearing disturbances, wheezing, paresthesia, diaphoresis, chills

Rare

Dizziness, urticaria, photosensitivity, nightmares

PRECAUTIONS AND CONTRAINDICATIONS

Angle-closure glaucoma, GI or GU obstruction, severe CNS depression or coma

Caution:

Increased intraocular pressure, renal disease, cardiac disease, hypertension, bronchial asthma, seizure disorder, stenosed peptic ulcers, hyperthyroidism, prostatic hypertrophy, bladder neck obstruction

DRUG INTERACTIONS OF CONCERN TO DENTISTRY

• Increased CNS depression: alcohol, all CNS depressants
• Hypotension: general anesthetics
• Increased effect of anticholinergic drugs

SERIOUS REACTIONS

❗ Children may experience paradoxical reactions, such as excitation, nervousness, tremor, hyperactive reflexes, and seizures.
❗ Infants and young children have experienced CNS depression manifested as respiratory depression, sleep apnea, and sudden infant death syndrome.
❗ Long-term therapy may produce extrapyramidal symptoms, such as dystonia (abnormal movements), pronounced motor restlessness (most frequently in children), and parkinsonian symptoms (most frequently in elderly patients).
❗ Blood dyscrasias, particularly agranulocytosis, occur rarely.

DENTAL CONSIDERATIONS

General:

• Determine why the patient is taking the drug.
• Patients on chronic drug therapy may rarely have symptoms of blood dyscrasias, which can include infection, bleeding, and poor healing.
• Monitor vital signs at every appointment because of cardiovascular side effects.
• Assess salivary flow as a factor in caries, periodontal disease, and candidiasis.
• Assess vital signs q30min after use as sedative.

Teach Patient/Family to:

• When chronic dry mouth occurs, advise patient to:
  • Avoid mouth rinses with high alcohol content because of drying effects.
  • Use daily home fluoride products to prevent caries.
  • Use sugarless gum, frequent sips of water, or saliva substitutes.

propafenone hydrochloride

proe-**pah**′-eh-none
high-droh-**klor**′-ide
(Rythmol, Rythmol SR)

CATEGORY AND SCHEDULE

Pregnancy Risk Category: C

Drug Class: Antidysrhythmic
(class Ic)

MECHANISM OF ACTION

An antidysrhythmic that decreases
the fast sodium current in Purkinje
or myocardial cells. Decreases
excitability and automaticity;
prolongs conduction velocity and
the refractory period.
Therapeutic Effect: Suppresses
dysrhythmias.

USES

Treatment of documented life-
threatening dysrhythmias;
unapproved: sustained ventricular
tachycardia

PHARMACOKINETICS

Peak 3–5 hr. *Half-life:* 2–10 hr;
metabolized in liver; excreted in
urine (metabolite).

INDICATIONS AND DOSAGES

▸ **Documented, Life-Threatening
Ventricular Arrhythmias, such as
Sustained Ventricular Tachycardia**
PO (Prompt-Release)
Adults, Elderly. Initially, 150 mg
q8h; may increase at 3- to 4-day
intervals to 225 mg q8h, then to
300 mg q8h. Maximum: 900 mg/
day.
PO (Extended-Release)
Adults, Elderly. Initially, 225 mg
q12h. May increase at 5-day
intervals. Maximum: 425 mg q12h.

SIDE EFFECTS/ADVERSE REACTIONS

Frequent
Dizziness, nausea, vomiting, altered
taste, constipation
Occasional
Headache, dyspnea, blurred vision,
dyspepsia (heartburn, indigestion,
epigastric pain)
Rare
Rash, weakness, dry mouth,
diarrhea, edema, hot flashes

PRECAUTIONS AND CONTRAINDICATIONS

Bradycardia; bronchospastic
disorders; cardiogenic shock;
electrolyte imbalance; sinoatrial, AV,
and intraventricular impulse
generation or conduction disorders,
such as sick sinus syndrome or AV
block, without the presence of a
pacemaker; uncontrolled CHF
Caution:
CHF, hypokalemia, hyperkalemia,
recent MI, nonallergic
bronchospasm, lactation, children,
hepatic or renal disease

DRUG INTERACTIONS OF CONCERN TO DENTISTRY

• No specific interactions are
reported; however, any drug that
could affect the cardiac action of
propafenone (other local anesthetics,
vasoconstrictors, anticholinergics)
should be used in the lowest
effective dose.

SERIOUS REACTIONS

! Propafenone may produce or
worsen existing arrhythmias.
! Overdose may produce
hypotension, somnolence,
bradycardia, and atrioventricular
conduction disturbances.

P

DENTAL CONSIDERATIONS

General:
• Monitor vital signs at every appointment because of cardiovascular side effects.
• Avoid or limit dose of vasoconstrictor.
• Patients on chronic drug therapy may rarely have symptoms of blood dyscrasias, which can include infection, bleeding, and poor healing.
• Assess salivary flow as a factor in caries, periodontal disease, and candidiasis.
• Stress from dental procedures may compromise cardiovascular function; determine patient risk and consider a stress-reduction protocol.
• Consider semisupine chair position for patients with respiratory distress.

Consultations:
• In a patient with symptoms of blood dyscrasias, request a medical consultation for blood studies and postpone dental treatment until normal values are reestablished.
• Medical consultation may be required to assess disease control and patient's ability to tolerate stress.

Teach Patient/Family to:
• Encourage effective oral hygiene to prevent soft tissue inflammation.
• Use caution to prevent injury when using oral hygiene aids.
• When chronic dry mouth occurs, advise patient to:
  • Avoid mouth rinses with high alcohol content because of drying effects.
  • Use daily home fluoride products to prevent caries.
  • Use sugarless gum, frequent sips of water, or saliva substitutes.

propantheline
proe-**pan**′-the-leen
(Pro-Banthine, Propanthl[CAN])

CATEGORY AND SCHEDULE
Pregnancy Risk Category: C

Drug Class: Anticholinergic

MECHANISM OF ACTION
A quaternary ammonium compound which has anticholinergic properties and that inhibits action of acetylcholine at postganglionic parasympathetic sites.
Therapeutic Effect: Reduces gastric secretions and urinary frequency, urgency and urge incontinence.

USES
Treatment of peptic ulcer disease, irritable bowel syndrome, duodenography, urinary incontinence; unapproved: reduction in salivary flow

PHARMACOKINETICS
Onset occurs within 90 min. but less than 50% is absorbed from GI tract. Extensive hepatic metabolism. Excreted in the urine and feces.
Half-life: 2.9 hr.

INDICATIONS AND DOSAGES
▸ **Peptic Ulcer**
PO
Adults, Elderly. 15 mg 3 times a day 30 min. before meals and 30 mg at bedtime.
Children. 1–2 mg/kg/day, divided q4–6h and at bedtime.

SIDE EFFECTS/ADVERSE REACTIONS
Frequent
Dry mouth, decreased sweating, constipation, hyperthermia

Occasional
Blurred vision, intolerance to light,
urinary hesitancy, drowsiness,
agitation, excitement
Rare
Confusion, increased intraocular
pressure, orthostatic hypotension,
tachycardia

PRECAUTIONS AND CONTRAINDICATIONS

GI or GU obstruction, myasthenia
gravis, narrow-angle glaucoma, toxic
megacolon, severe ulcerative colitis,
unstable cardiovascular adjustment
in acute hemorrhage,
hypersensitivity to propantheline or
other anticholinergics
Caution:
Hyperthyroidism, CAD,
dysrhythmias, CHF, ulcerative
colitis, hypertension, hiatal hernia,
hepatic disease, renal disease,
pregnancy category C, urinary
retention, prostatic hypertrophy

DRUG INTERACTIONS OF CONCERN TO DENTISTRY

• Increased anticholinergic effect:
other anticholinergic drugs
• Constipation, urinary retention:
opioid analgesics
• Decreased absorption of
ketoconazole; take doses 2 hr apart

SERIOUS REACTIONS

! Overdosage may produce
temporary paralysis of ciliary
muscle, pupillary dilation,
tachycardia, palpitations, hot, dry, or
flushed skin, absence of bowel
sounds, hyperthermia, increased
respiratory rate, ECG abnormalities,
nausea, vomiting, rash over face or
upper trunk, CNS stimulation, and
psychosis, marked by agitation,
restlessness, rambling speech, visual
hallucinations, paranoid behavior,
and delusions, followed by
depression.

DENTAL CONSIDERATIONS

General:
• Assess salivary flow as a factor in
caries, periodontal disease, and
candidiasis.
• Avoid dental light in patient's eyes;
offer dark glasses for patient
comfort.
• Place on frequent recall because of
oral side effects.
• Avoid prescribing aspirin-
containing products.
• Consider semisupine chair position
for patient comfort because of GI
effects of disease.
• Caution against exercise or
exposure to heat or bright light
while taking.
Consultations:
• Physician should be informed if
significant xerostomic side effects
occur (e.g., increased caries, sore
tongue, problems eating or
swallowing, difficulty wearing
prosthesis) so that a medication
change can be considered.
Teach Patient/Family to:
• When chronic dry mouth occurs,
advise patient to:
  • Avoid mouth rinses with high
  alcohol content because of
  drying effects.
  • Use daily home fluoride
  products to prevent caries.
  • Use sugarless gum, frequent
  sips of water, or saliva
  substitutes.

P

propofol
pro-poe-**fall'**
(Diprivan, Recofol[AUS])

CATEGORY AND SCHEDULE
Pregnancy Risk Category: B

Drug Class: General anesthetic

MECHANISM OF ACTION
A rapidly acting general anesthetic that inhibits sympathetic vasoconstrictor nerve activity and decreases vascular resistance. *Therapeutic Effect:* Produces hypnosis rapidly.

USES
Induction or maintenance of anesthesia as part of balanced anesthetic technique, in-patient sedation

PHARMACOKINETICS

Route	Onset	Peak	Duration
IV	40 sec	N/A	3–10 min

Rapidly and extensively distributed. Protein binding: 97%–99%. Metabolized in the liver. Primarily excreted in urine. Unknown if removed by hemodialysis. *Half-life:* 3–12 hr.

INDICATIONS AND DOSAGES
▸ **Intensive Care Unit Sedation**
IV
Adults, Elderly. Initially, 0.3 mg/kg/hr. May increase by 0.3–0.6 mg/kg/hr q5–10 min until desired effect is obtained. Maintenance: 0.3–3 mg/kg/h.
▸ **Anesthesia**
IV
Adults, American Society of Anesthesiologists (ASA) I and II patients. 2–2.5 mg/kg (about 40 mg q10sec until onset of anesthesia). Maintenance: 0.1–0.2 mg/kg/min. *Elderly, Debilitated, Hypovolemic, ASA III or IV patients.* 1–1.5 mg/kg (about 20 mg q10sec until onset of anesthesia). Maintenance: 0.05–0.1 mg/kg/min. *Children 3 yr and older, ASA I or II patients.* 2.5–3.5 mg/kg (lower dosage for ASA III or IV patients). *Children 2 mo–16 yr.* Maintenance dose: 0.125–0.15 mg/kg/min.

SIDE EFFECTS/ADVERSE REACTIONS
Frequent
Involuntary muscle movements, apnea (common during induction; lasts longer than 60 sec), hypotension, nausea, vomiting, IV site burning or stinging
Occasional
Twitching, bucking, jerking, thrashing, headache, dizziness, bradycardia, hypertension, fever, abdominal cramps, paresthesia, coldness, cough, hiccups, facial flushing, greenish-colored urine
Rare
Rash, dry mouth, agitation, confusion, myalgia, thrombophlebitis

PRECAUTIONS AND CONTRAINDICATIONS
Impaired cerebral circulation, increased intracranial pressure
Caution:
Elderly, debilitated, respiratory depression, severe respiratory disorders, cardiac dysrhythmias, pregnancy category B, labor and delivery, lactation, children younger than 3 yr, epilepsy

DRUG INTERACTIONS OF CONCERN TO DENTISTRY
• Increased CNS depression: alcohol, narcotics,

sedative-hypnotics, antipsychotics, skeletal muscle relaxants, inhalational anesthetics

SERIOUS REACTIONS

❗ A continuous infusion or repeated intermittent infusions of propofol may result in extreme somnolence, respiratory depression, and circulatory depression.

❗ Too-rapid IV administration may produce severe hypotension, respiratory depression, and involuntary muscle movements.

❗ The patient may experience an acute allergic reaction, characterized by abdominal pain, anxiety, restlessness, dyspnea, erythema, hypotension, pruritus, rhinitis, and urticaria.

DENTAL CONSIDERATIONS

General:
• Monitor vital signs at regular intervals during recovery after use as anesthetic.
• Have someone escort patient to and from dental office if used for general anesthesia.
• Geriatric patients are more susceptible to drug effects; use lower dose.
• Use only with resuscitative equipment available and only by qualified persons trained in anesthesia.
• Monitor:
  • Injection site: phlebitis, burning/stinging.
  • ECG for changes: PVC, PAC, ST-segment changes.
  • Allergic reactions: hives.
• Administer:
  • After diluting with D5W, use only glass containers when mixing; not stable in plastic.
  • By IV injection only.

• Alone; do not mix with other agents before using.
• Perform/provide:
  • Storage in light-resistant area at room temperature.
  • Coughing, turning, deep breathing for postoperative patients.
  • Safety measures: side rails, night light, call bell within reach.
• Evaluate:
  • CNS changes: movement, jerking, tremors, dizziness, LOC, pupil reaction.
  • Respiratory dysfunction: respiratory depression, character, rate, rhythm; notify physician if respirations are <10/min.
  • Treatment of overdose: discontinue drug, artificial ventilation, administer vasopressor agents or anticholinergics.

propranolol hydrochloride

proe-**pran′**-oh-lole
high-droh-**klor′**-ide
(Apo-Propranolol[CAN], Deralin[AUS], Inderal, Inderal LA, InnoPran XL, Nu-Propranolol[CAN], Propranolol Intensol)
Do not confuse Inderal with Adderall or Isordil, or propranolol with Pravachol.

CATEGORY AND SCHEDULE

Pregnancy Risk Category: C (D if used in second or third trimester)

Drug Class: Nonselective β-adrenergic blocker

MECHANISM OF ACTION

An antihypertensive, antianginal, antiarrhythmic, and antimigraine agent that blocks β_1- and β_2-adrenergic receptors. Decreases oxygen requirements. Slows AV conduction and increases refractory period in AV node. Large doses increase airway resistance.
Therapeutic Effect: Slows sinus heart rate; decreases cardiac output, B/P, and myocardial ischemia severity. Exhibits antiarrhythmic activity.

USES

Treatment of chronic stable angina pectoris, hypertension, supraventricular dysrhythmias (class II), migraine, MI prophylaxis, pheochromocytoma, essential tremor, hypertrophic cardiomyopathy, anxiety

PHARMACOKINETICS

Route	Onset	Peak	Duration
PO	1–2 hr	N/A	6 hr

Well absorbed from the GI tract. Protein binding: 93%. Widely distributed. Metabolized in the liver. Primarily excreted in urine. Not removed by hemodialysis. *Half-life:* 3–5 hr.

INDICATIONS AND DOSAGES
▸ **Hypertension**
PO
Adults, Elderly. Initially, 40 mg twice a day. May increase dose q3–7 days. Range: Up to 320 mg/day in divided doses. Maximum: 640 mg/day.
Children. Initially, 0.5–1 mg/kg/day in divided doses q6–12h. May increase at 3- to 5-day intervals.

Usual dose: 1–5 mg/kg/day.
Maximum: 16 mg/kg/day.
▸ **Angina**
PO
Adults, Elderly. 80–320 mg/day in divided doses. Long acting: Initially, 80 mg/day. Maximum: 320 mg/day.
▸ **Arrhythmias**
IV
Adults, Elderly. 1 mg/dose. May repeat q5min. Maximum: 5 mg total dose.
Children. 0.01–0.1 mg/kg.
Maximum: infants, 1 mg; children, 3 mg.
PO
Adults, Elderly. Initially, 10–20 mg q6–8h. May gradually increase dose. Range: 40–320 mg/day.
Children. Initially, 0.5–1 mg/kg/day in divided doses q6–8h. May increase q3–5 days. Usual dosage: 2–4 mg/kg/day. Maximum: 16 mg/kg/day or 60 mg/day.
▸ **Life-Threatening Arrhythmias**
IV
Adults, Elderly. 0.5–3 mg. Repeat once in 2 min. Give additional doses at intervals of at least 4 hr.
Children. 0.01–0.1 mg/kg.
▸ **Hypertrophic Subaortic Stenosis**
PO
Adults, Elderly. 20–40 mg in 3–4 divided doses. Or 80–160 mg/day as extended-release capsule.
▸ **Adjunct to α-Blocking Agents to Treat Pheochromocytoma**
PO
Adults, Elderly. 60 mg/day in divided doses with α-blocker for 3 days before surgery. Maintenance (inoperable tumor): 30 mg/day with α-blocker.
▸ **Migraine Headache**
PO
Adults, Elderly. 80 mg/day in divided doses. Or 80 mg once daily as extended-release capsule. Increase

up to 160–240 mg/day in divided doses.
Children. 0.6–1.5 mg/kg/day in divided doses q8h. Maximum: 4 mg/kg/day.

▸ **Reduction of Cardiovascular Mortality and Reinfarction in Patients with Previous MI**
PO
Adults, Elderly. 180–240 mg/day in divided doses.

▸ **Essential Tremor**
PO
Adults, Elderly. Initially, 40 mg twice a day increased up to 120–320 mg/day in 3 divided doses.

SIDE EFFECTS/ADVERSE REACTIONS
Frequent
Diminished sexual ability, drowsiness, difficulty sleeping, unusual fatigue or weakness
Occasional
Bradycardia, depression, sensation of coldness in extremities, diarrhea, constipation, anxiety, nasal congestion, nausea, vomiting
Rare
Altered taste, dry eyes, pruritus, paraesthesia

PRECAUTIONS AND CONTRAINDICATIONS
Asthma, bradycardia, cardiogenic shock, COPD, heart block, Raynaud's syndrome, uncompensated CHF
Caution:
Diabetes mellitus, renal disease, lactation, hyperthyroidism, COPD, hepatic disease, children, myasthenia gravis, peripheral vascular disease, hypotension

DRUG INTERACTIONS OF CONCERN TO DENTISTRY
• Decreased hypotensive effect: indomethacin, NSAIDs

• Increased hypotension, myocardial depression: hydrocarbon inhalation anesthetics
• Hypertension, bradycardia: sympathomimetics (epinephrine, ephedrine)
• Suspected increase in plasma levels: diphenhydramine
• Slow metabolism of lidocaine
• Decreased effects: didanosine (take 2 hr before didanosine tabs)

SERIOUS REACTIONS
! Overdose may produce profound bradycardia and hypotension.
! Abrupt withdrawal may result in sweating, palpitations, headache, and tremors.
! Propranolol administration may precipitate CHF and MI in patients with cardiac disease, thyroid storm in those with thyrotoxicosis, and peripheral ischemia in those with existing peripheral vascular disease.
! Hypoglycemia may occur in patients with previously controlled diabetes.

DENTAL CONSIDERATIONS

General:
• Monitor vital signs at every appointment because of cardiovascular side effects.
• Patients on chronic drug therapy may rarely have symptoms of blood dyscrasias, which can include infection, bleeding, and poor healing.
• Limit use of sodium-containing products, such as saline IV fluids, for patients with a dietary salt restriction.
• Assess salivary flow as a factor in caries, periodontal disease, and candidiasis.
• After supine positioning, have patient sit upright for at least 2 min

before standing to avoid orthostatic hypotension.

• Stress from dental procedures may compromise cardiovascular function; determine patient risk.

• Short appointments and a stress-reduction protocol may be required for anxious patients.

• Consider semisupine chair position for patients with respiratory distress.

• Use vasoconstrictors with caution, in low doses, and with careful aspiration. Avoid use of gingival retraction cord with epinephrine.

Consultations:

• In a patient with symptoms of blood dyscrasias, request a medical consultation for blood studies and postpone dental treatment until normal values are reestablished.

• Medical consultation may be required to assess disease control and patient's ability to tolerate stress.

Teach Patient/Family to:

• Use caution to prevent injury when using oral hygiene aids.

• Encourage effective oral hygiene to prevent soft tissue inflammation.

• When chronic dry mouth occurs, advise patient to:

• Avoid mouth rinses with high alcohol content because of drying effects.

• Use daily home fluoride products to prevent caries.

• Use sugarless gum, frequent sips of water, or saliva substitutes.

propylthiouracil

proe-pill-thye-oh-**yoor**′-ah-sill
(Propylthiouracil,
Propyl-Thyracil[CAN])

CATEGORY AND SCHEDULE
Pregnancy Risk Category: D

Drug Class: Thyroid hormone antagonist

MECHANISM OF ACTION
A thiourea derivative that blocks oxidation of iodine in the thyroid gland and blocks synthesis of thyroxine and triiodothyronine. *Therapeutic Effect:* Inhibits synthesis of thyroid hormone.

USES
Preparation for thyroidectomy, thyrotoxic crisis, hyperthyroidism, thyroid storm

PHARMACOKINETICS
PO: Onset 30–40 min, duration 2–4 hr. *Half-life:* 1–2 hr; excreted in urine, bile, breast milk; crosses placenta.

INDICATIONS AND DOSAGES
▶ Hyperthyroidism
PO
Adults, Elderly. Initially: 300–450 mg/day in divided doses q8h. Maintenance: 100–150 mg/day in divided doses q8–12h.
Children. Initially: 5–7 mg/kg/day in divided doses q8h. Maintenance: 33%–66% of initial dose in divided doses q8–12h.
Neonates. 5–10 mg/kg/day in divided doses q8h.

SIDE EFFECTS/ADVERSE REACTIONS
Frequent
Urticaria, rash, pruritus, nausea, skin pigmentation, hair loss, headache, paraesthesia
Occasional
Somnolence, lymphadenopathy, vertigo
Rare
Drug fever, lupus-like syndrome

PRECAUTIONS AND CONTRAINDICATIONS
Infection, bone marrow depression, hepatic disease
Caution:
Infection, bone marrow depression, hepatic disease

DRUG INTERACTIONS OF CONCERN TO DENTISTRY
• Increased cardiovascular side effects in uncontrolled patients: anticholinergics and sympathomimetics
• Patients with uncontrolled hyperthyroidism are at risk when vasoconstrictors are used
• Patients with uncontrolled hypothyroidism may be more responsive to CNS depressants

SERIOUS REACTIONS
! Agranulocytosis as long as 4 mo after therapy, pancytopenia, and fatal hepatitis have occurred.

DENTAL CONSIDERATIONS
General:
• Patients on chronic drug therapy may rarely have symptoms of blood dyscrasias, which can include infection, bleeding, and poor healing.
• Patients with uncontrolled hyperthyroidism should not be treated in the dental office until thyroid values are normalized.

• Uncontrolled patients should be referred for medical evaluation and treatment.
• Monitor vital signs at every appointment because of cardiovascular side effects.
• Consider semisupine chair position for patient comfort if GI side effects occur, and stress-reduction protocol.
Consultations:
• Medical consultation may be required to assess disease control and patient's ability to tolerate stress.

protein C, human
(Ceprotin)

CATEGORY AND SCHEDULE
Pregnancy Risk Category: C

Drug Class: Vitamin K antagonist, anticoagulant

MECHANISM OF ACTION
Protein C is a precursor of a vitamin K-dependent anticoagulant glycoprotein. Once activated, protein C inactivates factors V and VIII resulting in decreased thrombin formation. Protein C also has profibrinolytic effects.
Therapeutic Effect: Decrease in thrombin formation.

USES
Severe congenital Protein C deficiency for the prevention and treatment of venous thrombosis and purpura fulminans, replacement therapy for pediatric and adult patients

PHARMACOKINETICS
Half-life: 4.9–14.7 hr, median of 9.8 hr.

INDICATIONS AND DOSAGES
▶ Severe Congenital Protein C Deficiency for the Prevention and Treatment of Venous Thrombosis and Purpura Fulminans, Replacement Therapy for Pediatric and Adult Patients

Injection, Powder for Reconstitution
Adults. Ceprotin dosing schedule for acute episodes, short-term prophylaxis, and long-term prophylaxis:

	Initial Dose	Subsequent Dose	Maintenance Dose
Acute episode/ short-term prophylaxis	100–120 IU/kg	60–80 IU/kg q6 hr	45–60 IU/kg q6 or 12 hr
Long-term prophylaxis	NA	NA	45–60 IU/kg q12 hr

SIDE EFFECTS/ADVERSE REACTIONS
Occasional
Bleeding, rash, itching and light-headedness

PRECAUTIONS AND CONTRAINDICATIONS
Hypersensitivity to protein C or any component of the formulation including mouse proteins and/or heparin
Caution:
Made from pooled human plasma; possibility of transmitting infectious agents may occur
Concurrent use with tPA and/or other anticoagulants
Renal impairment (contains sodium)
Elderly
Immunocompromised patients
Sodium-restricted patients (e.g., heart failure patients)

DRUG INTERACTIONS OF CONCERN TO DENTISTRY
• tPA and/or anticoagulants: may increase risk of bleeding

SERIOUS REACTIONS
! Hemothorax has been reported.
! Hypotension may occur.
! Contains heparin; if heparin-induced thrombocytopenia is suspected, check platelets.

DENTAL CONSIDERATIONS
General:
• Monitor vital signs at every appointment because of cardiovascular side effects.
• Assess salivary flow as a factor in caries, periodontal disease, and candidiasis.
• Stress from dental procedures may compromise cardiovascular function; determine patient risk.
Consultations:
• Medical consultation may be required to assess disease control.
Teach Patient/Family to:
• Report oral lesions, soreness, or bleeding to dentist.
• When chronic dry mouth occurs, advise patient to:
  • Avoid mouth rinses with high alcohol content because of drying effects.
  • Use daily home fluoride products for anticaries effect.
  • Use sugarless gum, frequent sips of water, or saliva substitutes.

protriptyline
proe-**trip**′-ti-leen
(Vivactil, Triptil[CAN])

CATEGORY AND SCHEDULE
Pregnancy Risk Category: C

Drug Class: Tricyclic
antidepressant

MECHANISM OF ACTION
A tricyclic antidepressant that
increases synaptic concentration of
norepinephrine and/or serotonin by
inhibiting their reuptake by
presynaptic membranes.
Therapeutic Effect: Produces
antidepressant effect.

USES
Depression; unapproved use:
adjunctive use in narcolepsy and
attention-deficit disorders

PHARMACOKINETICS
Well absorbed from the GI tract.
Protein binding: 92%. Widely
distributed. Extensively metabolized
in liver. Excreted in urine. Not
removed by hemodialysis. ***Half-life:***
54–92 hr.

INDICATIONS AND DOSAGES
▶ **Depression**
PO
Adults. 15–40 mg/day divided into
3–4 doses/day. Maximum: 600 mg/
day.
Elderly. 5 mg 3 times a day. May
increase gradually.

SIDE EFFECTS/ADVERSE REACTIONS
Frequent
Drowsiness, weight gain, fatigue,
dry mouth, blurred vision,
constipation, delayed micturition,
postural hypotension, diaphoresis,
disturbed concentration, increased
appetite, urinary retention
Occasional
GI disturbances, such as nausea,
diarrhea, GI distress, metallic taste
sensation
Rare
Paradoxical reaction, marked by
agitation, restlessness, nightmares,
insomnia, extrapyramidal symptoms,
particularly fine hand tremor

PRECAUTIONS AND CONTRAINDICATIONS
Acute recovery period after
myocardial infarction,
coadministration with cisapride, use
of MAOIs within 14 days,
hypersensitivity to protriptyline or
any component of the formulation
Caution:
Suicidal patients, severe depression,
increased intraocular pressure,
narrow-angle glaucoma, urinary
retention, cardiac disease, hepatic
disease, hyperthyroidism,
electroshock therapy, elective
surgery, MAOIs

DRUG INTERACTIONS OF CONCERN TO DENTISTRY
• Increased anticholinergic effects:
muscarinic blockers, antihistamines,
phenothiazines
• Increased effects of direct-acting
sympathomimetics (epinephrine,
levonordefrin)
• Possible risk of increased CNS
depression: alcohol, barbiturates,
benzodiazepines, and other CNS
depressants
• Decreased antihypertensive effects
of: clonidine, guanadrel,
guanethidine
• Avoid concurrent use with St.
John's wort (herb)

P

SERIOUS REACTIONS

! High dosage may produce confusion, seizures, severe drowsiness, arrhythmias, fever, hallucinations, agitation, shortness of breath, vomiting, and unusual tiredness or weakness.

! Abrupt withdrawal from prolonged therapy may produce severe headache, malaise, nausea, vomiting, and vivid dreams.

DENTAL CONSIDERATIONS

General:
• Monitor vital signs at every appointment because of cardiovascular side effects.
• Assess salivary flow as a factor in caries, periodontal disease, and candidiasis.
• Patients on chronic drug therapy may rarely have symptoms of blood dyscrasias, which can include infection, bleeding, and poor healing.
• After supine positioning, have patient sit upright for at least 2 min before standing to avoid orthostatic hypotension.
• Use vasoconstrictors with caution, in low doses, and with careful aspiration. Avoid use of gingival retraction cord with epinephrine.
• Place on frequent recall because of oral side effects.
Consultations:
• In a patient with symptoms of blood dyscrasias, request a medical consultation for blood studies and postpone dental treatment until normal values are reestablished.
• Medical consultation may be required to assess disease control.
• Physician should be informed if significant xerostomic side effects occur (e.g., increased caries, sore tongue, problems eating or swallowing, difficulty wearing

prosthesis) so that a medication change can be considered.
Teach Patient/Family to:
• Encourage effective oral hygiene to prevent soft tissue inflammation.
• Use caution to prevent injury when using oral hygiene aids.
• When chronic dry mouth occurs, advise patient to:
  • Avoid mouth rinses with high alcohol content because of drying effects.
  • Use daily home fluoride products to prevent caries.
  • Use sugarless gum, frequent sips of water, or saliva substitutes.

pseudoephedrine

soo-doe-eh-**fed**′-rin
(Balminil Decongestant[CAN], Bio Contac Cold 12 Hour Relief Non Drowsy[CAN], Decofed, Dimetapp 12 Hour Non Drowsy Extentabs, Dimetapp Decongestant, Dimetapp Sinus Liquid Caps[AUS], Genaphed, PMS-Pseudoephedrine[CAN], Robidrine[CAN], Sudafed, Sudafed 12h[AUS], Sudafed 12 Hour, Sudafed 24 Hour)

CATEGORY AND SCHEDULE
Pregnancy Risk Category: C
OTC

Drug Class: α-adrenergic agonist

MECHANISM OF ACTION
A sympathomimetic that directly stimulates α-adrenergic and β-adrenergic receptors.
Therapeutic Effect: Produces vasoconstriction of respiratory tract mucosa; shrinks nasal mucous

membranes; reduces edema and nasal congestion.

USES

Decongestant, treatment of nasal congestion

PHARMACOKINETICS

Route	Onset	Peak	Duration
PO	15–30 min	N/A	4–6 hr
PO	N/A	N/A	8–12 hr

Well absorbed from the GI tract. Partially metabolized in the liver. Primarily excreted in urine. Not removed by hemodialysis. *Half-life:* 9–16 hr (children, 3.1 hr).

INDICATIONS AND DOSAGES

▸ **Decongestant**
PO
Adults, Children 12 yr and older. 60 mg q4–6h. Maximum: 240 mg/ day.
Children 6–11 yr. 30 mg q6h. Maximum: 120 mg/day.
Children 2–5 yr. 15 mg q6h. Maximum: 60 mg/day.
Children younger than 2 yr. 4 mg/ kg/day in divided doses q6h.
Elderly. 30–60 mg q6h as needed.
PO (Extended Release)
Adults, Children 12 yr and older. 120 mg q12h.

SIDE EFFECTS/ADVERSE REACTIONS

Occasional
Nervousness, restlessness, insomnia, tremor, headache
Rare
Diaphoresis, weakness

PRECAUTIONS AND CONTRAINDICATIONS

Breast-feeding women, coronary artery disease, severe hypertension, use within 14 days of MAOIs

Caution:
Cardiac disorders, hyperthyroidism, diabetes mellitus, prostatic hypertrophy

DRUG INTERACTIONS OF CONCERN TO DENTISTRY

• Dysrhythmia: hydrocarbon inhalation anesthetics
• Increased CNS, cardiovascular effects: sympathomimetics

SERIOUS REACTIONS

❗ Large doses may produce tachycardia, palpitations (particularly in patients with cardiac disease), light-headedness, nausea, and vomiting.
❗ Overdose in patients older than 60 yr may result in hallucinations, CNS depression, and seizures.

DENTAL CONSIDERATIONS

General:
• Assess salivary flow as a factor in caries, periodontal disease, and candidiasis.
• Monitor vital signs at every appointment because of cardiovascular side effects.
• Consider semisupine chair position for patient comfort if GI side effects occur.
Teach Patient/Family to:
• Use powered tooth brush if patient has difficulty holding conventional devices.
• When chronic dry mouth occurs, advise patient to:
  • Avoid mouth rinses with high alcohol content because of drying effects.
  • Use daily home fluoride products to prevent caries.
  • Use sugarless gum, frequent sips of water, or saliva substitutes.

P

pyrazinamide

pye-ra-**zin**'-ah-mide
(Pyrazinamide, Tebrazid[CAN], Zinamide[AUS])

CATEGORY AND SCHEDULE

Pregnancy Risk Category: C

Drug Class: Antitubercular

MECHANISM OF ACTION

An antitubercular whose exact mechanism of action is unknown. *Therapeutic Effect:* Either bacteriostatic or bactericidal, depending on the drug's concentration at the infection site and the susceptibility of infecting bacteria.

USES

Treatment of tuberculosis (TB), as an adjunct with other drugs

PHARMACOKINETICS

PO: Peak 2 hr. *Half-life:* 9–10 hr; metabolized in liver, excreted in urine (metabolites/unchanged drug).

INDICATIONS AND DOSAGES

▸ **TB (in Combination with Other Antituberculars)**
PO
Adults. 15–30 mg/kg/day in 1–4 doses. Maximum: 3 g/day.
Children. 20–40 mg/kg/day in 1 or 2 doses. Maximum: 2 g/day.

SIDE EFFECTS/ADVERSE REACTIONS

Frequent
Arthralgia, myalgia (usually mild and self-limiting)
Rare
Hypersensitivity reaction (rash, pruritus, urticaria), photosensitivity, gouty arthritis

PRECAUTIONS AND CONTRAINDICATIONS

Severe hepatic dysfunction
Caution:
Children younger than 13 yr

DRUG INTERACTIONS OF CONCERN TO DENTISTRY

• None reported

SERIOUS REACTIONS

❗ Hepatotoxicity, gouty arthritis, thrombocytopenia, and anemia occur rarely.

DENTAL CONSIDERATIONS

General:
• Determine why the patient is taking the drug (for prophylaxis or active therapy).
• Determine that noninfectious status exists by ensuring that (1) anti-TB drugs have been taken for longer than 3 wk, (2) culture has confirmed TB susceptibility to antiinfectives, (3) patient has had three consecutive negative sputum smears, and (4) patient is not in the coughing stage.
• Do not treat patients with active tuberculosis.
Consultations:
• Medical consultation may be required to assess disease control.
Teach Patient/Family to:
• Take medications for full length of regimen to ensure effectiveness of treatment and to prevent the emergence of resistant strains.

pyridostigmine bromide

peer-id-oh-**stig**′-meen **broe**′-mide
(Mestinon, Mestinon SR[CAN],
Mestinon Timespan)
Do not confuse pyridostigmine
with physostigmine or Mesitonin
with Mesantoin or Metatensin.

CATEGORY AND SCHEDULE
Pregnancy Risk Category: C

Drug Class: Cholinergic

MECHANISM OF ACTION
A cholinergic that prevents
destruction of acetylcholine by
inhibiting the enzyme
acetylcholinesterase, thus enhancing
impulse transmission across the
myoneural junction.
Therapeutic Effect: Produces
miosis; increases tone of intestinal,
skeletal muscle; stimulates salivary
and sweat gland secretions.

USES
Nondepolarizing muscle relaxant
antagonist, myasthenia gravis

PHARMACOKINETICS
PO: Onset 20–30 min, duration
3–6 hr
IM/IV/Subcutaneous: Onset
2–15 min, duration 2.5–4 hr;
metabolized in liver, excreted in
urine

INDICATIONS AND DOSAGES
▶ **Myasthenia Gravis**
PO
Adults, Elderly. Initially, 60 mg 3
times a day. Dosage increased at
48-hr intervals. Maintenance:
60 mg–1.5 g a day.

PO (Extended-Release)
Adults, Elderly. 180–540 mg once or
twice a day with at least a 6 hr
interval between doses.
IV, IM
Adults, Elderly. 2 mg q2–3h.
Children, Neonates. 0.05–0.15 mg/
kg/dose. Maximum single dose:
10 mg.
▶ **Reversal of Nondepolarizing
Neuromuscular Blockade**
IV
Adults, Elderly. 10–20 mg with, or
shortly after, 0.6–1.2 mg atropine
sulfate or 0.3–0.6 mg glycopyrrolate.
Children. 0.1–0.25 mg/kg/dose
preceded by atropine or
glycopyrrolate.

SIDE EFFECTS/ADVERSE REACTIONS
Frequent
Miosis, increased GI and skeletal
muscle tone, bradycardia,
constriction of bronchi and ureters,
diaphoresis, increased salivation
Occasional
Headache, rash, temporary decrease
in diastolic B/P with mild reflex
tachycardia, short periods of atrial
fibrillation (in hyperthyroid
patients), marked drop in B/P (in
hypertensive patients)

PRECAUTIONS AND CONTRAINDICATIONS
Mechanical GI or urinary tract
obstruction
Caution:
Seizure disorders, bronchial asthma,
coronary occlusion,
hyperthyroidism, dysrhythmias,
peptic ulcer, megacolon, poor GI
motility, elderly, lactation

DRUG INTERACTIONS OF CONCERN TO DENTISTRY
• Decreased effects: atropine,
scopolamine, and other

P

anticholinergic drugs;
methocarbamol
• Reduced rate of metabolism of
ester local anesthetics
• Avoid anticholinergic drugs to
control excessive salivation

SERIOUS REACTIONS

! Overdose may produce a
cholinergic crisis, manifested as
increasingly severe muscle weakness
that appears first in muscles
involving chewing and swallowing
and is followed by muscle weakness
of the shoulder girdle and upper
extremities, respiratory muscle
paralysis, and pelvis girdle and leg
muscle paralysis. If overdose occurs,
stop all cholinergic drugs and
immediately administer 1–4 mg
atropine sulfate IV for adults or
0.01 mg/kg for infants and children
younger than 12 yr.

DENTAL CONSIDERATIONS

General:
• Monitor vital signs at every
appointment because of
cardiovascular and respiratory side
effects.
• After supine positioning, have
patient sit upright for at least 2 min
before standing to avoid orthostatic
hypotension.
• Schedule short appointments
because of effects of disease on oral
musculature.
• Avoid dental light in patient's eyes;
offer dark glasses for patient
comfort.
• Place on frequent recall because of
oral side effects.
• Consider semisupine chair position
for patient comfort if GI side effects
occur.
Consultations:
• Medical consultation may be
required to assess disease control.

• Consult with physician about
adjusting dose if excessive salivation
becomes a problem.
Teach Patient/Family to:
• Use powered tooth brush or other
oral hygiene aids if patient has
difficulty in maintaining oral
hygiene.
• Encourage effective oral hygiene
to prevent soft tissue inflammation.
• Prevent injury when using oral
hygiene aids.

pyridoxine hydrochloride (vitamin B$_6$)

peer-ih-**dox**′-een
high-droh-**klor**′-ide
(Aminoxin, Beesix, Doxine,
Nestrex, Pryi, Pyroxin[AUS],
Rodex, Vitabee 6)
Do not confuse pyridoxine with
paroxetine, pralidoxime, or
Pyridium.

CATEGORY AND SCHEDULE

Pregnancy Risk Category: A
OTC

Drug Class: Vitamin B$_6$,
water-soluble vitamin

MECHANISM OF ACTION

Acts as a coenzyme for various
metabolic functions, including
metabolism of proteins,
carbohydrates, and fats. Aids in the
breakdown of glycogen and in the
synthesis of gamma-aminobutyric
acid in the CNS.
Therapeutic Effect: Prevents
pyridoxine deficiency. Increases the
excretion of certain drugs, such as
isoniazid, that are pyridoxine
antagonists.

USES

Treatment of vitamin B_6 deficiency associated with inborn errors of metabolism, inadequate diet; unapproved: drug-induced deficiencies

PHARMACOKINETICS

Readily absorbed primarily in jejunum. Stored in the liver, muscle, and brain. Metabolized in the liver. Primarily excreted in urine. Removed by hemodialysis. *Half-life:* 15–20 days.

INDICATIONS AND DOSAGES

▸ **Pyridoxine Deficiency**
PO
Adults, Elderly. Initially, 2.5–10 mg/day; then 2.5 mg/day when clinical signs are corrected.
Children. Initially, 5–25 mg/day for 3 wk, then 1.5–2.5 mg/day.
▸ **Pyridoxine Dependent Seizures**
PO, IV, IM
Infants. Initially, 10–100 mg/day.
Maintenance: PO: 50–100 mg/day.
▸ **Drug-Induced Neuritis**
PO (Treatment)
Adults, Elderly. 100–300 mg/day in divided doses.
Children. 10–50 mg/day.
PO (Prophylaxis)
Adults, Elderly. 25–100 mg/day.
Children. 1–2 mg/kg/day.

SIDE EFFECTS/ADVERSE REACTIONS

Occasional
Stinging at IM injection site
Rare
Headache, nausea, somnolence; sensory neuropathy (paresthesia, unstable gait, clumsiness of hands) with high doses

PRECAUTIONS AND CONTRAINDICATIONS

Hypersensitivity, Parkinson's disease

DRUG INTERACTIONS OF CONCERN TO DENTISTRY

• Decreased effectiveness: levodopa
• Decreased serum levels of phenytoin, phenobarbital

SERIOUS REACTIONS

! Long-term megadoses (2–6 g over more than 2 mo) may produce sensory neuropathy (reduced deep tendon reflexes, profound impairment of sense of position in distal limbs, gradual sensory ataxia). Toxic symptoms subside when drug is discontinued.
! Seizures have occurred after IV megadoses.

DENTAL CONSIDERATIONS

General:
• Vitamin B deficiency and peripheral neuropathy may manifest with oral symptoms of glossitis and cheilosis.

pyrimethamine

P

pye-ri-**meth**′-ah-meen
(Daraprim, Malocide[FRANCE])
Do not confuse with Dantrium, Daranide.

CATEGORY AND SCHEDULE

Pregnancy Risk Category: C

Drug Class: Antimalarial

MECHANISM OF ACTION

An antiprotozoal with blood and some tissue schizonticidal activity against malaria parasites of humans. Highly selective activity against plasmodia and *Toxoplasma gondii*. *Therapeutic Effect:* Inhibition of tetrahydrofolic acid synthesis.

USES
Malaria prophylaxis

PHARMACOKINETICS
Well absorbed, peak levels occurring between 2 and 6 hr following administration. Protein binding: 87%. Eliminated slowly. *Half-life:* approximately 96 hr.

INDICATIONS AND DOSAGES
▶ **Toxoplasmosis**
PO
Adults. Initially, 50–75 mg daily, with 1–4 g daily of a sulfonamide of the sulfapyrimidine type (e.g., sulfadoxine). Continue for 1–3 wk, depending on response of patient and tolerance to therapy, then reduce dose to one-half that previously given for each drug and continue for additional 4–5 wk.
Children. 1 mg/kg/day divided into 2 equal daily doses; after 2–4 days reduce to one-half and continue for approximately 1 month. The usual pediatric sulfonamide dosage is used in conjunction with pyrimethamine.
▶ **Acute Malaria**
PO
Adults (in combination with sulfonamide). 25 mg daily for 2 days with a sulfonamide.
Adults (without concomitant sulfonamide). 50 mg for 2 days.
Children 4–10 yr. 25 mg daily for 2 days.
▶ **Chemoprophylaxis of Malaria**
PO
Adults and pediatric patients over 10 yr. 25 mg once a wk.
Children 4–10 yr. 12.5 mg once a wk.
Infants and children under 4 yr. 6.25 mg once a wk.

SIDE EFFECTS/ADVERSE REACTIONS
Frequent
Anorexia, vomiting
Occasional
Hypersensitivity reactions, Stevens-Johnson syndrome, toxic epidermal necrolysis, erythema multiforme, anaphylaxis, hyperphenylalaninemia, megaloblastic anemia, leukopenia, thrombocytopenia, pancytopenia, atrophic glossitis, hematuria, and disorders of cardiac rhythm
Rare
Pulmonary eosinophilia

PRECAUTIONS AND CONTRAINDICATIONS
Hypersensitivity to pyrimethamine, megaloblastic anemia due to folate deficiency, monotherapy for treatment of acute malaria

DRUG INTERACTIONS OF CONCERN TO DENTISTRY
• Possible mild hepatotoxicity: lorazepam

SERIOUS REACTIONS
! None known

DENTAL CONSIDERATIONS

General:
• Determine why patient is taking the drug.
• Consider semisupine chair position for patient comfort if GI side effects occur.
• Question patient about tolerance of NSAIDs or aspirin related to GI disease.
• Patient on chronic drug therapy may rarely present with symptoms of blood dyscrasias, which can include infection, bleeding, and poor healing. If dyscrasia is present, advise patient to prevent oral tissue

trauma when using oral hygiene aids.
• Determine why patient is taking drug (prophylaxis or active therapy).
Consultations:
• Medical consultation may be required to assess disease control and patient's ability to tolerate stress.
Teach Patient/Family to:
• Report sore throat, pallor, purpura, or glossitis, which may be symptoms of serious effects.

• Encourage effective oral hygiene to prevent soft tissue inflammation.
• Prevent trauma when using oral hygiene aids.
• Update health and medication history if physician makes any changes in evaluation or drug regimens; include OTC, herbal, and nonherbal drug in the update.

P

quazepam
kwaz'-eh-pam
(Doral)

CATEGORY AND SCHEDULE
Pregnancy Risk Category: X
Controlled Substance: Schedule
IV

Drug Class: Benzodiazepine,
sedative-hypnotic

MECHANISM OF ACTION
A BZ-1 receptor selective
benzodiazepine with sedative
properties.
Therapeutic Effect: Produces
sedative effect from its CNS
depressant action.

USES
Treatment of insomnia

PHARMACOKINETICS
Rapidly absorbed from GI tract.
Food increases absorption. Protein
binding: 95%. Extensively
metabolized in liver. Excreted in
urine and feces. Unknown if
removed by hemodialysis. *Half-life:*
25–41 hr.

INDICATIONS AND DOSAGES
▸ **Insomnia**
PO
Adults (older than 18 yr). Initially,
15 mg at bedtime. Adjust dose up or
down from 7.5 mg to 30 mg at
bedtime, depending on initial
response.
Elderly, debilitated, liver disease.
Initially, 7.5–15 mg at bedtime.
Adjust dose depending on initial
response.

SIDE EFFECTS/ADVERSE REACTIONS
Frequent
Muscular incoordination (ataxia),
light-headedness, transient mild
drowsiness, slurred speech
(particularly in elderly or debilitated
patients)
Occasional
Confusion, depression, blurred
vision, constipation, diarrhea, dry
mouth, headache, nausea
Rare
Behavioral problems such as anger,
impaired memory; paradoxic
reactions, such as insomnia,
nervousness, or irritability

PRECAUTIONS AND CONTRAINDICATIONS
Pregnancy, sleep apnea,
hypersensitivity to quazepam or any
component of the formulation
Caution:
Hepatic disease, renal disease,
suicidal individuals, drug abuse,
elderly, psychosis, children younger
than 18 yr, lactation, depression,
pulmonary insufficiency

DRUG INTERACTIONS OF CONCERN TO DENTISTRY
• Increased effects: CNS
depressants, alcohol
• Delayed elimination: erythromycin
• Contraindicated with saquinavir,
ritonavir
• Increased serum levels and
prolonged effect of benzodiazepines:
erythromycin, ketoconazole,
itraconazole, fluconazole,
miconazole (systemic)

SERIOUS REACTIONS
! Abrupt or too-rapid withdrawal
may result in pronounced
restlessness, irritability, insomnia,
hand tremors, abdominal and muscle

Q

cramps, sweating, vomiting, and seizures.

! Overdosage results in somnolence, confusion, diminished reflexes, and coma.

! Blood dyscrasias have been reported rarely.

DENTAL CONSIDERATIONS

General:

• Assess salivary flow as a factor in caries, periodontal disease, and candidiasis.

• Psychologic and physical dependence may occur with chronic administration.

• Geriatric patients are more susceptible to drug effects; use a lower dose.

• Avoid using this drug in a patient with a history of drug abuse or alcoholism.

Consultations:

• Medical consultation may be required to assess disease control.

Teach Patient/Family to:

• When chronic dry mouth occurs, advise patient to:
  • Avoid mouth rinses with high alcohol content because of drying effects.
  • Use daily home fluoride products to prevent caries.
  • Use sugarless gum, frequent sips of water, or saliva substitutes.

quetiapine
kwe-**tye**′-ah-peen
(Seroquel)

CATEGORY AND SCHEDULE
Pregnancy Risk Category: C

Drug Class: Antipsychotic, atypical

MECHANISM OF ACTION
A dibenzepin derivative that antagonizes dopamine, serotonin, histamine, and α_1-adrenergic receptors.

Therapeutic Effect: Diminishes manifestations of psychotic disorders. Produces moderate sedation, few extrapyramidal effects, and no anticholinergic effects.

USES
Treatment of schizophrenia

PHARMACOKINETICS
Well absorbed after PO administration. Protein binding: 83%. Widely distributed in tissues; CNS concentration exceeds plasma concentration. Undergoes extensive first-pass metabolism in the liver. Primarily excreted in urine.
Half-life: 6 hr.

INDICATIONS AND DOSAGES
▸ **To Manage Manifestations of Psychotic Disorders, Bipolar Disorder**
PO
Adults, Elderly. Initially, 25 mg twice a day, then 25–50 mg 2–3 times a day on the second and third days, up to 300–400 mg/day in divided doses 2–3 times a day by the fourth day. Further adjustments of 25–50 mg twice a day may be made at intervals of 2 days or longer. Maintenance: 300–800 mg/day (adults); 50–200 mg/day (elderly).
▸ **Dosage in Hepatic Impairment, Elderly or Debilitated Patients, and Those Predisposed to Hypotensive Reactions**
These patients should receive a lower initial dose and lower dosage increases.

Q

SIDE EFFECTS/ADVERSE REACTIONS

Frequent

Headache, somnolence, dizziness

Occasional

Constipation, orthostatic hypotension, tachycardia, dry mouth, dyspepsia, rash, asthenia, abdominal pain, rhinitis

Rare

Back pain, fever, weight gain

PRECAUTIONS AND CONTRAINDICATIONS

Renal impairment, hepatic impairment, cardiovascular disease, thyroid disease, hyperprolactinemia, neuromalignant syndrome, tardive dyskinesia, seizure disorders, cataracts, dementia, suicide tendency, lactation; patients should be monitored for signs and symptoms of diabetes mellitus, severe CNS depression

DRUG INTERACTIONS OF CONCERN TO DENTISTRY

• Risk of increased CNS depression: CNS depressants

SERIOUS REACTIONS

! Overdose may produce heart block, hypotension, hypokalemia, and tachycardia.

DENTAL CONSIDERATIONS

General:

• Monitor vital signs at every appointment because of cardiovascular and respiratory side effects.

• Assess salivary flow as factor in caries, periodontal disease, and candidiasis.

• Assess for presence of extrapyramidal motor symptoms, such as tardive dyskinesia and akathisia.

• Extrapyramidal motor activity may complicate dental treatment.

• After supine positioning, have patient sit upright for at least 2 min before standing to avoid orthostatic hypotension.

• Consider semisupine chair position for patient comfort if GI side effects occur.

• Patients on chronic drug therapy may rarely have symptoms of blood dyscrasias, which can include infection, bleeding, and poor healing.

• Place on frequent recall because of oral side effects.

Consultations:

• In a patient with symptoms of blood dyscrasias, request a medical consultation for blood studies and postpone treatment until normal values are reestablished.

• Medical consultation may be required to assess disease control and patient's ability to tolerate stress.

• If signs of tardive dyskinesia or akathisia are present, refer to physician.

• Consultation with physician may be necessary if sedation or general anesthesia is required.

• Physician should be informed if significant xerostomic side effects occur (e.g., increased caries, sore tongue, problems eating or swallowing, difficulty wearing prosthesis) so that a medication change can be considered.

Teach Patient/Family to:

• Use caution to prevent trauma when using oral hygiene aids.

• Use powered tooth brush if patient has difficulty holding conventional devices.

• Encourage effective oral hygiene to prevent soft tissue inflammation.

• Update health and drug history if physician makes any changes in evaluation or drug regimens; include OTC, herbal, and nonherbal drugs in the update.

• Be aware of oral side effects and potential sequelae.

• When chronic dry mouth occurs, advise patient to:

  • Avoid mouth rinses with high alcohol content because of drying effects.

  • Use daily home fluoride products for anticaries effect.

  • Use sugarless gum, frequent sips of water, or saliva substitutes.

quinapril
kwin′-ah-pril
(Accupril, Asig[AUS])
Do not confuse Accupril with Accolate or Accutane.

CATEGORY AND SCHEDULE
Pregnancy Risk Category: C (D if used in second or third trimester)

Drug Class: Angiotensin-converting enzyme (ACE) inhibitor

MECHANISM OF ACTION
An ACE inhibitor that suppresses the renin-angiotensin-aldosterone system and prevents the conversion of angiotensin I to angiotensin II, a potent vasoconstrictor; may also inhibit angiotensin II at local vascular and renal sites.
Therapeutic Effect: Reduces peripheral arterial resistance, B/P, and pulmonary capillary wedge pressure; improves cardiac output.

USES
Treatment of hypertension, alone or in combination with thiazide diuretics, heart failure

PHARMACOKINETICS

Route	Onset	Peak	Duration
PO	1 hr	N/A	24 hr

Readily absorbed from the GI tract. Protein binding: 97%. Metabolized in the liver, GI tract, and extravascular tissue to active metabolite. Primarily excreted in urine. Minimal removal by hemodialysis. *Half-life:* 1–2 hr; metabolite, 3 hr (increased in those with impaired renal function).

INDICATIONS AND DOSAGES
▶ **Hypertension (Monotherapy)**
PO
Adults. Initially, 10–20 mg/day. May adjust dosage at intervals of at least 2 wk or longer. Maintenance: 20–80 mg/day as single dose or 2 divided doses. Maximum: 80 mg/day.
Elderly. Initially, 2.5–5 mg/day. May increase by 2.5–5 mg q1–2wk.
▶ **Hypertension (Combination Therapy)**
PO
Adults. Initially, 5 mg/day titrated to patient's needs.
Elderly. Initially, 2.5–5 mg/day. May increase by 2.5–5 mg q1–2wk.
▶ **Adjunct to Manage Heart Failure**
PO
Adults, Elderly. Initially, 5 mg twice a day. Range: 20–40 mg/day.
▶ **Dosage in Renal Impairment**
Dosage is titrated to the patient's needs after the following initial doses:

Creatinine Clearance	Initial Dose
More than 60 ml/min	10 mg
30–60 ml/min	5 mg
10–29 ml/min	2.5 mg

Q

SIDE EFFECTS/ADVERSE REACTIONS

Frequent
Headache, dizziness
Occasional
Fatigue, vomiting, nausea, hypotension, chest pain, cough, syncope
Rare
Diarrhea, cough, dyspnea, rash, palpitations, impotence, insomnia, drowsiness, malaise

PRECAUTIONS AND CONTRAINDICATIONS

Bilateral renal artery stenosis
Caution:
Pregnancy category D, impaired renal/liver function, dialysis patients, hypovolemia, blood dyscrasias, CHF, COPD, asthma, elderly, lactation

DRUG INTERACTIONS OF CONCERN TO DENTISTRY

• Increased hypotension: alcohol, phenothiazines
• Decreased hypotensive effects: indomethacin and possibly other NSAIDs, sympathomimetics
• Suspected reduction in the antihypertensive and vasodilator effects by salicylates; monitor B/P if used concurrently

SERIOUS REACTIONS

! Excessive hypotension ("first-dose syncope") may occur in patients with CHF and in those who are severely salt or volume depleted.
! Angioedema and hyperkalemia occur rarely.
! Agranulocytosis and neutropenia may be noted in those with collagen vascular disease, including scleroderma and systemic lupus erythematosus, and impaired renal function.

! Nephrotic syndrome may be noted in those with history of renal disease.

DENTAL CONSIDERATIONS

General:
• Monitor vital signs at every appointment because of cardiovascular side effects.
• After supine positioning, have patient sit upright for at least 2 min before standing to avoid orthostatic hypotension.
• Patients on chronic drug therapy may rarely have symptoms of blood dyscrasias, which can include infection, bleeding, and poor healing.
• Assess salivary flow as a factor in caries, periodontal disease, and candidiasis.
• Limit use of sodium-containing products, such as saline IV fluids, for patients with a dietary salt restriction.
• Use vasoconstrictors with caution, in low doses, and with careful aspiration.
• Stress from dental procedures may compromise cardiovascular function; determine patient risk.
• Short appointments and a stress-reduction protocol may be required for anxious patients.
Consultations:
• Medical consultation may be required to assess disease control and patient's ability to tolerate stress.
• In a patient with symptoms of blood dyscrasias, request a medical consultation for blood studies and postpone dental treatment until normal values are reestablished.
• Take precautions if dental surgery is anticipated and sedation or general anesthesia is required; risk of hypotensive episode.

Teach Patient/Family to:
• Encourage effective oral hygiene to prevent soft tissue inflammation.
• Use caution to prevent injury when using oral hygiene aids.
• When chronic dry mouth occurs, advise patient to:
  • Avoid mouth rinses with high alcohol content because of drying effects.
  • Use daily home fluoride products to prevent caries.
  • Use sugarless gum, frequent sips of water, or saliva substitutes.

quinidine

kwin´-ih-deen
(Apo-Quin-G[CAN], Apo-Quinidine[CAN], BioQuin Durules[CAN], Kinidin Durules[AUS], Quinaglute Dura-Tabs, Quinate[CAN], Quinidex Extentabs)
Do not confuse quinidine with clonidine or quinine.

CATEGORY AND SCHEDULE

Pregnancy Risk Category: C

Drug Class: Antidysrhythmic (class Ia)

MECHANISM OF ACTION

An antidysrhythmic that decreases sodium influx during depolarization, potassium efflux during repolarization, and reduces calcium transport across the myocardial cell membrane. Decreases myocardial excitability, conduction velocity, and contractility.
Therapeutic Effect: Suppresses cardiac dysrhythmias.

USES

Treatment of premature ventricular contractions (PVCs), atrial flutter and fibrillation, PAT, ventricular tachycardia

PHARMACOKINETICS

PO: Peak 0.5–6 hr (depending on form given), duration 6–8 hr, *Half-life:* 6–7 hr; metabolized in liver; excreted unchanged by kidneys.

INDICATIONS AND DOSAGES

▶ **Maintenance of Normal Sinus Rhythm after Conversion of Atrial Fibrillation or Flutter; Prevention of Premature Atrial, AV, and Ventricular Contractions; Paroxysmal Atrial Tachycardia; Paroxysmal AV Junctional Rhythm; Atrial Fibrillation; Atrial Flutter; Paroxysmal Ventricular Tachycardia Not Associated with Complete Heart Block**
PO
Adults, Elderly. 100–600 mg q4–6h. Long-acting: 324–972 mg q8–12h.
Children. 30 mg/kg/day in divided doses q4–6h.
IV
Adults, Elderly. 200–400 mg.
Children. 2–10 mg/kg.

SIDE EFFECTS/ADVERSE REACTIONS

Frequent
Abdominal pain and cramps, nausea, diarrhea, vomiting (can be immediate, intense)
Occasional
Mild cinchonism (ringing in ears, blurred vision, hearing loss) or severe cinchonism (headache, vertigo, diaphoresis, light-headedness, photophobia, confusion, delirium)

Q

Rare

Hypotension (particularly with IV administration), hypersensitivity reaction (fever, anaphylaxis, photosensitivity reaction)

PRECAUTIONS AND CONTRAINDICATIONS

Complete AV block, intraventricular conduction defects (widening of QRS complex)

Caution:

Lactation, children, renal disease, potassium imbalance, liver disease, CHF, respiratory depression

DRUG INTERACTIONS OF CONCERN TO DENTISTRY

• May decrease effects of quinidine: barbiturates
• Increased anticholinergic effect: anticholinergic drugs
• Increased effects of neuromuscular blockers, tricyclic antidepressants
• Contraindicated with itraconazole
• Prevention of action: cholinergics

SERIOUS REACTIONS

! Cardiotoxic effects occur most commonly with IV administration, particularly at high concentrations, and are observed as conduction changes (50% widening of QRS complex, prolonged QT interval, flattened T waves, and disappearance of P wave), ventricular tachycardia or flutter, frequent PVCs, or complete AV block.
! Quinidine-induced syncope may occur with the usual dosage.
! Severe hypotension may result from high dosages.
! Patients with atrial flutter and fibrillation may experience a paradoxical, extremely rapid ventricular rate that may be prevented by prior digitalization.

! Hepatotoxicity with jaundice caused by drug hypersensitivity may occur.

DENTAL CONSIDERATIONS

General:
• Monitor vital signs at every appointment because of cardiovascular and respiratory side effects.
• Minimize; use stress-reduction protocol.
• Patients on chronic drug therapy may rarely have symptoms of blood dyscrasias, which can include infection, bleeding, and poor healing.
• After supine positioning, have patient sit upright for at least 2 min before standing to avoid orthostatic hypotension.
• Use vasoconstrictors with caution, in low doses, and with careful aspiration. Avoid use of gingival retraction cord with epinephrine.
• Consider semisupine chair position for patient comfort if GI side effects occur.

Consultations:
• In a patient with symptoms of blood dyscrasias, request a medical consultation for blood studies and postpone dental treatment until normal values are reestablished.
• Medical consultation may be required to assess patient's ability to tolerate stress.

Teach Patient/Family to:
• Encourage effective oral hygiene to prevent soft tissue inflammation.

quinine
kwye´-nine
(Quinine)
Do not confuse with quinidine.

CATEGORY AND SCHEDULE
Pregnancy Risk Category: X

Drug Class: Antimalarial

MECHANISM OF ACTION
A cinchona alkaloid that relaxes skeletal muscle by increasing the refractory period, decreasing excitability of motor end plates (curare-like), and affecting distribution of calcium with muscle fiber. Antimalarial: Depresses oxygen uptake, carbohydrate metabolism, elevates pH in intracellular organelles of parasites. *Therapeutic Effect:* Relaxes skeletal muscle; produces parasite death.

USES
Treatment of *P. falciparum* malaria, nocturnal leg cramps

PHARMACOKINETICS
Rapidly absorbed mainly from upper small intestine. Protein binding: 70%–95%. Metabolized in liver. Excreted in feces, saliva, and urine. *Half-life:* 8–14 hr (adults), 6–12 hr (children).

INDICATIONS AND DOSAGES
▸ **Nocturnal Leg Cramps**
PO
Adults, Elderly. 260–300 mg at bedtime as needed.
▸ **Treatment of Malaria**
PO
Adults, Elderly. 260–650 mg 3 times a day for 6–12 days.
Children. 10 mg/kg q8h for 5–7 days.

▸ **Dosage in Renal Impairment**

Creatinine Clearance	Dosage Interval
10–50 ml/min	75% of normal dose or q12h
Less than 10 ml/min	30%–50% of normal dose or q24h

SIDE EFFECTS/ADVERSE REACTIONS
Frequent
Nausea, headache, tinnitus, slight visual disturbances (mild cinchonism)
Occasional
Extreme flushing of skin with intense generalized pruritus is most typical hypersensitivity reaction; also rash, wheezing, dyspnea, angioedema
Prolonged therapy: cardiac conduction disturbances, decreased hearing

PRECAUTIONS AND CONTRAINDICATIONS
Hypersensitivity to quinine (possible cross-sensitivity to quinidine), G-6-PD deficiency, tinnitus, optic neuritis, history of thrombocytopenia during previous quinine therapy, blackwater fever
Caution:
Blood dyscrasias, severe GI disease, neurologic disease, severe hepatic disease, psoriasis, cardiac dysrhythmias, tinnitus

DRUG INTERACTIONS OF CONCERN TO DENTISTRY
• Decreased absorption: magnesium or aluminum salts
• Prolonged duration of neuromuscular blocking drugs

SERIOUS REACTIONS
! Overdosage (severe cinchonism) may result in cardiovascular effects,

Q

severe headache, intestinal cramps with vomiting and diarrhea, apprehension, confusion, seizures, blindness, and respiratory depression.

! Hypoprothrombinemia, thrombocytopenic purpura, hemoglobinuria, asthma, agranulocytosis, hypoglycemia, deafness, and optic atrophy occur rarely.

DENTAL CONSIDERATIONS

General:
• Patients on chronic drug therapy rarely may have symptoms of blood dyscrasias, which can include infection, bleeding, and poor healing.
• Avoid dental light in patient's eyes; offer dark glasses for patient comfort.

• Monitor vital signs at every appointment because of cardiovascular side effects.
• Consider semisupine chair position for patient comfort if GI side effects occur.

Consultations:
• Medical consultation may be required to assess disease control.
• In a patient with symptoms of blood dyscrasias, request a medical consultation for blood studies and postpone dental treatment until normal values are reestablished.

Teach Patient/Family to:
• Encourage effective oral hygiene to prevent soft tissue inflammation.

rabeprazole sodium
rah-**bep**'-rah-zole **soe**'-dee-um
(AcipHex, Pariet[CAN])
Do not confuse AcipHex with
Accupril or Aricept.

CATEGORY AND SCHEDULE
Pregnancy Risk Category: B

Drug Class: Antisecretory,
proton pump inhibitor

MECHANISM OF ACTION
A proton pump inhibitor that
converts to active metabolites that
irreversibly bind to and inhibit
hydrogen-potassium adenosine
triphosphate, an enzyme on the
surface of gastric parietal cells.
Actively secretes hydrogen ions for
potassium ions, resulting in an
accumulation of hydrogen ions in
gastric lumen.
Therapeutic Effect: Increases
gastric pH, reducing gastric acid
production.

USES
Treatment of gastroesophageal reflux
disease (GERD), duodenal ulcers,
and hypersecretory conditions
(Zollinger-Ellison disease);
eradication of *Helicobacter pylori*
infection (with amoxicillin and
clarithromycin), *H. pylori*
eradication to reduce risk of
duodenal ulcer

PHARMACOKINETICS
Rapidly absorbed from the GI tract
after passing through the stomach
relatively intact. Protein binding:
96%. Metabolized extensively in the
liver. Primarily excreted in urine.
Unknown if removed by
hemodialysis. *Half-life:* 1–2 hr
(increased with hepatic impairment).

INDICATIONS AND DOSAGES
▶ **GERD**
PO
Adults, Elderly. 20 mg/day for
4–8 wk. Maintenance: 20 mg/day.
▶ **Duodenal Ulcer**
PO
Adults, Elderly. 20 mg/day after
morning meal for 4 wk.
▶ **NSAID-Induced Ulcer**
PO
Adults, Elderly. 20 mg/day.
▶ **Pathologic Hypersecretory
Conditions**
PO
Adults, Elderly. Initially, 60 mg/day.
May increase to 60 mg twice a day.
▶ *Helicobacter pylori* **Infection**
PO
Adults, Elderly. 20 mg twice a day
for 7 days (given with amoxicillin
1000 mg and clarithromycin
500 mg).

SIDE EFFECTS/ADVERSE REACTIONS
Rare
Headache, nausea, dizziness, rash,
diarrhea, malaise

PRECAUTIONS AND CONTRAINDICATIONS
Hypersensitivity
Caution:
Do not break, crush, or chew tablets,
avoid nursing, pediatric use not
studied

DRUG INTERACTIONS OF CONCERN TO DENTISTRY
• None reported

SERIOUS REACTIONS
! Hyperglycemia, hypokalemia,
hyponatremia, and hyperlipemia
occur rarely.

R

DENTAL CONSIDERATIONS

General:
• Assess salivary flow as a factor in caries, periodontal disease, and candidiasis.
• Consider semisupine chair position for patient comfort because of GI side effects of disease.
• Patients with gastroesophageal reflux may have oral symptoms, including burning mouth, secondary candidiasis, and signs of tooth erosion.
• Question the patient about tolerance of NSAIDs or aspirin related to GI problems.

Teach Patient/Family to:
• Prevent trauma when using oral hygiene aids.
• When chronic dry mouth occurs, advise patient to:
  • Avoid mouth rinses with high alcohol content because of drying effects.
  • Use daily home fluoride products for anticaries effect.
  • Use sugarless gum, frequent sips of water, or saliva substitutes.

raloxifene
ra-lox′-ih-feen
(Evista)

CATEGORY AND SCHEDULE
Pregnancy Risk Category: X

Drug Class: Synthetic estrogen

MECHANISM OF ACTION
A selective estrogen receptor modulator that affects some receptors like estrogen.

Therapeutic Effect: Like estrogen, prevents bone loss and improves lipid profiles.

USES
Prevention and treatment of osteoporosis in postmenopausal women, supplemented with calcium as based on need

PHARMACOKINETICS
Rapidly absorbed after PO administration. Highly bound to plasma proteins (>95%) and albumin. Undergoes extensive first-pass metabolism in liver. Excreted mainly in feces and, to a lesser extent, in urine. Unknown if removed by hemodialysis. *Half-life:* 27.7 hr.

INDICATIONS AND DOSAGES
▶ **Prevention or Treatment of Osteoporosis**
PO
Adults, Elderly. 60 mg/day.

SIDE EFFECTS/ADVERSE REACTIONS
Frequent
Hot flashes, flu-like symptoms, arthralgia, sinusitis
Occasional
Weight gain, nausea, myalgia, pharyngitis, cough, dyspepsia, leg cramps, rash, depression
Rare
Vaginitis, UTI, peripheral edema, flatulence, vomiting, fever, migraine, diaphoresis

PRECAUTIONS AND CONTRAINDICATIONS
Active or history of venous thromboembolic events, such as deep vein thrombosis, pulmonary embolism, and retinal vein thrombosis; women who are or may become pregnant.

Caution:
Hepatic impairment, risk of thromboembolic events, pregnancy category X, lactation

DRUG INTERACTIONS OF CONCERN TO DENTISTRY
• Reduced absorption: ampicillin
• Risk of potential drug interactions with other highly plasma protein–bound drugs, such as NSAIDs, aspirin, and diazepam, is unknown

SERIOUS REACTIONS
! Pneumonia, gastroenteritis, chest pain, vaginal bleeding, and breast pain occur rarely.

DENTAL CONSIDERATIONS

General:
• Drug should be discontinued 72 hr before prolonged immobilization, such as hospitalization, postsurgical recovery, and bed rest.
• Consider short appointments and dental chair position if needed for patient comfort.
Consultations:
• Medical consultation may be required to assess disease control and patient's ability to tolerate stress.

raltegravir
ral-**teg**′-ra-veer
(Isentress)

CATEGORY AND SCHEDULE
Pregnancy Risk Category: C

Drug Class: Antiretroviral agent, integrase inhibitor

MECHANISM OF ACTION
Inhibits the catalytic activity of HIV-1 integrase, an HIV-1–encoded enzyme required for viral replication.

USES
HIV-1 infection, multidrug resistance, in combination with other antiretroviral agents

PHARMACOKINETICS
Absorption: 19% increase in AUC after a high-fat meal. Protein binding: 83%. Primarily metabolized by glucuronidation mediated by UGT1A1. **Half-life:** 9 hr. Excreted in the feces (51%) and urine (32%).

INDICATIONS AND DOSAGES
▶ HIV Infection
PO
Adults. 400 mg twice a day.
Adolescents (16 yr). 400 mg twice a day.

SIDE EFFECTS/ADVERSE REACTIONS
▶ Adult
Frequent
Increased total cholesterol
Occasional
Hypertension, fatigue, dizziness, insomnia, rash, pruritus, folliculitis, increased glucose (<250 mg/dl: 9%), increased LDL-cholesterol, hypertriglyceridemia, hyperbilirubinemia, increased AST, increased ALT, increased alkaline phosphatase, arthralgia, extremity pain, increased creatine kinase, increased creatinine, nasopharyngitis, cough, influenza, sinusitis, herpes zoster, lymphadenopathy, anogenital warts

PRECAUTIONS AND CONTRAINDICATIONS
Use with caution in patients taking medications that cause rhabdomyolysis or other risk factors for creatine kinase elevations and/or

R

skeletal muscle abnormalities due to the risk of myopathy (e.g., statins). Immune reconstitution syndrome (occurrence of an inflammatory response to an indolent or residual opportunistic infection) may occur. Use with caution when combining with UGT1A1 glucuronidation inducers, such as rifampin and inhibitors such as atazanavir.

DRUG INTERACTIONS OF CONCERN TO DENTISTRY

• None reported

SERIOUS REACTIONS

! Myopathy and rhabdomyolysis have been reported.
! Immune reconstitution syndrome has been reported.

DENTAL CONSIDERATIONS

General:
• Examine for oral manifestations of opportunistic infections.
• Patients on chronic drug therapy may rarely have symptoms of blood dyscrasias, which can include infection, bleeding, and poor healing.
• Palliative medication may be required for management of oral side effects.
Consultations:
• Medical consultation may be required to assess disease control and ability of patient to tolerate dental treatment.
• In a patient with symptoms of blood dyscrasias, request a medical consultation for blood studies and postpone dental treatment until normal values are reestablished.
Teach Patient/Family to:
• Encourage effective oral hygiene to prevent soft tissue inflammation.
• Use caution to prevent trauma when using oral hygiene aids.

• See dentist immediately if secondary oral infection occurs.

ramipril

ram′-ih-pril
(Altace, Ramace[AUS], Tritace[AUS])
Do not confuse Altace with Alteplase or Artane.

CATEGORY AND SCHEDULE

Pregnancy Risk Category: C (D if used in second or third trimester)

Drug Class: Angiotensin-converting enzyme (ACE) inhibitor

MECHANISM OF ACTION

An ACE inhibitor that suppresses the renin-angiotensin-aldosterone system. Decreases plasma angiotensin II, increases plasma renin activity, and decreases aldosterone secretion.
Therapeutic Effect: Reduces peripheral arterial resistance and B/P.

USES

Treatment of hypertension; alone or in combination with thiazide diuretics; CHF immediately after MI; reduce risk of MI, stroke, and death from cardiovascular causes

PHARMACOKINETICS

Route	Onset	Peak	Duration
PO	1–2 hr	3–6 hr	24 hr

Well absorbed from the GI tract. Protein binding: 73%. Metabolized in the liver to active metabolite. Primarily excreted in urine. Not removed by hemodialysis. *Half-life:* 5.1 hr.

INDICATIONS AND DOSAGES
▶ **Hypertension (Monotherapy)**
PO
Adults, Elderly. Initially, 2.5 mg/day. Maintenance: 2.5–20 mg/day as single dose or in 2 divided doses.
▶ **Hypertension (in Combination with Other Antihypertensives)**
PO
Adults, Elderly. Initially, 1.25 mg/day titrated to patient's needs.
▶ **CHF**
PO
Adults, Elderly. Initially, 1.25–2.5 mg twice a day. Maximum: 5 mg twice a day.
▶ **Risk Reduction for MI Stroke**
PO
Adults, Elderly. Initially, 2.5 mg/day for 7 days, then 5 mg/day for 21 days, then 10 mg/day as a single dose or in divided doses.
▶ **Dosage in Renal Impairment**
Creatinine clearance 40 ml/min or less. 25% of normal dose.
Hypertension. Initially, 1.25 mg/day titrated upward.
CHF. Initially, 1.25 mg/day, titrated up to 2.5 mg twice a day.

SIDE EFFECTS/ADVERSE REACTIONS
Frequent
Cough, headache
Occasional
Dizziness, fatigue, nausea, asthenia (loss of strength)
Rare
Palpitations, insomnia, nervousness, malaise, abdominal pain, myalgia

PRECAUTIONS AND CONTRAINDICATIONS
Bilateral renal artery stenosis

Caution:
Impaired renal/liver function, dialysis patients, hypovolemia, blood dyscrasias, CHF, COPD, asthma, elderly

DRUG INTERACTIONS OF CONCERN TO DENTISTRY
• Increased hypotension: alcohol, phenothiazines
• Decreased hypotensive effects: indomethacin and possibly other NSAIDs, sympathomimetics
• Suspected reduction in the antihypertensive and vasodilator effects by salicylates; monitor B/P if used concurrently

SERIOUS REACTIONS
! Excessive hypotension ("first-dose syncope") may occur in patients with CHF and in those who are severely salt or volume depleted.
! Angioedema and hyperkalemia occur rarely.
! Agranulocytosis and neutropenia may be noted in those with collagen vascular disease, including scleroderma and systemic lupus erythematosus, and impaired renal function.
! Nephrotic syndrome may be noted in those with history of renal disease.

DENTAL CONSIDERATIONS

General:
• Monitor vital signs at every appointment because of cardiovascular and respiratory side effects.
• After supine positioning, have patient sit upright for at least 2 min before standing to avoid orthostatic hypotension.
• Patients on chronic drug therapy may rarely have symptoms of blood dyscrasias, which can include

R

infection, bleeding, and poor healing.

• Assess salivary flow as a factor in caries, periodontal disease, and candidiasis.

• Limit use of sodium-containing products, such as saline IV fluids, for patients with a dietary salt restriction.

• Use vasoconstrictors with caution, in low doses, and with careful aspiration.

• Stress from dental procedures may compromise cardiovascular function; determine patient risk.

• Short appointments and a stress-reduction protocol may be required for anxious patients.

Consultations:

• Medical consultation may be required to assess patient's ability to tolerate stress.

• In a patient with symptoms of blood dyscrasias, request a medical consultation for blood studies and postpone dental treatment until normal values are reestablished.

• Take precautions if dental surgery is anticipated and sedation or general anesthesia is required; risk of hypotensive episode.

Teach Patient/Family to:

• Encourage effective oral hygiene to prevent soft tissue inflammation.

• Use caution to prevent injury when using oral hygiene aids.

• When chronic dry mouth occurs, advise patient to:

  • Avoid mouth rinses with high alcohol content because of drying effects.

  • Use daily home fluoride products to prevent caries.

  • Use sugarless gum, frequent sips of water, or saliva substitutes.

ranitidine hydrochloride/ ranitidine bismuth citrate

ra-**ni**′-ti-deen high-droh-**klor**′-ide/ ra-**ni**′-ti-deen **biss**′-mooth **sih**′-trate

(ranitidine hydrochloride: Apo-Ranitidine[CAN], Ausran[AUS], Novo-Ranitidine[CAN], Rani-2[AUS], Ranihexal[AUS], Zantac, Zantac-75, Zantac-150, Zantac-300, Zantac EFFERdose, Zantac-25 EFFERdose, Zantac-150 EFFERdose, Zantac-150 Maximum Strength; ranitidine bismuth citrate: Pylorid[AUS], Tritec)

Do not confuse Zantac with Xanax, Ziac, or Zyrtec.

CATEGORY AND SCHEDULE

Pregnancy Risk Category: B

OTC (75 mg tablets)

Drug Class: H_2 histamine receptor antagonist

MECHANISM OF ACTION

An antiulcer agent that inhibits histamine action at histamine 2 receptors of gastric parietal cells.

Therapeutic Effect: Inhibits gastric acid secretion when fasting, at night, or when stimulated by food, caffeine, or insulin. Reduces volume and hydrogen ion concentration of gastric juice.

USES

Treatment of duodenal ulcer, Zollinger-Ellison syndrome, benign gastric ulcers, hypersecretory conditions, gastroesophageal reflux disease, erosive esophagitis, stress ulcers; unapproved: treatment of GI

symptoms associated with NSAID
use in rheumatoid arthritis

PHARMACOKINETICS
Rapidly absorbed from the GI tract.
Protein binding: 15%. Widely
distributed. Metabolized in the liver.
Primarily excreted in urine. Not
removed by hemodialysis. *Half-life:*
PO, 2.5 hr; IV, 2–2.5 hr (increased
with impaired renal function).

INDICATIONS AND DOSAGES
▸ **Duodenal Ulcers, Gastric Ulcers,
Gastroesophageal Reflux Disease**
PO
Adults, Elderly. 150 mg twice a day
or 300 mg at bedtime. Maintenance:
150 mg at bedtime.
Children. 2–4 mg/kg/day in divided
doses twice a day. Maximum:
300 mg/day.
▸ **Duodenal Ulcers Associated with
H. pylori Infection**
PO
Adults, Elderly. 400 mg twice a day
for 4 wk in combination with
clarithromycin 500 mg 2–3 times a
day for the first 2 wk.
▸ **Erosive Esophagitis**
PO
Adults, Elderly. 150 mg 4 times a
day. Maintenance: 150 mg twice a
day or 300 mg at bedtime.
Children. 4–10 mg/kg/day in 2
divided doses. Maximum: 600 mg/
day.
▸ **Hypersecretory Conditions**
PO
Adults, Elderly. 150 mg twice a day.
May increase up to 6 g/day.
▸ **OTC Use**
PO
Adults, Elderly. 75 mg 30–60 min
before eating food or drinking
beverages that cause heartburn.
Maximum: 150 mg per 24-hr period
and/or longer than 14 days.

▸ **Usual Parenteral Dosage**
IV, IM
Adults, Elderly. 50 mg/dose q6–8h.
Maximum: 400 mg/day.
Children. 2–4 mg/kg/day in divided
doses q6–8h. Maximum: 200 mg/
day.
▸ **Usual Neonatal Dosage**
PO
Neonates. 2 mg/kg/day in divided
doses q12h.
IV
Neonates. Initially, 1.5 mg/kg/dose;
then 1.5–2 mg/kg/day in divided
doses q12h.
▸ **Dosage in Renal Impairment**
For patients with creatinine
clearance less than 50 ml/min, give
150 mg PO q24h or 50 mg IV or IM
q18–24h.

SIDE EFFECTS/ADVERSE REACTIONS
Occasional
Diarrhea
Rare
Constipation, headache (may be
severe)

PRECAUTIONS AND CONTRAINDICATIONS
History of acute porphyria
Caution:
Pregnancy category B, lactation,
children younger than 12 yr, hepatic
disease, renal disease

DRUG INTERACTIONS OF CONCERN TO DENTISTRY
• Decreased absorption of diazepam,
anticholinergics, ketoconazole (take
doses 2 hr apart)

SERIOUS REACTIONS
! Reversible hepatitis and blood
dyscrasias occur rarely.

General:

• Avoid prescribing aspirin-containing products in patients with active GI disease.

• Consider semisupine chair position for patient comfort because of GI effects of disease.

rasagiline
rah-sa'-ji-leen
(Azilect)

CATEGORY AND SCHEDULE
Pregnancy Risk Category: C

Drug Class: Monoamine oxidase inhibitor

MECHANISM OF ACTION
An antiparkinson agent that irreversibly inhibits monoamine oxidase type B (more selective for MOA type B than type A).
Therapeutic Effect: Relieves signs and symptoms of Parkinson's disease.

USES
Parkinson's disease, monotherapy or adjunct therapy

PHARMACOKINETICS
Rapidly absorbed after PO administration. Protein binding: 88%–94%. Extensively metabolized in liver, primarily by CYP1A2. Less than 1% is excreted unchanged in the urine. **Half-life:** 1.34 hr.

INDICATIONS AND DOSAGES
▶ **Parkinson's Disease, Monotherapy**
PO
Adults. 1 mg a day.

▶ **Parkinson's Disease, Adjunct**
PO
Adults. 0.5 mg a day. May increase to 1 mg a day if clinical response is not achieved.

▶ **Hepatic Impairment**
Mild to moderate. 0.5 mg a day.
Severe hepatic impairment. Not recommended.

SIDE EFFECTS/ADVERSE REACTIONS
Frequent
Headache, orthostatic hypotension, rash, weight loss, GI upset, arthralgia, dyspepsia, depression, fall, flu syndrome, vertigo
Occasional
Conjunctivitis, fever, gastroenteritis, rhinitis, arthritis, ecchymosis, malaise, neck pain, paresthesia

PRECAUTIONS AND CONTRAINDICATIONS
Hypersensitivity to rasagiline or its components
Concurrent use with meperidine, tramadol, propoxyphene, dextromethorphan, St. John's wort, cyclobenzaprine, or other MAO inhibitors
Caution:
Hepatic impairment
Concurrent use with sympathomimetics, tyramine-containing foods, CYP1A2 inhibitors
Melanoma

DRUG INTERACTIONS OF CONCERN TO DENTISTRY
• Opioids (particularly meperidine): fatal interaction; serotonin syndrome; contraindicated
• St. John's wort, cyclobenzaprine: contraindicated
• Dextromethorphan: concurrent use may cause psychosis or bizarre behavior; contraindicated

• MOA inhibitors: may increase the risk of hypertensive crisis; contraindicated
• Potent CYP1A2 inhibitors (cimetidine, ciprofloxacin, fluvoxamine): may increase levels of rasagiline
• CYP inducers: may reduce rasagiline levels
• Sympathomimetics, tyramine-containing foods: may increase the risk of hypertensive crisis
• Antidepressants (SSRIs, SNRIs, TCAs): increased risk of serotonin syndrome

SERIOUS REACTIONS

! Rasagiline may cause low blood pressure; increased risk of postural hypotension.
! May cause or exacerbate hallucinations and psychotic behavior.
! Symptoms of overdose may vary from CNS depression, characterized by sedation, apnea, cardiovascular collapse, and death, to severe paradoxical reactions, such as hallucinations, tremor, and seizures.
! Other serious effects may include involuntary movements, impaired motor coordination, loss of balance, blepharospasm, facial grimaces, feeling of heaviness in the lower extremities, depression, nightmares, delusions, overstimulation, sleep disturbance, and anger.

DENTAL CONSIDERATIONS

General:
• Monitor vital signs at every appointment because of cardiovascular side effects.
• After supine positioning, have patient sit upright for at least 2 min before standing to avoid orthostatic hypotension.

• Assess for presence of extrapyramidal motor symptoms, such as tardive dyskinesia and akathisia. Extrapyramidal motor activity may complicate dental treatment.
• Assess salivary flow as a factor in caries, periodontal disease, and candidiasis.
• Consider semisupine chair position for patient comfort if GI side effects occur.
Consultations:
• Medical consultation may be required to assess disease control and patient's ability to tolerate stress.
• If signs of tardive dyskinesia or akathisia present, refer to physician.
Teach Patient/Family to:
• When chronic dry mouth occurs, advise patient to:
  • Avoid mouth rinses with high alcohol content because of drying effects.
  • Use daily home fluoride products for anticaries effect.
  • Use sugarless gum, frequent sips of water, or saliva substitutes.

R

repaglinide
re-**pag**'-lih-nide
(GlucoNorm[CAN], Novo Norm[AUS], Prandin)

CATEGORY AND SCHEDULE
Pregnancy Risk Category: C

Drug Class: Oral antidiabetic, meglitinide class

MECHANISM OF ACTION
An antihyperglycemic that stimulates release of insulin from

beta cells of the pancreas by depolarizing beta cells, leading to an opening of calcium channels. Resulting calcium influx induces insulin secretion.
Therapeutic Effect: Lowers blood glucose concentration.

USES
Treatment of Type 2 diabetes mellitus when hyperglycemia cannot be controlled by diet and exercise; may also be used in combination with metformin, rosiglitazone maleate, or pioglitazone HCl

PHARMACOKINETICS
Rapidly, completely absorbed from the GI tract. Protein binding: 98%. Metabolized in the liver to inactive metabolites. Excreted primarily in feces with a lesser amount in urine. Unknown if removed by hemodialysis. *Half-life:* 1 hr.

INDICATIONS AND DOSAGES
▶ **Diabetes Mellitus**
PO
Adults, Elderly. 0.5–4 mg 2–4 times a day. Maximum: 16 mg/day.

SIDE EFFECTS/ADVERSE REACTIONS
Frequent
Upper respiratory tract infection, headache, rhinitis, bronchitis, back pain
Occasional
Diarrhea, dyspepsia, sinusitis, nausea, arthralgia, UTI
Rare
Constipation, vomiting, paresthesia, allergy

PRECAUTIONS AND CONTRAINDICATIONS
Diabetic ketoacidosis, type 1 diabetes mellitus

Caution:
Increased cardiac mortality risk, hypoglycemia, hypoglycemia in patients taking adrenergic blockers, monitor laboratory values, lactation, pediatric patients

DRUG INTERACTIONS OF CONCERN TO DENTISTRY
• Clinical studies have not been completed; metabolism may be inhibited by ketoconazole, miconazole, erythromycin
• Risk of increased hypoglycemia: NSAIDs, salicylates
• Suspected increase in plasma levels: clarithromycin, erythromycin

SERIOUS REACTIONS
! Hypoglycemia occurs in 16% of patients.
! Chest pain occurs rarely.

DENTAL CONSIDERATIONS

General:
• If dentist prescribes any of the drugs listed in the drug interactions section, monitor patient blood sugar levels.
• Consider semisupine chair position for patient comfort because of GI side effects of drug.
• Ensure that patient is following prescribed diet and regularly takes medication.
• Place on frequent recall to evaluate healing response.
• Short appointments and a stress-reduction protocol may be required.
• Diabetics may be more susceptible to infection and have delayed wound healing.
Consultations:
• Medical consultation may include data from patient's blood glucose monitoring, including glycosylated hemoglobin or HbA_{1c} testing.

- Medical consultation may be required to assess disease control and patient's ability to tolerate stress.

Teach Patient/Family to:
- Prevent trauma when using oral hygiene aids.
- Update health and drug history if physician makes any changes in evaluation or drug regimens; include OTC, herbal, and nonherbal drugs in the update.

reserpine
reh-**zer**'-peen
(Serpalan, Maviserpin[MEX],
Novoreserpine[CAN],
Rauserpine[TAIWAN],
Rauverid[PHILIPPINES],
Reserfia[CAN], Serpasil[CAN,
INDONESIA], Serpasol[SPAIN])
Do not confuse with Risperdal, risperidone

CATEGORY AND SCHEDULE
Pregnancy Risk Category: C

Drug Class: Antiadrenergic agent, antihypertensive

MECHANISM OF ACTION
An antihypertensive that depletes stores of catecholamines and 5-hydroxytryptamine in many organs, including the brain and adrenal medulla. Depression of sympathetic nerve function results in a decreased heart rate and a lowering of arterial B/P. Depletion of catecholamines and 5-hydroxytryptamine from the brain is thought to be the mechanism of the sedative and tranquilizing properties.
Therapeutic Effects: Decrease B/P and heart rate; sedation.

USES
Treatment of refractory hypertension

PHARMACOKINETICS
Characterized by slow onset of action and sustained effects. Both cardiovascular and CNS effects may persist for a period of time following withdrawal of the drug. Mean maximum plasma levels were attained after a median of 3.5 hr. Bioavailability was approximately 50% of that of a corresponding intravenous dose. Protein binding: 96%. **Half-life:** 33 hr.

INDICATIONS AND DOSAGES
▸ **Hypertension**
PO
Adults. Usual initial dosage 0.5 mg/day for 1 or 2 wk. For maintenance, reduce to 0.1–0.25 mg/day.
Children. Reserpine is not recommended for use in children. If it is to be used in treating a child, the usual recommended starting dose is 20 mcg/kg daily. The maximum recommended dose is 0.25 mg (total) daily.
▸ **Psychiatric Disorders**
PO
Adults. Initial dosage 0.5 mg/day, may range from 0.1 to 1.0 mg. Adjust dosage upward or downward according to response.

SIDE EFFECTS/ADVERSE REACTIONS
Occasional
Burning in the stomach, nausea, vomiting, diarrhea, dry mouth, nosebleed, stuffy nose, dizziness, headache, nervousness, nightmares, drowsiness, muscle aches, weight gain, redness of the eyes
Rare
Irregular heart beat, difficulty breathing, heart problems, feeling

R

faint, swelling, gynecomastia, decreased libido

PRECAUTIONS AND CONTRAINDICATIONS

Hypersensitivity, mental depression or history of mental depression (especially with suicidal tendencies), active peptic ulcer, ulcerative colitis, patients receiving electroconvulsive therapy

Caution:
Lactation, seizure disorders, renal disease

DRUG INTERACTIONS OF CONCERN TO DENTISTRY

• Increased CNS depression: barbiturates, alcohol, opioids
• Increased pressor effects: epinephrine
• Decreased pressor effects: ephedrine, tricyclic antidepressants
• Decreased hypotensive effect: NSAIDs

SERIOUS REACTIONS

! None known

DENTAL CONSIDERATIONS

General:
• After supine positioning, have patient sit upright for at least 2 min before standing to avoid orthostatic hypotension.
  • Use vasoconstrictors with caution, in low doses, and with careful aspiration.
  • Avoid stress; consider a stress-reduction protocol.
Consultations:
• Medical consultation may be required to assess disease control.
Teach Patient/Family to:
• Encourage effective oral hygiene to prevent soft tissue inflammation.
• When chronic dry mouth occurs, advise patient to:

• Avoid mouth rinses with high alcohol content because of drying effects.
• Use daily home fluoride products to prevent caries.
• Use sugarless gum, frequent sips of water, or saliva substitutes.

retapamulin
ee-te-**pam**′-ue-lin
(Altabax)

CATEGORY AND SCHEDULE
Pregnancy Risk Category: B

Drug Class: Antibiotic

MECHANISM OF ACTION

Bacteriostatic binds to protein L2 on the ribosomal 50S subunit, inhibits peptidyl transfer and blocks P-site interaction to prevent formation of this subunit; therefore, inhibits bacterial protein biosynthesis.

USES

Impetigo caused by *Staphylococcus aureus* or *Streptococcus pyogenes*

PHARMACOKINETICS

When applied topically, low systemic absorption. Absorption increased when applied to abraded skin. Protein binding is 94%. Extensively metabolized in the liver via CYP 3A4.

INDICATIONS AND DOSAGES
▸ **Impetigo Caused by**
Staphylococcus aureus **or**
Streptococcus pyogenes
Topical
Adults. Apply to the affected area (up to 100 cm² in total area) twice a day for 5 days.

Children (9 mo or older). Apply to the affected area (2% total body surface area) twice a day for 5 days.

SIDE EFFECTS/ADVERSE REACTIONS
Occasional
▸ **Adults**
Headache, application site irritation, diarrhea, nausea, nasopharyngitis, increased creatinine phosphokinase.
▸ **Children**
Application site pruritus, diarrhea, nasopharyngitis, pruritus, eczema, headache, pyrexia.

PRECAUTIONS AND CONTRAINDICATIONS
Contraindicated in patients with hypersensitivity to retapamulin or components of the formulation. Sensitization or severe local irritation may occur.
Retapamulin is for external use only and has not been proven for intranasal, intravaginal, ophthalmic, oral, or mucosal application.

DRUG INTERACTIONS OF CONCERN TO DENTISTRY
• None reported

SERIOUS REACTIONS
! Superinfections may result from altered bacterial balance.

DENTAL CONSIDERATIONS
General:
• Consider semisupine chair position for patient comfort if GI side effects occur.
Consultations:
• Medical consultation may be required to assess disease control.
Teach Patient/Family to:
• Encourage effective oral hygiene to prevent soft tissue inflammation.
• Use caution to prevent injury when using oral hygiene aids.

reteplase, recombinant
reh′-te-place
(Rapilysin[AUS], Retavase)
Do not confuse reteplase or Retavase with Restasis.

CATEGORY AND SCHEDULE
Pregnancy Risk Category: C

Drug Class: Thrombolytic

MECHANISM OF ACTION
A tissue plasminogen activator that activates the fibrinolytic system by directly cleaving plasminogen to generate plasmin, an enzyme that degrades the fibrin of the thrombus. *Therapeutic Effect:* Exerts thrombolytic action.

USES
Dissolving of blood clots that have formed in certain blood vessels

PHARMACOKINETICS
Rapidly cleared from plasma. Eliminated primarily by the liver and kidney. *Half-life:* 13–16 min.

INDICATIONS AND DOSAGES
▸ **Acute MI, CHF**
IV Bolus
Adults, Elderly. 10 units over 2 min; repeat in 30 min.

SIDE EFFECTS/ADVERSE REACTIONS
Frequent
Bleeding at superficial sites, such as venous injection sites, catheter insertion sites, venous cutdowns, arterial punctures, and sites of recent surgical procedures, gingival bleeding

R

PRECAUTIONS AND CONTRAINDICATIONS

Active internal bleeding, AV malformation or aneurysm, bleeding diathesis, history of cerebrovascular accident, intracranial neoplasm, recent intracranial or intraspinal surgery or trauma, severe uncontrolled hypertension

DRUG INTERACTIONS OF CONCERN TO DENTISTRY

• Increased risk of bleeding: drugs that interfere with coagulation or platelet function, such as NSAIDs or aspirin

SERIOUS REACTIONS

! Bleeding at internal sites may occur, including intracranial, retroperitoneal, GI, GU, and respiratory sites.
! Lysis or coronary thrombi may produce atrial or ventricular arrhythmias and stroke.

DENTAL CONSIDERATIONS

General:
• Acute-use drug for use in hospitals or emergency rooms.
• Patients are at risk for bleeding, check for oral signs.
• Monitor and record vital signs.
• Avoid products that affect platelet function, such as aspirin and NSAIDs.
• Patients who have been treated with this drug may present with cardiovascular disease or stroke, review medical and drug history.
Consultations:
• Medical consultation should include routine blood counts including platelet counts and bleeding time.
• In a patient with symptoms of blood dyscrasias, request a medical consultation for blood studies and

postpone treatment until normal values are reestablished.
• Medical consultation may be required to assess disease control and patient's ability to tolerate stress.
Teach Patient/Family to:
• Use soft tooth brush to reduce risk of bleeding.
• Encourage effective oral hygiene to prevent soft tissue inflammation.
• Report oral lesions, soreness, or bleeding to dentist.
• Prevent trauma when using oral hygiene aids.
• Update health and medication history if physician makes any changes in evaluation or drug regimens; include OTC, herbal, and nonherbal remedies in the update.

ribavirin

rye-ba-**vye′**-rin
(Copegus, Rebetol, Rebetron, Virazole)
Do not confuse ribavirin with riboflavin.

CATEGORY AND SCHEDULE

Pregnancy Risk Category: X

Drug Class: Antiviral

MECHANISM OF ACTION

A synthetic nucleoside that inhibits influenza virus RNA polymerase activity and interferes with expression of messenger RNA.
Therapeutic Effect: Inhibits viral protein synthesis and replication of viral RNA and DNA.

USES

Treatment of adults and children with chronic hepatitis C but only in combination with interferon alfa-2b or peginterferon alfa-2a; patients must have compensated liver disease and not previously been treated with interferons; respiratory syncytial virus (RSV) in hospitalized infants and young children, unapproved use in influenza A or B or in lower respiratory tract pneumonia associated with an adenovirus

PHARMACOKINETICS

Rapidly absorbed from the GI tract following oral administration. A small amount is systemically absorbed following inhalation. Primarily excreted in urine.
Half-life: 298 hr (oral); 9.5 hr (inhalation).

INDICATIONS AND DOSAGES
▸ **Chronic Hepatitis C**
PO (Capsule or Oral Solution in Combination with Interferon Alfa-2b)
Adults, Elderly. 1000–1200 mg/day in 2 divided doses.
Children weighing 60 kg or more. Use adult dosage. (51–60 kg): 400 mg twice a day. (37–50 kg): 200 mg in morning, 400 mg in evening. (24–36 kg): 200 mg twice a day.
PO (Capsules in Combination with Peginterferon Alfa-2b)
Adults, Elderly. 800 mg/day in 2 divided doses.
PO (Tablets in Combination with Peginterferon Alfa-2b)
Adults, Elderly. 800–1200 mg/day in 2 divided doses.
▸ **Severe Lower Respiratory Tract Infection Caused by RSV**
Inhalation
Children, Infants. Use with Vivatek small-particle aerosol generator at a concentration of 20 mg/ml (6 g reconstituted with 300 ml sterile water) over 12–18 hr/day for 3–7 days.

SIDE EFFECTS/ADVERSE REACTIONS
Frequent
Dizziness, headache, fatigue, fever, insomnia, irritability, depression, emotional lability, impaired concentration, alopecia, rash, pruritus, nausea, anorexia, dyspepsia, vomiting, decreased hemoglobin, hemolysis, arthralgia, musculoskeletal pain, dyspnea, sinusitis, flu-like symptoms
Occasional
Nervousness, altered taste, weakness

PRECAUTIONS AND CONTRAINDICATIONS
Autoimmune hepatitis, creatinine clearance less than 50 ml/min, hemoglobinopathies, hepatic decompensation, hypersensitivity to ribavirin products, pregnancy, significant or unstable cardiac disease, women of childbearing age who will not use contraception reliably
Caution:
Must not be used alone for hepatitis C, severe side effects occur, pregnancy category X, aggravation of sarcoidosis, stop therapy if pancreatitis occurs, use aerosol only for RSV, extra contraception required to prevent pregnancy during use and for up to 6 mo after discontinuing use

DRUG INTERACTIONS OF CONCERN TO DENTISTRY
• None reported

SERIOUS REACTIONS
! Cardiac arrest, apnea, and ventilator dependence, bacterial pneumonia, pneumonia, and pneumothorax occur rarely.
! Anemia may occur if ribavirin therapy exceeds 7 days.

R

DENTAL CONSIDERATIONS

General:
• Patients taking this drug will also be taking an interferon drug; be sure to conduct a thorough drug history.
• Assess salivary flow as a factor in caries, periodontal disease, and candidiasis.
• Patients on chronic drug therapy may rarely have symptoms of blood dyscrasias, which can include infection, bleeding, and poor healing.
• Consider semisupine chair position for patient comfort if GI side effects occur.
• Examine for oral manifestation of opportunistic infection.
• Take precautions if dental surgery is anticipated and general anesthesia is required.
• Monitor vital signs at every appointment because of cardiovascular side effects.

Consultations:
• In a patient with symptoms of blood dyscrasias, request a medical consultation for blood studies and postpone treatment until normal values are reestablished.
• Medical consultation may be required to assess disease control and patient's ability to tolerate stress.
• Consultation with physician may be necessary if sedation or general anesthesia is required.

Teach Patient/Family to:
• Update health and drug history if physician makes any changes in evaluation or drug regimens; include OTC, herbal, and nonherbal drugs in the update.
• Encourage effective oral hygiene to prevent soft tissue inflammation.
• Prevent trauma when using oral hygiene aids.

• When chronic dry mouth occurs, advise patient to:
  • Avoid mouth rinses with high alcohol content because of drying effects.
  • Use daily home fluoride products for anticaries effect.
  • Use sugarless gum, frequent sips of water, or saliva substitutes.

rifabutin

rif′-ah-byoo-ten
(Mycobutin)
Do not confuse rifabutin with rifampin.

CATEGORY AND SCHEDULE
Pregnancy Risk Category: B

Drug Class: Antimycobacterial

MECHANISM OF ACTION
An antitubercular that inhibits DNA-dependent RNA polymerase, an enzyme in susceptible strains of *Escherichia coli* and *Bacillus subtilis*. Rifabutin has a broad spectrum of antimicrobial activity, including against mycobacteria such as *Mycobacterium avium* complex (MAC).
Therapeutic Effect: Prevents MAC disease.

USES
Prevention of disseminated MAC disease with advanced HIV infection

PHARMACOKINETICS
Readily absorbed from the GI tract (high-fat meals delay absorption). Protein binding: 85%. Widely distributed. Crosses the blood-brain barrier. Extensive intracellular tissue

uptake. Metabolized in the liver to active metabolite. Excreted in urine; eliminated in feces. Unknown if removed by hemodialysis. *Half-life:* 16–69 hr.

INDICATIONS AND DOSAGES
▶ **Prevention of MAC Disease (First Episode)**
PO
Adults, Elderly. 300 mg as a single dose or in 2 divided doses if GI upset occurs.
▶ **Prevention of Recurrent MAC Disease**
PO
Adults, Elderly. 300 mg/day (in combination).
▶ **Dosage in Renal Impairment**
Dosage is modified on the basis of creatinine clearance. If creatinine clearance is less than 30 ml/min, reduce dosage by 50%.

SIDE EFFECTS/ADVERSE REACTIONS
Frequent
Red-orange or red-brown discoloration of urine, feces, saliva, skin, sputum, sweat, or tears
Occasional
Rash, nausea, abdominal pain, diarrhea, dyspepsia, belching, headache, altered taste, uveitis, corneal deposits
Rare
Anorexia, flatulence, fever, myalgia, vomiting, insomnia

PRECAUTIONS AND CONTRAINDICATIONS
Active tuberculosis; hypersensitivity to other rifamycins, including rifampin
Caution:
Pregnancy category B, lactation, concurrent corticosteroid therapy

DRUG INTERACTIONS OF CONCERN TO DENTISTRY
• Decreases plasma concentrations of corticosteroids; may be significant
• May induce CYP3A4 isoenzymes, possible reduction in action of ketoconazole, itraconazole, benzodiazepines, doxycycline, erythromycin, clarithromycin

SERIOUS REACTIONS
! Hepatitis and thrombocytopenia occur rarely. Anemia and neutropenia may also occur.

DENTAL CONSIDERATIONS
General:
• Examine for evidence of oral signs of opportunistic disease.
• Determine why the patient is taking the drug.
• Patients on chronic drug therapy may rarely have symptoms of blood dyscrasias, which can include infection, bleeding, and poor healing.
Consultations:
• Medical consultation may be required to assess patient's ability to tolerate stress.
• In a patient with symptoms of blood dyscrasias, request a medical consultation for blood studies and postpone dental treatment until normal values are reestablished.
Teach Patient/Family to:
• Avoid mouth rinses with high alcohol content because of drying effects.
• Encourage effective oral hygiene to prevent soft tissue inflammation.

R

rifampin

rye′-fam-pin
(Rifadin, Rimactane, Rimycin[AUS], Rofact[CAN])
Do not confuse rifampin with rifabutin, Rifamate, rifapentine, or Ritalin.

CATEGORY AND SCHEDULE
Pregnancy Risk Category: C

Drug Class: Antitubercular antiinfective

MECHANISM OF ACTION
An antitubercular that interferes with bacterial RNA synthesis by binding to DNA-dependent RNA polymerase, thus preventing its attachment to DNA and blocking RNA transcription.
Therapeutic Effect: Bactericidal in susceptible microorganisms.

USES
Pulmonary tuberculosis (TB), meningococcal carriers (prevention); unapproved: leprosy and atypical mycobacterial infections

PHARMACOKINETICS
Well absorbed from the GI tract (food delays absorption). Protein binding: 80%. Widely distributed. Metabolized in the liver to active metabolite. Primarily eliminated by the biliary system. Not removed by hemodialysis. *Half-life:* 3–5 hr (increased in hepatic impairment).

INDICATIONS AND DOSAGES
▸ **Tuberculosis**
PO, IV
Adults, Elderly. 10 mg/kg/day. Maximum: 600 mg/day.
Children. 10–20 mg/kg/day in divided doses q12–24h.

▸ **Prevention of Meningococcal Infections**
PO, IV
Adults, Elderly. 600 mg q12h for 2 days.
Children 1 mo and older. 20 mg/kg/day in divided doses q12–24h. Maximum: 600 mg/dose.
Infants younger than 1 mo. 10 mg/kg/day in divided doses q12h for 2 days.

▸ **Staphylococcal Infections**
PO, IV
Adults, Elderly. 600 mg/day.
Children. 15 mg/kg/day in divided doses q12h.

▸ *Staphylococcus aureus* **Infections (in Combination with Other Antiinfectives)**
PO
Adults, Elderly. 300–600 mg twice a day.
Neonates. 5–20 mg/kg/day in divided doses q12h.

▸ **Prevention of** *Haemophilus influenzae* **Infection**
PO
Adults, Elderly. 600 mg/day for 4 days.
Children 1 mo and older. 20 mg/kg/day in divided doses q12h for 5–10 days.
Children younger than 1 mo. 10 mg/kg/day in divided doses q12h for 2 days.

SIDE EFFECTS/ADVERSE REACTIONS
Expected
Red-orange or red-brown discoloration of urine, feces, saliva, skin, sputum, sweat, or tears
Occasional
Hypersensitivity reaction (such as flushing, pruritus, or rash)
Rare
Diarrhea, dyspepsia, nausea, candida as evidenced by sore mouth or tongue

PRECAUTIONS AND CONTRAINDICATIONS

Concomitant therapy with amprenavir, hypersensitivity to rifampin or any other rifamycins

Caution:

Lactation, hepatic disease, blood dyscrasias, concurrent therapy with corticosteroids

Reduced effectiveness of oral contraceptives

DRUG INTERACTIONS OF CONCERN TO DENTISTRY

• Increased risk of hepatotoxicity: acetaminophen (chronic use and high doses), alcohol, hydrocarbon inhalation anesthetics (except isoflurane)

• Decreased effects of corticosteroids, dapsone, ketoconazole, fluconazole, itraconazole, oral contraceptives, benzodiazepines, doxycycline, erythromycin, clarithromycin, opioid analgesics

• Suspected decrease in fexofenadine effects

• Induces CYP450 isoenzymes

SERIOUS REACTIONS

! Rare reactions include hepatotoxicity (risk is increased when rifampin is taken with isoniazid), hepatitis, blood dyscrasias, Stevens-Johnson syndrome, and antibiotic-associated colitis.

DENTAL CONSIDERATIONS

General:

• Examine for oral manifestation of opportunistic infections.

• Do not treat patients with active tuberculosis.

• Patients on chronic drug therapy may rarely have symptoms of blood dyscrasias, which can include infection, bleeding, and poor healing.

• Determine why the patient is taking the drug (prophylaxis or active therapy).

• Determine that noninfectious status exists by ensuring that (1) anti-TB drugs have been taken for longer than 3 wk, (2) culture has confirmed TB susceptibility to antiinfectives, (3) patient has had three consecutive negative sputum smears, and (4) patient is not in the coughing stage.

Consultations:

• Medical consultation may be required to assess patient's ability to tolerate stress.

• In a patient with symptoms of blood dyscrasias, request a medical consultation for blood studies and postpone dental treatment until normal values are reestablished.

Teach Patient/Family to:

• Avoid mouth rinses with high alcohol content because of drying effects.

• Encourage effective oral hygiene to prevent soft tissue inflammation.

• Take medications for full length of regimen to ensure effectiveness of treatment and to prevent the emergence of resistant strains.

R

rifapentine

rif-ah-**pen**′-teen

(Priftin)

Do not confuse rifapentine with rifampin.

CATEGORY AND SCHEDULE

Pregnancy Risk Category: C

Drug Class: Antimycobacterial

MECHANISM OF ACTION

An antitubercular that inhibits bacterial RNA synthesis by binding to DNA-dependent RNA polymerase in *Mycobacterium tuberculosis*. This action prevents the enzyme from attaching to DNA, thereby blocking RNA transcription.
Therapeutic Effect: Bactericidal.

USES

Treatment of pulmonary tuberculosis (TB) in combination with other anti-TB drugs; unlabeled use includes prophylaxis of *Mycobacterium avium* complex (MAC) in patients with AIDS

PHARMACOKINETICS

PO: Slow absorption, peak levels 5–6 hr, highly plasma protein bound (97%–93%), hepatic metabolism, 25-desacetylrifapentine is active metabolite, hepatic metabolism, excreted in feces (70%) and urine (17%).

INDICATIONS AND DOSAGES

▸ **TB**
PO
Adults, Elderly. Intensive phase: 600 mg twice a wk for 2 mo (interval between doses no less than 3 days). Continuation phase: 600 mg/wk for 4 mo.

SIDE EFFECTS/ADVERSE REACTIONS

Rare
Red-orange or red-brown discoloration of urine, feces, saliva, skin, sputum, sweat, or tears; arthralgia, pain, nausea, vomiting, headache, dyspepsia, hypertension, dizziness, diarrhea

PRECAUTIONS AND CONTRAINDICATIONS

Hypersensitivity to rifampin, rifabutin
Caution:
Significant hepatic dysfunction, induces hepatic microsomal enzymes, pregnancy category C, lactation, children younger than 12 yr

DRUG INTERACTIONS OF CONCERN TO DENTISTRY

• May accelerate metabolism of clarithromycin, doxycycline, ciprofloxacin, fluconazole, ketoconazole, itraconazole, diazepam, barbiturates, corticosteroids, opioids, zolpidem, sildenafil, tricyclic antidepressants
• Inducer of CYP3A4 and CYP2C8/9 isoenzymes may cause drug interactions

SERIOUS REACTIONS

! Hyperuricemia, neutropenia, proteinuria, hematuria, and hepatitis occur rarely.

DENTAL CONSIDERATIONS

General:
• Determine why patient is taking the drug (prophylaxis or active therapy).
• Examine for oral manifestation of opportunistic infections.
• Do not treat patients with active tuberculosis.
• Patients on chronic drug therapy may rarely have symptoms of blood dyscrasias, which can include infection, bleeding, and poor healing.
• Determine that noninfectious status exists by ensuring that (1) anti-TB drugs have been taken for longer than 3 wk, (2) culture has confirmed TB susceptibility to

antiinfectives, (3) patient has had three consecutive negative sputum smears, and (4) patient is not in the coughing stage.

• Consider semisupine chair position for patient comfort because of GI side effects of drug.

Consultations:

• Medical consultation may be required to assess disease control and patient's ability to tolerate stress.

• In a patient with symptoms of blood dyscrasias, request a medical consultation for blood studies and postpone treatment until normal values are reestablished.

Teach Patient/Family to:

• Avoid mouth rinses with high alcohol content because of drying effects.

• Prevent trauma when using oral hygiene aids.

• Encourage effective oral hygiene to prevent soft tissue inflammation.

• Take medication for full length of regimen to ensure effectiveness of treatment and prevent emergence of resistant strains.

• Be aware of potential for extrinsic oral staining side effect.

---

rifaximin
rye-fax′-ih-min
(Xifaxan)
Do not confuse with rifampin.

CATEGORY AND SCHEDULE
Pregnancy Risk Category: C

Drug Class: Antibiotic

MECHANISM OF ACTION
An anti-infective that inhibits bacterial RNA synthesis by binding to the beta subunit of bacterial DNA-dependent RNA polymerase. Resulting in inhibition of bacterial RNA synthesis.
Therapeutic Effect: Bactericidal.

USES
Traveler's diarrhea
Hepatic encephalopathy

PHARMACOKINETICS
Less than 0.4% absorbed after PO administration. Protein binding: 62%–67.5%. Primarily eliminated in feces; minimal excretion in urine.
Half-life: 1.8–4.8 hr.

INDICATIONS AND DOSAGES
▶ **Traveler's Diarrhea**
PO
Adults, Elderly, Children 12 yr and older. 200 mg 3 times a day for 3 days.
▶ **Hepatic Encephalopathy**
PO
Adults, Elderly. One 550 mg tablet 2 times/day.

SIDE EFFECTS/ADVERSE REACTIONS
Frequent
Diarrhea, peripheral edema, nausea, dizziness, fatigue, ascites (HE), headache, flatulence, muscle spasms, pruritus, abdominal pain, abdominal distension, anemia
Occasional
Rectal tenesmus, defecation urgency, cough, depression, insomnia, nasopharyngitis, arthralgia, back pain, constipation, dyspnea
Rare
Rash, fever, vomiting, immuno-hypersensitivity reaction

PRECAUTIONS AND CONTRAINDICATIONS
Hypersensitivity to rifaximin, other rifamycin antibiotics, or any component of the formulation

R

Caution:
Hepatic impairment, severe
Clostridium difficile-associated
diarrhea
Pseudomembranous colitis
Use only if *E. coli* is the causative
pathogen

DRUG INTERACTIONS OF CONCERN TO DENTISTRY
• None reported

SERIOUS REACTIONS
! Hypersensitivity reactions,
including dermatitis, angioneurotic
edema, pruritus, rash, and urticaria
may occur.
! Superinfection occurs rarely.

DENTAL CONSIDERATIONS
General:
• Assess salivary flow as a factor in
caries, periodontal disease, and
candidiasis.
• Determine why the patient is
taking the drug.
• Examine for evidence oral signs of
opportunistic infection.
Consultations:
• Medical consultation may be
required to assess disease control.
Teach Patient/Family to:
• Report oral lesions, soreness, or
bleeding to dentist.
• When chronic dry mouth occurs,
advise patient to:
  • Avoid mouth rinses with high
  alcohol content because of
  drying effects.
  • Use daily home fluoride
  products for anticaries effect.
  • Use sugarless gum, frequent
  sips of water, or saliva
  substitutes.

riluzole
rye′-loo-zole
(Rilutek)

CATEGORY AND SCHEDULE
Pregnancy Risk Category: C

Drug Class: Glutamate
antagonist

MECHANISM OF ACTION
An amyotrophic lateral sclerosis
(ALS) agent that inhibits presynaptic
glutamate release in the CNS and
interferes postsynaptically with the
effects of excitatory amino acids.
Therapeutic Effect: Extends
survival of ALS patients.

USES
Treatment of ALS (Lou Gehrig's
disease)

PHARMACOKINETICS
PO: Well absorbed, extensively
metabolized by liver (CYP1A2
isoenzymes), excreted in urine/feces.

INDICATIONS AND DOSAGES
▶ ALS
PO
Adults, Elderly. 50 mg q12h.

SIDE EFFECTS/ADVERSE REACTIONS
Frequent
Nausea, asthenia, reduced
respiratory function
Occasional
Edema, tachycardia, headache,
dizziness, somnolence, depression,
vertigo, tremor, pruritus, alopecia,
abdominal pain, diarrhea, anorexia,
dyspepsia, vomiting, stomatitis,
increased cough

PRECAUTIONS AND CONTRAINDICATIONS
Hypersensitivity, hepatic impairment, renal impairment, hypertension, other CNS disorders, pregnancy category C, lactation, children

DRUG INTERACTIONS OF CONCERN TO DENTISTRY
• No data reported with dental drugs, but use with caution when given with inducers or inhibitors of CYP1A2 isoenzymes

SERIOUS REACTIONS
! None known

DENTAL CONSIDERATIONS

General:
• Short appointments may be required because of nature of disease process.
• Monitor vital signs at every appointment because of cardiovascular and respiratory side effects.
• Consider semisupine chair position for patient comfort.
• Assess salivary flow as factor in caries, periodontal disease, and candidiasis.
• Examine for oral manifestation of opportunistic infection.
• Patients on chronic drug therapy may rarely have symptoms of blood dyscrasias, which can include infection, bleeding, and poor healing.
• After supine positioning, have patient sit upright for at least 2 min before standing to avoid orthostatic hypotension.
Consultations:
• Medical consultation may be required to assess disease control.
• In a patient with symptoms of blood dyscrasias, request a medical

consultation for blood studies and postpone treatment until normal values are reestablished.
Teach Patient/Family to:
• Encourage effective oral hygiene, including use of powered tooth brush if patient has difficulty holding conventional devices or directions for caregiver.
• Use caution to prevent trauma when using oral hygiene aids.
• When chronic dry mouth occurs, advise patient to:
  • Avoid mouth rinses with high alcohol content because of drying effects.
  • Use daily home fluoride products for anticaries effect.
  • Use sugarless gum, frequent sips of water, or saliva substitutes.

rimantadine hydrochloride
ri-**man**'-ta-deen
high-droh-**klor**'-ide
(Flumadine)
Do not confuse rimantadine with ranitidine or Flumadine with flunisolide or flutamide.

CATEGORY AND SCHEDULE
Pregnancy Risk Category: C

Drug Class: Antiviral

MECHANISM OF ACTION
An antiviral that appears to exert an inhibitory effect early in the viral replication cycle. May inhibit uncoating of the virus.
Therapeutic Effect: Prevents replication of influenza A virus.

USES

Adult: prophylaxis and treatment of illnesses caused by strains of influenza A virus; children: prophylaxis against influenza A virus

PHARMACOKINETICS

PO: Peak plasma levels 6 hr; 40% plasma protein binding; hepatic metabolism; renal excretion.

INDICATIONS AND DOSAGES

▸ **Influenza A Virus**
PO
Adults, Elderly. 100 mg twice a day for 7 days.
Elderly nursing home patients, Patients with severe hepatic or renal impairment. 100 mg/day for 7 days.
▸ **Prevention of Influenza A Virus**
PO
Adults, Elderly, Children 10 yr and older. 100 mg twice a day for at least 10 days after known exposure (usually for 6–8 wk).
Children younger than 10 yr. 5 mg/kg/day. Maximum: 150 mg.
Elderly nursing home patients, Patients with severe hepatic or renal impairment. 100 mg/day.

SIDE EFFECTS/ADVERSE REACTIONS

Occasional
Insomnia, nausea, nervousness, impaired concentration, dizziness
Rare
Vomiting, anorexia, dry mouth, abdominal pain, asthenia, fatigue

PRECAUTIONS AND CONTRAINDICATIONS

Hypersensitivity to amantadine or rimantadine
Caution:
Pregnancy category C, elderly, epilepsy, hepatic or renal

impairment, emergence of resistant viral strains

DRUG INTERACTIONS OF CONCERN TO DENTISTRY

• Reduced peak plasma levels: aspirin, acetaminophen

SERIOUS REACTIONS

! None known

DENTAL CONSIDERATIONS

General:
• Monitor vital signs at every appointment because of cardiovascular side effects.
• Determine why the patient is taking the drug (probably will be used only during peak seasons for influenza).
• Assess salivary flow as a factor in caries, periodontal disease, and candidiasis.
Teach Patient/Family to:
• Encourage effective oral hygiene to prevent soft tissue inflammation.
• When chronic dry mouth occurs, advise patient to:
   • Avoid mouth rinses with high alcohol content because of drying effects.
   • Use daily home fluoride products to prevent caries.
   • Use sugarless gum, frequent sips of water, or saliva substitutes.

---

rimexolone
rye-**mex**′-oh-lone
(Vexol)
Do not confuse with riluzole.

CATEGORY AND SCHEDULE

Pregnancy Risk Category: C

Drug Class: Corticosteroid

MECHANISM OF ACTION
An ophthalmic agent that suppresses migration of polymorphonuclear leukocytes and reverses increased capillary permeability.
Therapeutic Effect: Decreases inflammation.

USES
Treatment of inflammation of the eye associated with ocular surgery and uveitis

PHARMACOKINETICS
Absorbed through aqueous humor. Metabolized in liver. Excreted in urine and feces.

INDICATIONS AND DOSAGES
▶ **Inflammation after Ocular Surgery, Treatment of Anterior Uveitis**
Ophthalmic
Adults, Elderly. Instill 1 drop 2–4 times a day up to q4h. May use q1–2h during the first 1–2 days.

SIDE EFFECTS/ADVERSE REACTIONS
Occasional
Temporary mild blurred vision

PRECAUTIONS AND CONTRAINDICATIONS
Fungal, viral, or untreated pus-forming bacterial ocular infections, hypersensitivity to rimexolone or any component of the formulation
Caution:
Increased intraocular pressure, lactation, children, secondary ocular infections

DRUG INTERACTIONS OF CONCERN TO DENTISTRY
• None reported

SERIOUS REACTIONS
! Prolonged use has been associated with the development of corneal or scleral perforation and posterior subcapsular cataracts.
! Cataracts, corneal thinning, glaucoma, increased intraocular pressure, optic nerve damage, secondary ocular infection, and visual acuity defects occur rarely.

DENTAL CONSIDERATIONS
General:
• Determine why the patient is taking the drug.
• Avoid dental light in patient's eyes; offer dark glasses for patient comfort.

risedronate sodium
rye-seh-**droe'**-nate **soe'**-dee-um
(Actonel)

CATEGORY AND SCHEDULE
Pregnancy Risk Category: C

Drug Class: Bisphosphonate

MECHANISM OF ACTION
A bisphosphonate that binds to bone hydroxyapatite and inhibits osteoclasts.
Therapeutic Effect: Reduces bone turnover (the number of sites at which bone is remodeled) and bone resorption.

USES
Treatment of Paget's disease of bone; treatment and prevention of osteoporosis in postmenopausal women and glucocorticoid-induced osteoporosis

INDICATIONS AND DOSAGES

▶ **Paget's Disease**

PO

Adults, Elderly. 30 mg/day for 2 mo. Retreatment may occur after 2-mo posttreatment observation period.

▶ **Prevention and Treatment of Postmenopausal Osteoporosis**

PO

Adults, Elderly. 5 mg/day or 35 mg once a wk.

▶ **Glucocorticoid-Induced Osteoporosis**

PO

Adults, Elderly. 5 mg/day.

SIDE EFFECTS/ADVERSE REACTIONS

Frequent

Arthralgia

Occasional

Rash, flu-like symptoms, peripheral edema

Rare

Bone pain, sinusitis, asthenia, dry eye, tinnitus

PRECAUTIONS AND CONTRAINDICATIONS

Hypersensitivity to other bisphosphonates, including etidronate, tiludronate, risedronate, and alendronate; hypocalcemia; inability to stand or sit upright for at least 20 min; renal impairment when serum creatinine clearance is greater than 5 mg/dl

Caution:

Upper GI disease, avoid use in significant renal impairment, pregnancy category C, lactation, pediatric patients

DRUG INTERACTIONS OF CONCERN TO DENTISTRY

• Retarded absorption: calcium, antacids, medications with divalent cations

• Increased GI side effects: NSAIDs, aspirin

SERIOUS REACTIONS

! Overdose causes hypocalcemia, hypophosphatemia, and significant GI disturbances.

DENTAL CONSIDERATIONS

General:

• Bisphosphonates may increase the risk of osteonecrosis of the jaw.

• Be aware of the oral manifestations of Paget's disease (macrognathia, alveolar pain).

• Consider semisupine chair position for patient comfort because of GI side effects of drug.

• Short appointments may be required for patient comfort.

Consultations:

• Medical consultation may be required to assess disease control.

Teach Patient/Family to:

• Observe regular recall schedule and practice effective oral hygiene to minimize risk of osteonecrosis of the jaw.

• Use powered tooth brush if patient has difficulty holding conventional devices.

risperidone

ris-**per**′-ih-done
(Risperdal, Risperdal Consta, Risperdal M-Tabs)
Do not confuse risperidone with reserpine.

CATEGORY AND SCHEDULE

Pregnancy Risk Category: C

Drug Class: Antipsychotic (benzisoxazole derivative)

MECHANISM OF ACTION

A benzisoxazole derivative that may antagonize dopamine and serotonin receptors.
Therapeutic Effect: Suppresses psychotic behavior.

USES

Treatment of schizophrenia

PHARMACOKINETICS

Well absorbed from the GI tract; unaffected by food. Protein binding: 90%. Extensively metabolized in the liver to active metabolite. Primarily excreted in urine. ***Half-life:*** 3–20 hr; metabolite: 21–30 hr (increased in elderly).

INDICATIONS AND DOSAGES
▸ **Psychotic Disorder**
PO
Adults. 0.5–1 mg twice a day. May increase dosage slowly. Range: 2–6 mg/day.
Elderly. Initially, 0.25–2 mg/day in 2 divided doses. May increase dosage slowly. Range: 2–6 mg/day.
IM
Adults, Elderly. 25 mg q2wk. Maximum: 50 mg q2wk.
▸ **Mania**
PO
Adults, Elderly. Initially, 2–3 mg as a single daily dose. May increase at 24-hr intervals of 1 mg/day. Range: 2–6 mg/day.
▸ **Dosage in Renal Impairment**
Initial dosage for adults and elderly patients is 0.25–0.5 mg twice a day. Dosage is titrated slowly to desired effect.

SIDE EFFECTS/ADVERSE REACTIONS
Frequent
Agitation, anxiety, insomnia, headache, constipation

Occasional
Dyspepsia, rhinitis, somnolence, dizziness, nausea, vomiting, rash, abdominal pain, dry skin, tachycardia
Rare
Visual disturbances, fever, back pain, pharyngitis, cough, arthralgia, angina, aggressive behavior, orthostatic hypotension, breast swelling

PRECAUTIONS AND CONTRAINDICATIONS

Hypersensitivity, pregnancy category C, lactation, seizures, suicidal patients, cardiac diseases, renal or hepatic impairment, elderly; patients should be monitored for signs and symptoms of diabetes mellitus

DRUG INTERACTIONS OF CONCERN TO DENTISTRY

• Increased excretion: chronic use of carbamazepine
• Increased sedation: other CNS depressants, alcohol, barbiturate anesthesia, opioid analgesics
• Increased extrapyramidal effects: phenothiazines and related drugs (haloperidol, droperidol), metoclopramide
• Additive photosensitization: tetracyclines
• Increased anticholinergic effects: anticholinergics, such as atropine and scopolamine

SERIOUS REACTIONS

! Rare reactions include tardive dyskinesia (characterized by tongue protrusion, puffing of the cheeks, and chewing or puckering of the mouth) and neuroleptic malignant syndrome (marked by hyperpyrexia, muscle rigidity, change in mental status, irregular pulse or B/P, tachycardia, diaphoresis, cardiac

R

arrhythmias, rhabdomyolysis, and acute renal failure).

DENTAL CONSIDERATIONS

General:
• Monitor vital signs at every appointment because of cardiovascular side effects.
• Patients on chronic drug therapy may rarely have symptoms of blood dyscrasias, which can include infection, bleeding, and poor healing.
• After supine positioning, have patient sit upright for at least 2 min before standing to avoid orthostatic hypotension.
• Assess salivary flow as a factor in caries, periodontal disease, and candidiasis.
• Consider semisupine chair position for patient comfort because of GI effects of drug.
• Assess for presence of extrapyramidal motor symptoms, such as tardive dyskinesia and akathisia. Extrapyramidal motor activity may complicate dental treatment.
• Use vasoconstrictors with caution, in low doses, and with careful aspiration; avoid use of gingival retraction cord with epinephrine.
Consultations:
• In a patient with symptoms of blood dyscrasias, request a medical consultation for blood studies and postpone dental treatment until normal values are reestablished.
• Take precautions if dental surgery is anticipated and anesthesia is required.
• If signs of tardive dyskinesia or other extrapyramidal symptoms are present, refer to physician.
• Physician should be informed if significant xerostomic side effects occur (e.g., increased caries, sore

tongue, problems eating or swallowing, difficulty wearing prosthesis) so that a medication change can be considered.
Teach Patient/Family to:
• Encourage effective oral hygiene to prevent soft tissue inflammation.
• Use caution to prevent injury when using oral hygiene aids.
• Use powered tooth brush if patient has difficulty holding conventional devices.
• When chronic dry mouth occurs, advise patient to:
  • Avoid mouth rinses with high alcohol content because of drying effects.
  • Use daily home fluoride products for anticaries effect.
  • Use sugarless gum, frequent sips of water, or saliva substitutes.

ritonavir

ri-**tone**′-ah-veer
(Norvir, Norvisec[CAN])
Do not confuse ritonavir with Retrovir.

CATEGORY AND SCHEDULE
Pregnancy Risk Category: B

Drug Class: Antiviral, protease inhibitor

MECHANISM OF ACTION
Inhibits HIV-1 and HIV-2 proteases, rendering these enzymes incapable of processing the polypeptide precursors; this results in the production of noninfectious, immature HIV particles.
Therapeutic Effect: Impedes HIV replication, slowing the progression of HIV infection.

USES
Treatment of HIV infection in adults and children as single-drug therapy or in combination with nucleoside analogs

PHARMACOKINETICS
Well absorbed after PO administration (absorption increased with food). Protein binding: 98%–99%. Extensively metabolized in the liver to active metabolite. Primarily eliminated in feces. Unknown if removed by hemodialysis. *Half-life:* 2.7–5 hr.

INDICATIONS AND DOSAGES
▸ **HIV Infection**
PO
Adults, Children 12 yr and older. 600 mg twice a day. If nausea occurs at this dosage, give 300 mg twice a day for 1 day, 400 mg twice a day for 2 days, 500 mg twice a day for 1 day, then 600 mg twice a day thereafter.
Children younger than 12 yr. Initially, 250 mg/m^2/dose twice a day. Increase by 50 mg/m^2/dose up to 400 mg/m^2/dose. Maximum: 600 mg/dose twice a day.

SIDE EFFECTS/ADVERSE REACTIONS
Frequent
GI disturbances (abdominal pain, anorexia, diarrhea, nausea, vomiting), circumoral and peripheral paresthesias, altered taste, headache, dizziness, fatigue, asthenia
Occasional
Allergic reaction, flu-like symptoms, hypotension
Rare
Diabetes mellitus, hyperglycemia

PRECAUTIONS AND CONTRAINDICATIONS
Concurrent use of amiodarone, astemizole, bepridil, bupropion, cisapride, clozapine, encainide, flecainide, meperidine, piroxicam, propafenone, propoxyphene, quinidine, rifabutin, or terfenadine (increased risk of serious or life-threatening drug interactions, such as arrhythmias, hematologic abnormalities, and seizures); concurrent use of alprazolam, clorazepate, diazepam, estazolam, flurazepam, midazolam, triazolam, or zolpidem (may produce extreme sedation and respiratory depression)
Caution:
Hepatic impairment, lactation, children younger than 12 yr, alters lab chemistry values (triglycerides, ALT, AST, GGT, CPK, uric acid)

DRUG INTERACTIONS OF CONCERN TO DENTISTRY
• Contraindicated with alprazolam, clorazepate, diazepam, bupropion, estazolam, flurazepam, midazolam, triazolam, zolpidem, meperidine, piroxicam, propoxyphene, chlordiazepoxide, halazepam, quazepam
• Increased plasma level drugs metabolized by CYP 3A4: (clarithromycin, fluconazole), macrolide antibiotics, azole antifungals
• Possible alcohol–disulfiram reaction: metronidazole, disulfiram
• Decreased plasma levels with carbamazepine, dexamethasone, phenobarbital, St. John's wort (herb)
• Increased plasma levels of fentanyl

SERIOUS REACTIONS
! None known

R

DENTAL CONSIDERATIONS

General:
• Monitor vital signs at every appointment because of cardiovascular side effects.
• Examine for oral manifestation of opportunistic infection.
• Place on frequent recall to evaluate healing response.
• Assess salivary flow as a factor in caries, periodontal disease, and candidiasis.
• Consider semisupine chair position for patient comfort because of GI effects of drug.

Consultations:
• Medical consultation may be required to assess disease control.

Teach Patient/Family to:
• Encourage effective oral hygiene to prevent soft tissue inflammation.
• See dentist immediately if secondary oral infection occurs.
• When chronic dry mouth occurs, advise patient to:
  • Avoid mouth rinses with high alcohol content because of drying effects.
  • Use daily home fluoride products for anticaries effect.
  • Use sugarless gum, frequent sips of water, or saliva substitutes.

rituximab
rye-**tucks'**-ih-mab
(Mabthera[AUS], Rituxan)

CATEGORY AND SCHEDULE
Pregnancy Risk Category: C

Drug Class: Antineoplastics, monoclonal antibodies

MECHANISM OF ACTION
Binds to CD20, the antigen found on the surface of B lymphocytes and B-cell non-Hodgkin's lymphomas. ***Therapeutic Effect:*** Produces cytotoxicity, reducing tumor size.

USES
Treatment of a type of cancer called non-Hodgkin's lymphoma. It can be used alone or with other cancer medicines or chemotherapy.

PHARMACOKINETICS
Rapidly depletes B cells. ***Half-life:*** 59.8 hr after first infusion and 174 hr after fourth infusion.

INDICATIONS AND DOSAGES
▶ **Non-Hodgkin's Lymphoma**
IV
Adults. 375 mg/m^2 once a wk for 4–8 wk. May administer a second 4-wk course.

SIDE EFFECTS/ADVERSE REACTIONS
Frequent
Fever, chills, nausea, asthenia, headache, angioedema, hypotension, rash or pruritus
Occasional
Myalgia, dizziness, abdominal pain, throat irritation, vomiting, neutropenia, rhinitis, bronchospasm, urticaria

PRECAUTIONS AND CONTRAINDICATIONS
Hypersensitivity to murine proteins

DRUG INTERACTIONS OF CONCERN TO DENTISTRY
• None reported

SERIOUS REACTIONS
! A hypersensitivity reaction marked by hypotension, bronchospasm, and angioedema may occur.

! Arrhythmias may occur, particularly in those with a history of preexisting cardiac conditions.

DENTAL CONSIDERATIONS

General:
• Monitor and record vital signs.
• If additional analgesia is required for dental pain, consider alternative analgesics (NSAIDs) in patients taking narcotics for acute or chronic pain.
• After supine positioning, have patient sit upright for at least 2 min before standing to avoid orthostatic hypotension.
• Patient on chronic drug therapy may rarely present with symptoms of blood dyscrasias, which can include infection, bleeding, and poor healing. If dyscrasia is present, caution patient to prevent oral tissue trauma when using oral hygiene aids.
• Provide emergency dental care only during drug use.
• Hypersensitivity reactions may occur.
• Oral infections should be eliminated and treated aggressively.

Consultations:
• Medical consultation should include routine blood counts including platelet counts and bleeding time.
• Consult physician; prophylactic or therapeutic antiinfectives may be indicated if surgery or periodontal treatment is required.
• Medical consultation may be required to assess immunologic status during cancer chemotherapy and determine safety risk, if any, posed by the required dental treatment.
• Medical consultation may be required to assess disease control and patient's ability to tolerate stress.

Teach Patient/Family to:
• Encourage effective oral hygiene to prevent soft tissue inflammation.
• Report oral lesions, soreness, or bleeding to dentist.
• Prevent trauma when using oral hygiene aids.
• Update health and medication history if physician makes any changes in evaluation or drug regimens; include OTC, herbal, and nonherbal remedies in the update.

rivastigmine tartrate
riv-ah-**stig**'-meen **tar**'-trate
(Exelon)

CATEGORY AND SCHEDULE
Pregnancy Risk Category: B

Drug Class: Reversible cholinesterase inhibitor

MECHANISM OF ACTION
A cholinesterase inhibitor that inhibits the enzyme acetylcholinesterase, thus increasing the concentration of acetylcholine at cholinergic synapses and enhancing cholinergic function in the CNS. **Therapeutic Effect:** Slows the progression of symptoms of Alzheimer's disease.

PHARMACOKINETICS
Rapidly and completely absorbed. Protein binding: 60%. Widely distributed throughout the body. Rapidly and extensively metabolized. Primarily excreted in urine. **Half-life:** 1.5 hr.

INDICATIONS AND DOSAGES
▶ Alzheimer's Disease
PO
Adults, Elderly. Initially, 1.5 mg twice a day. May increase at intervals of least 2 wk to 3 mg twice a day, then 4.5 mg twice a day, and finally 6 mg twice a day. Maximum: 6 mg twice a day.

SIDE EFFECTS/ADVERSE REACTIONS
Frequent
Nausea, vomiting, dizziness, diarrhea, headache, anorexia
Occasional
Abdominal pain, insomnia, dyspepsia (heartburn, indigestion, epigastric pain), confusion, UTI, depression
Rare
Anxiety, somnolence, constipation, malaise, hallucinations, tremor, flatulence, rhinitis, hypertension, flu-like symptoms, weight loss, syncope

PRECAUTIONS AND CONTRAINDICATIONS
Hypersensitivity to this drug or other carbamate derivatives
Caution:
Significant GI reactions, nausea, vomiting, and weight-loss occur; history of GI ulcers or GI bleeding, patients taking NSAIDs, seizures, asthma, COPD, lactation, pediatric patients (no studies); smoking increases renal clearance

DRUG INTERACTIONS OF CONCERN TO DENTISTRY
• Caution in use of NSAIDs if GI side effects are significant
• Decreased response to neuromuscular blocking agents used in general anesthesia
• Increased cholinergic response: other cholinergic drugs

• Decreased cholinergic response: anticholinergics or other drugs with anticholinergic actions

SERIOUS REACTIONS
! Overdose may result in cholinergic crisis, characterized by severe nausea and vomiting, increased salivation, diaphoresis, bradycardia, hypotension, respiratory depression, and seizures.

DENTAL CONSIDERATIONS
General:
• Determine why patient is taking the drug.
• Monitor vital signs at every appointment because of cardiovascular side effects.
• Drug is used early in the disease; ensure that patient or caregiver understands informed consent.
• Place on frequent recall because early attention to dental health is important for Alzheimer's patients.
• Assess salivary flow as a factor in caries, periodontal disease, and candidiasis.
• Use precaution if sedation or general anesthesia is required; risk of hypotensive episode.
• Consider semisupine chair position for patient comfort if GI side effects occur.
• Patients on chronic drug therapy may rarely have symptoms of blood dyscrasias, which can include infection, bleeding, and poor healing.
Consultations:
• Consultation with physician may be necessary if sedation or general anesthesia is required.
• In a patient with symptoms of blood dyscrasias, request a medical consultation for blood studies and postpone treatment until normal values are reestablished.

• Medical consultation may be required to assess disease control and patient's ability to tolerate stress.

Teach Patient/Family to:
• Use powered tooth brush if patient has difficulty holding conventional devices.
• Prevent trauma when using oral hygiene aids.
• Encourage effective oral hygiene to prevent soft tissue inflammation.

rizatriptan benzoate
rize-ah-**trip**'-tan **ben**'-zoe-ate
(Maxalt, Maxalt-MLT)

CATEGORY AND SCHEDULE
Pregnancy Risk Category: C

Drug Class: Serotonin agonist

MECHANISM OF ACTION
A serotonin receptor agonist that binds selectively to vascular receptors, producing a vasoconstrictive effect on cranial blood vessels.
Therapeutic Effect: Relieves migraine headache.

USES
Acute treatment of migraine attacks with or without aura

PHARMACOKINETICS
Well absorbed after PO administration. Protein binding: 14%. Crosses the blood-brain barrier. Metabolized by the liver to inactive metabolite. Eliminated primarily in urine and, to a lesser extent, in feces. *Half-life:* 2–3 hr.

INDICATIONS AND DOSAGES
▸ **Acute Migraine Attack**
PO
Adults older than 18 yr, Elderly.
5–10 mg. If headache improves, but then returns, dose may be repeated after 2 hr. Maximum: 30 mg/24 hr.

SIDE EFFECTS/ADVERSE REACTIONS
Frequent
Dizziness, somnolence, paraesthesia, fatigue
Occasional
Nausea, chest pressure, dry mouth
Rare
Headache; neck, throat, or jaw pressure; photosensitivity

PRECAUTIONS AND CONTRAINDICATIONS
Basilar or hemiplegic migraine, coronary artery disease, ischemic heart disease (including angina pectoris, history of MI, silent ischemia, and Prinzmetal's angina), uncontrolled hypertension, use within 24 hr of ergotamine-containing preparations or another serotonin receptor agonist, use within 14 days of MAOIs
Caution:
Risk of serious cardiovascular events, renal/hepatic impairment, SSRI antidepressants, lactation, use in children not established, orally disintegrating tabs contain aspartame

DRUG INTERACTIONS OF CONCERN TO DENTISTRY
• No specific interactions with dental drugs reported
• Increased plasma levels: propranolol
• Should not be used within 24 hr of another 5-HT agonist

R

SERIOUS REACTIONS

! Cardiac reactions (such as ischemia, coronary artery vasospasm, and MI) and noncardiac vasospasm-related reactions (including hemorrhage and CVA) occur rarely, particularly in patients with hypertension, diabetes, or a strong family history of coronary artery disease; obese patients; smokers; males older than 40 yr; and postmenopausal women.

DENTAL CONSIDERATIONS

General:
• This is an acute-use drug; it is doubtful that patients will be treated in the office if acute migraine is present.
• Be aware of patient's disease, its severity, and its frequency, when known.
• Avoid dental light in patient's eyes; offer dark glasses for patient comfort.
• Short appointments and a stress-reduction protocol may be required for anxious patients.
• After supine positioning, have patient sit upright for at least 2 min before standing to avoid orthostatic hypotension.

Consultations:
• If treating chronic orofacial pain, consult with physician of record.
• Medical consultation may be required to assess disease control and patient's ability to tolerate stress.

Teach Patient/Family to:
• Update health and drug history if physician makes any changes in evaluation or drug regimens; include OTC, herbal, and nonherbal drugs in the update.

ropinirole hydrochloride

roe-**pin**′-ih-role
high-droh-**klor**′-ide
(Requip)

CATEGORY AND SCHEDULE

Pregnancy Risk Category: C

Drug Class: Antiparkinson agent

MECHANISM OF ACTION

An antiparkinson agent that stimulates dopamine receptors in the striatum.
Therapeutic Effect: Relieves signs and symptoms of Parkinson's disease.

USES

Treatment of Parkinson's disease

PHARMACOKINETICS

Rapidly absorbed after PO administration. Protein binding: 40%. Extensively distributed throughout the body. Extensively metabolized. Steady-state concentrations achieved within 2 days. Eliminated in urine. Unknown if removed by hemodialysis.
Half-life: 6 hr.

INDICATIONS AND DOSAGES
▸ Parkinson's Disease
PO
Adults, Elderly. Initially, 0.25 mg 3 times a day. May increase dosage every 7 days.

SIDE EFFECTS/ADVERSE REACTIONS

Frequent
Nausea, dizziness, somnolence
Occasional
Syncope, vomiting, fatigue, viral infection, dyspepsia, diaphoresis,

asthenia, orthostatic hypotension, abdominal discomfort, pharyngitis, abnormal vision, dry mouth, hypertension, hallucinations, confusion

Rare

Anorexia, peripheral edema, memory loss, rhinitis, sinusitis, palpitations, impotence

PRECAUTIONS AND CONTRAINDICATIONS: HYPERSENSITIVITY

Cardiovascular disease, severely impaired renal or hepatic function, lactation, pregnancy category C, syncope, hypotension

DRUG INTERACTIONS OF CONCERN TO DENTISTRY

• Possible increase in sedation with all CNS depressants
• Possible diminished effects: dopamine antagonists, phenothiazines, haloperidol, droperidol, and metoclopramide

SERIOUS REACTIONS

! None known

DENTAL CONSIDERATIONS

General:
• Monitor vital signs at every appointment because of cardiovascular side effects.
• Assess salivary flow as factor in caries, periodontal disease, and candidiasis.
• After supine positioning, have patient sit upright for at least 2 min before standing to avoid orthostatic hypotension.
• Patients on chronic drug therapy may rarely have symptoms of blood dyscrasias, which can include infection, bleeding, and poor healing.

• Consider semisupine chair position for patient comfort if GI side effects occur.

Consultations:
• In a patient with symptoms of blood dyscrasias, request a medical consultation for blood studies and postpone treatment until normal values are reestablished.
• Medical consultation may be required to assess disease control and patient's ability to tolerate stress.

Teach Patient/Family to:
• Use caution to prevent trauma when using oral hygiene aids.
• Use powered tooth brush if patient has difficulty holding conventional devices.
• Encourage effective oral hygiene to prevent soft tissue inflammation.
• Update health and drug history if physician makes any changes in evaluation or drug regimens; include OTC, herbal, and nonherbal drugs in the update.
• When chronic dry mouth occurs, advise patient to:
  • Avoid mouth rinses with high alcohol content because of drying effects.
  • Use daily home fluoride products for anticaries effect.
  • Use sugarless gum, frequent sips of water, or saliva substitutes.

R

rosiglitazone maleate

roz-ih-**gli**′-tah-zone **mal**′-ee-ate (Avandia)

Do not confuse Avandia with Avalide, Avinza, or Prandin.

CATEGORY AND SCHEDULE

Pregnancy Risk Category: C

Drug Class: Oral antidiabetic

MECHANISM OF ACTION

An antidiabetic that improves target-cell response to insulin without increasing pancreatic insulin secretion. Decreases hepatic glucose output and increases insulin-dependent glucose utilization in skeletal muscle.
Therapeutic Effect: Lowers blood glucose concentration.

USES

Monotherapy, as an adjunct to diet and exercise in patients with Type 2 diabetes mellitus; may also be used with metformin when metformin, diet, and exercise are not adequate for control

PHARMACOKINETICS

Rapidly absorbed. Protein binding: 99%. Metabolized in the liver. Excreted primarily in urine, with a lesser amount in feces. Not removed by hemodialysis. *Half-life:* 3–4 hr.

INDICATIONS AND DOSAGES
▶ **Diabetes Mellitus, Combination Therapy**
PO
Adults, Elderly. Initially, 4 mg as a single daily dose or in divided doses twice a day. May increase to 8 mg/day after 12 wk of therapy if fasting glucose level is not adequately controlled.
▶ **Diabetes Mellitus, Monotherapy**
Adults, Elderly. Initially, 4 mg as single daily dose or in divided doses twice a day. May increase to 8 mg/day after 12 wk of therapy.

SIDE EFFECTS/ADVERSE REACTIONS

Frequent
Upper respiratory tract infection
Occasional
Headache, edema, back pain, fatigue, sinusitis, diarrhea

PRECAUTIONS AND CONTRAINDICATIONS

Active hepatic disease, diabetic ketoacidosis, increased serum transaminase levels, including ALT (SGPT) greater than 2.5 times the normal serum level, Type 1 diabetes mellitus
Caution:
May cause resumption of ovulation in premenopausal anovulatory women (risk of pregnancy), patients with edema, advanced heart failure, hepatic impairment, monitor liver enzymes, lactation

DRUG INTERACTIONS OF CONCERN TO DENTISTRY

• None reported

SERIOUS REACTIONS

! None known

DENTAL CONSIDERATIONS

General:
• Ensure that patient is following prescribed diet and regularly takes medication.
• Place on frequent recall to evaluate healing response.
• Short appointments and a stress-reduction protocol may be required for anxious patients.
• Diabetics may be more susceptible to infection and have delayed wound healing.
• Question patient about self-monitoring of drug's antidiabetic effect, including blood glucose values or finger-stick records.
Consultations:
• Medical consultation may include data from patient's blood glucose monitoring, including glycosylated hemoglobin or HbA$_{1c}$ testing.
• Medical consultation may be required to assess disease control and patient's ability to tolerate stress.

Teach Patient/Family to:
• Prevent trauma when using oral hygiene aids.
• Update health and drug history if physician makes any changes in evaluation or drug regimens; include OTC, herbal, and nonherbal drugs in the update.

rosuvastatin calcium
ross-uh-vah-**stah'**-tin **kal'**-see-um
(Crestor)

CATEGORY AND SCHEDULE
Pregnancy Risk Category: X

Drug Class: Antihyperlipidemic

MECHANISM OF ACTION
An antihyperlipidemic that interferes with cholesterol biosynthesis by inhibiting the conversion of the enzyme HMG-CoA to mevalonate, a precursor to cholesterol.
Therapeutic Effect: Decreases low-density lipoprotein (LDL) cholesterol, very low-density lipoprotein (VLDL), and plasma triglyceride levels; increases high-density lipoprotein (HDL) concentration.

USES
An adjunct to diet in primary hypercholesterolemia, mixed lipidemia (Fredricksen types IIa and IIb), and homozygous familial hypercholesterolemia and to lower triglycerides in Fredrickson type IV hyperlipidemia

PHARMACOKINETICS
Protein binding: 88%. Minimal hepatic metabolism. Primarily eliminated in the feces. **Half-life:** 19 hr (increased in patients with severe renal dysfunction).

INDICATIONS AND DOSAGES
▸ **Hyperlipidemia, Dyslipidemia**
PO
Adults, Elderly. 5 to 40 mg/day. Usual starting dosage is 10 mg/day, with adjustments based on lipid levels; monitor q2–4wk until desired level is achieved.
▸ **Renal Impairment (Creatinine Clearance <30 ml/min)**
PO
Adults, Elderly. 5 mg/day; do not exceed 10 mg/day.
▸ **Concurrent Cyclosporine Use**
PO
Adults, Elderly. 5 mg/day.
▸ **Concurrent Lipid-Lowering Therapy**
PO
Adults, Elderly. 10 mg/day.

SIDE EFFECTS/ADVERSE REACTIONS
Rosuvastatin is generally well tolerated. Side effects are usually mild and transient.
Occasional
Pharyngitis, headache, diarrhea, dyspepsia, including heartburn and epigastric distress, nausea
Rare
Myalgia, asthenia or unusual fatigue and weakness, back pain

PRECAUTIONS AND CONTRAINDICATIONS
Active hepatic disease, breast-feeding, pregnancy, unexplained, persistent elevations of serum transaminase levels
Caution:
Severe renal impairment, hepatic impairment, pregnancy category X, liver function test recommended, alcoholics, efficacy and safety in pediatric patients unknown

R

DRUG INTERACTIONS OF CONCERN TO DENTISTRY
• No dental drug interactions reported; however, interactions with cyclosporine, warfarin, and gemfibrozil are noted
• Does not inhibit CYP3A4

SERIOUS REACTIONS
! Lens opacities may occur.
! Hypersensitivity reaction and hepatitis occur rarely.

DENTAL CONSIDERATIONS

General:
• Monitor vital signs because patients with high cholesterol levels are predisposed to cardiovascular disease.
• Consider semisupine chair position for patient comfort if GI side effects occur.

---

rotigotine
roe-**tig**′-oh-teen
(Neupro)

CATEGORY AND SCHEDULE
Pregnancy Risk Category: C

Drug Class: Anti-Parkinson's agent, dopamine agonist

MECHANISM OF ACTION
Non-ergotinic dopamine agonists that specifically binds to D_3, D_2, and D_1 receptors. Stimulates postsynaptic D_2 receptors within the substantia nigra in the brain, resulting in improved dopaminergic transmission in the motor areas of the basal ganglia. Rotigotine is also known to have specificity for dopamine D_3 and D_1 receptors.

USES
Used for the treatment of signs and symptoms of Parkinson's disease.

PHARMACOKINETICS
Protein binding: 90%. Extensively metabolized through conjugation and N-dealkylation. *Half-life* (after patch removal): 5–7 hr. Excreted in the urine (71%) and feces (11%).

INDICATIONS AND DOSAGES
Patients receiving the patches should begin downward titration. Sudden discontinuation of rotigotine may result in a syndrome resembling neuroleptic malignant syndrome or akinetic crisis.
▶ **Parkinson's Disease**
Topical: Transdermal
Adults. Apply 2 mg/24 hr patch once daily initially, may increase by 2 mg/24 hr weekly. Maximum: 6 mg/24 hr.
Discontinue by decreasing or tapering the dose in 2 mg/24 hr increments

SIDE EFFECTS/ADVERSE REACTIONS
Adult
Frequent
Somnolence, dizziness, headache, insomnia, nausea, vomiting, application site reactions.
Occasional
Sinus tachycardia, peripheral edema, orthostatic hypotension, fatigue, abnormal dreams, hallucination, vertigo, erythematous rash, hypoglycemia, constipation, dyspepsia, anorexia, xerostomia, weight gain, weight loss, urinary tract infection, back pain, arthralgia, myalgia, vision changes, sinusitis, accident, increased diaphoresis.

PRECAUTIONS AND CONTRAINDICATIONS

Contraindicated in patients with hypersensitivity to rotigotine and its components.

May cause hallucinations. Use with caution because rotigotine can cause impulsive control disorders as well as melanoma in some cases.

Use with caution in patients with likely risk of hypotension because rotigotine can cause orthostatic hypotension and in patients using other CNS depressants or psychoactive agents due to somnolence risk associating with rotigotine use.

Use with caution in patients with predisposing dyskinesia and cardiovascular diseases.

DRUG INTERACTIONS OF CONCERN TO DENTISTRY

• CNS depressants: May enhance adverse effects of somnolence of rotigotine

SERIOUS REACTIONS

❗ Prolong use of rotigotine can lead to pleural, retroperitoneal fibrosis and/or cardiac valvulopathy in rare cases.

❗ Somnolence may occur. Patients falling asleep during daytime activities have been reported.

❗ Some cases resulted in accidents.

DENTAL CONSIDERATIONS

General:
• Xerostomia may complicate oral hygiene and dental treatment.

• Patients should be carefully assisted from the chair and observed for signs of orthostatic hypotension. After supine positioning, have patient sit upright for 2 min before standing.

• Understand limitations of Parkinson's disease on dental treatment (e.g., dyskinesias).

• Consider semisupine chair position for patient comfort if gastrointestinal (GI) side effects occur.

Consultations:
• Medical consultation may be required to assess disease control and ability of patient to tolerate dental treatment.

Teach Patient/Family to:
• Be alert for the possibility of xerostomia and the need to be consulted by a dentist if dry mouth occurs.

• Avoid mouth rinse with high alcohol content because of dryness effects.

• If dry mouth occurs, use sugarless gum, frequent sips of water, or saliva substitutes.

• Help patient with effective dental home care to minimize oral diseases if patient lacks adequate motor coordination.

• Understand importance of good oral hygiene to prevent soft tissue inflammation.

• Prevent trauma when using oral hygiene aids.

R

salmeterol
sal-**me**'-teh-rol
(Serevent Diskus, Serevent Inhaler and Disks[AUS])
Do not confuse Serevent with Serentil.

CATEGORY AND SCHEDULE
Pregnancy Risk Category: C

Drug Class: Long-acting selective β$_2$-adrenergic receptor agonist

MECHANISM OF ACTION
An adrenergic agonist that stimulates β$_2$-adrenergic receptors in the lungs, resulting in relaxation of bronchial smooth muscle.
Therapeutic Effect: Relieves bronchospasm and reduces airway resistance.

USES
Treatment of bronchospasm associated with COPD, maintenance treatment of bronchospasm associated with COPD, asthma, and exercise-induced bronchospasm

PHARMACOKINETICS

Route	Onset	Peak	Duration
Inhalation	10–20 min	3 hr	12 hr

Low systemic absorption; acts primarily in the lungs. Protein binding: 95%. Metabolized by hydroxylation. Primarily eliminated in feces. *Half-life:* 3–4 hr.

INDICATIONS AND DOSAGES
▶ **Prevention and Maintenance Treatment of Asthma**
Inhalation (Diskus)
Adults, Elderly, Children 4 yr and older. 1 inhalation (50 mcg) q12h.

▶ **Prevention of Exercise-Induced Bronchospasm**
Inhalation
Adults, Elderly, Children 4 yr and older. 1 inhalation at least 30 min before exercise.
▶ **COPD**
Inhalation
Adults, Elderly. 1 inhalation q12h.

SIDE EFFECTS/ADVERSE REACTIONS
Frequent
Headache
Occasional
Cough, tremor, dizziness, vertigo, throat dryness or irritation, pharyngitis
Rare
Palpitations, tachycardia, nausea, heartburn, GI distress, diarrhea

PRECAUTIONS AND CONTRAINDICATIONS
History of hypersensitivity to sympathomimetics
Caution:
Lactation, children younger than 12 yr, hepatic impairment, coronary insufficiency, dysrhythmias, hypertension, convulsive disorders; not for acute symptoms, not to exceed recommended dose, paradoxic bronchospasm may occur with use; not recommended for use with a spacer or other aerosol device

DRUG INTERACTIONS OF CONCERN TO DENTISTRY
• Increased cardiovascular effects: tricyclic antidepressants

SERIOUS REACTIONS
❗ Salmeterol may prolong the QT interval, which may precipitate ventricular arrhythmias.
❗ Hypokalemia and hyperglycemia may occur.

DENTAL CONSIDERATIONS

General:
• Monitor vital signs at every appointment because of cardiovascular and respiratory side effects.
• Be aware that aspirin or sulfite preservatives in vasoconstrictor-containing products can exacerbate asthma.
• Acute asthmatic episodes may be precipitated in the dental office. Rapid-acting sympathomimetic inhalants should be available for emergency use. Salmeterol is not a rapid-acting drug and is not intended for use in acute asthmatic attacks.
• Consider semisupine chair position for patients with respiratory disease.
• Midmorning appointments and a stress reduction protocol may be required for anxious patients.
Consultations:
• Medical consultation may be required to assess disease control and patient's ability to tolerate stress.
Teach Patient/Family to:
• Encourage effective oral hygiene to prevent soft tissue inflammation.

salsalate
sal'-sa-late
(Amigesic, Disalcid, Mono-Gesic, Salflex)

CATEGORY AND SCHEDULE
Pregnancy Risk Category: C

Drug Class: Salicylate, nonnarcotic analgesic

MECHANISM OF ACTION
An NSAID that inhibits prostaglandin synthesis, reducing the inflammatory response and the intensity of pain stimuli reaching the sensory nerve endings.
Therapeutic Effect: Produces analgesic and antiinflammatory effects.

USES
Treatment of mild-to-moderate pain or fever, including arthritis, juvenile rheumatoid arthritis

PHARMACOKINETICS
Half-life: 7–8 hr.

INDICATIONS AND DOSAGES
▶ Rheumatoid Arthritis, Osteoarthritis Pain
PO
Adults, Elderly. Initially, 3 g/day in 2–3 divided doses. Maintenance: 2–4 g/day.

SIDE EFFECTS/ADVERSE REACTIONS
Occasional
Nausea, dyspepsia (including heartburn, indigestion, and epigastric pain)

PRECAUTIONS AND CONTRAINDICATIONS
Bleeding disorders, hypersensitivity to salicylates or NSAIDs
Caution:
Anemia, hepatic disease, renal disease, Hodgkin's disease, lactation

DRUG INTERACTIONS OF CONCERN TO DENTISTRY
• Increased risk of GI complaints and occult blood loss: alcohol, NSAIDs, corticosteroids
• Increased risk of bleeding: oral anticoagulants, valproic acid, dipyridamole
• Avoid prolonged or concurrent use with NSAIDs, corticosteroids, acetaminophen

S

• Increased risk of hypoglycemia: oral antidiabetics
• Increased risk of toxicity: methotrexate, lithium, zidovudine
• Decreased effects of probenecid, sulfinpyrazone
• Suspected reduction in the antihypertensive and vasodilator effects of ACE inhibitors; monitor B/P if used concurrently

SERIOUS REACTIONS

! Tinnitus may be the first indication that the serum salicylic acid concentration is reaching or exceeding the upper therapeutic range.
! Salsalate use may also produce vertigo, headache, confusion, drowsiness, diaphoresis, hyperventilation, vomiting, and diarrhea.
! Reye's syndrome may occur in children with chickenpox or the flu.
! Severe overdose may result in electrolyte imbalance, hyperthermia, dehydration, and blood pH imbalance.
! GI bleeding, peptic ulcer, and Reye's syndrome rarely occur.

DENTAL CONSIDERATIONS

General:
• Patients on chronic drug therapy rarely have symptoms of blood dyscrasias, which can include infection, bleeding, and poor healing.
• Potential cross-allergies with other salicylates such as aspirin.
• Consider semisupine chair position for patients with inflammatory joint diseases.
• Avoid prescribing aspirin-containing products because this drug is a salicylate.
• If used for dental patients, take with food or milk to decrease GI

complaints; give 30 min before meals or 2 hr after meals; take with a full glass of water.
• Severe stomach bleeding may occur in patients who regularly use NSAIDs in recommended doses, when the patient is also taking another NSAID, a blood thinning, or steroid drug, if the patient has GI or peptic ulcer disease, if they are 60 yr or older, or when NSAIDs are taken longer than directed. Warn patients of the potential for severe stomach bleeding.
Consultations:
• In a patient with symptoms of blood dyscrasias, request a medical consultation for blood studies and postpone dental treatment until normal values are reestablished.
• Medical consultation may be required to assess disease control.
Teach Patient/Family to:
• Not place directly on a tooth or oral mucosa because of risk of chemical burns.
• Not exceed recommended dosage; acute toxicity may result.
• Read label on other OTC drugs; many contain aspirin.
• Avoid alcohol ingestion; GI bleeding may occur.
• Encourage effective oral hygiene to prevent soft tissue inflammation.
• Use caution to prevent injury when using oral hygiene aids.
• Warn patient of potential risks of increased GI adverse effects of NSAIDs.

S

sapropterin
sa-**prop**´-ter-in
(Kuvan)

CATEGORY AND SCHEDULE
Pregnancy Risk Category: C

Drug Class: Synthetic enzyme
cofactor

MECHANISM OF ACTION
Promotes action of phenylalanine-4-
hydroxylase as a cofactor for the
enzyme.
Therapeutic Effect: Replaces
tetrahydrobiopterin in
phenylketonuria (PKU) to reduce
blood phenylalanine levels.

USES
Treatment of hyperphenylalanemia
(PKU), in conjunction with a
phenylalanine-restricted diet

PHARMACOKINETICS
Absorbed after oral administration.
Metabolized primarily in the liver
(CYP 3A4); metabolites excreted in
urine

INDICATIONS AND DOSAGES
▶ **Management of Phenylketonuria**
Adult. PO 10 mg/kg/day for a period
of up to 1 month (may be increased
up to 20 mg/kg/day if phenylalanine
levels do not decrease from
baseline).

SIDE EFFECTS/ADVERSE REACTIONS
Frequent
Headache, peripheral edema,
arthralgia, polyuria, agitation,
dizziness, upper respiratory tract
infection, diarrhea, abdominal pain,
upper respiratory tract infection,
pharyngolaryngeal pain, nausea,
vomiting

Occasional
Confusion, rash, nasal congestion

PRECAUTIONS AND CONTRAINDICATIONS
Hypersensitivity
Blood phenylalanine levels need to
be monitored carefully during
therapy
Nonresponders to therapy need to be
identified
Monitor carefully in the presence of
hepatic impairment
Use with caution with inhibitors of
folate metabolism (e.g.,
methotrexate)
Possible hypotension if used with
PDE-5 inhibitors (e.g., sildenafil,
vardenafil)
Use with caution in patients taking
levodopa (seizures, overstimulation)

DRUG INTERACTIONS OF CONCERN TO DENTISTRY
• None reported

SERIOUS REACTIONS
! Gastritis, spinal cord injury,
streptococcal infection
! Testicular carcinoma, urinary tract
infection, neutropenia
! Convulsions
! Dizziness
! GI bleeding, postprocedural
bleeding, headache, irritability, MI,
overstimulation and respiratory tract
infection
! Safety during nursing is not
known

DENTAL CONSIDERATIONS
General:
• Monitor patient carefully for
adverse reactions/side effects of
drug.
• Phenylketonuric patients frequently
exhibit manifestations of neurologic
injury, including mental retardation

S

and must be managed accordingly, including knowledge of the patient's dietary restrictions.

• Early-morning appointments and stress-reduction protocol may be needed for anxious patients.

• Position patient for comfort if GI adverse effects occur.

Consultations:

• Consult with physician to determine disease control, dietary restrictions and ability to tolerate dental procedures.

Teach Patient/Family to:

• Avoid recommending artificially sweetened products that may otherwise be recommended in routine oral hygiene programs.

• Use home fluoride products for anticaries effect.

• Encourage effective oral hygiene measures to prevent soft tissue inflammation.

saquinavir
sa-kwin′-ah-veer
(Fortovase, Invirase)
Do not confuse saquinavir with Sinequan.

CATEGORY AND SCHEDULE
Pregnancy Risk Category: B

Drug Class: Antiviral

MECHANISM OF ACTION
Inhibits HIV protease, rendering the enzyme incapable of processing the polyprotein precursors needed to generate functional proteins in HIV-infected cells.

Therapeutic Effect: Interferes with HIV replication, slowing the progression of HIV infection.

USES
Treatment of AIDS in combination with nucleoside analogs, zidovudine, or zalcitabine

PHARMACOKINETICS
Poorly absorbed after PO administration (absorption increased with high-calorie and high-fat meals). Protein binding: 99%. Metabolized in the liver to inactive metabolite. Primarily eliminated in feces. Unknown if removed by hemodialysis. **Half-life:** 13 hr.

INDICATIONS AND DOSAGES
▶ **HIV Infection in Combination with Other Antiretrovirals**
PO
Adults, Elderly. 1200 mg Fortovase 3 times a day or 600 mg Invirase 3 times a day within 2 hr after a full meal.
▶ **Dosage Adjustments When Given in Combination Therapy**
Delavirdine: Fortovase 800 mg 3 times a day.
Lopinavir/ritonavir: Fortovase 800 mg 2 times a day.
Nelfinavir: Fortovase 800 mg 3 times/day or 1200 mg 2 times a day.
Ritonavir: Fortovase or Invirase 1000 mg 2 times a day.

SIDE EFFECTS/ADVERSE REACTIONS
Occasional
Diarrhea, abdominal discomfort and pain, nausea, photosensitivity, stomatitis
Rare
Confusion, ataxia, asthenia, headache, rash

PRECAUTIONS AND CONTRAINDICATIONS
Clinically significant hypersensitivity to saquinavir; concurrent use with

ergot medications, lovastatin, midazolam, simvastatin, or triazolam
Caution:
Hepatic impairment, children younger than 16 yr, pregnancy category B, lactation (unknown), bone marrow suppression, renal impairment

DRUG INTERACTIONS OF CONCERN TO DENTISTRY
• Increased plasma levels of clindamycin, troleandomycin, ketoconazole, itraconazole, fentanyl, clarithromycin, midazolam, triazolam
• Increased metabolism of carbamazepine, dexamethasone, phenobarbital
• Inhibits CYP3A4 isoenzymes: use with caution or avoid use with drugs metabolized by these enzymes (e.g. macrolide antibiotics)

SERIOUS REACTIONS
! Ketoacidosis occurs rarely.

DENTAL CONSIDERATIONS
General:
• Examine for oral manifestations of opportunistic infections.
• Patients on chronic drug therapy may rarely have symptoms of blood dyscrasias, which can include infection, bleeding, and poor healing.
• Palliative medication may be required for management of oral side effects.
Consultations:
• Medical consultation may be required to assess disease control.
• In a patient with symptoms of blood dyscrasias, request a medical consultation for blood studies and postpone dental treatment until normal values are reestablished.

Teach Patient/Family to:
• Encourage effective oral hygiene to prevent soft tissue inflammation.
• Use caution to prevent trauma when using oral hygiene aids.
• See dentist immediately if secondary oral infection occurs.
• Update medical/drug history if physician makes any changes in evaluation or drug regimen; include OTC, herbal, and nonherbal drugs in the update.

sargramostim (granulocyte macrophage colony-stimulating factor, GM-CSF)
sar-gra-**moh'**-stim
(Leukine)
Do not confuse Leukine with Leukeran.

CATEGORY AND SCHEDULE
Pregnancy Risk Category: C

Drug Class: Chemotherapeutic

MECHANISM OF ACTION
A colony-stimulating factor that stimulates proliferation and differentiation of hematopoietic cells to activate mature granulocytes and macrophages.
Therapeutic Effect: Assists bone marrow in making new WBCs and increases their chemotactic, antifungal, and antiparasitic activity. Increases cytoneoplastic cells and activates neutrophils to inhibit tumor cell growth.

USES
Acute myelogenous leukemia; myeloid reconstitution after bone marrow transplantation

S

PHARMACOKINETICS

Effect	Onset	Peak	Duration
Increase WBCs	7–14 days	N/A	1 wk

Detected in serum within 5 min after subcutaneous administration.
Half-life: IV, 1 hr; subcutaneous, 3 hr.

INDICATIONS AND DOSAGES
▸ **Myeloid Recovery Following Bone Marrow Transplant (BMT)**
IV Infusion
Adults, Elderly. Usual parenteral dosage: 250 mcg/m^2/day for 21 days (as 2-hr infusion). Begin 2–4 hr after autologous bone marrow infusion and not less than 24 hr after last dose of chemotherapy or not less than 12 hr after last radiation treatment. Discontinue if blast cells appear or underlying disease progresses.
▸ **BMT Failure, Engraftment Delay**
IV Infusion
Adults, Elderly. 250 mcg/m^2/day for 14 days. Infuse over 2 hr. May repeat after 7 days off therapy if engraftment has not occurred with 500 mcg/m^2/day for 14 days.
▸ **Stem Cell Transplant**
IV, Subcutaneous
Adults. 250 mcg/m^2/day.

SIDE EFFECTS/ADVERSE REACTIONS
Frequent
GI disturbances, including nausea, diarrhea, vomiting, stomatitis, anorexia, and abdominal pain; arthralgia or myalgia; headache; malaise; rash; pruritus
Occasional
Peripheral edema, weight gain, dyspnea, asthenia, fever, leukocytosis, capillary leak syndrome (such as fluid retention, irritation at local injection site, and peripheral edema)
Rare
Rapid or irregular heartbeat, thrombophlebitis

PRECAUTIONS AND CONTRAINDICATIONS
Use 12 hr before or after radiation therapy; 24 hr before or after chemotherapy; excessive leukemic myeloid blasts in bone marrow or peripheral blood (10%); known hypersensitivity to GM-CSF, yeast-derived products, or components of drug

DRUG INTERACTIONS OF CONCERN TO DENTISTRY
• Potentiation of myeloproliferative effects: corticosteroids

SERIOUS REACTIONS
! Pleural or pericardial effusion occurs rarely after infusion.

DENTAL CONSIDERATIONS

General:
• Caution: graft patients or myelosuppressed patients may be at high risk for infection.
• Provide palliative care for dental emergencies only.
• Oral infections should be eliminated and/or treated aggressively.
• If additional analgesia is required for dental pain, consider alternative analgesics (NSAIDs) in patients taking narcotics for acute or chronic pain.
• Monitor and record vital signs.
• Avoid products that affect platelet function, such as aspirin and NSAIDs.
• Patient on chronic drug therapy may rarely present with symptoms of blood dyscrasias, which can include

infection, bleeding, and poor healing. If dyscrasia is present, caution patient to prevent oral tissue trauma when using oral hygiene aids.
• Examine for oral manifestation of opportunistic infection.
• Palliative medication may be required for management of oral side effects.
Consultations:
• Medical consultation should include routine blood counts, including platelet counts and bleeding time.
• Consult physician; prophylactic or therapeutic antiinfectives may be indicated if surgery or periodontal treatment is required.
• In a patient with symptoms of blood dyscrasias, request a medical consultation for blood studies and postpone treatment until normal values are reestablished.
• Medical consultation may be required to assess disease control and patient's ability to tolerate stress.
Teach Patient/Family to:
• Use soft tooth brush to reduce risk of bleeding.
• Encourage effective oral hygiene to prevent soft tissue inflammation.
• Prevent trauma when using oral hygiene aids.
• Report oral lesions, soreness, or bleeding to dentist.

saxagliptin
sax´-a-glip´-tin
(Onglyza)
Do not confused with sitagliptin or sumatriptan.

CATEGORY AND SCHEDULE
Pregnancy Risk Category: B

Drug Class: Antidiabetic agent, Dipeptidyl peptidase 4 inhibitors

MECHANISM OF ACTION
A competitive inhibitor of dipeptidyl peptidase (DPP4) that delays the inactivation of incretin hormones.
Therapeutic Effect: Reduces fasting and postprandial glucose concentrations.

USES
Type 2 diabetes mellitus

PHARMACOKINETICS
Rapidly and well absorbed following PO administration. Protein binding: negligible. Metabolized in by CYP3A4/5. Partial excretion in feces, partial excretion in urine.
Half-life: 2.5 hr; 3.1 hr (active metabolite).

INDICATIONS AND DOSAGES
▸ **Type 2 Diabetes Mellitus**
PO
Adults. 2.5–5 mg a day.
Concurrent use with strong CYP3A4/5 inhibitors. 2.5 mg a day.
▸ **Dosage in Renal Impairment**
Mild impairment (CrCl greater than 50 ml/min). No adjustment needed.
Moderate to severe impairment (CrCl 50 ml/min or less). 2.5 mg a day.
ESRD requiring dialysis. 2.5 mg a day after dialysis.

SIDE EFFECTS/ADVERSE REACTIONS
Frequent
Headache, urinary tract infection, hypoglycemia, peripheral edema, upper respiratory tract infection, nasopharyngitis
Occasional
Sinusitis, abdominal pain, gastroenteritis, vomiting, decrease lymphocyte count, hypersensitivity reaction
Rare
Lymphopenia

S

PRECAUTIONS AND CONTRAINDICATIONS
Hypersensitivity to saxigliptin or its components
Caution:
Renal impairment
Concurrent use with insulin secretagogues; increase risk of hypoglycemia

DRUG INTERACTIONS OF CONCERN TO DENTISTRY
• Antacids: May decrease the levels and effects of saxagliptin
• CYP3A4 inducers: May decrease the levels and effects of saxagliptin
• CYP3A4 inhibitors: May increase the levels and effects of saxagliptin
• Insulin secretagogues; increase risk of hypoglycemia

SERIOUS REACTIONS
! A hypersensitivity reaction may be life threatening. Signs and symptoms include fever, rash, fatigue, intractable nausea and vomiting, severe diarrhea, abdominal pain, cough, pharyngitis, and dyspnea.
! Overdose or insufficient food intake may produce hypoglycemia, especially with increased glucose demands.
! Bone fracture has been reported.

DENTAL CONSIDERATIONS
General:
• Short appointments and a stress-reduction protocol may be required for anxious patients.
• Diabetics may be more susceptible to infection and have delayed wound healing.
• Question the patient about self-monitoring of drug's antidiabetic effect including blood glucose values or finger-stick records.

• Avoid prescribing aspiring-containing products.
• Consider semisupine chair position for patient comfort if GI side effects occur.
Consultations:
• Medical consultation may include data from patient's blood glucose monitoring, including glycosylated hemoglobin or HbA$_{1c}$ testing.
• Medical consultation may be required to assess disease control.
Teach Patient/Family to:
• Encourage effective oral hygiene to prevent soft tissue inflammation.
• Prevent trauma when using oral hygiene aids.
• Avoid mouth rinses with high alcohol content because of drying effects.

scopolamine
skoe-**pol**′-ah-meen
(Trans-Derm Scop, Transderm-V)

CATEGORY AND SCHEDULE
Pregnancy Risk Category: C

Drug Class: Antiemetic, anticholinergic

MECHANISM OF ACTION
An anticholinergic that reduces excitability of labyrinthine receptors, depressing conduction in the vestibular cerebellar pathway.
Therapeutic Effect: Prevents motion-induced nausea and vomiting.

USES
Prevention of motion sickness; prevention of nausea, vomiting associated with anesthesia or opiate analgesia

PHARMACOKINETICS
Patch: Onset 4–5 hr, duration 72 hr.

INDICATIONS AND DOSAGES
▸ **Prevention of Motion Sickness**
Transdermal
Adults. 1 system q72h.
▸ **Postoperative Nausea or Vomiting**
Transdermal
Adults, Elderly. 1 system no sooner than 1 hr before surgery and removed 24 hr after surgery.

SIDE EFFECTS/ADVERSE REACTIONS
Frequent
Dry mouth, somnolence, blurred vision
Rare
Dizziness, restlessness, hallucinations, confusion, difficulty urinating, rash

PRECAUTIONS AND CONTRAINDICATIONS
Angle-closure glaucoma, GI or GU obstruction, myasthenia gravis, paralytic ileus, tachycardia, thyrotoxicosis
Caution:
Children, elderly, pyloric, urinary, bladder neck, intestinal obstruction; liver, kidney disease

DRUG INTERACTIONS OF CONCERN TO DENTISTRY
• Increased anticholinergic effects: propantheline and other anticholinergic drugs
• Increased risk of CNS depression: alcohol, all CNS depressants

SERIOUS REACTIONS
! None known

DENTAL CONSIDERATIONS
General:
• Avoid dental light in patient's eyes; offer dark glasses for patient comfort.

• Caution patients about driving or performing other tasks requiring mental alertness.
Teach Patient/Family to:
• Avoid mouth rinses with high alcohol content because of drying effects.
• Avoid exposure to heat or exercise while taking.

---

secobarbital
see-koe-**bar**′-bih-tal
Schedule II
(Seconal)

CATEGORY AND SCHEDULE
Pregnancy Risk Category: D
Controlled Substance: Schedule II

Drug Class: Sedative-hypnotic barbiturate

MECHANISM OF ACTION
A barbiturate that depresses the CNS activity by binding to barbiturate site at the gamma-aminobutyric acid (GABA)-receptor complex, enhancing GABA activity and depressing the reticular activity system.
Therapeutic Effect: Produces hypnotic effect due to CNS depression.

S

USES
Treatment of insomnia, sedation, preoperative medication, status epilepticus, acute tetanus convulsions

PHARMACOKINETICS
Well absorbed from the GI tract. Protein binding: 52%–57%. Crosses blood-brain barrier. Widely distributed. Metabolized in liver by microsomal enzyme system to inactive and active metabolites.

Primarily excreted in urine. Not removed by hemodialysis. *Half-life:* 15–40 hr.

INDICATIONS AND DOSAGES
▸ **Insomnia**
PO
Adults. 100 mg at bedtime.
▸ **Preoperative Sedation**
PO
Adults. 100–300 mg 1–2 hr. before procedure.
Children. 2–6 mg/kg 1–2 hr. before procedure. Maximum: 100 mg/dose.
▸ **Sedation, Daytime**
PO
Adults. 30–50 mg 3–4 times a day.
Children. 2 mg/kg 3 times a day.

SIDE EFFECTS/ADVERSE REACTIONS
Frequent
Somnolence
Occasional
Agitation, confusion, hyperkinesia, ataxia, CNS depression, nightmares, nervousness, psychiatric disturbance, hallucinations, insomnia, anxiety, dizziness, abnormality in thinking, hypoventilation, apnea, bradycardia, hypotension, syncope, nausea, vomiting, constipation, headache
Rare
Hypersensitivity reactions, fever, liver damage, megaloblastic anemia

PRECAUTIONS AND CONTRAINDICATIONS
History of manifest or latent porphyria, marked liver dysfunction, marked respiratory disease in which dyspnea or obstruction is evident, and hypersensitivity to secobarbital or barbiturates
Caution:
Anemia, lactation, hepatic disease, renal disease, hypertension, elderly, acute/chronic pain

DRUG INTERACTIONS OF CONCERN TO DENTISTRY
• Hepatotoxicity: halogenated hydrocarbon anesthetics
• Increased CNS depression: alcohol, all CNS depressants
• Increased metabolism of carbamazepine, tricyclic antidepressants, corticosteroids
• Decreased half-life of doxycycline

SERIOUS REACTIONS
❗ Agranulocytosis, megaloblastic anemia, apnea, hypoventilation, bradycardia, hypotension, syncope, hepatic damage, and Stevens-Johnson syndrome rarely occur.
❗ Tolerance and physical dependence may occur with repeated use.

DENTAL CONSIDERATIONS

General:
• Determine why the patient is taking the drug.
• Monitor vital signs at every appointment because of cardiovascular side effects. Evaluate respiration characteristics and rate.
• Patients on chronic drug therapy may rarely have symptoms of blood dyscrasias, which can include infection, bleeding, and poor healing.
• When used for sedation in dentistry:
  • Assess vital signs before and after use as sedative.
  • Observe respiratory dysfunction: respiratory depression, character, rate, rhythm; hold drug if respirations are less than 10/min or if pupils are dilated.
• After supine positioning, have patient sit upright for at least 2 min before standing to avoid orthostatic hypotension.

- Have someone drive patient to and from dental office when drug used for conscious sedation.
- Barbiturates induce liver microsomal enzymes, which alter the metabolism of other drugs.
- Geriatric patients are more susceptible to drug effects; use a lower dose.

Consultations:
- In a patient with symptoms of blood dyscrasias, request a medical consultation for blood studies and postpone dental treatment until normal values are reestablished.

Teach Patient/Family to:
- Avoid driving or other activities requiring mental alertness.
- Avoid alcohol ingestion and CNS depressants; serious CNS depression may result.
- Use caution when using OTC preparations (antihistamines, cold remedies) that contain CNS depressants.

selegiline hydrochloride

seh-**ledge'**-ill-ene high-droh-**klor'**-ide
(Apo-Selegiline[CAN], Eldepryl, Novo-Selegiline[CAN], Selgene[AUS])
Do not confuse selegiline with Stelazine, or Eldepryl with enalapril.

CATEGORY AND SCHEDULE
Pregnancy Risk Category: C

Drug Class: Antiparkinson agent

MECHANISM OF ACTION
An antiparkinson agent that irreversibly inhibits the activity of monoamine oxidase type B, the enzyme that breaks down dopamine, thereby increasing dopaminergic action.
Therapeutic Effect: Relieves signs and symptoms of Parkinson's disease.

USES
Adjunct management of Parkinson's disease in patients being treated with levodopa or carbidopa

PHARMACOKINETICS
Rapidly absorbed from the GI tract. Crosses the blood-brain barrier. Metabolized in the liver to the active metabolites. Primarily excreted in urine. *Half-life:* 17 hr (amphetamine), 20 hr (methamphetamine).

INDICATIONS AND DOSAGES
▶ Adjunctive Treatment for Parkinsonism
PO
Adults. 10 mg/day in divided doses, such as 5 mg at breakfast and lunch, given concomitantly with each dose of carbidopa and levodopa.
Elderly. Initially, 5 mg in the morning. May increase up to 10 mg/day.

SIDE EFFECTS/ADVERSE REACTIONS
Frequent
Nausea, dizziness, light-headedness, syncope, abdominal discomfort
Occasional
Confusion, hallucinations, dry mouth, vivid dreams, dyskinesia
Rare
Headache, myalgia, anxiety, diarrhea, insomnia

PRECAUTIONS AND CONTRAINDICATIONS
Hypersensitivity: fluoxetine, meperidine

Caution:
Lactation, children

DRUG INTERACTIONS OF CONCERN TO DENTISTRY

• Fatal interaction: opioids (especially meperidine); do not administer together
• Risk of serotonin syndrome: serotonin uptake inhibitors (fluoxetine, sertraline, paroxetine)

SERIOUS REACTIONS

! Symptoms of overdose may vary from CNS depression, characterized by sedation, apnea, cardiovascular collapse, and death, to severe paradoxic reactions, such as hallucinations, tremor, and seizures.
! Other serious effects may include involuntary movements, impaired motor coordination, loss of balance, blepharospasm, facial grimaces, feeling of heaviness in the lower extremities, depression, nightmares, delusions, overstimulation, sleep disturbance, and anger.

DENTAL CONSIDERATIONS

General:
• Monitor vital signs at every appointment because of cardiovascular side effects.
• After supine positioning, have patient sit upright for at least 2 min before standing to avoid orthostatic hypotension.
• Assess for presence of extrapyramidal motor symptoms, such as tardive dyskinesia and akathisia. Extrapyramidal motor activity may complicate dental treatment.
• Assess salivary flow as a factor in caries, periodontal disease, and candidiasis.

Consultations:
• Medical consultation may be required to assess disease control and patient's ability to tolerate stress.
• If signs of tardive dyskinesia or akathisia are present, refer to physician.

Teach Patient/Family to:
• Use powered tooth brush if patient has difficulty holding conventional devices.
• When chronic dry mouth occurs, advise patient to:
  • Avoid mouth rinses with high alcohol content because of drying effects.
  • Use daily home fluoride products to prevent caries.
  • Use sugarless gum, frequent sips of water, or saliva substitutes.

sertaconazole
sir-tah-**con**´-ah-zole
(Ertaczo)

CATEGORY AND SCHEDULE
Pregnancy Risk Category: C

Drug Class: Antifungal

MECHANISM OF ACTION
An imidazole derivative that inhibits synthesis of ergosterol, a vital component of fungal cell formation. *Therapeutic Effect:* Damages the fungal cell membrane, altering its function.

USES
Fungal infections

PHARMACOKINETICS
Half-life: 60 hr.

INDICATIONS AND DOSAGES
▸ **Tinea Pedis**
Topical
Adults, Elderly, Children 12 yr and older. Apply to affected area twice a day for 4 wk.

SIDE EFFECTS/ADVERSE REACTIONS
Rare
Burning, tenderness, erythema, dryness, pruritus, hyperpigmentation, and contact dermatitis at application site

PRECAUTIONS AND CONTRAINDICATIONS
None known

DRUG INTERACTIONS OF CONCERN TO DENTISTRY
• None reported

SERIOUS REACTIONS
! None known

DENTAL CONSIDERATIONS

General:
• Determine why patient is taking this drug.

---

sertraline
sir′-trall-een
(Apo-Sertraline[CAN], Novo-Sertraline[CAN], PMS-Sertraline[CAN], Zoloft)
Do not confuse sertraline with Serentil.

CATEGORY AND SCHEDULE
Pregnancy Risk Category: B

Drug Class: Antidepressant

MECHANISM OF ACTION
An antidepressant, anxiolytic, and obsessive-compulsive disorder adjunct that blocks the reuptake of the neurotransmitter serotonin at CNS neuronal presynaptic membranes, increasing its availability at postsynaptic receptor sites.
Therapeutic Effect: Relieves depression, reduces obsessive-compulsive behavior, decreases anxiety.

USES
Treatment of major depression, obsessive-compulsive disorder (OCD), panic disorder, posttraumatic stress disorder, premenstrual dysphoric mood disorder, social anxiety disorder

PHARMACOKINETICS
Incompletely and slowly absorbed from the GI tract; food increases absorption. Protein binding: 98%. Widely distributed. Undergoes extensive first-pass metabolism in the liver to active compound. Excreted in urine and feces. Not removed by hemodialysis. *Half-life:* 26 hr.

INDICATIONS AND DOSAGES
▸ **Depression**
PO
Adults. Initially, 50 mg/day. May increase by 50 mg/day at 7-day intervals up to 200 mg/day.
Elderly. Initially, 25 mg/day. May increase by 25–50 mg/day at 7-day intervals up to 200 mg/day.
▸ **OCD**
PO
Adults, Children 13–17 yr. Initially, 50 mg/day with morning or evening meal. May increase by 50 mg/day at 7-day intervals.

S

Elderly, Children 6–12 yr. Initially, 25 mg/day. May increase by 25–50 mg/day at 7-day intervals. Maximum: 200 mg/day.

▸ **Panic Disorder, Posttraumatic Stress Disorder, Social Anxiety Disorder**

PO

Adults, Elderly. Initially, 25 mg/day. May increase by 50 mg/day at 7-day intervals. Range: 50–200 mg/day. Maximum: 200 mg/day.

▸ **Premenstrual Dysphoric Disorder**

PO

Adults. Initially, 50 mg/day. May increase up to 150 mg/day in 50-mg increments.

SIDE EFFECTS/ADVERSE REACTIONS

Frequent

Headache, nausea, diarrhea, insomnia, somnolence, dizziness, fatigue, rash, dry mouth

Occasional

Anxiety, nervousness, agitation, tremor, dyspepsia, diaphoresis, vomiting, constipation, abnormal ejaculation, visual disturbances, altered taste

Rare

Flatulence, urinary frequency, paraesthesia, hot flashes, chills

PRECAUTIONS AND CONTRAINDICATIONS

Use within 14 days of MAOIs

Caution:

Lactation, elderly, hepatic/renal disease, epilepsy

DRUG INTERACTIONS OF CONCERN TO DENTISTRY

• Increased CNS depression: alcohol, CNS depressants, St. John's wort (herb)

• Increased side effects: highly protein-bound drugs (aspirin), tricyclic antidepressants

• Increased half-life of diazepam

• Possible inhibition of sertraline metabolism: erythromycin, clarithromycin

• Potent inhibitor of CYP2D6 isoenzymes; use drugs metabolized by the enzyme only with caution

• Possible risk of serotonin syndrome with tramadol, oxycodone

• Decreased effects: carbamazepine

• NSAIDs: increased risk of GI side effects

SERIOUS REACTIONS

! None known

DENTAL CONSIDERATIONS

General:

• Monitor vital signs at every appointment because of cardiovascular side effects.

• After supine positioning, have patient sit upright for at least 2 min before standing to avoid orthostatic hypotension.

• Assess salivary flow as a factor in caries, periodontal disease, and candidiasis.

• Avoid dental light in patient's eyes; offer dark glasses for patient comfort.

• Consider semisupine chair position for patient comfort if GI side effects occur.

Consultations:

• Medical consultation may be required to assess patient's ability to tolerate stress.

• Physician should be informed if significant xerostomic side effects occur (e.g., increased caries, sore tongue, problems eating or swallowing, difficulty wearing prosthesis) so that a medication change can be considered.

Teach Patient/Family to:
• Use powered tooth brush if patient has difficulty holding conventional devices.
• When chronic dry mouth occurs, advise patient to:
  • Avoid mouth rinses with high alcohol content because of drying effects.
  • Use daily home fluoride products to prevent caries.
  • Use sugarless gum, frequent sips of water, or saliva substitutes.

sevelamer hydrochloride
seh-**vel**′-ah-mer
high-droh-**klor**′-ide
(Renagel)
Do not confuse Renagel with Reglan or Regonol.

CATEGORY AND SCHEDULE
Pregnancy Risk Category: C

Drug Class: Chelating agent

MECHANISM OF ACTION
An antihyperphosphatemic agent that binds with dietary phosphorus in the GI tract, thus allowing phosphorus to be eliminated through the normal digestive process and decreasing the serum phosphorus level.
Therapeutic Effect: Decreases incidence of hypercalcemic episodes in patients receiving calcium acetate treatment.

USES
Adjunct to peritoneal dialysis

PHARMACOKINETICS
Not absorbed systemically.
Unknown if removed by hemodialysis.

INDICATIONS AND DOSAGES
▸ **Hyperphosphatemia**
PO
Adults, Elderly. 800–1600 mg with each meal, depending on severity of hyperphosphatemia.

SIDE EFFECTS/ADVERSE REACTIONS
Frequent
Infection, pain, hypotension, diarrhea, dyspepsia, nausea, vomiting
Occasional
Headache, constipation, hypertension, thrombosis, increased cough

PRECAUTIONS AND CONTRAINDICATIONS
Bowel obstruction, hypophosphatemia

DRUG INTERACTIONS OF CONCERN TO DENTISTRY
• Possible decrease in bioavailability: orally administered, rapidly absorbed drugs; give at least 1 hr before or 3 hr after sevelamer doses.

SERIOUS REACTIONS
! None known

DENTAL CONSIDERATIONS
General:
• Patients taking this drug may be undergoing renal dialysis; confirm the medical and drug history to plan appropriate management.
• If you prescribe medications for dental needs, have patient take medication 1 hr before or 3 hr after sevelamer doses.

- Monitor and record vital signs.
- Consider semisupine chair position for patient comfort if GI side effects occur.
- Patient may need assistance getting into and out of dental chair. Adjust chair position for patient comfort.
- Consultation with physician may be necessary if sedation or general anesthesia is required.

Consultations:
- Medical consultation may be required to assess disease control and patient's ability to tolerate stress.

Teach Patient/Family to:
- Report oral lesions, soreness, or bleeding to dentist.
- Encourage effective oral hygiene to prevent soft tissue inflammation.
- Prevent trauma when using oral hygiene aids.
- Update health and medication history if physician makes any changes in evaluation or drug regimens; include OTC, herbal, and nonherbal remedies in the update.

sibutramine
sih-**byoo**′-tra-meen
(Meridia)

CATEGORY AND SCHEDULE
Pregnancy Risk Category: C
Controlled Substance: Schedule IV

Drug Class: Amphetamine analog anorexiant

MECHANISM OF ACTION
A CNS stimulant that inhibits reuptake of serotonin (enhancing satiety) and norepinephrine (raises metabolic rate) centrally.

Therapeutic Effect: Induces and maintains weight loss.

USES
Treatment of obesity

PHARMACOKINETICS
Rapidly absorbed from the GI tract. Protein binding: 95%–97%. Metabolized in liver, undergoes first-pass metabolism. Primarily excreted in urine, minimal elimination in feces. *Half-life:* 1.1 hr.

INDICATIONS AND DOSAGES
▶ **Weight Loss**
PO
Adults 16 yr and older. Initially, 10 mg/day. May increase up to 15 mg/day. Maximum: 20 mg/day.

SIDE EFFECTS/ADVERSE REACTIONS
Frequent
Headache, dry mouth, anorexia, constipation, insomnia, rhinitis, pharyngitis
Occasional
Back pain, flu syndrome, dizziness, nausea, asthenia (loss of strength, energy), arthralgia, nervousness, dyspepsia, sinusitis, abdominal pain, anxiety, dysmenorrhea
Rare
Depression, rash, cough, sweating, tachycardia, migraine, increased B/P, paresthesia, altered taste

PRECAUTIONS AND CONTRAINDICATIONS
Anorexia nervosa, concomitant MAOI use, concomitant use of centrally acting appetite suppressants, hypersensitivity to sibutramine or any component of the formulation

Caution:
Requires monitoring of B/P, risk of serotonin syndrome with other serotonin reuptake inhibitors, glaucoma, lactation, children younger than 16 yr, elderly, seizures

DRUG INTERACTIONS OF CONCERN TO DENTISTRY

• Avoid use of meperidine: risk of serotonin syndrome

SERIOUS REACTIONS

! Seizures, thrombocytopenia, and deaths have been reported.
! Serotonin syndrome can occur with concomitant use of drugs that increase serotonin.
! Large doses may produce extreme nervousness and tachycardia.

DENTAL CONSIDERATIONS

General:
• Monitor vital signs at every appointment because of cardiovascular side effects.
• Avoid or limit dose of vasoconstrictor.
• Assess salivary flow as factor in caries, periodontal disease, and candidiasis.
• Information on any abuse liability is unknown.
• Determine why patient is taking the drug.
Teach Patient/Family:
• When chronic dry mouth occurs, advise patient to:
  • Avoid mouth rinses with high alcohol content because of drying effects.
  • Use daily home fluoride products to prevent caries.
  • Use sugarless gum, frequent sips of water, or saliva substitutes.

sildenafil citrate
sill-**den′**-ah-fill **sih′**-trate
(Viagra)
Do not confuse Viagra with Vaniqa.

CATEGORY AND SCHEDULE
Pregnancy Risk Category: B

Drug Class: Impotence therapy

MECHANISM OF ACTION
An erectile dysfunction agent that inhibits phosphodiesterase type 5, the enzyme responsible for degrading cyclic guanosine monophosphate in the corpus cavernosum of the penis, resulting in smooth muscle relaxation and increased blood flow.
Therapeutic Effect: Facilitates an erection.

USES
Treatment of male erectile dysfunction

PHARMACOKINETICS
PO: Rapid oral absorption, bioavailability 40%, peak plasma levels 30 min–2 hr, hepatic metabolism by CYP3A4 (major) and CYP2C9 (minor) isoenzymes, active metabolite, highly plasma protein bound (96%), major excretion route in feces, lesser route in urine.

INDICATIONS AND DOSAGES
▸ **Erectile Dysfunction**
PO
Adults. 50 mg (30 min–4 hr before sexual activity). Range: 25–100 mg. Maximum dosing frequency is once daily.
Elderly older than 65 yr. Consider starting dose of 25 mg.

S

SIDE EFFECTS/ADVERSE REACTIONS
Frequent
Headache, flushing
Occasional
Dyspepsia, nasal congestion, UTI, abnormal vision, diarrhea
Rare
Dizziness, rash

PRECAUTIONS AND CONTRAINDICATIONS
Concurrent use of sodium nitroprusside or nitrates in any form
Caution:
Complete medical and physical exam to determine cause of erectile dysfunction; because of cardiac risk associated with sexual activity, cardiovascular status should be evaluated; anatomic deformation of penis, conditions predisposing to priapism (sickle cell anemia, anemia, multiple myeloma, leukemia), retinitis pigmentosa, not indicated for women, children, or newborns, pregnancy category B; hepatic or renal impairment, men 65 yr or older

DRUG INTERACTIONS OF CONCERN TO DENTISTRY
• Avoid use of nitroglycerin within 24 hr
• Increased plasma levels caused by interference with metabolism: cimetidine, erythromycin, ketoconazole, itraconazole
• Inhibitors of CYP3A4 or CYP2C9 isoenzymes: should be used with caution

SERIOUS REACTIONS
! Prolonged erections (lasting over 4 hr) and priapism (painful erections lasting over 6 hr) occur rarely.

DENTAL CONSIDERATIONS

General:
• This is an acute-use drug intended to be taken just before sexual activity, and the reported incidence of oral side effects does not differ from a placebo. However, the potential interacting drugs should be avoided.

silver sulfadiazine
sul-fah-**dye**′-ah-zeen
(Flamazine[CAN], SSD, SSD AF, Silvadene)

CATEGORY AND SCHEDULE
Pregnancy Risk Category: B

Drug Class: Antimicrobial

MECHANISM OF ACTION
An antiinfective that acts upon the cell wall and cell membrane. Releases silver slowly in concentrations selectively toxic to bacteria.
Therapeutic Effect: Bactericidal.

USES
Treatment of urinary tract infections

PHARMACOKINETICS
Variably absorbed. Significant systemic absorption may occur if applied to extensive burns. Absorbed medication excreted unchanged in urine. ***Half-life:*** 10 hr (half-life increased with impaired renal function).

INDICATIONS AND DOSAGES
▶ **Burns**
Topical
Adults, Elderly, Children. Apply 1–2 times daily.

SIDE EFFECTS/ADVERSE REACTIONS

Side effects characteristic of all sulfonamides may occur when systemically absorbed, such as extensive burn areas, anorexia, nausea, vomiting, headache, diarrhea, dizziness, photosensitivity, joint pain
Frequent
Burning feeling at treatment site
Occasional
Brown-gray skin discoloration, rash, itching
Rare
Increased sensitivity of skin to sunlight

PRECAUTIONS AND CONTRAINDICATIONS

Hypersensitivity to silver sulfadiazine or any component of the formulation

DRUG INTERACTIONS OF CONCERN TO DENTISTRY

• None reported

SERIOUS REACTIONS

! If significant systemic absorption occurs, less often but serious are hemolytic anemia, hypoglycemia, diuresis, peripheral neuropathy, Stevens-Johnson syndrome, agranulocytosis, disseminated lupus erythematosus, anaphylaxis, hepatitis, and toxic nephrosis.
! Fungal superinfections may occur.
! Interstitial nephritis occurs rarely.

DENTAL CONSIDERATIONS

General:
• Dental management depends on extent and severity of burns and patient's ability to cooperate; above all use aseptic techniques.
• Provide palliative dental care for dental emergencies only.

Consultations:
• Medical consultation may be required to assess disease control and patient's ability to tolerate stress.
• Consult patient's physician if an acute dental infection occurs and another antiinfective is required.
Teach Patient/Family to:
• Encourage effective oral hygiene to prevent soft tissue inflammation.
• Prevent trauma when using oral hygiene aids.

simethicone
sih-**meth**'-ih-kone
(Alka-Seltzer Gas Relief, Gas-X, Genasyme, Infant Mylicon, Mylanta Gas, Ovol[CAN], Phazyme)

CATEGORY AND SCHEDULE
Pregnancy Risk Category: C
OTC

Drug Class: Antiflatulent

MECHANISM OF ACTION
An antiflatulent that changes surface tension of gas bubbles, allowing easier elimination of gas.
Therapeutic Effect: Prevents formation of gas pockets in the GI tract.

USES
Relief of bloating, discomfort, and pain caused by excessive gas in the stomach

PHARMACOKINETICS
Does not appear to be absorbed from GI tract. Excreted unchanged in feces.

S

INDICATIONS AND DOSAGES

▶ **Antiflatulent**

PO

Adults, Elderly, Children 12 yr and older. 40–250 mg after meals and at bedtime. Maximum: 500 mg/day.
Children 2–11 yr. 40 mg 4 times a day.
Children younger than 2 yr. 20 mg 4 times a day.

SIDE EFFECTS/ADVERSE REACTIONS

None known

PRECAUTIONS AND CONTRAINDICATIONS

None known

DRUG INTERACTIONS OF CONCERN TO DENTISTRY

• None reported

SERIOUS REACTIONS

! None known

DENTAL CONSIDERATIONS

General:

• Determine why patient is taking the drug.
• Consider semisupine chair position for patient comfort because of GI effects of disease.
• Question patient about tolerance of NSAIDs or aspirin related to GI disease.
• Patients with gastroesophageal reflux may present with oral symptoms, including burning mouth, secondary candidiasis, and signs of tooth erosion.
• Patients using this drug may have GI disease; review medical and drug history.

Teach Patient/Family to:

• Update health and medication history if physician makes any changes in evaluation or drug

regimens; include OTC, herbal, and nonherbal remedies in the update.
• Encourage effective oral hygiene to prevent soft tissue inflammation.

simvastatin

sim′-vah-sta-tin
(Apo-Simvastatin[CAN],
Lipex[AUS], Zocor)
Do not confuse Zocor with
Cozaar.

CATEGORY AND SCHEDULE

Pregnancy Risk Category: X

Drug Class: Antihyperlipidemic

MECHANISM OF ACTION

A HMG-CoA reductase inhibitor that interferes with cholesterol biosynthesis by inhibiting the conversion of the enzyme HMG-CoA to mevalonate.
Therapeutic Effect: Decreases serum low-density lipoproteins (LDLs), cholesterol, very low-density lipoproteins (VLDLs), and plasma triglyceride levels; slightly increases serum high-density lipoprotein (HDL) concentration.

USES

An adjunct in homozygous familial hypercholesterolemia, mixed hyperlipidemia, elevated serum triglyceride levels, and type IV hyperproteinemia; also reduces total cholesterol LDL-C, apo B, and triglyceride levels; patient should first be placed on cholesterol-lowering diet; effective in reducing risk of heart attacks and strokes

PHARMACOKINETICS

Route	Onset	Peak	Duration
PO to reduce cholesterol	3 days	14 days	N/A

Well absorbed from the GI tract. Protein binding: 95%. Undergoes extensive first-pass metabolism. Hydrolyzed to active metabolite. Primarily eliminated in feces. Unknown if removed by hemodialysis.

INDICATIONS AND DOSAGES
▸ **Adjunct to Diet to Decrease Heterozygous Familial Hypercholesterolemia in Adolescents 10–17 Yr of Age (Girls at Least 1-Yr Post-menarche) Heterozygous Familial Hypercholesterolemia**
PO
Pediatric. 10 mg once daily in evening. Range: 10–40 mg/day. Maximum: 40 mg/day.
▸ **To Decrease Elevated Total and LDL Cholesterol in Hypercholesterolemia (Types IIA and IIIB), Lower Triglyceride Levels, and Increase HDL Levels; to Reduce Risk of Death and Prevent MI in Patients with Heart Disease and Elevated Cholesterol Level; to Reduce Risk of Revascularization Procedures; to Decrease Risk of Stroke or Transient Ischemic Attack; to Prevent Cardiovascular Events**
PO
Adults. Initially, 10–40 mg/day in evening. Dosage adjusted at 4-wk intervals.
Elderly. Initially, 10 mg/day. May increase by 5–10 mg/day q4wk. Range: 5–80 mg/day. Maximum: 80 mg/day.

SIDE EFFECTS/ADVERSE REACTIONS
Simvastatin is generally well tolerated; side effects are usually mild and transient
Occasional
Headache, abdominal pain or cramps, constipation, upper respiratory tract infection
Rare
Diarrhea, flatulence, asthenia (loss of strength and energy), nausea or vomiting

PRECAUTIONS AND CONTRAINDICATIONS
Active hepatic disease or unexplained, persistent elevations of liver function test results, age younger than 18 yr, pregnancy
Caution:
Past liver disease, alcoholics (first-pass metabolism with CYP3A4 isoenzymes); severe acute infections, trauma, hypotension, uncontrolled seizure disorders, severe metabolic disorders, electrolyte imbalances

DRUG INTERACTIONS OF CONCERN TO DENTISTRY
• Increased myalgia, myositis: erythromycin, cyclosporine, itraconazole, ketoconazole
• Caution with use of drugs that are strong inhibitors of CYP3A4 isoenzymes

SERIOUS REACTIONS
! Lens opacities may occur.
! Hypersensitivity reaction and hepatitis occur rarely.

DENTAL CONSIDERATIONS
General:
• Consider semisupine chair position for patient comfort because of GI side effects.
• Assess patient for possible cardiovascular disease.

S

sirolimus
sir-oh-**leem**′-us
(Rapamune)

CATEGORY AND SCHEDULE
Pregnancy Risk Category: C

Drug Class: Immunosuppressant

MECHANISM OF ACTION
An immunosuppressant that inhibits T-lymphocyte proliferation induced by stimulation of cell surface receptors, mitogens, alloantigens, and lymphokines. Prevents activation of the enzyme target of rapamycin, a key regulatory kinase in cell cycle progression.
Therapeutic Effect: Inhibits proliferation of T and B cells, essential components of the immune response; prevents organ transplant rejection.

USES
Adjunct to organ transplantation

PHARMACOKINETICS
Rapidly absorbed from the GI tract. Peak levels 1 hr (inhibited by food). Protein binding: 92%. Extensively metabolized by the CYP3A4 isoenzyme in the intestinal wall and liver. Primarily excreted in feces.

INDICATIONS AND DOSAGES
▸ **Prevention of Organ Transplant Rejection**
PO
Adults. Loading dose: 6 mg. Maintenance: 2 mg/day.
Children 13 yr and older weighing less than 40 kg. Loading dose: 3 mg/m^2. Maintenance: 1 mg/m^2/day.

SIDE EFFECTS/ADVERSE REACTIONS
Occasional
Hypercholesterolemia, hyperlipidemia, hypertension, rash; with high doses (5 mg/day): anemia, arthralgia, diarrhea, hypokalemia, and thrombocytopenia

PRECAUTIONS AND CONTRAINDICATIONS
Hypersensitivity to sirolimus, malignancy

DRUG INTERACTIONS OF CONCERN TO DENTISTRY
• Increased blood levels: potent inhibitors of CYP3A4 isoenzymes (clarithromycin, clotrimazole, erythromycin, fluconazole, itraconazole, ritonavir, indinavir, grapefruit juice)
• Decreased blood levels: potent inducers of CYP3A4 isoenzymes (phenobarbital, carbamazepine, St. John's wort [herb])

SERIOUS REACTIONS
! None known

DENTAL CONSIDERATIONS

General:
• Caution: patients on immunosuppressive therapy may be at high risk for infection.
• Provide palliative dental care for dental emergencies only.
• Oral infections should be eliminated and/or treated aggressively.
• Patients may be at risk for bleeding; check oral signs.
• Examine for evidence of oral candidiasis. Topically acting antifungals may be preferred: note potential drug interactions.
• Monitor and record vital signs.

• Avoid products that affect platelet function, such as aspirin and NSAIDs.

• Patient on chronic drug therapy may rarely present with symptoms of blood dyscrasias, which can include infection, bleeding, and poor healing. If dyscrasia is present, caution patient to prevent oral tissue trauma when using oral hygiene aids.

• Consider local hemostasis measures to prevent excessive bleeding.

Consultations:

• Medical consultation should include routine blood counts, including platelet counts and bleeding time.

• Consult physician; prophylactic or therapeutic antiinfectives may be indicated if surgery or periodontal treatment is required.

• In a patient with symptoms of blood dyscrasias, request a medical consultation for blood studies and postpone treatment until normal values are reestablished.

• Medical consultation may be required to assess disease control and patient's ability to tolerate stress.

Teach Patient/Family to:

• Use soft tooth brush to reduce risk of bleeding.

• Encourage effective oral hygiene to prevent soft tissue inflammation.

• Prevent trauma when using oral hygiene aids.

• Report oral lesions, soreness, or bleeding to dentist.

• Use powered tooth brush if patient has difficulty holding conventional devices.

sitagliptin
sit-ah-**glip**′-tin
(Januvia)

CATEGORY AND SCHEDULE
Pregnancy Risk Category: B

Drug Class: Antihyperglycemic (Type-2 diabetes mellitus)

MECHANISM OF ACTION
Therapeutic Effect: Increases and prolongs active incretin levels, thereby increasing insulin release and decreasing glucagon levels in the circulation in a glucose-dependent manner

USES
Improves glycemic control in Type 2 diabetes mellitus in combination with metformin or a PPAR-gamma agonist (e.g., thiazolidinediones) when the single agent alone, with diet and exercise, does not provide adequate glycemic control

PHARMACOKINETICS
Rapidly absorbed after oral administration. Protein binding: 38%. Primarily excreted unchanged in the urine (79%) by active tubular secretion, minor fraction metabolized in the liver (CYP3A4, 2C8)

INDICATIONS AND DOSAGES
▸ **Monotherapy of Type 2 Diabetes Mellitus (or Combination Therapy with Metformin or a PPAR-gamma Agonist)**
PO
Adult. 100 mg once daily.

S

SIDE EFFECTS/ADVERSE REACTIONS

Frequent

Hypoglycemia, nasopharyngitis, upper respiratory tract infection, headache

Occasional

Abdominal pain, nausea, diarrhea

Rare

Anaphylaxis, angioedema, rash, urticaria, exfoliative skin reactions

PRECAUTIONS AND CONTRAINDICATIONS

Hypersensitivity

Renal insufficiency (requires dosage adjustment)

Safety is nursing not established

Increased possibility of hypoglycemia when used with other antidiabetic agents

DRUG INTERACTIONS OF CONCERN TO DENTISTRY

- None reported

SERIOUS REACTIONS

! Anaphylaxis, angioedema, Stevens-Johnson syndrome

DENTAL CONSIDERATIONS

General:

- Short appointments and a stress-reduction protocol may be required for anxious patients.
- Question patient about self-monitoring of blood glucose values.
- Ensure that patient is following prescribed diet and medication regimen.
- Consider semisupine chair position for patient comfort if GI side/adverse effects occur.
- Diabetics may be more susceptible to infection and have delayed wound healing.
- Place on frequent recall to evaluate oral hygiene and healing response.

Consultations:

- Consult with physician to determine disease control and ability to tolerate dental procedures.
- Notify physician immediately if symptoms of lactic acidosis are observed (myalgia, respiratory distress, weakness, diarrhea, malaise, muscle cramps, somnolence).
- Medical consultation may include data from patient's blood glucose monitoring, including glycosylated hemoglobin or HbA$_{1c}$ testing.
- Oral and maxillofacial surgical procedures associated with significantly restricted food intake require a medical consultation and may require physician adjusting medication regimen.

Teach Patient/Family to:

- Encourage effective oral hygiene to prevent soft-tissue inflammation.
- Update medical history when disease status/glycemic control or medication regimen change.

sodium fluoride

soe′-dee-um **flor**′-ide
(Fluoritab, Flura-Drops, Fluor-A-Day, Fluotic, Fluoridex Karidium, Luride Lozi-Tabs, Pediaflor, PediDent, Solu-Flur; also found in pediatric vitamin formulas)

CATEGORY AND SCHEDULE

Pregnancy Risk Category: Not established

Drug Class: Fluoride ion

MECHANISM OF ACTION

Interacts with tooth structure to increase resistance to acid dissolution; promotes enamel remineralization and inhibits dental plaque microorganisms.

USES
Prevention of dental caries

PHARMACOKINETICS
PO: Efficient oral absorption (75%–90%); distributed to calcified tissues (bones and teeth); excreted in urine, feces; crosses placenta, excreted in breast milk.

INDICATIONS AND DOSAGES
▶ Prevention of Dental Caries
Topical
Adult, Children older than 12 yr.
10 ml 0.2% solution daily after brushing teeth; rinse mouth for at least 1 min with solution. Do not swallow.
PO
Children 6–12 yr. 5 ml 0.2% solution. Must ascertain fluoride concentration in patient's drinking water before prescribing, as shown in the following tables:
▶ USA—Fluoride Supplementation Schedule
Drinking Water [F⁻]

Child's Age	Less than 0.3 ppm	0.3– 0.6 ppm	More than 0.6 ppm
Birth– 6 mo	0	0	0
6 mo– 3 yr	0.25 mg/ day	***	0
3–6 yr	0.50 mg/ day	0.25 mg/day	0
6–16 yr	1.0 mg/day	0.50 mg/day	0

Canada-Fluoride Supplementation Schedule

Age	Canadian Paediatric Society (Applies to all Children)	Canadian Dental Association (Applies to Children with High Risk of Caries)
6 mo– 2 yr	0.25 mg/day	0
3–5 yr	0.50 mg/day	0.25 mg/day (0.5 mg/day if fluoridated toothpaste is not used regularly)
6–12 yr	Not applicable	1.00 mg/day
6–16 yr	1.0 mg/day	Not applicable

SIDE EFFECTS/ADVERSE REACTIONS
Occasional
Mottled, stained enamel (chronic use), stomatitis
Acute overdose: Black tarry stools, bloody vomit, diarrhea, decreased respiration, increased salivation, watery eyes
Chronic overdose: Hypocalcemia, tetany, respiratory arrest, constipation, loss of appetite, nausea, vomiting, weight loss

PRECAUTIONS AND CONTRAINDICATIONS
Hypersensitivity, renal insufficiency, GI ulcerations
Caution:
Children younger than 6 yr (must evaluate total fluoride ingestion)

DRUG INTERACTIONS OF CONCERN TO DENTISTRY
• Avoid use with dairy products and gastric alkalinizers

S

SERIOUS REACTIONS
! Cardiac arrhythmias, renal failure

DENTAL CONSIDERATIONS

General:
• Determine fluoride concentration in water supply, and then calculate dosage.
• Recommended dose should not be exceeded or dental fluorosis and osseous changes may occur.
• To reduce risk of accidental ingestion and overdosage, ADA recommends that a limit of 264 mg sodium fluoride be dispensed in prepackaged containers.
• Give drops after meals with fluids or undiluted tablets; may be chewed; do not swallow whole; may be given with water or juice; avoid milk.
• Systemic fluoride use during pregnancy has not been shown to prevent tooth decay in children.
• Treatment of acute overdose:
  • Gastric lavage with calcium chloride or calcium hydroxide solution to precipitate fluoride.
  • Maintenance of high urine output.
  • Refer to hospital emergency facility.

Teach Patient/Family to:
• Monitor children using gel or rinse; not to be swallowed.
• Not drink, eat, or rinse mouth for at least 0.5 hr after topical use.
• Apply after brushing and flossing at bedtime.
• Store out of children's reach.

sodium fluoride (topical)
soe′-dee-um **flor**′-ide
(nonabrasive: Karigel, NeutraCare, PreviDent; with abrasive: PreviDent 5000 Plus)

CATEGORY AND SCHEDULE
Pregnancy Risk Category: Not established

Drug Class: Fluoride ion

MECHANISM OF ACTION
Interacts with enamel surface to increase resistance to acid dissolution; promotes enamel remineralization and inhibits dental plaque microorganisms

USES
Prevention of dental caries, hypersensitive root surfaces

PHARMACOKINETICS
PO: Efficient oral absorption (75%–90%); distributed to calcified tissues (bones and teeth); excreted in urine, feces; crosses placenta, excreted in breast milk.

INDICATIONS AND DOSAGES
▸ Prevention of Dental Caries
Topical
Adults, Children older than 6 yr.
Nonabrasive gels—use daily; apply thin ribbon to tooth brush for at least 1 min after regular brushing, preferably at bedtime; expectorate and refrain from eating, drinking, and rinsing; children should use under parental supervision.
Available forms include: Gel or cream 2 oz (56 g) squeeze tube 0.5% (as 1.1% sodium fluoride) with and without mild abrasive.

Other fluoride topical products include the following daily-use gels. 1.1% APF (Thera-Flur); 0.4% Sn F2 (Control, Easy-Gel, Flocare, Flo-Gel, Florentine, Gel-Kam, Gel-Pro, Gel-Tin, Perfect Choice, Quick-Gel, Stan-Gard, Stop Gel). Rinses: 0.05% APF daily use (NaFrinse, Phos-Flur) and 0.2% NaF weekly use (NaFrinse, Point-Two, Preventive, PreviDent).

Product Strength	F-Ion (%)	ppm F Equivalence
1.1% NaF	0.5	4950
0.4% SnF2	0.10	970
0.2 % NaF	0.10	910
0.05% NaF	0.02	230

SIDE EFFECTS
Occasional
Mottled, stained enamel (chronic use), stomatitis
Acute overdose: Black tarry stools, bloody vomit, diarrhea, decreased respiration, increased salivation, watery eyes
Chronic overdose: Hypocalcemia, tetany, respiratory arrest, constipation, loss of appetite, nausea, vomiting, weight loss

PRECAUTIONS AND CONTRAINDICATIONS
Hypersensitivity; may be used in areas of fluoridated drinking water
Caution:
Children younger than 6 yr (repeated swallowing of agent could cause dental fluorosis); do not use in pediatric patients younger than 6 yr, infants. Supervise children younger than 6 yr. A 2-oz tube of 1.1% NaF contains 250 mg fluoride, more than twice the amount that the ADA recommends to be dispensed in 1 container. Ingestion of as little as

0.29 oz could cause acute toxicity in a 1-yr-old child. Repeated swallowing could cause fluorosis.

DRUG INTERACTIONS OF CONCERN TO DENTISTRY
• None reported

SERIOUS REACTIONS
! Cardiac arrhythmias, renal failure

DENTAL CONSIDERATIONS
General:
• Neutral sodium fluoride preparations are recommended for patients with exposed root surfaces, which may be hypersensitive.
Teach Patient/Family to:
• Apply daily a thin ribbon of dental cream or gel to tooth brush and brush thoroughly for 2 min, preferably at bedtime.
• Expectorate after use and not to eat, drink, or rinse for 30 min.
• Have children use under parental supervision.

somatropin
soe-mah-**troe**′-pin
(Accretropin; Genotropin, Genotropin MiniQuick, Humatrope, Norditropin, Norditropin Cartridge, Nutropin, Nutropin AQ, Nutropin Depot, Saizen, Serostim, Zorbtive)

S

CATEGORY AND SCHEDULE
Pregnancy Risk Category: C

Drug Class: Growth hormone

MECHANISM OF ACTION
Somatotropin, a purified polypeptide hormone of recombinant DNA origin, contains the identical

sequence of amino acids found in human growth hormone that stimulates growth of linear bone, skeletal muscle, and organs. Human growth hormone also stimulates erythropoietin, which increases red blood cell mass, exerts both insulin-like and diabetogenic effects, and enhances the transmucosal transport of water, electrolytes, and nutrients across the gut.

USES

Growth hormone deficiency
Turner syndrome
AIDS-related wasting
Short bowel syndrome

PHARMACOKINETICS

Bioavailability: 70% when administered subcutaneously. Metabolized in the liver and kidneys. *Half life*: IV, 20–30 min; subcutaneous, IM, 3–5 hr.

INDICATIONS AND DOSAGES
▸ **Growth Hormone Deficiency**
SC (Accretropin)
Children. 0.18 to 0.3 mg/kg body weight divided 6 or 7 times per week.
SC (Humatrope)
Adults. 0.006 mg/kg once daily.
Children. 0.18–0.3 mg/kg weekly divided into alternate-day doses or 6 doses/wk.
SC (Nutropin)
Adults. 0.006 mg/kg once daily.
Children. 0.3–0.7 mg/kg weekly divided into daily doses.
SC (Nutropin AQ)
Adults. 0.006 mg/kg once daily.
SC (Genotropin)
Adults. 0.04–0.08 mg/kg weekly divided into 6–7 equal doses/wk.
Children. 0.16–0.24 mg/kg weekly divided into daily doses.
SC (Protopine)

Children. 0.3 mg/kg weekly divided into daily doses.
SC (Norditropin)
Children. 0.024–0.036 mg/kg/dose 6–7 times a week.
SC (Saizen)
Children. 0.06 mg/kg 3 times a week.
SC only (Nutropin Depot)
Children. 0.75 mg/kg twice monthly or 1.5 mg/kg once monthly.
▸ **Turner Syndrome**
SC (Accretropin)
Children. 0.36 mg/kg divided in doses of 6 or 7 times a week.
SC (Humatrope, Nutropin, Nutropin AQ)
Children. 0.375 mg/kg weekly divided into equal doses 3–7 times a week.
▸ **AIDS-Related Wasting**
SC
Adults weighing more than 55 kg. 6 mg once a day at bedtime.
Adults weighing 45–55 kg. 5 mg once a day at bedtime.
Adults weighing 35–44 kg. 4 mg once a day at bedtime.
Adults weighing less than 35 kg. 0.1 mg/kg once a day at bedtime.
▸ **Short Bowel Syndrome**
SC (Zorbtive)
Adults. 0.1 mg/kg/day. Maximum: 8 mg/day.

SIDE EFFECTS/ADVERSE REACTIONS
Frequent
Bruising, erythema, hemorrhage, edema, pain, pruritus, rash, swelling, injection site reaction
Occasional
Nausea, headache, fatigue, scoliosis

PRECAUTIONS AND CONTRAINDICATIONS
Hypersensitivity to growth hormone, *E. coli* or any component of the formulation

Closed epiphyses (Accretropin)
Local or systemic allergic reaction
may occur
Use with caution in patients with
intracranial hypertension
Progression of scoliosis may occur
Use with caution in patients with
risk factors for diabetes since
somatropin may decrease insulin
sensitivity
Use with caution in patients with
hypopituitarism, hypothyroidism,
and preexisting tumors or growth
hormone deficiency secondary to an
intracranial lesion

DRUG INTERACTIONS OF CONCERN TO DENTISTRY
• Corticosteroids: May inhibit
growth response.

SERIOUS REACTIONS
! Intracranial hypertension with
papilledema, visual changes,
headache, nausea, and/ or vomiting
may occur.
! Glucose intolerance can occur
with overdosage. Long-term
overdosage with growth hormone
could result in signs and symptoms
of acromegaly.

DENTAL CONSIDERATIONS
General:
• Consider semisupine chair position
for patient comfort if GI side effects
occur.
• Avoid dental light in patient's eyes;
offer dark glasses for patient
comfort.
Consultations:
• Medical consultation may be
required to assess disease control.
Teach Patient/Family to:
• Encourage effective oral hygiene
to prevent soft tissue inflammation.
• Use caution to prevent injury when
using oral hygiene aids.

sotalol hydrochloride
soe'-tah-lole high-droh-**klor'**-ide
(Apo-Sotalol[CAN], Betapace,
Betapace AF, Cardol[AUS],
Novo-Sotalol[CAN], PMS-
Sotalol[CAN], Solavert[AUS],
Sorine, Sotab[AUS], Sotacor[AUS],
Sotahexal[AUS])
Do not confuse sotalol with
Stadol.

CATEGORY AND SCHEDULE
Pregnancy Risk Category: B (D if
used in second or third trimester)

Drug Class: Nonselective
β-adrenergic blocker

MECHANISM OF ACTION
A β-adrenergic blocking agent that
prolongs action potential, effective
refractory period, and QT interval.
Decreases heart rate and AV node
conduction; increases AV node
refractoriness.
Therapeutic Effect: Produces
antiarrhythmic activity.

USES
Treatment of life-threatening
ventricular dysrhythmias (class II),
atrial fibrillation (Betapace AF
only), mild-to-moderate heart failure

PHARMACOKINETICS
Well absorbed from the GI tract.
Protein binding: None. Widely
distributed. Primarily excreted
unchanged in urine. Removed by
hemodialysis. *Half-life:* 12 hr
(increased in the elderly and patients
with impaired renal function).

INDICATIONS AND DOSAGES
▸ Documented, Life-Threatening Arrhythmias
PO
Adults, Elderly. Initially, 80 mg twice a day. May increase gradually at 2- to 3-day intervals. Range: 240–320 mg/day.
▸ Dosage in Renal Impairment
Dosage interval is modified on the basis of creatinine clearance.

Creatinine Clearance	Dosage Interval
31–60 ml/min	24 hr
10–30 ml/min	36–48 hr
Less than 10 ml/min	Individualized

SIDE EFFECTS/ADVERSE REACTIONS
Frequent
Diminished sexual function, drowsiness, insomnia, unusual fatigue or weakness
Occasional
Depression, cold hands or feet, diarrhea, constipation, anxiety, nasal congestion, nausea, vomiting
Rare
Altered taste, dry eyes, itching, numbness of fingers, toes, or scalp

PRECAUTIONS AND CONTRAINDICATIONS
Bronchial asthma, cardiogenic shock, prolonged QT syndrome (unless functioning pacemaker is present), second- and third-degree heart block, sinus bradycardia, uncontrolled cardiac failure
Caution:
Lactation, diabetes mellitus, renal disease. Before initiating doses, place patient in cardiac care facility to monitor for drug-induced arrhythmia

DRUG INTERACTIONS OF CONCERN TO DENTISTRY
• Decreased hypotensive effect: NSAIDs, indomethacin
• Increased hypotension, myocardial depression: hydrocarbon inhalation anesthetics
• Hypertension, bradycardia: sympathomimetics
• Slow metabolism of lidocaine

SERIOUS REACTIONS
! Bradycardia, CHF, hypotension, bronchospasm, hypoglycemia, prolonged QT interval, torsades de pointes, ventricular tachycardia, and premature ventricular complexes may occur.

DENTAL CONSIDERATIONS
General:
• Monitor vital signs at every appointment because of cardiovascular side effects.
• After supine positioning, have patient sit upright for at least 2 min before standing to avoid orthostatic hypotension.
• Stress from dental procedures may compromise cardiovascular function; determine patient risk.
• Use vasoconstrictors with caution, in low doses, and with careful aspiration. Avoid use of gingival retraction cord with epinephrine.
• Short appointments and a stress-reduction protocol may be required for anxious patients.
Consultations:
• Medical consultation should be made to assess disease control and patient's ability to tolerate stress.

S

spironolactone

speer-on-oh-**lak′**-tone
(Aldactone, Novo-Spiroton[CAN],
Spiractin[AUS])
Do not confuse Aldactone with
Aldactazide.

CATEGORY AND SCHEDULE

Pregnancy Risk Category: C (D if
used in pregnancy-induced
hypertension)

Drug Class: Potassium-sparing
diuretic

MECHANISM OF ACTION

A potassium-sparing diuretic that
interferes with sodium reabsorption
by competitively inhibiting the
action of aldosterone in the distal
tubule, thus promoting sodium and
water excretion and increasing
potassium retention.
Therapeutic Effect: Produces
diuresis; lowers B/P; diagnostic aid
for primary aldosteronism.

USES

Edema, hypertension, diuretic-
induced hypokalemia, primary
hyperaldosteronism (diagnosis,
short-term treatment, long-term
treatment), nephrotic syndrome,
cirrhosis of the liver with ascites

PHARMACOKINETICS

Route	Onset	Peak	Duration
PO	24–48 hr	48–72 hr	48–72 hr

Well absorbed from the GI tract
(absorption increased with food).
Protein binding: 91%–98%.
Metabolized in the liver to active
metabolite. Primarily excreted in
urine. Unknown if removed by
hemodialysis. *Half-life:* 0–24 hr
(metabolite, 13–24 hr).

INDICATIONS AND DOSAGES
▸ **Edema**
PO
Adults, Elderly. 25–200 mg/day as a
single dose or in 2 divided doses.
Children. 1.5–3.3 mg/kg/day in
divided doses.
Neonates. 1–3 mg/kg/day in 1–2
divided doses.
▸ **Hypertension**
PO
Adults, Elderly. 25–50 mg/day in
1–2 doses/day.
Children. 1.5–3.3 mg/kg/day in
divided doses.
▸ **Hypokalemia**
PO
Adults, Elderly. 25–200 mg/day as a
single dose or in 2 divided doses.
▸ **Male Hirsutism**
PO
Adults, Elderly. 50–200 mg/day as a
single dose or in 2 divided doses.
▸ **Primary Aldosteronism**
PO
Adults, Elderly. 100–400 mg/day as
a single dose or in 2 divided doses.
Children. 100–400 mg/m^2/day as a
single dose or in 2 divided doses.
▸ **Dosage in Renal Impairment**
Dosage interval is modified on the
basis of creatinine clearance.

Creatinine Clearance	Interval
10–50 ml/min	Usual dose q12h–24h
Less than 10 ml/min	Avoid use

SIDE EFFECTS/ADVERSE REACTIONS
Frequent
Hyperkalemia (in patients with renal
insufficiency and those taking

S

potassium supplements),
dehydration, hyponatremia, lethargy
Occasional
Nausea, vomiting, anorexia,
abdominal cramps, diarrhea,
headache, ataxia, somnolence,
confusion, fever
Male: Gynecomastia, impotence,
decreased libido
Female: Menstrual irregularities
(including amenorrhea and
postmenopausal bleeding), breast
tenderness
Rare
Rash, urticaria, hirsutism

PRECAUTIONS AND CONTRAINDICATIONS

Acute renal insufficiency, anuria,
BUN and serum creatinine levels
more than twice normal values,
hyperkalemia
Caution:
Dehydration, hepatic disease,
lactation, hyponatremia

DRUG INTERACTIONS OF CONCERN TO DENTISTRY

• Nephrotoxicity: indomethacin and
possibly other NSAIDs
• Decreased antihypertensive effect:
indomethacin and possibly other
NSAIDs

SERIOUS REACTIONS

! Severe hyperkalemia may produce
arrhythmias, bradycardia, and ECG
changes (tented T waves, widening
QRS complex and ST segment
depression). These may proceed to
cardiac standstill or ventricular
fibrillation.
! Cirrhosis patients are at risk for
hepatic decompensation if
dehydration or hyponatremia occurs.
! Patients with primary
aldosteronism may experience rapid
weight loss and severe fatigue
during high-dose therapy.

DENTAL CONSIDERATIONS

General:
• Monitor vital signs at every
appointment because of
cardiovascular side effects.
• Assess salivary flow as a factor in
caries, periodontal disease, and
candidiasis.
• If dry mouth occurs, follow usual
preventive and palliative measures,
but consider hyponatremia as a
contributing factor.
• Consider semisupine chair position
for patient comfort if GI side effects
occur.
Consultations:
• Medical consultation may be
required to assess disease control
and patient's ability to tolerate
stress.
Teach Patient/Family:
• When chronic dry mouth occurs,
advise patient to:
  • Avoid mouth rinses with high
  alcohol content because of
  drying effects.
  • Use daily home fluoride
  products to prevent caries.
  • Use sugarless gum, frequent
  sips of water, or saliva
  substitutes.

streptomycin
strep-toe-**mye'**-sin

CATEGORY AND SCHEDULE
Pregnancy Risk Category: D

Drug Class: Antibiotics,
aminoglycosides, antitubercular
agent

MECHANISM OF ACTION
An aminoglycoside that binds
directly to the 30S ribosomal
subunits causing a faulty peptide

sequence to form in the protein chain.
Therapeutic Effect: Inhibits bacterial protein synthesis.

USES

Tuberculosis, brucellosis, endocarditis, mycobacterium avium complex (adjunct), plague, tularemia, gram-negative bacteremia (adjunct)

PHARMACOKINETICS

Protein binding: 34%–35%. Excreted in urine by glomerular filtration. **Half-life:** 2.5 hr.

INDICATIONS AND DOSAGES
▸ **Tuberculosis**
IM
Adults. 15 mg/kg/day. Maximum: 1 g/day.
Elderly. 10 mg/kg/day. Maximum: 750 mg/day.
Children. 20–40 mg/kg/day. Maximum: 1 g/day.
▸ **Bacterial Endocarditis**
IM
▸ **Streptococcal**
Adults. 1 g twice daily for the first week, and 500 mg twice daily for the second week.
Elderly (over 60 yr of age). 500 mg twice daily for the entire 2-wk period.
▸ **Enterococcal**
Adults. 1 g twice daily for 2 wk and 500 mg twice daily for an additional 4 wk concomitantly with penicillin. Ototoxicity may require early termination.
▸ **Plague**
IM
Adults. 2 g in two divided doses for a minimum of 10 days.

▸ **Tularemia**
IM
Adults. 1 to 2 g daily in divided doses for 7–10 days or until patient is afebrile for 5–7 days.
Dosage in Renal Impairment

GFR (mL/min)	Dosage Interval
Greater than 50	24 hr
10–50	24–72 hr
Less than 10	72–96 hr

SIDE EFFECTS/ADVERSE REACTIONS
Frequent
Vestibular ototoxicity (nausea, vomiting, and vertigo), paresthesia of face, rash, fever, urticaria, angioneurotic edema, and eosinophilia
Less Frequent
Deafness, exfoliative dermatitis, anaphylaxis, azotemia, leucopenia, thrombocytopenia, pancytopenia, hemolytic anemia, muscular weakness, and amblyopia

PRECAUTIONS AND CONTRAINDICATIONS
Hypersensitivity to streptomycin, other aminoglycosides, or sulfites
Caution:
Antibiotic hypersensitivity
Preexisting kidney or auditory impairment
Concomitant nephrotoxic, ototoxic, or neurotoxic drugs
Concomitant anesthesia or certain muscle relaxing drugs because of the risk of neuromuscular blockade

DRUG INTERACTIONS OF CONCERN TO DENTISTRY
• Increased risk of nephrotoxicity: amphotericin, loop diuretics

S

• May increase the effects of streptomycin: neuromuscular blockers

SERIOUS REACTIONS

! Nephrotoxicity (as evidenced by increased BUN and serum creatinine levels and decreased creatinine clearance) may be reversible if the drug is stopped at the first sign of nephrotoxic symptoms.

! Irreversible ototoxicity (manifested as tinnitus, dizziness, ringing or roaring in the ears, and impaired hearing) and neurotoxicity (as evidenced by headache, dizziness, lethargy, tremor, and visual disturbances) occur occasionally. Symptoms of ototoxicity, nephrotoxicity, and neuromuscular toxicity may occur.

! Superinfections, particularly with fungal infections, may result from bacterial imbalance.

DENTAL CONSIDERATIONS

General:
• Caution patient regarding allergy to medication.
• Do not treat patients with active tuberculosis.
• Determine why the patient is using this medication.
• Determine if the patient is pregnant.
Consultation:
• Laboratory tests may be required to assess hearing, kidney function, and streptomycin blood levels.
Teach Patient/Family to:
• Advise the patient to report any ringing in the ears, hearing loss, balance problems, or changes in vision.

sucralfate

soo-**kral**′-fate
(Apo-Sucralate[CAN], Carafate, Novo-Sucralate[CAN], Ulcyte[AUS])
Do not confuse Carafate with Cafergot.

CATEGORY AND SCHEDULE

Pregnancy Risk Category: B

Drug Class: Protectant, aluminum salt of a sulfated sucrose

MECHANISM OF ACTION

An antiulcer agent that forms an ulcer-adherent complex with proteinaceous exudate, such as albumin, at ulcer site. Also forms a viscous adhesive barrier on the surface of intact mucosa of the stomach or duodenum.
Therapeutic Effect: Protects damaged mucosa from further destruction by absorbing gastric acid, pepsin, and bile salts.

USES

Treatment of duodenal ulcer

PHARMACOKINETICS

Minimally absorbed from the GI tract. Eliminated in feces, with small amount excreted in urine. Not removed by hemodialysis.

INDICATIONS AND DOSAGES

▸ Active Duodenal Ulcers
PO
Adults, Elderly. 1 g 4 times a day (before meals and at bedtime) for up to 8 wk.
▸ Maintenance Therapy after Healing of Acute Duodenal Ulcers
PO
Adults, Elderly. 1 g twice a day.

SIDE EFFECTS/ADVERSE REACTIONS
Frequent
Constipation
Occasional
Dry mouth, backache, diarrhea, dizziness, somnolence, nausea, indigestion, rash, hives, itching, abdominal discomfort

PRECAUTIONS AND CONTRAINDICATIONS
Caution:
Lactation, children

DRUG INTERACTIONS OF CONCERN TO DENTISTRY
- Gastric irritation: chloral hydrate
- Decreased absorption of tetracyclines, fluoroquinolones
- Decreased effects of diclofenac, ketoconazole

SERIOUS REACTIONS
! None known

DENTAL CONSIDERATIONS

General:
- Prescribe acetaminophen for analgesia if needed. ASA and NSAIDs are contraindicated in active upper GI disease.
- Consider semisupine chair position for patient comfort because of GI effects of disease.
- Tetracycline doses should be given 2 hr before or after the sucralfate dose.
Teach Patient/Family to:
- Avoid mouth rinses with high alcohol content because of drying effects.

---

sulconazole nitrate
sul-**kon**′-ah-zole **nye**′-trate
(Exelderm)

CATEGORY AND SCHEDULE
Pregnancy Risk Category: C

Drug Class: Topical antifungal

MECHANISM OF ACTION
An imidazole derivative that inhibits synthesis of ergosterol (a vital component of fungal cell formation), the damaging cell membrane.
Therapeutic Effect: Fungistatic.

USES
Treatment of tinea pedis, tinea corporis, tinea cruris, tinea versicolor; unapproved: cutaneous candidiasis

PHARMACOKINETICS
Minimal systemic absorption following topical administration. Excreted in urine. *Half-life:* Unknown.

INDICATIONS AND DOSAGES
▶ **Tinea Pedis**
Topical
Adults, Elderly, Children 12 yr and older. Apply 2 times a day until signs and symptoms significantly improve.
▶ **Tinea Corporis, Tinea Cruris, Tinea Versicolor**
Topical
Adults, Elderly, Children 12 yr and older. Apply 1–2 times a day until signs and symptoms significantly improve.

SIDE EFFECTS/ADVERSE REACTIONS
Occasional
Headache, nausea

S

Rare
Burning or stinging, pruritus, redness

PRECAUTIONS AND CONTRAINDICATIONS

Hypersensitivity to sulconazole nitrate or any component of the formulation
Caution:
Pregnancy Category: C

DRUG INTERACTIONS OF CONCERN TO DENTISTRY

• None reported

SERIOUS REACTIONS

! None known

DENTAL CONSIDERATIONS

General:
• There are no significant dental considerations. One possible concern is the few patients with topical candidiasis, in whom broad-spectrum antiinfectives could potentially contribute to a suprainfection.

sulfacetamide

sul-fa-**see**′-ta-mide
(AK-Sulf, Bleph-10, Isopto Cetamide, Diosulf[CAN], Ophthacet, Sodium Sulamyd, Sulfair)

CATEGORY AND SCHEDULE

Pregnancy Risk Category: C

Drug Class: Antibacterial sulfonamide

MECHANISM OF ACTION

Interferes with synthesis of folic acid that bacteria require for growth.

Therapeutic Effect: Prevents further bacterial growth. Bacteriostatic.

USES

Treatment of conjunctivitis, superficial eye infections, corneal ulcers, trachoma

PHARMACOKINETICS

Small amounts may be absorbed into the cornea. Excreted rapidly in urine. *Half-life:* 7–13 hr.

INDICATIONS AND DOSAGES

▶ Treatment of Corneal Ulcers, Conjunctivitis, and Other Superficial Infections of the Eye, Prophylaxis after Injuries to the Eye/Removal of Foreign Bodies, Adjunctive Therapy for Trachoma and Inclusion Conjunctivitis
Ophthalmic
Adults, Elderly. Ointment: Apply small amount in lower conjunctival sac 1–4 times a day and at bedtime. Solution: 1–3 drops to lower conjunctival sac q2–3h. Seborrheic dermatitis, seborrheic sicca (dandruff), secondary bacterial skin infections.
Topical
Adults, Elderly. Apply 1–4 times a day.

SIDE EFFECTS/ADVERSE REACTIONS

Frequent
Transient ophthalmic burning, stinging
Occasional
Headache
Rare
Hypersensitivity (erythema, rash, itching, swelling, photosensitivity)

PRECAUTIONS AND CONTRAINDICATIONS

Hypersensitivity to sulfonamides or any component of preparation (some

products contain sulfite), use in combination with silver-containing products
Caution:
Cross-sensitivity with other sulfas; pregnancy category C

DRUG INTERACTIONS OF CONCERN TO DENTISTRY
• None reported

SERIOUS REACTIONS
! Superinfection, drug-induced lupus erythematosus, Stevens-Johnson syndrome occur rarely; nephrotoxicity with high dermatologic concentrations.

DENTAL CONSIDERATIONS
General:
• Avoid dental light in patient's eyes; offer dark glasses for patient comfort.

sulfasalazine
sul-fa-**sal**′-ah-zeen
(Alti-Sulfasalazine[CAN], Azulfidine, Azulfidine EN-tabs, Pyralin EN[AUS], Salazopyrin[CAN], Salazopyrin EN[AUS], Salazopyrin EN-Tabs[CAN])
Do not confuse Azulfidine with azathioprine, or sulfasalazine with sulfadiazine or sulfisoxazole.

CATEGORY AND SCHEDULE
Pregnancy Risk Category: B (D if given near term)

Drug Class: Sulfonamide derivative with antiinflammatory action

MECHANISM OF ACTION
A sulfonamide that inhibits prostaglandin synthesis, acting locally in the colon.
Therapeutic Effect: Decreases inflammatory response, interferes with GI secretion.

USES
Treatment of ulcerative colitis, Crohn's disease, rheumatoid arthritis, juvenile rheumatoid arthritis; unapproved: ankylosing spondylitis

PHARMACOKINETICS
Poorly absorbed from the GI tract. Cleaved in colon by intestinal bacteria, forming sulfapyridine and mesalamine (5-ASA). Absorbed in colon. Widely distributed. Metabolized in the liver. Primarily excreted in urine. *Half-life:* sulfapyridine, 6–14 hr; 5-ASA, 0.6–1.4 hr.

INDICATIONS AND DOSAGES
▶ **Ulcerative Colitis**
PO
Adults, Elderly. 1 g 3–4 times a day in divided doses q4–6h.
Maintenance: 2 g/day in divided doses q6–12h. Maximum: 6 g/day.
Children. 40–75 mg/kg/day in divided doses q4–6h. Maintenance: 30–50 mg/kg/day in divided doses q4–8h. Maximum: 2 g/day. Maximum: 6 g/day.
▶ **Rheumatoid Arthritis**
PO
Adults, Elderly. Initially, 0.5–1 g/day for 1 wk. Increase by 0.5 g/wk, up to 3 g/day.
▶ **Juvenile Rheumatoid Arthritis**
PO
Children. Initially, 10 mg/kg/day. May increase by 10 mg/kg/day at weekly intervals. Range: 30–50 mg/kg/day. Maximum: 2 g/day.

S

SIDE EFFECTS/ADVERSE REACTIONS

Frequent
Anorexia, nausea, vomiting, headache, oligospermia (generally reversed by withdrawal of drug)
Occasional
Hypersensitivity reaction (rash, urticaria, pruritus, fever, anemia)
Rare
Tinnitus, hypoglycemia, diuresis, photosensitivity

PRECAUTIONS AND CONTRAINDICATIONS

Children younger than 2 yr; hypersensitivity to carbonic anhydrase inhibitors, local anesthetics, salicylates, sulfonamides, sulfonylureas, sunscreens containing PABA, or thiazide or loop diuretics; intestinal or urinary tract obstruction; porphyria; pregnancy at term; severe hepatic or renal dysfunction
Caution:
Lactation, impaired hepatic function, severe allergy, bronchial asthma, impaired renal function, intolerance to aspirin

DRUG INTERACTIONS OF CONCERN TO DENTISTRY

• Increased photosensitizing effects: tetracycline
• Decreased absorption: folic acid

SERIOUS REACTIONS

! Anaphylaxis, Stevens-Johnson syndrome, hematologic toxicity (leukopenia, agranulocytosis), hepatotoxicity, and nephrotoxicity occur rarely.

DENTAL CONSIDERATIONS

General:
• Patients on chronic drug therapy may rarely have symptoms of blood dyscrasias, which can include infection, bleeding, and poor healing.
• Question patient about response to antibiotics to avoid responses that might provoke pseudomembranous colitis.
• Palliative medication may be required for management of oral side effects.
• Consider semisupine chair position for patient comfort because of GI effects of disease.
Consultations:
• Medical consultation may be required to assess disease control and patient's ability to tolerate stress.
• In a patient with symptoms of blood dyscrasias, request a medical consultation for blood studies and postpone dental treatment until normal values are reestablished.
Teach Patient/Family to:
• Use caution to prevent injury when using oral hygiene aids.

sulfinpyrazone

sul-fin-**pyr**'-ah-zone
(Anturane, Apo-Sulfinpyrazone[CAN], Nu-Sulfinpyrazone[CAN])
Do not confuse with Accutane.

CATEGORY AND SCHEDULE

Pregnancy Risk Category: C/D (near term)

Drug Class: Uricosuric

MECHANISM OF ACTION

A uricosuric that increases urinary excretion of uric acid, thereby decreasing blood urate levels.

Therapeutic Effect: Promotes uric acid excretion and reduces serum uric acid levels.

USES
Treatment of chronic gouty arthritis

PHARMACOKINETICS
Rapidly and completely absorbed from GI tract. Widely distributed. Metabolized in liver to 2 active metabolites, *p*-hydroxy-sulfinpyrazone and a sulfide analog. Excreted primarily in urine. Not removed by hemodialysis. *Half-life:* 2.7–6 hr.

INDICATIONS AND DOSAGES
▶ **Gout**
PO
Adults, Elderly. 100–200 mg 2 times a day. Maximum: 800 mg/day.

SIDE EFFECTS/ADVERSE REACTIONS
Frequent
Nausea, vomiting, stomach pain
Occasional
Flushed face, headache, dizziness, frequent urge to urinate, rash
Rare
Increased bleeding time, hepatic necrosis, nephrotic syndrome, uric acid stones

PRECAUTIONS AND CONTRAINDICATIONS
Active peptic ulcer, blood dyscrasias, GI inflammation, pregnancy (near term), hypersensitivity to sulfinpyrazone or any of its components, phenylbutazone, or other pyrazoles

DRUG INTERACTIONS OF CONCERN TO DENTISTRY
• Increased bleeding: NSAIDs, aspirin
• Decreased effects of salicylates

SERIOUS REACTIONS
❗ Hematological toxicity including anemia, leucopenia, agranulocytosis, thrombocytopenia, and aplastic anemia occur rarely.
❗ Overdose causes a drowsiness, dizziness, anorexia, abdominal pain, hemolytic anemia, acidosis, jaundice, fever, and agranulocytosis.

DENTAL CONSIDERATIONS
General:
• Consider local hemostasis measures to prevent excessive bleeding.
• Avoid prescribing aspirin-containing products.
• Patients on chronic drug therapy may rarely have symptoms of blood dyscrasias, which can include infection, bleeding, and poor healing.
• Consider semisupine chair position for patient comfort if GI side effects occur.
• Evaluate respiration characteristics and rate.
Consultations:
• In a patient with symptoms of blood dyscrasias, request a medical consultation for blood studies and postpone dental treatment until normal values are reestablished.
Teach Patient/Family to:
• Use caution to prevent injury when using oral hygiene aids.

S

sulfisoxazole

sul-fi-**sox**'-ah-zole
(Gantrisin, Novo-Soxazole[CAN], Sulfizole[CAN], Truxazole)
Do not confuse with sulfadiazine, sulfamethoxazole, sulfasalazine, Gastrosed

CATEGORY AND SCHEDULE

Pregnancy risk category: B/D (near term)

Drug Class: Sulfonamide, antiinfective

MECHANISM OF ACTION

An antibacterial sulfonamide that inhibits bacterial synthesis of dihydrofolic acid by preventing condensation of pteridine with aminobenzoic acid through competitive inhibition of the enzyme dihydropteroate synthetase.
Therapeutic Effect: Bacteriostatic.

USES

Treatment of urinary tract, systemic infections; chancroid; trachoma; toxoplasmosis; acute otitis media; lymphogranuloma venereum; eye infections

PHARMACOKINETICS

Rapidly and completely absorbed. Small intestine is major site of absorption, but some absorption occurs in the stomach. Exists in the blood as unbound, protein-bound, and conjugated forms. Sulfisoxazole is metabolized primarily by acetylation and oxidation in the liver. The free form is considered to be the therapeutically active form. Protein binding: 85%. *Half-life:* 5–8 hr.

INDICATIONS AND DOSAGES

▶ **Acute, Recurrent or Chronic UTI, Meningococcal Meningitis, Acute Otitis Media Caused by** *Haemophilus influenzae*
PO
Infants older than 2 mo, Children. One-half of the 24-hr dose initially then 150 mg/kg daily or 4 g/m² daily for maintenance divided q4–6h.
Maximum dose: 6 g daily.
Adults. 2–4 g initially, then 4–8 g daily divided q4–6h.

SIDE EFFECTS/ADVERSE REACTIONS

Anaphylaxis, erythema multiforme (Stevens-Johnson syndrome), toxic epidermal necrolysis, exfoliative dermatitis, angioedema, arteritis and vasculitis, allergic myocarditis, serum sickness, rash, urticaria, pruritus, photosensitivity, conjunctival and scleral injection, generalized allergic reactions, generalized skin eruptions, tachycardia, palpitations, syncope, cyanosis, goiter, diuresis, hypoglycemia, arthralgia, myalgia, headache, dizziness, peripheral neuritis, paresthesia, convulsions, tinnitus, vertigo, ataxia, intracranial hypertension, cough, shortness of breath, pulmonary infiltrates

PRECAUTIONS AND CONTRAINDICATIONS

Patients with a known hypersensitivity to sulfonamides, children younger than 2 mo (except in the treatment of congenital toxoplasmosis as adjunctive therapy with pyrimethamine), pregnant women at term, and mothers nursing infants younger than 2 mo of age
Caution:
Lactation, impaired hepatic function, severe allergy, bronchial asthma

DRUG INTERACTIONS OF CONCERN TO DENTISTRY

• Decreased effect: ester-type local anesthetics (procaine, tetracaine)
• Increased photosensitizing effect: tetracycline
• Decreased effect of penicillins, cephalosporins

SERIOUS REACTIONS

! Fatalities associated with the administration of sulfonamides, including Stevens-Johnson syndrome toxic epidermal necrolysis; fulminant hepatic necrosis, agranulocytosis, aplastic anemia, and other blood dyscrasias occur rarely.

! Clinical signs, such as rash, sore throat, fever, arthralgia, pallor, purpura, or jaundice, may be early indications of serious reactions.

DENTAL CONSIDERATIONS

General:
• Patients on chronic drug therapy may rarely have symptoms of blood dyscrasias, which can include infection, bleeding, and poor healing.
• Determine why the patient is taking the drug.
• Palliative medication may be required for management of oral side effects.
• Consider semisupine chair position for patient comfort if GI side effects occur.
Consultations:
• Medical consultation may be required to assess disease control.
• In a patient with symptoms of blood dyscrasias, request a medical consultation for blood studies and postpone dental treatment until normal values are reestablished.
Teach Patient/Family to:
• Encourage effective oral hygiene to prevent soft tissue inflammation.

sulindac
sul-**in′**-dak
(Aclin[AUS], Apo-Sulin[CAN], Clinoril, Novo Sundac[CAN])
Do not confuse Clinoril with Clozaril.

CATEGORY AND SCHEDULE
Pregnancy Risk Category: B (D if used in third trimester or near delivery)

Drug Class: Nonsteroidal antiinflammatory

MECHANISM OF ACTION
An NSAID that produces analgesic and antiinflammatory effects by inhibiting prostaglandin synthesis.
Therapeutic Effect: Reduces inflammatory response and intensity of pain.

USES
Treatment of osteoarthritis, rheumatoid arthritis, acute gouty arthritis, tendinitis, bursitis, ankylosing spondylitis

PHARMACOKINETICS

Route	Onset	Peak	Duration
PO (Anti-rheumatic)	7 days	2–3 wk	N/A

Well absorbed from the GI tract. Metabolized in liver to active metabolite. Primarily excreted in urine. Not removed by hemodialysis.
Half-life: 7.8 hr; metabolite: 16.4 hr.

S

INDICATIONS AND DOSAGES
▸ **Rheumatoid Arthritis, Osteoarthritis, Ankylosing Spondylitis**
PO
Adults, Elderly. Initially, 150 mg twice a day; may increase up to 400 mg/day.
▸ **Acute Shoulder Pain, Gouty Arthritis, Bursitis, Tendinitis**
PO
Adults, Elderly 200 mg twice a day.

SIDE EFFECTS/ADVERSE REACTIONS
Frequent
Diarrhea or constipation, indigestion, nausea, maculopapular rash, dermatitis, dizziness, headache
Occasional
Anorexia, abdominal cramps, flatulence

PRECAUTIONS AND CONTRAINDICATIONS
Active peptic ulcer disease, chronic inflammation of GI tract, GI bleeding or ulceration, history of hypersensitivity to aspirin or NSAIDs
Caution:
Lactation, children, bleeding disorders, GI disorders, cardiac disorders, hypersensitivity to other NSAIDs, geriatric patients

DRUG INTERACTIONS OF CONCERN TO DENTISTRY
• Increased bleeding, GI effects: alcohol, aspirin, steroids, other NSAIDs
• Renal toxicity: acetaminophen (prolonged use)
• Possible risk of decreased renal function: cyclosporine
• Increased photosensitizing effect: tetracycline
• Increased toxicity of methotrexate, cyclosporine

• Decreased plasma levels: diflunisal
• SSRIs: increased risk of GI side effects

SERIOUS REACTIONS
! Rare reactions with long-term use include peptic ulcer disease
! GI bleeding, gastritis, nephrotoxicity (glomerular nephritis, interstitial nephritis, nephrotic syndrome), severe hepatic reactions (cholestasis, jaundice), and severe hypersensitivity reactions (fever, chills, and joint pain)

DENTAL CONSIDERATIONS

General:
• Patients on chronic drug therapy may rarely have symptoms of blood dyscrasias, which can include infection, bleeding, and poor healing.
• Assess salivary flow as a factor in caries, periodontal disease, and candidiasis.
• Avoid prescribing in last trimester of pregnancy.
• Should oral inflammation or lesions occur, refer to physician and consider palliative treatment for the lesions.
• Consider semisupine chair position for patient comfort because of GI side effects.
Consultations:
• Medical consultation may be required to assess disease control.
• In a patient with symptoms of blood dyscrasias, request a medical consultation for blood studies and postpone dental treatment until normal values are reestablished.
Teach Patient/Family to:
• Report oral lesions, soreness, or bleeding to dentist.
• Use caution to prevent injury in use of oral hygiene aids.
• Encourage effective oral hygiene to prevent soft tissue inflammation.

- When chronic dry mouth occurs, advise patient to:
  - Avoid mouth rinses with high alcohol content because of drying effects.
  - Use daily home fluoride products to prevent caries.
  - Use sugarless gum, frequent sips of water, or saliva substitutes.

sumatriptan

soo-ma-**trip**′-tan
(Imigran[AUS], Imitrex,
Suvalan[AUS])
Do not confuse sumatriptan with
somatropin.

CATEGORY AND SCHEDULE
Pregnancy Risk Category: C

Drug Class: Serotonin agonist

MECHANISM OF ACTION
A serotonin receptor agonist that binds selectively to vascular receptors, producing a vasoconstrictive effect on cranial blood vessels.
Therapeutic Effect: Relieves migraine headache.

USES
Treatment of migraine headaches; cluster headaches

PHARMACOKINETICS

Route	Onset	Peak	Duration
Nasal	15 min	N/A	24–48 hr
PO	30 min	2 hr	24–48 hr
Subcutaneous	10 min	1 hr	24–48 hr

Rapidly absorbed after subcutaneous administration. Absorption after PO administration is incomplete, with significant amounts undergoing hepatic metabolism, resulting in low bioavailability (about 14%). Protein binding: 10%–21%. Widely distributed. Undergoes first-pass metabolism in the liver. Excreted in urine. *Half-life:* 2 hr.

INDICATIONS AND DOSAGES
▸ **Acute Migraine Attack**
PO
Adults, Elderly. 25–50 mg. Dose may be repeated after at least 2 hr. Maximum: 100 mg/single dose; 200 mg/24 hr.
Subcutaneous
Adults, Elderly. 6 mg. Maximum: Two 6-mg injections/24 hr (separated by at least 1 hr).
Intranasal
Adults, Elderly. 5–20 mg; may repeat in 2 hr. Maximum: 40 mg/24 hr.

SIDE EFFECTS/ADVERSE REACTIONS
Frequent
Oral: Tingling, nasal discomfort
Subcutaneous: Injection site reactions, tingling, warm or hot sensation, dizziness, vertigo
Nasal: Bad or unusual taste, nausea, vomiting
Occasional
Oral: Flushing, asthenia, visual disturbances
Subcutaneous: Burning sensation, numbness, chest discomfort, drowsiness, asthenia
Nasal: Nasopharyngeal discomfort, dizziness
Rare
Oral: Agitation, eye irritation, dysuria
Subcutaneous: Anxiety, fatigue, diaphoresis, muscle cramps, myalgia
Nasal: Burning sensation

S

PRECAUTIONS AND CONTRAINDICATIONS

CVA, ischemic heart disease (including angina pectoris, history of MI, silent ischemia, and Prinzmetal's angina), severe hepatic impairment, transient ischemic attack, uncontrolled hypertension, use within 14 days of MAOIs, use within 24 hr of ergotamine preparations

Caution:
Hepatic and renal impairment, elderly, lactation, children

DRUG INTERACTIONS OF CONCERN TO DENTISTRY

• None reported; avoid ergot-containing medications.

SERIOUS REACTIONS

! Excessive dosage may produce tremor, red extremities, reduced respirations, cyanosis, seizures, and paralysis.
! Serious arrhythmias occur rarely, especially in patients with hypertension, diabetes, or a strong family history of coronary artery disease; obese patients; and smokers.

DENTAL CONSIDERATIONS

S

General
• Be aware of the patient's disease, its severity, and its frequency, when known.
• Monitor vital signs at every appointment because of cardiovascular side effects.
• Avoid dental light in patient's eyes; offer dark glasses for patient comfort.

Consultations:
• If treating chronic orofacial pain, consult with physician of record.

Teach Patient/Family:
• That oral symptoms rarely occur and will disappear when drug is discontinued.

---

sunitinib
soo-**nih′**-tih-nib
(Sutent)

CATEGORY AND SCHEDULE
Pregnancy Risk Category: D

Drug Class: Antineoplastic (tyrosine kinase inhibitor)

MECHANISM OF ACTION

An antineoplastic agent that inhibits multiple receptor tyrosine kinases (RTK) inducing platelet-derived growth factor (PDGF), vascular endothelial growth factor receptors (VEGFR1, VEGFR2, and VEGFR3), stem cell factor receptor (KIT), FMS-like tyrosine kinase-3 (FLT3), colony stimulation factor receptor Type 1 (CSF-1R), and glial cell-line derived neurotrophic factor receptor (RET).

Therapeutic Effect: Decreases tumor cell growth.

USES

Treatment of GI stromal tumor after disease progression on or intolerance to imatinib; also used for treatment of advanced renal cell carcinoma

PHARMACOKINETICS

Protein binding: 90%–95% (primary metabolite). Primarily metabolized in liver by CYP450 3A4. Primarily eliminated in feces (61%); partial excretion in urine (16%). ***Half-life:*** 40–60 hr; 80–110 hr (primary metabolite).

INDICATIONS AND DOSAGES
▶ **GI Stromal Tumor after Disease Progression on or Intolerance to Imatinib**
PO

Adults. 50 mg once a day, on a schedule of 4 wk on treatment followed by 2 wk off.

▶ **Renal Cell Carcinoma, Advanced**
PO

Adults. 50 mg once a day, on a schedule of 4 wk on treatment followed by 2 wk off.

▶ **Dosage Adjustment**
Concurrent CYP3A4 inhibitor (such as ketoconazole). Reduce sunitinib to a minimum of 37.5 mg daily. Concurrent CYP3A4 inducer (such as rifampin). Increase sunitinib to a maximum of 87.5 mg daily.

SIDE EFFECTS/ADVERSE REACTIONS
Frequent

Fatigue, diarrhea, nausea, mucositis/stomatitis, neutropenia, dyspepsia, taste perversion, AST/ALT increased, lymphopenia, rash, thrombocytopenia, vomiting, constipation, anorexia, hyperpigmentation, abdominal pain, hypertension, arthralgia, dyspnea, bleeding, anemia, hyperlipasemia, headache, alkaline phosphatase increased, weakness, limb pain, fever, edema, dry skin, myalgia, back pain, cough, hair color changes, amylase increased, dizziness, hyperbilirubinemia, glossodynia, hyperuricemia, flatulence, hand-foot syndrome, hypokalemia, creatinine increased, alopecia, dehydration, hypernatremia, neuropathy, hypophosphatemia, LVEF decreased
Occasional

Appetite disturbance, skin blistering, periorbital edema, hypothyroidism, lacrimation increased, oral pain, hyperkalemia, hyponatremia, DVT
Rare

Myocardial ischemia, pulmonary embolism

PRECAUTIONS AND CONTRAINDICATIONS
Hypersensitivity to sunitinib or its components
Caution:

Do not breast-feed, left ventricular dysfunction, hypertension

DRUG INTERACTIONS OF CONCERN TO DENTISTRY
• CYP3A4 inducers: may decrease the levels and effects of sunitinib.
• CYP3A4 inhibitors (e.g., macrolide antibiotics, azole antifungal agents): may increase the blood levels and effects of sunitinib.

SERIOUS REACTIONS
❗ Severe GI complications have been reported.
❗ Hemorrhagic events have been reported.
❗ Hypertension may occur.
❗ Left ventricular dysfunction has been reported.
❗ Adrenal toxicities have been noted.

DENTAL CONSIDERATIONS
General:

• Avoid aspirin and NSAIDs to prevent GI irritation and excessive bleeding.
• Examine patient carefully for signs of opportunistic infections, mucositis, blood dyscrasias, stomatitis and bleeding.
• Confirm patient's disease status and treatment regimen.
• Chlorhexidine mouth rinse prior to and during chemotherapy may reduce severity of oral inflammation.

• Palliative medication may be required for management of oral adverse effects of drug.
• Patient may be taking prophylactic antiinfective drug.
• Place patient on frequent recall because of adverse oral effects of drug.

Consultations:
• Consult physician to determine control of disease and ability of patient to tolerate dental procedures.
• Consult physician to determine need for prophylactic or therapeutic antiinfective medications if oral surgery or periodontal treatment is planned.
• Consult physician to determine patient's immunologic and

coagulation status and determine safety risk, if any, posed by the required dental treatment.

Teach Patient/Family to:
• Be aware of oral adverse effects of drugs.
• Use effective, atraumatic oral hygiene measures to prevent soft tissue inflammation.
• Report oral lesions, soreness, or bleeding to dentist.
• Update health and medication history if physician makes any changes in evaluation or drug regimen; include OTC, herbal, and nonherbal drugs in update.

tacrine hydrochloride
tack'-rin high-droh-**klor'**-ide
(Cognex)

CATEGORY AND SCHEDULE
Pregnancy Risk Category: C

Drug Class: Cholinesterase
Inhibitor

MECHANISM OF ACTION
A cholinesterase inhibitor that
inhibits the enzyme
acetylcholinesterase, thus increasing
the concentration of acetylcholine at
cholinergic synapses and enhancing
cholinergic function in the CNS.
Therapeutic Effect: Slows the
progression of Alzheimer's disease.

USES
Treatment of mild-to-moderate
cognitive defects associated with
Alzheimer's disease

PHARMACOKINETICS
PO: Peak plasma levels 1–2 hr;
plasma levels are higher in females;
hepatic metabolism (CYP1A2
isoenzymes); renal excretion.

INDICATIONS AND DOSAGES
▸ **Alzheimer's Disease**
PO
Adults, Elderly. Initially, 10 mg 4
times a day for 6 wk, followed by
20 mg 4 times a day for 6 wk,
30 mg 4 times a day for 12 wk, then
40 mg 4 times a day if needed.
▸ **Dosage in Hepatic Impairment**
For patients with ALT (SGPT)
greater than 3–5 times normal,
decrease the dose by 40 mg/day and
resume the normal dose when ALT
(SGPT) returns to normal. For
patients with ALT (SGPT) greater

than 5 times normal, stop treatment
and resume it when ALT (SGPT)
returns to normal.

SIDE EFFECTS/ADVERSE REACTIONS
Frequent
Headache, nausea, vomiting,
diarrhea, dizziness
Occasional
Fatigue, chest pain, dyspepsia,
anorexia, abdominal pain, flatulence,
constipation, confusion, agitation,
rash, depression, ataxia, insomnia,
rhinitis, myalgia
Rare
Weight loss, anxiety, cough, facial
flushing, urinary frequency, back
pain, tremor

PRECAUTIONS AND CONTRAINDICATIONS
Known hypersensitivity to tacrine,
patients previously treated with
tacrine who developed jaundice
Caution:
Cardiovascular disease, GI ulcers,
general anesthesia, smokers, liver
disease, seizures, asthma, lactation,
children, decrease in absolute
neutrophil count; liver enzyme
monitoring required

DRUG INTERACTIONS OF CONCERN TO DENTISTRY
• Potential increase in GI
complaints: NSAIDs
• Action inhibited by anticholinergic
drugs
• Increased effects with
succinylcholine and other
cholinergic agonists

SERIOUS REACTIONS
! Overdose can cause cholinergic
crisis, marked by increased
salivation, lacrimation, bradycardia,
respiratory depression, hypotension,
and increased muscle weakness.

T

1238 Individual Drug Monographs

Treatment usually consists of supportive measures and an anticholinergic, such as atropine.

DENTAL CONSIDERATIONS

General:
• Patients on chronic drug therapy may rarely have symptoms of blood dyscrasias, which can include infection, bleeding, and poor healing.
• Monitor vital signs at every appointment because of cardiovascular and respiratory side effects.
• After supine positioning, have patient sit upright for at least 2 min before standing to avoid orthostatic hypotension.
• Assess salivary flow as a factor in caries, periodontal disease, and candidiasis.
• Take precautions if dental surgery is anticipated and anesthesia is required.
• Consider semisupine chair position for patient comfort because of GI effects of drug.
• Place on frequent recall because early attention to dental health is important for Alzheimer's patients.
Consultations:
• Medical consultation may be required to assess disease control.
• In a patient with symptoms of blood dyscrasias, request a medical consultation for blood studies and postpone dental treatment until normal values are reestablished.
Teach Patient/Family to:
• Encourage effective oral hygiene to prevent soft tissue inflammation.
• Prevent injury when using oral hygiene aids.
• Use powered tooth brush if patient has difficulty holding conventional devices.
• When chronic dry mouth occurs, advise patient to:

• Avoid mouth rinses with high alcohol content because of drying effects.
• Use daily home fluoride to prevent caries.
• Use sugarless gum, frequent sips of water, or saliva substitutes.

tacrolimus
tak-roe-**leem**′-us
(Prograf, Protopic)
Do not confuse Protopic with Protonix, Protopam, Protropin.

CATEGORY AND SCHEDULE
Pregnancy Risk Category: C

Drug Class: Immunosuppressant

MECHANISM OF ACTION
An immunologic agent that inhibits T-lymphocyte activation by binding to intracellular proteins, forming a complex and inhibiting phosphatase activity.
Therapeutic Effect: Suppresses the immunologically mediated inflammatory response; prevents organ transplant rejection.

USES
Treatment of short-term and intermittent long-term treatment of moderate-to-severe atopic dermatitis in patients not able to use or who do not respond to alternative, conventional therapies.

PHARMACOKINETICS
Variably absorbed after PO administration (food reduces absorption). Protein binding: 75%–97%. Extensively metabolized in the liver. Excreted in urine. Not removed by hemodialysis. *Half-life:* 11.7 hr.

INDICATIONS AND DOSAGES
▸ **Prevention of Liver Transplant Rejection**
PO
Adults, Elderly. 0.1–0.15 mg/kg/day in 2 divided doses 12 hr apart.
Children. 0.15–0.2 mg/kg/day in 2 divided doses 12 hr apart.
IV
Adults, Elderly, Children. 0.03–0.15 mg/kg/day as a continuous infusion.
▸ **Prevention of Kidney Transplant Rejection**
PO
Adults, Elderly. 0.2 mg/kg/day in 2 divided doses 12 hr apart.
IV
Adults, Elderly. 0.03–0.15 mg/kg/day as continuous infusion.
▸ **Atopic Dermatitis**
Topical
Adults, Elderly, Children 2 yr and older. Apply 0.03% ointment to affected area twice a day. 0.1% ointment may be used in adults and the elderly. Continue until 1 wk after symptoms have cleared.

SIDE EFFECTS/ADVERSE REACTIONS
Frequent
Headache, tremor, insomnia, paresthesia, diarrhea, nausea, constipation, vomiting, abdominal pain, hypertension
Occasional
Rash, pruritus, anorexia, asthenia, peripheral edema, photosensitivity

PRECAUTIONS AND CONTRAINDICATIONS
Concurrent use with cyclosporine (increases the risk of nephrotoxicity), hypersensitivity to HCO-60 polyoxyl 60 hydrogenated castor oil (used in solution for injection), hypersensitivity to tacrolimus

Caution:
Infections at treatment site; lymphadenopathy, acute infections, mononucleosis, reduce exposure to sunlight or artificial sunlight, lactation, use has not been established in children younger than 2 yr

DRUG INTERACTIONS OF CONCERN TO DENTISTRY
Topical
• No drug interactions are documented, but use with caution in patients taking CYP3A4 isoenzyme inhibitors: erythromycin, itraconazole, ketoconazole, fluconazole tacrolimus (FK506)
• No confirmed studies to date: avoid drugs with potential for renal impairment
• Risk of increased blood levels with clotrimazole, fluconazole, ketoconazole, clarithromycin, erythromycin, and methylprednisolone
• Risk of decreased blood levels with carbamazepine, phenobarbital, St. John's wort (herb)

SERIOUS REACTIONS
! Nephrotoxicity (characterized by increased serum creatinine level and decreased urine output), neurotoxicity (including tremor, headache, and mental status changes), and pleural effusion are common adverse reactions. Thrombocytopenia, leukocytosis, anemia, atelectasis, sepsis, and infection occur occasionally.

DENTAL CONSIDERATIONS
Topical
General:
• Advise patient if dental drugs prescribed have a potential for photosensitivity.

FK506

General:
- Patients on immunosuppressant therapy have increased susceptibility to infection.
- Patients on chronic drug therapy may rarely have symptoms of blood dyscrasias, which can include infection, bleeding, and poor healing.
- Monitor vital signs at every appointment because of cardiovascular side effects.
- Prophylactic antibiotics may be indicated to prevent infection if surgery or deep scaling is planned.
- Examine for evidence of oral candidiasis. Topically acting antifungals may be preferred.

Consultations:
- Medical consultation may be required to assess disease control.
- In a patient with symptoms of blood dyscrasias, request a medical consultation for blood studies and postpone dental treatment until normal values are reestablished.
- Consult with patient's physician for recommendations on possible antibiotic prophylaxis before dental treatment or when considering use of systemic antifungals.

Teach Patient/Family to:
- Encourage effective oral hygiene to prevent soft tissue inflammation.
- Use caution to prevent injury when using oral hygiene aids.
- Use powered tooth brush if patient has difficulty holding conventional devices.
- See dentist immediately if secondary oral infection occurs.
- Report oral lesions, soreness, or bleeding to dentist.

tadalafil
tah-**dal**′-ah-fill
(Cialis)

CATEGORY AND SCHEDULE
Pregnancy Risk Category: B

Drug Class: Impotence therapy

MECHANISM OF ACTION
An erectile dysfunction agent that inhibits phosphodiesterase type 5, the enzyme responsible for degrading cyclic guanosine monophosphate in the corpus cavernosum of the penis, resulting in smooth muscle relaxation and increased blood flow.
Therapeutic Effect: Facilitates an erection.

USES
Treatment of male erectile dysfunction

PHARMACOKINETICS

Route	Onset	Peak	Duration
PO	16 min	2 hr	36 hr

Rapidly absorbed after PO administration. Drug has no effect on penile blood flow without sexual stimulation. **Half-life:** 17.5 hr.

INDICATIONS AND DOSAGES
▶ **Erectile Dysfunction**
PO
Adults, Elderly. 10 mg 30 min before sexual activity. Dose may be increased to 20 mg or decreased to 5 mg based on patient tolerance. Maximum dosing frequency is once daily.

▶ **Dosage in Renal Impairment**
For patients with a creatinine clearance of 31–50 ml/min, the

starting dose is 5 mg before sexual activity once a day and the maximum dose is 10 mg no more frequently than once q48h.

For patients with a creatinine clearance of less than 31 ml/min, the starting dose is 5 mg before sexual activity once a day.

▶ **Dosage in Mild or Moderate Hepatic Impairment**

Patients with Child-Pugh class A or B hepatic impairment should take no more than 10 mg once a day.

SIDE EFFECTS/ADVERSE REACTIONS

Occasional

Headache, dyspepsia, back pain, myalgia, nasal congestion, flushing

PRECAUTIONS AND CONTRAINDICATIONS

Concurrent use of α-adrenergic blockers (other than the minimum dose tamsulosin), concurrent use of sodium nitroprusside or nitrates in any form, severe hepatic impairment

Caution:

Renal impairment, hepatic dysfunction, risk of hypotension in cardiovascular disease, ischemic heart disease, patients at risk of priapism, penile deformities, safety and efficacy for use in women not established

DRUG INTERACTIONS OF CONCERN TO DENTISTRY

• Maximum dose in patients taking CYP3A4 isoenzyme inhibitors is 10 mg: includes ketoconazole, erythromycin, itraconazole, and other potent inhibitors of CYP3A4.

• Avoid use of nitroglycerin within 24–36 hr.

SERIOUS REACTIONS

! Prolonged erections (lasting longer than 4 hr) and priapism (painful

erections lasting longer than 6 hr) occur rarely.

DENTAL CONSIDERATIONS

General:

• This is an acute-use drug intended to be taken just before sexual activity. Be mindful of the drug interactions when prescribing potent inhibitors of CYP3A4 isoenzymes and warn patient.

tamoxifen citrate

ta-**mox**′-ih-fen **sih**′-trate

(Apo-Tamox[CAN], Genox[AUS], Istubol, Nolvadex, Nolvadex-D[CAN], Novo-Tamoxifen[CAN], Tamofen[CAN], Tamosin[AUS])

CATEGORY AND SCHEDULE

Pregnancy Risk Category: D

Drug Class: Antineoplastic, antiestrogen hormone

MECHANISM OF ACTION

A nonsteroidal antiestrogen that competes with estradiol for estrogen-receptor binding sites in the breasts, uterus, and vagina.

Therapeutic Effect: Inhibits DNA synthesis and estrogen response.

USES

Advanced breast carcinoma that has not responded to other therapy in estrogen receptor-positive patients (usually postmenopausal), to reduce the incidence of breast cancer in healthy women with high risk of developing the disease; ductal carcinoma in situ

PHARMACOKINETICS

Well absorbed from the GI tract. Metabolized in the liver. Primarily

T

eliminated in feces by biliary system. *Half-life:* 7 days.

INDICATIONS AND DOSAGES
▶ **Adjunctive Treatment of Breast Cancer**
PO
Adults, Elderly. 20–40 mg/day. Give doses greater than 20 mg/day in divided doses.
▶ **Prevention of Breast Cancer in High-Risk Women**
PO
Adults, Elderly. 20 mg/day.

SIDE EFFECTS/ADVERSE REACTIONS
Frequent
Women: Hot flashes, nausea, vomiting
Occasional
Women: Changes in menstruation, genital itching, vaginal discharge, endometrial hyperplasia or polyps
Men: Impotence, decreased libido
Men and women: Headache, nausea, vomiting, rash, bone pain, confusion, weakness, somnolence

PRECAUTIONS AND CONTRAINDICATIONS
Concomitant coumarin-type therapy when used in the treatment of breast cancer in high-risk women, history of deep vein thrombosis or pulmonary embolism in high-risk women, pregnancy
Caution:
Leukopenia, thrombocytopenia, lactation, cataracts, risk of stroke, pulmonary emboli, and uterine malignancy

DRUG INTERACTIONS OF CONCERN TO DENTISTRY
• None reported

SERIOUS REACTIONS
❗ Retinopathy, corneal opacity, and decreased visual acuity have been noted in patients receiving extremely high dosages (240–320 mg/day) for longer than 17 mo.
❗ There has been an increased number of incidences of endometrial changes, thromboembolic events, and uterine malignancies while using tamoxifen.

DENTAL CONSIDERATIONS
General:
• Patients on chronic drug therapy may rarely have symptoms of blood dyscrasias, which can include infection, bleeding, and poor healing.
• Consider semisupine chair position for patient comfort if GI side effects occur.
Consultations:
• Medical consultation may be required to assess disease control.
• In a patient with symptoms of blood dyscrasias, request a medical consultation for blood studies and postpone dental treatment until normal values are reestablished.
Teach Patient/Family:
• Importance of good oral hygiene to prevent soft tissue inflammation.

tamsulosin hydrochloride
tam-**sool**′-oh-sin
high-droh-**klor**′-ide
(Flomax)
Do not confuse Flomax with Fosamax or Volmax.

CATEGORY AND SCHEDULE
Pregnancy Risk Category: B (not indicated for use in women)

Drug Class: Adrenoreceptor antagonist

MECHANISM OF ACTION

An α_1 antagonist that targets receptors around bladder neck and prostate capsule.
Therapeutic Effect: Relaxes smooth muscle and improves urinary flow and symptoms of prostatic hypertrophy.

USES

Treatment of benign prostatic hyperplasia (BPH)

PHARMACOKINETICS

Well absorbed and widely distributed. Protein binding: 94%–99%. Metabolized in the liver. Primarily excreted in urine. Unknown if removed by hemodialysis. *Half-life:* 9–13 hr.

INDICATIONS AND DOSAGES
▸ BPH
PO
Adults. 0.4 mg once a day, approximately 30 min after same meal each day. May increase dosage to 0.8 mg if inadequate response in 2–4 wk.

SIDE EFFECTS/ADVERSE REACTIONS

Frequent
Dizziness, somnolence
Occasional
Headache, anxiety, insomnia, orthostatic hypotension
Rare
Nasal congestion, pharyngitis, rhinitis, nausea, vertigo, impotence

PRECAUTIONS AND CONTRAINDICATIONS

History of sensitivity to tamsulosin
Caution:
Potential syncope risk caused by hypotension, vertigo, dizziness, carcinoma of prostate; avoid use with other-adrenoreceptor antagonists; not for use in women, children; lactation

DRUG INTERACTIONS OF CONCERN TO DENTISTRY

• No interactions reported with usual dental drugs; it is possible but not known whether risk of orthostatic hypotension could be increased with conscious sedation techniques.
• Opioids and anticholinergic drugs may enhance urinary retention; use alternative analgesics (NSAIDs).
• Caution in use or avoid concurrent use with other adrenergic antagonists.

SERIOUS REACTIONS

! First-dose syncope (hypotension with sudden loss of consciousness) may occur within 30–90 min after administration of initial dose and may be preceded by tachycardia (pulse rate of 120–160 beats/min).

DENTAL CONSIDERATIONS

General:
• Monitor vital signs at every appointment because of cardiovascular and respiratory side effects.
• Consider semisupine chair position for patient comfort when GI side effects occur.
• After supine positioning, have patient sit upright for at least 2 min before standing to avoid orthostatic hypotension.

T

tapentadol hydrochloride

tay-**pen**-tah-dole hi-dro-**klor**-ide
(Nucynta)
Do not confuse with tramadol.

CATEGORY AND SCHEDULE

Pregnancy Risk Category: C
Controlled Substance: Schedule II

Drug Class: Analgesic

MECHANISM OF ACTION

Centrally-acting analgesic, mu
opioid receptor agonist and inhibitor
of norepinephrine reuptake.
Therapeutic Effect: reduces
perception of pain in CNS.

USES

Moderate to severe acute pain

PHARMACOKINETICS

Limited oral bioavailability (32%)
due to extensive hepatic first-pass
metabolism. Peak concentration
reached at 1.25 hr, widely
distributed. Protein binding: 20%.
Metabolized in the liver, primarily
by glucuronide conjugation.
Half-life: 4 hr. 99% excreted by the
kidneys. No active metabolites.

INDICATIONS AND DOSAGES
▶ **Analgesia**
PO
Adults, Elderly. 50–100 mg every 4
to 6 hr, 700 mg total dose on first
day of therapy, 600 mg/day
subsequently.

SIDE EFFECTS/ADVERSE REACTIONS

Frequent
Dizziness, nausea, vomiting,
somnolence, constipation

Occasional
Fatigue, insomnia, pruritus,
hyperhidrosis, dry mouth, dyspepsia,
decreased appetite

RARE

Hypotension, bradycardia,
tachycardia, agitation, ataxia,
euphoria, depressed consciousness,
restlessness, syncope, seizures,
delayed gastric emptying, urinary
retention, involuntary muscle
contractions, cough, dyspnea, drug
withdrawal, hypersensitivity

PRECAUTIONS AND CONTRAINDICATIONS

Hypersensitivity to tapentadol
hydrochloride or its ingredients,
children under the age of 18
Caution:
Respiratory depression, CNS
depression, head injury/increased
intracranial pressure, seizures,
serotonin syndrome risk, pancreatic/
biliary tract disease, renal function
impairment, moderate to severe
hepatic impairment, drug abuse/
dependence, hazardous tasks,
pregnancy/lactation

DRUG INTERACTIONS OF CONCERN TO DENTISTRY

• Increased risk of CNS depression:
all CNS depressants, alcohol. May
potentiate mental impairment and
somnolence, respiratory depression,
hypotension (avoid alcohol)
• MAOIs: increased toxicity of
tapentadol
• SSRIs (e.g., fluoxetine): potentially
life-threatening serotonin syndrome

SERIOUS REACTIONS

! CNS depression with or without
respiratory depression
! Serotonin syndrome (agitation,
coma, autonomic instability
including tachycardia,

neuromuscular abnormalities, diarrhea, nausea, vomiting)
! Drug abuse, withdrawal syndrome with abrupt discontinuation of prolonged use

General:
• Assess salivary flow as a factor in caries, periodontal disease, and candidiasis.
• Geriatric patients may be more susceptible to adverse effects.
• Avoid or reduce doses of co-adminsistered sedatives.
• Avoid in patients taking MAOIs or selective serotonin reuptake inhibitors (SSRIs).
Teach Patient/Family to:
• Avoid mouth rinses with high alcohol content because of drying effect.
• Use home fluoride products for anticaries effect.
• Use sugarless/xylitol gum, frequent sips of water, or saliva substitutes if dry mouth occurs.

tegaserod
teh-**gas**′-er-od
(Zelnorm)

CATEGORY AND SCHEDULE
Pregnancy Risk Category: B

Drug Class: Serotonin agonist, a prokinetic drug

MECHANISM OF ACTION
An anti-irritable bowel syndrome agent that binds to 5-HT4 receptors in the GI tract.
Therapeutic Effect: Triggers a peristaltic reflex in the gut, increasing bowel motility.

USES
Short-term treatment of irritable bowel syndrome in women whose primary bowel symptom is constipation

PHARMACOKINETICS
Rapidly absorbed. Widely distributed. Protein binding: 98%. Metabolized by hydrolysis in the stomach and by oxidation and conjugation of the primary metabolite. Primarily excreted in feces. *Half-life:* 11 hr.

INDICATIONS AND DOSAGES
▸ **Irritable Bowel Syndrome**
PO
Adults, Elderly women. 6 mg twice a day for 4–6 wk.
▸ **Chronic Constipation**
PO
Adults. 6 mg twice a day.

SIDE EFFECTS/ADVERSE REACTIONS
Frequent
Headache, abdominal pain, diarrhea, nausea, flatulence
Occasional
Dizziness, migraine, back pain, extremity pain

PRECAUTIONS AND CONTRAINDICATIONS
Abdominal adhesions, diarrhea, history of bowel obstruction, moderate to severe hepatic impairment, severe renal impairment, suspected sphincter of Oddi dysfunction, symptomatic gallbladder disease
Caution:
Avoid use in patients with diarrhea, pregnancy category B, lactation (discontinue drug or discontinue nursing), safety and usefulness in children younger than 18 yr not established

T

DRUG INTERACTIONS OF CONCERN TO DENTISTRY

• No dental drug interactions reported; does not induce CYP450 isoenzymes.
• Avoid use of drugs (opioids, anticholinergics) that could lead to risk of constipation.
• Use NSAIDs or acetaminophen for mild or moderate pain.

SERIOUS REACTIONS

! None known

DENTAL CONSIDERATIONS

General:
• Monitor vital signs at every appointment because of cardiovascular side effects.
• Consider semisupine chair position for patient comfort if GI side effects occur.
• Short appointments and a stress-reduction protocol may be required for anxious patients.
• Avoid drugs with anticholinergic activity, such as antihistamines, opioids, benzodiazepines, propantheline, atropine, and scopolamine.
• Question patient about tolerance of NSAIDs or aspirin related to GI disease.
Consultations:
• Consult with physician before prescribing drugs that can cause constipation (opioids).
• Consultation with physician may be necessary if sedation or general anesthesia is required.
• Medical consultation may be required to assess disease control and patient's ability to tolerate stress.
Teach Patient/Family to:
• Update health and drug history if physician makes any changes in evaluation or drug regimens; include OTC, herbal, and nonherbal drugs in the update.

telmisartan

tel-meh-**sar′**-tan
(Micardis, Pritor[AUS])

CATEGORY AND SCHEDULE

Pregnancy Risk Category: C (D if used in second or third trimester)

Drug Class: Angiotensin II (AT1) receptor antagonist

MECHANISM OF ACTION

An angiotensin II receptor, type AT1, antagonist that blocks vasoconstrictor and aldosterone-secreting effects of angiotensin II, inhibiting the binding of angiotensin II to the AT1 receptors.
Therapeutic Effect: Causes vasodilation, decreases peripheral resistance, and decreases B/P.

USES

Treatment of hypertension as a single drug or in combination with other antihypertensives

PHARMACOKINETICS

Rapidly and completely absorbed after PO administration. Protein binding: greater than 99%. Undergoes metabolism in the liver to inactive metabolite. Excreted in feces. Unknown if removed by hemodialysis. *Half-life:* 24 hr.

INDICATIONS AND DOSAGES
▸ Hypertension
PO
Adults, Elderly. 40 mg once a day. Range: 20–80 mg/day.

SIDE EFFECTS/ADVERSE REACTIONS
Occasional
Upper respiratory tract infection, sinusitis, back or leg pain, diarrhea
Rare
Dizziness, headache, fatigue, nausea, heartburn, myalgia, cough, peripheral edema

PRECAUTIONS AND CONTRAINDICATIONS
Hypersensitivity, discontinue if pregnancy occurs, risk of fetal and neonatal injury, correct volume depletion if present, hepatic impairment, impaired renal function
Caution:
Discontinue if pregnancy occurs, risk of fetal and neonatal injury, correct volume depletion if present, hepatic impairment, impaired renal function; lactation

DRUG INTERACTIONS OF CONCERN TO DENTISTRY
• None reported; CYP450 isoenzymes are not involved with metabolism of this drug.

SERIOUS REACTIONS
! Overdosage may manifest as hypotension and tachycardia. Bradycardia occurs less often.

DENTAL CONSIDERATIONS
General:
• Monitor vital signs at every appointment because of cardiovascular side effects.
• Stress from dental procedures may compromise cardiovascular function; determine patient risk.
• Use precaution if sedation or general anesthesia is required; risk of hypotensive episode.

• Short appointments and a stress-reduction protocol may be required for anxious patients.
• Limit use of sodium-containing products, such as saline IV fluids, for patients with a dietary salt restriction.
Consultations:
• Medical consultation may be required to assess disease control and patient's ability to tolerate stress.

temazepam
te-**maz**'-eh-pam
(Apo-Temazepam[CAN], Novo-Temazepam[CAN], PMS-Temazepam[CAN], Restoril)
Do not confuse Restoril with Vistaril or Zestril.

CATEGORY AND SCHEDULE
Pregnancy Risk Category: X
Controlled Substance: Schedule IV

Drug Class: Benzodiazepine, sedative-hypnotic

MECHANISM OF ACTION
A benzodiazepine that enhances the action of the inhibitory neurotransmitter gamma-aminobutyric acid (GABA), resulting in CNS depression.
Therapeutic Effect: Induces sleep.

USES
A sedative and hypnotic for treatment of insomnia

PHARMACOKINETICS
Well absorbed from the GI tract. Protein binding: 96%. Widely distributed. Crosses the blood-brain barrier. Metabolized in the liver.

T

Primarily excreted in urine. Not removed by hemodialysis. *Half-life:* 4–18 hr.

INDICATIONS AND DOSAGES
▶ **Insomnia**
PO
Adults, Children 18 yr and older. 15–30 mg at bedtime.
Elderly, Debilitated. 7.5–15 mg at bedtime.

SIDE EFFECTS/ADVERSE REACTIONS
Frequent
Somnolence, sedation, rebound insomnia (may occur for 1–2 nights after drug is discontinued), dizziness, confusion, euphoria
Occasional
Asthenia, anorexia, diarrhea
Rare
Paradoxic CNS excitement or restlessness (particularly in elderly or debilitated patients)

PRECAUTIONS AND CONTRAINDICATIONS
Angle-closure glaucoma; CNS depression; pregnancy or breast-feeding; severe, uncontrolled pain; sleep apnea
Caution:
Anemia, hepatic disease, renal disease, suicidal individuals, drug abuse, elderly, psychosis, children younger than 18 yr, acute narrow-angle glaucoma

DRUG INTERACTIONS OF CONCERN TO DENTISTRY
• Increased action: alcohol, all CNS depressants
• Increased bioavailability: macrolide antibiotics

SERIOUS REACTIONS
! Abrupt or too-rapid withdrawal may result in pronounced restlessness, irritability, insomnia, hand tremor, abdominal or muscle cramps, vomiting, diaphoresis, and seizures. Overdose results in somnolence, confusion, diminished reflexes, respiratory depression, and coma.

DENTAL CONSIDERATIONS
General:
• Psychologic and physical dependence may occur with chronic administration.
• Geriatric patients are more susceptible to drug effects; use lower dose.
Teach Patient/Family to:
• Encourage effective oral hygiene to prevent soft tissue inflammation.

temozolomide
teh-moe-**zoll**'-oh-mide
(Temodal[AUS], Temodar)

CATEGORY AND SCHEDULE
Pregnancy Risk Category: D

Drug Class: Antineoplastic

MECHANISM OF ACTION
An imidazotetrazine derivative that acts as a prodrug and is converted to a highly active cytotoxic metabolite. Its cytotoxic effect is associated with methylation of DNA.
Therapeutic Effect: Inhibits DNA replication, causing cell death.

USES
Treatment of specific types of cancer of the brain

PHARMACOKINETICS
Rapidly and completely absorbed after PO administration. Protein

binding: 15%. Peak plasma concentration occurs in 1 hr. Penetrates the blood-brain barrier. Eliminated primarily in urine and, to a much lesser extent, in feces. *Half-life:* 1.6–1.8 hr.

INDICATIONS AND DOSAGES
▸ **Anaplastic Astrocytoma**
PO
Adults, Elderly. Initially, 150 mg/m²/day for 5 consecutive days of a 28-day treatment cycle. Subsequent doses based on platelet count and ANC during previous cycle. ANC greater than 1500 per microliter and platelet: more than 100,000 per microliter. Maintenance: 200 mg/m²/day for 5 days q4wk. Minimum: 100 mg/m²/day for 5 days q4wk.

SIDE EFFECTS/ADVERSE REACTIONS
Frequent
Nausea, vomiting, headache, fatigue, constipation
Occasional
Diarrhea, asthenia, fever, dizziness, peripheral edema, incoordination, insomnia
Rare
Paraesthesia, drowsiness, anorexia, urinary incontinence, anxiety, pharyngitis, cough

PRECAUTIONS AND CONTRAINDICATIONS
Hypersensitivity to dacarbazine, pregnancy

DRUG INTERACTIONS OF CONCERN TO DENTISTRY
• None reported

SERIOUS REACTIONS
! Elderly patients and women are at increased risk for developing severe myelosuppression, characterized by neutropenia and thrombocytopenia

and usually occurring within the first few cycles. Neutrophil and platelet counts reach their nadirs approximately 26–28 days after administration and recover within 14 days of the nadir.

DENTAL CONSIDERATIONS
General:
• Caution: patients may be at high risk for infection.
• Provide palliative dental care for dental emergencies only.
• Oral infections should be eliminated and/or treated aggressively.
• Patients may be at risk for bleeding; check oral signs.
• Caution: potential drug interactions with drugs used in dentistry.
• Monitor and record vital signs.
• If additional analgesia is required for dental pain, consider alternative analgesics (NSAIDs) in patients taking narcotics for acute or chronic pain.
• Avoid products that affect platelet function, such as aspirin and NSAIDs.
• Patient on chronic drug therapy may rarely present with symptoms of blood dyscrasias, which can include infection, bleeding, and poor healing. If dyscrasia is present, caution patient to prevent oral tissue trauma when using oral hygiene aids.
• Consider local hemostasis measures to prevent excessive bleeding.
• Consider semisupine chair position for patient comfort if GI side effects occur.
Consultations:
• Medical consultation should include routine blood counts including platelet counts and bleeding time.

T

- Consult physician; prophylactic or therapeutic antiinfectives may be indicated if surgery or periodontal treatment is required.
- In a patient with symptoms of blood dyscrasias, request a medical consultation for blood studies and postpone treatment until normal values are reestablished.
- Medical consultation may be required to assess disease control and patient's ability to tolerate stress.

Teach Patient/Family to:
- Use soft tooth brush to reduce risk of bleeding.
- Encourage effective oral hygiene to prevent soft tissue inflammation.
- Prevent trauma when using oral hygiene aids.
- Report oral lesions, soreness, or bleeding to dentist.
- Use powered tooth brush if patient has difficulty holding conventional devices.

temsirolimus
tem-sir-**oh**′-lee-mus
(Torisel)

CATEGORY AND SCHEDULE
Pregnancy Risk Category: D

Drug Class: Antineoplastic agent, mTOR kinase inhibitor

MECHANISM OF ACTION
Temsirolimus and sirolimus, its active metabolite, bind to FKBP-12, an intracellular protein, to form a complex that blocks the effects of mTOR (an enzyme that regulates the synthesis of proteins that control cell division). Inhibition of mTOR results in stopping the cell cycle at the G1 phase in tumor cells. When

mTOR is inhibited, the process of p70S6k and S6 ribosomal protein phosphorylation, induced by mTOR, is in turn blocked.

USES
Renal cell cancer (RCC), advanced

PHARMACOKINETICS
Metabolized in the liver via CYP3A4 to sirolimus and other minor metabolites. **Half-life:** 17 hr for temsirolimus and 55 hr for sirolimus. Excreted in the feces (78%) and urine (5%).

INDICATIONS AND DOSAGES
▸ **Advanced Renal Cell Cancer**
IV
Adults. 25 mg infused over a 20–60 min period once a week.
Note: Patients should be given prophylactic IV diphenhydramine 25–50 mg (or similar antihistamine) about 30 min before the start of each dose.
Avoid concomitant use of CYP3A4 inhibitors. If these drugs are necessary, a dose adjustment of 12.5 mg/week of temsirolimus may be considered. If the CYP3A4 inhibitor is discontinued, allow for a washout period of 1 wk before administering temsirolimus.
Avoid concomitant use of CYP3A4 inducers. If these drugs are necessary, a dose adjustment from 25 mg/week up to 50 mg/week may be considered. If the CYP3A4 inducer is discontinued, the temsirolimus dose should be returned to the dose used prior to initiation of CYP3A4 inducer.
Dose adjustment for toxicity:
ANC <1000/mm³, platelet count <75,000/mm³, or NCI CTCAE grade 3 or greater, stop temsirolimus. Consider restart with the dose reduced by 5 mg/week to a dose no

lower than 15 mg/week only if toxicities come back to grade 2 or less.

SIDE EFFECTS/ADVERSE REACTIONS
Adult
Frequent
Edema, peripheral edema, chest pain, pain, fever, headache, insomnia, rash, pruritus, nail disorder/thinning, dry skin, hypoglycemia, hypercholesterolemia, hyperlipidemia, hypophosphatemia, hypokalemia, mucositis, nausea, anorexia, diarrhea, abdominal pain, constipation, stomatitis, taste disturbance, vomiting, weight loss, urinary tract infection, anemia, lymphopenia, thrombocytopenia, leukopenia, neutropenia, increased alkaline phosphatase, increased AST, weakness, back pain, arthralgia, increased creatinine, dyspnea, cough, epistaxis, pharyngitis, infection
Occasional
Hypertension, venous thromboembolism, thrombophlebitis, chills, depression, acne, impaired wound healing, bowel perforation, hyperbilirubinemia, myalgia, conjunctivitis, rhinitis, pneumonia, upper respiratory tract infection, interstitial lung disease, allergic/hypersensitivity reaction

PRECAUTIONS AND CONTRAINDICATIONS
Handle and dispose with caution since temsirolimus is a hazardous agent.
Hypersensitivity to temsirolimus, sirolimus, or any other components of the formulation. Hypersensitivity reactions may occur. Symptoms include anaphylaxis, dyspnea, flushing, and chest pain.

Fatal cases of renal failure, bowel perforation, and interstitial lung disease have occurred.
Avoid live vaccines.
Infection may occur as a result of immunosuppression.

DRUG INTERACTIONS OF CONCERN TO DENTISTRY
• CYP3A4 inhibitors (e.g., macrolide antibiotics and azole antifungals): May increase the effects of sirolimus (active metabolite).

SERIOUS REACTIONS
! Renal failure, sometimes fatal, has occurred. Monitor renal function at baseline and while on temsirolimus.
! Angioedema, asthenia, anemia, dyspnea, immunosuppression, interstitial lung disease, hyperglycemia, hyperlipidemia, bowel perforation (fatal), wound healing complications, and intracerebral hemorrhage have been reported.

DENTAL CONSIDERATIONS

General:
• Mucositis, stomatitis, and taste disturbances may complicate oral hygiene and dental treatment.
• Examine for oral manifestation of infections.
• Consider semisupine chair position for patient comfort if gastrointestinal (GI) side effects occur.
Consultations:
• Medical consultation may be required to assess disease control and ability of patient to tolerate dental treatment.
Teach Patient/Family to:
• Be alert for the possibility of mucositis, stomatitis, and taste disturbances and the need to be

T

consulted by a dentist if any signs and symptoms occur.
• Encourage effective oral hygiene to prevent soft tissue inflammation.
• Prevent trauma when using oral hygiene aids.

(kg)	(mg)	(ml)
90 or more	50	10
80 to less than 90	45	9
70 to less than 80	40	8
60 to less than 70	35	7
Less than 60	30	6

tenecteplase
ten-**eck**′-teh-place
(Metalyse[AUS], TNKase)

CATEGORY AND SCHEDULE
Pregnancy Risk Category: C

Drug Class: Thrombolytic

MECHANISM OF ACTION
A tissue plasminogen activator produced by recombinant DNA that binds to fibrin and converts plasminogen to plasmin. Initiates fibrinolysis by degrading fibrin clots, fibrinogen, other plasma proteins.
Therapeutic Effect: Exerts thrombolytic action.

USES
Dissolving blood clots

PHARMACOKINETICS
Extensively distributed to tissues. Completely eliminated by hepatic metabolism. **Half-life:** 11–20 min.

INDICATIONS AND DOSAGES
▸ Acute MI
IV
Adults. Dosage is based on patient's weight. Treatment should be initiated as soon as possible after onset of symptoms.
Weight

SIDE EFFECTS/ADVERSE REACTIONS
Frequent
Bleeding (major, 4.7%; minor, 21.8%)

PRECAUTIONS AND CONTRAINDICATIONS
Active internal bleeding, aneurysm, AV malformation, bleeding diathesis, history of cerebrovascular accident, intracranial or intraspinal surgery or trauma within past 2 mo, intracranial neoplasm, severe uncontrolled hypertension

DRUG INTERACTIONS OF CONCERN TO DENTISTRY
• Increased risk of bleeding: drugs that interfere with coagulation or platelet function, such as NSAIDs and aspirin, ginkgo biloba (herb)

SERIOUS REACTIONS
! Bleeding at internal sites may occur, including intracranial, retroperitoneal, GI, GU, and respiratory sites. Lysis or coronary thrombi may produce atrial or ventricular arrhythmias and stroke.

DENTAL CONSIDERATIONS
General:
• An acute use drug for use in hospitals or emergency departments.
• Patients are at risk for bleeding; check for oral signs.

- Avoid products that affect platelet function, such as aspirin and NSAIDs.
- Monitor and record vital signs.
- Review medical and drug history.

Consultations:
- Medical consultation should include routine blood counts, including platelet counts and bleeding time.
- In a patient with symptoms of blood dyscrasias, request a medical consultation for blood studies and postpone treatment until normal values are reestablished.
- Medical consultation may be required to assess disease control and patient's ability to tolerate stress.

Teach Patient/Family to:
- Use soft tooth brush to reduce risk of bleeding.
- Encourage effective oral hygiene to prevent soft tissue inflammation.
- Report oral lesions, soreness, or bleeding to dentist.
- Prevent trauma when using oral hygiene aids.
- Update health and medication history if physician makes any changes in evaluation or drug regimens; include OTC, herbal, and nonherbal remedies in the update.

teniposide
ten-ih´-poe-side
(Vumon)

CATEGORY AND SCHEDULE
Pregnancy Risk Category: D

Drug Class: Antineoplastics, epipodophyllotoxins

MECHANISM OF ACTION
An epipodophyllotoxin that induces single- and double-strand breaks in DNA, inhibiting or altering DNA synthesis. Acts in the late S and early G2 phases of cell cycle.
Therapeutic Effect: Prevents cells from entering mitosis.

USES
Treatment of childhood acute lymphocytic leukemia

PHARMACOKINETICS
Plasma levels decline biexponentially over 1–2.5 hr, with a mean terminal half-life of 5 hr. Protein binding: >99%, excreted in the urine, primarily as metabolites.

INDICATIONS AND DOSAGES
▶ Induction Therapy in Patients with Refractory Childhood Acute Lymphoblastic Leukemia (in Combination with Other Antineoplastic Agents)
Children. Dosage is individualized on the basis of the patient's clinical response and tolerance of the drug's adverse effects. When used in combination therapy, consult specific protocols for optimum dosage or sequence of drug administration.

SIDE EFFECTS/ADVERSE REACTIONS
Frequent
Mucositis, nausea, vomiting, diarrhea, anemia
Occasional
Alopecia, rash
Rare
Hepatic dysfunction, fever, renal dysfunction, peripheral neurotoxicity

PRECAUTIONS AND CONTRAINDICATIONS
Absolute neutrophil count less than 500/mm^3; hypersensitivity to

T

Cremophor EL (polyoxyethylated castor oil), etoposide, or teniposide; platelet count less than 50,000/mm³

DRUG INTERACTIONS OF CONCERN TO DENTISTRY
• None reported

SERIOUS REACTIONS
! Myelosuppression manifested as hematologic toxicity (principally leukopenia, neutropenia, and thrombocytopenia) may be severe and may increase the risk of infection or bleeding. Hypersensitivity reaction may include anaphylaxis (marked by chills, fever, tachycardia, bronchospasm, dyspnea, and facial flushing).

DENTAL CONSIDERATIONS
General:
• If additional analgesia is required for dental pain, consider alternative analgesics (NSAIDs) in patients taking opioids for acute or chronic pain.
• Examine for oral manifestation of opportunistic infection.
• Avoid products that affect platelet function, such as aspirin and NSAIDs.
• This drug may be used in the hospital or on an outpatient basis. Confirm the patient's disease and treatment status.
• Chlorhexidine mouth rinse prior to and during chemotherapy may reduce severity of mucositis.
• Patient on chronic drug therapy may rarely present with symptoms of blood dyscrasias, which can include infection, bleeding, and poor healing. If dyscrasia is present, caution patient to prevent oral tissue trauma when using oral hygiene aids.

• Palliative medication may be required for management of oral side effects.
• Short appointments and a stress reduction protocol may be required for anxious patients.
• Consider semisupine chair position for patient comfort if GI side effects occur.
• Caution: patients may be at high risk for infection.
• Patients may be at risk for bleeding; check oral signs.
• Oral infections should be eliminated and/or treated aggressively.
Consultations:
• Medical consultation should include routine blood counts, including platelet counts and bleeding time.
• Consult physician; prophylactic or therapeutic antiinfectives may be indicated if surgery or periodontal treatment is required.
• Medical consultation may be required to assess immunologic status during cancer chemotherapy and determine safety risk, if any, posed by the required dental treatment.
• Medical consultation may be required to assess disease control and patient's ability to tolerate stress.
• In a patient with symptoms of blood dyscrasias, request a medical consultation for blood studies and postpone treatment until normal values are reestablished.
Teach Patient/Family to:
• See dentist immediately if secondary oral infection occurs.
• Be aware of oral side effects.
• Encourage effective oral hygiene to prevent soft tissue inflammation.
• Report oral lesions, soreness, or bleeding to dentist.

• Prevent trauma when using oral hygiene aids.
• Update health and medication history if physician makes any changes in evaluation or drug regimens; include OTC, herbal, and nonherbal remedies in the update.

tenofovir
ten-**oh**′-foh-veer
(Viread)

CATEGORY AND SCHEDULE
Pregnancy Risk Category: B

Drug Class: Antiviral

MECHANISM OF ACTION
A nucleotide analog that inhibits HIV reverse transcriptase by being incorporated into viral DNA, resulting in DNA chain termination. **Therapeutic Effect:** Slows HIV replication and reduces HIV RNA levels (viral load).

USES
Treatment of HIV-1 infection in combination with other antiretroviral drugs

PHARMACOKINETICS
PO: Bioavailability 5% (improves with meal); maximum serum levels 0.6–1.4 hr; low plasma protein binding less than 7%; minimal systemic metabolism; excreted by glomerular filtration and active tubular secretion; use in children not evaluated.

INDICATIONS AND DOSAGES
▶ **HIV Infection (in combination with other antiretrovirals)**
PO
Adults, Elderly, Children 18 yr and older. 300 mg once a day.

SIDE EFFECTS/ADVERSE REACTIONS
Occasional
GI disturbances (diarrhea, flatulence, nausea, vomiting)

PRECAUTIONS AND CONTRAINDICATIONS
Hypersensitivity; avoid breast-feeding; obesity and prolonged nucleoside use; risk of lactic acidosis/severe hepatomegaly with steatosis; no data on hepatic impairment; redistribution of body fat
Caution:
Obesity and prolonged nucleoside use; risk of lactic acidosis/severe hepatomegaly with steatosis; no data on hepatic impairment; redistribution of body fat

DRUG INTERACTIONS OF CONCERN TO DENTISTRY
• Potential for competition for renal clearance: acyclovir, valacyclovir

SERIOUS REACTIONS
! Lactic acidosis and hepatomegaly with steatosis occur rarely but may be severe.

DENTAL CONSIDERATIONS
General:
• Examine for oral manifestation of opportunistic infection.
Consultations:
• Medical consultation may be required to assess disease control and patient's ability to tolerate stress.

Teach Patient/Family to:
• Encourage effective oral hygiene to prevent soft tissue inflammation/infection.

terazosin hydrochloride
ter-**ah**′-zoe-sin
high-droh-**klor**′-ide
(Apo-Terazosin[CAN], Hytrin, Novo-Terazosin[CAN])

CATEGORY AND SCHEDULE
Pregnancy Risk Category: C

Drug Class: Antihypertensive, antiadrenergic

MECHANISM OF ACTION
An antihypertensive and benign prostatic hypertrophy agent that blocks α-adrenergic receptors. Produces vasodilation, decreases peripheral resistance, and targets receptors around bladder neck and prostate.
Therapeutic Effect: In hypertension, decreases B/P. In benign prostatic hyperplasia, relaxes smooth muscle and improves urine flow.

USES
Treatment of hypertension as a single agent or in combination with diuretics or β-blockers; benign prostatic hypertrophy

PHARMACOKINETICS
Rapidly, completely absorbed from the GI tract. Protein binding: 90%–94%. Metabolized in the liver to active metabolite. Primarily eliminated in feces via biliary system; excreted in urine. Not removed by hemodialysis. *Half-life:* 12 hr.

Route	Onset	Peak	Duration
PO	15 min	1–2 hr	12–24 hr

INDICATIONS AND DOSAGES
▶ **Mild-to-Moderate Hypertension**
PO
Adults, Elderly. Initially, 1 mg at bedtime. Slowly increase dosage to desired levels. Range: 1–5 mg/day as single or 2 divided doses. Maximum: 20 mg.
▶ **Benign Prostatic Hyperplasia**
PO
Adults, Elderly. Initially, 1 mg at bedtime. May increase up to 10 mg/day. Maximum: 20 mg/day.

SIDE EFFECTS/ADVERSE REACTIONS
Frequent
Dizziness, headache, unusual tiredness
Rare
Peripheral edema, orthostatic hypotension, myalgia, arthralgia, blurred vision, nausea, vomiting, nasal congestion, somnolence

PRECAUTIONS AND CONTRAINDICATIONS
Hypersensitivity, children, lactation

DRUG INTERACTIONS OF CONCERN TO DENTISTRY
• Decreased antihypertensive effects: NSAIDs, indomethacin

SERIOUS REACTIONS
! First-dose syncope (hypotension with sudden loss of consciousness) may occur 30–90 min after initial dose of 2 mg or more, a too-rapid increase in dosage, or addition of another antihypertensive agent to therapy. First-dose syncope may be preceded by tachycardia (pulse rate of 120–160 beats/min).

General:
• Monitor vital signs at every appointment because of cardiovascular side effects.
• After supine positioning, have patient sit upright for at least 2 min before standing to avoid orthostatic hypotension.
• Assess salivary flow as a factor in caries, periodontal disease, and candidiasis.
• Limit use of sodium-containing products, such as saline IV fluids, for patients with a dietary salt restriction.
• Consider semisupine chair position for patient comfort if GI side effects occur.

Teach Patient/Family:
• When chronic dry mouth occurs, advise patient to:
  • Avoid mouth rinses with high alcohol content because of drying effects.
  • Use daily home fluoride to prevent caries.
  • Use sugarless gum, frequent sips of water, or saliva substitutes.

terbinafine hydrochloride

ter-**been**′-ah-feen
high-droh-**klor**′-ide
(Apo-Terbinafine[CAN], Lamisil, Lamisil AT, Novo-Terbinafine [CAN])
Do not confuse terbinafine with terbutaline or Lamisil with Lamictal.

CATEGORY AND SCHEDULE
Pregnancy Risk Category: B

Drug Class: Antifungal

MECHANISM OF ACTION
A fungicidal antifungal that inhibits the enzyme squalene epoxidase, thereby interfering with fungal biosynthesis.
Therapeutic Effect: Fungicidal.

USES
Treatment of tinea pedis, tinea cruris, tinea corporis; unapproved uses: treatment of cutaneous candidiasis, tinea versicolor; treatment of onychomycosis of the toenail or fingernail caused by dermatophytes (tinea unguium)

PHARMACOKINETICS
PO: Bioavailability 40%, peak plasma levels approximately 2 hr; highly plasma protein bound (99%), extensive metabolism, excreted in urine (70%).

INDICATIONS AND DOSAGES
▸ **Tinea Pedis**
Topical
Adults, Elderly, Children 12 yr and older. Apply twice a day until signs and symptoms significantly improve.
▸ **Tinea Cruris, Tinea Corporis**
Topical
Adults, Elderly, Children 12 yr and older. Apply 1–2 times a day until signs and symptoms significantly improve.
▸ **Onychomycosis**
PO
Adults, Elderly, Children 12 yr and older. 250 mg/day for 6 wk (fingernails) or 12 wk (toenails).
▸ **Tinea Versicolor**
Topical Solution
Adults, Elderly. Apply to the affected area twice a day for 7 days.
▸ **Systemic Mycosis**
PO
Adults, Elderly. 250–500 mg/day for up to 16 mo.

T

SIDE EFFECTS/ADVERSE REACTIONS
Frequent
Oral: Headache
Occasional
Oral: Diarrhea, rash, dyspepsia, pruritus, taste disturbance, nausea, abdominal pain, flatulence, urticaria, visual disturbance
Topical: Irritation, burning, pruritus, dryness

PRECAUTIONS AND CONTRAINDICATIONS
Oral: Children younger than 12 yr, preexisting hepatic or renal impairment (creatinine clearance of less than 50 ml/min)
Caution:
Preexisting liver or renal disease, use not recommended during nursing, pediatric patients

DRUG INTERACTIONS OF CONCERN TO DENTISTRY
• None reported

SERIOUS REACTIONS
! Hepatobiliary dysfunction (including cholestatic hepatitis), serious skin reactions, and severe neutropenia occur rarely. Ocular lens and retinal changes have been noted.

DENTAL CONSIDERATIONS
General:
• Determine why patient is taking the drug.
• Consider semisupine chair position for patient comfort if GI side effects occur.
• Patients on chronic drug therapy may rarely have symptoms of blood dyscrasias, which can include infection, bleeding, and poor healing.

Consultations:
• In a patient with symptoms of blood dyscrasias, request a medical consultation for blood studies and postpone treatment until normal values are reestablished.
Teach Patient/Family to:
• Encourage effective oral hygiene to prevent soft tissue inflammation.
• Prevent trauma when using oral hygiene aids.

terconazole
ter-**kon**′-ah-zole
(Terazol[CAN], Terazol 3, Terazol 7)

CATEGORY AND SCHEDULE
Pregnancy Risk Category: C

Drug Class: Local antifungal

MECHANISM OF ACTION
An antifungal that disrupts fungal cell membrane permeability.
Therapeutic Effect: Fungicidal.

USES
Treatment of vaginal, vulval, vulvovaginal candidiasis (moniliasis)

PHARMACOKINETICS
Extent of systemic absorption after vaginal administration may be dependent on presence of a uterus, 5%–8% in women who had a hysterectomy versus 12%–16% in nonhysterectomy women.

INDICATIONS AND DOSAGES
▶ Vulvovaginal Candidiasis
Intravaginal
Adults, Elderly. 1 suppository vaginally at bedtime for 3 days.
Adults, Elderly. 1 applicatorful at bedtime for 7 days (0.4% cream) or for 3 days (0.8% cream).

SIDE EFFECTS/ADVERSE REACTIONS
Frequent
Headache, vulvovaginal burning
Occasional
Dysmenorrhea, pain in female genitalia, abdominal pain, fever, itching
Rare
Chills

PRECAUTIONS AND CONTRAINDICATIONS
Hypersensitivity to terconazole or any component of the formulation
Caution:
Children younger than 2 yr, pregnancy, lactation

DRUG INTERACTIONS OF CONCERN TO DENTISTRY
• None reported

SERIOUS REACTIONS
! Flu-like syndrome has been reported.

DENTAL CONSIDERATIONS
General:
• Broad-spectrum antibiotics can exacerbate vaginal candidiasis.

teriparatide
ter-ih-**par'**-ah-tide
(Forteo)

CATEGORY AND SCHEDULE
Pregnancy Risk Category: C

Drug Class: Bone resorption inhibitor (a synthetic polypeptide of rDNA origin, contains recombinant human parathyroid hormone [rhPTH(1–34)])

MECHANISM OF ACTION
A synthetic polypeptide hormone that acts on bone to mobilize calcium; also acts on kidney to reduce calcium clearance, increase phosphate excretion.
Therapeutic Effect: Promotes an increased rate of release of calcium from bone into blood, stimulates new bone formation.

USES
Treatment of postmenopausal women with osteoporosis at high risk for fracture; to increase bone mass in men with primary or hypogonadal osteoporosis at high risk for fracture

PHARMACOKINETICS
Subcutaneous: Absolute bioavailability 95%, peak serum levels 30 min. **Half-life:** 1 hr, no excretion or metabolism studies have been done, may be the same as PTH with hepatic metabolism and renal excretion.

INDICATIONS AND DOSAGES
▸ **Osteoporosis**
Subcutaneous
Adults, Elderly. 20 mcg once daily into the thigh or abdominal wall.

SIDE EFFECTS/ADVERSE REACTIONS
Occasional
Leg cramps, nausea, dizziness, headache, orthostatic hypotension, increased heart rate

PRECAUTIONS AND CONTRAINDICATIONS
Serum calcium above normal level, those at increased risk for osteosarcoma (Paget's disease, unexplained elevations of alkaline phosphatase, open epiphyses, prior radiation therapy that includes the

T

skeleton), hypercalcemic disorder (e.g., hyperparathyroidism), hypersensitivity to teriparatide or any of the components of the formulation

Caution:
Active or recent urolithiasis, use longer than 2 yr, postinjection orthostatic hypotension, symptoms of hypercalcemia, pregnancy category C, avoid in nursing mothers, not for use in children

DRUG INTERACTIONS OF CONCERN TO DENTISTRY
• None reported

SERIOUS REACTIONS
! None known

DENTAL CONSIDERATIONS
General:
• Patients with osteoporosis and risk of fracture should be asked if they use this drug; otherwise, some patients may not report its use.
• Patients may need special assistance in the dental office to avoid risk of falling.

Teach Patient/Family to:
• Update health and drug history, reporting changes in health status, drug regimen, or disease/treatment status.
• Contact physician if symptoms of hypercalcemia appear (nausea, vomiting, constipation, lethargy, muscle weakness).

testosterone
tess-**toss**´-ter-one
(Andriol[CAN], Androderm, AndroGel, Andropository[CAN], Delatestryl, Depotest[CAN], Depo-Testosterone, Everone[CAN], Striant, Testim, Testoderm, Testopel, Virilon IM[CAN])
Do not confuse testosterone with testolactone.

CATEGORY AND SCHEDULE
Pregnancy Risk Category: X
Controlled Substance: Schedule III

Drug Class: Androgen, anabolic steroid

MECHANISM OF ACTION
A primary endogenous androgen that promotes growth and development of male sex organs and maintains secondary sex characteristics in androgen-deficient males.
Therapeutic Effect: Helps relieve androgen deficiency.

USES
Treatment of androgen deficiency, delayed puberty, female breast cancer, certain anemias, gender changes, hypogonadism, cryptorchidism

PHARMACOKINETICS
Well absorbed after IM administration. Protein binding: 98%. Undergoes first-pass metabolism in the liver. Primarily excreted in urine. Unknown if removed by hemodialysis. *Half-life:* 10–20 min.

INDICATIONS AND DOSAGES
▶ **Male Hypogonadism**
IM
Adults. 50–400 mg q2–4wk.
Adolescents. Initially, 40–50 mg/m²/dose monthly until growth rate falls to prepubertal levels. 100 mg/m²/dose until growth ceases. Maintenance virilizing dose: 100 mg/m²/dose twice a mo.
Subcutaneous (Pellets)
Adults, Adolescents. 150–450 mg q3–6mo.
Transdermal (Patch [Testoderm])
Adults, Elderly. Start therapy with 6 mg/day patch. Apply patch to scrotal skin.
Transdermal (Patch [Testoderm TTS])
Adults, Elderly. Apply TTS patch to arm, back, or upper buttocks.
Transdermal (Patch [Androderm])
Adults, Elderly. Start therapy with 5 mg/day patch applied at night. Apply patch to abdomen, back, thighs, or upper arms.
Transdermal (Gel [AndroGel])
Adults, Elderly. Initial dose of 5 mg delivers 50 mg testosterone and is applied once daily to the abdomen, shoulders, or upper arms. May increase to 7.5 g, then to 10 g, if necessary.
Transdermal (Gel [Testim])
Adults, Elderly. Initial dose of 5 g delivers 50 mg testosterone and is applied once a day to the shoulders or upper arms. May increase to 10 g.
Buccal System (Striant)
Adults, Elderly. 30 mg q12h.
▶ **Delayed Puberty**
IM
Adults. 50–200 mg q2–4wk.
Adolescents. 40–50 mg/m²/dose every mo for 6 mo.
Subcutaneous (Pellets)
Adults, Adolescents. 150–450 mg q3–6mo.

▶ **Breast Carcinoma**
IM (Testosterone Aqueous)
Adults. 50–100 mg 3 times a wk.
IM (Testosterone Cypionate or Testosterone Ethanate)
Adults. 200–400 mg q2–4wk.
IM (Testosterone Propionate)
Adults. 50–100 mg 3 times a wk.

SIDE EFFECTS/ADVERSE REACTIONS
Frequent
Gynecomastia, acne
Females: Hirsutism, amenorrhea or other menstrual irregularities, deepening of voice, clitoral enlargement that may not be reversible when drug is discontinued
Occasional
Edema, nausea, insomnia, oligospermia, priapism, male-pattern baldness, bladder irritability, hypercalcemia (in immobilized patients or those with breast cancer), hypercholesterolemia, inflammation and pain at IM injection site
Transdermal: Pruritus, erythema, skin irritation
Rare
Polycythemia (with high dosage), hypersensitivity

PRECAUTIONS AND CONTRAINDICATIONS
Cardiac impairment, hypercalcemia, pregnancy, prostate or breast cancer in males, severe hepatic or renal disease
Caution:
Diabetes mellitus, cardiovascular disease, MI, increased risk of prostatic hypertrophy, prostatic carcinoma, virilization (women), increased PT

DRUG INTERACTIONS OF CONCERN TO DENTISTRY
• Edema: ACTH, adrenal steroids

T

SERIOUS REACTIONS

! Peliosis hepatitis (presence of blood-filled cysts in parenchyma of liver), hepatic neoplasms, and hepatocellular carcinoma have been associated with prolonged high-dose therapy. Anaphylactic reactions occur rarely.

DENTAL CONSIDERATIONS

General:
• Determine why the patient is taking the drug.
• Consider local hemostasis measures to prevent excessive bleeding.
• Short appointments and a stress-reduction protocol may be required for anxious patients.
• Prophylactic antibiotics may be indicated to prevent infection if surgery or deep scaling is planned.
Consultations:
• Physician consultation may be required if signs of anemia are observed in oral tissues.
• Medical consultation may be required to assess disease control and patient's ability to tolerate stress.
• Medical consultation should include PPT or PT.
Teach Patient/Family to:
• Encourage effective oral hygiene to prevent soft tissue inflammation.
• Be aware of the possibility of secondary oral infection and the need to see dentist immediately if infection occurs.

tetrabenazine
tet′-ra-**ben**′-a-zeen
(Xenazine)

CATEGORY AND SCHEDULE
Pregnancy Risk Category: C

Drug Class: CNS agent, monoamine depleter

MECHANISM OF ACTION
A monoamine depleter that inhibits the human vesicular monoamine transporter type 2 (VMAT2), resulting in decreased uptake of monoamines into synaptic vesicles and depletion of monoamine stores; depletes stores of dopamine, serotonin, and noradrenalin.
Therapeutic Effect: Reduces uncontrolled muscle movements.

USES
Chorea associated with Huntington's disease

PHARMACOKINETICS
Well absorbed following PO administration. Protein binding: 82%–85%. Metabolized in liver, primarily by CYP2D6. Primarily excreted in urine; minimal elimination in feces. *Half-life:* 2–8 hr.

INDICATIONS AND DOSAGES
▸ **Chorea Associated with Huntington's Disease**
PO
Adults. 12.5 mg a day given once in the morning. After 1 wk, the dose should be increased to 25 mg a day given as 12.5 mg twice a day. Titrate slowly at weekly intervals by 12.5 mg. If a dose of 37.5 to 50 mg per day is needed, give in a three

times a day regimen. Maximum single dose: 25 mg.

SIDE EFFECTS/ADVERSE REACTIONS
Frequent
Extrapyramidal events, sedation, fatigue, insomnia, akathisia, depression, anxiety, difficulty balancing, bradykinesia, nausea, dysphagia, upper respiratory tract infection, falling, parkinsonism
Occasional
Irritability, decreased appetite, dizziness, dysarthria, headache, obsessive reaction, unsteady gait, vomiting, dysuria, ecchymosis, bronchitis, shortness of breath, head laceration, hyperprolactinemia, orthostatic hypotension
Rare
Neuroleptic malignant syndrome, QT prolongation

PRECAUTIONS AND CONTRAINDICATIONS
Hypersensitivity to tetrabenazine or its components
Hepatic impairment
Concurrent use with monoamine oxidase inhibitors or reserpine; initiation of tetrabenazine less than 20 days after discontinuation of reserpine
Use in suicidal or depressed patients (not treated or inadequately treated)
Caution:
Concurrent use with CYP2D6 inhibitors and inducers
History of depression or suicidal behavior
History of cardiac arrhythmias
Congenital ong QTc syndrome
Hypokalemia and/or hypomagnesemia

DRUG INTERACTIONS OF CONCERN TO DENTISTRY
• Strong CYP2D6 inhibitors (fluoxetine, paroxetine, quinidine): May increase tetrabenazine levels; reduce dose by half
• Alcohol, CNS depressants: Additive CNS depressant effects
• Drugs that prolong QT interval: Increased risk of arrhythmias
• Neuroleptic agents: May increase the risk of tetrabenazine adverse effects
• Monoamine oxidase inhibitors, reserpine: Contraindicated

SERIOUS REACTIONS
! Black box warning: May increase the risk of depression and suicidal thoughts or behavior.
! Neuroleptic malignant syndrome (NMS), akathisia, agitation, parkinsonism, dysphagia, and QT prolongation–related arrhythmias have been reported.

DENTAL CONSIDERATIONS
General:
• Examine for oral manifestation of opportunistic infection.
• Patient on chronic drug therapy may rarely have symptoms of blood dyscrasias, which include infection, bleeding, and poor healing.
• Avoid dental light in patient's eyes; offer dark glasses for patient comfort.
• Place on frequent recall because of oral side effects.
• Consider semisupine chair position for patient comfort if GI side effects occur.
Consultations:
• In a patient with symptoms of blood dyscrasias, request a medical consultation for blood studies and postpone treatment until normal values are reestablished.

T

• Medical consultation may be required to assess disease control.

Teach Patient/Family to:

• Encourage effective oral hygiene to prevent soft tissue inflammation.
• Prevent trauma when using oral hygiene aids.
• Be alert for the possibility of secondary oral infection and the need to see dentist immediately if signs of infection occur.

---

tetracaine
tet´-ra-cane
(AK-T Caine, Cepacol, Opticaine, Pontocaine, Viractin)
Do not confuse with procaine, lidocaine.

CATEGORY AND SCHEDULE
Pregnancy Risk Category: C

Drug Class: Topical anesthetic (ester group)

MECHANISM OF ACTION
Tetracaine causes a reversible blockade of nerve conduction by decreasing nerve membrane permeability to sodium.
Therapeutic Effect: Local anesthetic.

USES
Local anesthesia of mucous membranes, pruritus, sunburn, sore throat, cold sores, oral pain, rectal pain and irritation, control of gagging

PHARMACOKINETICS
Systemic absorption of tetracaine is variable. Metabolized by plasma pseudocholinesterases. Excreted in the urine.

INDICATIONS AND DOSAGES
▶ **Anesthetize Lower Abdomen**
Spinal
Adults. 3–4 ml (9–12 mg) of a 0.3% solution.
▶ **Anesthetize Perineum**
Spinal
Adults. 1–2 ml (3–6 mg) of a 0.3% solution.
▶ **Anesthetize Upper Abdomen**
Spinal
Adults. 5 ml (15 mg) of a 0.3% solution.
▶ **Obstetric Anesthesia, Low Spinal (Saddle Block) Anesthesia**
Spinal
Adults. 1–2 ml (2–14 mg) of a 0.2% solution.
▶ **Anesthesia of the Perineum**
Intrathecal
Adults. 0.5 ml (5 mg) as a 1% solution, diluted with equal amount of CSF or 10% dextrose injection.
▶ **Anesthesia of the Perineum and Lower Extremities**
Intrathecal
Adults. 1 ml (10 mg) as a 1% solution, diluted with equal amount of CSF or 10% dextrose injection.
▶ **Anesthesia up to the Costal Margin**
Intrathecal
Adults. 1.5–2 ml (15–20 mg) as a 1% solution, diluted with equal amount of CSF.
▶ **Topical Anesthesia**
Topical
Adults. Apply to the affected areas as needed. Maximum dosage is 28 g/24 hr.
Children. Apply to the affected areas as needed. Maximum dosage is 7 g in a 24-hr period.

▸ **Topical Anesthesia of Nose and Throat, Abolish Laryngeal and Esophageal Reflexes Prior to Diagnostic Procedure**
Topical
Adults. Direct application of a 0.25% or 0.5% topical solution or by oral inhalation of a nebulized 0.5% solution. Total dose should not exceed 20 mg.
▸ **Mild Pain, Burning, and/or Pruritus Associated with Herpes Labialis (Cold Sores or Fever Blisters)**
Topical
Adults, Children 2 yr and older. Apply to the affected area no more than 3–4 times a day.
▸ **Ophthalmic Anesthesia**
Topical
Adults. 1–2 drops of a 0.5% solution.

SIDE EFFECTS/ADVERSE REACTIONS
Frequent
Burning, stinging, or tenderness; skin rash; itching, redness, or inflammation; numbness or tingling of the face or mouth; pain at the injection site; sensitivity to light; swelling of the eye or eyelid; watering of the eyes; acute ocular pain and ocular irritation (burning, stinging, or redness)
Occasional
Paresthesias, weakness and paralysis of lower extremity, hypotension, high or total spinal block, urinary retention or incontinence, fecal incontinence, headache, back pain, septic meningitis, meningismus, arachnoiditis, shivering, cranial nerve palsies due to traction on nerves from loss of CSF, and loss of perineal sensation and sexual function
Rare
Anxiety; restlessness; difficulty breathing; shortness of breath;

dizziness; drowsiness; light-headedness; nausea; vomiting; seizures (convulsions); slow, irregular heartbeat (palpitations); swelling of the face or mouth; skin rash; itching (hives); tremors; visual impairment

PRECAUTIONS AND CONTRAINDICATIONS
Hypersensitivity to ester local anesthetics, sulfites, PABA; infection or inflammation at the injection site, bacteremia, platelet abnormalities, thrombocytopenia, increased bleeding time, uncontrolled coagulopathy, anticoagulant therapy, sulfonamide therapy
Caution:
Children younger than 12 yr, sepsis, lactation, local infection, geriatric, debilitated patient

DRUG INTERACTIONS OF CONCERN TO DENTISTRY
• Specific drug interactions are not listed; it would be wise to use with caution in patients taking tocainide, mexiletine; significant systemic absorption could lead to synergistic and potentially toxic effects.

SERIOUS REACTIONS
! Tetracaine-induced CNS toxicity usually presents with symptoms of CNS stimulation, such as anxiety, apprehension, restlessness, nervousness, disorientation, confusion, dizziness, tinnitus, blurred vision, tremor, and/or seizures. Subsequently, depressive symptoms may occur, including drowsiness, respiratory arrest, or coma.
! Depression or cardiac excitability and contractility may cause AV block, ventricular arrhythmias, or cardiac arrest. Symptoms of local anesthetic CNS toxicity, such as dizziness, tongue numbness, visual

impairment or disturbances, and muscular twitching appear to occur before cardiotoxic effects. Cardiotoxic effects include angina, QT prolongation, PR prolongation, atrial fibrillation, sinus bradycardia, hypotension, palpitations, and cardiovascular collapse. Maternal seizures and cardiovascular collapse may occur following paracervical block in early pregnancy due to rapid systemic absorption.

Alert

! Tetracaine is more likely than any other topical anesthetic to cause contact reactions, including skin rash (unspecified), mucous membrane irritation, erythema, pruritus, urticaria, burning, stinging, edema, or tenderness.

Alert

! During labor and obstetric delivery, local anesthetics can cause varying degrees of maternal, fetal, and neonatal toxicities. Fetal heart rate should be monitored continuously because fetal bradycardia may occur in patients receiving tetracaine anesthesia and may be associated with fetal acidosis. Maternal hypotension can result from regional anesthesia; patient position can alleviate this problem. Spinal tetracaine may cause decreased uterine contractility or maternal expulsion efforts and alter the forces of parturition.

DENTAL CONSIDERATIONS

General:

• Apply smallest effective dose; apply to small area because significant absorption can occur, especially from denuded areas.
• Absorption of excessive amounts of drug may lead to signs of local anesthetic toxicity; with correct use, toxicity is a rare event.

• Use for topical anesthesia or temporary relief of symptoms; reevaluate if symptoms persist.
• Toxic amounts can be absorbed from denuded mucosa or skin.
• Apply with cotton-tipped applicator by pressing, not rubbing, paste on lesion.

Teach Patient/Family to:

• Apply correctly.
• Not chew gum or eat while numbness is present after dental treatment.
• Recognize the symptoms of systemic toxicity, which can include nervousness, nausea, excitement followed by drowsiness, convulsions, and cardiac and respiratory depression.
• Be aware that symptoms may vary because they depend on the amount of drug actually absorbed.

tetracycline hydrochloride

tet-ra-**sye**′-kleen
high-droh-**klor**′-ide
(Apo-Tetra[CAN], Latycin[AUS], Mysteclin[AUS], Novotetra[CAN], Nu-Tetra[CAN], Sumycin, Tetrex[AUS])

CATEGORY AND SCHEDULE

Pregnancy Risk Category: D (B with topical form)

Drug Class: Tetracycline, broad-spectrum antibiotic

MECHANISM OF ACTION

A tetracycline antibiotic that inhibits bacterial protein synthesis by binding to ribosomes.
Therapeutic Effect: Bacteriostatic.

USES

Treatment of syphilis, *C. trachomatis,* gonorrhea, lymphogranuloma venereum, *M. pneumoniae,* rickettsial infections, acne, actinomycosis, anthrax, bronchitis, GU infections, sinusitis, and many other infections produced by susceptible organisms; *H. pylori*–associated duodenal ulcer

PHARMACOKINETICS

Readily absorbed from the GI tract. Protein binding: 30%–60%. Widely distributed. Excreted in urine; eliminated in feces through biliary system. Not removed by hemodialysis. *Half-life:* 6–11 hr (increased in impaired renal function).

INDICATIONS AND DOSAGES

▶ **Inflammatory Acne Vulgaris, Lyme Disease, Mycoplasmal Disease, Legionella Infections, Rocky Mountain Spotted Fever, Chlamydial Infections in Patients with Gonorrhea**
PO
Adults, Elderly. 250–500 mg q6–12h.
Children 8 yr and older. 25–50 mg/kg/day in 4 divided doses. Maximum: 3 g/day.
▶ **H. pylori Infections**
PO
Adults, Elderly. 500 mg 2–4 times a day (in combination).
Topical
Adults, Elderly. Apply twice a day (once in the morning, once in the evening).
▶ **Dosage in Renal Impairment**
Dosage interval is modified on the basis of creatinine clearance.

Creatinine Clearance	Dosage Interval
50–80 ml/min	Usual dose q8–12h
10–50 ml/min	Usual dose q12–24h
Less than 10 ml/min	Usual dose q24h

SIDE EFFECTS/ADVERSE REACTIONS

Frequent
Dizziness, light-headedness, diarrhea, nausea, vomiting, abdominal cramps, possibly severe photosensitivity
Topical: Dry, scaly skin; stinging or burning sensation
Occasional
Pigmentation of skin or mucous membranes, rectal or genital pruritus, stomatitis
Topical: Pain, redness, swelling, or other skin irritation.

PRECAUTIONS AND CONTRAINDICATIONS

Children 8 yr and younger, hypersensitivity to tetracyclines or sulfites.
The use of tetracycline drugs during tooth development (last half of pregnancy, infancy, and childhood up to the age of 8 may cause permanent discoloration of the teeth (yellow-gray-brown). Enamel hypoplasia has also been reported. May also cause retardation of skeletal development and deformations.
Caution:
Renal disease, hepatic disease

DRUG INTERACTIONS OF CONCERN TO DENTISTRY

• Decreased absorption: $NaHCO_3$, other antacids
• Decreased effect of penicillins, cephalosporins
• Possible increase in serum levels of methotrexate

T

• Suspected increase in effects of warfarin, theophylline

SERIOUS REACTIONS
! Superinfection (especially fungal), anaphylaxis, and benign intracranial hypertension may occur. Bulging fontanelles occur rarely in infants.

DENTAL CONSIDERATIONS
General:
• Determine why the patient is taking tetracycline.
• Broad-spectrum antibiotics may be a factor in oral or vaginal *Candida* infections.
• Advise patient if dental drugs prescribed have a potential for photosensitivity.
• Dental staining or enamel hypoplasia may be associated with exposure to this drug before birth or up to the age of 8. Tetracycline stains may be extremely resistant to ordinary tooth-whitening procedures.
Consultations:
• Medical consultation may be required to assess disease control.
Teach Patient/Family to:
• Encourage effective oral hygiene to prevent soft tissue inflammation.
• Prevent injury when using oral hygiene aids.
• Avoid milk products; to take with a full glass of water.
• Take tetracycline doses 1 hr before or 2 hr after air polishing device (Prophy-Jet), if used.
• When used for dental infection, advise patient to:
  • Use additional method of contraception for duration of cycle if taking birth control pill.
  • Report sore throat, oral burning sensation, fever, fatigue, any of which could indicate superinfection.

• Take at prescribed intervals and complete dosage regimen.
• Immediately notify the dentist if signs or symptoms of infection increase.

tetracycline periodontal fiber
tet-ra-**sye**′-kleen pare-ee-oh-**don**′-tal **fye**′-ber
(Actisite)

CATEGORY AND SCHEDULE
Pregnancy Risk Category: C

Drug Class: Tetracycline, broad-spectrum antiinfective

MECHANISM OF ACTION
Antimicrobial effect related to inhibition of protein synthesis; decreases incidence of postsurgical inflammation and edema; suppresses bacteria and acts as a barrier to bacterial entry; acts on cementum or fibroblasts to enhance periodontal ligament regeneration.

USES
Adjunctive treatment in adult periodontitis.

PHARMACOKINETICS
Topical: In vitro release rate 2 mcg/cm/hr; gingival concentration maintained over 10 days; plasma levels below detectable limits

INDICATIONS AND DOSAGES
Fiber: Adjust length to fit pocket depth and contour of teeth treated; fiber should contact base of pocket; apply cyanoacrylate adhesive to secure fiber for 10 days; replace if lost before 7 days; up to 11 teeth can be treated.

T

SIDE EFFECTS/ADVERSE REACTIONS

Oral: Gingival inflammation and pain, glossitis, local erythema, candidiasis, staining of tongue
EENT: Minor throat irritation
INTEG: Photosensitivity

PRECAUTIONS AND CONTRAINDICATIONS

Hypersensitivity, children younger than 8 yr, acutely abscessed periodontal pocket
Caution:
Lactation, children, superinfection, patients with predisposition to candidiasis; must remove fibers after 10 days

DRUG INTERACTIONS OF CONCERN TO DENTISTRY

• It is not known if the tetracycline fiber will decrease the effectiveness of oral contraceptives; however, manufacturer recommends suggesting the use of an alternative form of contraception during the remaining cycle to female patients taking oral contraceptives.

SERIOUS REACTIONS

! Serious systemic toxicity unlikely by this route of administration.

DENTAL CONSIDERATIONS

General:
• Take precautions regarding allergy to tetracyclines.
• Examine oral mucosa for candidiasis before placing fiber.
Teach Patient/Family to:
• Not chew hard, crusty, or sticky foods.
• Not brush or floss near treated area but clean other teeth.
• Avoid other oral hygienic practices that could dislodge fibers, such as the use of toothpicks.

• Do not irritate the treated area.
• Notify dentist if fiber dislodges or falls out.
• Notify dentist if pain, swelling, or other symptoms occur.

---

thalidomide
thah-**lid**'-owe-mide
(Thalomid)

CATEGORY AND SCHEDULE
Pregnancy Risk Category: X

Drug Class: Immunomodulators, tumor necrosis factor modulators

MECHANISM OF ACTION
An immunomodulator whose exact mechanism is unknown. Has sedative, antiinflammatory, and immunosuppressive activity, which may be caused by selective inhibition of the production of tumor necrosis factor-α.
Therapeutic Effect: Improves muscle wasting in HIV patients; reduces local and systemic effects of leprosy.

USES
Treatment of and prevention of erythema nodosum leprosum (ENL)

PHARMACOKINETICS
Slowly absorbed from GI tract; peak blood level in 2.9–5.7 hr. Protein binding 55%–66%; metabolized in plasma. *Half-life:* 5–7 hr; elimination in urine and by other routes.

INDICATIONS AND DOSAGES
▸ AIDS-Related Muscle Wasting
PO
Adults. 100–300 mg a day.

T

▶ **Leprosy**

PO

Adults, Elderly. Initially, 100–300 mg/day as single bedtime dose, at least 1 hr after the evening meal. Continue until active reaction subsides, then reduce dose q2–4 wk in 50 mg increments.

SIDE EFFECTS/ADVERSE REACTIONS

Frequent

Somnolence, dizziness, mood changes, constipation, dry mouth, peripheral neuropathy

Occasional

Increased appetite, weight gain, headache, loss of libido, edema of face and limbs, nausea, alopecia, dry skin, rash, hypothyroidism

PRECAUTIONS AND CONTRAINDICATIONS

Neutropenia, peripheral neuropathy; pregnancy, sensitivity to thalidomide

DRUG INTERACTIONS OF CONCERN TO DENTISTRY

• Increased sedative effects of: alcohol, barbiturates, phenothiazines
• Increased risk of peripheral neuropathy: metronidazole
• May interfere with hormonal contraceptives: patient must use two alternative methods of contraception

SERIOUS REACTIONS

! Neutropenia, peripheral neuropathy, and thromboembolism occur rarely.

DENTAL CONSIDERATIONS

General:
• Determine why patient is taking the drug.
• Consider semisupine chair position for patient comfort if GI side effects occur.

• Assess salivary flow as a factor in caries, periodontal disease, and candidiasis.
• Examine for oral manifestation of opportunistic infection.
• Patient on chronic drug therapy may rarely present with symptoms of blood dyscrasias, which can include infection, bleeding, and poor healing. If dyscrasia is present, caution patient to prevent oral tissue trauma when using oral hygiene aids.
• After supine positioning, have patient sit upright for at least 2 min before standing to avoid orthostatic hypotension.
• Can be prescribed only by S.T.E.P.S. (System for Thalidomide Education and Prescribing Safety) registered prescribers.
• Absolutely contraindicated in pregnancy.

Consultations:
• Refer patients to attending physician if symptoms of peripheral neuropathy are present (numbness, tingling or pain in hands or feet).
• Consultation with physician may be necessary if sedation or general anesthesia is required.
• Medical consultation may be required to assess disease control and patient's ability to tolerate stress.
• In a patient with symptoms of blood dyscrasias, request a medical consultation for blood studies and postpone treatment until normal values are reestablished.
• Precaution if dental surgery is anticipated or general anesthesia required.

Teach Patient/Family to:
• Not drive or perform other tasks requiring mental alertness.
• When chronic dry mouth occurs, advise patient to:

• Avoid mouth rinses with high alcohol content due to drying effects.
• Use daily home fluoride products for anticaries effect.
• Use sugarless gum, frequent sips of water, or saliva substitutes.
• Encourage effective oral hygiene to prevent soft tissue inflammation.
• Prevent trauma when using oral hygiene aids.
• Report oral lesions, soreness, or bleeding to dentist.
• Update health and medication history if physician makes any changes in evaluation or drug regimens; include OTC, herbal, and nonherbal remedies in the update.

theophylline
thee-**off**'-ih-lin
(Accurbron, Aquaphyllin, Asmalix, Bronkodyl, Elixomin, Elixophyllin, Lanophyllin, Quibron-T, Respbid, Slo-Bid, Slo-Phyllin, Sustaire, T-Phyl, Theobid, Theoclear LA, Theolair, Theo-Dur, Theo-24, Theolair-24, Theochron, Theo-Sav, Theovent, Theo-X, Uni-Dur, Uniphyl)

CATEGORY AND SCHEDULE
Pregnancy Risk Category: C

Drug Class: Xanthine

MECHANISM OF ACTION
An antiasthmatic medication with two distinct actions in the airways of patients with reversible obstruction; smooth muscle relaxation and suppression of the response of airways to stimuli. Mechanisms of action are not known with certainty.

It is known that theophylline increases force of contraction of diaphragmatic muscles by enhancing calcium uptake through adenosine-mediated channels.
Therapeutic Effect: Bronchodilation and decreased airway reactivity.

USES
Treatment of bronchial asthma, bronchospasm of COPD, chronic bronchitis; unapproved use: apnea in the neonate

PHARMACOKINETICS
The pharmacokinetics of theophylline vary widely among similar patients and cannot be predicted by age, sex, body weight or other characteristics. Rapidly and completely absorbed after oral administration in solution or immediate-release solid oral dosage form. Distributed freely into fat-free tissues. Extensively metabolized in liver. *Half-life:* 4–8 hr.

INDICATIONS AND DOSAGES
▶ **Chronic Asthma/Lung Diseases**
PO
Adults. Acute symptoms: 5 mg/kg as a loading dose, maintenance 3 mg/kg every 8 hr (nonsmokers), 3 mg/kg every 6 hr (smokers), 2 mg/kg every 8 hr (older patients), 1–2 mg/kg every 12 hr (CHF); IV 5 mg/kg load over 20 min, maintenance 0.2 mg/kg/hr (CHF, elderly), 0.43 mg/kg/hr (nonsmokers), 0.7 mg/kg/hr (young adult smokers). Slow titration. Initial dose 16 mg/kg/day or 400 mg daily, whichever is less, doses divided every 6–8 hr.

SIDE EFFECTS/ADVERSE REACTIONS
Anxiety, dizziness, headache, insomnia, light-headedness, muscle twitching, restlessness, seizures,

T

dysrhythmias, fluid retention with tachycardia, hypotension, palpitations, pounding heartbeat, sinus tachycardia, anorexia, bitter taste, diarrhea, dyspepsia, gastroesophageal reflux, nausea, vomiting, urinary frequency, increased respiratory rate, flushing, urticaria

PRECAUTIONS AND CONTRAINDICATIONS

Hypersensitivity to theophylline or any component of the formulation, active peptic ulcer disease, underlying seizure disorders unless receiving appropriate anticonvulsant medication

Caution:
Elderly, CHF, cor pulmonale, hepatic disease, active peptic ulcer disease, diabetes mellitus, hyperthyroidism, hypertension, children

DRUG INTERACTIONS OF CONCERN TO DENTISTRY

• Increased action: erythromycin, ciprofloxacin, glucocorticoids
• Increased risk of cardiac dysrhythmia: halothane inhalation anesthesia, CNS stimulants
• Decreased effect: barbiturates, carbamazepine, ketoconazole
• May decrease sedative effects of benzodiazepines

SERIOUS REACTIONS

! Severe toxicity from theophylline overdose is a relatively rare event.

DENTAL CONSIDERATIONS

General:
• Consider semisupine chair position for patients with respiratory disease.
• Monitor vital signs at every appointment because of cardiovascular side effects.

• Assess salivary flow as a factor in caries, periodontal disease, and candidiasis.
• Be aware that aspirin or sulfite preservatives in vasoconstrictor-containing products can exacerbate asthma.
• Acute asthmatic episodes may be precipitated in the dental office. Sympathomimetic inhalants should be available for emergency use.
• Midday appointments and a stress-reduction protocol may be required for anxious patients.

Consultations:
• Medical consultation may be required to assess disease control.

Teach Patient/Family:
• When chronic dry mouth occurs, advise patient to:
  • Avoid mouth rinses with high alcohol content because of drying effects.
  • Use daily home fluoride products to prevent caries.
  • Use sugarless gum, frequent sips of water, or saliva substitutes.

thiabendazole
thye-ah-**ben**′-da-zole
(Mintezol)

CATEGORY AND SCHEDULE
Pregnancy Risk Category: C

Drug Class: Anthelmintic, systemic

MECHANISM OF ACTION
An anthelmintic agent that inhibits helminth-specific mitochondrial fumarate reductase.
Therapeutic Effect: Suppresses parasite production.

USES
Treatment of worm infections

PHARMACOKINETICS
Rapidly and well absorbed from the GI tract. Rapidly metabolized in liver. Primarily excreted in urine; partially eliminated in feces.
Half-life: 1.2 hr.

INDICATIONS AND DOSAGES
Dose is based on patient's body weight.
▸ **Cutaneous Lava Migrans (Creeping Eruption)**
PO
Adults, Elderly, Children. 50 mg/kg/day q12h for 2 days. Maximum: 3 g/day.
▸ **Intestinal Roundworms**
PO
Adults, Elderly, Children. 50 mg/kg/day q12h for 2 days. Maximum: 3 g/day.
▸ **Strongyloidiasis (Thread Worms)**
PO
Adults, Elderly, Children. 50 mg/kg/day q12h for 2 days. Maximum: 3 g/day.
▸ **Trichinosis**
PO
Adults, Elderly, Children. 50 mg/kg/day q12h for 2–4 days. Maximum: 3 g/day.
▸ **Visceral Larva Migrans**
PO
Adults, Elderly, Children. 50 mg/kg/day q12h for 7 days. Maximum: 3 g/day.

SIDE EFFECTS/ADVERSE REACTIONS
Occasional
Dizziness, drowsiness, nausea, vomiting, diarrhea
Rare
Erythema multiform, liver damage

PRECAUTIONS AND CONTRAINDICATIONS
Prophylactic treatment of pinworm infestation, hypersensitivity to thiabendazole or its components

DRUG INTERACTIONS OF CONCERN TO DENTISTRY
• Suspected interference with xanthine metabolism

SERIOUS REACTIONS
❗ Overdose includes symptoms of altered mental status and visual problems. Erythema multiform, liver damage, and Stevens-Johnson syndrome occur rarely.

DENTAL CONSIDERATIONS
General:
• Determine why patient is taking the drug.
• Patient on chronic drug therapy may rarely present with symptoms of blood dyscrasias, which can include infection, bleeding, and poor healing. If dyscrasia is present, caution patient to prevent oral tissue trauma when using oral hygiene aids.
• Assess salivary flow as a factor in caries, periodontal disease, and candidiasis.
• Pinworm infections are easily spread to persons in close contact.
• Question patients about other drugs they may be using.
Consultations:
• In a patient with symptoms of blood dyscrasias, request a medical consultation for blood studies and postpone treatment until normal values are reestablished.
• Medical consultation may be required to assess disease control in the patient.

T

Teach Patient/Family:

• When chronic dry mouth occurs, advise patient to:

  • Avoid mouth rinses with high alcohol content because of drying effects.

  • Use daily home fluoride products for anticaries effect.

  • Use sugarless gum, frequent sips of water, or saliva substitutes.

thiamine hydrochloride (vitamin B₁)

thy′-ah-min high-droh-**klor**′-ide
(Beta-Sol[AUS], Betaxin[CAN], Thiamilate)

CATEGORY AND SCHEDULE

Pregnancy Risk Category: A (C if used in doses above recommended daily allowance)
OTC (tablets)

Drug Class: Vitamin B₁, water soluble

MECHANISM OF ACTION

A water-soluble vitamin that combines with adenosine triphosphate in the liver, kidneys, and leukocytes to form thiamine diphosphate, a coenzyme that is necessary for carbohydrate metabolism.
Therapeutic Effect: Prevents and reverses thiamine deficiency.

USES

Treatment of vitamin B₁ deficiency or prophylaxis, beriberi, Wernicke-Korsakoff syndrome

PHARMACOKINETICS

Readily absorbed from the GI tract, primarily in duodenum, after IM administration. Widely distributed. Metabolized in the liver. Primarily excreted in urine.

INDICATIONS AND DOSAGES

▶ **Dietary Supplement**
PO
Adults, Elderly. 1–2 mg/day.
Children. 0.5–1 mg/day.
Infants. 0.3–0.5 mg/day.

▶ **Thiamine Deficiency**
PO
Adults, Elderly. 5–30 mg/day, as a single dose or in 3 divided doses, for 1 mo.
Children. 10–50 mg/day in 3 divided doses.

▶ **Thiamine Deficiency on Patients Who Are Critically Ill or Have Malabsorption Syndrome**
IV, IM
Adults, Elderly. 5–100 mg, 3 times a day.
Children. 10–25 mg/day.

▶ **Metabolic Disorders**
PO
Adults, Elderly, Children. 10–20 mg/day; increased up to 4 g/day in divided doses.

SIDE EFFECTS/ADVERSE REACTIONS

Frequent
Pain, induration, and tenderness at IM injection site

PRECAUTIONS AND CONTRAINDICATIONS

Sensitivity to thiamin, Wernicke's encephalopathy

DRUG INTERACTIONS OF CONCERN TO DENTISTRY

• None reported

SERIOUS REACTIONS

! IV administration may result in a rare, severe hypersensitivity reaction marked by a feeling of warmth, pruritus, urticaria, weakness, diaphoresis, nausea, restlessness, tightness in throat, angioedema, cyanosis, pulmonary edema, GI tract bleeding, and cardiovascular collapse.

DENTAL CONSIDERATIONS

General:
• Determine why the patient is taking this vitamin.
Teach Patient/Family:
• Food sources to be included in diet: yeast, whole grain, beef, liver, legumes.

thiethylperazine
thye-eth-il-**per**′-ah-zeen
(Torecan)
Do not confuse with thioridazine.

CATEGORY AND SCHEDULE
Pregnancy Risk Category: X

Drug Class: Phenothiazine-type antiemetic

MECHANISM OF ACTION
A piperazine phenothiazine that acts centrally to block dopamine receptors in chemoreceptor trigger zone (CTZ) in CNS.
Therapeutic Effect: Relieves nausea and vomiting.

USES
Treatment of nausea, vomiting

PHARMACOKINETICS
PO: Onset 45–60 min. Rectal: Onset 45–60 min. Metabolized by liver; excreted by kidneys; crosses placenta; excreted in breast milk.

INDICATIONS AND DOSAGES
▸ **Nausea or Vomiting**
PO/Rectal/IM
Adults, Elderly. 10 mg 1–3 times a day.

SIDE EFFECTS/ADVERSE REACTIONS
Frequent
Drowsiness, dizziness
Occasional
Blurred vision, decreased color/night vision, fever, headache, orthostatic hypotension, rash, ringing in ears, constipation, dry mouth, decreased sweating

PRECAUTIONS AND CONTRAINDICATIONS
Comatose states, severe CNS depression, pregnancy, hypersensitivity to phenothiazines
Caution:
Children younger than 12 yr, elderly

DRUG INTERACTIONS OF CONCERN TO DENTISTRY
• Increased anticholinergic action: anticholinergics
• Increased CNS depression, hypotension: alcohol, CNS depressants

SERIOUS REACTIONS
! Extrapyramidal symptoms manifested as torticollis (neck muscle spasm), oculogyric crisis (rolling back of eyes), and akathisia (motor restlessness, anxiety) occur rarely.

DENTAL CONSIDERATIONS
General:
• Postpone elective dental treatment when symptoms are present.

Consultations:
• Medical consultation may be required to assess disease control.

thioridazine

thye-oh-**rid**′-ah-zeen
(Aldazine[AUS], Apo-Thioridazine [CAN], Mellaril, Mellaril [AUS], Thioridazine Intensol)
Do not confuse thioridazine with thiothixene or Thorazine, or Mellaril with Mebaral.

CATEGORY AND SCHEDULE
Pregnancy Risk Category: C

Drug Class: Phenothiazine antipsychotic

MECHANISM OF ACTION
A phenothiazine that blocks dopamine at postsynaptic receptor sites. Possesses strong anticholinergic and sedative effects. **Therapeutic Effect:** Suppresses behavioral response in psychosis; reduces locomotor activity and aggressiveness.

USES
Treatment of psychotic disorders, schizophrenia, behavioral problems in children, alcohol withdrawal as adjunct, anxiety, major depressive disorders, organic brain syndrome

PHARMACOKINETICS
PO: Onset erratic, peak 2–4 hr. **Half-life:** 26–36 hr; metabolized by liver; excreted in urine; crosses placenta; excreted in breast milk.

INDICATIONS AND DOSAGES
▸ **Psychosis**
PO
Adults, Elderly, Children 12 yr and older. Initially, 25–100 mg 3 times a day; dosage increased gradually. Maximum: 800 mg/day.
Children 2–11 yr. Initially, 0.5 mg/ kg/day in 2–3 divided doses. Maximum: 3 mg/kg/day.

SIDE EFFECTS/ADVERSE REACTIONS
Occasional
Drowsiness during early therapy, dry mouth, blurred vision, lethargy, constipation or diarrhea, nasal congestion, peripheral edema, urine retention
Rare
Ocular changes, altered skin pigmentation (in those taking high doses for prolonged periods), photosensitivity, darkening of urine

PRECAUTIONS AND CONTRAINDICATIONS
Angle-closure glaucoma, blood dyscrasias, cardiac arrhythmias, cardiac or hepatic impairment, concurrent use of drugs that prolong QT interval, severe CNS depression
Caution:
Lactation, seizure disorders, hypertension, hepatic disease, cardiac disease

DRUG INTERACTIONS OF CONCERN TO DENTISTRY
• Increased sedation: other CNS depressants, alcohol, barbiturate anesthetics, opioid analgesics
• Hypotension, tachycardia: epinephrine (systemic)
• Increased extrapyramidal effects: phenothiazines and related drugs (haloperidol, droperidol), metoclopramide
• Additive photosensitization: tetracyclines
• Increased anticholinergic effects: anticholinergics

SERIOUS REACTIONS

! Prolonged QT interval may produce torsades de pointes, a form of ventricular tachycardia, and sudden death.

DENTAL CONSIDERATIONS

General:
• Monitor vital signs at every appointment because of cardiovascular side effects.
• Patients on chronic drug therapy may rarely have symptoms of blood dyscrasias, which can include infection, bleeding, and poor healing.
• After supine positioning, have patient sit upright for at least 2 min before standing to avoid orthostatic hypotension.
• Assess salivary flow as a factor in caries, periodontal disease, and candidiasis.
• Avoid dental light in patient's eyes; offer dark glasses for patient comfort.
• Assess for presence of extrapyramidal motor symptoms, such as tardive dyskinesia and akathisia. Extrapyramidal motor activity may complicate dental treatment.
• Geriatric patients are more susceptible to drug effects; use lower dose.
• Use vasoconstrictors with caution, in low doses, and with careful aspiration.
Consultations:
• In a patient with symptoms of blood dyscrasias, request a medical consultation for blood studies and postpone dental treatment until normal values are reestablished.
• Take precautions if dental surgery is anticipated and anesthesia is required.
• Refer to physician if signs of tardive dyskinesia or akathisia are present.

• Physician should be informed if significant xerostomic side effects occur (e.g., increased caries, sore tongue, problems eating or swallowing, difficulty wearing prosthesis) so that a medication change can be considered.
Teach Patient/Family to:
• Encourage effective oral hygiene to prevent soft tissue inflammation.
• Use caution to prevent injury when using oral hygiene aids.
• Use powered tooth brush if patient has difficulty holding conventional devices.
• When chronic dry mouth occurs, advise patient to:
  • Avoid mouth rinses with high alcohol content because of drying effects.
  • Use daily home fluoride products to prevent caries.
  • Use sugarless gum, frequent sips of water, or saliva substitutes.

thiotepa
thigh-oh-**teh**′-pah
(Thioplex)

CATEGORY AND SCHEDULE
Pregnancy Risk Category: D

Drug Class: Antineoplastic

MECHANISM OF ACTION
An alkylating agent that inhibits DNA and RNA protein synthesis by cross-linking with DNA and RNA strands, preventing cell growth. Cell cycle–phase nonspecific.
Therapeutic Effect: Interferes with DNA and RNA function.

USES
Treatment of some kinds of cancer

PHARMACOKINETICS

Peak serum levels reached rapidly; elimination half-life of 2.4 hr. Excreted in urine primarily as TEPA metabolite and parent drug.

INDICATIONS AND DOSAGES

▸ **Adenocarcinoma of Breast and Ovary, Hodgkin's Disease, Lymphosarcoma, Superficial Papillary Carcinoma of Urinary Bladder**

IV

Adults, Elderly. Initially, 0.3–0.4 mg/kg every 1–4 wk. Maintenance dose adjusted weekly on the basis of blood counts.
Children. 25–65 mg/m^2 as a single dose every 3–4 wk.

▸ **Control of Pericardial, Peritoneal, or Pleural Effusions Caused by Metastatic Tumors**

Intracavitary Injection
Adults, Elderly. 0.6–0.8 mg/kg every 1–4 wk.

SIDE EFFECTS/ADVERSE REACTIONS

Occasional
Pain at injection site, headache, dizziness, urticaria, rash, nausea, vomiting, anorexia, stomatitis
Rare
Alopecia, cystitis, hematuria (after intravesical dose)

PRECAUTIONS AND CONTRAINDICATIONS

Pregnancy, severe myelosuppression (leukocyte count less than 3000/mm^3 or platelet count less than 150,000/mm^3)

DRUG INTERACTIONS OF CONCERN TO DENTISTRY

• Suspected decrease in effects: probenecid
• Prolonged neuromuscular blockade: pancuronium

SERIOUS REACTIONS

! Hematologic toxicity, manifested as leukopenia, anemia, thrombocytopenia, and pancytopenia, may occur from bone marrow depression. Although the WBC count falls to its lowest point 10–14 days after initial therapy, the initial effects on bone marrow may not be evident for 30 days. Stomatitis and ulceration of intestinal mucosa may occur.

DENTAL CONSIDERATIONS

General:
• If additional analgesia is required for dental pain, consider alternative analgesics (NSAIDs) in patients taking narcotics for acute or chronic pain.
• Examine for oral manifestation of opportunistic infection.
• Avoid products that affect platelet function, such as aspirin and NSAIDs.
• This drug may be used in the hospital or on an outpatient basis. Confirm the patient's disease and treatment status.
• Patient on chronic drug therapy may rarely present with symptoms of blood dyscrasias, which can include infection, bleeding, and poor healing. If dyscrasia is present, caution patient to prevent oral tissue trauma when using oral hygiene aids.
• Palliative medication may be required for management of oral side effects.
• Patient may need assistance in getting into and out of dental chair. Adjust chair position for patient comfort.
• Consider semisupine chair position for patient comfort if GI side effects occur.
• Caution: patients may be at high risk for infection.

• Patients may be at risk for bleeding; check oral signs.
• Oral infections should be eliminated and/or treated aggressively.

Consultations:

• Medical consultation should include routine blood counts including platelet counts and bleeding time.
• In a patient with symptoms of blood dyscrasias, request a medical consultation for blood studies and postpone treatment until normal values are reestablished.
• Consult physician; prophylactic or therapeutic antiinfectives may be indicated if surgery or periodontal treatment is required.
• Medical consultation may be required to assess immunologic status during cancer chemotherapy and determine safety risk, if any, posed by the required dental treatment.
• Medical consultation may be required to assess disease control and patient's ability to tolerate stress.

Teach Patient/Family to:

• Encourage effective oral hygiene to prevent soft tissue inflammation.
• Report oral lesions, soreness, or bleeding to dentist.
• Prevent trauma when using oral hygiene aids.
• Update health and medication history if physician makes any changes in evaluation or drug regimen; include OTC, herbal, and nonherbal remedies in the update.

thiothixene
thye-oh-**thix**′-een
(Navane)
Do not confuse thiothixene with thioridazine.

CATEGORY AND SCHEDULE
Pregnancy Risk Category: C

Drug Class: Thioxanthene/antipsychotic

MECHANISM OF ACTION
An antipsychotic that blocks postsynaptic dopamine receptor sites in brain. Has α-adrenergic blocking effects, and depresses the release of hypothalamic and hypophyseal hormones.
Therapeutic Effect: Suppresses psychotic behavior.

USES
Treatment of psychotic disorders, schizophrenia, acute agitation

PHARMACOKINETICS
Well absorbed from the GI tract after IM administration. Widely distributed. Metabolized in the liver. Primarily excreted in urine. Unknown if removed by hemodialysis. ***Half-life:*** 34 hr.

INDICATIONS AND DOSAGES
▸ **Psychosis**
PO
Adults, Elderly, Children older than 12 yr. Initially, 2 mg 3 times a day. Maximum: 60 mg/day.
IM
Adults, Elderly, Children older than 12 yr. Initially, 4 mg 2–4 times a day. Maximum: 30 mg/day.

T

SIDE EFFECTS/ADVERSE REACTIONS

Expected

Hypotension, dizziness, syncope (occur frequently after first injection, occasionally after subsequent injections, and rarely with oral form)

Frequent

Transient drowsiness, dry mouth, constipation, blurred vision, nasal congestion

Occasional

Diarrhea, peripheral edema, urine retention, nausea

Rare

Ocular changes, altered skin pigmentation (in those taking high doses for prolonged periods), photosensitivity

PRECAUTIONS AND CONTRAINDICATIONS

Blood dyscrasias, circulatory collapse, CNS depression, coma, history of seizures

Caution:

Lactation, seizure disorders, hypertension, hepatic disease

DRUG INTERACTIONS OF CONCERN TO DENTISTRY

• Increased sedation: other CNS depressants, alcohol, barbiturate anesthetics, opioid analgesics
• Hypotension, tachycardia: epinephrine (systemic)
• Increased extrapyramidal effects: phenothiazines and related drugs (haloperidol, droperidol), metoclopramide
• Additive photosensitization: tetracyclines
• Increased anticholinergic effects: anticholinergics

SERIOUS REACTIONS

! The most common extrapyramidal reaction is akathisia, characterized by motor restlessness and anxiety.

Akinesia, marked by rigidity, tremor, increased salivation, mask-like facial expression, and reduced voluntary movements, occurs less frequently. Dystonias, including torticollis, opisthotonos, and oculogyric crisis, occur rarely. Tardive dyskinesia, characterized by tongue protrusion, puffing of the cheeks, and chewing or puckering of the mouth, occurs rarely but may be irreversible. Elderly female patients have a greater risk of developing this reaction. Grand mal seizures may occur in epileptic patients, especially those receiving the drug by IM administration. Neuroleptic malignant syndrome occurs rarely.

DENTAL CONSIDERATIONS

General:

• Monitor vital signs at every appointment because of cardiovascular side effects.
• Patients on chronic drug therapy may rarely have symptoms of blood dyscrasias, which can include infection, bleeding, and poor healing.
• After supine positioning, have patient sit upright for at least 2 min before standing to avoid orthostatic hypotension.
• Assess salivary flow as a factor in caries, periodontal disease, and candidiasis.
• Assess for presence of extrapyramidal motor symptoms, such as tardive dyskinesia and akathisia. Extrapyramidal motor activity may complicate dental treatment.
• Use vasoconstrictors with caution, in low doses, and with careful aspiration.
• Avoid dental light in patient's eyes; offer dark glasses for patient comfort.

• Geriatric patients are more susceptible to drug effects; use lower dose.

Consultations:

• In a patient with symptoms of blood dyscrasias, request a medical consultation for blood studies and postpone dental treatment until normal values are reestablished.

• Take precautions if dental surgery is anticipated and anesthesia is required.

• If signs of tardive dyskinesia or akathisia are present, refer to physician.

Teach Patient/Family to:

• Encourage effective oral hygiene to prevent soft tissue inflammation.

• Use caution to prevent injury when using oral hygiene aids.

• Use powered tooth brush if patient has difficulty holding conventional devices.

• When chronic dry mouth occurs, advise patient to:

  • Avoid mouth rinses with high alcohol content because of drying effects.

  • Use daily home fluoride products to prevent caries.

  • Use sugarless gum, frequent sips of water, or saliva substitutes.

---

thrombin, topical (thrombinar, thrombin-JMI, thrombostat, etc.)
throm´-bin

CATEGORY AND SCHEDULE
Pregnancy Risk Category: C

Drug Class: Thrombolytic

MECHANISM OF ACTION
A protein substance produced through a conversion reaction in which prothrombin of bovine origin is activated by tissue thromboplastin in the presence of calcium chloride. It directly clots fibrinogen in the blood.
Therapeutic Effect: Controls bleeding.

USES
Hemostasis

PHARMACOKINETICS
The speed with which thrombin clots blood is dependent upon the concentration of both thrombin and fibrinogen.

INDICATIONS AND DOSAGES
▸ **Hemorrhage, Mild**
Topical
Adults. Apply 100 units/ml as needed.
▸ **Hemorrhage, Severe**
Topical
Adults. Apply 1000 units/ml as needed.

SIDE EFFECTS/ADVERSE REACTIONS
Occasional
Allergic reaction

PRECAUTIONS AND CONTRAINDICATIONS
Sensitivity to thrombin, any of its components and/or to material of bovine origin

DRUG INTERACTIONS OF CONCERN TO DENTISTRY
• None reported

SERIOUS REACTIONS
! Because of its action in the clotting mechanism, thrombin must

not be injected or otherwise allowed to enter large blood vessels. Extensive intravascular clotting and even death may result.

DENTAL CONSIDERATIONS

General:
• Solutions (approximately 100 U/ml) are prepared with sterile normal saline or sterile distilled water.
• Can be used with absorbable gelatin sponge but not microfibrillar collagen.

Teach Patient/Family to:
• Report oral lesions, soreness, or bleeding to dentist.

thyroid
thye'-roid
(Armour Thyroid, Nature-Throid NT, Westhroid)

CATEGORY AND SCHEDULE
Pregnancy Risk Category: A

Drug Class: Thyroid hormone

MECHANISM OF ACTION
A natural hormone derived from animal sources, usually beef or pork, that is involved in normal metabolism, growth, and development, especially the CNS of infants. Possesses catabolic and anabolic effects. Provides both levothyroxine and liothyronine hormones.
Therapeutic Effect: Increases basal metabolic rate, enhances gluconeogenesis, stimulates protein synthesis.

USES
Treatment of hypothyroidism, cretinism, myxedema

PHARMACOKINETICS
Partially absorbed from the GI tract. Protein binding: 99%. Widely distributed. Metabolized in liver to active liothyronine (T3), and inactive reverse triiodothyronine (rT3), metabolites. Eliminated by biliary excretion. *Half-life:* 2–7 days.

INDICATIONS AND DOSAGES
▶ Hypothyroidism
PO
Adults, Elderly. Initially, 15–30 mg. May increase by 15 mg increments q2–4wk. Maintenance: 60–120 mcg/day. Use 15 mg in patients with cardiovascular disease or myxedema.
Children 12 yr and older. 90 mg/day.
Children 6–12 yr. 60–90 mg/day.
Children older than 1 yr–5 yr. 45–60 mg/day.
Children older than 6–12 mo. 30–45 mg/day.
Children 3 mo and younger. 15–30 mg/day.

SIDE EFFECTS/ADVERSE REACTIONS
Rare
Dry skin, GI intolerance, skin rash, hives, severe headache

PRECAUTIONS AND CONTRAINDICATIONS
Uncontrolled adrenal cortical insufficiency, untreated thyrotoxicosis, treatment of obesity, uncontrolled angina, uncontrolled hypertension, uncontrolled MI, and hypersensitivity to any component of the formulations
Caution:
Lactation, seizure disorders, hypertension, hepatic disease

DRUG INTERACTIONS OF CONCERN TO DENTISTRY
• Increased effects of sympathomimetics when thyroid doses are not carefully monitored or with coronary artery disease

SERIOUS REACTIONS
! Excessive dosage produces signs and symptoms of hyperthyroidism including weight loss, palpitations, increased appetite, tremors, nervousness, tachycardia, hypertension, headache, insomnia, and menstrual irregularities. Cardiac arrhythmias occur rarely.

DENTAL CONSIDERATIONS
General:
• Increased nervousness, excitability, sweating, or tachycardia may indicate uncontrolled hyperthyroidism or a dose of medication that is too high. Uncontrolled patients should be referred for medical treatment.
• Use vasoconstrictors with caution and at low doses.
Consultations:
• Medical consultation may be required to assess disease control.

tiagabine
tih-ah-**ga**′-bean
(Gabitril)

CATEGORY AND SCHEDULE
Pregnancy Risk Category: C

Drug Class: Anticonvulsant

MECHANISM OF ACTION
An anticonvulsant that enhances the activity of gamma-aminobutyric acid, the major inhibitory neurotransmitter in the CNS.

Therapeutic Effect: Inhibits seizures.

USES
Adjunctive therapy for partial seizures

PHARMACOKINETICS
PO: Rapid absorption, peak plasma levels 0.5–1 hr; highly plasma protein bound (95%), hepatic metabolism (CYP 3A isoenzymes), some enterohepatic circulation

INDICATIONS AND DOSAGES
▶ **Adjunctive Treatment of Partial Seizures**
PO
Adults, Elderly. Initially, 4 mg once a day. May increase by 4–8 mg/day at weekly intervals. Maximum: 56 mg/day.
Children 12–18 yr. Initially, 4 mg once a day. May increase by 4 mg at wk 2 and by 4–8 mg at weekly intervals thereafter. Maximum: 32 mg/day.

SIDE EFFECTS/ADVERSE REACTIONS
Frequent
Dizziness, asthenia, somnolence, nervousness, confusion, headache, infection, tremor
Occasional
Nausea, diarrhea, abdominal pain, impaired concentration

PRECAUTIONS AND CONTRAINDICATIONS
Hepatic disease, Alzheimer's disease, dementia, organic brain disease, stroke

DRUG INTERACTIONS OF CONCERN TO DENTISTRY
• Increased tiagabine clearance: carbamazepine, phenobarbital

T

• Use CNS depressants with caution because of possible additional effects

SERIOUS REACTIONS
! Overdose is characterized by agitation, confusion, hostility, and weakness. Full recovery occurs within 24 hr.

DENTAL CONSIDERATIONS
General:
• Monitor vital signs at every appointment because of cardiovascular and respiratory side effects.
• Consider semisupine chair position for patient comfort when GI side effects occur.
• Short appointments and a stress reduction protocol may be required for anxious patients.
• Determine type of epilepsy, seizure frequency, and quality of seizure control.
• Assess salivary flow as factor in caries, periodontal disease, and candidiasis.
• Place on frequent recall if oral side effects occur.
Consultations:
• Consultation with physician may be necessary if sedation or general anesthesia is required.
Teach Patient/Family to:
• Use caution to prevent trauma when using oral hygiene aids.
• Use powered tooth brush if patient has difficulty holding conventional devices.
• Encourage effective oral hygiene to prevent soft tissue inflammation.
• Update health and drug history if physician makes any changes in evaluation or drug regimens; include OTC, herbal, and nonherbal drugs in the update.

• Be aware of oral side effects and potential sequelae.
• When chronic dry mouth occurs, advise patient to:
  • Avoid mouth rinses with high alcohol content because of drying effects.
  • Use daily home fluoride products for anticaries effect.
  • Use sugarless gum, frequent sips of water, or saliva substitutes.

ticarcillin
tye-kar-**sill**'-in
(Ticar)

CATEGORY AND SCHEDULE
Pregnancy Risk Category: B

Drug Class: Antibiotic, penicillin

MECHANISM OF ACTION
Binds to bacterial cell wall, inhibiting bacterial cell wall synthesis.
Therapeutic Effect: Bactericidal.

USES
Treatment of infections caused by bacteria

PHARMACOKINETICS
Well absorbed. Widely distributed. Protein binding: 45%–60%. Minimal metabolism in liver. Primarily excreted unchanged in urine. Moderately dialyzable. *Half-life:* 1.2 hr (half-life is increased in those with impaired renal function).

INDICATIONS AND DOSAGES
▶ **Septicemia; Skin and Skin-Structure, Bone, Joint, and Lower Respiratory Tract Infections; and Endometriosis**
IV

Adults, Elderly, Children over 40 kg. 200–300 mg/kg/day q4–6h or 3 g q4h or 4 g q6h. Maximum: 18 g/day.
Children and infants under 40 kg. 200–300 mg/kg/day q4–6h. Maximum: 18 g/day.
Neonates over 2000 g. 75 mg/kg IV q8h under 7 days old; 100 mg/kg IV q8h over 7 old.
Neonates under 2000 g. 75 mg/kg IV q12h under 7 days old; 75 mg/kg q8h over 7 days old.
▶ **UTI, Complicated**
IV

Adults, Elderly, Children over 40 kg. 150–200 mg/kg/day divided q4–6h or 3 g q6h.
Children under 40 kg. 150–200 mg/kg/day in divided doses q6–8h.
▶ **UTI, Uncomplicated**
IV/IM

Adults, Elderly, Children over 40 kg. 1 g q6h.
Children under 40 kg. 50–100 mg/kg/day in divided doses q6–8h.
Dosage in Renal Impairment

Creatinine Clearance	Dosage Interval
30–60 ml/min	2 g q4h
10–30 ml/min	2 g q8h
Less than 10 ml/min	2 g q12h

SIDE EFFECTS/ADVERSE REACTIONS
Frequent
Phlebitis, thrombophlebitis with IV dose, rash, urticaria, pruritus, smell or taste disturbances
Occasional
Nausea, diarrhea, vomiting

Rare
Headache, fatigue, hallucinations, bleeding or bruising

PRECAUTIONS AND CONTRAINDICATIONS
Hypersensitivity to any penicillin

DRUG INTERACTIONS OF CONCERN TO DENTISTRY
• Possible increase in bleeding: anticoagulants, thrombolytic drugs, diflunisal (high doses), platelet aggregation inhibitors
• Decreased antimicrobial effectiveness: erythromycins, sulfonamides, tetracyclines
• Possible increase in methotrexate toxicity
• Increased or prolonged plasma levels: probenecid

SERIOUS REACTIONS
❗ Overdosage may produce seizures and neurologic reactions. Superinfections including potentially fatal antibiotic-associated colitis; may result from bacterial imbalance. Severe hypersensitivity reactions, including anaphylaxis, occur rarely.

DENTAL CONSIDERATIONS
General:
• For selected infections in the hospital setting; provide emergency dental treatment only.
• Caution regarding allergy to medication.
• Examine for oral manifestation of opportunistic infection.
• Determine why patient is taking the drug.
Consultations:
• Medical consultation may be required to assess disease control.
Teach Patient/Family to:
• Encourage effective oral hygiene to prevent soft tissue inflammation.

• Report oral lesions, soreness, or bleeding to dentist.
• Prevent trauma when using oral hygiene aids.

ticarcillin disodium/ clavulanate potassium

tie-car-**sill'**-in dye-**soe'**-dee-um/ klah-view-**lan'**-ate poh-**tass'**-ee-um
(Timentin)

CATEGORY AND SCHEDULE
Pregnancy Risk Category: B

Drug Class: Antibiotics, penicillin

MECHANISM OF ACTION
Ticarcillin binds to bacterial cell walls, inhibiting cell wall synthesis. Clavulanate inhibits the action of bacterial β-lactamase.
Therapeutic Effect: Bactericidal. Clavulanate protects ticarcillin from enzymatic degradation.

USES
Treatment of infections caused by bacteria

PHARMACOKINETICS
Widely distributed. Protein binding: ticarcillin 45%–60%, clavulanate 9%–30%. Minimally metabolized in the liver. Primarily excreted unchanged in urine. Removed by hemodialysis. **Half-life:** 1–1.2 hr (increased in impaired renal function).

INDICATIONS AND DOSAGES
▶ **Skin and Skin-Structure, Bone, Joint, and Lower Respiratory Tract Infections; Septicemia; Endometriosis**
IV
Adults, Elderly. 3.1 g (3 g ticarcillin) q4–6h. Maximum: 18–24 g/day.
Children 3 mo and older. 200–300 mg (as ticarcillin) q4–6h.
▶ **UTIs**
IV
Adults, Elderly. 3.1 g q6–8h.
▶ **Dosage in Renal Impairment**
Dosage interval is modified on the basis of creatinine clearance.

Creatinine Clearance	Dosage Interval
10–30 ml/min	Usual dose q8h
Less than 10 ml/min	Usual dose q12h

SIDE EFFECTS/ADVERSE REACTIONS
Frequent
Phlebitis or thrombophlebitis (with IV dose), rash, urticaria, pruritus, altered smell or taste
Occasional
Nausea, diarrhea, vomiting
Rare
Headache, fatigue, hallucinations, bleeding, or ecchymosis

PRECAUTIONS AND CONTRAINDICATIONS
Hypersensitivity to any penicillin

DRUG INTERACTIONS OF CONCERN TO DENTISTRY
• Possible increase in bleeding: anticoagulants, thrombolytic drugs, diflunisal (high doses), platelet aggregation inhibitors

• Decreased antimicrobial effectiveness: erythromycins, sulfonamides, tetracyclines
• Possible increase in methotrexate toxicity
• Increased or prolonged plasma levels: probenecid

SERIOUS REACTIONS

! Overdosage may produce seizures and other neurologic reactions. Antibiotic-associated colitis and other superinfections may result from bacterial imbalance. Severe hypersensitivity reactions including anaphylaxis occur rarely.

DENTAL CONSIDERATIONS

General:
• For selected infections in the hospital setting; provide emergency dental treatment only.
• Caution regarding allergy to medication.
• Examine for oral manifestation of opportunistic infection.
• Determine why patient is taking the drug.

Consultations:
• Medical consultation may be required to assess disease control.

Teach Patient/Family to:
• Encourage effective oral hygiene to prevent soft tissue inflammation.
• Report oral lesions, soreness, or bleeding to dentist.
• Prevent trauma when using oral hygiene aids.

ticlopidine hydrochloride

tye-**klo**′-pa-deen
high-droh-**klor**′-ide
(Apo-Ticlopidine[CAN], Ticlid,
Tilodene[AUS])

CATEGORY AND SCHEDULE

Pregnancy Risk Category: B

Drug Class: Platelet aggregation inhibitor

MECHANISM OF ACTION

An aggregation inhibitor that inhibits the release of adenosine diphosphate from activated platelets, which prevents fibrinogen from binding to glycoprotein IIb/IIIa receptors on the surface of activated platelets.
Therapeutic Effect: Inhibits platelet aggregation and thrombus formation.

USES

Reduction of the risk of stroke in high-risk patients

PHARMACOKINETICS

Peak 1–3 hr, half-life increases with repeated dosing; metabolized by the liver; excreted in urine, feces.

INDICATIONS AND DOSAGES

▶ **Prevention of Stroke**
PO
Adults, Elderly. 250 mg twice a day.

SIDE EFFECTS/ADVERSE REACTIONS

Frequent
Diarrhea, nausea, dyspepsia including heartburn, indigestion GI discomfort, and bloating
Rare
Vomiting, flatulence, pruritus, dizziness

PRECAUTIONS AND CONTRAINDICATIONS
Active pathologic bleeding, such as bleeding peptic ulcer and intracranial bleeding, hematopoietic disorders including neutropenia and thrombocytopenia; presence of hemostatic disorder; severe hepatic impairment
Caution:
Past liver disease, renal disease, elderly, lactation, children; increased bleeding risk requires hematologic monitoring every 2 wk for the first 3 mo of therapy

DRUG INTERACTIONS OF CONCERN TO DENTISTRY
• Increased bleeding tendencies: aspirin, NSAIDs

SERIOUS REACTIONS
! Neutropenia occurs in approximately 2% of patients. Thrombotic thrombocytopenia purpura, agranulocytosis, hepatitis, cholestatic jaundice, and tinnitus occur rarely.

DENTAL CONSIDERATIONS
General:
• Patients on chronic drug therapy may rarely have symptoms of blood dyscrasias, which can include infection, bleeding, and poor healing.
• Consider local hemostatic measures to prevent excessive bleeding.
• Do not arbitrarily discontinue.
Consultations:
• Medical consultation may be required to assess disease control and patient's ability to tolerate stress. Consultation should include data on hematologic profile.
Teach Patient/Family to:
• Prevent injury when using oral hygiene aids.

tiludronate
ti-**loo**′-dro-nate
(Skelid)

CATEGORY AND SCHEDULE
Pregnancy Risk Category: C

Drug Class: Bisphosphonate derivative

MECHANISM OF ACTION
A calcium regulator that inhibits functioning osteoclasts through disruption of cytoskeletal ring structure and inhibition of osteoclastic proton pump.
Therapeutic Effect: Inhibits bone resorption.

USES
Treatment of Paget's disease of bone in patients with twice normal upper limit values for serum alkaline phosphatase (SAP) and who are symptomatic and at risk for future complications

PHARMACOKINETICS
PO: Rapid but incomplete absorption, bioavailability 6% (fasted), peak plasma levels 2 hr, little or no metabolism, excreted in urine.

INDICATIONS AND DOSAGES
▶ Paget's Disease
PO
Adults, Elderly. 400 mg once a day for 3 mo. Must take with 6–8 oz plain water. Do not give within 2 hr of food intake. Avoid giving aspirin, calcium supplements, mineral supplements, or antacids within 2 hr of tiludronate administration.

SIDE EFFECTS/ADVERSE REACTIONS

Frequent

Nausea, diarrhea, generalized body pain, back pain, headache

Occasional

Rash, dyspepsia, vomiting, rhinitis, sinusitis, dizziness

PRECAUTIONS AND CONTRAINDICATIONS

GI disease, such as dysphagia and gastric ulcer, impaired renal function

Caution:

Lactation, safety in children younger than 18 yr not established

DRUG INTERACTIONS OF CONCERN TO DENTISTRY

• Bioavailability decreased by calcium, food, aluminum or magnesium antacids.

• Do not take indomethacin, aspirin, or calcium supplements 2 hr before or after tiludronate.

SERIOUS REACTIONS

! Acute renal failure associated with hypocalcemia

DENTAL CONSIDERATIONS

General:

• Potential for osteonecrosis of the jaw (emphasize preventive care and avoid invasive procedures).

• Be aware of oral manifestations of Paget's disease (macrognathia, alveolar pain).

• Consider semisupine chair position for patient comfort when GI side effects occur.

• Consider short appointments for patient comfort.

• Assess salivary flow as a factor in caries, periodontal disease, and candidiasis.

Consultations:

• Medical consultation may be required to assess disease control.

Teach Patient/Family to:

• Use caution to prevent trauma when using oral hygiene aids.

• Encourage effective oral hygiene to prevent soft tissue inflammation.

• Update health and drug history if physician makes any changes in evaluation or drug regimens; include OTC, herbal, and nonherbal drugs in the update.

• When chronic dry mouth occurs, advise patient to:

• Avoid mouth rinses with high alcohol content because of drying effects.

• Use daily home fluoride products for anticaries effect.

• Use sugarless gum, frequent sips of water, or saliva substitutes.

timolol maleate

tim´-oh-lole **mal**´-ee-ate
(Apo-Timol[CAN], Apo-Timop[CAN], Betimol, Blocadren, Gen-Timolol[CAN], Istalol, Optimol[AUS], PMS-Timolol[CAN], Tenopt[AUS], Timoptic, Timoptic Ocudose, Timoptic XE, Timoptol[AUS], Timoptol XE[AUS])
Do not confuse timolol with atenolol, or Timoptic with Viroptic.

CATEGORY AND SCHEDULE

Pregnancy Risk Category: C (D if used in second or third trimester)

Drug Class: Nonselective β-adrenergic blocker

MECHANISM OF ACTION

An antihypertensive, antimigraine, and antiglaucoma agent that blocks β_1- and β_2-adrenergic receptors.
Therapeutic Effect: Reduces intraocular pressure (IOP) by

reducing aqueous humor production, lowers B/P, slows the heart rate, and decreases myocardial contractility.

USES

Treatment of mild-to-moderate hypertension, reduction of mortality risk after MI, migraine prophylaxis; unapproved uses: essential tremors, angina, cardiac dysrhythmias, anxiety, mild-to-moderate heart failure

PHARMACOKINETICS

Route	Onset	Peak	Duration
PO	15–45 min	0.5–2.5 hr	4 hr
Ophthalmic	30 min	1–2 hr	12–24 hr

Well absorbed from the GI tract. Protein binding: 60%. Minimal absorption after ophthalmic administration. Metabolized in the liver. Primarily excreted in urine. Not removed by hemodialysis. *Half-life:* 4 hr. Systemic absorption may occur with ophthalmic administration.

INDICATIONS AND DOSAGES
▸ **Mild-to-Moderate Hypertension**
PO
Adults, Elderly. Initially, 10 mg twice a day, alone or in combination with other therapy. Gradually increase at intervals of not less than 1 wk. Maintenance: 20–60 mg/day in 2 divided doses.
▸ **Reduction of Cardiovascular Mortality in Definite or Suspected Acute MI**
PO
Adults, Elderly. 10 mg twice a day, beginning 1–4 wk after infarction.
▸ **Migraine Prevention**
PO
Adults, Elderly. Initially, 10 mg twice a day. Range: 10–30 mg/day.

▸ **Reduction of IOP in Open-Angle Glaucoma, Aphakic Glaucoma, Ocular Hypertension, and Secondary Glaucoma**
Ophthalmic
Adults, Elderly, Children. 1 drop of 0.25% solution in affected eye(s) twice a day. May be increased to 1 drop of 0.5% solution in affected eye(s) twice a day. When IOP is controlled, dosage may be reduced to 1 drop once a day. If patient is switched to timolol from another antiglaucoma agent, administer concurrently for 1 day. Discontinue other agent on following day.
Ophthalmic (Timoptic XE)
Adults, Elderly. 1 drop/day.
Ophthalmic (Istalol)
Adults, Elderly. Apply once a day.

SIDE EFFECTS/ADVERSE REACTIONS
Frequent
Diminished sexual function, drowsiness, difficulty sleeping, unusual tiredness or weakness
Ophthalmic: Eye irritation, visual disturbances
Occasional
Depression, cold hands or feet, diarrhea, constipation, anxiety, nasal congestion, nausea, vomiting
Rare
Altered taste, dry eyes, itching, numbness of fingers, toes, or scalp

PRECAUTIONS AND CONTRAINDICATIONS
Bronchial asthma, cardiogenic shock, CHF unless secondary to tachyarrhythmias, COPD, patients receiving MAOI therapy, second- or third-degree heart block, sinus bradycardia, uncontrolled cardiac failure
Caution:
Major surgery, lactation, diabetes mellitus, renal disease, thyroid

disease, COPD, well-compensated heart failure, CAD, nonallergic bronchospasm

DRUG INTERACTIONS OF CONCERN TO DENTISTRY

• Increased hypotension, bradycardia: anticholinergics, sympathomimetics (epinephrine)
• Decreased antihypertensive effects: indomethacin and other NSAIDs
• Suspected increase in plasma levels: diphenhydramine
• May slow metabolism of lidocaine
Optic
• Avoid use of anticholinergic drugs, atropine-like drugs, propantheline, and diazepam (benzodiazepines)

SERIOUS REACTIONS

! Overdose may produce profound bradycardia, hypotension, and bronchospasm.
! Abrupt withdrawal may result in diaphoresis, palpitations, headache, and tremors.
! Timolol administration may precipitate CHF and MI in patients with cardiac disease, thyroid storm in those with thyrotoxicosis, and peripheral ischemia in those with existing peripheral vascular disease. Hypoglycemia may occur in patients with previously controlled diabetes.
! Ophthalmic overdose may produce bradycardia, hypotension, bronchospasm, and acute cardiac failure.

DENTAL CONSIDERATIONS

General:
• Potentially reduced effectiveness of epinephrine administered for anaphylaxis.
• Monitor vital signs at every appointment because of cardiovascular side effects.
• Patients on chronic drug therapy may rarely have symptoms of blood

dyscrasias, which can include infection, bleeding, and poor healing.
• Assess salivary flow as a factor in caries, periodontal disease, and candidiasis.
• Limit use of sodium-containing products, such as saline IV fluids, for patients with a dietary salt restriction.
• After supine positioning, have patient sit upright for at least 2 min before standing to avoid orthostatic hypotension.
• Stress from dental procedures may compromise cardiovascular function; determine patient risk.
• Short appointments and a stress-reduction protocol may be required for anxious patients.
• Consider semisupine chair position for patients with nausea or respiratory distress.
Consultations:
• In a patient with symptoms of blood dyscrasias, request a medical consultation for blood studies and postpone dental treatment until normal values are reestablished.
• Medical consultation may be required to assess disease control and patient's ability to tolerate stress.
Teach Patient/Family to:
• Encourage effective oral hygiene to prevent soft tissue inflammation.
• Use caution to prevent injury when using oral hygiene aids.
• When chronic dry mouth occurs, advise patient to:
  • Avoid mouth rinses with high alcohol content because of drying effects.
  • Use daily home fluoride products to prevent caries.
  • Use sugarless gum, frequent sips of water, or saliva substitutes.

T

Optic

General:
• Check compliance of patient with prescribed drug regimen for glaucoma.
• Avoid dental light in patient's eyes; offer dark glasses for patient comfort.
Consultations:
• Consultation with physician may be necessary if sedation or anesthesia is required.

tinzaparin sodium
tin-**za**′-pair-in **soe**′-dee-um
(Innohep)

CATEGORY AND SCHEDULE
Pregnancy Risk Category: B

Drug Class: Anticoagulant

MECHANISM OF ACTION
A low-molecular-weight heparin that inhibits factor Xa. Causes less inactivation of thrombin, inhibition of platelets, and bleeding than standard heparin. Does not significantly influence bleeding time, PT, aPTT.
Therapeutic Effect: Anticoagulant.

USES
Prevention and/or treatment of deep venous thrombosis (DVT), a condition in which harmful blood clots form in the blood vessels of the legs

PHARMACOKINETICS
Well absorbed after subcutaneous administration. Primarily eliminated in urine. ***Half-life:*** 3–4 hr.

INDICATIONS AND DOSAGES
▸ **DVT**
Subcutaneous

Adults, Elderly. 175 anti-Xa international units/kg once a day. Continue for at least 6 days and until patient is sufficiently anticoagulated with warfarin (INR of 2 or more for 2 consecutive days).

SIDE EFFECTS/ADVERSE REACTIONS
Frequent
Injection site reaction, such as inflammation, oozing, nodules, and skin necrosis
Rare
Nausea, asthenia, constipation, epistaxis

PRECAUTIONS AND CONTRAINDICATIONS
Active major bleeding, concurrent heparin therapy, hypersensitivity to heparin or pork products, thrombocytopenia associated with positive in vitro test for antiplatelet antibody

DRUG INTERACTIONS OF CONCERN TO DENTISTRY
• Increased risk of bleeding: drugs that interfere with coagulation or platelet function, such as NSAIDs and aspirin

SERIOUS REACTIONS
❗ Overdose may lead to bleeding complications ranging from local ecchymoses to major hemorrhage. Antidote: Dose of protamine sulfate (1% solution) should be equal to dose of tinzaparin injected. 1 mg protamine sulfate neutralizes 100 units of tinzaparin. A second dose of 0.5 mg tinzaparin per 1 mg protamine sulfate may be given if aPTT tested 2–4 hr after the initial infusion remains prolonged.

General:
• Determine why patient is taking the drug.
• Consider local hemostasis measures to prevent excessive bleeding.
• Avoid products that affect platelet function, such as aspirin and NSAIDs.
• Antibiotic prophylaxis prior to dental treatment may be required for joint prosthesis.
• Patient may need assistance in getting into and out of dental chair. Adjust chair position for patient comfort.
• Product may be used in outpatient therapy. Delay elective dental treatment until patient completes tinzaparin therapy.
Consultations:
• Medical consultation should include routine blood counts including platelet counts and bleeding time.
Teach Patient/Family to:
• Prevent trauma when using oral hygiene aids.
• Report oral lesions, soreness, or bleeding to dentist.
• Encourage effective oral hygiene to prevent soft tissue inflammation.

tioconazole
tyo-**con**′-ah-zole
(Gynecure[CAN], Monistat-1, Trosyd[CAN], Vagistat)

CATEGORY AND SCHEDULE
Pregnancy Risk Category: C

Drug Class: Antifungals, topical, dermatologics

MECHANISM OF ACTION
An imidazole derivative that inhibits synthesis of ergosterol (vital component of fungal cell formation). *Therapeutic Effect:* Fungistatic.

USES
Treatment of infections caused by a fungus or yeast

PHARMACOKINETICS
Negligible absorption from vaginal application.

INDICATIONS AND DOSAGES
▶ **Vulvovaginal Candidiasis**
Intravaginal
Adults, Elderly. 1 applicatorful just before bedtime as a single dose.

SIDE EFFECTS/ADVERSE REACTIONS
Frequent
Headache
Occasional
Burning, itching
Rare
Irritation, vaginal pain, dysuria, dryness of vaginal secretions, vulvar edema/swelling

PRECAUTIONS AND CONTRAINDICATIONS
Hypersensitivity to tioconazole or other imidazole antifungal agents

DRUG INTERACTIONS OF CONCERN TO DENTISTRY
• None reported

SERIOUS REACTIONS
! None reported

General:
• Be aware that broad-spectrum antibiotics can exacerbate vaginal candidiasis.

T

tiotropium bromide
tee-oh-**trow**′-pea-um **broe**′-mide
(Spiriva)

CATEGORY AND SCHEDULE
Pregnancy Risk Category: C

Drug Class: Anticholinergics,
bronchodilators

MECHANISM OF ACTION
An anticholinergic that binds to
recombinant human muscarinic
receptors at the smooth muscle,
resulting in long-acting bronchial
smooth-muscle relaxation.
Therapeutic Effect: Relieves
bronchospasm.

USES
Treatment of bronchospasm
(wheezing or difficulty in breathing)
that is associated with chronic
obstructive pulmonary disease
(COPD)

PHARMACOKINETICS

Route	Onset	Peak	Duration
Inhalation	N/A	N/A	24–36 hr

Binds extensively to tissue. Protein
binding: 72%. Metabolized by
oxidation. Excreted in urine.
Half-life: 5–6 days.

INDICATIONS AND DOSAGES
▶ COPD
Inhalation
Adults, Elderly. 18 mcg (1 capsule)/
day via HandiHaler inhalation
device.

SIDE EFFECTS/ADVERSE
REACTIONS
Frequent
Dry mouth, sinusitis, pharyngitis,
dyspepsia, UTI, rhinitis

Occasional
Abdominal pain, peripheral edema,
constipation, epistaxis, vomiting,
myalgia, rash, oral candidiasis

PRECAUTIONS AND
CONTRAINDICATIONS
History of hypersensitivity to
atropine or its derivatives, including
ipratropium

DRUG INTERACTIONS OF
CONCERN TO DENTISTRY
• Dental drug interactions have not
been studied.

SERIOUS REACTIONS
❗ Angina pectoris, depression, and
flu-like symptoms occur rarely.

DENTAL CONSIDERATIONS

General:
• Monitor vital signs, especially
respiration.
• Ask patient about exercise and
activity tolerance.
• Caution: Not for acute episodes or
emergency use.
• Assess salivary flow as a factor in
caries, periodontal disease, and
candidiasis.
• Place on frequent recall due to
oral side effects.
• Acute asthmatic episodes may be
precipitated in the dental office. A
rapid-acting sympathomimetic
inhalant (rescue inhaler) should be
available for emergency use. Many
patients may already have a
prescribed rescue inhaler they
normally use for acute asthmatic
events.
• Consider semisupine chair position
for patients with respiratory disease.
Consultations:
• Medical consultation may be
required to assess disease control and
patient's ability to tolerate stress.

Teach Patient/Family to:
• Gargle, rinse mouth with water, and expectorate after each aerosol dose.
• When chronic dry mouth occurs, advise patient to:
  • Avoid mouth rinses with high alcohol content due to drying effects.
  • Use daily home fluoride products for anticaries effect.
  • Use sugarless gum, frequent sips of water, or saliva substitutes.

tirofiban
tye-roe-**fye′**-ban
(Aggrastat)
Do not confuse Aggrastat with Aggrenox.

CATEGORY AND SCHEDULE
Pregnancy Risk Category: B

Drug Class: Platelet inhibitor

MECHANISM OF ACTION
An antiplatelet and antithrombotic agent that binds to platelet receptor glycoprotein IIb/IIIa, preventing binding of fibrinogen.
Therapeutic Effect: Inhibits platelet aggregation and thrombus formation.

USES
An antiplatelet in combination with heparin, treatment of acute coronary syndrome, including those to be managed medically and those undergoing percutaneous transluminal coronary angioplasty (PTCA) or atherectomy

PHARMACOKINETICS
Poorly bound to plasma proteins; unbound fraction in plasma: 35%. Limited metabolism. Primarily eliminated in the urine (65%) and, to

a lesser amount, in the feces. Removed by hemodialysis. *Half-life:* 2 hr. Clearance is significantly decreased in severe renal impairment (creatinine clearance less than 30 ml/min).

INDICATIONS AND DOSAGES
▶ **Inhibition of Platelet Aggregation**
IV
Adults, Elderly. Initially, 0.4 mcg/kg/min for 30 min; then continue at 0.1 mcg/kg/min through procedure and for 12–24 hr after procedure.
▶ **Severe Renal Insufficiency (Creatinine Clearance Less Than 30 ml/min)**
Adults, Elderly. Half the usual rate of IV infusion.

SIDE EFFECTS/ADVERSE REACTIONS
Occasional
Pelvis pain, bradycardia, dizziness, leg pain
Rare
Edema and swelling, vasovagal reaction, diaphoresis, nausea, fever, headache

PRECAUTIONS AND CONTRAINDICATIONS
Active internal bleeding or a history of bleeding diathesis within previous 30 days, arteriovenous malformation or aneurysm, history of intracranial hemorrhage, history of thrombocytopenia after prior exposure to tirofiban, intracranial neoplasm, major surgical procedure within previous 30 days, severe hypertension, stroke

DRUG INTERACTIONS OF CONCERN TO DENTISTRY
• Increased risk of bleeding: drugs that interfere with coagulation or platelet function, such as NSAIDs and aspirin

SERIOUS REACTIONS

! Signs and symptoms of overdose include generally minor mucocutaneous bleeding and bleeding at the femoral artery access site. Thrombocytopenia occurs rarely.

DENTAL CONSIDERATIONS

General:

• An acute-use drug for use in hospitals or emergency departments. If a patient should report this drug in his/her medical history, question about cardiovascular disease and drugs he or she may be taking.

• Patients are at risk for bleeding while receiving this drug; provide palliative dental care for dental emergencies only.

• Avoid products that affect platelet function, such as aspirin and NSAIDs.

Consultations:

• Medical consultation should include routine blood counts, including platelet counts and bleeding time.

• Medical consultation may be required to assess disease control and patient's ability to tolerate stress.

Teach Patient/Family:

• To inform dentist of unusual bleeding episodes following dental treatment.

tobramycin

toe-bra-**mye**′-sin
(Nebcin, Nebcin Pediatric, TOBI)

CATEGORY AND SCHEDULE

Pregnancy Risk Category: C

Drug Class: Antiinfective

MECHANISM OF ACTION

An aminoglycoside antibiotic that irreversibly binds to protein on bacterial ribosomes.
Therapeutic Effect: Interferes in protein synthesis of susceptible microorganisms.

USES

Treatment of serious bacterial infections

PHARMACOKINETICS

Rapid, complete absorption after IM administration. Protein binding: less than 30%. Widely distributed but does not cross the blood-brain barrier and is in low concentrations in CSF. Excreted unchanged in urine. Removed by hemodialysis.
Half-life: 2 hr. Half-life is increased with impaired renal function and in neonates. Half-life is decreased in cystic fibrosis, febrile, or burn patients.

INDICATIONS AND DOSAGES

▶ Skin/Skin-Structure, Bone, Joint, Respiratory Tract, Postoperative, Burn, Intraabdominal Infections; Complicated UTI; Septicemia; Meningitis

IM/IV

Adults, Elderly. 3 mg/kg/day in 3 divided doses. May use up to 5 mg/kg/day in 3 to 4 equal doses.

▶ Cystic Fibrosis

Inhalation

Adult, Elderly, Children 6 yr and older. 1 ampule (300 mg) via nebulizer twice daily (28 days on, 28 days off). Consider starting elderly patients at 3 mg/kg IV q8h.

▶ Dosage in Renal Impairment

Dosage and frequency are modified on the basis of degree of renal impairment and the serum concentration of the drug. After a loading dose of 1–2 mg/kg, the maintenance dose and frequency are based on serum creatinine levels and creatinine clearance. Dosage should be reduced to 3 mg/kg/day as soon as clinically indicated. Dosage should not exceed 5 mg/kg/day.

SIDE EFFECTS/ADVERSE REACTIONS

Occasional
IM: Pain, induration at IM injection site
IV: Phlebitis, thrombophlebitis
Rare
Hypotension, nausea, vomiting

PRECAUTIONS AND CONTRAINDICATIONS

Hypersensitivity to aminoglycosides (cross-sensitivity)

DRUG INTERACTIONS OF CONCERN TO DENTISTRY

• Increased risk of nephrotoxicity: cephalosporins, enflurane, vancomycin
• Increased neuromuscular blocking effects: neuromuscular blockers

SERIOUS REACTIONS

! Nephrotoxicity, as evidenced by increased BUN and serum creatinine and decreased creatinine clearance, may be reversible if the drug is stopped at the first sign of nephrotoxic symptoms.
! Irreversible ototoxicity, manifested as tinnitus, dizziness, ringing or roaring in ears, impaired hearing and neurotoxicity, as evidenced by headache, dizziness, lethargy, tremors, and visual disturbances, occur occasionally. The risk of irreversible neurotoxicity and ototoxicity is greater with higher dosages, prolonged therapy, or if the solution is applied directly to the mucosa.

! Superinfections, particularly with fungi, may result from bacterial imbalance with any route of administration. Anaphylaxis may occur.

DENTAL CONSIDERATIONS

General:
• For selected infections in the hospital setting; provide emergency dental treatment only.
• Caution regarding allergy to medication.
• Examine for oral manifestation of opportunistic infection.
• Determine why patient is taking the drug.
Consultations:
• Medical consultation may be required to assess disease control in the patient.
Teach Patient/Family to:
• Encourage effective oral hygiene to prevent soft tissue inflammation.
• Report oral lesions, soreness, or bleeding to dentist.
• Prevent trauma when using oral hygiene aids.

tobramycin sulfate
tow-bra-**my**′-sin **sull**′-fate
(AK-Tob, Apo-Tobramycin[CAN], Nebcin, PMS-Tobramycin, TOBI, Tobrex)

CATEGORY AND SCHEDULE

Pregnancy Risk Category: C (B, ophthalmic form)

Drug Class: Antiinfective

MECHANISM OF ACTION

An aminoglycoside antibiotic that irreversibly binds to protein on bacterial ribosomes.

Therapeutic Effect: Interferes with protein synthesis of susceptible microorganisms.

USES
Treatment of serious bacterial infections

PHARMACOKINETICS
Rapid, complete absorption after IM administration. Protein binding: less than 30%. Widely distributed (doesn't cross the blood-brain barrier; low concentrations in CSF). Excreted unchanged in urine. Removed by hemodialysis. ***Half-life:*** 2–4 hr (increased in impaired renal function and neonates; decreased in cystic fibrosis and febrile or burn patients).

INDICATIONS AND DOSAGES
▶ **Skin and Skin-Structure, Bone, Joint, Respiratory Tract, Postoperative, Intraabdominal, and Burn Wound Infections; Complicated UTIs; Septicemia; Meningitis**
IV, IM
Adults, Elderly. 3–6 mg/kg/day in 3 divided doses or 4–6.6 mg/kg once a day.
▶ **Superficial Eye Infections Including Blepharitis, Conjunctivitis, Keratitis, and Corneal Ulcers**
Ophthalmic Ointment
Adults, Elderly. Usual dosage, apply a thin strip to conjunctiva q8–12h (q3–4h for severe infections).
Ophthalmic Solution
Adults, Elderly. Usual dosage, 1–2 drops in affected eye q4h (2 drops/hr for severe infections).
▶ **Bronchopulmonary Infections in Patients with Cystic Fibrosis**
Inhalation Solution
Adults. Usual dosage, 60–80 mg twice a day for 28 days, then off for 28 days.

Children. 40–80 mg 2–3 times a day.
▶ **Dosage in Renal Impairment**
Dosage and frequency are modified on the basis of the degree of renal impairment and the serum drug concentration. After a loading dose of 1–2 mg/kg, the maintenance dose and frequency are based on serum creatinine levels and creatinine clearance.

SIDE EFFECTS/ADVERSE REACTIONS
Occasional
IM: Pain, induration
IV: Phlebitis, thrombophlebitis
Topical: Hypersensitivity reaction (fever, pruritus, rash, urticaria)
Ophthalmic: Tearing, itching, redness, eyelid swelling
Rare
Hypotension, nausea, vomiting

PRECAUTIONS AND CONTRAINDICATIONS
Hypersensitivity to tobramycin, other aminoglycosides (cross-sensitivity), and their components

DRUG INTERACTIONS OF CONCERN TO DENTISTRY
• Antibiotics: potentially reduced effectiveness

SERIOUS REACTIONS
! Nephrotoxicity (as evidenced by increased BUN and serum creatinine levels and decreased creatinine clearance) may be reversible if the drug is stopped at the first sign of nephrotoxic symptoms. Irreversible ototoxicity (manifested as tinnitus, dizziness, ringing or roaring in ears, and hearing loss) and neurotoxicity (manifested as headache, dizziness, lethargy, tremor, and visual disturbances) occur occasionally. The risk of these reactions increases

with higher dosages or prolonged therapy and when the solution is applied directly to the mucosa. Superinfections, particularly fungal infections, may result from bacterial imbalance with any administration route.

! Anaphylaxis may occur.

DENTAL CONSIDERATIONS

General:
• Avoid directing dental light into patient's eyes; provide dark glasses during treatment to avoid irritation.
• Protect patient's eyes from accidental spatter during dental treatment.

tocainide hydrochloride
toe'-kay-nide high-droh-**klor'**-ide
(Tonocard)

CATEGORY AND SCHEDULE
Pregnancy Risk Category: C

Drug Class: Antidysrhythmic (class IB), lidocaine analog

MECHANISM OF ACTION
An amide-type local anesthetic that shortens the action potential duration and decreases the effective refractory period and automaticity in the His-Purkinje system of the myocardium by blocking sodium transport across myocardial cell membranes.
Therapeutic Effect: Suppresses ventricular dysrhythmias.

USES
Treatment of documented life-threatening ventricular dysrhythmias

PHARMACOKINETICS
PO: Peak 0.5–3 hr. *Half-life:* 10–17 hr; metabolized by liver; excreted in urine.

INDICATIONS AND DOSAGES
▸ **Suppression and Prevention of Ventricular Arrhythmias**
PO
Adults, Elderly. Initially, 400 mg q8h. Maintenance: 1.2–1.8 g/day in divided doses q8h. Maximum: 2400 mg/day.

SIDE EFFECTS/ADVERSE REACTIONS
Tocainide is generally well tolerated.
Frequent
Minor, transient light-headedness, dizziness, nausea, paraesthesia, rash, tremor
Occasional
Clammy skin, night sweats, myalgia
Rare
Restlessness, nervousness, disorientation, mood changes, ataxia (muscular incoordination), visual disturbances

PRECAUTIONS AND CONTRAINDICATIONS
Hypersensitivity to local anesthetics, second- or third-degree AV block
Caution:
Lactation, children, renal disease, liver disease, CHF, respiratory depression, myasthenia gravis, blood dyscrasias

DRUG INTERACTIONS OF CONCERN TO DENTISTRY
• No specific interactions are reported with dental drugs; however, any drug that could affect the cardiac action of tocainide (local anesthetics, vasoconstrictors, and anticholinergics) should be used in the least effective dose.

T

SERIOUS REACTIONS

! High dosage may produce bradycardia or tachycardia, hypotension, palpitations, increased ventricular arrhythmias, premature ventricular contractions (PVCs), chest pain, and exacerbation of CHF.

DENTAL CONSIDERATIONS

General:
• Monitor vital signs at every appointment because of cardiovascular and respiratory side effects.
• After supine positioning, have patient sit upright for at least 2 min before standing to avoid orthostatic hypotension.
• Patients on chronic drug therapy may rarely have symptoms of blood dyscrasias, which can include infection, bleeding, and poor healing.
• Assess salivary flow as a factor in caries, periodontal disease, and candidiasis.
• Stress from dental procedures may compromise cardiovascular function; determine patient risk.
Consultations:
• In a patient with symptoms of blood dyscrasias, request a medical consultation for blood studies and postpone dental treatment until normal values are reestablished.
• Medical consultation may be required to assess disease control and patient's ability to tolerate stress.
Teach Patient/Family to:
• Encourage effective oral hygiene to prevent soft tissue inflammation.
• Use caution to prevent injury when using oral hygiene aids.
• When chronic dry mouth occurs, advise patient to:
  • Avoid mouth rinses with high alcohol content because of drying effects.

• Use daily home fluoride products to prevent caries.
• Use sugarless gum, frequent sips of water, or saliva substitutes.

tolazamide

tole-**az**´-ah-mide
(Tolinase)
Do not confuse with tolbutamide, tocainide, or tolazine.

CATEGORY AND SCHEDULE

Pregnancy Risk Category: D

Drug Class: Sulfonylurea (first-generation) oral antidiabetic

MECHANISM OF ACTION

A first-generation sulfonylurea that promotes release of insulin from beta cells of pancreas.
Therapeutic Effect: Lowers blood glucose concentration.

USES

Treatment of Type 2 diabetes mellitus

PHARMACOKINETICS

Well absorbed from the GI tract. Extensively metabolized in liver to five metabolites, three of which are active. Primarily excreted in urine. Unknown if removed by hemodialysis. *Half-life:* 7 hr.

INDICATIONS AND DOSAGES
▸ Diabetes Mellitus
PO
Adults, Elderly. Initially, 100–250 mg once a day, with breakfast or first main meal. Maintenance: 100–1000 mg once a day. May increase by increments of

100–250 mg weekly on the basis of blood glucose response. May increase by 100–250 mg/day at weekly intervals. Maximum: 1000 mg/day. Doses more than 500 mg/day should be given in 2 divided doses with meals.

SIDE EFFECTS/ADVERSE REACTIONS

Frequent
Altered taste sensation, dizziness, drowsiness, weight gain, constipation, diarrhea, heartburn, nausea, vomiting, stomach fullness, headache

Occasional
Increased sensitivity of skin to sunlight, peeling of skin, itching, rash

PRECAUTIONS AND CONTRAINDICATIONS

Diabetic complications, such as ketosis, acidosis, and diabetic coma, sole therapy for Type 1 diabetes mellitus, hypersensitivity to tolazamide or its components

Caution:
Elderly, cardiac disease, thyroid disease, severe hypoglycemic reactions, renal disease, hepatic disease

DRUG INTERACTIONS OF CONCERN TO DENTISTRY

• Increased hypoglycemic reaction: NSAIDs, salicylates, ketoconazole, miconazole
• Decreased action of tolazamide: corticosteroids, sympathomimetics (epinephrine)

SERIOUS REACTIONS

❗ Severe hypoglycemia may occur due to overdosage and insufficient food intake, especially with increased glucose demands.
❗ GI hemorrhage, cholestatic hepatic jaundice, leukopenia, thrombocytopenia, pancytopenia, agranulocytosis, and aplastic or hemolytic anemia occur rarely.

DENTAL CONSIDERATIONS

General:
• Patients on chronic drug therapy may rarely have symptoms of blood dyscrasias, which can include infection, bleeding, and poor healing.
• Place on frequent recall to evaluate healing response.
• Short appointments and a stress-reduction protocol may be required for anxious patients.
• Diabetics may be more susceptible to infection and have delayed wound healing.
• Anticipate possible hypoglycemic episodes.
• Ensure that patient is following prescribed diet and regularly takes medication.
• Question patient about self-monitoring of drug's antidiabetic effect.
• Avoid prescribing aspirin-containing products.

Consultations:
• In a patient with symptoms of blood dyscrasias, request a medical consultation for blood studies and postpone dental treatment until normal values are reestablished.
• Medical consultation may be required to assess disease control.

Teach Patient/Family to:
• Encourage effective oral hygiene to prevent soft tissue inflammation.
• Avoid mouth rinses with high alcohol content because of drying effects.

T

tolbutamide

tole-**byoo'**-ta-mide
(Apo-Tolbutamide[CAN], Orinase,
Orinase Diagnostic,
Rastinon[AUS], Tol-Tab)
Do not confuse with tolazamide,
tocainide, or tolazine.

CATEGORY AND SCHEDULE

Pregnancy Risk Category: C

Drug Class: Sulfonylurea
(first-generation) oral antidiabetic

MECHANISM OF ACTION

A first-generation sulfonylurea that
promotes the release of insulin from
β cells of pancreas.
Therapeutic Effect: Lowers blood
glucose concentration.

USES

Treatment of Type 2 diabetes
mellitus

PHARMACOKINETICS

Route	Onset	Peak	Duration
PO	1 hr	5–8 hr	12–24 hr
IV	N/A	30–45 min	90–180 min

Well absorbed from the GI tract.
Protein binding: 80%–99%.
Extensively metabolized in liver to
two inactive metabolites, primarily
via oxidation. Excreted in urine.
Removed by hemodialysis. **Half-life:**
4.5–6.5 hr.

INDICATIONS AND DOSAGES
▶ Diabetes Mellitus
PO
Adults. Initially, 1 g daily, with
breakfast or first main meal, or in
divided doses. Maintenance:
0.25–3 g once a day. After dose of

2 g is reached, dosage should be
increased in increments of up to
2 mg q1–2wk, based on blood
glucose response. Maximum: 3 g/
day.
▶ Endocrine Tumor Diagnosis
IV
Adults. 1 g infused over 2–3 min.

SIDE EFFECTS/ADVERSE REACTIONS
Frequent
Increased sensitivity of skin to
sunlight, peeling of skin, itching,
rash, dizziness, drowsiness, weight
gain, constipation, diarrhea,
heartburn, nausea, headache, pain at
injection site, oral lichenoid reaction
Occasional
Altered taste sensation, constipation,
vomiting, stomach fullness

PRECAUTIONS AND CONTRAINDICATIONS
Diabetic ketoacidosis with or
without coma, sole therapy for Type
1 diabetes mellitus, use in children,
hypersensitivity to tolbutamide or
any component of its formulation
Caution:
Elderly, cardiac disease, thyroid
disease, severe hypoglycemic
reactions, renal disease, hepatic
disease

DRUG INTERACTIONS OF CONCERN TO DENTISTRY
• Increased hypoglycemic reactions:
NSAIDs, salicylates, ketoconazole,
miconazole
• Decreased effects: corticosteroids,
sympathomimetics

SERIOUS REACTIONS
! Severe hypoglycemia may occur
because of overdosage or insufficient
food intake, especially with
increased glucose demands.
Cardiovascular mortality has been

reported higher in patients treated with tolbutamide. GI hemorrhage, cholestatic hepatic jaundice, leukopenia, thrombocytopenia, pancytopenia, agranulocytosis, and aplastic or hemolytic anemia occur rarely.

DENTAL CONSIDERATIONS

General:
• Patients on chronic drug therapy may rarely have symptoms of blood dyscrasias, which can include infection, bleeding, and poor healing.
• Ensure that patient is following prescribed diet and regularly takes medication.
• Question patient about self-monitoring of drug's antidiabetic effect including blood glucose values or finger-stick records.
• Anticipate possible hypoglycemic episodes.
• Place on frequent recall to evaluate healing response.
• Short appointments and a stress-reduction protocol may be required for anxious patients.
• Diabetics may be more susceptible to infection and have delayed wound healing.
• Avoid prescribing aspirin-containing products.
Consultations:
• In a patient with symptoms of blood dyscrasias, request a medical consultation for blood studies and postpone dental treatment until normal values are reestablished.
• Medical consultation may be required to assess disease control.
• Medical consultation may include data from patient's blood glucose monitoring including glycosylated hemoglobin or HbA$_{1c}$ testing.
Teach Patient/Family to:
• Encourage effective oral hygiene to prevent soft tissue inflammation.

• Avoid mouth rinses with high alcohol content because of drying effects.

tolcapone
toll′-ka-pone
(Tasmar)

CATEGORY AND SCHEDULE
Pregnancy Risk Category: C

Drug Class: Antiparkinsonian

MECHANISM OF ACTION
An antiparkinson agent that inhibits the enzyme catechol-O-methyltransferase (COMT), potentiating dopamine activity and increasing the duration of action of levodopa.
Therapeutic Effect: Relieves signs and symptoms of Parkinson's disease.

USES
An adjunct to levodopa and carbidopa in the treatment of Parkinson's disease

PHARMACOKINETICS
Rapidly absorbed after PO administration. Protein binding: 99%. Metabolized in the liver. Eliminated primarily in urine (60%) and, to a lesser extent, in feces (40%). Unknown if removed by hemodialysis. *Half-life:* 2–3 hr.

INDICATIONS AND DOSAGES
▸ Adjunctive Treatment of Parkinson's Disease
PO
Adults, Elderly. Initially, 100–200 mg 3 times a day concomitantly with each dose of carbidopa and levodopa. Maximum: 600 mg/day.

▶ **Dosage in Hepatic Impairment**
Patients with moderate to severe cirrhosis should not receive more than 200 mg tolcapone 3 times a day.

SIDE EFFECTS/ADVERSE REACTIONS
Alert
Frequency of side effects increases with dosage. The following effects are based on a 200-mg dose.
Frequent
Nausea, insomnia, somnolence, anorexia, diarrhea, muscle cramps, orthostatic hypotension, excessive dreaming, dry mouth
Occasional
Headache, vomiting, confusion, hallucinations, constipation, diaphoresis, bright yellow urine, dry eyes, abdominal pain, dizziness, flatulence
Rare
Dyspepsia, neck pain, hypotension, fatigue, chest discomfort

PRECAUTIONS AND CONTRAINDICATIONS
Hypersensitivity, patients with SGPT/ALT and SGOT/AST exceeding upper limit of normal or other signs of hepatic impairment; informed consent required; history of nontraumatic rhabdomyolysis, hyperpyrexia, and confusion related to medication
Caution:
Discontinue drug with signs of hepatocellular injury, MAOIs, hypotension, dyskinesia, lactation

DRUG INTERACTIONS OF CONCERN TO DENTISTRY
• Increased sedation: alcohol and all CNS depressants
• No other data for dental drugs reported

SERIOUS REACTIONS
! Upper respiratory tract infection and UTI occur in 5%–7% of patients. Too-rapid withdrawal from therapy may produce withdrawal-emergent hyperpyrexia, characterized by fever, muscular rigidity, and altered LOC. Dyskinesia and dystonia occur frequently.

DENTAL CONSIDERATIONS
General:
• Notify physician immediately if symptoms of liver failure are observed (bleeding, jaundice, etc.).
• Assess salivary flow as a factor in caries, periodontal disease, and candidiasis.
• After supine positioning, have patient sit upright for at least 2 min before standing to avoid orthostatic hypotension.
• Consider semisupine chair position for patient comfort because of GI side effects of drug.
Consultations:
• Medical consultation may be required to assess disease control.
• Take precaution if dental surgery is anticipated and general anesthesia is required.
Teach Patient/Family to:
• Use powered tooth brush if patient has difficulty holding conventional devices.
• When chronic dry mouth occurs, advise patient to:
  • Avoid mouth rinses with high alcohol content because of drying effects.
  • Use daily home fluoride products for anticaries effect.
  • Use sugarless gum, frequent sips of water, or saliva substitutes.

tolmetin
tole′-met-in
(Novo-Tolmetin[CAN], Tolectin,
Tolectin DS)

CATEGORY AND SCHEDULE
Pregnancy Risk Category: C (D if
used in third trimester or near
delivery)

Drug Class: Nonsteroidal
antiinflammatory

MECHANISM OF ACTION
A nonsteroidal antiinflammatory that
produces analgesic and
antiinflammatory effects by
inhibiting prostaglandin synthesis.
Therapeutic Effect: Reduces
inflammatory response and intensity
of pain stimulus reaching sensory
nerve endings.

USES
Treatment of osteoarthritis,
rheumatoid arthritis, juvenile
rheumatoid arthritis

PHARMACOKINETICS
Rapidly absorbed from the GI tract.
Metabolized in liver. Excreted in
urine. Minimally removed by
hemodialysis. *Half-life:* 5 hr.

INDICATIONS AND DOSAGES
▶ **Rheumatoid Arthritis,
Osteoarthritis**
PO
Adults, Elderly. Initially, 400 mg 3
times a day (including 1 dose upon
arising, 1 dose at bedtime). Adjust
dose at 1- to 2-wk intervals.
Maintenance: 600–1800 mg/day in
3–4 divided doses.
▶ **Juvenile Rheumatoid Arthritis**
PO
Children more than 2 yr. Initially,
20 mg/kg/day in 3–4 divided doses.

Maintenance: 15–30 mg/kg/day in
3–4 divided doses.

SIDE EFFECTS/ADVERSE
REACTIONS
Occasional
Nausea, vomiting, diarrhea,
abdominal cramping, dyspepsia
(heartburn, indigestion, epigastric
pain), flatulence, dizziness,
headache, weight decrease or
increase
Rare
Constipation, anorexia, rash, pruritus

PRECAUTIONS AND
CONTRAINDICATIONS
Severely incapacitated, bedridden,
wheelchair bound, hypersensitivity
to aspirin or other NSAIDs
Caution:
Lactation, children, bleeding
disorders, GI disorders, cardiac
disorders, hypersensitivity to aspirin,
NSAIDs, peptic ulcer disease,
geriatric patients

DRUG INTERACTIONS OF
CONCERN TO DENTISTRY
• Increased risk of GI side effects:
ASA, NSAIDs, ethanol (alcohol)
• Nephrotoxicity: acetaminophen
(prolonged use and high doses)
• Possible risk of decreased renal
function: cyclosporine
• Decreased antihypertensive effect
of diuretics, α-adrenergic blockers,
and ACE inhibitors
• SSRIs: increased risk of GI side
effects

SERIOUS REACTIONS
! Peptic ulcer, GI bleeding, gastritis,
and severe hepatic reaction
(cholestasis, jaundice) occur rarely.
Nephrotoxicity (dysuria, hematuria,
proteinuria, nephrotic syndrome)
and severe hypersensitivity reaction

T

(fever, chills, bronchospasm) occur rarely.

DENTAL CONSIDERATIONS

General:
- Patients on chronic drug therapy may rarely have symptoms of blood dyscrasias, which can include infection, bleeding, and poor healing.
- Monitor vital signs at every appointment because of cardiovascular side effects.
- Assess salivary flow as a factor in caries, periodontal disease, and candidiasis.
- Avoid prescribing in last trimester of pregnancy.
- Possibility of cross-allergenicity when patient is allergic to aspirin.

Consultations:
- Medical consultation may be required to assess disease control.
- In a patient with symptoms of blood dyscrasias, request a medical consultation for blood studies and postpone dental treatment until normal values are reestablished.

Teach Patient/Family to:
- Encourage effective oral hygiene to prevent soft tissue inflammation.
- Use caution to prevent injury when using oral hygiene aids.
- When chronic dry mouth occurs, advise patient to:
  - Avoid mouth rinses with high alcohol content because of drying effects.
  - Use daily home fluoride products to prevent caries.
  - Use sugarless gum, frequent sips of water, or saliva substitutes.

tolterodine tartrate
tol-**tare**'-oh-deen **tar**'-trate
(Detrol, Detrol LA)

CATEGORY AND SCHEDULE
Pregnancy Risk Category: C

Drug Class: Antispasmodic

MECHANISM OF ACTION
An antispasmodic that exhibits potent antimuscarinic activity by interceding via cholinergic muscarinic receptors, thereby inhibiting urinary bladder contraction.
Therapeutic Effect: Decreases urinary frequency, urgency.

USES
Treatment of overactive bladder with symptoms of urinary frequency or incontinence

PHARMACOKINETICS
Rapidly and well absorbed after PO administration. Protein binding: 96%. Extensively metabolized in the liver to active metabolite. Primarily excreted in urine. Unknown if removed by hemodialysis. **Half-life:** 1.9–3.7 hr.

INDICATIONS AND DOSAGES
▸ **Overactive Bladder**
PO
Adults, Elderly. 1–2 mg twice a day.
▸ **Dosage in Severe Renal or Hepatic Impairment**
PO
Adults, Elderly. 1 mg twice a day.
PO (Extended-Release)
Adults, Elderly. 2–4 mg once a day.

SIDE EFFECTS/ADVERSE REACTIONS

Frequent
Dry mouth
Occasional
Headache, dizziness, fatigue, constipation, dyspepsia (heartburn, indigestion, epigastric discomfort), upper respiratory tract infection, UTI, dry eyes, abnormal vision (accommodation problems), nausea, diarrhea
Rare
Somnolence, chest or back pain, arthralgia, rash, weight gain, dry skin

PRECAUTIONS AND CONTRAINDICATIONS

Uncontrolled angle-closure glaucoma, urine retention
Caution:
Bladder obstruction, pyloric stenosis, GI obstructive disorders, treated narrow-angle glaucoma, significant hepatic dysfunction, renal impairment, lactation, pediatric use

DRUG INTERACTIONS OF CONCERN TO DENTISTRY

• Studies not available; however, drugs that inhibit cytochrome P-450 3A4 enzymes, such as erythromycin, clarithromycin, ketoconazole, itraconazole, and fluoxetine, require a dose reduction to 1 mg twice daily
• Increased anticholinergic effects: possibly with other anticholinergic drugs

SERIOUS REACTIONS

! Overdose can result in severe anticholinergic effects including abdominal cramps, facial warmth, excessive salivation or lacrimation, diaphoresis, pallor, urinary urgency, blurred vision, and prolonged QT interval.

DENTAL CONSIDERATIONS

General:
• Assess salivary flow as a factor in caries, periodontal disease, and candidiasis.
• Consider semisupine chair position for patient comfort because of GI side effects of drug.
• Avoid dental light in patient's eyes; offer dark glasses for patient comfort.
• Avoid drugs with anticholinergic activity, such as antihistamines, opioids, benzodiazepines, propantheline, atropine, and scopolamine.
Consultations:
• Physician should be informed if significant xerostomic side effects occur (e.g., increased caries, sore tongue, problems eating or swallowing, difficulty wearing prosthesis) so that a medication change can be considered.
Teach Patient/Family to:
• Encourage effective oral hygiene to prevent soft tissue inflammation.
• When chronic dry mouth occurs, advise patient to:
  • Avoid mouth rinses with high alcohol content because of drying effects.
  • Use daily home fluoride products for anticaries effect.
  • Use sugarless gum, frequent sips of water, or saliva substitutes.

T

tolvaptan
tol-**vap**′-tan
(Samsca)

CATEGORY AND SCHEDULE
Pregnancy Risk Category: C

Drug Class: Vasopressin receptor antagonist

MECHANISM OF ACTION

A non-peptide vasopressin V(2)-receptor antagonist that blocks the effect of vasopressin. *Therapeutic Effect:* Increases urine water excretion; results in aquaresis (free water clearance), decrease in urine osmolality, increase in serum sodium concentrations.

USES

Hyponatremia (serum sodium <125 mEq/L or less marked hyponatremia that is symptomatic and resistant to fluid restriction)

PHARMACOKINETICS

Well absorbed after PO administration. Bioavailability: ~40%. Protein binding: 99%. Metabolized in liver, primarily by CYP3A; substrate and inhibitor of P-glycoprotein. Eliminated via nonrenal routes. *Half-life:* 12 hr.

INDICATIONS AND DOSAGES

▸ **Hyponatremia**

PO

Adults. 15 mg a day, without regard to meals. Increase dose to 30 mg a day, after at least 24 hr, to a maximum of 60 mg a day, as needed to achieve the desired level of serum sodium.

SIDE EFFECTS/ADVERSE REACTIONS

Frequent

Nausea, xerostomia, pollakiuria or polyuria, thirst

Occasional

Asthenia, constipation, anorexia, hyperglycemia, pyrexia, dehydration

Rare

Deep vein thrombosis, disseminated intravascular coagulation, intracardiac thrombus, ventricular fibrillation, respiratory failure, cerebrovascular accident, ischemic colitis, vaginal hemorrhage, diabetic ketoacidosis, rhabdomyolysis, pulmonary embolism, prolonged prothrombin time, urethral hemorrhage

PRECAUTIONS AND CONTRAINDICATIONS

Hypersensitivity to tolvaptan or its components

Alcoholism—Black Box Warning

Malnutrition—Black Box Warning

Hepatic disease—Black Box Warning

Anuria

Urgent need to raise serum sodium acutely

Inability of the patient to sense or appropriately respond to thirst

Hypovolemic hyponatremia

Concurrent use with strong CYP3A inhibitors (e.g., atazanavir, ritonavir, nelfinavir, indinavir, saquinavir, itraconazole, ketoconazole, clarithromycin, telithromycin, nefazodone)

Caution:

Renal or hepatic impairment

Chronic alcoholics, SIADH (increase risk for overly rapid correction of hyponatremia)

DRUG INTERACTIONS OF CONCERN TO DENTISTRY

• CYP3A inducers: May reduce the effectiveness of tolvaptan

• CYP3A inhibitors: May increase tolvaptan concentrations; avoid use with strong CYP3A inhibitors

• Drugs that increase potassium: May increase the risk of hyperkalemia

• Hypertonic solutions: not recommended

• P-glycoprotein inhibitors: May increase tolvaptan exposure; consider dose reduction

SERIOUS REACTIONS

! Dehydration and hypovolemia can occur, especially in potentially volume-depleted patients receiving diuretic or those on fluid restrictions.
! Rapid correction of hyponatremia may cause osmotic demyelination resulting in dysarthria, mutism, dysphagia, lethargy, affective changes, spastic quadriparesis, seizures, coma, and death.

DENTAL CONSIDERATIONS

General:
• Monitor vital signs at every appointment.
• Patients taking this medication are treated on an inpatient basis.
• Assess salivary flow as a factor in caries, periodontal disease, and candidiasis.
Consultations:
• Consult physician to determine disease control and ability of patient to tolerate dental procedures, if needed while receiving drug.
Teach Patient/Family to:
• Report signs and symptoms of dry mouth.

topiramate
toe-**peer**′-ah-mate
(Topamax)
Do not confuse topiramate or Topamax with Toprol XL.

CATEGORY AND SCHEDULE
Pregnancy Risk Category: C

Drug Class: Anticonvulsant

MECHANISM OF ACTION
An anticonvulsant that blocks repetitive, sustained firing of neurons by enhancing the ability of gamma-aminobutyric acid to induce an influx of chloride ions into the neurons; may also block sodium channels.
Therapeutic Effect: Decreases seizure activity.

USES
Adjunctive therapy for adult patients with partial-onset seizures or for primary generalized tonic-clonic seizures; Lennox-Gastaut syndrome

PHARMACOKINETICS
Rapidly absorbed after PO administration. Protein binding: 13%–17%. Not extensively metabolized. Primarily excreted unchanged in urine. Removed by hemodialysis. **Half-life:** 21 hr.

INDICATIONS AND DOSAGES
▶ **Adjunctive Treatment of Partial Seizures, Lennox-Gestant Syndrome**
PO
Adults, Elderly, Children older than 17 yr. Initially, 25–50 mg for 1 wk. May increase by 25–50 mg/day at weekly intervals. Maximum: 1600 mg/day.
Children 2–16 yr. Initially, 1–3 mg/kg/day to maximum of 25 mg. May increase by 1–3 mg/kg/day at weekly intervals. Maintenance: 5–9 mg/kg/day in 2 divided doses.
▶ **Tonic-Clonic Seizures**
PO
Adults, Elderly, Children. Dosage is individualized and titrated.
▶ **Migraine Prevention**
PO
Adults, Elderly. 100 mg/day in 2 divided doses.
▶ **Dosage in Renal Impairment**
Expect to reduce drug dosage by 50% in patients with tonic-clonic seizures who have a creatinine clearance of less than 70 ml/min.

SIDE EFFECTS/ADVERSE REACTIONS

Frequent

Somnolence, dizziness, ataxia, nervousness, nystagmus, diplopia, paresthesia, nausea, tremor

Occasional

Confusion, breast pain, dysmenorrhea, dyspepsia, depression, asthenia, pharyngitis, weight loss, anorexia, rash, musculoskeletal pain, abdominal pain, difficulty with coordination, sinusitis, agitation, flu-like symptoms

Rare

Mood disturbances, such as irritability and depression; dry mouth; aggressive behavior

PRECAUTIONS AND CONTRAINDICATIONS

Renal impairment, hepatic impairment, rapid drug withdrawal, kidney stones, lactation, children

Caution:

Renal impairment, hepatic impairment, rapid drug withdrawal, kidney stones, lactation, children

DRUG INTERACTIONS OF CONCERN TO DENTISTRY

• Increased CNS depression: opioids, sedatives, ethanol, and other CNS depressants

• Decreased serum levels: carbamazepine

SERIOUS REACTIONS

! Psychomotor slowing, impaired concentration, language problems (such as word-finding difficulties), and memory disturbances occur occasionally. These reactions are generally mild to moderate but may be severe enough to require discontinuation of drug therapy.

DENTAL CONSIDERATIONS

General:

• Patients on chronic drug therapy may rarely have symptoms of blood dyscrasias, which can include infection, bleeding, and poor healing.

• Short appointments and a stress-reduction protocol may be required for anxious patients.

• Assess salivary flow as factor in caries, periodontal disease, and candidiasis.

• Avoid dental light in patient's eyes; offer dark glasses for patient comfort.

• Determine type of epilepsy, seizure frequency, and quality of seizure control. A stress reduction protocol may be required.

Consultations:

• In a patient with symptoms of blood dyscrasias, request a medical consultation for blood studies and postpone dental treatment until normal values are reestablished.

• Medical consultation may be required to assess disease control.

Teach Patient/Family to:

• Encourage effective oral hygiene to prevent soft tissue inflammation.

• Use caution to prevent trauma when using oral hygiene aids.

• Use powered tooth brush if patient has difficulty holding conventional devices.

• Update health and drug history if physician makes any changes in evaluation or drug regimens; include OTC, herbal, and nonherbal drugs in the update.

• When chronic dry mouth occurs, advise patient to:

• Avoid mouth rinses with high alcohol content because of drying effects.

• Use daily home fluoride products for anticaries effect.

• Use sugarless gum, frequent sips of water, or saliva substitutes.

topotecan
toe-**poh**´-teh-can
(Hycamtin)

CATEGORY AND SCHEDULE
Pregnancy Risk Category: D

Drug Class: Antineoplastic

MECHANISM OF ACTION
A DNA topoisomerase inhibitor that interacts with topoisomerase I, an enzyme that allows DNA replication by producing reversible single-strand breaks in DNA that relieve torsional strain. Topotecan prevents relegation of the DNA strand, resulting in damage to double-strand DNA and cell death.
Therapeutic Effect: Kills cancer cells.

USES
Treatment of breast cancer that has spread to other parts of the body

PHARMACOKINETICS
Hydrolyzed to active form after IV administration. Protein binding: 35%. Excreted in urine. *Half-life:* 2–3 hr (increased in impaired renal function).

INDICATIONS AND DOSAGES
▸ **Ovarian Carcinoma, Small-Cell Lung Cancer**
IV
Adults, Elderly. 1.5 mg/m²/day over 30 min for 5 consecutive days, beginning on day 1 of a 21-day course. Minimum of 4 courses recommended. If severe neutropenia (neutrophil count less than 1500/ mm²) occurs during treatment, reduce dose for subsequent courses by 0.25 mg/m² or administer filgrastim (G-CSF) no sooner than 24 hr after the last dose of topotecan.
▸ **Dosage in Renal Impairment**
No dosage adjustment is necessary in patients with mild renal impairment (creatinine clearance of 40–60 ml/min). For moderate renal impairment (creatinine clearance of 20–39 ml/min), give 0.75 mg/m².

SIDE EFFECTS/ADVERSE REACTIONS
Frequent
Nausea, vomiting, diarrhea, total alopecia, headache, dyspnea
Occasional
Paraesthesia, constipation, abdominal pain
Rare
Anorexia, malaise, arthralgia, asthenia, myalgia

PRECAUTIONS AND CONTRAINDICATIONS
Baseline neutrophil count less than 1500 cells/mm³, breast-feeding, pregnancy, severe myelosuppression

DRUG INTERACTIONS OF CONCERN TO DENTISTRY
• None reported

SERIOUS REACTIONS
! Severe neutropenia (neutrophil count less than 500 cells/mm³) occurs in 60% of patients, usually during the first course of therapy. The neutrophil nadir usually occurs at a median of 11 days after starting therapy. Thrombocytopenia (platelet count less than 25,000/mm³) occurs in 26% of patients, and severe anemia (RBC count less than 8 g/dl) occurs in 40% of patients. The platelet and RBC nadirs usually occur at a median of 15 days after starting the first course of therapy.

T

DENTAL CONSIDERATIONS

General:
• If additional analgesia is required for dental pain, consider alternative analgesics (NSAIDs) in patients taking narcotics for acute or chronic pain.
• Examine for oral manifestations of opportunistic infection.
• This drug may be used in the hospital or on an outpatient basis. Confirm the patient's disease and treatment status.
• Chlorhexidine mouth rinse prior to and during chemotherapy may reduce severity of mucositis.
• Patient on chronic drug therapy may rarely present with symptoms of blood dyscrasias, which can include infection, bleeding, and poor healing. If dyscrasia is present, caution patient to prevent oral tissue trauma when using oral hygiene aids.
• Palliative medication may be required for management of oral side effects.
• Short appointments and a stress-reduction protocol may be required for anxious patients.
• Consider semisupine chair position for patient comfort if GI side effects occur.
• Caution: patients may be at high risk for infection.
• Patients may have received other chemotherapy or radiation; confirm medical and drug history.
• Oral infections should be eliminated and/or treated aggressively.

Consultations:
• Medical consultation should include routine blood counts including platelet counts and bleeding time.
• Consult physician; prophylactic or therapeutic antiinfectives may be indicated if surgery or periodontal treatment is required.
• Medical consultation may be required to assess immunologic status during cancer chemotherapy and determine safety risk, if any, posed by the required dental treatment.
• Medical consultation may be required to assess disease control and patient's ability to tolerate stress.
• In a patient with symptoms of blood dyscrasias, request a medical consultation for blood studies and postpone treatment until normal values are reestablished.

Teach Patient/Family to:
• See dentist immediately if secondary oral infection occurs.
• Be aware of oral side effects.
• Encourage effective oral hygiene to prevent soft tissue inflammation.
• Report oral lesions, soreness, or bleeding to dentist.
• Prevent trauma when using oral hygiene aids.
• Update health and medication history if physician makes any changes in evaluation or drug regimens; include OTC, herbal, and nonherbal remedies in the update.
• Use soft tooth brush to reduce risk of bleeding.

toremifene citrate
tor-**eh**′-mih-feen **sih**′-trate
(Fareston)

CATEGORY AND SCHEDULE
Pregnancy Risk Category: D

Drug Class: Antineoplastic, antiestrogen agent

MECHANISM OF ACTION

A nonsteroidal antiestrogen and antineoplastic agent that binds to estrogen receptors on tumors, producing a complex that decreases DNA synthesis and inhibits estrogen effects.
Therapeutic Effect: Blocks growth-stimulating effects of estrogen in breast cancer.

USES

Treatment of metastatic breast cancer in postmenopausal women with estrogen receptor-positive or unknown tumors

PHARMACOKINETICS

Well absorbed after PO administration. Metabolized in the liver. Eliminated in feces. *Half-life:* Approximately 5 days.

INDICATIONS AND DOSAGES
▸ **Breast Cancer**
PO
Adults. 60 mg/day until disease progression is observed.

SIDE EFFECTS/ADVERSE REACTIONS
Frequent
Hot flashes, diaphoresis, nausea, vaginal discharge, dizziness, dry eyes
Occasional
Edema, vomiting, vaginal bleeding
Rare
Fatigue, depression, lethargy, anorexia

PRECAUTIONS AND CONTRAINDICATIONS
History of thromboembolic disease
Caution:
Thromboembolic diseases, endometrial hyperplasia, hypercalcemia with bone metastases,

monitor leukocyte and platelet counts, tumor flare

DRUG INTERACTIONS OF CONCERN TO DENTISTRY
• None reported

SERIOUS REACTIONS
! Ocular toxicity (cataracts, glaucoma, decreased visual acuity) and hypercalcemia may occur.

DENTAL CONSIDERATIONS
General:
• Patients on chronic drug therapy may rarely have symptoms of blood dyscrasias, which can include infection, bleeding, and poor healing.
• Consider semisupine chair position for patient comfort because of GI side effects of drug.
Consultations:
• Medical consultation may be required to assess disease control.
Teach Patient/Family to:
• Encourage effective oral hygiene to prevent soft tissue inflammation.

torsemide
tor′-se-mide
(Demadex)
Do not confuse torsemide with furosemide.

CATEGORY AND SCHEDULE
Pregnancy Risk Category: B

Drug Class: Loop diuretic

MECHANISM OF ACTION
A loop diuretic that enhances excretion of sodium, chloride, potassium, and water at the ascending limb of the loop of Henle; also reduces plasma and extracellular fluid volume.

Therapeutic Effect: Produces diuresis; lowers B/P.

USES

Treatment of hypertension and edema associated with CHF, liver disease, chronic renal failure

PHARMACOKINETICS

Route	Onset	Peak	Duration
PO	1 hr	1–2 hr	6–8 hr
IV	10 min	1 hr	6–8 hr

Rapidly and well absorbed from the GI tract. Protein binding: 97%–99%. Metabolized in the liver. Primarily excreted in urine. Not removed by hemodialysis. ***Half-life:*** 3.3 hr.

INDICATIONS AND DOSAGES

▶ **Hypertension**

PO

Adults, Elderly. Initially, 5 mg/day. May increase to 10 mg/day if no response in 4–6 wk. If no response, additional antihypertensive added.

▶ **CHF**

PO, IV

Adults, Elderly. Initially, 10–20 mg/day. May increase by approximately doubling dose until desired therapeutic effect is attained. Doses greater than 200 mg have not been adequately studied.

▶ **Chronic Renal Failure**

PO, IV

Adults, Elderly. Initially, 20 mg/day. May increase by approximately doubling dose until desired therapeutic effect is attained. Doses greater than 200 mg have not been adequately studied.

▶ **Hepatic Cirrhosis**

PO, IV

Adults, Elderly. Initially, 5 mg/day given with aldosterone antagonist or potassium-sparing diuretic. May increase by approximately doubling dose until desired therapeutic effect is attained. Doses greater than 40 mg have not been adequately studied.

SIDE EFFECTS/ADVERSE REACTIONS

Frequent

Headache, dizziness, rhinitis

Occasional

Asthenia, insomnia, nervousness, diarrhea, constipation, nausea, dyspepsia, edema, ECG changes, pharyngitis, cough, arthralgia, myalgia

Rare

Syncope, hypotension, arrhythmias

PRECAUTIONS AND CONTRAINDICATIONS

Anuria, hepatic coma, severe electrolyte depletion

Caution:

Lactation, children younger than 18 yr, dehydration, systemic lupus erythematosus, ototoxicity, electrolyte imbalance

DRUG INTERACTIONS OF CONCERN TO DENTISTRY

• Increased electrolyte imbalance: systemic corticosteroids
• Masked ototoxicity: phenothiazines
• Decreased antihypertensive effects: NSAIDs
• Increased sweating, hot flashes, weakness, cardiovascular symptoms: chloral hydrate (rare)

SERIOUS REACTIONS

! Ototoxicity may occur with high doses or a too-rapid IV administration. Overdose produces acute, profound water loss; volume and electrolyte depletion; dehydration; decreased blood volume; and circulatory collapse.

DENTAL CONSIDERATIONS

General:
• Monitor vital signs at every appointment because of cardiovascular side effects.
• After supine positioning, have patient sit upright for at least 2 min before standing to avoid orthostatic hypotension.
• Patients on high-potency loop diuretics should be questioned about serum potassium levels or potassium supplement use.
• Short appointments and a stress-reduction protocol may be required for anxious patients.
• Consider semisupine chair position for patient comfort if GI side effects occur.

Consultations:
• Medical consultation may be required to assess disease control and patient's ability to tolerate stress.

Teach Patient/Family to:
• Update health history/drug record if physician makes any changes in evaluation or drug regimens; include OTC, herbal, and nonherbal drugs in the update.

tramadol hydrochloride

tram´-ah-dole high-droh-**klor**´-ide
(Tramal[AUS], Tramal SR[AUS], Ultram, Zydol[AUS])
Do not confuse tramadol with Toradol, or Ultram with Ultane.

CATEGORY AND SCHEDULE
Pregnancy Risk Category: C

Drug Class: Synthetic opioid analgesic

MECHANISM OF ACTION
An analgesic that binds to μ-opioid receptors and inhibits reuptake of norepinephrine and serotonin. Reduces the intensity of pain stimuli reaching sensory nerve endings. ***Therapeutic Effect:*** Alters the perception of and emotional response to pain.

USES
Treatment of moderate-to-severe pain

PHARMACOKINETICS

Route	Onset	Peak	Duration
PO	Less than 1 hr	2–3 hr	4–6 hr

Rapidly and almost completely absorbed after PO administration. Protein binding: 20%. Extensively metabolized in the liver to active metabolite (reduced in patients with advanced cirrhosis). Primarily excreted in urine. Minimally removed by hemodialysis. ***Half-life:*** 6–7 hr.

INDICATIONS AND DOSAGES
▸ **Moderate to Moderately Severe Pain**
PO
Adults, Elderly. 50–100 mg q4–6h. Maximum: 400 mg/day for patients 75 yr and younger; 300 mg/day for patients older than 75 yr.
▸ **Dosage in Renal Impairment**
For patients with creatinine clearance of less than 30 ml/min, increase dosing interval to q12h. Maximum: 200 mg/day.
▸ **Dosage in Hepatic Impairment**
Dosage is decreased to 50 mg q12h.

SIDE EFFECTS/ADVERSE REACTIONS

Frequent
Dizziness or vertigo, nausea, constipation, headache, somnolence

Occasional
Vomiting, pruritus, CNS stimulation (such as nervousness, anxiety, agitation, tremor, euphoria, mood swings, and hallucinations), asthenia, diaphoresis, dyspepsia, dry mouth, diarrhea

Rare
Malaise, vasodilation, anorexia, flatulence, rash, blurred vision, urine retention or urinary frequency, menopausal symptoms

PRECAUTIONS AND CONTRAINDICATIONS
Acute alcohol intoxication; concurrent use of centrally acting analgesics, hypnotics, opioids, or psychotropic drugs

Caution:
Not a controlled substance, but dependence and abuse are possible

DRUG INTERACTIONS OF CONCERN TO DENTISTRY
• Increased risk of respiratory depression: anesthetics, alcohol
• Significant increase in metabolism: carbamazepine
• Increased serum concentrations: quinidine
• Increased risk of seizures: MAOIs, tricyclic antidepressants, selective serotonin reuptake inhibitors
• Increased risk of sedation: other CNS depressant drugs, alcohol

SERIOUS REACTIONS
! Overdose results in respiratory depression and seizures. Tramadol may have a prolonged duration of action and cumulative effect in patients with hepatic or renal impairment.

DENTAL CONSIDERATIONS

General:
• Determine why the patient is taking the drug.
• Patients taking opioids for acute or chronic pain should be given alternative analgesics for dental pain.
• Geriatric patients are more susceptible to drug effects; use lower dose.
• Assess salivary flow as a factor in caries, periodontal disease, and candidiasis.
• Take precautions if dental surgery is anticipated and general anesthesia is required.
• Risk of cross-hypersensitivity to other opioid analgesics.

Teach Patient/Family to:
• Use caution to prevent trauma when using oral hygiene aids.
• Use caution when driving or operating complex equipment.
• When chronic dry mouth occurs, advise patient to:
  • Avoid mouth rinses with high alcohol content because of drying effects.
  • Use daily home fluoride products for anticaries effect.
  • Use sugarless gum, frequent sips of water, or saliva substitutes.

trandolapril
tran-**doe′**-la-pril
(Gopten[AUS], Mavik, Odrik[AUS])
Do not confuse trandolapril with tramadol.

CATEGORY AND SCHEDULE
Pregnancy Risk Category: C (D if used in second or third trimester)

Drug Class: Angiotensin-converting enzyme (ACE) inhibitor

MECHANISM OF ACTION

An ACE inhibitor that suppresses the renin-angiotensin-aldosterone system and prevents the conversion of angiotensin I to angiotensin II, a potent vasoconstrictor; may also inhibit angiotensin II at local vascular and renal sites. Decreases plasma angiotensin II, increases plasma renin activity, and decreases aldosterone secretion.
Therapeutic Effect: Reduces peripheral arterial resistance and pulmonary capillary wedge pressure; improves cardiac output and exercise tolerance.

USES

Treatment of hypertension alone or in combination with other antihypertensive medications; maintenance therapy to prevent CHF after MI; ventricular dysfunction after MI

PHARMACOKINETICS

Slowly absorbed from the GI tract. Protein binding: 80%. Metabolized in the liver and GI mucosa to active metabolite. Primarily excreted in urine. Removed by hemodialysis.
Half-life: 24 hr.

INDICATIONS AND DOSAGES
▶ **Hypertension (Without Diuretic)**
PO
Adults, Elderly. Initially, 1 mg once a day in nonblack patients, 2 mg once a day in African-American patients. Adjust dosage at least at 7-day intervals. Maintenance: 2–4 mg/day. Maximum: 8 mg/day.
▶ **CHF**
PO
Adults, Elderly. Initially, 0.5–1 mg, titrated to target dose of 4 mg/day.

SIDE EFFECTS/ADVERSE REACTIONS
Frequent
Dizziness, cough
Occasional
Hypotension, dyspepsia (heartburn, epigastric pain, indigestion), syncope, asthenia (loss of strength), tinnitus
Rare
Palpitations, insomnia, drowsiness, nausea, vomiting, constipation, flushed skin

PRECAUTIONS AND CONTRAINDICATIONS
History of angioedema from previous treatment with ACE inhibitors
Caution:
Angioedema (higher rate in African-American patients), CHF, ischemic heart disease, aortic stenosis, cerebrovascular disease, monitor WBC count in SLE or scleroderma, impaired renal function, hyperkalemia, pediatric patients, potassium-sparing diuretics

DRUG INTERACTIONS OF CONCERN TO DENTISTRY
• Decreased absorption of tetracycline
• Drugs that lower B/P could possibly exaggerate hypotensive effects

SERIOUS REACTIONS
! Excessive hypotension ("first-dose syncope") may occur in patients with CHF and in those who are severely salt or volume depleted.
! Angioedema and hyperkalemia occur rarely.
! Agranulocytosis and neutropenia may be noted in those with collagen vascular disease including scleroderma and systemic lupus erythematosus and impaired renal function.

T

! Nephrotic syndrome may be noted
in those with history of renal disease.

DENTAL CONSIDERATIONS

General:
• Monitor vital signs at every
appointment because of
cardiovascular disease.
• Limit use of sodium-containing
products, such as saline IV fluids,
for patients with a dietary salt
restriction.
• Stress from dental procedures may
compromise cardiovascular function;
determine patient risk.
• Short appointments and a
stress-reduction protocol may be
required for anxious patients.
• Use precaution if sedation or
general anesthesia is required; risk
of hypotensive episode.
• After supine positioning, have
patient sit upright for at least 2 min
before standing to avoid orthostatic
hypotension.
• Consider semisupine chair position
for patient comfort because of
respiratory side effects of drug.
• Patients on chronic drug therapy
may rarely have symptoms of blood
dyscrasias, which can include
infection, bleeding, and poor
healing.
Consultations:
• Medical consultation may be
required to assess disease control and
patient's ability to tolerate stress.
Teach Patient/Family to:
• Encourage effective oral hygiene
to prevent soft tissue inflammation.
• Use caution to prevent trauma
when using oral hygiene aids.
• Update health and drug history if
physician makes any changes in
evaluation or drug regimens; include
OTC, herbal, and nonherbal drugs in
the update.

tranexamic acid
tran-ex-**am**′-ik ass-id
(Cyklokapron)

CATEGORY AND SCHEDULE
Pregnancy Risk Category: B

Drug Class: Hemostatic,
antithrombolytic

MECHANISM OF ACTION
A competitive inhibitor of
plasminogen activation and, at much
higher concentrations, a
noncompetitive inhibitor of plasmin
(i.e., actions similar to aminocaproic
acid), which exerts its
antifibrinolytic effects primarily by
forming a reversible complex with a
modified plasminogen.
Therapeutic Effect: Prevents fibrin
clots from forming.

USES
Prophylaxis and treatment of
hemophilia patients to reduce or
prevent hemorrhage during and after
extractions; unapproved uses: in
hyperfibrinolysis-induced
hemorrhage, angioedema; oral rinse
(with systemic therapy) to reduce
bleeding in oral surgery patients
who are also taking anticoagulants

PHARMACOKINETICS
Absorption after PO administration
represents 30%–50% of the ingested
dose, and bioavailability is not
affected by food intake. Protein
binding: 3%. Site of metabolism is
not established. Excreted in urine.
Half-life: Unknown.

INDICATIONS AND DOSAGES
▶ **Hemorrhage Prophylaxis, Tooth Extraction**
IV/PO
Adults, Children. 10 mg/kg body weight immediately before dental extraction. Following surgery, a dose of 25 mg/kg body weight can be given orally 3 or 4 times daily for 2–8 days. Alternatively, tranexamic acid can be administered entirely orally, 25 mg/kg body weight 3–4 times per day beginning 1 day before surgery.

Dosage in Renal Impairment

Serum Creatinine	IV Dosage	Tablets
120–250 µmol/L (1.36–2.83 mg/dl)	10 mg/kg twice daily	15 mg/kg twice daily
250–500 µmol/L (2.83–5.66 mg/dl)	10 mg/kg daily	15 mg/kg daily
More than 500 µmol/L (2–5.66 mg/dl)	10 mg/kg q48h or 5 mg/kg q24h	15 mg/kg q48h or 7.5 mg/kg q24h

SIDE EFFECTS/ADVERSE REACTIONS
Occasional
Hypotension, diarrhea, nausea, vomiting, dizziness

PRECAUTIONS AND CONTRAINDICATIONS
Acquired defective color vision, subarachnoid hemorrhage, active intravascular clotting process, hypersensitivity to tranexamic acid or any component of the formulation
Caution:
Lactation, reduce dose in renal impairment, limited use experience in children

DRUG INTERACTIONS OF CONCERN TO DENTISTRY
• Increased risk of bleeding: drugs that affect coagulation
• Factor IX complex: increased risk of thrombotic complications when used concurrently

SERIOUS REACTIONS
! Thromboembolic events (e.g., deep vein thrombosis, pulmonary embolism, cerebral thrombosis, acute renal cortical necrosis, central retinal artery and vein obstruction) have been reported.

DENTAL CONSIDERATIONS
General:
• Used as an antifibrinolytic mouthwash following oral surgery to prevent hemorrhage in patients taking oral anticoagulants.
Consultations:
• Hematologist consultation is strongly recommended.
Teach Patient/Family to:
• Update health and drug history if physician makes any changes in evaluation or drug regimens; include OTC, herbal, and nonherbal drugs in the update.
• Report hemorrhage or bleeding not responding to postsurgical hemostasis.
• Use caution to prevent trauma when using oral hygiene aids.

tranylcypromine sulfate
tran-ill-**sip**′-roe-meen **sull**′-fate
(Parnate)

CATEGORY AND SCHEDULE
Pregnancy Risk Category: C

Drug Class: Antidepressant, MAOI

T

MECHANISM OF ACTION

An MAOI that inhibits the activity of the enzyme monoamine oxidase at CNS storage sites, leading to increased levels of the neurotransmitters epinephrine, norepinephrine, serotonin, and dopamine at neuronal receptor sites. *Therapeutic Effect:* Relieves depression.

USES

Treatment of depression (when uncontrolled by other means)

PHARMACOKINETICS

Well absorbed from GI tract. Metabolized in the liver. Primarily excreted in urine. Removed by hemodialysis. *Half-life:* 1.5–3.5 hr.

INDICATIONS AND DOSAGES

▸ **Depression Refractory to or Intolerant of Other Therapy**
PO
Adults, Elderly. Initially, 10 mg twice a day. May increase by 10 mg/day at 1- to 3-wk intervals up to 60 mg/day in divided doses.

SIDE EFFECTS/ADVERSE REACTIONS

Frequent
Orthostatic hypotension, restlessness, GI upset, insomnia, dizziness, lethargy, weakness, dry mouth, peripheral edema
Occasional
Flushing, diaphoresis, rash, urinary frequency, increased appetite, transient impotence
Rare
Visual disturbances

PRECAUTIONS AND CONTRAINDICATIONS

CHF, children younger than 16 yr, pheochromocytoma, severe hepatic or renal impairment, uncontrolled hypertension
Caution:
Suicidal patients, convulsive disorders, severe depression, schizophrenia, hyperactivity, diabetes mellitus

DRUG INTERACTIONS OF CONCERN TO DENTISTRY

• Increased pressor effects: indirect-acting sympathomimetics (ephedrine)
• Hyperpyretic crisis, convulsions, hypertensive episode, and death: carbamazepine, meperidine, and possibly other opioids
• Increased anticholinergic effects: anticholinergics and antihistamines
• Increased effects of alcohol, barbiturates, benzodiazepines, CNS depressants, fluoxetine, tricyclic antidepressants

SERIOUS REACTIONS

❗ Hypertensive crisis occurs rarely and is marked by severe hypertension, occipital headache radiating frontally, neck stiffness or soreness, nausea, vomiting, diaphoresis, fever or chills, clammy skin, dilated pupils, palpitations, tachycardia or bradycardia, and constricting chest pain.
❗ Intracranial bleeding has been reported in association with severe hypertension.

DENTAL CONSIDERATIONS

General:
• After supine positioning, have patient sit upright for at least 2 min before standing to avoid orthostatic hypotension.
• Monitor vital signs at every appointment because of cardiovascular side effects.

• Assess salivary flow as a factor in caries, periodontal disease, and candidiasis.

• Hypertensive episodes are possible even though there are no specific contraindications to vasoconstrictor use in local anesthetics.

Consultations:

• Medical consultation may be required to assess patient's ability to tolerate stress.

Teach Patient/Family to:

• Use powered tooth brush if patient has difficulty holding conventional devices.

• When chronic dry mouth occurs, advise patient to:

  • Avoid mouth rinses with high alcohol content because of drying effects.

  • Use daily home fluoride products to prevent caries.

  • Use sugarless gum, frequent sips of water, or saliva substitutes.

---

trastuzumab
traz-**two**′-zoo-mab
(Herceptin)

CATEGORY AND SCHEDULE
Pregnancy Risk Category: B

Drug Class: Antineoplastic, monoclonal antibody

MECHANISM OF ACTION
Binds to the HER-2 protein, which is overexpressed in 25%–30% of primary breast cancers, thereby inhibiting proliferation of tumor cells.
Therapeutic Effect: Inhibits the growth of tumor cells and mediates antibody-dependent cellular cytotoxicity.

USES
Treatment of breast cancer that has spread to other parts of the body

PHARMACOKINETICS
Half-life: 5.8 days (range: 1–32 days).

INDICATIONS AND DOSAGES
▸ **Breast Cancer**
IV
Adults, Elderly. Initially, 4 mg/kg as a 30- to 90-min infusion, then 2 mg/kg weekly as a 30-min infusion.

SIDE EFFECTS/ADVERSE REACTIONS
Frequent
Pain, asthenia, fever, chills, headache, abdominal pain, back pain, infection, nausea, diarrhea, vomiting, cough, dyspnea
Occasional
Tachycardia, CHF, flu-like symptoms, anorexia, edema, bone pain, arthralgia, insomnia, dizziness, paresthesia, depression, rhinitis, pharyngitis, sinusitis
Rare
Allergic reaction, anemia, leukopenia, neuropathy, herpes simplex

PRECAUTIONS AND CONTRAINDICATIONS
Preexisting cardiac disease

DRUG INTERACTIONS OF CONCERN TO DENTISTRY
• Dental drug interactions have not been studied.

SERIOUS REACTIONS
! Cardiomyopathy, ventricular dysfunction, and CHF occur rarely.
! Pancytopenia may occur.

T

DENTAL CONSIDERATIONS

General:

• If additional analgesia is required for dental pain, consider alternative analgesics (NSAIDs) in patients taking narcotics for acute or chronic pain.

• Monitor and record vital signs.

• Avoid products that affect platelet function, such as aspirin and NSAIDs.

• This drug may be used in the hospital or on an outpatient basis. Confirm the patient's disease and treatment status.

• Patient on chronic drug therapy may rarely present with symptoms of blood dyscrasias, which can include infection, bleeding, and poor healing. If dyscrasia is present, caution patient to prevent oral tissue trauma when using oral hygiene aids.

• Consider semisupine chair position for patient comfort if GI side effects occur.

• Caution: patients may be at high risk for infection.

• Patients may be at risk for bleeding; check oral signs.

• Oral infections should be eliminated and/or treated aggressively.

Consultations:

• Medical consultation should include routine blood counts including platelet counts and bleeding time.

• In a patient with symptoms of blood dyscrasias, request a medical consultation for blood studies and postpone treatment until normal values are reestablished.

• Consult physician; prophylactic or therapeutic antiinfectives may be indicated if surgery or periodontal treatment is required.

• Medical consultation may be required to assess immunologic status during cancer chemotherapy and determine safety risk, if any, posed by the required dental treatment.

• Medical consultation may be required to assess disease control and patient's ability to tolerate stress.

Teach Patient/Family to:

• Inform dentist of unusual bleeding episodes following dental treatment.

• See dentist immediately if secondary oral infection occurs.

• Encourage effective oral hygiene to prevent soft tissue inflammation.

• Report oral lesions, soreness, or bleeding to dentist.

• Prevent trauma when using oral hygiene aids.

• Update health and medication history if physician makes any changes in evaluation or drug regimens; include OTC, herbal, and nonherbal remedies in the update.

travoprost
tra′-voe-prost
(Apo-Timop[CAN], Gen-Timolol[CAN], Optimol[AUS], Tenopt[AUS], Travatan)

CATEGORY AND SCHEDULE
Pregnancy Risk Category: C

Drug Class: Synthetic prostaglandin F_2-α analog

MECHANISM OF ACTION
An ophthalmic agent that is a prostanoid-selective FP receptor agonist.

Therapeutic Effect: Reduces intraocular pressure (IOP) by reducing aqueous humor production.

USES

Reduction of elevated IOP in patients with open-angle glaucoma or ocular hypertension in patients intolerant to, or who show insufficient response to, other IOP-reducing drugs

PHARMACOKINETICS

Absorbed through the cornea and hydrolyzed to the active free acid form. Metabolized in cornea and liver. Metabolites are inactive. Excreted in urine. *Half-life:* 17–86 min.

INDICATIONS AND DOSAGES
▸ **Open-Angle Glaucoma, Ocular Hypertension**
Ophthalmic
Adults, Elderly. 1 drop in affected eye(s) once daily, in the evening.

SIDE EFFECTS/ADVERSE REACTIONS
Frequent
Ocular hyperemia
Occasional
Ocular pain, pruritus, eye discomfort, decreased visual acuity, foreign body sensation
Rare
Abnormal vision, cataract, conjunctivitis, dry eye, eye disorder, flare, iris discoloration, keratitis, lid margin crusting, photophobia, subconjunctival hemorrhage, and tearing

PRECAUTIONS AND CONTRAINDICATIONS

Hypersensitivity to travoprost or benzalkonium chloride, or any other component of the formulation
Caution:
May cause changes in pigmented tissues (iris, eyelid) and growth of eyelashes (length, thickness, color); do not administer with contact lens in place; renal or hepatic impairment, lactation, pediatric use, macular edema

DRUG INTERACTIONS OF CONCERN TO DENTISTRY
• None reported

SERIOUS REACTIONS

! Ocular adverse events including accidental injury, angina pectoris, anxiety, arthritis, back pain, bradycardia, bronchitis, chest pain, cold syndrome, depression, dyspepsia, gastrointestinal disorder, headache, hypercholesterolemia, hypertension, hypotension, infection, pain, prostate disorder, sinusitis, urinary incontinence, and UTI, occur rarely.

DENTAL CONSIDERATIONS

General:
• Monitor vital signs at every appointment because of cardiovascular and respiratory side effects and question patient about occurrence of cardiovascular side effects.
• Avoid drugs with anticholinergic activity, such as antihistamines, opioids, benzodiazepines, propantheline, atropine, and scopolamine.
• Protect patient's eyes from accidental spatter during dental treatment.
• Avoid dental light in patient's eyes; offer dark glasses for patient comfort.
Consultations:
• Medical consultation may be required to assess disease control.
Teach Patient/Family to:
• Update health and drug history if physician makes any changes in evaluation or drug regimens.

T

trazodone hydrochloride

trah′-zoe-done
high-droh-**klor′**-ide
(Apo-Trazodone[CAN], Desyrel,
Novo-Trazodone[CAN],
PMS-Trazodone[CAN])
Do not confuse Desyrel with
Delsym or Zestril.

CATEGORY AND SCHEDULE
Pregnancy Risk Category: C

Drug Class: Antidepressant

MECHANISM OF ACTION
An antidepressant that blocks the
reuptake of serotonin at neuronal
presynaptic membranes, increasing
its availability at postsynaptic
receptor sites.
Therapeutic Effect: Antidepressant.

USES
Treatment of depression

PHARMACOKINETICS
Well absorbed from the GI tract.
Protein binding: 85%–95%.
Metabolized in the liver. Primarily
excreted in urine. Unknown if
removed by hemodialysis. *Half-life:*
5–9 hr.

INDICATIONS AND DOSAGES
▶ Depression
PO
Adults. Initially, 150 mg/day in
equally divided doses. Increase by
50 mg/day at 3- to 4-day intervals
until therapeutic response is
achieved. Maximum: 600 mg/day.
Elderly. Initially, 25–50 mg at
bedtime. May increase by 25–50 mg
every 3–7 days. Range: 75–150 mg/
day.

Children 6–18 yr. Initially,
1.5–2 mg/kg/day in divided doses.
May increase gradually to 6 mg/kg/
day in 3 divided doses.

SIDE EFFECTS/ADVERSE REACTIONS
Frequent
Somnolence, dry mouth, light-
headedness, dizziness, headache,
blurred vision, nausea, vomiting
Occasional
Nervousness, fatigue, constipation,
generalized aches and pains, mild
hypotension
Rare
Photosensitivity reaction

PRECAUTIONS AND CONTRAINDICATIONS
Hypersensitivity to tricyclic
antidepressants, recovery phase of
MI, convulsive disorders, prostatic
hypertrophy
Caution:
Suicidal patients, severe depression,
increased intraocular pressure,
narrow-angle glaucoma, urinary
retention, cardiac disease, hepatic
disease, hyperthyroidism,
electroshock therapy, elective surgery

DRUG INTERACTIONS OF CONCERN TO DENTISTRY
• Increased anticholinergic effects:
anticholinergic drugs
• Increased CNS depression:
alcohol, all other CNS depressants

SERIOUS REACTIONS
! Priapism, diminished or improved
libido, retrograde ejaculation, and
impotence occur rarely.
! Trazodone appears to be less
cardiotoxic than other
antidepressants, although
arrhythmias may occur in patients
with preexisting cardiac disease.

T

DENTAL CONSIDERATIONS

General:
• Monitor vital signs at every appointment because of cardiovascular side effects.
• Patients on chronic drug therapy may rarely have symptoms of blood dyscrasias, which can include infection, bleeding, and poor healing.
• Assess salivary flow as a factor in caries, periodontal disease, and candidiasis.
• After supine positioning, have patient sit upright for at least 2 min before standing to avoid orthostatic hypotension.

Consultations:
• In a patient with symptoms of blood dyscrasias, request a medical consultation for blood studies and postpone dental treatment until normal values are reestablished.
• Medical consultation may be required to assess disease control.
• Physician should be informed if significant xerostomic side effects occur (e.g., increased caries, sore tongue, problems eating or swallowing, difficulty wearing prosthesis) so that a medication change can be considered.

Teach Patient/Family to:
• Report oral lesions, soreness, or bleeding to dentist.
• When chronic dry mouth occurs, advise patient to:
  • Avoid mouth rinses with high alcohol content because of drying effects.
  • Use daily home fluoride products to prevent caries.
  • Use sugarless gum, frequent sips of water, or saliva substitutes.

treprostinil sodium
treh-**prost**′-in-ill **soe**′-dee-um
(Remodulin)

CATEGORY AND SCHEDULE
Pregnancy Risk Category: B

Drug Class: Antihypertensive (pulmonary), vasodilator

MECHANISM OF ACTION
An antiplatelet that directly dilates pulmonary and systemic arterial vascular beds, inhibiting platelet aggregation.
Therapeutic Effect: Reduces symptoms of pulmonary arterial hypertension associated with exercise.

USES
Treatment of the symptoms of primary pulmonary hypertension or high B/P

PHARMACOKINETICS
Rapidly, completely absorbed after subcutaneous infusion; 91% bound to plasma protein. Metabolized by the liver. Excreted mainly in the urine with a lesser amount eliminated in the feces. *Half-life:* 2–4 hr.

INDICATIONS AND DOSAGES
▶ **Pulmonary Arterial Hypertension**
Continuous Subcutaneous Infusion
Adults, Elderly. Initially, 1.25 ng/kg/min. Reduce infusion rate to 0.625 ng/kg/min if initial dose cannot be tolerated. Increase infusion rate in increments of no more than 1.25 ng/kg/min per week for the first 4 wk and then no more than 2.5 ng/kg/min per wk for the duration of infusion.

▶ **Hepatic Impairment (Mild to Moderate)**

Adults, Elderly. Decrease the initial dose to 0.625 ng/kg/min on the basis of ideal body weight and increase cautiously.

SIDE EFFECTS/ADVERSE REACTIONS

Frequent
Infusion site pain, erythema, induration, rash
Occasional
Headache, diarrhea, jaw pain, vasodilation, nausea
Rare
Dizziness, hypotension, pruritus, edema

PRECAUTIONS AND CONTRAINDICATIONS

None known

DRUG INTERACTIONS OF CONCERN TO DENTISTRY

• Increased risk of bleeding: drugs that interfere with coagulation or platelet function, such as NSAIDs and aspirin

SERIOUS REACTIONS

! Abrupt withdrawal or sudden large reductions in dosage may result in worsening of pulmonary arterial hypertension symptoms.

DENTAL CONSIDERATIONS

General:
• An acute use drug for use in hospitals or emergency departments.
• If a patient reports this drug in his or her medical history, question about cardiovascular disease and drugs he or she may be taking.
• Patients are at risk for bleeding while receiving this drug; provide palliative dental care for dental emergencies only.

• Avoid products that affect platelet function, such as aspirin and NSAIDs.
Consultations:
• Medical consultation should include routine blood counts including platelet counts and bleeding time.
• Medical consultation may be required to assess disease control and patient's ability to tolerate stress.
Teach Patient/Family to:
• Inform dentist of unusual bleeding episodes following dental treatment.

tretinoin

tret'-ih-noyn
(Altinac, Avita, Renova, Retin-A, Retin-A Micro, Vesanoid)

CATEGORY AND SCHEDULE
Pregnancy Risk Category: D (oral), C (topical)

Drug Class: Vitamin A acid

MECHANISM OF ACTION

A retinoid that decreases cohesiveness of follicular epithelial cells. Increases turnover of follicular epithelial cells. Bacterial skin counts are not altered. Transdermal: Exerts its effects on growth and differentiation of epithelial cells. Antineoplastic: Induces maturation, decreases proliferation of acute promyelocytic leukemia (APL) cells. ***Therapeutic Effect:*** Causes expulsion of blackheads; alleviates fine wrinkles, hyperpigmentation; causes repopulation of bone marrow and blood by normal hematopoietic cells.

USES

Treatment of acne vulgaris, reducing fine facial wrinkles associated with

sun exposure and aging; unlabeled
uses: skin cancer, lichen planus
(Renova: not for use in acne)

PHARMACOKINETICS

Topical: Minimally absorbed. Oral:
Well absorbed following oral
administration. Protein binding:
95%. Metabolized in liver. Primarily
excreted in urine, minimal excretion
in feces. *Half-life:* 0.5–2 hr.

INDICATIONS AND DOSAGES
▸ **Acne**
Topical
Adults. Apply once daily at bedtime.
Transdermal
Adults. Apply to face once daily at
bedtime.
▸ **Acute Promyelocytic Leukemia**
PO
Adults. 45 mg/m^2/day given as two
evenly divided doses until complete
remission is documented.
Discontinue therapy 30 days after
complete remission or after 90 days
of treatment, whichever comes first.

SIDE EFFECTS/ADVERSE
REACTIONS
Expected
Topical: Temporary change in
pigmentation, photosensitivity. Local
inflammatory reactions (peeling, dry
skin, stinging, erythema, pruritus)
are to be expected and are reversible
with discontinuation of tretinoin
Frequent
PO: Headache, fever, dry skin/oral
mucosa, bone pain, nausea,
vomiting, rash
Occasional
PO: Mucositis, earache or feeling of
fullness in ears, flushing, pruritus,
increased sweating, visual
disturbances, hypo-/hypertension,
dizziness, anxiety, insomnia,
alopecia, skin changes

Rare
PO: Change in visual acuity,
temporary hearing loss

PRECAUTIONS AND
CONTRAINDICATIONS
Sensitivity to parabens (used as
preservative in gelatin capsule)
Caution:
Pregnancy category C, lactation,
eczema, sunburn

DRUG INTERACTIONS OF
CONCERN TO DENTISTRY
• Increased peeling: medication-
containing agents, such as alcohol or
astringents
• Avoid concurrent use with
photosensitizing drugs: tetracycline,
fluoroquinolones, sulfonamides

SERIOUS REACTIONS
PO
! Retinoic acid syndrome (fever,
dyspnea, weight gain, abnormal
chest auscultatory findings, episodic
hypotension) occurs commonly, as
does leukocytosis. Syndrome
generally occurs during first month
of therapy (sometimes occurs
following first dose).
! Pseudotumor cerebri may be
noted, especially in children
(headache, nausea, vomiting, visual
disturbances).
! Possible tumorigenic potential
when combined with ultraviolet
radiation.
Topical
! Possible tumorigenic potential
when combined with ultraviolet
radiation.

DENTAL CONSIDERATIONS
General:
• May cause dry, peeling skin if
used around lips; provide lip
lubricant for patient comfort during
dental treatment.

• Advise patient if dental drugs prescribed have a potential for photosensitivity.
Teach Patient/Family to:
• Avoid application on normal skin or getting cream in eyes, mouth, or other mucous membranes.

triamcinolone/ triamcinolone acetonide/ triamcinolone diacetate/ triamcinolone hexacetonide

trye-am-**sin**′-oh-lone/trye-am-**sin**′-oh-lone ah-**set**′-oh-nide/ trye-am-**sin**′-oh-lone dye-**ass**′-ih-tate/trye-am-**sin**′-oh-lone hex-ah-**set**′-oh-nide
triamcinolone (Aristocort) triamcinolone acetonide: (Aristocort, Azmacort, Kenacort A[AUS], Kenalog, Kenalog in Orabase[AUS], Nasacort AQ, Triaderm[CAN]) triamcinolone diacetate: (Amcort, Aristocort Intralesional) triamcinolone hexacetonide: (Aristospan)
Do not confuse triamcinolone with Triaminicin or Triaminicol.

CATEGORY AND SCHEDULE
Pregnancy Risk Category: C (D if used in first trimester)

Drug Class: Glucocorticoid, intermediate-acting

MECHANISM OF ACTION
An adrenocortical steroid that inhibits accumulation of inflammatory cells at inflammation sites, phagocytosis, lysosomal enzyme release and synthesis, and release of mediators of inflammation.
Therapeutic Effect: Prevents or suppresses cell-mediated immune reactions. Decreases or prevents tissue response to inflammatory process.

USES
Maintenance treatment of chronic asthma

PHARMACOKINETICS
PO/IM: Peak 1–2 hr. *Half-life:* 2–5 hr.

INDICATIONS AND DOSAGES
▶ **Immunosuppression, Relief of Acute Inflammation**
PO
Adults, Elderly. 4–60 mg/day.
IM (Triamcinolone Acetonide)
Adults, Elderly. Initially, 2.5–60 mg/day.
IM (Triamcinolone Diacetate)
Adults, Elderly. 40 mg/wk.
IM (Triamcinolone Hexacetonide)
Adults, Elderly. Initially, 2.5–40 mg up to 100 mg; 2–20 mg.
Intraarticular, Intralesional
Adults, Elderly. 5–40 mg.
▶ **Control of Bronchial Asthma**
Inhalation
Adults, Elderly. 2 inhalations 3–4 times a day.
Children 6–12 yr. 1–2 inhalations 3–4 times a day. Maximum: 12 inhalations/day.
▶ **Rhinitis**
Intranasal
Adults, Children 6 yr and older. 2 sprays each nostril each day.
▶ **Relief of Inflammation or Pruritus Associated with Corticoid-Responsive Dermatoses**
Topical
Adults, Elderly. 2–4 times a day. May give 1–2 times a day or as intermittent therapy.

SIDE EFFECTS/ADVERSE REACTIONS

Frequent

Insomnia, dry mouth, heartburn, nervousness, abdominal distention, diaphoresis, acne, mood swings, increased appetite, facial flushing, delayed wound healing, increased susceptibility to infection, diarrhea or constipation

Occasional

Headache, edema, change in skin color, frequent urination

Rare

Tachycardia, allergic reaction (including rash and hives), mental changes, hallucinations, depression
Topical: Allergic contact dermatitis

PRECAUTIONS AND CONTRAINDICATIONS

Administration of live-virus vaccines, especially smallpox vaccine; hypersensitivity to corticosteroids or tartrazine; IM injection or oral inhalation in children younger than 6 yr; peptic ulcer disease (except life-threatening situations); systemic fungal infection
Topical: Marked circulation impairment

Caution:

Tuberculosis; untreated fungal, bacterial or viral infections of respiratory tract; lactation, children younger than 6 yr; different doses may be required for patients on systemic glucocorticoids or patients with chickenpox, measles; transfer from systemic glucocorticoid therapy to inhalation must be done cautiously to avoid adrenal insufficiency response

DRUG INTERACTIONS OF CONCERN TO DENTISTRY

Triamcinolone/Triamcinolone Acetonide/Triamcinolone Hexacetonide

• Decreased action: barbiturates, rifampin, rifabutin
• Increased GI side effects: alcohol, salicylates, NSAIDs
• Increased action: ketoconazole, macrolide antibiotics

SERIOUS REACTIONS

! Long-term therapy may cause muscle wasting in the arms or legs, osteoporosis, spontaneous fractures, amenorrhea, cataracts, glaucoma, peptic ulcer disease, and CHF.
! Abruptly withdrawing the drug following long-term therapy may cause anorexia, nausea, fever, headache, arthralgia, rebound inflammation, fatigue, weakness, lethargy, dizziness, and orthostatic hypotension.
! Anaphylaxis occurs rarely with parenteral administration.
! Suddenly discontinuing triamcinolone may be fatal.
! Blindness has occurred rarely after intralesional injection around face and head.

DENTAL CONSIDERATIONS

General:

• Place on frequent recall because of oral side effects.
• Evaluate respiration characteristics and rate.
• Midday appointments and a stress-reduction protocol may be required for anxious patients.
• Acute asthmatic episodes may be precipitated in the dental office. Rapid-acting sympathomimetic inhalants should be available for emergency use. Triamcinolone is not a rapid-acting drug and is not

intended for use in acute asthmatic attacks.
• Be aware that aspirin or sulfite preservatives in vasoconstrictor-containing products can exacerbate asthma.
• Examine for oral manifestation of opportunistic infection.

Consultations:
• Medical consultation may be required to assess disease control.

Teach Patient/Family to:
• Encourage effective oral hygiene to prevent soft tissue inflammation.
• Gargle, rinse mouth with water, and expectorate after each aerosol dose.

DENTAL CONSIDERATIONS

Triamcinolone/Triamcinolone Acetonide/Triamcinolone Diacetate/Triamcinolone Hexacetonide

General:
• Symptoms of oral infections may be masked.
• Examine for oral manifestation of opportunistic infections.
• Oral side effects may be more common with inhalation products; significant steroid side effects are more likely to occur with chronic systemic doses.
• Acute asthmatic episodes may be precipitated in the dental office. Rapid-acting sympathomimetic inhalants should be available for emergency use. A stress reduction protocol may be required.
• Monitor vital signs at every appointment because of cardiovascular side effects.
• Assess salivary flow as a factor in caries, periodontal disease, and candidiasis.
• Place on frequent recall to monitor healing response.

• Determine dose and duration of steroid therapy for each patient to assess risk for stress tolerance and immunosuppression.
• Be aware that aspirin or sulfite preservatives in vasoconstrictor-containing products can exacerbate asthma.
• Patients who have been or are currently on chronic steroid therapy may require supplemental steroids for dental treatment.

Consultations:
• Medical consultation may be required to assess disease control.
• Consultation may be required to confirm steroid dose and duration of use.

Teach Patient/Family to:
• Encourage effective oral hygiene to prevent soft tissue inflammation.
• Report oral lesions, soreness, or bleeding to dentist.
• When chronic dry mouth occurs, advise patient to:
  • Avoid mouth rinses with high alcohol content because of drying effects.
  • Use daily home fluoride products for anticaries effect.
  • Use sugarless gum, frequent sips of water, or saliva substitutes.

Triamcinolone Acetonide (Topical)

General:
• Apply approximately 0.25 inch; measure with cotton-tipped applicator; press on lesion, do not rub. Use after brushing and eating and at bedtime for optimal effect.
• When used for oral lesions, return for oral evaluation if response of oral tissues has not occurred in 7–14 days.

triamterene
try-**am**′-ter-een
(Dyrenium)
Do not confuse triamterene with
trimipramine.

CATEGORY AND SCHEDULE
Pregnancy Risk Category: C (D if
used in pregnancy-induced
hypertension)

Drug Class: Potassium-sparing
diuretic

MECHANISM OF ACTION
A potassium-sparing diuretic that
inhibits sodium, potassium, ATPase.
Interferes with sodium and
potassium exchange in distal tubule,
cortical collecting tubule, and
collecting duct. Increases sodium
and decreases potassium excretion.
Also increases magnesium,
decreases calcium loss.
Therapeutic Effect: Produces
diuresis and lowers B/P.

USES
Edema; hypertension; more
commonly used in combination with
a thiazide diuretic

PHARMACOKINETICS

Route	Onset	Peak	Duration
PO	2–4 hr	N/A	7–9 hr

Incompletely absorbed from the GI
tract. Widely distributed.
Metabolized in the liver. Primarily
eliminated in feces via biliary route.

Half-life: 1.5–2.5 hr (increased in
renal impairment).

INDICATIONS AND DOSAGES
▸ **Edema, Hypertension**
PO
Adults, Elderly. 25–100 mg/day as a
single dose or in 2 divided doses.
Maximum: 300 mg/day.
Children. 2–4 mg/kg/day as a single
dose or in 2 divided doses.
Maximum: 6 mg/kg/day or 300 mg/
day.

SIDE EFFECTS/ADVERSE REACTIONS
Occasional
Fatigue, nausea, diarrhea, abdominal
pain, leg cramps, headache
Rare
Anorexia, asthenia, rash, dizziness

PRECAUTIONS AND CONTRAINDICATIONS
Drug-induced or preexisting
hyperkalemia, progressive or severe
renal disease, severe hepatic disease
Caution:
Dehydration, hepatic disease,
lactation, CHF, renal disease,
cirrhosis

DRUG INTERACTIONS OF CONCERN TO DENTISTRY
• Nephrotoxicity: possible risk with
NSAIDs
• Decreased antihypertensive effect:
possible risk with NSAIDs,
indomethacin
• Decreased effect of folic acid

SERIOUS REACTIONS
! Triamterene use may result in
hyponatremia (somnolence, dry
mouth, increased thirst, lack of
energy) or severe hyperkalemia
(irritability, anxiety, heaviness of
legs, paresthesia, hypotension,
bradycardia, ECG changes [tented T

T

waves, widening QRS complex, ST segment depression]).

! Agranulocytosis, nephrolithiasis, and thrombocytopenia occur rarely.

DENTAL CONSIDERATIONS

General:

• Limit use of sodium-containing products, such as saline IV fluids, for patients with a dietary salt restriction.

• Assess salivary flow as a factor in caries, periodontal disease, and candidiasis.

• Monitor vital signs at every appointment because of cardiovascular effects and possible hyperkalemia.

• Patients on chronic drug therapy may rarely have symptoms of blood dyscrasias, which can include infection, bleeding, and poor healing.

Consultations:

• In a patient with symptoms of blood dyscrasias, request a medical consultation for blood studies and postpone dental treatment until normal values are reestablished.

• Medical consultation may be required to assess disease control.

Teach Patient/Family to:

• Encourage effective oral hygiene to prevent soft tissue inflammation.

• Use caution to prevent injury when using oral hygiene aids.

• Report oral lesions, soreness, or bleeding to dentist.

• When chronic dry mouth occurs, advise patient to:

 • Avoid mouth rinses with high alcohol content because of drying effects.

 • Use daily home fluoride products to prevent caries.

 • Use sugarless gum, frequent sips of water, or saliva substitutes.

triazolam

trye-**ay**′-zoe-lam
(Apo-Triazo[CAN], Halcion)
Do not confuse Halcion with
Haldol or Healon.

CATEGORY AND SCHEDULE
Pregnancy Risk Category: X
Controlled Substance: Schedule
IV

Drug Class: Benzodiazepine,
sedative-hypnotic

MECHANISM OF ACTION
A benzodiazepine that enhances the action of the inhibitory neurotransmitter gamma-aminobutyric acid, resulting in CNS depression.
Therapeutic Effect: Induces sleep.

USES
Treatment of insomnia, preoperative sedation (unapproved)

PHARMACOKINETICS
PO: Onset 30–45 min, duration 6–8 hr. **Half-life:** 2–3 hr; metabolized by liver (CYP3A4 isoenzymes); excreted by kidneys (inactive metabolites); crosses placenta; excreted in breast milk.

INDICATIONS AND DOSAGES
▸ **Insomnia**
PO
Adults, Children 18 yr and older.
0.125–0.5 mg at bedtime.
Elderly. 0.0625–0.125 mg at bedtime.

SIDE EFFECTS/ADVERSE REACTIONS
Frequent
Somnolence, sedation, dry mouth, headache, dizziness, nervousness,

light-headedness, incoordination, nausea, rebound insomnia (may occur for 1–2 nights after drug is discontinued)

Occasional
Euphoria, tachycardia, abdominal cramps, visual disturbances

Rare
Paradoxic CNS excitement or restlessness (particularly in elderly or debilitated patients)

PRECAUTIONS AND CONTRAINDICATIONS
Angle-closure glaucoma; CNS depression; pregnancy or breast-feeding; severe, uncontrolled pain; sleep apnea

Caution:
Anemia, hepatic disease, renal disease, suicidal individuals, drug abuse, elderly, psychosis, children younger than 15 yr, acute narrow-angle glaucoma, seizure disorders

DRUG INTERACTIONS OF CONCERN TO DENTISTRY
• Increased effects: erythromycin, clarithromycin
• Increased sedation: alcohol, CNS depressants, opioid analgesics, diltiazem, anesthetics
• Avoid use with ketoconazole, itraconazole, ritonavir, indinavir, nelfinavir
• Caution if used with fluvoxamine, reduce dose by 50%
• Caution when used with drugs that are strong inhibitors of CYP3A4 isoenzymes (e.g., erythromycin)

SERIOUS REACTIONS
! Abrupt or too-rapid withdrawal may result in pronounced restlessness, irritability, insomnia, hand tremors, abdominal or muscle cramps, vomiting, diaphoresis, and seizures.

! Overdose results in somnolence, confusion, diminished reflexes, respiratory depression, and coma.

DENTAL CONSIDERATIONS

General:
• Assess salivary flow as a factor in caries, periodontal disease, and candidiasis.
• If dizziness occurs, provide assistance when escorting patient to and from dental chair.
• When used for conscious sedation, have someone drive patient to and from dental office.
• Avoid the use of this drug in a patient with a history of drug abuse or alcoholism.
• Geriatric patients are more susceptible to drug effects; use a lower dose.
• Psychologic and physical dependence may occur with chronic administration.
• Determine why the patient is taking the drug.
• Patients on chronic drug therapy may rarely have symptoms of blood dyscrasias, which can include infection, bleeding, and poor healing.

Teach Patient/Family:
• When chronic dry mouth occurs, advise patient to:
  • Avoid mouth rinses with high alcohol content because of drying effects.
  • Use daily home fluoride products to prevent caries.
  • Use sugarless gum, frequent sips of water, or saliva substitutes.

T

trifluoperazine hydrochloride

trye-floo-oh-**per′**-ah-zeen
high-droh-**klor′**-ide
(Apo-Trifluoperazine[CAN],
Nono-Trifluzine[CAN], PMS-
Trifluoperazine[CAN], Stelazine)
Do not confuse trifluoperazine
with triflupromazine, or Stelazine
with selegiline.

CATEGORY AND SCHEDULE
Pregnancy Risk Category: C

Drug Class: Phenothiazine
antipsychotic

MECHANISM OF ACTION
A phenothiazine derivative that
blocks dopamine at postsynaptic
receptor sites. Possesses strong
extrapyramidal and antiemetic
effects and weak anticholinergic and
sedative effects.
Therapeutic Effect: Suppresses
behavioral response in psychosis;
reduces locomotor activity and
aggressiveness.

USES
Treatment of psychotic disorders,
nonpsychotic anxiety, schizophrenia

PHARMACOKINETICS
PO: Onset rapid, peak 2–3 hr,
duration 12 hr. IM: Onset
immediate, peak 1 hr, duration
12 hr. Metabolized by liver, excreted
in urine, crosses placenta, excreted
in breast milk.

INDICATIONS AND DOSAGES
▸ **Psychotic Disorders**
PO
*Adults, Elderly, Children 12 yr and
older.* Initially, 2–5 mg once or twice
a day. Range: 15–20 mg/day.
Maximum: 40 mg/day.
Children 6–11 yr. Initially, 1 mg
once or twice a day. Maintenance:
Up to 15 mg/day.
IM
Adults. 1–2 mg q4–6h. Maximum:
10 mg/24h.
Elderly. 1 mg q4–6h. Maximum:
6 mg/24h.
Children. 1 mg 2 times a day.

SIDE EFFECTS/ADVERSE REACTIONS
Frequent
Hypotension, dizziness, and syncope
(occur frequently after first injection,
occasionally after subsequent
injections, and rarely with oral form)
Occasional
Drowsiness during early therapy, dry
mouth, blurred vision, lethargy,
constipation or diarrhea, nasal
congestion, peripheral edema, urine
retention
Rare
Ocular changes, altered skin
pigmentation (in those taking high
doses for prolonged periods),
photosensitivity

PRECAUTIONS AND CONTRAINDICATIONS
Angle-closure glaucoma, circulatory
collapse, myelosuppression, severe
cardiac or hepatic disease, severe
hypertension or hypotension
Caution:
Breast cancer, seizure disorders,
lactation, diabetes mellitus,
respiratory conditions, prostatic
hypertrophy

DRUG INTERACTIONS OF CONCERN TO DENTISTRY
• Increased sedation: other CNS
depressants, alcohol, barbiturate
anesthetics, opioid analgesics

• Hypotension, tachycardia: epinephrine
• Increased extrapyramidal effects: phenothiazines and related drugs (haloperidol, droperidol), metoclopramide
• Additive photosensitization: tetracyclines
• Increased anticholinergic effects: anticholinergics

SERIOUS REACTIONS

! Extrapyramidal symptoms appear to be dose related (particularly high doses) and are divided into 3 categories: akathisia (inability to sit still, tapping of feet), parkinsonian symptoms (such as mask-like face, tremors, shuffling gait, and hypersalivation), and acute dystonias (such as torticollis, opisthotonos, and oculogyric crisis). Dystonic reactions may also produce diaphoresis and pallor.
! Tardive dyskinesia, marked by tongue protrusion, puffing of the cheeks, and chewing or puckering of the mouth, occurs rarely but may be irreversible.
! Abrupt withdrawal after long-term therapy may precipitate nausea, vomiting, gastritis, dizziness, and tremors.
! Blood dyscrasias, particularly agranulocytosis, and mild leukopenia may occur.
! Trifluoperazine may lower the seizure threshold.

DENTAL CONSIDERATIONS

General:
• Monitor vital signs at every appointment because of cardiovascular side effects.
• Patients on chronic drug therapy may rarely have symptoms of blood dyscrasias, which can include infection, bleeding, and poor healing.

• After supine positioning, have patient sit upright for at least 2 min before standing to avoid orthostatic hypotension.
• Assess salivary flow as a factor in caries, periodontal disease, and candidiasis.
• Avoid dental light in patient's eyes; offer dark glasses for patient comfort.
• Assess for presence of extrapyramidal motor symptoms, such as tardive dyskinesia and akathisia. Extrapyramidal motor activity may complicate dental treatment.
• Geriatric patients are more susceptible to drug effects; use lower dose.
• Use vasoconstrictors with caution, in low doses, and with careful aspiration.
Consultations:
• In a patient with symptoms of blood dyscrasias, request a medical consultation for blood studies and postpone dental treatment until normal values are reestablished.
• Take precautions if dental surgery is anticipated and anesthesia is required.
• Physician should be informed if significant xerostomic side effects occur (e.g., increased caries, sore tongue, problems eating or swallowing, difficulty wearing prosthesis) so that a medication change can be considered.
• If signs of tardive dyskinesia or akathisia are present, refer to physician.
Teach Patient/Family to:
• Encourage effective oral hygiene to prevent soft tissue inflammation.
• Use caution to prevent injury when using oral hygiene aids.
• Use powered tooth brush if patient has difficulty holding conventional devices.

• When chronic dry mouth occurs, advise patient to:
  • Use daily home fluoride products for anticaries effect.
  • Avoid mouth rinses with high alcohol content because of drying effects.
  • Use sugarless gum, frequent sips of water, or saliva substitutes.

trifluridine

trye-**flure**′-ih-deen
(Viroptic)
Do not confuse with Zostrix.

CATEGORY AND SCHEDULE

Pregnancy Risk Category: C

Drug Class: Antiviral

MECHANISM OF ACTION

An antiviral agent that incorporates into DNS causing increased rate of mutation and errors in protein formation.
Therapeutic Effect: Prevents viral replication.

USES

Treatment of primary keratoconjunctivitis, recurring epithelial keratitis, keratitis associated with human herpes virus types 1 and 2, and vacciniavirus

PHARMACOKINETICS

Intraocular solution is undetectable in serum. *Half-life:* 12 min.

INDICATIONS AND DOSAGES
▸ **Herpes Simplex Virus Ocular Infections**
Ophthalmic
Adults, Elderly, Children older than 6 yr. 1 drop onto cornea q2h while awake. Maximum: 9 drops/day. Continue until corneal ulcer has completely reepithelialized, then 1 drop q4h while awake (minimum: 5 drops/day) for an additional 7 days.

SIDE EFFECTS/ADVERSE REACTIONS
Frequent
Transient stinging or burning with instillation
Occasional
Edema of eyelid
Rare
Hypersensitivity reaction

PRECAUTIONS AND CONTRAINDICATIONS
Hypersensitivity to trifluridine or any component of the formulation
Caution:
Antibiotic hypersensitivity

DRUG INTERACTIONS OF CONCERN TO DENTISTRY
• None reported

SERIOUS REACTIONS
! Ocular toxicity may occur if used longer than 21 days.

DENTAL CONSIDERATIONS

General:
• Avoid dental light in patient's eyes; offer dark glasses for patient comfort.
• Evaluate:
  • Therapeutic response: absence of redness, inflammation, tearing.
  • Allergy: itching, lacrimation, redness, swelling.

trihexyphenidyl
trye-hex-ee-**fen**′-ih-dill
(Artane, Apo-Trihex[CAN])

CATEGORY AND SCHEDULE
Pregnancy Risk Category: C

Drug Class: Antiparkinsonian, anticholinergic

MECHANISM OF ACTION
An anticholinergic agent that blocks central cholinergic receptors (aids in balancing cholinergic and dopaminergic activity).
Therapeutic Effect: Decreases salivation, relaxes smooth muscle.

USES
Treatment of Parkinson symptoms

PHARMACOKINETICS
Well absorbed from GI tract. Primarily excreted in urine.
Half-life: 3.3–4.1 hr.

INDICATIONS AND DOSAGES
▸ **Parkinsonism**
PO
Adults, Elderly. Initially, 1 mg on first day. May increase by 2 mg/day at 3–5-day intervals up to 6–10 mg/day (12–15 mg/day in patients with postencephalitic parkinsonism).
▸ **Drug-Induced Extrapyramidal Symptoms**
PO
Adults, Elderly. Initially, 1 mg/day. Range: 5–15 mg/day.

SIDE EFFECTS/ADVERSE REACTIONS
Elderly (older than 60 yr) tend to develop mental confusion, disorientation, agitation, psychotic-like symptoms

Frequent
Drowsiness, dry mouth
Occasional
Blurred vision, urinary retention, constipation, dizziness, headache, muscle cramps
Rare
Seizures, depression, rash

PRECAUTIONS AND CONTRAINDICATIONS
Angle closure glaucoma, GI obstruction, paralytic ileus, intestinal atony, severe ulcerative colitis, prostatic hypertrophy, myasthenia gravis, megacolon, hypersensitivity to trihexyphenidyl or any component of the formulation
Caution:
Children, gastric ulcer

DRUG INTERACTIONS OF CONCERN TO DENTISTRY
• Increased anticholinergic effects: scopolamine, atropine, phenothiazines, antihistamines, and other anticholinergics
• Increased CNS depression: alcohol, CNS depressants
• Decreased effects of phenothiazines

SERIOUS REACTIONS
❗ Hypersensitivity reaction (eczema, pruritus, rash, cardiac disturbances, photosensitivity) may occur.
❗ Overdosage may vary from CNS depression (sedation, apnea, cardiovascular collapse, death) to severe paradoxic reaction (hallucinations, tremor, seizures).

T

DENTAL CONSIDERATIONS
General:
• Assess salivary flow as a factor in caries, periodontal disease, and candidiasis.
• Place on frequent recall because of oral side effects.

• After supine positioning, have patient sit upright for at least 2 min before standing to avoid orthostatic hypotension.

• Avoid dental light in patient's eyes; offer dark glasses for patient comfort.

Teach Patient/Family to:

• Encourage effective oral hygiene to prevent soft tissue inflammation.

• Use powered tooth brush if patient has difficulty holding conventional devices.

• When chronic dry mouth occurs, advise patient to:

  • Avoid mouth rinses with high alcohol content because of drying effects.

  • Use daily home fluoride products to prevent caries.

  • Use sugarless gum, frequent sips of water, or saliva substitutes.

trimethobenzamide hydrochloride
trye-meth-oh-**ben**'-za-mide
high-droh-**klor**'-ide
(Tigan)

CATEGORY AND SCHEDULE
Pregnancy Risk Category: C

Drug Class: Antiemetic

MECHANISM OF ACTION
An anticholinergic that acts at the chemoreceptor trigger zone in the medulla oblongata.
Therapeutic Effect: Relieves nausea and vomiting.

USES
Treatment of nausea, vomiting

PHARMACOKINETICS

Route	Onset	Peak	Duration
PO	10–40 min	N/A	3–4 hr
IM	15–30 min	N/A	2–3 hr

Partially absorbed from the GI tract. Distributed primarily to the liver. Metabolic fate unknown. Excreted in urine. ***Half-life:*** 7–9 hr.

INDICATIONS AND DOSAGES
▸ **Nausea and Vomiting**
PO
Adults, Elderly. 300 mg 3–4 times a day.
Children weighing 30–100 lb. 100–200 mg 3–4 times a day.
IM
Adults, Elderly. 200 mg 3–4 times a day.
Rectal
Adults, Elderly. 200 mg 3–4 times a day.
Children weighing 30–100 lb. 100–200 mg 3–4 times a day.
Children weighing less than 30 lb. 100 mg 3–4 times a day.

SIDE EFFECTS/ADVERSE REACTIONS
Frequent
Somnolence
Occasional
Blurred vision, diarrhea, dizziness, headache, muscle cramps
Rare
Rash, seizures, depression, opisthotonos, parkinsonian syndrome, Reye's syndrome (marked by vomiting, seizures)

PRECAUTIONS AND CONTRAINDICATIONS
Hypersensitivity to benzocaine or similar local anesthetics; use of parenteral form in children or

suppositories in premature infants or neonates

Caution:
Children, cardiac dysrhythmias, elderly, asthma, prostatic hypertrophy, bladder neck obstruction, narrow-angle glaucoma, stenosing peptic ulcer, pyloroduodenal obstruction

DRUG INTERACTIONS OF CONCERN TO DENTISTRY
• Increased effect: CNS depressants
• May mask ototoxic symptoms associated with antibiotics or large doses of salicylates

SERIOUS REACTIONS
! A hypersensitivity reaction, manifested as extrapyramidal symptoms such as muscle rigidity and allergic skin reactions, occurs rarely.
! Children may experience paradoxic reactions, marked by restlessness, insomnia, euphoria, nervousness, and tremor.
! Overdose may produce CNS depression (manifested as sedation, apnea, cardiovascular collapse, and death) or severe paradoxic reactions (such as hallucinations, tremor, and seizures).

DENTAL CONSIDERATIONS

General:
• Nausea and vomiting may be accompanied by dehydration and electrolyte imbalance and should be corrected as part of treatment.
• Postpone elective dental treatment when symptoms are present.

trimetrexate
try-meh-**trex**′-ate
(NeuTrexin)
Do not confuse with Amicar.

CATEGORY AND SCHEDULE
Pregnancy Risk Category: D

Drug Class: Folate antagonist

MECHANISM OF ACTION
A folate antagonist that inhibits the enzyme dihydrofolate reductase (DHFR).
Therapeutic Effect: Disrupts purine, DNA, RNA, protein synthesis, with consequent cell death.

USES
Alternative therapy for *P. carinii* pneumonia (PCP) in immunocompromised patients, including patients with AIDS; unapproved uses: treatment of lung, prostate, colon cancer

PHARMACOKINETICS
Following IV administration, distributed readily into ascitic fluid. Metabolized in liver. Eliminated in urine. *Half-life:* 11–20 hr.

INDICATIONS AND DOSAGES
▶ PCP
IV Infusion
Adults. Trimetrexate: 45 mg/m² once daily over 60–90 min. Leucovorin: 20 mg/m² over 5–10 min q6h for total daily dose of 80 mg/m², or orally as 4 doses of 20 mg/m² spaced equally throughout the day. Round up the oral dose to the next higher 25-mg increment. Recommended course of therapy: 21 days trimetrexate, 24 days leucovorin.

SIDE EFFECTS/ADVERSE REACTIONS

Occasional
Fever, rash, pruritus, nausea, vomiting, confusion
Rare
Fatigue

PRECAUTIONS AND CONTRAINDICATIONS

Clinically significant hypersensitivity to trimetrexate, leucovorin, or methotrexate
Caution:
Lactation, children younger than 18 yr; impaired hematologic, renal, or hepatic function; serious bone marrow depression can occur if leucovorin is not used concurrently

DRUG INTERACTIONS OF CONCERN TO DENTISTRY

• Alteration of plasma levels: concurrent use with erythromycin, ketoconazole, and fluconazole
• Alteration in trimetrexate metabolites: acetaminophen
• Caution with use of drugs that are strong inhibitors of CYP3A4 isoenzymes

SERIOUS REACTIONS

❗ Trimetrexate given without concurrent leucovorin may result in serious or fatal hematologic, hepatic, and/or renal complications, including bone marrow suppression, oral and GI mucosal ulceration, and renal and hepatic dysfunction.
❗ In event of overdose, stop trimetrexate and give leucovorin 40 mg/m^2 q6h for 3 days.
❗ Anaphylaxis occurs rarely.

DENTAL CONSIDERATIONS

General:
• Examine for evidence of oral manifestations of blood dyscrasia (infection, bleeding, poor healing).

• Place on frequent recall because of oral side effects.
• Determine why the patient is taking the drug.
• Examine for oral manifestations of opportunistic infections.
• Consider local hemostasis measures to prevent excessive bleeding.
• Palliative treatment may be required for stomatitis.
• Refer to physician if oral ulcerative lesions occur.
• Consider semisupine chair position for patient comfort because of GI effects of disease.
Consultations:
• Obtain a medical consultation for blood studies (CBC) because leukopenic or thrombocytopenic side effects may result in infection, delayed healing, and excessive bleeding. Postpone elective dental treatment until normal values are maintained.
• Medical consultation may be required to assess disease control.
Teach Patient/Family to:
• Encourage effective oral hygiene to prevent soft tissue inflammation.
• Use caution to prevent injury when using oral hygiene aids.
• See dentist immediately if secondary oral infection occurs.

trimipramine

trye-**mih'**-pra-meen
(Apo-Trimip[CAN], Novo-Tripramine[CAN], Nu-Trimipramine[CAN], Rhotrimine[CAN], Surmontil)
Do not confuse with desipramine.

CATEGORY AND SCHEDULE

Pregnancy Risk Category: C

Drug Class:
Antidepressant-tricyclic

MECHANISM OF ACTION

A tricyclic antibulimic, anticataplectic, antidepressant, antinarcoleptic, antineuralgic, antineuritic, and antipanic agent that blocks the reuptake of neurotransmitters, such as norepinephrine and serotonin, at presynaptic membranes, increasing their concentration at postsynaptic receptor sites. May demonstrate less autonomic toxicity than other tricyclic antidepressants.
Therapeutic Effect: Results in antidepressant effect. Anticholinergic effect controls nocturnal enuresis.

USES

Treatment of depression

PHARMACOKINETICS

Rapidly, completely absorbed after PO administration, and not affected by food. Protein binding: 95%. Metabolized in liver (significant first-pass effect). Primarily excreted in urine. Not removed by hemodialysis. *Half-life:* 16–40 hr.

INDICATIONS AND DOSAGES
▸ **Depression**
PO
Adults. 50–150 mg/day at bedtime. Maximum: 200 mg/day for outpatients, 300 mg/day for inpatients.
Elderly. Initially, 25 mg/day at bedtime. May increase by 25 mg q3–7days. Maximum: 100 mg/day.

SIDE EFFECTS/ADVERSE REACTIONS
Frequent
Drowsiness, fatigue, dry mouth, blurred vision, constipation, delayed micturition, postural hypotension, diaphoresis, disturbed concentration, increased appetite, urinary retention, photosensitivity

Occasional
GI disturbances, such as nausea, and a metallic taste sensation
Rare
Paradoxic reaction marked by agitation and restlessness, nightmares, insomnia, and extrapyramidal symptoms, particularly fine hand tremors

PRECAUTIONS AND CONTRAINDICATIONS

Acute recovery period after MI, within 14 days of MAOI ingestion, hypersensitivity to trimipramine or any component of the formulation
Caution:
Suicidal patients, severe depression, increased intraocular pressure, narrow-angle glaucoma, urinary retention, cardiac disease, hepatic disease, hyperthyroidism, electroshock therapy, elective surgery, MAOIs

DRUG INTERACTIONS OF CONCERN TO DENTISTRY

• Increased anticholinergic effects: muscarinic blockers, antihistamines, phenothiazines
• Increased effects of direct-acting sympathomimetics (epinephrine, levonordefrin)
• Possible risk of increased CNS depression: alcohol, barbiturates, benzodiazepines, and other CNS depressants
• Decreased antihypertensive effects: clonidine, guanadrel, guanethidine

SERIOUS REACTIONS

! High dosage may produce cardiovascular effects, such as severe postural hypotension, dizziness, tachycardia, palpitations, arrhythmias and seizures. High dosage may also result in altered temperature regulation, including hyperpyrexia or hypothermia.

! Abrupt withdrawal from prolonged therapy may produce headache, malaise, nausea, vomiting, and vivid dreams.

DENTAL CONSIDERATIONS

General:

• Monitor vital signs at every appointment because of cardiovascular side effects.

• Assess salivary flow as a factor in caries, periodontal disease, and candidiasis.

• Patients on chronic drug therapy may rarely have symptoms of blood dyscrasias, which can include infection, bleeding, and poor healing.

• After supine positioning, have patient sit upright for at least 2 min before standing to avoid orthostatic hypotension.

• Use vasoconstrictors with caution, in low doses, and with careful aspiration. Avoid use of gingival retraction cord with epinephrine.

• Place on frequent recall because of oral side effects.

Consultations:

• In a patient with symptoms of blood dyscrasias, request a medical consultation for blood studies and postpone dental treatment until normal values are reestablished.

• Medical consultation may be required to assess disease control.

• Physician should be informed if significant xerostomic side effects occur (e.g., increased caries, sore tongue, problems eating or swallowing, difficulty wearing prosthesis) so that a medication change can be considered.

Teach Patient/Family:

• Importance of good oral hygiene to prevent soft tissue inflammation.

• To use caution to prevent injury when using oral hygiene aids.

• When chronic dry mouth occurs, advise patient:

  • To avoid mouth rinses with high alcohol content because of drying effects.

  • To use daily home fluoride products to prevent caries.

  • To use sugarless gum, frequent sips of water, or saliva substitutes.

---

triptorelin pamoate
trip-toe-**ree**′-linn **pam**′-oh-ate
(Trelstar Depot, Trelstar LA)

CATEGORY AND SCHEDULE
Pregnancy Risk Category: X

Drug Class: Antineoplastic

MECHANISM OF ACTION
A gonadotropin-releasing hormone (GnRH) analog and antineoplastic agent that inhibits gonadotropin hormone secretion through a negative feedback mechanism. Circulating levels of luteinizing hormone, follicle-stimulating hormone, testosterone, and estradiol rise initially, then subside with continued therapy.
Therapeutic Effect: Suppresses growth of abnormal prostate tissue.

USES
Decreasing testosterone levels

PHARMACOKINETICS
Metabolism may be by CYP450, eliminated by liver, kidneys; terminal half-life is 3 hr in healthy males.

INDICATIONS AND DOSAGES
▶ **Prostate Cancer**
IM (Trelstar Depot)
Adults, Elderly. 3.75 mg once q28 days.
IM (Trelstar LA)
Adults, Elderly. 11.25 mg q84 days.

SIDE EFFECTS/ADVERSE REACTIONS
Frequent
Hot flashes, skeletal pain, headache, impotence
Occasional
Insomnia, vomiting, leg pain, fatigue
Rare
Dizziness, emotional lability, diarrhea, urine retention, UTIs, anemia, pruritus

PRECAUTIONS AND CONTRAINDICATIONS
Hypersensitivity to luteinizing hormone-releasing hormone (LHRH) or LHRH agonists

DRUG INTERACTIONS OF CONCERN TO DENTISTRY
• Dental drug interactions have not been studied.

SERIOUS REACTIONS
! Bladder outlet obstruction, skeletal pain, hematuria, and spinal cord compression (with weakness or paralysis of the lower extremities) may occur.

DENTAL CONSIDERATIONS
General:
• If additional analgesia is required for dental pain, consider alternative analgesics (NSAIDs) in patients taking opioids for acute or chronic pain.
• This drug may be used in the hospital or on an outpatient basis. Confirm the patient's disease and treatment status.

• Patients may have received other chemotherapy or radiation; confirm medical and drug history.
• When urinary retention is a problem, use anticholinergic drugs with care.
Consultations:
• Consult patient's physician if an acute dental infection occurs and another antiinfective is required.
• Medical consultation may be required to assess disease control and patient's ability to tolerate stress.
Teach Patient/Family to:
• Encourage effective oral hygiene to prevent soft tissue inflammation.
• Prevent trauma when using oral hygiene aids.
• Update health and medication history if physician makes any changes in evaluation or drug regimen; include OTC, herbal, and nonherbal remedies in the update.

tropicamide
troe-**pik**′-ah-mide
(Diotrope[CAN], Mydriacyl, Opticyl, Tropicacyl)

CATEGORY AND SCHEDULE
Pregnancy Risk Category: C

Drug Class: Mydriatic, cycloplegic

T

MECHANISM OF ACTION
An antimuscarinic agent that produces competitive antagonism of the actions of acetylcholine.
Therapeutic Effect: Produces dilation of pupil (mydriasis); produces paralysis of accommodation (cycloplegia).

USES
Dilation of the pupil

PHARMACOKINETICS
Onset of action occurs within 20–40 min. The duration is about 6 hr.

INDICATIONS AND DOSAGES
▶ **Ocular Diagnostic Procedure, Examination of Fundus**
Ophthalmic
Adults, Elderly, Children. 1–2 drops in the eye(s) 15–20 min prior to exam.
▶ **Ocular Diagnostic Procedure, Refractive Procedures**
Ophthalmic
Adults, Elderly, Children. 1–2 drops in the eye(s). May be repeated in 5 min.

SIDE EFFECTS/ADVERSE REACTIONS
Occasional
Blurred vision, ocular irritation, headache
Rare
Photophobia, increased intraocular pressure

PRECAUTIONS AND CONTRAINDICATIONS
Primary glaucoma or tendency toward glaucoma, hypersensitivity to tropicamide or any component of the formulation

DRUG INTERACTIONS OF CONCERN TO DENTISTRY
• None reported

SERIOUS REACTIONS
! Cardiorespiratory collapse has been reported.
! Systemic absorption, including behavioral disturbances, confusion, dry mouth, fast heartbeat, and psychotic reactions, occurs rarely.

DENTAL CONSIDERATIONS

General:
• An acute use drug for diagnostic purposes.
• Protect patient's eyes from accidental spatter during dental treatment.
• Avoid dental light in patient's eyes; offer dark glasses for patient comfort.

trovafloxacin mesylate/ alatrofloxacin mesylate
troe-va-**flox**′-ah-sin **meh**′-sil-ate/
ala-troe-**flox**′-ah-sin **meh**′-sil-ate
Trovafloxacin mesylate oral: (Trovan) Alatrofloxacin mesylate injection: (Trovan I.V.)

CATEGORY AND SCHEDULE
Pregnancy Risk Category: C

Drug Class: Antibiotic fluoronaphthyridone antiinfective (related to the fluoroquinolones)

MECHANISM OF ACTION
A broad-spectrum bactericidal agent that inhibits the enzymes topoisomerase II (DNA gyrase) and topoisomerase IV required for bacterial DNA replication, transcription repair, and recombination.
Therapeutic Effect: Antibacterial.

USES
Treatment of infections caused by susceptible microorganisms in nosocomial pneumonia, community-acquired pneumonia, acute bacterial exacerbated chronic bronchitis, acute sinusitis, abdominal infections, gynecologic infections, UTI, bacterial prostatitis, skin and

skin-structure infections, and selected STDs

PHARMACOKINETICS

PO: Good oral absorption, bioavailability 88%, can be administered with food, peak serum levels 1.7 hr, plasma protein binding 76%, wide tissue distribution, excreted in breast milk, hepatic metabolism, excretion in feces and urine, 50% of dose is excreted unchanged in feces. IV: Alatrofloxacin is a prodrug converted to trovafloxacin.

INDICATIONS AND DOSAGES

PO: Skin Infections
Adults older than 18 yr. Dose depends on type of infection; 200 mg daily for 1–14 days.
IV: Nosocomial Pneumonia
Adults older than 18 yr. IV dose depends on type of infection; range 300 mg daily; single IV doses can be followed by appropriate oral doses for 10–14 days.

SIDE EFFECTS/ADVERSE REACTIONS

Oral: Dry mouth, stomatitis, angular cheilitis
CNS: Dizziness, headache, light-headedness, confusion, anxiety, hallucinations
CV: Hypotension, palpitation, flushing, peripheral edema, chest pain
GI: Vomiting, nausea, diarrhea, abdominal pain, flatulence, antibiotic-associated pseudomembranous colitis, hepatic toxicity
Resp: Dyspnea, bronchospasm, coughing
Hema: Anemia, leukopenia, thrombocytopenia
GU: Vaginitis, frequency of urination, abnormal renal function

EENT: Rhinitis, sinusitis
Integ: Pruritus, rash, photosensitization
Meta: Increased liver enzymes
MS: Arthralgia, myalgia, muscle cramps
Misc: Pain on injection, increased sweating, fatigue, fever, anaphylaxis

PRECAUTIONS AND CONTRAINDICATIONS

Hypersensitivity and allergy to the fluoroquinolones
Serious liver injury
Caution:
Children younger than 18 yr, mild to moderate cirrhosis, potential for liver damage, exposure to sunlight, visible or ultraviolet radiation, seizure disorders, cerebral atherosclerosis, lactation, warning associated with possible serious hepatic injury leading to death or transplant

DRUG INTERACTIONS OF CONCERN TO DENTISTRY

• Reduction in absorption: magnesium or aluminum antacid products, iron salts, sucralfate, and morphine within 30 min of oral trovafloxacin; separate doses by at least 2 hr
• Increases serum levels of caffeine

SERIOUS REACTIONS

! Serious liver injury

DENTAL CONSIDERATIONS

General:
• Determine why patient is taking the drug; specific infection.
• Do not use ingestible sodium bicarbonate products, such as the air polishing system Prophy-Jet, within 2 hr of drug use.
• Examine for oral manifestation of opportunistic infection.

• Avoid dental light in patient's eyes; offer dark glasses for patient comfort.
• Use caution in prescribing caffeine-containing analgesics.

Consultations:
• Medical consultation may be required to assess disease control in the patient.
• Consult with patient's physician if an acute dental infection occurs and another antiinfective is required.

Teach Patient/Family to:
• Prevent trauma when using oral hygiene aids.
• Encourage effective oral hygiene to prevent soft tissue inflammation.
• Avoid mouth rinses with high alcohol content because of drying effects.

unoprostone isopropyl

yoo-noh-**prost**'-ohn
eye-seh-**pro**'-pel
(Rescula)

CATEGORY AND SCHEDULE
Pregnancy Risk Category: C

Drug Class: Prostaglandin agonist

MECHANISM OF ACTION
An ophthalmic agent that increases the outflow of aqueous humor. *Therapeutic Effect:* Decreases intraocular pressure.

USES
Indicated for lowering intraocular pressure (IOP) in patients with open-angle glaucoma or ocular hypertension who are intolerant to other medications or who failed to achieve a targeted IOP

PHARMACOKINETICS
Peak response occurs in 4–8 wk. The duration of a single dose is about 10 hr. Hydrolyzed to unoprostone free acid form in the cornea. Rapidly eliminated from plasma. Excreted as metabolites in urine. *Half-life:* 14 min.

INDICATIONS AND DOSAGES
▸ **Glaucoma, Ocular Hypertension**
Ophthalmic
Adults, Elderly. Instill 1 drop in affected eye(s) 2 times a day.

SIDE EFFECTS/ADVERSE REACTIONS
Frequent
Burning, stinging, dry eyes, itching, increased eyelash length and redness
Occasional
Abnormal vision, eyelid disorder, foreign body sensation

PRECAUTIONS AND CONTRAINDICATIONS
Hypersensitivity to unoprostone isopropyl, benzalkonium chloride, or any other component of the formulation
Caution:
Permanent changes in pigmented tissues of eye, bacterial keratitis, do not use while wearing contact lens, no data on use in renal or hepatic failure or pediatric patients

DRUG INTERACTIONS OF CONCERN TO DENTISTRY
• None reported; avoid use of anticholinergic drugs: atropine-like drugs, propantheline, diazepam, other benzodiazepines.

SERIOUS REACTIONS
❗ Elevated IOP occurs rarely.

DENTAL CONSIDERATIONS
General:
• Check compliance of patient with prescribed drug regimen for glaucoma.
• Avoid dental light in patient's eyes; offer dark glasses for patient comfort.
Consultations:
• Medical consultation may be required to assess disease control.

U

ursodiol
your-**soo'**-dee-ol
(Actigall, Urso)

CATEGORY AND SCHEDULE
Pregnancy Risk Category: B

Drug Class: Gallstone
solubilizing agent

MECHANISM OF ACTION
A gallstone solubilizing agent that
suppresses hepatic synthesis and
secretion of cholesterol; inhibits
intestinal absorption of cholesterol.
Therapeutic Effect: Changes the
bile of patients with gallstones from
precipitating (capable of forming
crystals) to cholesterol solubilizing
(capable of being dissolved).

USES
Dissolution of radiolucent,
noncalcified gallbladder stones
(<20 mm in diameter) in which
surgery is not indicated; prevent
gallstones in obese patients
experiencing rapid weight loss

INDICATIONS AND DOSAGES
▶ **Dissolution of Radiolucent,
Noncalcified Gallstones When
Cholecystectomy Is Not
Recommended; Treatment of Biliary
Cirrhosis**
PO
Adults, Elderly. 8–10 mg/kg/day in
2–3 divided doses. Treatment may
require months. Obtain ultrasound
image of gallbladder at 6-mo
intervals for first yr. If gallstones

have dissolved, continue therapy and
repeat ultrasound within 1–3 mo.
▶ **Prevention of Gallstones**
PO
Adults, Elderly. 300 mg twice a day.

SIDE EFFECTS/ADVERSE REACTIONS
Occasional
Diarrhea

PRECAUTIONS AND CONTRAINDICATIONS
Allergy to bile acids, calcified
cholesterol stones, chronic hepatic
disease, radiolucent bile pigment
stones, radiopaque stones
Caution:
Lactation, children

DRUG INTERACTIONS OF CONCERN TO DENTISTRY
• Reduced action: aluminum-based
antacids

SERIOUS REACTIONS
! None significant

DENTAL CONSIDERATIONS
General:
• Consider semisupine chair position
for patient comfort because of GI
effects of disease.
• Some opioids can cause spasm of
bile duct leading to epigastric
distress. Use caution in use for
sedation or pain control. NSAIDs
may be better choice for pain
control.
• Consider drug as a factor in the
diagnosis of altered taste.

U

valacyclovir
val-ah-**sye'**-kloe-ver
(Valtrex)

CATEGORY AND SCHEDULE
Pregnancy Risk Category: B

Drug Class: Antiviral

MECHANISM OF ACTION
A virustatic antiviral that is converted to acyclovir triphosphate, becoming part of the viral DNA chain.
Therapeutic Effect: Interferes with DNA synthesis and replication of herpes simplex virus and varicella-zoster virus, antiviral.

USES
Treatment of herpes zoster in immunocompetent patients, genital herpes, recurrent genital herpes; treatment of herpes labialis

PHARMACOKINETICS
Rapidly absorbed after PO administration. Protein binding: 13%–18%. Rapidly converted by hydrolysis to the active compound acyclovir. Widely distributed to tissues and body fluids (including CSF). Primarily eliminated in urine. Removed by hemodialysis. *Half-life:* 2.5–3.3 hr (increased in impaired renal function).

INDICATIONS AND DOSAGES
▶ **Herpes Zoster (shingles)**
PO
Adults, Elderly. 1 g 3 times a day for 7 days.
▶ **Herpes Simplex (cold sores)**
PO
Adults, Elderly. 2 g twice a day for 1 day.

▶ **Initial Episode of Genital Herpes**
PO
Adults, Elderly. 1 g twice a day for 10 days.
▶ **Recurrent Episodes of Genital Herpes**
PO
Adults, Elderly. 500 mg twice a day for 3 days.
▶ **Prevention of Genital Herpes**
PO
Adults, Elderly. 500–1000 mg/day.
▶ **Dosage in Renal Impairment**
Dosage and frequency are modified on the basis of creatinine clearance.

Creatinine Clearance	Herpes Zoster	Genital Herpes
50 ml/min or higher	1 g q8h	500 mg q12h
30–49 ml/min	1 g q12h	500 mg q12h
10–29 ml/min	1 g q24h	500 mg q24h
Less than 10 ml/min	500 mg q24h	500 mg q24h

SIDE EFFECTS/ADVERSE REACTIONS
Frequent
Herpes zoster: Nausea, headache
Genital herpes: Headache
Occasional
Herpes zoster: Vomiting, diarrhea, constipation (50 yr and older), asthenia, dizziness (50 yr and older)
Genital herpes: Nausea, diarrhea, dizziness
Rare
Herpes zoster: Abdominal pain, anorexia
Genital herpes: Asthenia, abdominal pain

PRECAUTIONS AND CONTRAINDICATIONS
Hypersensitivity to or intolerance of acyclovir, valacyclovir, or their components

V

Caution:
Renal impairment, lactation, children; reduce dose in renal impairment

DRUG INTERACTIONS OF CONCERN TO DENTISTRY
• None reported in otherwise uncompromised patients

SERIOUS REACTIONS
! None known

DENTAL CONSIDERATIONS
General:
• Determine why the patient is taking the drug.
• Be aware of general discomfort associated with shingles; acute symptoms may preclude patient's routine dental visit or mandate short appointments.
• Patients on chronic drug therapy may rarely have symptoms of blood dyscrasias, which can include infection, bleeding, and poor healing.
Consultations:
• Medical consultation may be required to assess disease control.
• In a patient with symptoms of blood dyscrasias, request a medical consultation for blood studies and postpone dental treatment until normal values are reestablished.
Teach Patient/Family to:
• Encourage effective oral hygiene to prevent soft tissue inflammation.
• Use caution to prevent trauma when using oral hygiene aids.

valganciclovir hydrochloride
val-gan-**sye′**-kloh-veer
high-droh-**klor′**-ide
(Valcyte)

CATEGORY AND SCHEDULE
Pregnancy Risk Category: C

Drug Class: Antiviral

MECHANISM OF ACTION
A synthetic nucleoside that competes with viral DNA esterases and is incorporated directly into growing viral DNA chains.
Therapeutic Effect: Interferes with DNA synthesis and viral replication.

USES
Treatment of cytomegalovirus (CMV) retinitis in patients with AIDS

PHARMACOKINETICS
Well absorbed and rapidly converted to ganciclovir by intestinal and hepatic enzymes. Widely distributed. Slowly metabolized intracellularly. Primarily excreted unchanged in urine. Removed by hemodialysis.
Half-life: 18 hr (increased in impaired renal function).

INDICATIONS AND DOSAGES
▶ **CMV Retinitis in Patients with Normal Renal Function**
PO
Adults. Initially, 900 mg (two 450-mg tablets) twice a day for 21 days. Maintenance: 900 mg once a day.
▶ **Prevention of CMV after Transplant**
PO
Adults, Elderly. 900 mg once a day beginning within 10 days of

transplant and continuing until 100 days posttransplant.

▸ **Dosage in Renal Impairment**

Dosage and frequency are modified on the basis of creatinine clearance.

Creatinine Clearance	Induction Dosage	Maintenance Dosage
60 ml/min or more	900 mg twice a day	900 mg once a day
40–59 ml/min	450 mg twice a day	450 mg once a day
25–36 ml/min	450 mg once a day	450 mg every 2 days
10–24 ml/min	450 mg every 2 days	450 mg twice a wk

PRECAUTIONS AND CONTRAINDICATIONS

Hypersensitivity to acyclovir or ganciclovir

Caution:

Renal impairment (requires dose adjustment), preexisting cytopenias, cannot be substituted for ganciclovir capsules on a one-to-one basis, patients older than 65 yr, pediatric use

DRUG INTERACTIONS OF CONCERN TO DENTISTRY

• Increased risk of blood dyscrasias: dapsone, carbamazepine, phenothiazines
• Increased risk of seizures: imipenem/cilastatin (Primaxin)
• Low platelet counts may prevent the use of aspirin, NSAIDs

SERIOUS REACTIONS

! Hematologic toxicity including severe neutropenia (most common), anemia, and thrombocytopenia may occur.

! Retinal detachment occurs rarely.
! An overdose may result in renal toxicity.
! Valganciclovir may decrease sperm production and fertility.

DENTAL CONSIDERATIONS

General:
• Patients on chronic drug therapy may rarely have symptoms of blood dyscrasias, which can include infection, bleeding, and poor healing.
• Examine for oral manifestation of opportunistic infection.
• Place on frequent recall to evaluate healing response.
• Consider local hemostasis measures to control excessive bleeding.

Consultations:
• Medical consultation for blood studies (CBC); leukopenic or thrombocytopenic side effects may result in infection, delayed healing, and excessive bleeding. Postpone elective dental treatment until normal values are maintained.
• Medical consultation may be required to assess disease control.

Teach Patient/Family to:
• Prevent trauma when using oral hygiene aids.
• See dentist immediately if signs of secondary oral infection occur.
• Encourage effective oral hygiene to prevent soft tissue inflammation.

V

valproic acid/ valproate sodium/ divalproex sodium

val-pro'-ick
valproic acid
(Depakene)
valproate sodium
(Depakene syrup, Epilim[AUS]
Valpro[AUS])
divalproex sodium
(Depacon, Depakote, Depakote
ER, Depakote Sprinkle)

CATEGORY AND SCHEDULE
Pregnancy Risk Category: D

Drug Class: Anticonvulsant

MECHANISM OF ACTION
An anticonvulsant, antimanic, and antimigraine agent that directly increases concentration of the inhibitory neurotransmitter gamma-aminobutyric acid.
Therapeutic Effect: Reduces seizure activity.

USES
Treatment of simple, complex (petit mal) absence, mixed seizures; divalproex for manic episodes in bipolar disorder, complex partial seizures, migraine prophylaxis; unapproved: tonic-clonic (grand mal) seizures

PHARMACOKINETICS
Well absorbed from the GI tract. Protein binding: 80%–90%. Metabolized in the liver. Primarily excreted in urine. Not removed by hemodialysis. *Half-life:* 6–16 hr (may be increased in hepatic impairment, the elderly, and children younger than 18 mo).

INDICATIONS AND DOSAGES
▸ **Seizures**
PO
Adults, Elderly, Children 10 yr and older. Initially, 10–15 mg/kg/day in 1–3 divided doses. May increase by 5–10 mg/kg/day at weekly intervals up to 30–60 mg/kg/day. Usual adult dosage: 1000–2500 mg/day.
IV
Adults, Elderly, Children. Same as oral dose but given q6h.
▸ **Manic Episodes**
PO
Adults, Elderly. Initially, 750 mg/day in divided doses. Maximum: 60 mg/kg/day.
▸ **Prevention of Migraine Headaches**
PO (Extended Release)
Adults, Elderly. Initially, 500 mg/day for 7 days. May increase up to 1000 mg/day.
PO (Delayed Release)
Adults, Elderly. Initially, 250 mg twice a day. May increase up to 1000 mg/day.

SIDE EFFECTS/ADVERSE REACTIONS
Frequent
Epilepsy: Abdominal pain, irregular menses, diarrhea, transient alopecia, indigestion, nausea, vomiting, tremors, weight gain or loss
Mania: Nausea, somnolence
Occasional
Epilepsy: Constipation, dizziness, drowsiness, headache, skin rash, unusual excitement, restlessness
Mania: Asthenia, abdominal pain, dyspepsia (heartburn, indigestion, epigastric distress), rash
Rare
Epilepsy: Mood changes, diplopia, nystagmus, spots before eyes, unusual bleeding or ecchymosis

V

PRECAUTIONS AND CONTRAINDICATIONS

Active hepatic disease
Caution:
MI (recovery phase), hepatic disease, renal disease, Addison's disease, pancreatitis, lactation, children younger than 2 yr have higher risk for hepatotoxicity, urea cycle disorders, thrombocytopenia, acute head injury

DRUG INTERACTIONS OF CONCERN TO DENTISTRY

• Increased effects: CNS depressants; carbamazepine, phenobarbital levels may be increased; phenothiazines can lower the seizure threshold
• Increased bleeding and toxicity: salicylates, NSAIDs
• Increased blood levels: erythromycin
• Increased serum levels of amitriptyline, nortriptyline (start with low dose and monitor)
• Decreased effects of diazepam

SERIOUS REACTIONS

! Hepatotoxicity may occur, particularly in the first 6 months of valproic acid therapy. It may be preceded by loss of seizure control, malaise, weakness, lethargy, anorexia, and vomiting rather than abnormal serum liver function test results. Blood dyscrasias may occur.

DENTAL CONSIDERATIONS

General:
• Patients on chronic drug therapy may rarely have symptoms of blood dyscrasias, which can include infection, bleeding, and poor healing.
• Evaluate for clotting ability during gingival instrumentation because

inhibition of platelet aggregation may occur.
• Consider semisupine chair position for patient comfort if GI side effects occur.
• Place on frequent recall if gingival overgrowth occurs.
• Ask about type of epilepsy, seizure frequency, and quality of seizure control.
Consultations:
• In a patient with symptoms of blood dyscrasias, request a medical consultation for blood studies and postpone dental treatment until normal values are reestablished.
• Medical consultation may be required to assess disease control.
Teach Patient/Family to:
• Encourage effective oral hygiene to prevent soft tissue inflammation and minimize gingival overgrowth.
• Use caution to prevent injury when using oral hygiene aids.
• Use powered tooth brush if patient has difficulty holding conventional devices.
• Schedule frequent oral prophylaxis if gingival overgrowth occurs.
• Report oral lesions, soreness, or bleeding to dentist.

valrubicin

val-**rue**′-bih-sin
(VaHaxan[CAN], Valstar)
Do not confuse valrubicin with valsartan.

CATEGORY AND SCHEDULE

Pregnancy Risk Category: C

Drug Class: Antineoplastic

MECHANISM OF ACTION

An anthracycline antibiotic that inhibits incorporation of nucleosides

V

into nucleic acids after penetrating cells.

Therapeutic Effect: Causes chromosomal damage, arresting cells in the G_2 phase of cell division, and interferes with DNA synthesis.

USES

Treatment of bladder cancer

PHARMACOKINETICS

Concentrated in bladder wall; not absorbed into circulation. Excreted in urine.

INDICATIONS AND DOSAGES

▶ **Bladder Cancer**

Intravesical

Adults, Elderly. 800 mg once weekly for 6 wk.

SIDE EFFECTS/ADVERSE REACTIONS

Frequent

Local intravesical reaction: Local bladder symptoms, urinary frequency or urgency, dysuria, hematuria, bladder pain, cystitis, bladder spasms

Systemic: Abdominal pain, nausea, UTI

Occasional

Local intravesical reaction: Nocturia, local burning, urethral pain, pelvic pain, gross hematuria

Systemic: Diarrhea, vomiting, urine retention, microscopic hematuria, asthenia, headache, malaise, back pain, chest pain, dizziness, rash, anemia, fever, vasodilation

Rare

Systemic: Flatus, peripheral edema, hyperglycemia, pneumonia, myalgia

PRECAUTIONS AND CONTRAINDICATIONS

Perforated bladder, sensitivity to valrubicin, severe irritated bladder, small bladder capacity, UTI

DRUG INTERACTIONS OF CONCERN TO DENTISTRY

• None reported

SERIOUS REACTIONS

! Serious systemic toxicity if bladder wall perforated

DENTAL CONSIDERATIONS

General:

• If additional analgesia is required for dental pain, consider alternative analgesics (NSAIDs) in patients taking narcotics for acute or chronic pain.

• This drug may be used in the hospital or on an outpatient basis. Confirm the patient's disease and treatment status.

• Offer patient frequent breaks if urinary frequency is a concern.

• Avoid prescribing drugs that could cause urinary retention, such as drugs with anticholinergic activity.

Consultations:

• Medical consultation may be required to assess disease control and patient's ability to tolerate stress.

Teach Patient/Family to:

• Encourage effective oral hygiene to prevent soft tissue inflammation.

• Update health and medication history if physician makes any changes in evaluation or drug regimens; include OTC, herbal, and nonherbal remedies in the update.

valsartan
val-**sar**′-tan
(Diovan)
Do not confuse valsartan with
Valstan.

CATEGORY AND SCHEDULE
Pregnancy Risk Category: C (D if
used in second or third trimester)

Drug Class: Angiotensin II
receptor (AT1) antagonist

MECHANISM OF ACTION
An angiotensin II receptor, type AT_1,
antagonist that blocks
vasoconstrictor and aldosterone-
secreting effects of angiotensin II,
inhibiting the binding of angiotensin
II to the AT_1 receptors.
Therapeutic Effect: Causes
vasodilation, decreases peripheral
resistance, and decreases B/P.

USES
Treatment of hypertension as a
single drug or in combination with
other antihypertensive medications,
heart failure

PHARMACOKINETICS
Poorly absorbed after PO
administration. Food decreases peak
plasma concentration. Protein
binding: 95%. Metabolized in the
liver. Recovered primarily in feces
and, to a lesser extent, in urine.
Unknown if removed by
hemodialysis. *Half-life:* 6 hr.

INDICATIONS AND DOSAGES
▸ **Hypertension**
PO
Adults, Elderly. Initially, 80–160 mg/
day in patients who are not volume
depleted. May increase up to a
maximum of 320 mg/day.

▸ **CHF**
PO
Adults, Elderly. Initially, 40 mg
twice a day. May increase up to
160 mg twice a day. Maximum:
320 mg/day.

SIDE EFFECTS/ADVERSE REACTIONS
Rare
Insomnia, fatigue, heartburn,
abdominal pain, dizziness, headache,
diarrhea, nausea, vomiting,
arthralgia, edema

PRECAUTIONS AND CONTRAINDICATIONS
Bilateral renal artery stenosis,
biliary cirrhosis or obstruction,
hypoaldosteronism, severe hepatic
impairment
Caution:
Volume depletion, less effect in
African Americans, liver
impairment, lactation, children
younger than 18 yr, elevated labs for
liver function, BUN, and potassium

DRUG INTERACTIONS OF CONCERN TO DENTISTRY
• Possible reduction in effect:
ketoconazole

SERIOUS REACTIONS
! Overdosage may manifest as
hypotension and tachycardia.
Bradycardia occurs less often. Viral
infection and upper respiratory tract
infection (cough, pharyngitis,
sinusitis, rhinitis) occur rarely.

DENTAL CONSIDERATIONS
General:
• Monitor vital signs at every
appointment because of
cardiovascular side effects.
• Limit use of sodium-containing
products, such as saline IV fluids,

V

for patients with a dietary salt restriction.

• Stress from dental procedures may compromise cardiovascular function; determine patient risk.

• Short appointments and a stress-reduction protocol may be required for anxious patients.

• Use precaution if sedation or general anesthesia is required; risk of hypotensive episode.

Consultations:

• Medical consultation may be required to assess disease control and patient's ability to tolerate stress.

vancomycin hydrochloride

van-koe-**mye'**-sin
high-droh-**klor'**-ide
(Vancocin, Vancocin CP[AUS], Vancocin HCl Pulvules[AUS])

CATEGORY AND SCHEDULE
Pregnancy Risk Category: B

Drug Class: Glycopeptide-type antiinfective

MECHANISM OF ACTION
A tricyclic glycopeptide antibiotic that binds to bacterial cell walls, altering cell membrane permeability and inhibiting RNA synthesis. **Therapeutic Effect:** Bactericidal.

USES
Treatment of resistant staphylococcal infections, pseudomembranous colitis, staphylococcal enterocolitis, endocarditis

PHARMACOKINETICS
PO: Poorly absorbed from the GI tract. Primarily eliminated in feces.

Parenteral: Widely distributed. Protein binding: 55%. Primarily excreted unchanged in urine. Not removed by hemodialysis. **Half-life:** 4–11 hr (increased in impaired renal function).

INDICATIONS AND DOSAGES
▸ **Treatment of Bone, Respiratory Tract, Skin, and Soft Tissue Infections; Endocarditis, Peritonitis, and Septicemia; Prevention of Bacterial Endocarditis in Those at Risk (If Penicillin Is Contraindicated) When Undergoing Biliary, Dental, GI, GU, or Respiratory Surgery or Invasive Procedures**
IV
Adults, Elderly. 500 mg q6h or 1 g q12h.
Children older than 1 mo. 40 mg/kg/day in divided doses q6–8h.
Maximum: 3–4 g/day.
Neonates. Initially, 15 mg/kg, then 10 mg/kg q8–12h.
▸ **Staphylococcal Enterocolitis, Antibiotic-Associated Pseudomembranous Colitis Caused by *Clostridium Difficile***
PO
Adults, Elderly. 0.5–2 g/day in 3–4 divided doses for 7–10 days.
Children. 40 mg/kg/day in 3–4 divided doses for 7–10 days.
Maximum: 2 g/day.
▸ **Dosage in Renal Impairment**
After a loading dose, subsequent dosages and frequency are modified on the basis of creatinine clearance, the severity of the infection, and the serum concentration of the drug.

SIDE EFFECTS/ADVERSE REACTIONS
Frequent
PO: Bitter or unpleasant taste, nausea, vomiting, mouth irritation (with oral solution)

Rare
Parenteral: Phlebitis,
thrombophlebitis, or pain at
peripheral IV site; dizziness;
vertigo; tinnitus; chills; fever; rash;
necrosis with extravasation
PO: Rash

PRECAUTIONS AND CONTRAINDICATIONS
Hypersensitivity, decreased hearing
Caution:
Renal disease, lactation, elderly

DRUG INTERACTIONS OF CONCERN TO DENTISTRY
• Ototoxicity or nephrotoxicity:
aminoglycosides and high-dose
salicylates
• Increased effects of
nondepolarizing muscle relaxants

SERIOUS REACTIONS
! Nephrotoxicity and ototoxicity
may occur. "Red-neck" syndrome
(redness on face, neck, arms, and
back; chills; fever; tachycardia;
nausea or vomiting; pruritus; rash;
unpleasant taste) may result from
too-rapid injection.

DENTAL CONSIDERATIONS
General:
• Monitor vital signs at every
appointment because of
cardiovascular side effects.
• Administer IV slowly over 1 hr;
administration that is too rapid can
lead to a fall in B/P (monitor) and a
red rash on the face, neck, and chest
caused by local histamine release.
No specific treatment is required for
this reaction; evaluate recovery
progress.
• Determine why the patient is
taking the drug.
Consultations:
• Medical consultation may be
required to assess disease control.

vardenafil
var-**den**′-ah-fill
(Levitra)
Do not confuse Levitra with
Lexiva.

CATEGORY AND SCHEDULE
Pregnancy Risk Category: B

Drug Class: Impotence therapy

MECHANISM OF ACTION
An erectile dysfunction agent that
inhibits phosphodiesterase type 5,
the enzyme responsible for
degrading cyclic guanosine
monophosphate in the corpus
cavernosum of the penis, resulting in
smooth muscle relaxation and
increased blood flow.
Therapeutic Effect: Facilitates an
erection.

USES
Treatment of male erectile
dysfunction

PHARMACOKINETICS
Rapidly absorbed after PO
administration. Extensive tissue
distribution. Protein binding: 95%.
Metabolized in the liver. Excreted
primarily in feces; a lesser amount
eliminated in urine. Drug has no
effect on penile blood flow without
sexual stimulation. **Half-life:** 4–5 hr.

INDICATIONS AND DOSAGES
▸ Erectile Dysfunction
PO
Adults. 10 mg approximately 1 hr
before sexual activity. Dose may be
increased to 20 mg or decreased to
5 mg, based on patient tolerance.
Maximum dosing frequency is once
daily.
Elderly, older than 65 yr. 5 mg.

▸ **Dosage in Moderate Hepatic Impairment**
PO
For patients with Child-Pugh class B hepatic impairment. 5 mg 60 min before sexual activity.
▸ **Dosage with Concurrent Ritonavir**
PO
Adults. 2.5 mg in a 72-hr period.
▸ **Dosage with Concurrent Ketoconazole or Itraconazole (at 400 mg/day), or Indinavir**
PO
Adults. 2.5 mg in a 24-hr period.
▸ **Dosage with Concurrent Ketoconazole or Itraconazole (at 200 mg/day), or Erythromycin**
PO
Adults. 5 mg in a 24-hr period.

SIDE EFFECTS/ADVERSE REACTIONS
Occasional
Headache, flushing, rhinitis, indigestion
Rare
Dizziness, changes in color vision, blurred vision

PRECAUTIONS AND CONTRAINDICATIONS
Concurrent use of α-adrenergic blockers, sodium nitroprusside, or nitrates in any form
Caution:
Men with cardiovascular disease in whom sexual activity is not recommended, left ventricular outflow destruction, vasodilator effects on B/P, strong inhibitors of CYP3A4 isoenzymes, anatomic deformation of penis, not approved for use in women or children

DRUG INTERACTIONS OF CONCERN TO DENTISTRY
• Dose adjustments caused by potential drug interactions—do not

exceed the maximum single dose of 2.5 mg in a 72-hr period: ritonavir
• Do not exceed 2.5 mg in a 24-hr period: indinavir, ketoconazole (400 mg), itraconazole (400 mg)
• Do not exceed 5 mg in a 24-hr period: ketoconazole (200 mg), itraconazole (200 mg), erythromycin
• Increased plasma levels: drugs that are potent inhibitors of CYP3A4 isoenzymes (e.g., erythromycin, ketoconazole)
• Avoid nitroglycerin within a 24-hr period

SERIOUS REACTIONS
! Prolonged erections (lasting longer than 4 hr) and priapism (painful erections lasting longer than 6 hr) occur rarely.

DENTAL CONSIDERATIONS
General:
• This is an acute-use drug intended to be taken just before sexual activity. Be sure to include drug use in medical history and avoid use of potentially interacting drugs or warn patient of the interaction when CYP3A4 isoenzyme inhibitors are required (e.g., clarithromycin, azole antifungals).
• If signs of angina pectoris occur during dental treatment, do not use sublingual nitroglycerin.

varenicline
var-in-**eh**-klin
(Chantix)
Do not confuse with venlafaxine.

CATEGORY AND SCHEDULE
Pregnancy Risk Category: C

Drug Class: Nicotine receptor agonist

MECHANISM OF ACTION
Binds to neuronal nicotinic acetylcholine receptors and blocks nicotine binding, reducing central effects of smoking

USES
Smoking cessation treatment

PHARMACOKINETICS
Well absorbed following oral administration, peak levels in 3–4 hr. Protein binding: 20%. *Half-life:* 24 hr. Excreted primarily unchanged in the urine.

INDICATIONS AND DOSAGES
▸ **Aid to Smoking Cessation**
Adult. PO 0.5 mg per day on days 1–3, PO 0.5 mg twice daily on days 4–7, PO 1 mg twice daily day 8 until end of treatment (up to 24 weeks).

SIDE EFFECTS/ADVERSE REACTIONS
Frequent
Dry mouth, taste alterations, gingivitis, dizziness, headache, insomnia, sleep disturbances, abnormal dreams, anxiety, depression, disturbance in attention, irritability, restlessness, emotional changes, flushing, hypertension, nausea, vomiting, constipation, gastric reflux, flatulence, abnormal liver function test values
Occasional
Epistaxis, respiratory disorders, rhinorrhea, polyuria, menstrual disorders, pruritus, rash, sweating
Rare
Arthralgia, back pain, muscle cramps, myalgia, increased or decreased appetite, chest pain, flu symptoms, edema, fatigue, lethargy, malaise, thirst, weight gain, allergy

PRECAUTIONS AND CONTRAINDICATIONS
Hypersensitivity, nausea, altered metabolism of some drugs due to smoking cessation

DRUG INTERACTIONS OF CONCERN TO DENTISTRY
• None reported

DENTAL CONSIDERATIONS
General:
• Assess salivary flow as a factor in caries, periodontal disease, and candidiasis.
• Take vital signs at every appointment because of cardiovascular side effects.
• Differentiate taste changes due to drug from those associated with restorative materials or preventive aids (e.g., chlorhexidine).
• Consider semisupine chair position to minimize nausea.
• Avoid or use with caution drugs that provoke nausea (e.g., opioids).
Consultations:
• Consult with individual guiding smoking cessation program to assist with compliance and reinforcement of importance of tobacco cessation.
Teach Patient/Family to:
• Avoid mouth rinses with high alcohol content because of drying effect.
• Use home fluoride products to prevent caries.
• Use sugarless gum, frequent sips of water, or saliva substitutes if dry mouth occurs.
Teach Patient/Family to:
• When used in conjunction with a smoking-cessation program in the dental office, be familiar with all aspects of drug use, including drug package insert ("Information for Patients").

V

• Stop smoking 1 wk after beginning drug therapy.

vasopressin
vay-soe-**press**'-in
(Pitressin, Pressyn[CAN])
Do not confuse Pitressin with Pitocin.

CATEGORY AND SCHEDULE
Pregnancy Risk Category: B

Drug Class: Antidiuretic

MECHANISM OF ACTION
A posterior pituitary hormone that increases reabsorption of water by the renal tubules. Increases water permeability at the distal tubule and collecting duct. Directly stimulates smooth muscle in the GI tract.
Therapeutic Effect: Peristalsis and vasoconstriction.

USES
Control of frequent urination, increased thirst, and loss of water associated with diabetes insipidus

PHARMACOKINETICS

Route	Onset	Peak	Duration
IV	N/A	N/A	0.5–1 hr
IM, Subcutaneous	1–2 hr	N/A	2–8 hr

Distributed throughout extracellular fluid. Metabolized in the liver and kidney. Primarily excreted in urine.
Half-life: 10–20 min.

INDICATIONS AND DOSAGES
▸ **Cardiac Arrest**
IV
Adults, Elderly. 40 units as a one-time bolus.

▸ **Diabetes Insipidus**
IV Infusion
Adults, Children. 0.5 m Units/kg/hr. May double dose q30min. Maximum: 10 m Units/kg/hr.
IM, Subcutaneous
Adults, Elderly. 5–10 units 2–4 times a day. Range: 5–60 unit/day.
Children. 2.5–10 units, 2–4 times a day.

▸ **Abdominal Distention, Intestinal Paresis**
IM
Adults, Elderly. Initially, 5 units. Subsequent doses, 10 units q3–4h.

▸ **GI Hemorrhage**
IV Infusion
Adults, Elderly. Initially, 0.2–0.4 unit/min progressively increased to 0.9 unit/min.
Children. 0.002–0.005 unit/kg/min. Titrate as needed. Maximum: 0.01 unit/kg/min.

▸ **Vasodilatory Shock**
IV
Adults, Elderly. Initially, 0.04–0.1 unit/min. Titrate to desired effect.

SIDE EFFECTS/ADVERSE REACTIONS
Frequent
Pain at injection site (with vasopressin tannate)
Occasional
Abdominal cramps, nausea, vomiting, diarrhea, dizziness, diaphoresis, pale skin, circumoral pallor, tremors, headache, eructation, flatulence
Rare
Chest pain; confusion; allergic reaction, including rash or hives, pruritus, wheezing or difficulty breathing, facial and peripheral edema; sterile abscess (with vasopressin tannate)

PRECAUTIONS AND CONTRAINDICATIONS

Hypersensitivity, patients taking nitrates or β-adrenergic blockers, unstable cardiovascular disease, severe hepatic impairment, ESRD, degenerative retinal disorders Men with cardiovascular disease in whom sexual activity is not recommended, left ventricular outflow destruction, vasodilator effects on B/P, strong inhibitors of CYP3A4 isoenzymes, anatomic deformation of penis, not approved for use in women or children

DRUG INTERACTIONS OF CONCERN TO DENTISTRY

• Decreased effects: demeclocycline, alcohol
• Increased effects: carbamazepine

SERIOUS REACTIONS

! Anaphylaxis, MI, and water intoxication have occurred. The elderly and very young are at higher risk for water intoxication.

DENTAL CONSIDERATIONS

General:
• Normally for acute use in the hospital or emergency department setting.
• Determine why patient is taking the drug.
Consultations:
• Medical consultation may be required to assess disease control and patient's ability to tolerate stress.

venlafaxine
ven-la-**fax**′-een
(Effexor, Effexor XR)

CATEGORY AND SCHEDULE
Pregnancy Risk Category: C

Drug Class: Bicyclic antidepressant

MECHANISM OF ACTION

A phenethylamine derivative that potentiates CNS neurotransmitter activity by inhibiting the reuptake of serotonin, norepinephrine and, to a lesser degree, dopamine.
Therapeutic Effect: Relieves depression.

USES

Treatment of depression, prevention of major depressive disorder relapse; generalized anxiety disorder (XR product only)

PHARMACOKINETICS

Well absorbed from the GI tract. Protein binding: 25%–30%. Metabolized in the liver to active metabolite. Primarily excreted in urine. Not removed by hemodialysis. **Half-life:** 3–7 hr; metabolite, 9–13 hr (increased in hepatic or renal impairment).

INDICATIONS AND DOSAGES
▶ Depression
PO
Adults, Elderly. Initially, 75 mg/day in 2–3 divided doses with food. May increase by 75 mg/day at intervals of 4 days or longer. Maximum: 375 mg/day in 3 divided doses.
PO (Extended-Release)
Adults, Elderly. 75 mg/day as a single dose with food. May increase

V

by 75 mg/day at intervals of 4 days or longer. Maximum: 225 mg/day.

▸ **Anxiety Disorder**
PO (Extended-Release)
Adults. 37.5–225 mg/day.

▸ **Dosage in Renal and Hepatic Impairment**
Expect to decrease venlafaxine dosage by 50% in patients with moderate hepatic impairment, 25% in patients with mild to moderate renal impairment, and 50% in patients on dialysis (withhold dose until completion of dialysis).

SIDE EFFECTS/ADVERSE REACTIONS

Frequent
Nausea, somnolence, headache, dry mouth

Occasional
Dizziness, insomnia, constipation, diaphoresis, nervousness, asthenia, ejaculatory disturbance, anorexia

Rare
Anxiety, blurred vision, diarrhea, vomiting, tremor, abnormal dreams, impotence

PRECAUTIONS AND CONTRAINDICATIONS

Use within 14 days of MAOIs
Caution:
Lactation, children younger than 18 yr, sustained hypertension with use, renal or hepatic impairment, elderly, long-term use (longer than 4–6 wk), history of seizures, suicidal patients, mania, hyperthyroidism, impairment of driving, avoid use of alcohol

DRUG INTERACTIONS OF CONCERN TO DENTISTRY

• None reported; however, because this drug is similar in action to other antidepressants, it would be wise to avoid excessive amounts of

vasoconstrictors, especially in gingival retraction cords.
• Increased CNS depression: all CNS depressants
• Risk of serotonin syndrome: St. John's wort (herb)

SERIOUS REACTIONS

❗ A sustained increase in diastolic B/P of 10–15 mm Hg occurs occasionally.

DENTAL CONSIDERATIONS

General:
• Monitor vital signs at every appointment because of cardiovascular side effects.
• After supine positioning, have patient sit upright for at least 2 min before standing to avoid orthostatic hypotension.
• Assess salivary flow as a factor in caries, periodontal disease, and candidiasis.
• Examine for evidence of oral manifestations of blood dyscrasias (infection, bleeding, poor healing).
• Place on frequent recall to evaluate healing response.
• Consider semisupine chair position for patient comfort because of GI effects of disease.
Consultations:
• Medical consultation may be required to assess disease control.
• Physician should be informed if significant xerostomic side effects occur (e.g., increased caries, sore tongue, problems eating or swallowing, difficulty wearing prosthesis) so that a medication change can be considered.
• Obtain a medical consultation for blood studies (CBC) because leukopenic or thrombocytopenic side effects may result in infection, delayed healing, and excessive bleeding. Postpone elective dental

treatment until normal values are maintained.

Teach Patient/Family to:
• Encourage effective oral hygiene to prevent soft tissue inflammation.
• Use caution to prevent injury when using oral hygiene aids.
• When chronic dry mouth occurs, advise patient to:
 • Avoid mouth rinses with high alcohol content because of drying effects.
 • Use home fluoride products daily to prevent caries.
 • Use sugarless gum, frequent sips of water, or saliva substitutes.

verapamil hydrochloride

ver-**ap′**-ah-mill
high-droh-**klor′**-ide
(Anpec[AUS], Apo-Verap[CAN], Calan, Calan SR, Chronovera[CAN], Cordilox SR[AUS], Covera-HS, Isoptin[AUS], Isoptin SR, Novo-Veramil[CAN], Novo-Veramil SR[CAN], Veracaps SR[AUS], Verahexal[AUS], Verelan, Verelan PM)
Do not confuse Isoptin with Intropin, or Verelan with Virilon, Vivarin, or Voltaren.

CATEGORY AND SCHEDULE
Pregnancy Risk Category: C

Drug Class: Calcium channel blocker

MECHANISM OF ACTION
A calcium channel blocker and antianginal, antiarrhythmic, and antihypertensive agent that inhibits calcium ion entry across cardiac and vascular smooth-muscle cell membranes. This action causes the dilation of coronary arteries, peripheral arteries, and arterioles. *Therapeutic Effect:* Decreases heart rate and myocardial contractility and slows SA and AV conduction. Decreases total peripheral vascular resistance by vasodilation.

USES
Treatment of chronic stable angina pectoris, vasospastic angina, dysrhythmias (class IV), hypertension; unapproved: migraine headache, cardiomyopathy

PHARMACOKINETICS

Route	Onset	Peak	Duration
PO	30 min	1–2 hr	6–8 hr
PO (extended release)	30 min	N/A	N/A
IV	1–2 min	3–5 min	10–60 min

Well absorbed from the GI tract. Protein binding: 90% (60% in neonates). Undergoes first-pass metabolism in the liver to active metabolite. Primarily excreted in urine. Not removed by hemodialysis. *Half-life:* 2–8 hr.

INDICATIONS AND DOSAGES
▸ **Supraventricular Tachyarrhythmias, Temporary Control of Rapid Ventricular Rate with Atrial Fibrillation or Flutter**
IV
Adults, Elderly. Initially, 5–10 mg; repeat in 30 min with 10-mg dose. *Children 1–15 yr.* 0.1 mg/kg. May repeat in 30 min up to a maximum second dose of 10 mg. Not recommended in children younger than 1 yr.

V

▸ **Arrhythmias, Including Prevention of Recurrent Paroxysmal Supraventricular Tachycardia and Control of Ventricular Resting Rate in Chronic Atrial Fibrillation or Flutter (with Digoxin)**
PO
Adults, Elderly. 240–480 mg/day in 3–4 divided doses.

▸ **Vasospastic Angina (Prinzmetal's Variant), Unstable (Crescendo or Preinfarction) Angina, Chronic Stable (Effort-Associated) Angina**
PO
Adults. Initially, 80–120 mg 3 times a day. For elderly patients and those with hepatic dysfunction, 40 mg 3 times a day. Titrate to optimal dose. Maintenance: 240–480 mg/day in 3–4 divided doses.
PO (Covera-HS)
Adults, Elderly. 180–480 mg/day at bedtime.

▸ **Hypertension**
PO
Adults, Elderly. Initially, 40–80 mg 3 times a day. Maintenance: 480 mg or less a day.
PO (Covera-HS)
Adults, Elderly. 180–480 mg/day at bedtime.
PO (Extended-Release)
Adults, Elderly. 120–240 mg/day. May give 480 mg or less a day in 2 divided doses.
PO (Verelan PM)
Adults, Elderly. 100–300 mg/day.

SIDE EFFECTS/ADVERSE REACTIONS
Frequent
Constipation
Occasional
Dizziness, light-headedness, headache, asthenia (loss of strength, energy), nausea, peripheral edema, hypotension, possible gingival enlargement

Rare
Bradycardia, dermatitis, or rash

PRECAUTIONS AND CONTRAINDICATIONS
Atrial fibrillation or flutter and an accessory bypass tract, cardiogenic shock, heart block, sinus bradycardia, ventricular tachycardia
Caution:
CHF, hypotension, hepatic injury, lactation, children, renal disease, concomitant blocker therapy

DRUG INTERACTIONS OF CONCERN TO DENTISTRY
• Decreased effect: indomethacin, possibly other NSAIDs, phenobarbital
• Increased effect: parenteral and inhalation general anesthetics or other drugs with hypotensive actions, benzodiazepines
• Increased effects of nondepolarizing muscle relaxants
• Increased effects of carbamazepine
• Caution in use of strong inhibitors of CYP3A4 isoenzymes, e.g., itraconazole

SERIOUS REACTIONS
! Rapid ventricular rate in atrial flutter or fibrillation, marked hypotension, extreme bradycardia, CHF, asystole, and second- and third-degree AV block occur rarely.

DENTAL CONSIDERATIONS
General:
• Monitor cardiac status; take vital signs at every appointment because of cardiovascular side effects. Consider a stress-reduction protocol to prevent angina during the dental appointment.

• After supine positioning, have patient sit upright for at least 2 min before standing to avoid orthostatic hypotension.

• Place on frequent recall to monitor gingival condition for possible enlargement.

• Limit use of sodium-containing products, such as saline IV fluids, for patients with a dietary salt restriction.

• Assess salivary flow as a factor in caries, periodontal disease, and candidiasis.

• Use vasoconstrictors with caution, in low doses, and with careful aspiration. Avoid use of gingival retraction cord with epinephrine.

Consultations:

• In a patient with symptoms of blood dyscrasias, request a medical consultation for blood studies and postpone dental treatment until normal values are reestablished.

• Medical consultation may be required to assess disease control and patient's ability to tolerate stress.

Teach Patient/Family to:

• Encourage effective oral hygiene to prevent soft tissue inflammation and minimize gingival overgrowth.

• Schedule frequent oral prophylaxis if gingival overgrowth occurs.

• When chronic dry mouth occurs, advise patient to:

  • Avoid mouth rinses with high alcohol content because of drying effects.

  • Use daily home fluoride products to prevent caries.

  • Use sugarless gum, frequent sips of water, or saliva substitutes.

vidarabine
vye-**dare**'-ah-been
(Ara-A, Vira-A)
Do not confuse with Zostrix.

CATEGORY AND SCHEDULE
Pregnancy Risk Category: C

Drug Class: Antiviral

MECHANISM OF ACTION
An antiviral agent that appears to interfere with viral DNS synthesis. *Therapeutic Effect:* Regenerates corneal epithelium.

USES
Treatment of keratoconjunctivitis caused by human herpes virus, recurrent epithelial keratitis

PHARMACOKINETICS
None reported

INDICATIONS AND DOSAGES
▸ **Treatment of Keratitis, Keratoconjunctivitis Caused by Human Herpes Virus, Types 1 and 2**
Ophthalmic
Adults, Elderly. Apply 0.5 inch into lower conjunctival sac 5 times a day at 3-hr intervals. After reepithelialization, treat for additional 7 days at dosage of 2 times a day.

SIDE EFFECTS/ADVERSE REACTIONS
Frequent
Burning, itching, irritation
Occasional
Foreign body sensation, tearing, sensitivity to light, pain, photophobia

V

PRECAUTIONS AND CONTRAINDICATIONS

Hypersensitivity to vidarabine or any component of the formulation
Caution:
Antibiotic hypersensitivity

DRUG INTERACTIONS OF CONCERN TO DENTISTRY

• None reported

SERIOUS REACTIONS

! None significant

DENTAL CONSIDERATIONS

General:
• Avoid dental light in patient's eyes; offer dark glasses for patient comfort.
Teach Patient/Family to:
• Seek evaluation if healing has not occurred in 7–10 days.

vigabatrin
vig-ah-**bat**-trin
Sabril
Do not confuse with Vigamox.

CATEGORY AND SCHEDULE
Pregnancy Risk Category: C

Drug Class: Anticonvulsant

MECHANISM OF ACTION

An anticonvulsant whose exact mechanism is unknown but may be the result of increased levels of gamma-aminobutyric acid (GABA). Vigabatrin irreversibly inhibits GABA transaminase, the enzyme responsible for GABA inactivation.

USES

Adjunctive therapy of refractory complex partial seizures in adults

for whom the potential benefits outweigh the risk of vision loss

PHARMACOKINETICS

Extensively absorbed following oral administration (100%), can be taken with food. Peak plasma concentrations reached in 1 hr, widely distributed. Does not bind to plasma proteins. Undergoes hepatic metabolism (CYP 2C19). *Half-life:* 7.5 hr. Excreted primarily (65%) by the kidneys as unchanged drug.

INDICATIONS AND DOSAGES
▸ Partial-Onset Seizures
Adult. PO 500 mg twice daily initially, may be increased by 500 mg/day, up to 2–4 g/day, based on response and tolerability

SIDE EFFECTS/ADVERSE REACTIONS

Frequent
Permanent vision loss, headache, fatigue, somnolence, nystagmus, tremor, blurred vision, memory loss, weight gain, arthralgia, abnormal coordination, confusion
Occasional
Cough

PRECAUTIONS AND CONTRAINDICATIONS

Progressive and permanent bilateral visual field constriction and reduced visual acuity (30% or more of patients, ranging in severity from mild to severe)
Increased risk of suicidal thoughts and behavior

DRUG INTERACTIONS OF CONCERN TO DENTISTRY

• None reported

SERIOUS REACTIONS

! Hypersensitivity, loss of vision

DENTAL CONSIDERATIONS

General:
• Early-morning appointments and stress-reduction protocol may be needed for anxious patients.
• Be prepared to manage seizures and/or nausea.
• After supine positioning, allow patient to sit upright for 2 min to avoid occurrence of dizziness.
• Do not interrupt drug therapy (requires gradual discontinuation by physician).

Consultations:
• Consult with physician to determine seizure control and ability to tolerate dental procedures.

Teach Patient/Family to:
• Update medical and drug history when physician determines change in disease status or alters drug regimen.
• Report changes in vision.

vinblastine sulfate
vin-**blass**'-teen **sull**'-fate
(Oncovin[AUS], Velban, Velbe[AUS])
Do not confuse vinblastine with vincristine or vinorelbine.

CATEGORY AND SCHEDULE
Pregnancy Risk Category: D

Drug Class: Antineoplastic

MECHANISM OF ACTION
A vinca alkaloid that binds to microtubular protein of mitotic spindle, causing metaphase arrest. *Therapeutic Effect:* Inhibits cell division.

USES
Treatment of certain kinds of cancer, including lymphoma and cancer of the breast or testicles

PHARMACOKINETICS
Does not cross the blood-brain barrier. Protein binding: 75%. Metabolized in the liver to active metabolite. Primarily eliminated in feces by biliary system. *Half-life:* 24.8 hr.

INDICATIONS AND DOSAGES
▶ **Remission Induction in Advanced Testicular Carcinoma, Advanced Mycosis Fungoides, Breast Carcinoma, Choriocarcinoma, Disseminated Hodgkin's Disease, Non-Hodgkin's Lymphoma, Kaposi's Sarcoma (KS), or Letterer-Siwe Disease**
IV
Adults, Elderly. Initially, 3.7 mg/m^2 as a single dose. Increase dose by about 1.8 mg/m^2 at weekly intervals until desired therapeutic response is attained, WBC count falls below 3000/mm^3, or maximum weekly dose of 18.5 mg/m^2 is reached.
Children. Initially, 2.5 mg/m^2 as a single dose. Increase dose by about 1.25 mg/m^2 at weekly intervals until desired therapeutic response is attained, WBC count falls below 3000/mm^3, or maximum weekly dose of 7.5–12.5 mg/m^2 is reached.
▶ **Maintenance Dose for Treatment of Advanced Testicular Carcinoma, Advanced Mycosis Fungoides, Breast Carcinoma, Choriocarcinoma, Disseminated Hodgkin's Disease, Non-Hodgkin's Lymphoma, KS, or Letterer-Siwe Disease**
IV
Adults, Elderly, Children.
Administer one increment less than dose required to produce WBC count of 3000/mm^3. Each

V

subsequent dose given when WBC count returns to 4000/mm³ and at least 7 days have elapsed since previous dose.

SIDE EFFECTS/ADVERSE REACTIONS

Frequent
Nausea, vomiting, alopecia

Occasional
Constipation or diarrhea, rectal bleeding, headache, paraesthesia (occur 4–6 hr after administration and persist for 2–10 hr); malaise; asthenia; dizziness; pain at tumor site; jaw or face pain; depression; dry mouth

Rare
Dermatitis, stomatitis, phototoxicity, hyperuricemia

PRECAUTIONS AND CONTRAINDICATIONS

Bacterial infection, severe leukopenia, significant granulocytopenia (unless it stems from disease being treated)

DRUG INTERACTIONS OF CONCERN TO DENTISTRY

• Suspected increase in metabolism: strong inhibitors of CYP3A4 isoenzymes (erythromycin, clarithromycin, fluconazole, itraconazole, ketoconazole, metronidazole)

SERIOUS REACTIONS

! Hematologic toxicity is manifested as leukopenia and, less commonly, anemia. The WBC count reaches its nadir 4–10 days after initial therapy and recovers within 7–14 days (21 days with high vinblastine dosages). Thrombocytopenia is usually mild and transient, with recovery occurring in a few days. Hepatic insufficiency may increase the risk of toxic drug effects. Acute

shortness of breath or bronchospasm may occur, particularly when vinblastine is administered concurrently with mitomycin.

DENTAL CONSIDERATIONS

General:
• If additional analgesia is required for dental pain, consider alternative analgesics (NSAIDs) in patients taking opioids for acute or chronic pain.
• This drug may be used in the hospital or on an outpatient basis. Confirm the patient's disease and treatment status.
• Short appointments and a stress reduction protocol may be required for anxious patients.
• Patient on chronic drug therapy may rarely present with symptoms of blood dyscrasias, which can include infection, bleeding, and poor healing. If dyscrasia is present, caution patient to prevent oral tissue trauma when using oral hygiene aids.
• Examine for oral manifestation of opportunistic infection.
• Palliative medication may be required for management of oral side effects.
• Chlorhexidine mouth rinse prior to and during chemotherapy may reduce severity of mucositis.
• Advise patient if dental drugs prescribed have a potential for photosensitivity.
• Assess salivary flow as a factor in caries, periodontal disease, and candidiasis.
• Patients may have received other chemotherapy and radiation; confirm medical and drug history.
• Patients presenting with KS also may be HIV positive.
• Patients may be at risk for infection.

Consultations:
• Medical consultation may be required to assess immunologic status during cancer chemotherapy and determine safety risk, if any, posed by the required dental treatment.
• Medical consultation may be required to assess disease control and patient's ability to tolerate stress.
• In a patient with symptoms of blood dyscrasias, request a medical consultation for blood studies and postpone treatment until normal values are reestablished.

Teach Patient/Family to:
• Maintain fastidious oral hygiene.
• Encourage effective oral hygiene to prevent soft tissue inflammation.
• Report oral lesions, soreness, or bleeding to dentist.
• Prevent trauma when using oral hygiene aids.
• When chronic dry mouth occurs, advise patient to:
  • Avoid mouth rinses with high alcohol content because of drying effects.
  • Use daily home fluoride products for anticaries effect.
  • Use sugarless gum, frequent sips of water or saliva substitutes.
• Update health and medication history if physician makes any changes in evaluation or drug regimens; include OTC, herbal, and nonherbal remedies in the update.

vincristine sulfate
vin-**cris**′-teen **sull**′-fate
(Oncovin, Vincasar PFS)
Do not confuse vincristine with vinblastine, or Oncovin with Ancobon.

CATEGORY AND SCHEDULE
Pregnancy Risk Category: D

Drug Class: Antineoplastic

MECHANISM OF ACTION
A vinca alkaloid that binds to microtubular protein of mitotic spindle, causing metaphase arrest. *Therapeutic Effect:* Inhibits cell division.

USES
Treatment of acute leukemia, advanced non-Hodgkin's lymphoma, disseminated Hodgkin's disease, neuroblastoma, rhabdomyosarcoma, Wilms' tumor

PHARMACOKINETICS
Does not cross the blood-brain barrier. Protein binding: 75%. Metabolized in the liver. Primarily eliminated in feces by biliary system. *Half-life:* 10–37 hr.

INDICATIONS AND DOSAGES
▶ **Acute Leukemia, Advanced Non-Hodgkin's Lymphoma, Disseminated Hodgkin's Disease, Neuroblastoma, Rhabdomyosarcoma, Wilms' Tumor**
IV
Adults, Elderly. 0.4–1.4 mg/m² once a wk.
Children. 1–2 mg/m² once a wk.
Children weighing less than 10 kg or with a body surface area less than 1 m² 0.05 mg/kg. Maximum: 2 mg.

V

▸ **Dosage in Hepatic Impairment**
Reduce dosage by 50% in patients
with a direct serum bilirubin
concentration more than 3 mg/dl.

SIDE EFFECTS/ADVERSE REACTIONS

Expected
Peripheral neuropathy (occurs in
nearly every patient; first clinical
sign is depression of Achilles tendon
reflex)

Frequent
Peripheral paraesthesia, alopecia,
constipation or obstipation (upper
colon impaction with empty
rectum), abdominal cramps,
headache, jaw pain, hoarseness,
diplopia, ptosis or drooping of
eyelid, urinary tract disturbances

Occasional
Nausea, vomiting, diarrhea,
abdominal distention, stomatitis,
fever

Rare
Mild leukopenia, mild anemia,
thrombocytopenia

PRECAUTIONS AND CONTRAINDICATIONS

Patients receiving radiation therapy
through ports that include the liver

DRUG INTERACTIONS OF CONCERN TO DENTISTRY

• None reported

SERIOUS REACTIONS

! Acute shortness of breath and
bronchospasm may occur, especially
when vincristine is administered
concurrently with mitomycin.
Prolonged or high-dose therapy may
produce foot or wrist drop, difficulty
walking, slapping gait, ataxia, and
muscle wasting. Acute uric acid
nephropathy may occur.

DENTAL CONSIDERATIONS

General:
• If additional analgesia is required
for dental pain, consider alternative
analgesics (NSAIDs) in patients
taking opioids for acute or chronic
pain.
• This drug may be used in the
hospital or on an outpatient basis.
Confirm the patient's disease and
treatment status.
• Short appointments and a stress
reduction protocol may be required
for anxious patients.
• Patient on chronic drug therapy
may rarely present with symptoms
of blood dyscrasias, which can
include infection, bleeding, and poor
healing. If dyscrasia is present,
caution patient to prevent oral tissue
trauma when using oral hygiene
aids.
• Examine for oral manifestation of
opportunistic infection.
• Assess salivary flow as a factor in
caries, periodontal disease, and
candidiasis.
• Palliative medication may be
required for management of oral
side effects.
• Chlorhexidine mouth rinse prior to
and during chemotherapy may
reduce severity of mucositis.
• Patients may have received other
chemotherapy or radiation; confirm
medical and drug history.
• Patients may be at risk for
infection.
Consultations:
• Medical consultation may be
required to assess immunologic
status during cancer chemotherapy
and determine safety risk, if any,
posed by the required dental
treatment.
• Medical consultation may be
required to assess disease control

and patient's ability to tolerate stress.

• In a patient with symptoms of blood dyscrasias, request a medical consultation for blood studies and postpone treatment until normal values are reestablished.

• Refer patients to attending physician if symptoms of peripheral neuropathy are present (numbness, tingling, or pain in hands or feet).

Teach Patient/Family to:

• Encourage effective oral hygiene to prevent soft tissue inflammation.

• Report oral lesions, soreness, or bleeding to dentist.

• Prevent trauma when using oral hygiene aids.

• Update health and medication history if physician makes any changes in evaluation or drug regimens; include OTC, herbal, and nonherbal remedies in the update.

• When chronic dry mouth occurs, advise patient to:

  • Avoid mouth rinses with high alcohol content due to drying effects.

  • Use daily home fluoride products for anticaries effect.

  • Use sugarless gum, frequent sips of water, or saliva substitutes.

---

vinorelbine

vin-oh-**rell**′-bean
(Navelbine)
Do not confuse vinorelbine with vinblastine.

CATEGORY AND SCHEDULE

Pregnancy Risk Category: D

Drug Class: Antineoplastic

MECHANISM OF ACTION

A semisynthetic vinca alkaloid that interferes with mitotic microtubule assembly.
Therapeutic Effect: Prevents cell division.

USES

Treatment of some kinds of lung cancer

PHARMACOKINETICS

Widely distributed after IV administration. Protein binding: 80%–90%. Metabolized in the liver. Primarily eliminated in feces by biliary system. ***Half-life:*** 28–43 hr.

INDICATIONS AND DOSAGES

▶ **Unresectable, Advanced Non–Small-Cell Lung Cancer (as Monotherapy or in Combination with Cisplatin)**
IV
Adults, Elderly. 30 mg/m^2 administered weekly over 6–10 min.
▶ **Dosage Adjustment Guidelines**
Dosage adjustments should be based on granulocyte count obtained on the day of treatment, as follows:

Granulocyte Count (cells/mm^3)	Dose on Day of Treatment
More than 1500	30 mg/m^2
1000–1499	15 mg/m^2
Less than 1000	Do not administer

▶ **Combination Therapy (with Cisplatin)**
IV Injection
Adults, Elderly. 25 mg/m^2 every wk or 30 mg/m^2 on days 1 and 29, then q6wk.

SIDE EFFECTS/ADVERSE REACTIONS

Frequent
Asthenia; mild or moderate nausea; constipation; erythema, pain, or vein

V

discoloration at injection site; fatigue; peripheral neuropathy manifested as paresthesia and hyperesthesia; diarrhea; alopecia
Occasional
Phlebitis, dyspnea, loss of deep tendon reflexes
Rare
Chest pain, jaw pain, myalgia, arthralgia, rash

PRECAUTIONS AND CONTRAINDICATIONS

Granulocyte count before treatment of fewer than 1000 cells/mm³

DRUG INTERACTIONS OF CONCERN TO DENTISTRY

- None reported

SERIOUS REACTIONS

! Bone marrow depression is manifested mainly as granulocytopenia, which may be severe. Other hematologic toxicities, including neutropenia, thrombocytopenia, leukopenia, and anemia, increase the risk of infection and bleeding. Acute shortness of breath and severe bronchospasm occur infrequently, particularly in patients with preexisting pulmonary dysfunction and in those receiving mitomycin concurrently.

DENTAL CONSIDERATIONS

General:
- If additional analgesia is required for dental pain, consider alternative analgesics in patients taking narcotics for acute or chronic pain (e.g., acetaminophen).
- Avoid products that affect platelet function, such as aspirin and NSAIDs.
- This drug may be used in the hospital or on an outpatient basis.

Confirm the patient's disease and treatment status.
- Patient on chronic drug therapy may rarely present with symptoms of blood dyscrasias, which can include infection, bleeding, and poor healing. If dyscrasia is present, caution patient to prevent oral tissue trauma when using oral hygiene aids.
- Consider semisupine chair position for patients with respiratory disease.
- Caution: patients may be at high risk for infection.
- Patient may have received other chemotherapy or radiation; confirm medical and drug history.
- Oral infections should be eliminated and/or treated aggressively.
Consultations:
- Medical consultation should include routine blood counts including platelet counts and bleeding time.
- Consult physician; prophylactic or therapeutic antiinfectives may be indicated if surgery or periodontal treatment is required.
- Medical consultation may be required to assess immunologic status during cancer chemotherapy and determine safety risk, if any, posed by the required dental treatment.
- Medical consultation may be required to assess disease control and patient's ability to tolerate stress.
Teach Patient/Family to:
- See dentist immediately if secondary oral infection occurs.
- Encourage effective oral hygiene to prevent soft tissue inflammation.
- Report oral lesions, soreness, or bleeding to dentist.
- Prevent trauma when using oral hygiene aids.

• Update health and medication history if physician makes any changes in evaluation or drug regimens; include OTC, herbal, and nonherbal remedies in the update.

vitamin A
vight'-ah-min A
(Aquasol A, Palmitate A)
Do not confuse Aquasol A with Anusol.

CATEGORY AND SCHEDULE
Pregnancy Risk Category: A (X if used in doses greater than recommended daily allowance)

Drug Class: Fat-soluble vitamin

MECHANISM OF ACTION
A fat-soluble vitamin that may act as a cofactor in biochemical reactions.
Therapeutic Effect: Is essential for normal function of retina, visual adaptation to darkness, bone growth, testicular and ovarian function, and embryonic development; preserves integrity of epithelial cells.

USES
Treatment of vitamin A deficiency

PHARMACOKINETICS
Rapidly absorbed from the GI tract if bile salts, pancreatic lipase, protein, and dietary fat are present. Transported in blood to the liver, where it is metabolized; stored in parenchymal hepatic cells, then transported in plasma as retinol, as needed. Excreted primarily in bile and, to a lesser extent, in urine.

INDICATIONS AND DOSAGES
▸ **Severe Vitamin A Deficiency**
PO
Adults, Elderly, Children 8 yr and older. 500,000 units/day for 3 days; then 50,000 units/day for 14 days, then 10,000–20,000 units/day for 2 mo.
Children 1–7 yr. 5000 units/kg/day for 5 days, then 5000–10,000 units/day for 2 mo.
Children younger than 1 yr. 5000–10,000 units/day for 2 mo.
IM
Adults, Elderly, Children 8 yr and older. 100,000 units/day for 3 days; then 50,000 units/day for 14 days.
Children 1–7 yr. 17,500–35,000 units/day for 10 days.
Children younger than 1 yr. 7500–15,000 units/day.
▸ **Malabsorption Syndrome**
PO
Adults, Elderly, Children 8 yr and older. 10,000–50,000 units/day.
▸ **Dietary Supplement**
PO
Adults, Elderly. 4000–5000 units/day.
Children 7–10 yr. 3300–3500 units/day.
Children 4–6 yr. 2500 units/day.
Children 6 mo–3 yr. 1500–2000 units/day.
Neonates younger than 5 mo. 1500 units/day.

SIDE EFFECTS/ADVERSE REACTIONS
None known

PRECAUTIONS AND CONTRAINDICATIONS
Hypervitaminosis A
Caution:
Impaired renal function; pregnancy category A (RDA doses), otherwise pregnancy category C

V

DRUG INTERACTIONS OF CONCERN TO DENTISTRY
• None listed

SERIOUS REACTIONS
! Chronic overdose produces malaise, nausea, vomiting, drying or cracking of skin or lips, inflammation of tongue or gums, irritability, alopecia, and night sweats. Bulging fontanelles have occurred in infants.

DENTAL CONSIDERATIONS
General:
• Oral manifestation of side effects could indicate hypervitaminosis.
• May cause dry or peeling skin around lips; provide lip lubricant for patient comfort during dental treatment.

vitamin D
vight'-ah-min D
(Calciferol, Drisdol, Ostoforte[CAN])

CATEGORY AND SCHEDULE
Pregnancy Risk Category: A (D if used in doses above recommended daily allowance)

Drug Class: Fat-soluble vitamin

MECHANISM OF ACTION
A fat-soluble vitamin that stimulates calcium and phosphate absorption from the small intestine, promotes secretion of calcium from bone to blood, and promotes resorption of phosphate in renal tubules; also acts on bone cells to stimulate skeletal growth and on parathyroid gland to suppress hormone synthesis and secretion.

Therapeutic Effect: Essential for absorption and utilization of calcium and phosphate and normal bone calcification. Reduces parathyroid hormone level. Improves phosphorus and calcium homeostasis in chronic renal failure.

USES
Varies with the type of vitamin D selected, but generally includes vitamin D deficiency, rickets, renal osteodystrophy, tetany, hypoparathyroidism, and hypophosphatemia; doxercalciferol is indicated for reduction of elevated intact parathyroid hormone (iPTH) levels for secondary hyperparathyroidism in patients receiving chronic renal dialysis

PHARMACOKINETICS
Readily absorbed from small intestine. Concentrated primarily in liver and fat deposits. Activated in the liver and kidneys. Eliminated by biliary system; excreted in urine. *Half-life:* 19–48 hr for ergocalciferol.

INDICATIONS AND DOSAGES
Alert
Oral dosing is preferred. Administer the drug IM only in patients with GI, hepatic, or biliary disease associated with malabsorption of vitamin D.
▶ Dietary Supplement
PO
Adults, Elderly, Children. 10 mcg (400 units)/day.
Neonates. 10–20 mcg (400–800 units)/day.
▶ Renal Failure
PO
Adults, Elderly. 0.5 mg/day.
Children. 0.1–1 mg/day.

▸ **Hypoparathyroidism**
PO
Adults, Elderly. 625 mcg–5 mg/day
(with calcium supplements).
Children. 1.25–5 mg/day (with
calcium supplements).
▸ **Nutritional Rickets, Osteomalacia**
PO
Adults, Elderly, Children. 25–
125 mcg/day for 8–12 wk.
*Adults, Elderly (with malabsorption
syndrome).* 250–7500 mcg/day.
*Children (with malabsorption
syndrome).* 250–625 mcg/day.
▸ **Vitamin D–Dependent Rickets**
PO
Adults, Elderly. 250 mcg–1.5 mg/
day.
Children. 75–125 mcg/day.
Maximum: 1500 mcg/day.
▸ **Vitamin D–Resistant Rickets**
PO
Adults, Elderly. 250–1500 mcg/day
(with phosphate supplements).
Children. Initially, 1000–2000 mcg/
day (with phosphate supplements).
May increase in 250- to 600-mcg
increments q3–4mo.

SIDE EFFECTS/ADVERSE REACTIONS
None known

PRECAUTIONS AND CONTRAINDICATIONS
Hypercalcemia, malabsorption
syndrome, vitamin D toxicity
Caution:
Cardiovascular disease, renal calculi,
hyperphosphatemia

DRUG INTERACTIONS OF CONCERN TO DENTISTRY
• Reduction in calcitriol levels:
ketoconazole

SERIOUS REACTIONS
! Early signs and symptoms of
overdose are weakness, headache,
somnolence, nausea, vomiting, dry
mouth, constipation, muscle and
bone pain, and metallic taste. Later
signs and symptoms of overdose
include polyuria, polydipsia,
anorexia, weight loss, nocturia,
photophobia, rhinorrhea, pruritus,
disorientation, hallucinations,
hyperthermia, hypertension, and
cardiac arrhythmias.

DENTAL CONSIDERATIONS
General:
• Sensitivity of eyes to dental light
may indicate late toxicity.
Teach Patient/Family to:
• Be aware that oral side effects are
associated with early symptoms of
overdose.

vitamin E
vight′-ah-min E
(Aqua Gem E, Aquasol E,
E-Gems, Key-E, Key-E Kaps)
Do not confuse Aquasol E with
Anusol.

CATEGORY AND SCHEDULE
Pregnancy Risk Category: A (C if
used in doses above recommended
daily allowance)
OTC

Drug Class: Vitamin E
(fat-soluble vitamin)

MECHANISM OF ACTION
An antioxidant that prevents
oxidation of vitamins A and C,
protects fatty acids from attack by
free radicals, and protects RBCs
from hemolysis by oxidizing
agents.
Therapeutic Effect: Prevents and
treats vitamin E deficiency.

V

USES
Treatment of vitamin E deficiency, hemolytic anemia in premature neonates, prevention of retrolental fibroplasia

PHARMACOKINETICS
Variably absorbed from the GI tract (requires bile salts, dietary fat, and normal pancreatic function). Primarily concentrated in adipose tissue. Metabolized in the liver. Primarily eliminated by biliary system.

INDICATIONS AND DOSAGES
▸ **Vitamin E Deficiency**
PO
Adults, Elderly. 60–75 units/day.
Children. 1 unit/kg/day.

SIDE EFFECTS/ADVERSE REACTIONS
CNS: Headache, fatigue
CV: Increased risk of thrombophlebitis
GI: Nausea, cramps, diarrhea
GU: Gonadal dysfunction
EENT: Blurred vision

Integ: Sterile abscess, contact dermatitis
MS: Weakness
Meta: Altered metabolism of hormones (thyroid, pituitary, adrenal), altered immunity

PRECAUTIONS AND CONTRAINDICATIONS
None significant

DRUG INTERACTIONS OF CONCERN TO DENTISTRY
• With doses greater than 400 international units: increased action of oral anticoagulants

SERIOUS REACTIONS
❗ Chronic overdose may produce fatigue, weakness, nausea, headache, blurred vision, flatulence, and diarrhea.

DENTAL CONSIDERATIONS

General:
• Determine why the patient is taking the drug.

V

warfarin sodium
war'-far-in **soe'**-dee-um
(Apo-Warfarin[CAN], Coumadin,
Gen-Warfarin[CAN], Jantoven,
Marevan[AUS],
Tar-Warfarin[CAN])
Do not confuse Coumadin with
Kemadrin.

CATEGORY AND SCHEDULE
Pregnancy Risk Category: D

Drug Class: Oral anticoagulant

MECHANISM OF ACTION
A coumarin derivative that interferes
with hepatic synthesis of vitamin
K–dependent clotting factors,
resulting in depletion of coagulation
factors II, VII, IX, and X.
Therapeutic Effect: Prevents further
extension of formed existing clot;
prevents new clot formation or
secondary thromboembolic
complications.

USES
Treatment of pulmonary emboli,
deep vein thrombosis (DVT), MI,
atrial dysrhythmias, to reduce risk of
recurrent MI and thromboembolic
events.

PHARMACOKINETICS

Route	Onset	Peak	Duration
PO	1.5–3 days	5–7 days	N/A

Well absorbed from the GI tract.
Metabolized in the liver. Primarily
excreted in urine. Not removed by
hemodialysis. *Half-life:* 1.5–2.5
days.

INDICATIONS AND DOSAGES
Anticoagulant
PO
Adults, Elderly. Initially, 5–15 mg/
day for 2–5 days; then adjust based
on INR. Maintenance: 2–10 mg/day.
Children. Initially, 0.1–0.2 mg/kg
(maximum 10 mg). Maintenance:
0.05–0.34 mg/kg/day.
Usual Elderly Dosage (Maintenance)
PO, IV
Elderly. 2–5 mg/day.

SIDE EFFECTS/ADVERSE REACTIONS
Occasional
GI distress, such as nausea,
anorexia, abdominal cramps,
diarrhea
Rare
Hypersensitivity reaction including
dermatitis and urticaria, especially
in those sensitive to aspirin

PRECAUTIONS AND CONTRAINDICATIONS
Neurosurgical procedures, open
wounds, pregnancy, severe
hypertension, severe hepatic or renal
damage, uncontrolled bleeding,
ulcers
Caution:
Alcoholism, elderly

DRUG INTERACTIONS OF CONCERN TO DENTISTRY
• Increased action: diflunisal,
salicylates, propoxyphene,
metronidazole, erythromycin,
clarithromycin, ketoconazole,
itraconazole, fluconazole, NSAIDs,
indomethacin, chloral hydrate,
tetracyclines, fluoroquinolones,
acetaminophen, ciprofloxacin,
levofloxacin
• Decreased action: barbiturates,
carbamazepine acetaminophen
(monitor INR levels)

W

• Herbal products with some anticoagulant activity: feverfew, garlic, ginger, ginkgo, ginseng

SERIOUS REACTIONS

! Bleeding complications ranging from local ecchymoses to major hemorrhage may occur. Drug should be discontinued immediately and vitamin K or phytonadione administered. Mild hemorrhage: 2.5–10 mg PO, IM, or IV. Severe hemorrhage: 10–15 mg IV and repeated q4h as necessary.

! Hepatotoxicity, blood dyscrasias, necrosis, vasculitis, and local thrombosis occur rarely.

DENTAL CONSIDERATIONS

General:

• Reports on concomitant use of acetaminophen and warfarin seem to suggest a possible increase in anticoagulant effects, especially in patients with other diseases or contributing factors (diarrhea, age, debilitation, etc.). Patients taking warfarin should be questioned about recent use of acetaminophen and current INR values. Acetaminophen has been shown to increase the INR, depending on the amount of acetaminophen taken and duration of use. A new INR value may be required if surgical procedures are planned.

• Patients on chronic drug therapy may rarely have symptoms of blood dyscrasias, which can include infection, bleeding, and poor healing.

• Consider local hemostasis measures to prevent excessive bleeding.

• Increased bleeding may occur with IM injections.

Consultations:

• Medical consultation should include current INR value.

• For dental surgical procedures that may result in excessive bleeding, consider requesting physician to make dose reduction before dental treatment so that INR is within appropriate therapeutic range.

• In a patient with symptoms of blood dyscrasias, request a medical consultation for blood studies and postpone dental treatment until normal values are reestablished.

Teach Patient/Family to:

• Encourage effective oral hygiene to prevent soft tissue inflammation.

• Use caution to prevent injury when using oral hygiene aids.

• Report oral lesions, soreness, or bleeding to dentist.

zafirlukast
za-**feer**′-loo-kast
(Accolate)
Do not confuse Accolate with
Accupril or Aclovate.

CATEGORY AND SCHEDULE
Pregnancy Risk Category: B

Drug Class: Selective
leukotriene receptor antagonist

MECHANISM OF ACTION
An antiasthmatic that binds to
leukotriene receptors, inhibiting
bronchoconstriction caused by sulfur
dioxide, cold air, and specific
antigens, such as grass, cat dander,
and ragweed.
Therapeutic Effect: Reduces airway
edema and smooth muscle
constriction; alters cellular activity
associated with the inflammatory
process.

USES
Prophylaxis and chronic treatment of
asthma

PHARMACOKINETICS
Rapidly absorbed after PO
administration (food reduces
absorption). Protein binding: 99%.
Extensively metabolized in the liver.
Primarily excreted in feces.
Unknown if removed by
hemodialysis. *Half-life:* 10 hr.

INDICATIONS AND DOSAGES
▶ Bronchial Asthma
PO
*Adults, Elderly, Children 12 yr and
older.* 20 mg twice a day.
Children 5–11 yr. 10 mg twice a
day.

SIDE EFFECTS/ADVERSE REACTIONS
Frequent
Headache
Occasional
Nausea, diarrhea
Rare
Generalized pain, asthenia,
myalgia, fever, dyspepsia, vomiting,
dizziness

PRECAUTIONS AND CONTRAINDICATIONS
Hypersensitivity, hepatic dysfunction
with prior use of zafirlukast
Caution:
Not for acute bronchospasm, food
decreases bioavailability, pregnancy
category B, lactation, patients
younger than 7 yr, hepatic
impairment, liver enzyme elevation,
elderly (increased infection); if liver
dysfunction suspected, discontinue
use and measure liver enzymes,
serum ALT (SPGT)

DRUG INTERACTIONS OF CONCERN TO DENTISTRY
• Increased PT with concurrent use
of warfarin
• Reduced plasma levels:
erythromycin, terfenadine,
theophylline
• Increased plasma levels with
aspirin
• Inhibits CYP2C9 and CYP3A4
isoenzymes: use with caution when
drugs metabolized by these enzymes
are used

SERIOUS REACTIONS
! Concurrent administration of
inhaled corticosteroids increases the
risk of upper respiratory tract
infection.

Z

DENTAL CONSIDERATIONS

General:
• Midday appointments and a stress-reduction protocol may be required for anxious patients.
• Avoid prescribing aspirin-containing products and NSAIDs.
• Acute asthmatic episodes may be precipitated in the dental office. Sympathomimetic inhalants should be available for emergency use. A stress-reduction protocol may be required.
• Be aware that aspirin or sulfite preservatives in vasoconstrictor-containing products can exacerbate asthma.
• Consider semisupine chair position for patients with respiratory disease or if GI side effects occur.
Consultations:
• Medical consultation may be required to assess disease control.
Teach Patient/Family to:
• Use powered tooth brush if patient has difficulty holding conventional devices.
• Update health and drug history if physician makes any changes in evaluation or drug regimens; include OTC, herbal, and nonherbal remedies in the update.

zalcitabine

zal-**site**′-ah-been
(Hivid)

CATEGORY AND SCHEDULE
Pregnancy Risk Category: C

Drug Class: Synthetic pyrimidine antiviral

MECHANISM OF ACTION
A nucleoside reverse transcriptase inhibitor that inhibits viral DNA synthesis.
Therapeutic Effect: Prevents replication of HIV-1.

USES
Treatment of advanced HIV infection in combination with zidovudine

PHARMACOKINETICS
Readily absorbed from the GI tract (absorption decreased by food). Protein binding: less than 4%. Undergoes phosphorylation intracellularly to the active metabolite. Primarily excreted in urine. Removed by hemodialysis.
Half-life: 1–3 hr; metabolite, 2.6–10 hr (increased in impaired renal function).

INDICATIONS AND DOSAGES
▸ **HIV Infection (in Combination with Other Antiretrovirals)**
PO
Adults, Children 13 yr and older.
0.75 mg q8h.
Children younger than 13 yr.
0.01 mg/kg q8h. Range: 0.005–0.01 mg/kg q8h.
▸ **Dosage in Renal Impairment**
Dosage and frequency are modified on the basis of creatinine clearance.

Creatinine Clearance	Dose
10–40 ml/min	0.75 mg q12h
Less than 10 ml/min	0.75 mg q24h

SIDE EFFECTS/ADVERSE REACTIONS
Frequent
Peripheral neuropathy, fever, fatigue, headache, rash

Z

Occasional

Diarrhea, abdominal pain, oral ulcers, cough, pruritus, myalgia, weight loss, nausea, vomiting

Rare

Nasal discharge, dysphagia, depression, night sweats, confusion

PRECAUTIONS AND CONTRAINDICATIONS

Moderate or severe peripheral neuropathy

Caution:

Lactation, children younger than 13 yr, renal impairment, hepatic impairment, risk of serious peripheral neuropathy, risk of severe hepatic impairment, CHF

DRUG INTERACTIONS OF CONCERN TO DENTISTRY

• Increased peripheral neuropathy: metronidazole, dapsone, or other drugs associated with peripheral neuropathy

SERIOUS REACTIONS

! Peripheral neuropathy (characterized by numbness, tingling, burning, and pain in the lower extremities) occurs in 17% to 31% of patients. These symptoms may be followed by sharp, shooting pain and progress to a severe, continuous, burning pain that may be irreversible if the drug is not discontinued in time.

! Pancreatitis, leukopenia, neutropenia, eosinophilia, and thrombocytopenia occur rarely.

DENTAL CONSIDERATIONS

General:

• Examine oral cavity for side effects if on long-term drug therapy.

• Monitor vital signs at every appointment because of cardiovascular side effects.

• Palliative medication may be required for management of oral side effects.

• Assess salivary flow as a factor in caries, periodontal disease, and candidiasis.

• Prophylactic antibiotics may be indicated to prevent infection if surgery or deep scaling is planned.

• Patients may be more susceptible to infection and have delayed wound healing.

Consultations:

• Medical consultation may be required to assess disease control and patient's ability to tolerate stress.

Teach Patient/Family to:

• Encourage effective oral hygiene to prevent soft tissue inflammation.

• Use caution to prevent injury when using oral hygiene aids.

• See dentist immediately if secondary oral infection occurs.

• When chronic dry mouth occurs, advise patient to:

  • Avoid mouth rinses with high alcohol content because of drying effects.

  • Use daily home fluoride products to prevent caries.

  • Use sugarless gum, frequent sips of water, or saliva substitutes.

zaleplon

zal'-eh-plon

(Sonata, Stamoc[CAN])

CATEGORY AND SCHEDULE

Pregnancy Risk Category: C

Controlled Substance Schedule IV

Drug Class: Hypnotic

Z

MECHANISM OF ACTION

A nonbenzodiazepine that enhances the action of the inhibitory neurotransmitter gamma-aminobutyric acid.
Therapeutic Effect: Induces sleep.

USES

Short-term treatment of insomnia

PHARMACOKINETICS

PO: Rapid absorption, bioavailability 30%, peak plasma levels 1 hr, wide tissue distribution, rapid hepatic metabolism (CYP3A4 minor pathway), excretion in urine; heavy, high-fat meal significantly delays absorption

INDICATIONS AND DOSAGES

▸ Insomnia

PO
Adults. 10 mg at bedtime. Range: 5–20 mg.
Elderly. 5 mg at bedtime.

SIDE EFFECTS/ADVERSE REACTIONS

Expected
Somnolence, sedation, mild rebound insomnia (on first night after drug is discontinued)
Frequent
Nausea, headache, myalgia, dizziness
Occasional
Abdominal pain, asthenia, dyspepsia, eye pain, paresthesia
Rare
Tremors, amnesia, hyperacusis (acute sense of hearing), fever, dysmenorrhea

PRECAUTIONS AND CONTRAINDICATIONS

Severe hepatic impairment
Caution:
Abuse potential similar to benzodiazepines, elderly, debilitated, smaller patients adjust dose downward; lactation, children

DRUG INTERACTIONS OF CONCERN TO DENTISTRY

• Caution when using dental drugs that inhibit or induce cytochrome. P-450 enzymes; this drug is a minor substrate for CYP3A4; however, use caution (see Appendix I).
• CNS depression: all CNS depressant drugs.

SERIOUS REACTIONS

! Zaleplon may produce altered concentration, behavior changes, and impaired memory.
! Taking the drug while up and about may result in adverse CNS effects, such as hallucinations, impaired coordination, dizziness, and light-headedness.
! Overdose results in somnolence, confusion, diminished reflexes, and coma.

DENTAL CONSIDERATIONS

General:
• Assess salivary flow as a factor in caries, periodontal disease, and candidiasis.
• Determine why patient is taking the drug.
• Consider semisupine chair position for patient comfort if GI side effects occur.
Consultations:
• Medical consultation may be required to assess disease control and patient's ability to tolerate stress.
Teach Patient/Family to:
• When chronic dry mouth occurs, advise patient to:
  • Avoid mouth rinses with high alcohol content because of drying effects.

Z

- Use daily home fluoride products for anticaries effect.
- Use sugarless gum, frequent sips of water, or saliva substitutes.

zanamivir
za-**na**′-mi-veer
(Relenza)

CATEGORY AND SCHEDULE
Pregnancy Risk Category: B

Drug Class: Antiviral

MECHANISM OF ACTION
An antiviral that appears to inhibit the influenza virus enzyme neuraminidase, which is essential for viral replication.
Therapeutic Effects: Prevents viral release from infected cells.

USES
Treatment of uncomplicated influenza in adults and children older than 7 yr with symptoms of no more than 2 days; more effective against influenza type A virus.

PHARMACOKINETICS
Inhalation: 4%–17% of inhaled dose is absorbed, peak serum levels 1–2 hr, low plasma protein binding (less than 10%), excreted unchanged in urine.

INDICATIONS AND DOSAGES
▶ **Influenza Virus**
Inhalation
Adults, Elderly, Children 7 yr and older. 2 inhalations (one 5-mg blister per inhalation for a total dose of 10 mg) twice a day (about 12 hr apart) for 5 days.

▶ **Prevention of Influenza Virus**
Inhalation
Adults, Elderly. 2 inhalations once a day for the duration of the exposure period.

SIDE EFFECTS/ADVERSE REACTIONS
Occasional
Diarrhea, sinusitis, nausea, bronchitis, cough, dizziness, headache
Rare
Malaise, fatigue, fever, abdominal pain, myalgia, arthralgia, urticaria

PRECAUTIONS AND CONTRAINDICATIONS
Hypersensitivity
Caution:
Teach use of inhaler to patient; chronic obstructive pulmonary disease or asthma does not preclude influenza vaccine, safety in children younger than 12 yr not established

DRUG INTERACTIONS OF CONCERN TO DENTISTRY
- None reported

SERIOUS REACTIONS
! Neutropenia may occur. Bronchospasm may occur in those with a history of COPD or bronchial asthma.

DENTAL CONSIDERATIONS
General:
- Acute influenza patients are unlikely to be seen in the dental office except for dental emergencies.

Z

ziconotide
zi-**koe'**-no-tide
(Prialt)

CATEGORY AND SCHEDULE
Pregnancy Risk Category: C

Drug Class: Analgesic

MECHANISM OF ACTION
A synthetic peptide that selectively binds to and blocks *N*-type voltage-sensitive calcium channels located on afferent nerves in the spinal cord.
Therapeutic Effect: Blocks excitatory neurotransmitter release, reducing sensitivity to painful stimuli.

USES
Reduction of chronic pain in the body

PHARMACOKINETICS
Elimination Half-life: 4.6 hr after intrathecal administration. 50% bound to plasma proteins; metabolized in multiple organs. Excreted in urine as proteolytic degradation products.

INDICATIONS AND DOSAGES
▸ **Pain Control**
Intrathecal
Adults, Elderly. Initially, 2.4 mcg/day (0.1 mcg/hr). May titrate to maximum of 19.2 mcg/day (0.8 mcg/hr).

SIDE EFFECTS/ADVERSE REACTIONS
Frequent
Dizziness, nausea, somnolence, weakness, diarrhea, confusion, ataxia, headache, vomiting, gait disturbance, memory impairment, hypertonia
Occasional
Anorexia, visual disturbances, anxiety, urinary retention, speech disorder, aphasia, nystagmus, paresthesia, fever, hallucinations, nervousness, vertigo
Rare
Insomnia, dry skin, constipation, arthralgia, myalgia, tremor

PRECAUTIONS AND CONTRAINDICATIONS
History of psychosis, presence of infection at the injection site, uncontrolled bleeding, or spinal canal obstruction that impairs CSF circulation, IV administration

DRUG INTERACTIONS OF CONCERN TO DENTISTRY
• Enhanced CNS depression: all CNS depressants

SERIOUS REACTIONS
! Atrial fibrillation, cerebral vascular accident, seizures, kidney failure (acute), myoclonus, and psychosis occur rarely.

DENTAL CONSIDERATIONS
General:
• Determine why patient is taking the drug.
• For use in the hospital setting.
Consultations:
• Medical consultation may be required to assess disease control and patient's ability to tolerate stress.
Teach Patient/Family to:
• Encourage effective oral hygiene to prevent soft tissue inflammation.
• Update health and medication history if physician makes any changes in evaluation or drug

Z

regimens; include OTC, herbal, and nonherbal remedies in the update.

zidovudine
zyde-**oh'**-vue-deen
(Apo-Zidovudine[CAN], AZT, Novo-AZT[CAN], Retrovir)
Do not confuse Retrovir with ritonavir.

CATEGORY AND SCHEDULE
Pregnancy Risk Category: C

Drug Class: Antiviral thymidine analog

MECHANISM OF ACTION
A nucleoside reverse transcriptase inhibitor that interferes with viral RNA-dependent DNA polymerase, an enzyme necessary for viral HIV replication.
Therapeutic Effect: Interferes with HIV replication, slowing the progression of HIV infection.

USES
Treatment of symptomatic HIV infections (AIDS, ARC), confirmed *P. carinii* pneumonia (PCP), or absolute CD4 lymphocytes less than 200/mm^3; prevention of maternal-fetal transmission.

PHARMACOKINETICS
Rapidly and completely absorbed from the GI tract. Protein binding: 25%–38%. Undergoes first-pass metabolism in the liver. Crosses the blood-brain barrier and is widely distributed, including to CSF. Primarily excreted in urine. Minimal removal by hemodialysis. *Half-life:* 0.8–1.2 hr (increased in impaired renal function).

INDICATIONS AND DOSAGES
▶ **HIV Infection**
PO
Adults, Elderly, Children older than 12 yr. 200 mg q8h or 300 mg q12h.
Children 12 yr and younger. 160 mg/m^2/dose q8h. Range: 90–180 mg/m^2/dose q6–8h.
Neonates. 2 mg/kg/dose q6h.
IV
Adults, Elderly, Children older than 12 yr. 1–2 mg/kg/dose q4h.
Children 12 yr and younger. 120 mg/m^2/dose q6h.
Neonates. 1.5 mg/kg/dose q6h.

SIDE EFFECTS/ADVERSE REACTIONS
Expected
Nausea, headache
Frequent
Abdominal pain, asthenia, rash, fever, acne
Occasional
Diarrhea, anorexia, malaise, myalgia, somnolence
Rare
Dizziness, paresthesia, vomiting, insomnia, dyspnea, altered taste

PRECAUTIONS AND CONTRAINDICATIONS
Life-threatening allergic reactions to zidovudine or its components
Caution:
Granulocyte count less than 1000/mm^3 or Hgb less than 9.5 g/dl, lactation, children, severe renal disease, severe hepatic function, risk of severe neutropenia and anemia

DRUG INTERACTIONS OF CONCERN TO DENTISTRY
• Decreased blood levels: acetaminophen, clarithromycin
• Increased serum levels: fluconazole

Z

SERIOUS REACTIONS

! Serious reactions include anemia, which occurs most commonly after 4–6 wk of therapy, and granulocytopenia; both effects are more likely to occur in patients who have a low Hgb level or granulocyte count before beginning therapy.

! Neurotoxicity (as evidenced by ataxia, fatigue, lethargy, nystagmus, and seizures) may occur.

DENTAL CONSIDERATIONS

General:

· Examine for oral manifestations of opportunistic infections.

· Patients on chronic drug therapy may rarely have symptoms of blood dyscrasias, which can include infection, bleeding, and poor healing.

· Avoid dental light in patient's eyes; offer dark glasses for patient comfort.

· Place on frequent recall because of oral side effects.

Consultations:

· In a patient with symptoms of blood dyscrasias, request a medical consultation for blood studies and postpone dental treatment until normal values are reestablished.

· Medical consultation may be required to assess disease control.

Teach Patient/Family to:

· Encourage effective oral hygiene to prevent soft tissue inflammation.

· Use caution to prevent injury when using oral hygiene aids.

· See dentist immediately if secondary oral infection occurs.

zileuton

zye-**lew**′-ton
(zyelo)
Do not confuse Zyflo with Zyban.

CATEGORY AND SCHEDULE

Pregnancy Risk Category: C

Drug Class: Leukotriene pathway inhibitor

MECHANISM OF ACTION

A leukotriene inhibitor that inhibits the enzyme responsible for producing inflammatory response. Prevents formation of leukotrienes (leukotrienes induce bronchoconstriction response, enhances vascular permeability, stimulates mucus secretion).
Therapeutic Effect: Prevents airway edema, smooth muscle contraction, and the inflammatory process, relieving signs and symptoms of bronchial asthma.

USES

Prophylaxis and chronic treatment of asthma

PHARMACOKINETICS

Rapidly absorbed from GI tract. Protein binding: 93%. Metabolized in liver. Primarily excreted in urine. Unknown if removed by hemodialysis. *Half-life:* 2.1–2.5 hr.

INDICATIONS AND DOSAGES

▶ Bronchial Asthma
PO
Adults, Elderly, Children 12 yr and older. 600 mg 4 times a day. Total daily dosage: 2400 mg.

Z

SIDE EFFECTS/ADVERSE REACTIONS
Frequent
Headache
Occasional
Dyspepsia, nausea, abdominal pain, asthenia (loss of strength), myalgia
Rare
Conjunctivitis, constipation, dizziness, flatulence, insomnia

PRECAUTIONS AND CONTRAINDICATIONS
Active liver disease, impaired liver function, hypersensitivity to zileuton or any component of the formulation
Caution:
Not for acute bronchospasm, status asthmaticus; theophylline, warfarin, propranolol; hepatic impairment, lactation, children younger than 12 yr, monitor ALT (SGPT) levels

DRUG INTERACTIONS OF CONCERN TO DENTISTRY
• Increased plasma levels of theophylline, propranolol
• Significant increase in PT when taking warfarin
• Use caution when prescribing dental drugs that are strong inhibitors of CYP1A2 isoenzymes

SERIOUS REACTIONS
! Liver dysfunction occurs rarely and may be manifested as right upper quadrant pain, nausea, fatigue, lethargy, pruritus, jaundice, or flu-like symptoms.

DENTAL CONSIDERATIONS
General:
• Consider semisupine chair position for patient comfort because of GI side effects of disease.
• Acute asthmatic episodes may be precipitated in the dental office.
• Avoid prescribing NSAIDs.

• Sympathomimetic inhalants should be available for emergency use.
• Midday appointments and a stress-reduction protocol may be required for anxious patients.
• Be aware that aspirin or sulfite preservatives in vasoconstrictor-containing products can exacerbate asthma.
Consultations:
• Medical consultation may be required to assess disease control.
Teach Patient/Family to:
• Update health and drug history if physician makes any changes in evaluation or drug regimens; include OTC, herbal, and nonherbal remedies in the update.

zinc oxide/zinc sulfate
zink′ ox′-eyed/zink′ sul′-fate
(zinc oxide: Balmex, Desitin; zinc sulfate: Orazinc, Zincaps[AUS])

CATEGORY AND SCHEDULE
Pregnancy Risk Category: C

Drug Class: Mineral

MECHANISM OF ACTION
A mineral that acts as a cofactor for enzymes that are important for protein and carbohydrate metabolism.
Therapeutic Effect: Zinc oxide acts as a mild astringent and skin protectant. Zinc sulfate helps maintain normal growth and tissue repair, as well as skin hydration.

USES
Treatment of zinc deficiency

Z

INDICATIONS AND DOSAGES
▶ **Mild Skin Irritations and Abrasions (e.g., Chapped Skin, Diaper Rash)**
Topical (Zinc Oxide)
Adults, Elderly, Children. Apply as needed.
▶ **Treatment and Prevention of Zinc Deficiency, Wound Healing**
PO (Zinc Sulfate)
Adults, Elderly. 220 mg 3 times a day.

SIDE EFFECTS/ADVERSE REACTIONS
None known

PRECAUTIONS AND CONTRAINDICATIONS
None known

DRUG INTERACTIONS OF CONCERN TO DENTISTRY
• Decreased absorption: tetracyclines, fluoroquinolones

SERIOUS REACTIONS
! None known

DENTAL CONSIDERATIONS

General:
• Determine why patient is taking the drug.

ziprasidone
zye-**pray'**-za-done
(Geodon)

CATEGORY AND SCHEDULE
Pregnancy Risk Category: C

Drug Class: Antipsychotic, atypical

MECHANISM OF ACTION
A piperazine derivative that antagonizes adrenergic, dopamine, histamine, and serotonin receptors; also inhibits reuptake of serotonin and norepinephrine.
Therapeutic Effect: Diminishes symptoms of schizophrenia and depression.

USES
Treatment of schizophrenia

PHARMACOKINETICS
Well absorbed after PO administration. Food increases bioavailability. Protein binding: 99%. Extensively metabolized in the liver. Not removed by hemodialysis.
Half-life: 7 hr.

INDICATIONS AND DOSAGES
▶ **Schizophrenia**
PO
Adults, Elderly. Initially, 20 mg twice a day with food. Titrate at intervals of no less than 2 days. Maximum: 80 mg twice a day.
IM
Adults, Elderly. 10 mg q2h or 20 mg q4h. Maximum: 40 mg/day.
▶ **Bipolar Mania**
PO
Adults, Elderly. 40 mg 2 times a day.

SIDE EFFECTS/ADVERSE REACTIONS
Frequent
Headache, somnolence, dizziness
Occasional
Rash, orthostatic hypotension, weight gain, restlessness, constipation, dyspepsia

PRECAUTIONS AND CONTRAINDICATIONS
Conditions that prolong the QT interval, such as congenital long QT syndrome

Z

Caution:
May antagonize levodopa, dopamine agonists; QT prolongation and risk of sudden death, bradycardia, hypokalemia, hypomagnesemia, electrolyte depletion caused by diarrhea, diuretics, or vomiting, neuromalignant syndrome, tardive dyskinesia, seizures, suicide, lactation, pediatric use

DRUG INTERACTIONS OF CONCERN TO DENTISTRY
• Avoid use of any drug that prolongs the QT interval
• Caution in use of other CNS depressants: increased risk of CNS depressant effects
• Reduced plasma levels: carbamazepine
• Increased plasma levels: ketoconazole and other strong inhibitors of CYP3A4 isoenzymes (see Appendix I)
• Drugs that lower B/P: increased risk of hypotension
• Increased extrapyramidal effects: phenothiazines and related drugs (haloperidol, droperidol), metoclopramide

SERIOUS REACTIONS
! Prolongation of QT interval may produce torsades de pointes, a form of ventricular tachycardia.
! Patients with bradycardia, hypokalemia, or hypomagnesemia are at increased risk.

DENTAL CONSIDERATIONS
General:
• Monitor vital signs at every appointment because of cardiovascular side effects.
• After supine positioning, have patient sit upright for at least 2 min before standing to avoid orthostatic hypotension.

• Assess salivary flow as a factor in caries, periodontal disease, and candidiasis.
• Consider semisupine chair position for patient comfort if GI side effects occur.
• Assess for presence of extrapyramidal motor symptoms, such as tardive dyskinesia and akathisia. Extrapyramidal motor activity may complicate dental treatment.
• Use vasoconstrictors with caution, in low doses, and with careful aspiration; avoid use of epinephrine-impregnated gingival retraction cord.
Consultations:
• Consultation with physician may be necessary if sedation or general anesthesia is required.
• Physician should be informed if significant xerostomic side effects occur (e.g., increased caries, sore tongue, problems eating or swallowing, difficulty wearing prosthesis) so that a medication change can be considered.
• Medical consultation may be required to assess disease control and patient's ability to tolerate stress.
Teach Patient/Family to:
• Encourage effective oral hygiene to prevent soft tissue inflammation.
• Prevent trauma when using oral hygiene aids.
• Use powered tooth brush if patient has difficulty holding conventional devices.
• When chronic dry mouth occurs, advise patient to:
  • Avoid mouth rinses with high alcohol content because of drying effects.
  • Use daily home fluoride products for anticaries effect.
  • Use sugarless gum, frequent sips of water, or saliva substitutes.

Z

zoledronic acid
zole-eh-**drone'**-ick **ass'**-id
(Zometa, Reclast)

CATEGORY AND SCHEDULE
Pregnancy Risk Category: C

Drug Class: Osteoporosis
therapy adjunct, bisphosphonate

MECHANISM OF ACTION
A bisphosphonate that inhibits the
resorption of mineralized bone and
cartilage; inhibits increased
osteoclastic activity and skeletal
calcium release induced by
stimulatory factors produced by
tumors.
Therapeutic Effect: Increases
urinary calcium and phosphorus
excretion; decreases serum calcium
and phosphorus levels.

USES
Treatment of hypercalcemia from
malignancy, bone metastases
associated with prostate and lung
cancer; multiple myeloma, bone
metastases from solid tumors

PHARMACOKINETICS
IV Infusion: Shows triphasic
half-life; plasma protein binding
22%; little to no metabolism;
excreted mainly in urine; a high
percentage of the dose remains
bound to bone

INDICATIONS AND DOSAGES
▸ **Hypercalcemia**
IV Infusion
Adults, Elderly. 4 mg IV infusion
given over no less than 15 min.
Retreatment may be considered, but
at least 7 days should elapse to
allow for full response to initial
dose.

▸ **Multiple Myeloma**
IV
Adults, Elderly. 4 mg q3–4wk.

SIDE EFFECTS/ADVERSE REACTIONS
Frequent
Fever, nausea, vomiting,
constipation
Occasional
Hypotension, anxiety, insomnia,
flu-like symptoms (fever, chills,
bone pain, myalgia, and arthralgia)
Rare
Conjunctivitis

PRECAUTIONS AND CONTRAINDICATIONS
Hypersensitivity to other
bisphosphonates, including
alendronate, etidronate, pamidronate,
risedronate, and tiludronate. Dental
implants are contraindicated for
patients taking this drug.
Caution:
Data for use in children not
available, monitor hypercalcemic
parameters, ensure good hydration,
renal impairment, bronchospasm
in aspirin-sensitive asthmatics,
hypocalcemia, hypoparathyroidism,
lactation

DRUG INTERACTIONS OF CONCERN TO DENTISTRY
• None reported

SERIOUS REACTIONS
❗ Renal toxicity may occur if IV
infusion is administered in less than
15 min.

DENTAL CONSIDERATIONS

General:
• Bisphosphonates may increase the
risk of osteonecrosis of the jaw.
• This drug is used only in oncology
units or hospitals.

Z

• Examine for oral manifestation of opportunistic infection.
• Consider semisupine chair position for patient comfort if GI side effects occur.
• Short appointments may be required.
• If oral candidiasis occurs, treat with suitable antifungal drug.
Consultations:
• Medical consultation may be required to assess disease control.
Teach Patient/Family to:
• Observe regular recall schedule and practice effective oral hygiene to minimize risk of osteonecrosis of the jaw.

zolmitriptan
zohl-mih-**trip**'-tan
(Zomig, Zomig Rapimelt[CAN], Zomig-ZMT)

CATEGORY AND SCHEDULE
Pregnancy Risk Category: C

Drug Class: Serotonin agonist

MECHANISM OF ACTION
A serotonin receptor agonist that binds selectively to vascular receptors, producing a vasoconstrictive effect on cranial blood vessels.
Therapeutic Effect: Relieves migraine headache.

USES
Acute treatment of migraine with or without aura in adults

PHARMACOKINETICS
Rapidly but incompletely absorbed after PO administration. Protein binding: 15%. Undergoes first-pass metabolism in the liver to active metabolite. Eliminated primarily in urine (60%) and, to a lesser extent, in feces (30%). *Half-life:* 3 hr.

INDICATIONS AND DOSAGES
▸ **Acute Migraine Attack**
PO
Adults, Elderly, Children older than 18 yr. Initially, 2.5 mg or less. If headache returns, may repeat dose in 2 hr. Maximum: 10 mg/24 hr.
Intranasal
Adults, Elderly. 5 mg. May repeat in 2 hr. Maximum: 10 mg/24 hr.

SIDE EFFECTS/ADVERSE REACTIONS
Frequent
Oral: Dizziness; tingling; neck, throat, or jaw pressure; somnolence
Nasal: Altered taste, paraesthesia
Occasional
Oral: Warm or hot sensation, asthenia, chest pressure
Nasal: Nausea, somnolence, nasal discomfort, dizziness, asthenia, dry mouth
Rare
Diaphoresis, myalgia, paresthesia

PRECAUTIONS AND CONTRAINDICATIONS
Arrhythmias associated with conduction disorders, basilar or hemiplegic migraine, coronary artery disease, ischemic heart disease (including angina pectoris, history of MI, silent ischemia, and Prinzmetal's angina), uncontrolled hypertension, use within 24 hr of ergotamine-containing preparations or another serotonin receptor agonist, use within 14 days of MAOIs, Wolff-Parkinson-White syndrome
Caution:
Renal impairment, hepatic impairment, may cause coronary

Z

vasospasm, lactation, children, elderly

DRUG INTERACTIONS OF CONCERN TO DENTISTRY

• Potential serotonin crises: selective serotonin reuptake inhibitors, ergot-containing drugs (avoid use within 24 hr of taking this drug)
• Decreased plasma levels: cimetidine

SERIOUS REACTIONS

! Cardiac reactions (including ischemia, coronary artery vasospasm, and MI) and noncardiac vasospasm-related reactions (e.g., hemorrhage and CVA) occur rarely, particularly in patients with hypertension, diabetes, or a strong family history of coronary artery disease; obese patients; smokers; males older than 40 yr; and postmenopausal women.

DENTAL CONSIDERATIONS

General:
• This is an acute-use drug; thus, it is doubtful that patients will come to the office if acute migraine is present.
• Be aware of patient's disease, its severity, and its frequency, when known.
• Advise patient if dental drugs prescribed have potential for photosensitivity.
Consultations:
• If treating chronic orofacial pain, consult with physician of record.
• Medical consultation may be required to assess disease control and patient's ability to tolerate stress.
Teach Patient/Family to:
• Be aware that dryness of the mouth may occur when taking this drug.

• Avoid mouth rinses with high alcohol content because of drying effects.
• Update health and drug history if physician makes any changes in evaluation or drug regimens; include OTC, herbal, and nonherbal remedies in the update.

---

zolpidem tartrate
zole-**pi**′-dem **tar**′-trate
(Ambien, Stilnox[AUS])
Do not confuse Ambien with Amen.

CATEGORY AND SCHEDULE
Pregnancy Risk Category: B
Controlled Substance: Schedule IV

Drug Class: Nonbarbiturate, nonbenzodiazepine sedative-hypnotic

---

MECHANISM OF ACTION
A nonbenzodiazepine that enhances the action of the inhibitory neurotransmitter gamma-aminobutyric acid.
Therapeutic Effect: Induces sleep and improves sleep quality.

USES
Treatment of insomnia

PHARMACOKINETICS

Route	Onset	Peak	Duration
PO	30 min	N/A	6–8 hr

Rapidly absorbed from the GI tract. Protein binding: 92%. Metabolized in the liver; excreted in urine. Not removed by hemodialysis. *Half-life:* 1.4–4.5 hr (increased in hepatic impairment).

Z

INDICATIONS AND DOSAGES
▸ **Insomnia**
PO
Adults. 10 mg at bedtime.
Elderly, Debilitated. 5 mg at bedtime.

SIDE EFFECTS/ADVERSE REACTIONS
Occasional
Headache
Rare
Dizziness, nausea, diarrhea, muscle pain

PRECAUTIONS AND CONTRAINDICATIONS
Hypersensitivity, ritonavir
Caution:
Discontinue if skin rash occurs, pediatric patients at risk for oligohidrosis, hyperthermia; seizures with abrupt withdrawal; use contraception in women of childbearing age; hepatic or renal dysfunction; lactation, kidney stones

DRUG INTERACTIONS OF CONCERN TO DENTISTRY
• Increased CNS depression: alcohol, all CNS depressants, fluconazole, ketoconazole, itraconazole

SERIOUS REACTIONS
❗ Overdose may produce severe ataxia, bradycardia, altered vision (e.g., diplopia), severe drowsiness, nausea and vomiting, difficulty breathing, and unconsciousness.
❗ Abrupt withdrawal of the drug after long-term use may produce asthenia, facial flushing, diaphoresis, vomiting, and tremor.
❗ Drug tolerance or dependence may occur with prolonged, high-dose therapy.

DENTAL CONSIDERATIONS
General:
• Assess salivary flow as a factor in caries, periodontal disease, and candidiasis.
• Monitor vital signs at every appointment because of cardiovascular side effects.
Consultations:
• Medical consultation may be required to assess disease control.
Teach Patient/Family to:
• When chronic dry mouth occurs, advise patient to:
  • Avoid mouth rinses with high alcohol content because of drying effects.
  • Use daily home fluoride products to prevent caries.
  • Use sugarless gum, frequent sips of water, or saliva substitutes.

zonisamide
zoh-**nis'**-ah-mide
(Zonegran)

CATEGORY AND SCHEDULE
Pregnancy Risk Category: C

Drug Class: Anticonvulsant (sulfonamide derivative)

MECHANISM OF ACTION
A succinimide that may stabilize neuronal membranes and suppress neuronal hypersynchronization by blocking sodium and calcium channels.
Therapeutic Effect: Reduces seizure activity.

USES
Adjunctive therapy in partial seizures in adults with epilepsy

Z

PHARMACOKINETICS

Well absorbed after PO administration. Extensively bound to RBCs. Protein binding: 40%. Primarily excreted in urine. *Half-life:* 63 hr (plasma), 105 hr (RBCs).

INDICATIONS AND DOSAGES
▸ **Partial Seizures**
PO
Adults, Elderly, Children older than 16 yr. Initially, 100 mg/day for 2 wk. May increase by 100 mg/day at intervals of 2 wk or longer. Range: 100–600 mg/day.

SIDE EFFECTS/ADVERSE REACTIONS
Frequent
Somnolence, dizziness, anorexia, headache, agitation, irritability, nausea
Occasional
Fatigue, ataxia, confusion, depression, impaired memory or concentration, insomnia, abdominal pain, diplopia, diarrhea, speech difficulty
Rare
Paresthesia, nystagmus, anxiety, rash, dyspepsia, weight loss

PRECAUTIONS AND CONTRAINDICATIONS
Allergy to sulfonamides
Caution:
Discontinue if skin rash occurs, pediatric patients at risk for oligohidrosis, hyperthermia; seizures with abrupt withdrawal; use contraception in women of childbearing age; hepatic or renal dysfunction; lactation, kidney stones

DRUG INTERACTIONS OF CONCERN TO DENTISTRY
• No dental drug interactions reported; it has been proposed that drugs which either induce or inhibit CYP3A4 enzymes may not significantly alter serum levels.
• Carbamazepine increases renal clearance.

SERIOUS REACTIONS
! Overdose is characterized by bradycardia, hypotension, respiratory depression, and coma.
! Leukopenia, anemia, and thrombocytopenia occur rarely.

DENTAL CONSIDERATIONS
General:
• Determine type of epilepsy, seizure frequency, and quality of seizure control.
• Patients on chronic drug therapy may rarely have symptoms of blood dyscrasias, which can include infection, bleeding, and poor healing.
• Short appointments and a stress-reduction protocol may be required for anxious patients.
• Place on frequent recall to evaluate gingival condition and self-care.
• Consider semisupine chair position for patient comfort if GI side effects occur.
• Warn patient of increased CNS side effects when sedation is used. Advise not to drive a car to and from dental appointment.
Consultations:
• Consultation with physician may be necessary if sedation or general anesthesia is required.
• In a patient with symptoms of blood dyscrasias, request a medical consultation for blood studies and postpone treatment until normal values are reestablished.
• Medical consultation may be required to assess disease control and patient's ability to tolerate stress.

Teach Patient/Family to:
• Encourage effective oral hygiene to prevent soft tissue inflammation.
• Prevent trauma when using oral hygiene aids.
• Update health and drug history if physician makes any changes in evaluation or drug regimens; include OTC, herbal, and nonherbal remedies in the update.
• See physician immediately if rash develops because of drug.

Z

Appendix A Abbreviations

aa   of each

ab   antibody

abd   abdomen

ABGs   arterial blood gases

ac   before meals (ante cibum)

ACE   angiotensin-converting enzyme

ACEI   angiotensin-converting enzyme inhibitor

ACh   acetylcholine

ACT   activated clotting time

ACTH   adrenocorticotropic hormone

ad lib   as desired

ADH   antidiuretic hormone

ADP   adenosine diphosphate

ADR   adverse drug reaction

AIDS   acquired immunodeficiency syndrome

aka   also known as

ALT   alanine aminotransferase, serum

ama   against medical advice

amb   ambulation

amp   ampule

ANA   antinuclear antibody

ant   anterior

ANUG   acute necrotizing ulcerative gingivitis

AP   anteroposterior

APAP   N-acetyl-para-aminophenol (acetaminophen)

APB   atrial premature beat

aPTT   activated partial thromboplastin time

ARC   AIDS-related complex

AROM   active range of motion

ASA   acetylsalicylic acid (aspirin)

asap   as soon as possible

ASHD   arteriosclerotic heart disease

AST   aspartate aminotransferase, serum

AV   atrioventricular

BAC   blood alcohol concentration

bid   twice per day (bis in die)

BM   bowel movement

BMR   basal metabolic rate

bol   bolus

B/P   blood pressure

BPH   benign prostatic hypertrophy

bpm   beats per minute

BS   blood sugar

BUN   blood urea nitrogen

Bx   biopsy

C   Celsius (centigrade)

C section   cesarean section

CA   cancer

Ca   calcium

CAD   coronary artery disease

cAMP   cyclic adenosine monophosphate

cap   capsule

cath   catheterization or catheterize

CBC   complete blood count

CC   chief complaint

cc   cubic centimeter

CCB   calcium channel blocker

cGMP   cyclic guanosine monophosphate

CHD   coronary heart disease

CHF   congestive heart failure

cm   centimeter

CML   chronic myeloid leukemia

CMV   cytomegalovirus I

CNS   central nervous system

CO   cardiac output

CO_2 carbon dioxide

CoA   coenzyme A

c/o   complains of

COMT   catechol-O-methyltransferase

con rel   controlled release

conc   concentration

COPD   chronic obstructive pulmonary disease

COX-1   cyclooxygenase-1

COX-2   cyclooxygenase-2

CPAP   continuous positive airway pressure

CPK   creatinine phosphokinase

CPR   cardiopulmonary resuscitation

CrCl   creatinine clearance

CRD   chronic respiratory disease

CRF   chronic renal failure

C&S   culture and sensitivity

CSF   cerebrospinal fluid

CTZ   chemoreceptor trigger zone

CV   cardiovascular

CVA   cerebrovascular accident

CVP   central venous pressure

$CysLT_1$ cysteinyl leukotriene receptor

D&C   dilation and curettage

del rel   delayed release

DIC   disseminated intravascular coagulation

DM   diabetes mellitus

DMARD   disease-modifying antirheumatic drug

DNA   deoxyribonucleic acid

DOB   date of birth

dr   dram

dsg   dressing

DVT   deep vein thrombosis

D_5W 5% glucose in distilled water

Dx   diagnosis

EBV   Epstein-Barr virus

ECG   electrocardiogram (EKG)

EEG   electroencephalogram

EENT   ear, eye, nose, and throat

elix   elixir, hydroalcoholic solution containing an active drug(s)

ENDO   endocrine systems

EPO   erythropoietin

EPS   extrapyramidal symptoms

ESR   erythrocyte sedimentation rate

ext rel   extended release

F   Fahrenheit

FBS   fasting blood sugar

FHT   fetal heart tones

FIO$_2$ inspired oxygen concentration

FSH   follicle-stimulating hormone

fx   fracture

g   gram

GABA   gamma-aminobutyric acid

gal   gallon

GERD   gastroesophageal reflux disease

GGTP   gamma-glutamyl transpeptidase

GHb   glycosylated hemoglobin

GI   gastrointestinal

G6PD   glucose-6-phosphate dehydrogenase

GR   glucocorticoid receptor

gr   grain

GTT   glucose tolerance test

gtt   drop

GU   genitourinary

Gyn   gynecology

HbA1c   laboratory test for glycosylated hemoglobin

HCG   human chorionic gonadotropin

Hct   hematocrit

HDL   high-density lipoprotein

HEMA   hematologic system

Hgb   hemoglobin

H&H   hematocrit and hemoglobin

5-HIAA   5-hydroxyindole-acetic acid

HIV   human immunodeficiency virus

HMG-CoA   3-hydroxy-3-methyl-glutaryl-coenzyme A reductase

H$_2$O   water

H&P   history and physical examination

HPA   hypothalamic-pituitary-adrenocortical axis

HR   heart rate

hr   hour(s)

HRT   hormone replacement therapy

hs   at bedtime

HSV   herpes simplex virus

HSV-2   herpes genitalis

5-HT   5-hydroxytryptamine (serotonin)

Hypo   hypodermically

Hx   history

IBS   irritable bowel syndrome

ICP   intracranial pressure

ICU   intensive care unit

I&D   incision and drainage

IDDM insulin-dependent diabetes mellitus

IgG immunoglobulin G

IL-2 interleukin-2

IM intramuscular

immed rel immediate release

inf infusion

inh inhalation

inj injection

INR international normalized ratio

INTEG relating to integumentary structures

IOP intraocular pressure

IPPB intermittent positive-pressure breathing

ITP idiopathic thrombocytopenic purpura

IU international unit

IUD intrauterine contraceptive device

IV intravenous

IVP intravenous piggyback

K potassium

kg kilogram

L or l left; liter

lat lateral

lb pound

LDH lactic dehydrogenase

LDL low-density lipoprotein

LDL-C low-density lipoprotein-cholesterol

LE lupus erythematosus

LFT liver function test

LH luteinizing hormone

LHRH luteinizing hormone-releasing hormone

liq liquid

LLQ left lower quadrant

LMP last menstrual period

LOC loss of consciousness

lot lotion

loz lozenge

LR lactated Ringer's solution

LRI lower respiratory infection

LVD left ventricular dysfunction

m meter

m² square meter

MAC *Mycobacterium avium* complex

MAO monoamine oxidase

MAOI monoamine oxidase inhibitor

max maximum

mEq milliequivalent

META metabolic

mg milligram

mcg microgram

MI myocardial infarction

min minute(s)

mixt mixture

ml milliliter

mm millimeter

mo month

MPA   mycophenolic acid

MS   musculoskeletal

MVA   motor vehicle accident

Na   sodium

NC   nasal cannula

neg   negative

ng   nanogram

NIDDM   non–insulin-dependent diabetes mellitus

NKA   no known allergies

NMDA   *N*-methyl-D-aspartate

NMI   no middle initial

noc   nocturnal (night)

NPH   neutral protamine Hagedorn

NPO   nothing by mouth (nil per os)

NS   normal saline

NSAID   nonsteroidal antiinflammatory drug

NV   neurovascular

O_2 oxygen

OBS   organic brain syndrome

OC   oral contraceptive

OD   right eye (oculus dexter)

oint   ointment

OOB   out of bed

Ophth   ophthalmic

OR   operating room

ORIF   open reduction, internal fixation

OS   left eye (ocular sinister)

OTC   over the counter

ou   each eye (oculus uterque)

oz   ounce

p̄   after (post)

p   pulse

PABA   para-aminobenzoic acid

PAC   premature atrial contraction

PAT   paroxysmal atrial tachycardia

PBI   protein-bound iodine

PBP   penicillin binding protein

pc   after meals (post cibum)

PCA   patient-controlled analgesia

PCN   penicillin

pCO_2 arterial carbon dioxide tension (pressure in mm Hg)

PE   physical examination

PG   prostaglandin

pH   hydrogen ion concentration

PMDD   premenstrual dysphoric disorder

PMS   premenstrual syndrome

PNS   peripheral nervous system

PO   by mouth (per os)

pO_2 arterial oxygen tension (pressure in mm Hg)

postop   postoperatively

PP   postprandial

ppm   parts per million

preop   preoperatively

prep   preparation

prn   as needed (pro re nata)

PSA prostate-specific antigen

PT prothrombin time

PTSD posttraumatic stress disorder

PTT partial thromboplastin time

PVC premature ventricular contraction

PVD peripheral vascular disease

q every

qAM every morning

qd every day

qh every hour

qid four times per day

qod every other day

qPM every night

qt quart

q2h every 2 hours

q3h every 3 hours

q4h every 4 hours

q6h every 6 hours

q12h every 12 hours

qwk every week

r right

rap disintegr rapidly disintegrating

RAR retinoic acid receptor

RBC red blood count or cell

RDA recommended dietary allowance

rec rectal

REM rapid eye movement

RESP respiratory system

rhPDGF-BB recombinant human platelet-derived growth factor

RNA ribonucleic acid

R/O rule out

ROAD reversible obstructive airway disease

ROM range of motion

RTI respiratory tract infection

Rx therapy, treatment, or prescription

s̄ without

SA sinoatrial

SAN sinoatrial node

SC subcutaneous

sec second

SERM selective estrogen receptor modulator

SGOT serum glutamic-oxaloacetic transaminase (now AST)

SGPT serum glutamic pyruvate transaminase (now ALT)

SIADH syndrome of inappropriate antidiuretic hormone

sig patient dosing instructions on prescription label

SL sublingual

SLE systemic lupus erythematosus

slow rel slow release

SMBG self-monitored blood glucose

SMZ sulfamethoxazole

SOB shortness of breath

sol   solution

ss   semis (one-half)

SSRI   selective serotonin reuptake inhibitor

stat   at once

STD   sexually transmitted disease

supp   suppository

surg   surgical

sus rel   sustained-release dose form

Sx   symptoms

syr   syrup, a highly concentrated sucrose solution containing a drug(s)

T   temperature

$T_{1/2}$ drug half-life

T_3 triiodothyronine

T_4 thyroxine

tab   tablet

TB   tuberculosis

TBG   thyroxine-binding globulin

tbsp   tablespoon

TCA   tricyclic antidepressant

TD   transdermal

temp   temperature

TG   total triglycerides

TIA   transient ischemic attack

tid   three times per day (ter in die)

time rel   time-release dose form

tinc   tincture, alcoholic solution of a drug

TMD   temporomandibular disorder

TMJ   temporomandibular joint

TMP   trimethoprim

TNF   tumor necrosis factor

top   topical

tPA   tissue plasminogen activator

TPN   total parenteral nutrition

TPR   temperature, pulse, respirations

TSH   thyroid-stimulating hormone

tsp   teaspoon

TT   thrombin time

Tx   treatment

U   unit

UA   urinalysis

ULDL   ultra-low-density lipoprotein

URI   upper respiratory infection

USP   United States Pharmacopeia

UTI   urinary tract infection

UV   ultraviolet

vag   vaginal

visc   viscous

VD   venereal disease

VHDL   very-high-density lipoprotein

VLDL   very-low-density lipoprotein

VO   verbal order

vol   volume

VPB	ventricular premature beat	yr	year(s)
VS	vital signs	>	greater than
WBC	white blood cell, white blood cell count	<	less than
		≠	not equal
WHO	World Health Organization	↑	increase
Wk	week	↓	decrease
WNL	within normal limits	2°	secondary
wt	weight		

Appendix B Anesthetics

ANESTHETICS: GENERAL

Uses

IV anesthetic agents are used to induce general anesthesia. The general anesthetic state consists of unconsciousness, amnesia, analgesia, immobility, and attenuation of autonomic responses to noxious stimuli.

Volatile inhalation agents produce all of the components of the anesthetic state but are administered through the lungs via an anesthesia machine. Agents for use include desflurane, enflurane, halothane, isoflurane, and sevoflurane. They are used in practice to maintain general anesthesia.

Mechanisms of Action

IV anesthetic agents act on the gamma-aminobutyric acid (GABA) receptor complex to produce CNS depression. GABA is the primary inhibitory neurotransmitter in the CNS. Ketamine produces dissociation between the thalamus and the limbic system.

The specific actions of volatile inhalation agents are not all fully understood but may disrupt neuronal transmission throughout the CNS. These agents may either block excitatory transmission or enhance inhibitory transmission through axons or synapses.

TABLE B–1

Anesthetics: General

Name	Availability	Uses	Dosage Range	Side Effects
Etomidate (Amidate)	I: 2 mg/ml	IV induction	0.2–0.6 mg/kg	Myoclonus, pain on injection, nausea, vomiting, respiratory depression
Ketamine (Ketalar)	I: 10 mg/ml, 50 mg/ml, 100 mg/ml	Analgesia, sedation, IV induction	1–4.5 mg/kg	Delirium, euphoria, nausea, vomiting
Methohexital (Brevital)	Powder for injection: 500 mg	IV induction, sedation	50–120 mg	Cardiovascular depression, myoclonus, nausea, vomiting, respiratory depression
Midazolam (Versed)	I: 1 mg/ml, 5 mg/ml	Anxiolytic, amnesic, sedation	1–5 mg titrated slowly	Respiratory depression
Propofol (Diprivan)	I: 10 mg/ml	Sedation IV induction maintenance	0.5 mg/kg 2–2.5 mg/kg 100–200 mcg/kg/min	Cardiovascular depression, delirium, euphoria, pain on injection, respiratory depression
Thiopental (Pentothal)	Powder for injection: 2.5% (25 mg/ml)	IV induction	Titrate vs. pt response. Average: 50–75 mg	Cardiovascular depression, nausea, vomiting, respiratory depression

I, injection; pt, patient.

ANESTHETICS: LOCAL

Uses

Local anesthetics suppress pain by blocking impulses along axons. When carefully administered, they do not cause generalized depression of the entire nervous system. Local anesthetics may be given topically and by injection (local infiltration, peripheral nerve block [axillary], IV regional [Bier block], epidural, and spinal).

Action

Most local anesthetics fall into one of two groups: esters or amides. Both provide anesthesia and analgesia by reversibly binding to and blocking sodium (Na) channels. This slows the rate of depolarization of the nerve action potential; thus, the electrical impulses needed for nerve conduction are blocked.

TABLE B–2

Anesthetics: Local

Name	Uses	Onset (min)	Duration (hr)	Side Effects
Esters				
Chloroprocaine (Nesacaine)	Local infiltration Nerve block Spinal	6–12	0.25–0.5	Excitation (e.g., seizures) followed by decreased level of consciousness (drowsiness to unconsciousness), bradycardia, heart block, decreased myocardial contractile force, hypotension, hypersensitivity reaction
Procaine (Novocaine)	Local infiltration Nerve block Spinal	2–5	0.25–1	Same as above
Tetracaine	Topical Spinal	15	2–3	Same as above
Amides				
Bupivacaine (Marcaine, Sensorcaine)	Local infiltration Nerve block Epidural Spinal	5	2–4	Same as above
Etidocaine (Duranest)	Nerve block Epidural	3–5	5–10	Same as above
Levobupivacaine (Chirocaine)	Nerve block Epidural	—	—	Same as above

TABLE B–2

Anesthetics: Local—cont'd

Name	Uses	Onset (min)	Duration (hr)	Side Effects
Lidocaine	Local infiltration Nerve block Spinal Epidural Topical IV regional	Less than 2	0.5–1	Same as above
Mepivacaine (Carbocaine, Polocaine)	Local infiltration Nerve block Epidural	3–5	0.75–1.5	Same as above
Ropivacaine (Naropin)	Local infiltration Nerve block Epidural Spinal	1–15	2–6	Same as above

Note: Most side effects are manifestations of excessive plasma concentrations.
From *Mosby's 2006 drug consult for nurses,* St. Louis, 2006, Mosby.

TABLE B-3
Contraindications for Local Anesthetics

Medical Problem	Drugs to Avoid	Type of Contraindication	Alternative Drug
Local anesthetic allergy, documented	All local anesthetics in same chemical class (e.g., esters)	Absolute	Local anesthetics in a different chemical class (e.g., amides)
Bisulfite allergy	Vasoconstrictor-containing local anesthetics	Absolute	Local anesthetic without vasoconstrictor
Atypical plasma cholinesterase	Esters	Relative	Amides
Methemoglobinemia, idiopathic or congenital	Prilocaine	Relative	Other amides or esters
Significant liver dysfunction (ASA III–IV)	Amides	Relative	Amides or esters, but judiciously
Significant renal dysfunction (ASA III–IV)	Amides or esters	Relative	Amides or esters, but judiciously
Significant cardiovascular disease (ASA III–IV)	High concentrations of vasoconstrictors	Relative	Local anesthetics with epinephrine concentrations of 1:200,000 or 1:100,000 or mepivacaine 3% or prilocaine 4% (nerve blocks)
Clinical hyperthyroidism (ASA III–IV)	High concentrations of vasoconstrictors	Relative	Local anesthetics with epinephrine concentrations of 1:200,000 or 1:100,000 or mepivacaine 3% or prilocaine 4% (nerve blocks)

ASA, American Society of Anesthesiologists' classification.
From Malamed SF: *Handbook of local anesthesia*, ed 5, St. Louis, 2004, Mosby.

TABLE B-4
Dental Local Anesthetic Preparations and Pharmacologic Characteristics

| Proprietary Name | Manufacturer | Percent Local Anesthetic | Vasoconstrictor | Duration of Analgesia (min) | | MRD^A | MRD^B |
				Pulpal	Soft Tissue		
Articaine hydrochloride							
(United States) Septocaine (Canada) Septanest SP Astracaine Ultracaine D–S forte Zorcaine	Septodont Septodont Dentsply Hoechst Kodak	4	Epinephrine 1:100,000	45–60	120–300	7 mg/kg 3.2 mg/lb 500 mg absolute maximum	
(Canada) Septanest N Astracaine Ultracaine D–S	Septodont Dentsply Hoechst	4	Epinephrine 1:200,000	45–60	120–300	7 mg/kg 3.2 mg/lb 500 mg absolute maximum	
Bupivacaine hydrochloride							
Marcaine	Kodak	0.5	Epinephrine 1:200,000	90–180	240–540 (reports up to 720)	1.3 mg/kg 0.6 mg/lb 90 mg absolute maximum	

(Continued)

TABLE B-4
Dental Local Anesthetic Preparations and Pharmacologic Characteristics—cont'd

Proprietary Name	Manufacturer	Percent Local Anesthetic	Vasoconstrictor	Duration of Analgesia (min)		MRD^A	MRD^B
				Pulpal	Soft Tissue		
Lidocaine hydrochloride							
Lidocaine HCl Alphacaine Xylocaine	Many generics Carlisle Labs Dentsply	2	—	5–10	60–120	4.4 mg/kg 2.0 mg/lb 300 mg absolute maximum	
Lidocaine HCl Alphacaine Lignospan Octocaine Xylocaine	Many generics Carlisle Labs Septodont Novocol Chemical Dentsply	2	Epinephrine 1:50,000	60	180–300	6.6 mg/kg 3.0 mg/lb 500 mg absolute maximum	4.4 mg/kg 2.0 mg/lb 300 mg absolute maximum
Mepivacaine hydrochloride							
Mepivacaine HCl Arestocaine Carbocaine Isocaine Polocaine Scandonest	Many generics Carlisle Labs Kodak Novocol Dentsply Septodont	3	—	20–40 (20 for infiltration; 40 for nerve block)	120–180	6.6 mg/kg 3.0 mg/lb 400 absolute maximum	4.4 mg/kg 2.0 mg/lb 300 absolute maximum

Drug	Manufacturer	%	Vasoconstrictor				
Mepivacaine HCl Arestocaine Isocaine Polocaine Scandonest Carbocaine	Many generics Carlisle Labs Dentsply Kodak Septodent Novocol	2	Levonordefrin 1:20,000 Neo-Cobefrin 1:20,000	60	180–300	6.6 mg/kg 3.0 mg/lb 400 absolute maximum	4.4 mg/kg 2.0 mg/lb 300 absolute maximum
Carbocaine	Kodak	2	Epinephrine 1:200,000	45–60	120–240	6.6 mg/kg 3.0 mg/lb 400 absolute maximum	4.4 mg/kg 2.0 mg/lb 300 absolute maximum
Scandonest 2% Special	Septodont	2	Epinephrine 1:200,000	60	120–300	6.6 mg/kg 3.0 mg/lb 400 absolute maximum	4.4 mg/kg 2.0 mg/lb 300 absolute maximum
Prilocaine hydrochloride							
Prilocaine HCl Citanest Plain	Generic Dentsply	4		10–15 (infiltration) 40–60 (nerve block)	90–120 (inf) 120–240 (nb)	6 mg/kg 2.7 mg/lb 400 mg absolute maximum	
Prilocaine HCl + epinephrine 1:200,000 Citanest Forte	Generic Dentsply	4	Epinephrine 1:200,000	60–90	180–480	6 mg/kg 2.7 mg/lb 400 mg absolute maximum	

MRD, manufacturer maximum recommended dose.
From Malamed SF: *Handbook of local anesthesia*, ed 5, St. Louis, 2004, Mosby.

TABLE B–5

Mandibular Teeth and Available Local Anesthetic Techniques

Teeth	Pulpal Anesthesia	Soft Tissue	
		Buccal	**Lingual**
Incisors	Incisive IANB GG VA PDL injection IS IO Inf	IANB GG VA IS Mental PDL injection Inf	IANB GG VA PDL injection IS Inf
Canines	IANB GG VA Inc PDL injection IS IO	IANB GG VA Inc PDL injection IS Mental Inf	IANB GG VA PDL injection IS Inf
Premolars	IANB GG VA Inc PDL injection IS IO	IANB GG VA Inc PDL injection IS Mental Inf	IANB GG VA PDL injection IS Inf
Molars	IANB GG VA PDL injection IS IO	IANB GG VA PDL injection IS Inf	IANB GG VA PDL injection IS Inf

GG, Gow–Gates; IANB, inferior alveolar; Inc, incisive; Inf, infiltration; IO, intraosseous; IS, intraseptal; PDL, periodontal ligament; VA, Vazirani-Akinosi.
From Malamed SF: *Handbook of local anesthesia,* ed 5, St. Louis, 2004, Mosby.

TABLE B–6

Maxillary Teeth and Available Local Anesthetic

Teeth	Pulpal Anesthesia	Soft Tissue	
		Buccal	Palatal
Incisors	IO Infiltration P–ASA V2	IO Infiltration P–ASA V2	Nasopalatine Infiltration P–ASA V2
Canines	Infraorbital Infiltration P–ASA V2	Infraorbital Infiltration P–ASA V2	Nasopalatine Infiltration P–ASA V2
Premolars	Infraorbital Infiltration MSA ASA V2	Infraorbital Infiltration MSA ASA V2	Greater palatine Infiltration AMSA V2
Molars	PSA Infiltration V2	PSA Infiltration V2	Greater palatine Infiltration V2

ASA, anterior superior alveolar; IO, infraorbital; PSA, posterior superior alveolar; MSA, middle superior alveolar; V2, maxillary division block.

From Malamed SF: *Handbook of local anesthesia,* ed 5, St. Louis, 2004, Mosby.

Appendix C   Combination Drugs by Trade Name

Many drugs are available in fixed combinations of two or more medications. Some of the most common trade names for combination drugs in the United States are listed, along with their generic components and classifications. The list is alphabetical by the brand name of the combination product. Brand names for identical drug combinations are listed together. When the patient's drug history includes one of these combination products, it can be easily accessed through the index.

Combination Product Name	Generic Components
AC Gel	Cocaine (an anesthetic)/epinephrine (a vasopressor)
Accuretic	Quinapril (an ACE inhibitor)/hydrochlorothiazide (a diuretic)
Activella	Estradiol (an estrogen)/norethindrone (a hormone)
Advair	Fluticasone (a corticosteroid)/salmeterol (a bronchodilator)
Advil Cold	Pseudoephedrine (a sympathomimetic)/ibuprofen (an NSAID)
Aggrenox	Aspirin (an antiplatelet and nonnarcotic analgesic)/dipyridamole (an antiplatelet)
Aldactazide	Spironolactone (a potassium-sparing diuretic)/hydrochlorothiazide (a diuretic)
Aldoril	Methyldopa (an antihypertensive)/hydrochlorothiazide (a diuretic)
Allegra-D	Fexofenadine (an antihistamine)/pseudoephedrine (a sympathomimetic nasal decongestant)
Allegra-D 24 Hour	Fexofenadine (an antihistamine)/pseudoephedrine (a sympathomimetic nasal decongestant)
Anexsia	Hydrocodone (a narcotic analgesic)/acetaminophen (a nonnarcotic analgesic)
Apresazide	Hydralazine (a vasodilator)/hydrochlorothiazide (a diuretic)
Arthrotec	Diclofenac (an NSAID)/misoprostol (an antisecretory gastric protectant)
Atacand HCT	Candesartan (an angiotensin II receptor antagonist)/hydrochlorothiazide (a diuretic)
Avalide	Irbesartan (an angiotensin II receptor antagonist)/hydrochlorothiazide (a diuretic)
Avandamet	Rosiglitazone (an antidiabetic)/metformin (an antidiabetic)
Bactrim	Sulfamethoxazole (a sulfonamide)/trimethoprim (an antiinfective)
Bellergal-S	Ergotamine (an antimigraine)/belladonna (an anticholinergic)/phenobarbital (an anticonvulsant)
Benicar HCT	Olmesartan (an angiotensin II receptor antagonist)/hydrochlorothiazide (a diuretic)

Combination Product Name	Generic Components
Bicillin CR	Penicillin G benzathine (a penicillin)/penicillin procaine (a penicillin)
Blephamide	Sulfacetamide (an antiinfective)/prednisolone (an adrenocortical steroid)
Caduet	Amlodipine (a calcium channel blocker)/atorvastatin (an antihyperlipidemic)
Caladryl	Calamine (an astringent)/diphenhydramine (an antihistamine)/camphor (a counterirritant)
Capital with Codeine	Acetaminophen (a nonnarcotic analgesic)/codeine (a narcotic analgesic)
Capozide	Captopril (an ACE inhibitor)/hydrochlorothiazide (a diuretic)
Children's Advil Cold	Ibuprofen (an NSAID)/pseudoephedrine (a sympathomimetic nasal decongestant)
Cipro HC Otic	Ciprofloxacin (an antiinfective)/hydrocortisone (an adrenocortical steroid)
Ciprodex Otic	Ciprofloxacin (an antiinfective)/dexamethasone (an adrenocortical steroid)
Claritin-D	Loratadine (an antihistamine)/pseudoephedrine (a nasal decongestant)
CombiPatch	Estradiol (an estrogen)/norethindrone (a hormone)
Combipres	Clonidine (an antihypertensive)/chlorthalidone (a diuretic)
Combivent	Ipratropium (a bronchodilator)/albuterol (a bronchodilator)
Combivir	Lamivudine (an antiretroviral)/zidovudine (an antiretroviral)
Combunox	Ibuprofen (an NSAID)/oxycodone (a narcotic analgesic)
Cortisporin	Neomycin (an antiinfective)/polymyxin B (an antiinfective)/hydrocortisone (an adrenocortical steroid)
Corzide	Nadolol (a β-blocker)/bendroflumethiazide (a diuretic)
Cosopt	Dorzolamide (a carbonic anhydrase inhibitor)/timolol (a β-blocker)
Dexacidin	Neomycin (an antiinfective)/polymyxin (an antiinfective)/dexamethasone (an adrenocortical steroid)
Dilantin with PB	Phenobarbital (an anticonvulsant)/phenytoin (an anticonvulsant)
Diovan HCT	Valsartan (an angiotensin II receptor antagonist)/hydrochlorothiazide (a diuretic)
Donnatal	Atropine (an anticholinergic)/hyoscyamine (an anticholinergic)/phenobarbital (a sedative)/scopolamine (an anticholinergic)
Duocet	Acetaminophen (a nonopioid analgesic)/hydrocodone (an opioid analgesic)

(Continued)

Combination Product Name	Generic Components
DuoNeb	Ipratropium (a bronchodilator)/albuterol base (a bronchodilator)
Dyazide	Triamterene (a potassium-sparing diuretic)/hydrochlorothiazide (a diuretic)
EMLA	Lidocaine (a local anesthetic)/prilocaine (an anesthetic)
Epzicom	Abacavir (an antiretroviral)/lamivudine (an antiretroviral)
Eryzole	Erythromycin (a macrolide)/sulfisoxazole (a sulfonamide)
Etrafon	Perphenazine (an antipsychotic)/amitriptyline (an antidepressant)
Exforge	Amlodipine (antianginal and antihypertensive agent) Losartan (an angiotensin II receptor, type AT1)
Extra Strength Maalox	Magnesium hydroxide (an antacid)/simethicone Maalox (an antiflatulent)
Femhrt	Norethindrone (a hormone)/estradiol (an estrogen)
Ferro-Sequels	Ferrous fumarate (a hematinic)/docusate (a laxative)
Fioricet	Butabarbital (a sedative-hypnotic)/acetaminophen (a nonnarcotic analgesic)/caffeine (a CNS stimulant)
Fiorinal	Butabarbital (a sedative-hypnotic)/aspirin (a nonnarcotic analgesic)/caffeine (a CNS stimulant)
Gaviscon (oral suspension)	Aluminum hydroxide (an antacid)/magnesium carbonate (an antacid)
Gaviscon (tablets)	Aluminum hydroxide (an antacid)/magnesium trisilicate (an antacid)
Gelusil	Aluminum hydroxide (an antacid)/magnesium hydroxide (a laxative)/simethicone (an antiflatulent)
Gentlax-S	Senna (a laxative)/docusate (a laxative)
Glucovance	Glyburide (an antidiabetic)/metformin (an antidiabetic)
Haley's M-O	Magnesium (a laxative)/mineral oil (a lubricant laxative)
Helidac	Bismuth (an antidiarrheal)/metronidazole (an antiinfective)/tetracycline (an antiinfective)
Humalog Mix 75/25	Insulin: lispro suspension 75% and lispro solution 25%
Humulin 50/50	Insulin: NPH 50% and regular 50%
Humulin 70/30	Insulin: NPH 70% and rapid-acting regular 30%
Hyzaar	Losartan (an angiotensin II receptor antagonist)/hydrochlorothiazide (a diuretic)
Imodium Advanced	Loperamide (an antidiarrheal)/simethicone (an antiflatulent)
Inderide	Propranolol (a β-blocker)/hydrochlorothiazide (a diuretic)
Inderide LA	Propranolol (a β-blocker)/hydrochlorothiazide (a diuretic)
Lexxel	Enalapril (an ACE inhibitor)/felodipine (a calcium channel blocker)

Combination Product Name	Generic Components
Librax	Chlordiazepoxide (an antianxiety agent)/clidinium (an anticholinergic)
Lidocaine with Epinephrine	Lidocaine (a local anesthetic)/epinephrine (a vasoconstrictor)
LidoSite	Epinephrine (a sympathomimetic)/lidocaine (an anesthetic)
Limbitrol	Chlordiazepoxide (an antianxiety agent)/amitriptyline (an antidepressant)
Lomotil	Diphenoxylate (an antidiarrheal)/atropine (an anticholinergic/antispasmodic)
Lopressor HCT	Metoprolol (a β-blocker)/hydrochlorothiazide (a diuretic)
Lorcet	Acetaminophen (a nonnarcotic analgesic)/hydrocodone (a narcotic analgesic)
Lortab	Hydrocodone (an opioid analgesic)/acetaminophen (a nonopioid analgesic)
Lortab Elixir	Hydrocodone (a narcotic analgesic)/acetaminophen (a nonopioid analgesic)
Lortab/ASA	Hydrocodone (a narcotic analgesic)/aspirin (a nonnarcotic analgesic)
Lotensin HCT	Benazepril (an ACE inhibitor)/hydrochlorothiazide (a diuretic)
Lotrel	Amlodipine (a calcium channel blocker)/benazepril (an ACE inhibitor)
Lotrisone	Clotrimazole (an antifungal)/betamethasone (an adrenocortical steroid)
Lunelle	Medroxyprogesterone (a progestin)/estradiol (an estrogen)
Maalox	Aluminum hydroxide (an antacid)/magnesium hydroxide (an antacid)
Maalox Plus	Aluminum hydroxide (an antacid)/magnesium hydroxide (an antacid)/simethicone (an antiflatulent)
Maxitrol	Neomycin (an antiinfective)/polymyxin (an antiinfective)/dexamethasone (an adrenocortical steroid)
Maxzide	Triamterene (a potassium-sparing diuretic)/hydrochlorothiazide (a diuretic)
Metaglip	Glipizide (an antidiabetic)/metformin (an antidiabetic)
Micardis HCT	Telmisartan (an angiotensin II receptor antagonist)/hydrochlorothiazide (a diuretic)
Minizide	Prazosin (an antihypertensive)/polythiazide (a diuretic)
Moduretic	Amiloride (a potassium-sparing diuretic)/hydrochlorothiazide (a diuretic)

(Continued)

Combination Product Name	Generic Components
Motrin Cold	Pseudoephedrine (a sympathomimetic nasal decongestant)/ibuprofen (an NSAID)
Mucinex D	Guaifenesin (an expectorant)/pseudoephedrine (a sympathomimetic nasal decongestant)
Mucinex DM	Guaifenesin (an expectorant)/dextromethorphan (an expectorant)
Mycitracin	Neomycin (an aminoglycoside)/polymyxin B (an antiinfective)/bacitracin (an antiinfective)
Myco II	Nystatin (an antifungal)/triamcinolone (an adrenocortical steroid)
Mycolog II	Nystatin (an antifungal)/triamcinolone (an adrenocortical steroid)
Myco-Triacet	Nystatin (an antifungal)/triamcinolone (an adrenocortical steroid)
Mylanta	Aluminum hydroxide (an antacid)/magnesium hydroxide (oral suspension) (an antacid)/simethicone (an antiflatulent)
Mylanta (tablets)	Calcium carbonate/magnesium hydroxide
Naphcon-A	Naphazoline (a nasal decongestant)/pheniramine (an antihistamine)
Neosporin GU	Neomycin (an aminoglycoside)/polymyxin B (an antiinfective)
Neosporin Ointment, Triple Antibiotic	Neomycin (an aminoglycoside)/polymyxin B (an antiinfective)/bacitracin (an antiinfective)
Norco	Hydrocodone (an opioid analgesic)/acetaminophen (a nonopioid analgesic)
Normozide	Labetalol (a β-blocker)/hydrochlorothiazide (a diuretic)
Novolin 70/30	Insulin: NPH 70% and rapid-acting regular 30%
NovoLog 70/30	Insulin: aspart suspension 70% and aspart solution 30%
Pediazole	Erythromycin (a macrolide)/sulfisoxazole (a sulfonamide)
Pepcid Complete	Famotidine (an H_2 antagonist)/calcium chloride (an antacid)/magnesium hydroxide (an antacid)
Percocet	Oxycodone (an opioid analgesic)/acetaminophen (a nonopioid analgesic)
Percodan	Oxycodone (an opioid analgesic)/aspirin (a nonopioid analgesic)
Phenergan with Codeine	Promethazine (an antihistamine)/codeine (a cough suppressant)
Phenergan VC	Promethazine (an antihistamine)/phenylephrine (a vasopressor)
Phenergan VC with Codeine	Promethazine (an antihistamine)/phenylephrine (a vasopressor)/codeine (a cough suppressant)
Polysporin	Polymyxin B (an antiinfective)/bacitracin (an antiinfective)
Pravigard	Aspirin (an antiplatelet)/pravastatin (an antihyperlipidemic)

Combination Product Name	Generic Components
Premphase	Conjugated estrogens (an estrogen)/medroxyprogesterone (an androgen)
Prempro	Conjugated estrogens (an estrogen)/medroxyprogesterone (an androgen)
Prevacid NapraPAC	Lansoprazole (a proton pump inhibitor)/naproxen (an NSAID)
Prinzide	Lisinopril (an ACE inhibitor)/hydrochlorothiazide (a diuretic)
Rebetron	Ribavirin (an antiviral)/interferon alfa 2b (an immunologic agent)
Reprexain CIII	Ibuprofen (an NSAID)/hydrocodone (an opioid analgesic)
Rifamate	Rifampin (an antitubercular)/isoniazid (an antitubercular)
Rifater	Rifampin (an antitubercular)/isoniazid (an antitubercular)/ pyrazinamide (an antitubercular)
Robitussin AC	Guaifenesin (an antitussive)/codeine (a narcotic analgesic)
Robitussin DM	Dextromethorphan (a cough suppressant)/guaifenesin (an antitussive)
Roxicet	Oxycodone (an opioid analgesic)/acetaminophen (a nonopioid analgesic)
Senokot-S	Senna (a laxative)/docusate (a laxative)
Septra	Sulfamethoxazole (a sulfonamide)/trimethoprim (an antiinfective)
Silain-Gel	Magnesium hydroxide (an antacid)/aluminum hydroxide (an antacid)/simethicone (an antiflatulent)
Stalevo	Carbidopa-levodopa (an antiparkinson agent)/entacapone (an antiparkinson agent)
Suboxone	Buprenorphine (a nonnarcotic analgesic)/naloxone (a narcotic antagonist)
Symbyax	Fluoxetine (an antidepressant)/olanzapine (an antipsychotic)
TAC	Tetracaine (an anesthetic)/epinephrine (a vasoconstrictor)/ cocaine (an anesthetic)
Tarka	Trandolapril (an ACE inhibitor)/verapamil (a calcium blocker)
Teczem	Enalapril (an ACE inhibitor)/diltiazem (a calcium channel blocker)
Tenoretic	Atenolol (a β-blocker)/chlorthalidone (a diuretic)
Teveten HCT	Eprosartan (an angiotensin II receptor antagonist)/ hydrochlorothiazide (a diuretic)
Thyrolar	Liothyronine (a thyroid agent)/levothyroxine (a thyroid agent)
Timolide	Timolol (a β-blocker)/hydrochlorothiazide (a diuretic)
TobraDex	Tobramycin (an aminoglycoside)/dexamethasone (an adrenocortical steroid)

(Continued)

Combination Product Name	**Generic Components**
Triavil	Perphenazine (an antipsychotic)/amitriptyline (an antidepressant)
Trizivir	Abacavir (an antiretroviral)/lamivudine (an antiretroviral)/ zidovudine (an antiretroviral)
Truvada	Emtricitabine (an antiretroviral)/tenofovir (an antiretroviral)
Tylenol with Codeine	Acetaminophen (a nonopioid analgesic)/codeine (an opioid analgesic)
Tylox	Acetaminophen (a nonopioid analgesic)/oxycodone (an opioid analgesic)
Ultracet	Tramadol (a nonopioid analgesic)/acetaminophen (a nonopioid analgesic)
Uniretic	Moexipril (an ACE inhibitor)/hydrochlorothiazide (a diuretic)
Vaseretic	Enalapril (an ACE inhibitor)/hydrochlorothiazide (a diuretic)
Vasocidin	Sulfacetamide (an antiinfective)/prednisolone (an adrenocortical steroid)
Vicodin	Hydrocodone (an opioid analgesic)/acetaminophen (a nonopioid analgesic)
Vicodin ES	Hydrocodone (an opioid analgesic)/acetaminophen (a nonopioid analgesic)
Vicodin HP	Hydrocodone (an opioid analgesic)/acetaminophen (a nonopioid analgesic)
Vicoprofen	Hydrocodone (an opioid analgesic)/ibuprofen (an NSAID)
Vytorin	Ezetimibe (an antihyperlipidemic)/simvastatin (an antihyperlipidemic)
Zestoretic	Lisinopril (an ACE inhibitor)/hydrochlorothiazide (a diuretic)
Ziac	Bisoprolol (a β-blocker)/hydrochlorothiazide (a diuretic)
Zotrim	Trimethoprim (an antiinfective)/sulfamethoxazole (a sulfonamide)/ phenazopyridine (a spasmolytic)
Zydone	Hydrocodone (an opioid analgesic)/acetaminophen (a nonopioid analgesic)
Zyrtec D 12 Hour Tablets	Cetirizine (an antihistamine)/pseudoephedrine (a nasal decongestant)

ACE, angiotensin-converting enzyme inhibitor.
From *Mosby's 2006 drug consult for nurses,* St. Louis, 2006, Mosby.

Appendix D   Controlled Substances Classes

Drugs	United States	Canada
Heroin, LSD, peyote, marijuana, mescaline, phencyclidine	Schedule I (CI)	Schedule H
Opium, fentanyl, morphine, meperidine, methadone, oxycodone (and its combinations), hydromorphone, codeine (single-drug entity), and cocaine	Schedule II (CII)	Schedule N
Short-acting barbiturates	Schedule II (CII)	Schedule C
Amphetamine and methylphenidate	Schedule II (CII)	Schedule G
Codeine combinations, hydrocodone combinations, glutethimide, paregoric, phendimetrazine, thiopental, testosterone, and other androgens	Schedule III (CIII)	Schedule F
Benzodiazepines (diazepam, midazolam, etc.), chloral hydrate, meprobamate, phenobarbital, propoxyphene (and combinations), pentazocine (and combinations), and methohexital	Schedule IV (CIV)	Schedule F
Antidiarrheals and antitussives with opioid derivatives	Schedule V (CV)	

Appendix E   Disorders and Conditions

TABLE E-1

Asthma Medications

Agent	Indication	Mechanism of Action	Example
Inhaled β₂-agonist (short-acting)	Acute exacerbation, used in all categories.	Bronchodilator: smooth muscle relaxation following adenylate cyclase activation, resulting in an increase in cAMP activating protein kinase A, which lowers needed intracellular calcium for smooth muscle contraction.	Albuterol Metaproterenol
Inhaled β₂-agonist (long-acting)	Longer-term prevention usually added to antiinflammatory therapy.	Bronchodilator (see above).	Salmeterol
Oral β₂-agonist (long-lasting)	Longer-term prevention usually added to antiinflammatory therapy.	Bronchodilator (see above).	Albuterol (sustained-release)
Inhaled corticosteroids	Longer-term prevention in all persistent forms. Daily medication. Low-, medium-, high-dose formulations depending on asthma severity/control.	Antiinflammatory: inhibits cytokine production and adhesion protein activation. Reserves β₂ down-regulation. Suppresses recruitment of airway eosinophils.	Beclomethasone Flunisolide Fluticasone Budesonide Triamcinolone

Systemic corticosteroids	Acute exacerbation, used in all categories. Long-term prevention in severe, persistent asthma.	Antiinflammatory (see above).	Methylprednisolone Prednisolone Prednisone
Anticholinergics	Acute exacerbation, used in patients intolerant to short-acting β_2-agonists.	Bronchodilator: competitive inhibition of muscarinic cholinergic receptors.	Ipratropium bromide Cromolyn Nedocromil Theophylline (sustained-release)
Leukotriene modifiers	Long-term control and prevention in Step 2 mild, persistent asthma.	Antiinflammatory: Leukotriene receptor antagonist (competitive inhibition) = Zafirlukast/Montelukast 5-Lipoxygenase inhibitor interfering with leukotriene synthesis = Zileuton.	Zafirlukast Montelukast Zileuton

All medications have side effects with which the dentist should be familiar.
Medication usage/discontinuance based on step-up, step-down fashion relating to symptoms.
Specific dosage/delivery of medication tailored to patient/severity.
Children younger than 5 years old have different regimens.
From Sollecito TP, Tino G: *Oral Surg Oral Med Oral Pathol Radiol Endod* 92:486-487, 2001.

TABLE E–2

Drugs Used for Treatment of Seizure Disorder

Drug	Pharmacologic Category	Adverse Effects
Carbamazepine (Epitol, Tegretol)	Anticonvulsant	Sedation, dizziness, fatigue, confusion, ataxia, nausea, blood dyscrasias, hepatotoxicity
Clonazepam (Klonopin)	Benzodiazepine	Tachycardia, drowsiness, fatigue, anxiety, ataxia, headache, dizziness, blurred vision, xerostomia
Ethosuximide (Zarontin)	Succinimide	Ataxia, sedation, dizziness, hallucinations, behavioral changes, headache, Stevens-Johnson syndrome, systemic lupus erythematosus, nausea, anorexia
Gabapentin (Neurontin)	Neurotransmitter	Somnolence, dizziness, ataxia, fatigue, nystagmus
Phenobarbital (Luminal, Solfoton)	Barbiturate	Dizziness, light-headedness, sedation, ataxia, impaired judgment, skin rashes
Phenytoin (Mysoline)	Barbiturate derivative	Drowsiness, vertigo, ataxia, behavioral changes, headache, nausea
Primidone (Mysoline)	Barbiturate derivative	Drowsiness, vertigo, ataxia, behavioral changes, headache, nausea
Topiramate (Topamax)	Sulfamate-substituted monosaccharide	Acidosis (may decrease serum bicarbonate concentrations), increased risk of kidney stones, hyperthermia, paresthesias, sedation, confusion, psychomotor slowing, mood disturbances
Valproic acid, sodium valproate (Depakene, Depakote)	Carboxylic acid	Anorexia, diarrhea, nausea, drowsiness, ataxia, irritability, confusion, headache, hepatotoxicity, leucopenia, thrombocytopenia resulting in prolonged bleeding time

From Hupp JR, Williams TP, Firriolo FJ: *Dental clinical advisor*, ed 1, St. Louis, 2006, Elsevier.

TABLE E–3

Drugs Used for Management of Oral Candidosis

Medication	Dosage and Directions*
Chlorhexidine 0.12% oral rinse (Peridex, PerioGard)† or 0.2% alcohol-free aqueous‡	15 ml mouth rinse and expectorate 3 times a day. NPO ½ hr after use.
Nystatin oral suspension 100,000 units/ml§¶	5 ml mouth rinse and 1 min expectorate 4 times a day (before breakfast and at bedtime). NPO ½ hr after use.
Clotrimazole 10 mg/ml suspension¶	Swab 1–2 ml on affected area 4 times a day (pc and hs). NPO ½ hr after use.
Ketoconazole 2% cream (Nizoral) or clotrimazole 1% cream (Lotrimin)	Apply thin film to inner surface of denture(s) and/or corners of mouth 4 times a day (before breakfast and at bedtime). NPO ½ hr after use.
Clotrimazole 200-mg vaginal tablets (Gyne-Lotrimin)	Dissolve ½ tablet slowly in mouth 2 times a day. NPO ½ hr after use.
Clotrimazole 10-mg oral troches (Nizoral)	Dissolve 1 troche slowly in mouth 5 times a day. NPO ½ hr after use.
Ketoconazole 200-mg tablets (Nizoral)	1 tablet PO 4 times a day for 7–10 days. Do not take antacids within 2 hr of this medication.**
Fluconazole 100-mg tablets (Diflucan)	1 tablet PO 2 times a day for first day, then 1 tablet PO 4 times a day for 10–14 days.

*In most patients, decreased frequency and dosages can be used if maintenance therapy is required.

†High alcohol content (11.6%) will irritate mucosa and enhance xerostomia. Should not be prescribed for recovering alcoholics.

‡Must be prepared by experienced compounding pharmacist. Many formulas include flavorings that decrease efficacy.

§High sucrose content. Not first-choice in high caries-risk patients.

¶May be swallowed for pharyngeal involvement.

**Acidic environment is required for absorption.

From Klienegger CL: Diseases of the mouth. In Rakel RE, Bope ET, editors: *Conn's current therapy 2002.* Philadelphia, 2002, WB Saunders.

Appendix F   Drugs Associated with Dry Mouth

Drug Category	Brand Name	Generic Name
Alcohol Abuse Deterrent	Campral	acamprosate calcium
Anorexiant	Adipex-P, Fastin, Ionamin	phentermine
	Anorex	phendimetrazine
	Mazanor, Sanorex	mazindol
	Tenuate, Tepanil	diethylpropion
Antiacne	Accutane	isotretinoin
Antianemic	Revlimid	lenalidomide
Antianxiety	Atarax, Vistaril	hydroxyzine
	Ativan	lorazepam
	BuSpar	buspirone
	Equanil, Miltown	meprobamate
	Librium	chlordiazepoxide
	Paxipam	halazepam
	Serax	oxazepam
	Sonata	zaleplon
	Valium	diazepam
	Xanax	alprazolam
Antiarthritic	Arava	leflunomide
Anticholinergic/ Antispasmodic	Anaspaz	hyoscyamine
	Sal-Tropine	atropine
	Bellergal	belladonna alkaloids
	Bentyl	dicyclomine
	Ditropan	oxybutynin
	Donnatal, Kinesed	hyoscyamine atropine, phenobarbital, scopolamine
	Librax	chlordiazepoxide, clidinium
	Pro-Banthine	propantheline
	Transderm-Scop	scopolamine
Anticonvulsant	Felbatol	felbamate
	Lamictal	lamotrigine
	Lyrica	pregabalin
	Neurontin	gabapentin
	Tegretol	carbamazepine
	Vimpat	lacosamide
	Premarin	pregabalin
Antidepressant	Anafranil	clomipramine
	Asendin	amoxapine
	Celexa	citalopram
	Cymbalta	duloxetine
	Effexor	venlafaxine
	Elavil	amitriptyline
	Luvox	fluvoxamine
	Marplan	isocarboxazid

Drug Category	Brand Name	Generic Name
	Nardil	phenelzine
	Norpramin	desipramine
	Parnate	tranylcypromine
	Paxil	paroxetine
	Prozac	fluoxetine
	Replax	eletriptan
	Sinequan	doxepin
	Tofranil	imipramine
	Wellbutrin, Zyban	bupropion
	Zoloft	sertraline
Antidiarrheal	Imodium AD	loperamide
	Lomotil	diphenoxylate, atropine
	Motofen	difenoxin
Antifungal	Noxafil	posaconazole
Antihistamine	Actifed	triprolidine with pseudoephedrine
	Atarax	hydroxyzine
	Benadryl	diphenhydramine
	Chlor-Trimeton	chlorpheniramine
	Claritin	loratadine
	Dimetapp	pseudoephedrine
	Levocetirizine	xyzal
	Phenergan	promethazine
Antihypertensive	Norvasc	amlodipine
	Capoten	captopril
	Catapres	clonidine
	Coreg	carvedilol
	Ismelin	guanethidine
	Aceon	perindopril
	Minipress	prazosin
	Serpasil	reserpine
	Wytensin	guanabenz
	Vasotec	enalapril
Antiinflammatory Analgesic	Celebrex	celecoxib
	Dolobid	diflunisal
	Feldene	piroxicam
	Motrin	ibuprofen
	Nalfon	fenoprofen
	Naprosyn	naproxen
	Vioxx	rofecoxib
Antiinflammatory GI	Colazal	balsalazide
Antinauseant	Antivert	meclizine
	Dramamine	dimenhydrinate
	Emend	aprepitant
	Marezine	cyclizine

(Continued)

Drug Category	Brand Name	Generic Name
Anti-parkinsonian	Akineton	biperiden
	Artane	trihexyphenidyl
	Cogentin	benztropine mesylate
	Larodopa	levodopa
	Peridol	ethopropazine
	Sinemet	carbidopa, levodopa
	Tasmar	tolcapone
Antipsychotic	Abilify	aripiprazole
	Clozaril	clozapine
	Compazine	prochlorperazine
	Eskalith	lithium
	Haldol	haloperidol
	Mellaril	thioridazine
	Navane	thiothixene
	Orap	pimozide
	Risperdal	risperidone
	Sparine	promazine
	Thorazine	chlorpromazine
	Triavil	amitriptyline, perphenazine
	Zyprexa	olanzapine
Antisecretory	AcipHex	rabeprazole
	Nexium	esomeprazole
Antispasmodic	Detrol	tolterodine
	Sanctura	trospium chloride
Antiviral	Copegus	ribavirin
	Sustiva	efavirenz
Bronchodilator	(generic)	ephedrine
	Isuprel	isoproterenol
	Proventil, Ventolin	albuterol
	Xopenex	levalbuterol
CNS Stimulant	Desoxyn	methamphetamine
	Dexedrine	dextroamphetamine
	Savella	milnacipran
Decongestant	Sudafed	pseudoephedrine
Diuretic	Aldactone	spironolactone
	Diuril	chlorothiazide
	Dyazide, Maxzide, Dyrenium	triamterene
	Esidrix, HydroDIURIL	hydrochlorothiazide
	Lasix	furosemide
	Midamor	amiloride
Migraine	Amerge	naratriptan
	Axert	almotriptan
	Frova	frovatriptan
	Maxalt	rizatriptan
	Replax	eletriptan

Drug Category	Brand Name	Generic Name
Multikinase Inhibitor	Nexavar	sorafenib
Muscle Relaxant	Flexeril Lioresal Norflex	cyclobenzaprine baclofen orphenadrine
Antinarcoleptic	Provigil	modafinil
Nicotine Receptor Agonist	Chantix	varenicline
Opioid Analgesic	Buprenex Demerol MS Contin Synalgos DC	buprenorphine meperidine morphine dihydrocodeine combinations
Ophthalmic	Azopt	brinzolamide
Sedative	Dalmane Halcion Lunesta Restoril	flurazepam triazolam eszopiclone temazepam

Appendix G   Drugs That Affect Taste

ALCOHOL DETOXIFICATION
disulfiram (Antabuse)

ALZHEIMER'S
donepezil (Aricept)

ANALGESICS (NSAIDs)
diclofenac (Voltaren)
etodolac (Lodine)
ketoprofen (Orudis)
meclofenamate (Meclofen)
sulindac (Clinoril)

ANESTHETICS (GENERAL)
midazolam (Versed)
propofol (Diprivan)

ANESTHETICS (LOCAL)
lidocaine transoral delivery system
    (DentiPatch)

ANOREXIANTS
diethylpropion (Tenuate)
mazindol (Mazanor)
phendimetrazine (Adipost)
phentermine (Ionamin)

ANTACIDS
aluminum hydroxide (Amphojel)
calcium carbonate (Tums)
lansoprazole (Prevacid)
magaldrate (Riopan)
omeprazole (Prilosec)
sucralfate (Carafate)

ANTAGONISTS
azelastine (Astelin)
cetirizine (Zyrtec)
famotidine (Pepcid)

ANTIANEMIC
lenalidomide (Revlimid)

ANTIANXIETY
buspirone (BuSpar)

ANTIARTHRITIC
leflunomide (Arava)

ANTICHOLINERGICS
clidinium (Quarzan)
mepenzolate (Cantil)
propantheline (Pro-Banthine)

ANTICONVULSANTS
fosphenytoin (Cerebyx)
phenytoin (Dilantin)
topiramate (Topamax)

ANTIDEPRESSANTS
amitriptyline (Elavil)
clomipramine (Anafranil)
desipramine (Norpramin)
doxepin (Sinequan)
fluoxetine (Prozac)
imipramine (Tofranil)
nefazodone (Serzone)
nortriptyline (Pamelor)
protriptyline (Vivactil)
sertraline (Zoloft)

ANTIDIABETICS
metformin (Glucophage)
tolbutamide (Orinase)

ANTIDIARRHEALS
bismuth subsalicylate
    (Pepto-Bismol)

ANTIEMETICS
aprepitant (Emend)
dolasetron mesylate (Anzemet)

ANTIFUNGALS
terbinafine (Lamisil)

ANTIGOUT
allopurinol (Zyloprim)
colchicine

ANTIHISTAMINE (H_1)

ANTIHISTAMINE (H_2)

ANTIHYPERLIPIDEMICS
clofibrate (Atromid-S)
fluvastatin (Lescol)

ANTIINFECTIVES

ciprofloxacin (Ciloxan)
daptomycin (Cubicin)
ethionamide (Trecator-SC)
gatifloxacin (Zymar)
gemifloxacin (Factive)
levofloxacin (Levaquin)
lincomycin (Lincocin)
metronidazole (Flagyl)
ofloxacin (Floxin)

ANTIINFLAMMATORY/ ANTIARTHRITIC

auranofin (Ridaura)
aurothioglucose (Solganal)
celecoxib (Celebrex)
sulfasalazine (Azulfidine)

ANTIMIGRAINE

almotriptan (Axert)
frovatriptan (Frova)

ANTIPARKINSON

apomorphine (Apokyn)
entacapone (Comtan)
levodopa (Larodopa)
levodopa-carbidopa (Sinemet)
pergolide (Permax)
pramipexole dihydrochloride
   (Mirapex)

ANTIPROTOZOAL

tinidazole (Tindamax)

ANTIPSYCHOTICS

lithium (Eskalith)
pimozide (Orap)
prochlorperazine (Compazine)
quetiapine fumarate (Seroquel)
risperidone (Risperdal)

ANTITHYROID

methimazole (Tapazole)
propylthiouracil

ANTIVIRALS

acyclovir (Zovirax)
amprenavir (Agenerase)
atazanavir (Reyataz)

delavirdine mesylate (Rescriptor)
didanosine (Videx)
efavirenz (Sustiva)
foscarnet (Foscavir)
indinavir (Crixivan)
penciclovir (Denavir)
ribavirin (Copegus)
rimantadine (Flumadine)
ritonavir (Norvir)
saquinavir (Invirase)
valacyclovir (Valtrex)
zidovudine (Retrovir)

ANXIOLYTIC/SEDATIVES

chloral hydrate
estazolam (ProSom)
quazepam (Doral)
zolpidem (Ambien)

ASTHMA PREVENTIVES

cromolyn (Intal)
nedocromil (Tilade)

BRONCHODILATORS

albuterol (Proventil)
bitolterol (Tornalate)
formoterol fumarate (Foradil)
ipratropium (Atrovent)
isoproterenol (Isuprel)
metaproterenol (Alupent)
pirbuterol (Maxair)
terbutaline (Brethine)

CALCIUM-AFFECTING DRUGS

alendronate (Fosamax)
calcitonin (Calcimar)
etidronate (Didronel)

CANCER CHEMOTHERAPEUTICS

capecitabine (Xeloda)
fluorouracil (Efudex)
levamisole (Ergamisol)
tamoxifen (Nolvadex)

CARDIOVASCULAR

amiodarone (Cordarone)
amlodipine (Norvasc)
bepridil (Vascor)
captopril (Capoten)

clonidine (Catapres)
diltiazem (Cardizem)
enalapril (Vasotec)
flecainide (Tambocor)
fosinopril (Monopril)
guanfacine (Tenex)
labetalol (Trandate)
losartan (Cozaar)
mecamylamine (Inversine)
mexiletine (Mexitil)
moricizine (Ethmozine)
nadolol (Corgard)
nifedipine (Procardia XL)
penbutolol (Levatol)
perindopril (Aceon)
propafenone (Rythmol)
quinidine (Cardioquin)
valsartan (Diovan)

CNS STIMULANTS
dextroamphetamine (Dexedrine)
methamphetamine (Desoxyn)

DECONGESTANT
phenylephrine (Neo-Synephrine)

DIURETICS
acetazolamide (Diamox)
methazolamide (Neptazane)
polythiazide (Renese)

GLUCOCORTICOIDS
budesonide (Rhinocort)
flunisolide (AeroBid)
rimexolone (Vexol)

GALLSTONE SOLUBILIZATION
ursodiol (Actigall)

HEMORHEOLOGIC
pentoxifylline (Trental)

IMMUNOMODULATORS
interferon alfa (Roferon-A)
levamisole (Ergamisol)
tacrolimus (Protopic)

IMMUNOSUPPRESSANTS
azathioprine (Imuran)

IRRITABLE BOWEL SYNDROME
alosetron (Lotronex)
telithromycin (Ketek)

MELATONIN RECEPTOR AGONIST HYPNOTIC
ramelteon (Rozerem)

METHYLXANTHINES
aminophylline (Somophyllin)
dyphylline (Dilor)
oxtriphylline (Choledyl)
theophylline (Theo-Dur)

NICOTINE CESSATION
nicotine polacrilex (Nicorette)
varenicline (Chantix)

OPHTHALMICS
apraclonidine (Iopidine)
brimonidine (Alphagan)
brinzolamide (Azopt)
dorzolamide (Trusopt)
olopatadine (Patanol)

PROTON PUMP INHIBITORS
esomeprazole (Nexium)
lansoprazole (Prevacid)
omeprazole (Prilosec)

RETINOID, SYSTEMIC
acitretin (Soriatane)

SALIVARY STIMULANT
pilocarpine (Salagen)

SEDATIVE-HYPNOTIC
eszopiclone (Lunesta)

SKELETAL MUSCLE RELAXANTS
baclofen (Lioresal)
cyclobenzaprine (Flexeril)
methocarbamol (Robaxin)

VITAMINS
calcifediol (vitamin D)
calcitriol (vitamin D)
dihydrotachysterol (vitamin D)
phytonadione (vitamin K)

Appendix H Complementary and Alternative Medications and Dietary Supplements

For Appendix H and more information on Complementary and Alternative Medications, see the Companion CD-ROM and the Evolve site.

Appendix I   Pregnancy and Pediatrics

TABLE I–1

FDA Drug Pregnancy Risk Category Descriptions

Pregnancy Risk Category	Description	Application in Dentistry
A	Drug has been studied in humans. Evidence supports its safe use. Remote possibility of fetal harm.	Can be appropriately administered during pregnancy.
B	Animal studies demonstrate no fetal risk. Inadequate studies in pregnant women. Slightly increased fetal risk.	Can be appropriately administered during pregnancy.
C	Teratogenic risk cannot be ruled out. Animal studies show potential adverse fetal effects. Potential benefits may outweigh risks.	Can be used with caution.
D	Drug demonstrates risk in humans. Potential benefits may outweigh risks.	Should be avoided.
X	Drug demonstrates harm in mother or fetus. Risk clearly outweighs benefit.	Contraindicated.

From Hupp JR, Williams TP, Firriolo FJ: *Dental clinical advisor,* ed 1, St. Louis, 2006, Elsevier.

TABLE I–2

FDA Drug Pregnancy Risk Category and Use during Breast-feeding

Generic Name	Brand Name	FDA Pregnancy Risk Category	Use during Breast-feeding
Antimicrobials			
Amoxicillin	Amoxil, Polymox	B	Yes
Amoxicillin clavulanic acid	Augmentin	B	Yes
Azithromycin	Zithromax	B	Yes
Cephalexin	Keflex	B	Yes
Chlorhexidine	Peridex	B	Yes
Clindamycin	Cleocin	B	Yes
Doxycycline	Doryx, Vibramycin, Atridox, Periostat	D	No
Erythromycin†	Ery-Tab, E-Mycin, E.E.S., PCE	B	Yes
Fluconazole	Diflucan	C	No
Ketoconazole	Nizoral	C	No
Metronidazole	Flagyl	B	Caution
Nystatin	Mycostatin	B	Yes
Penicillin V Potassium	V-Cillin K, V-Pen	B	Yes
Tetracycline	Actisite, Achromycin	D	No

TABLE I–2
FDA Drug Pregnancy Risk Category and Use during Breast-feeding—cont'd

Generic Name	Brand Name	FDA Pregnancy Risk Category	Use during Breast-feeding
Analgesics			
Acetaminophen	Tylenol	B	Yes
Aspirin	Bayer	C/D3	No
Celecoxib/Valdecoxib	Celebrex/Bextra	C/D3	Unknown
Codeine	Various combinations	C/D*	Yes
Hydrocodone	Various combinations	C/D*	Caution
Ibuprofen	Advil, Motrin	B/D3	Yes
Naproxen	Aleve, Anaprox	B/D3	Unknown
Oxycodone	Various combinations	C/D*	Caution
Sedatives			
Chloral hydrate	Somnote	C	Yes
Diazepam	Valium	D	No
Hydroxyzine	Atarax/Vistaril	C	Unknown
Lorazepam	Ativan	D	No
Midazolam	Versed	D	No
Nitrous oxide	N/A	None‡	Controversial
Triazolam	Halcion	X	No
Local anesthetics			
Articaine	Septocaine	C	Unknown
Bupivacaine	Marcaine	C	Yes
Etidocaine	Duranest	B	Yes
Lidocaine	Xylocaine	B	Yes
Mepivacaine	Carbocaine	C	Yes
Prilocaine	Citanest	B	Yes
Vasoconstrictors			
Epinephrine 1:100,000; 1:200,000	N/A	C*	Yes
Levonordefrin 1:20,000	Neo-Cobefrin	None	Yes
Topical anesthetics			
Benzocaine	Anbesol, Hurricaine	C	Yes
Lidocaine	Xylocaine, DentiPatch	B	Yes
Tetracaine	Pontocaine	C	Yes

C/D3, Pregnancy risk category D during the third trimester.
C/D*, Pregnancy risk category D in high doses at term or with prolonged use.
C*, Pregnancy risk category C in high doses.
†Avoid estolate form.
‡Best used in the second and third trimesters and for less than 30 min with at least 50% O$_2$; consult physician.
Modified from Hilgers K, Douglass J, Mathieu G: *Pediatr Dent* 25:459–467, 2003.

TABLE I–3

Drug Usage in Pediatric Dentistry

Drug	Route	Dose	Frequency	Notes
Antibiotics				
Amoxicillin	PO IV PO, IV	25–50 mg/kg/day 100–400 mg/kg/day 50 mg/kg up to adult dose 3g	3 times a day 3 times a day 30 min–1 hr before procedure	Syrup or chewable tablets for young children Endocarditis prophylaxis
Amoxicillin clavulanic acid	PO	20–40 mg/kg/day	3 times a day	For β-lactam resistant organisms only
Ampicillin	IV IV	50–100 mg/kg/day 50 mg/kg	4 times a day stat	Endocarditis prophylaxis
Benzylpenicillin	IV	15–350 mg/kg/day 20,000–500,000 Units/kg/day	4 times a day	IV drug of choice for odontogenic infections
Penicillin VK	PO	Younger than 5 yr 500 mg/day Older than 5 yr 1–2 kg/day	4 times a day	Give 1 hr before meals or 2 hr after meals
Cephalexin	PO	25–50 mg/kg/day	4 times a day	
Cephalothin IV	IV	40–80 mg/kg/day	4 times a day	Not in pregnancy
Cephazolin	IV	25–50 mg/kg/day		
Erythromycin	PO	25–40 mg/kg/day	4 times a day	Ethylsuccinate is readily absorbed
Metronidazole	IV PO	22.5 mg/kg/day 10–15 mg/kg/day	3 times a day 3 times a day	Not in pregnancy
Gentamicin	IV	2.5 mg/kg (children) up to 80 mg maximum	stat	Endocarditis prophylaxis, highly susceptible patients. In conjunction with ampicillin

TABLE I–3
Drug Usage in Pediatric Dentistry—cont'd

Drug	Route	Dose	Frequency	Notes
Antibiotics				
Clindamycin	PO, IV PO, IV	15–40 mg/kg/day 10 mg/kg up to adult dose 600 mg	4 times a day PO: 1 hr before, IV: stat	Risk of pseudomembranous colitis Endocarditis prophylaxis, susceptible patients Follow-up dose half initial dose, 6 hr later (5 mg/kg up to 300 mg)
Vancomycin	IV	20 mg/kg up to adult dose 1 g	infused over 1 hr	Endocarditis prophylaxis, susceptible patients allergic to penicillin
Antifungals				
Nystatin	Tablets Suspension	500,000 Units 100,000 Units/mL	tds every 6 hr	Apply to affected area
Amphotericin B	Lozenges Suspension Ointment	10 mg 100 mg/mL 3%	every 6 hr every 6 hr every 6 hr	Apply to affected area Apply to affected area Apply to affected area
Analgesics and sedatives				
Aspirin	PO	325–650 mg	every 4 hr	Should not be used in children younger than 12 yr because of the risk of Reye's syndrome
Paracetamol	PO, PR	15 mg/kg	every 4 hr	Hepatotoxic if overdose
Codeine phosphate	PO	1–1.5 mg/kg single dose 1–3 mg/kg/day	4–6 divided doses	Similar side effects to opioids, including nausea and constipation
Pethidine	IV, IM	1 mg/kg	every 3–4 hr	Maximum 100 mg
Morphine	IV, IM	0.1–0.2 mg/kg	every 6 hr	Should only be used in admitted patients
Naloxone	IM, IV	1–10 mcg/kg	Stat	May be repeated at 2–3 min intervals if necessary
Midazolam	IV, IM	0.1–0.2 mg/kg	single dose	Sedation, may be given intranasally

(Continued)

TABLE I–3
Drug Usage in Pediatric Dentistry—cont'd

Drug	Route	Dose	Frequency	Notes
Chloral hydrate	PO	30–50 mg/kg/ day, 15–20 mg/kg single dose	every 4–6 hr	Sedation
Trimeprazine	PO	3–4 mg/kg	single dose	Valergen, sedation
Metoclopramide	PO, IM	3–5 yr: 2 mg 5–9 yr: 2.5 mg 9–14 yr: 5 mg 15–19 yr: 10 mg	single dose	Single dose after narcotic if vomiting or nausea Maxolon. Dystonic reactions may occur
Other medications				
Kenalog in Orabase	Ointment	Triamcinolone 0.1%	every 4–6 hr	Recurrent severe oral ulceration in children; apply to ulcer but do not rub ointment in
ε-aminocaproic acid	IV	30 mg/kg		Antifibrinolytic; loading dose of 100 mg/kg
Tranexamic acid	PO	15–20 mg/kg	4 times a day	Antifibrinolytic
DDAVP	IV	0.3 mcg/kg		Infused over 1 hr before surgery
Heparin	IV	50–100 Units/kg	every 4–6 hr	Anticoagulant
Tetanus toxoid	IM	0.5 mL	single dose	If immunization protocol not complete, course should be given. Otherwise, a booster may be required for tetanus-prone wounds if longer than 2 yr since last booster

From Cameron AC, Widmer RP: *Handbook of pediatric dentistry,* ed 2, London, 2003, Mosby.
The table that forms Table K–2 is a guide to the administration of commonly used drugs in pediatric dentistry. Medications for children should always be prescribed in relation to weight. It is of utmost importance that clinicians understand the contraindications and precautions relevant to the drugs they are prescribing, and should consult prescribing information supplied by the pharmaceutical manufacturers and relevant pharmacopeia.
PR = per rectum; stat = immediately.

Appendix J Preventing Medication Errors and Improving Medication Safety

Medication safety is a high priority for the health care professional. Prevention of medication errors and improved safety for the patient are important, especially in today's health care environment, when today's patient is older and sometimes sicker and the drug therapy regimen can be more sophisticated and complex.

A medication error is defined by the National Coordinating Council for Medication Error Reporting and Prevention (NCC MERP) as "any preventable event that may cause or lead to inappropriate medication use or patient harm while the medication is in the control of the health care professional, patient, or consumer."

Most medication errors occur as a result of multiple compounding events as opposed to a single act by a single individual.

Use of the wrong medication, strength, or dose; confusion over sound-alike or look-alike drugs; administration of medications by the wrong route; miscalculations (especially when used in pediatric patients or when administering medications intravenously); and errors in prescribing and transcription all can contribute to compromising the safety of the patient. The potential for adverse events and medication errors is definitely a reality and is potentially tragic and costly in both human and economic terms.

Health care professionals must take the initiative to create and implement procedures to reduce, and hopefully prevent, medication errors. The first priority in preventing medication errors is to establish a multidisciplinary team to improve medication use. The goal for this team would be to assess medication safety and implement changes that would make it difficult or impossible for mistakes to reach the patient. Some important criteria in making improved medication safety successful include the following:
• Promote a nonpunitive approach to reducing medication errors.
• Increase the detection and the reporting of medication errors, near misses, and potentially hazardous situations that may result in medication errors.
• Determine root causes of medication errors.
• Educate about the causes of medication errors and ways to prevent these errors.
• Make recommendations to allow organization-wide, system-based changes to prevent medication errors.
• Learn from errors that occur in other organizations and take measures to prevent similar errors.

Some common causes and ways to prevent medication errors and improve safety include the following:

Communicating Prescription Information

Poor handwriting can make it difficult to distinguish between two medications with similar names. Also, many drug names sound similar, especially when the names are spoken over the telephone, poorly enunciated, or mispronounced.
• Take time to write legibly.
• Keep phone or verbal orders to a minimum to prevent misinterpretation.
• Repeat back orders taken over the telephone.

- When ordering a new or rarely used medication, print the name.
- Always specify the drug strength, even if only one strength exists.
- Print generic and brand names of look-alike or sound-alike medications.

Zeros and Decimal Points

Hastily written orders can present problems even if the name of the medication is clear.

- Always place a zero before a decimal point when the number is less than a whole unit (e.g., use 0.25 mg or 250 mcg, not .25 mg).
- Never have a trailing zero following a decimal point (e.g., use 2 mg, not 2.0 mg).

Abbreviations

Errors can occur because of a failure to standardize abbreviations. Establishing a list of abbreviations that should never be used is recommended.

- Never abbreviate unit as "U," spell out "unit."
- Do not abbreviate "once daily" as od or qd, or "every other day" as qod; spell it out.
- Do not use DC, because it may be misinterpreted as either discharge or discontinue.
- Do not abbreviate drug names; spell out the generic and/or brand names.

Ambiguous or Incomplete Orders

These types of orders can cause confusion or misinterpretation of the writer's intention. Examples include situations in which the route of administration, dose, or dosage form has not been specified.

- Do not use slash marks—they are read as the number one (1).
- When reviewing an unusual order, verify the order with the person writing the order to prevent any misunderstanding.
- Read over orders after writing.

- Encourage that the drug's indication for use be provided on medication orders.
- Provide complete medication orders—do not use "resume preop" or "continue previous meds."

High-Alert Medications

Medications in this category have an increased risk of causing significant patient harm when used in error. Mistakes with these medications may or may not be more common but may be more devastating to the patient if an error occurs. A list of high-alert medications can be obtained from the Institute for Safe Medication Practices (ISMP) at www.ismp.org.

Technologies available today that can be used to address and help to solve potential medication problems or errors include the following:

- Electronic prescribing systems— This refers to computerized prescriber order entry systems. Within these systems is the capability to incorporate medication safety alerts (e.g., maximum dose alerts, allergy screening). Additionally, these systems should be integrated or interfaced with pharmacy and laboratory systems to provide drug-drug and drug-disease interaction alerts and include clinical order screening capability.
- Bar codes—These systems are designed to use bar-code scanning devices to validate identity of patients, verify medications administered, document administration, and provide safety alerts.
- "Smart" infusion pumps—These pumps allow users to enter drug infusion protocols into a drug library along with predefined dosage limits. If a dosage is outside the limits established, an alarm is sounded and drug delivery is halted,

informing the clinician that the dose is outside the recommended range.

• Automated dispensing systems/ point-of-use dispensing systems— These systems should be integrated with information systems, especially pharmacy systems.

• Pharmacy order entry system— This should be fully integrated with an electronic prescribing system

with the capability of producing medication safety alerts. Additionally, the system should generate a computerized medication administration record (MAR), which would be used by a nursing staff while administering medications.

From *Mosby's 2006 drug consult for nurses,* St. Louis, 2006, Mosby.

Appendix K   Oral Contraceptives

Estrogens: ethinyl estradiol, mestranol
Progestins (progesterone derivatives): desogestrel, drospirenone, ethynodiol diacetate, etonorgestrel, levonorgestrel, norethindrone, norgestimate, norgestrel
Many products available in the following categories:
Monophasic products: Alesse, Apri, Aviane, Brevicon, Cryselle, Demulen 1/35, Demulen 1/50, Desogen, Kariva, Lessina, Levlite, Levlen, Levora, Loestrin 21, Loestrin Fe, Low-Ogestrel, Lo/Ovral, Mircette, Modicon, MonoNessa, Necon 0.5/35, Nelova 0.5/35^E, Nordette, Norethin 1/35E, Norinyl 1+50, Norinyl 1+35, Nortrel 1/35, Nortrel 0.5/35, Ogestrel 0.5/50, Ortho-Cept, Ortho-Cyclen, Ortho-Novum 1/35, Ortho-Novum 1/50, Ovcon 35, Ovcon-50, Ovral, Ovral-28, Portia, Sprintec, Zovia 1/35E, Zovia 1/50E, Yasmin, others
Biphasic products: Necon 10/11, Ortho-Novum 10/11
Triphasic products: Cyclessa, Enpresse, Estrostep-21, Estrostep Fe, Necon 7/7/7, Ortho Tri-Cyclen, Tri-Levlen, Tri-Norinyl, Triphasil, Trivora
Progestin-only: Aygestin, Camila, Errin, Jolivette, Micronor, Nor-QD, Nora-BE, Ortho Micronor, Ovrette, Norlutate [CAN]

CATEGORY AND SCHEDULE
Pregnancy Risk Category: X

Drug Class: Estrogen derivative, progesterone derivatives, combination oral contraceptives

MECHANISM OF ACTION
Prevents ovulation by suppression of the hypothalamic-pituitary system, decreasing the secretion of gonadotropin-releasing hormone (GnRH). Progestins blunt luteinizing hormone (LH) release and estrogens suppress follicle-stimulating hormone (FSH), ultimately inhibiting maturation and release of the dominant ovule.

USES
To prevent pregnancy, endometriosis, hypermenorrhea, hypogonadism; acne (Tri-Cyclen)

PHARMACOKINETICS
Readily absorbed from GI tract. Widely distributed, variable degrees of protein binding.
Extensively metabolized in liver by oxidation and conjugation; excreted in breast milk, urine, and feces. Estrogens undergo enterohepatic cycling via excretion in the bile. Half-life varies with individual agent.

INDICATIONS AND DOSAGES
▶ **Contraception**
PO
Adults. 1 tablet per day starting on day 5 of menstrual cycle (day 1 is first day of period).

20/21-TABLET PACKS
PO
Adults. 1 tablet per day starting on day 7 of menstrual cycle; then on for 20 or 21 days, off 7 days.

28-TABLET PACKS
PO
Adults. 1 tablet per day continuously.

BIPHASIC

PO

Adults. 1 tablet per day for 10 days, then next color 1 tablet for 11 days.

TRIPHASIC

PO

Adults. 1 tablet per day; consult package insert for detailed instructions.

▸ **Amenorrhea and Abnormal Uterine Bleeding**

PO

Adults. Follow dose for routine contraception for specific product. Treatment for 6–12 mo may be required.

▸ **Endometriosis**

PO

Adults and adolescent females. Follow dose for routine contraception for specific product; alternatively, the active tablets can be given continuously. Treatment for 6–9 mo may be needed to induce endometrial atrophy and reduce symptoms.

SIDE EFFECTS/ADVERSE REACTIONS

Occasional

Breast tenderness, dizziness, headache, breakthrough bleeding, amenorrhea, menstrual irregularity, nausea, weakness

Rare

Mental depression, fever, insomnia, rash, acne, weight gain/loss, cholestatic jaundice, increased blood pressure, thromboembolism, hypersensitivity reactions (rash, urticaria, pruritus, erythema multiforme), optic neuritis, decreased glucose tolerance, tumors of breast

PRECAUTIONS AND CONTRAINDICATIONS

Acute liver disease, benign or malignant liver tumors, hypersensitivity to estrogen and/or progesterone derivatives, known or suspected breast cancer, known or suspected pregnancy, undiagnosed vaginal bleeding

Caution:

Lactation, hypertension, asthma, blood dyscrasias, gallbladder disease, congestive circulatory failure, diabetes mellitus, bone diseases, depression, migraine, convulsive disorders, liver disease, kidney disease, family history of breast or reproductive tract cancer

DRUG INTERACTIONS OF CONCERN TO DENTISTRY

• Very low risk of decreased effectiveness with antibiotics (documented risk only with non-dental antibiotics, e.g., rifampin)

SERIOUS REACTIONS

! Thrombophlebitis, cerebrovascular disorders, retinal thrombosis, cholestatic jaundice, and pulmonary embolism occur rarely.

DENTAL CONSIDERATIONS

General:

• Place on regular recall to evaluate gingival inflammation, if present.

• Increased incidence of dry socket has been reported after tooth extraction.

• Monitor vital signs at each appointment because of potential cardiovascular adverse effects.

Teach Patient/Family to:

• Use effective oral hygiene to prevent periodontal inflammation.

• Advise patient of potential low risk of antibiotic interference with oral contraceptive effect.

Generic and Trade Name Index

Entries can be identified as follows: generic name, Trade Name/Trade Name [REGION].
The letter *t* indicates a table.

abacavir, 55
abarelix, 56
abatacept, 57
Abbocillin VK [AUS], 1036
abbreviations, 1397–1404
abciximab, 57
abdominal distention
  vasopressin, 1360
abdominal surgery
  dalteparin sodium, 396
Abelcet, 131, 133
Abeno [CAN], 65
Abilify, 154
Abraxane, 1006
Abreva, 466
absorbable gelatin sponge, 60
AC Gel, 1414t–1420t
acamprosate calcium, 61
acarbose, 62
Accolate, 1379
accommodative esotropia
  demecarium bromide, 413
  echothiophate iodide, 493
Accretropin, 1217
AccuNeb, 81
Accupril, 1145
Accurbron, 1271
Accuretic, 1414t–1420t
acebutolol, 63
Acenorm [AUS], 257
Aceon, 1048
Acetadote, 71
acetaminophen, 38t–46t, 65
acetaminophen overdose
  acetylcysteine, 71
acetazolamide, 67
acetohexamide, 69
Acetoxyl [CAN], 196
acetylcholine chloride, 71
acetylcysteine, 71
acetylsalicylic acid, 162
Achihexal [AUS], 75
Aciclovir-BC IV [AUS], 75
AcipHex, 1151
acitretin, 73
Aclin [AUS], 1231
Aclovate, 83
acne
  adapalene, 78
  azelaic acid, 177
  benzoyl peroxide, 196
  clindamycin, 348
  demeclocycline
    hydrochloride, 414
  erythromycin, 526
  minocycline hydrochloride,
    887
  tetracycline hydrochloride,
    1266

Acova, 153
acromegaly
  bromocriptine mesylate, 223
  lanreotide, 749
  octreotide acetate, 970
  pegvisomant, 1028
Act-3 [AUS], 682
Actacode [AUS], 369
Actigall, 1348
Actilyse [AUS], 102
Actimmune, 716
actinic (solar) cheilitis, 11–12
actinic keratoses
  diclofenac, 437
  fluorouracil, 591
Actiq, 568
Actisite, 1268
Activase, 102
Activella, 1414t–1420t
Actonel, 1175
Actos, 1075
Actrapid [AUS], 703
ACU-dyne, 1089
Acular, 739
Acular LS, 739
Acular PF, 739
acute coronary syndrome
  clopidogrel, 362
  eptifibatide, 520
acute dystonic reactions
  benztropine mesylate, 198
acute ischemic stroke
  alteplase, recombinant, 102
acute lymphocytic leukemia
    (ALL)
  clofarabine, 352
  cytarabine, 391
  dasatinib, 407
  mercaptopurine (6-MP), 832
  methotrexate sodium, 853
  teniposide, 1253
acute myelocytic leukemia
    (AML)
  etoposide, 548
  idarubicin hydrochloride,
    685
  sargramostim, 1195
acute myocardial infarction.
    See also myocardial
    infarction
  alteplase, recombinant, 102
  atenolol, 166
  reteplase, recombinant,
    1163
  tenecteplase, 1252
  timolol maleate, 1289
acute nonlymphocytic
    leukemia
  mitoxantrone, 895

acute pyelonephritis. *See*
    pyelonephritis
Acyclo-V [AUS], 75
acyclovir, 75
Adalat 5 [AUS], 947
Adalat 10 [AUS], 947
Adalat 20 [AUS], 947
Adalat CC, 947
Adalat Oros [AUS], 947
adalimumab, 77
adapalene, 78
Addison's disease, 31
  fludrocortisone, 583
adefovir, 79
adenocarcinoma
  thiotepa, 1277
Adipex-P, 1058
Adipost, 1052
adjunct to scaling/root planing
  chlorhexidine gluconate
    chip, 321
  doxycycline hyclate, 482
AD-Nephrin, 1061
Adoxa, 480
adrenal crisis, 31
adrenal insufficiency, 31–33
  cortisone acetate, 376
  hydrocortisone, 669
  methylprednisolone, 863
  prednisolone, 1095
  prednisone, 1103
Adrenalin, 509
Adrenaline Injection [AUS],
  509
adrenocortical carcinoma
  mitotane, 893
Adrucil, 591
Advair, 1414t–1420t
Advil, 682
Advil Cold, 1414t–1420t
Aerius [AUS], 419
AeroBid, 586
Aerodil [AUS], 532
Aerodine, 1089
Aerosporin, 1083
A-Fil, 147
Afinitor, 551
Afrin, 1003
Afrin 12-Hour, 1003
Afrin Children's Strength Nose
    Drops, 1003
Agenerase, 139
Aggrastat, 1295
Aggrenox, 1414t–1420t
AGON SR [AUS], 563
agoraphobia
  alprazolam, 99
Agrylin, 142
A-Hydrocort, 669

AIDS-related KS. *See* Kaposi's sarcoma
AIDS-related wasting
  somatropin, 1217
  thalidomide, 1269
Airomir [AUS], 81
Akamin [AUS], 887
AK-Beta, 766
AK-Cide, 1099
AK-Con, 924
AK-Dex, 427
AK-Dilate, 1061
Akineton HCl, 211
Akne-Mycin, 526
AK-Pentolate, 362
AK-Pred, 1095, 1097, 1101
AK-Sulf, 1226
AK-T Caine, 1264
AK-Tate [CAN], 1095
AK-Tob, 1297
Alamast, 1029
alatrofloxacin mesylate, 1344
Alavert, 796
Albalon, 924
albendazole, 80
Albenza, 80
Albert [CAN], 1046
albuterol, 81
alclometasone, 83
alcoholism
  acamprosate calcium, 61
  chlordiazepoxide, 318
  clonidine, 360
  clorazepate dipotassium, 363
  diazepam, 435
  disulfiram, 462
  oxazepam, 995
Alcomicin [CAN], 633
Aldactazide, 1414t–1420t
Aldactone, 1221
Aldara, 696
Aldazine, 1276
aldesleukin, 84
Aldomet, 859
Aldoril, 1414t–1420t
aldosteronism
  spironolactone, 1221
alefacept, 86
alemtuzumab, 87
alendronate sodium, 89
Alepam [AUS], 995
Alertec [CAN], 897
Aleve, 925
Alferon N, 715
alfuzosin, 90
alglucosidase alfa, 92
Alinia, 956
aliskiren, 93
alitretinoin, 94
Alka-Seltzer Gas Relief, 1209
Alkeran, 823
ALL. *See* acute lymphocytic leukemia (ALL)

Allegra, 572
Allegra-D, 1414t–1420t
Allegra-D 24 Hour, 1414t–1420t
Allegron [AUS], 966
Aller-Chlor, 326
Allerdryl [CAN], 455
allergic conjunctivitis. *See also* conjunctivitis
  emedastine, 497
  epinastine, 508
  ketorolac tromethamine, 739
  ketotifen fumarate, 741
  levocabastine, 767
  loteprednol, 801
  nedocromil sodium, 932
  olopatadine, 978
  pemirolast potassium, 1029
allergic rhinitis. *See also* rhinitis
  azatadine maleate, 174
  brompheniramine, 225
  carbinoxamine maleate, 263
  cetirizine, 313
  chlorpheniramine, 326
  ciclesonide, 334
  clemastine fumarate, 345
  cromolyn sodium, 378
  desloratadine, 419
  dexchlorpheniramine, 429
  diphenhydramine, 455
  fexofenadine hydrochloride, 572
  fluticasone propionate, 602
  loratadine, 796
  mometasone furoate monohydrate, 901
allergy symptoms
  brompheniramine, 225
  cyproheptadine, 389
  promethazine hydrochloride, 1121
Allermax Aqueous [AUS], 901
Allohexal [AUS], 95
allopurinol, 95
Allosig [AUS], 95
almotriptan malate, 96
Alocril, 932
Alomide, 789
Alophen, 213
Aloprim, 95
Alora, 532
alosetron, 98
Aloxi, 1009
Alpha-D, 1409t–1411t
Alphacaine [AUS], 95
Alphacin [AUS], 136
Alphagan P, 221
Alphapress [AUS], 662
Alphapril [AUS], 499
Alphatrex, 202
Alpovex [AUS], 134
alprazolam, 38t–46t, 99

alprostadil, 101
Alrex, 801
ALS. *See* amyotrophic lateral sclerosis (ALS)
Altabax, 1162
Altace, 1154
alteplase, recombinant, 102
Alti-Azathioprine, 175
Alti-Clobetasol [CAN], 350
Altinac, 1326
Alti-Sulfasalazine [CAN], 1227
Altoprev, 803
Alupent, 840
Alvesco, 334
alvimopan, 103
Alzheimer's disease
  donepezil hydrochloride, 470
  ergoloid mesylates, 521
  galantamine, 621
  memantine hydrochloride, 824
  rivastigmine tartrate, 1181
  tacrine hydrochloride, 1237
amantadine hydrochloride, 104
Amaryl, 637
Amatine, 882
Ambien, 1392
AmBisome, 131, 133
ambrisentan, 107
amcinonide, 108
Amcort, 1328
amebiasis
  chloroquine, 322
  intestinal, 1018
  metronidazole hydrochloride, 874
amenorrhea
  medroxyprogesterone acetate, 815
  norethindrone, 962
  progesterone, 1119
Amerge, 927
Americaine Anesthetic Lubricant, 193
Americaine Otic, 193
A-Methapred, 863
Amevive, 86
Amfamox [AUS], 559
Amficot, 134
Amidate, 1405t
amifostine, 109
Amigesic, 1191
amiloride hydrochloride, 111
aminoglutethimide, 113
aminophylline/theophylline, 114
aminosalicylic acid, 116
Aminoxin, 1138
amiodarone hydrochloride, 117
amitriptyline hydrochloride, 119
amlexanox, 121

amlodipine, 122
amoxapine, 124
amoxicillin, 125
amoxicillin/clavulanate
    potassium, 127
Amoxil, 125
amphetamine, 129
Amphocin, 131
Amphotec, 131, 133
amphotericin b, 131
amphotericin b, lipid-based,
    133
ampicillin, 134
ampicillin sodium, 136
ampicillin/sulbactam sodium,
    137
Amprace [AUS], 499
amprenavir, 139
Ampyra, 395
Amyl Nitrite, 140
amyl nitrite, 140
amyotrophic lateral sclerosis
    (ALS)
    riluzole, 1172
Anadrol, 1004
Anafranil, 356
anagrelide, 142
anakinra, 143
analgesia
    acetaminophen, 65
    aspirin, 162
    buprenorphine
        hydrochloride, 236
    butorphanol tartrate, 245
    codeine phosphate, 369
    diclofenac, 437
    etodolac, 546
    hydrocodone, 667
    hydrocodone bitartrate, 665
    hydromorphone
        hydrochloride, 672
    meperidine hydrochloride,
        825
    methadone hydrochloride,
        845
    morphine sulfate, 905
    nalbuphine hydrochloride,
        918
    oxycodone, 1002
    pentazocine, 1041
    tapentadol hydrochloride,
        1244
Anamorph [AUS], 905
Anandron [CAN], 950
anaplastic astrocytoma
    temozolomide, 1248
Anapolon [CAN], 1004
Anaprox, 925
Anaprox DS, 925
Anaspaz, 679
anastrozole, 144
Anbesol, 193
Anbesol Baby Gel, 193

Anbesol Maximum Strength,
    193
Ancef, 278
Ancobon, 580
Andrio [CAN], 1260
Androderm, 1260
AndroGel, 1260
Android, 865
Android-10, 865
Android-25, 865
Android-F, 594
Andropository [CAN], 1260
anemia
    darbepoetin alfa, 404
    epoetin alfa, 515
    methoxy polyethylene
        glycol-epoetin beta,
        855
    oxymetholone, 1004
anesthesia
    articaine hydrochloride,
        159
    benzocaine, 193
    bupivacaine, 232
    cocaine hydrochloride, 368
    droperidol, 487
    flumazenil, 585
    ketamine, 734
    lidocaine transoral delivery
        system, 776
    mepivacaine HCl, 829
    pentobarbital, 1042
    prilocaine hydrochloride,
        1106
    procaine, 1112
    propofol, 1126
    tetracaine, 1264
anesthetics, 2
    contradictions, 1408t
    dental preparations,
        1409t–1411t
    general, 1405
    local, 1406–1413
    mandibular teeth, 1412t
    maxillary teeth, 1413t
Anexate [CAN], 585
Anexsia, 667, 1414t–1420t
angina
    abciximab, 57
    amlodipine, 122
    amyl nitrite, 140
    atenolol, 166
    atorvastatin, 169
    bepridil, 200
    bivalirudin, 217
    dalteparin sodium, 396
    diltiazem hydrochloride,
        451
    enoxaparin sodium, 503
    felodipine, 563
    isosorbide, 724
    isosorbide dinitrate, 726
    metoprolol tartrate, 871

angina (Continued)
    nadolol, 914
    nicardipine hydrochloride,
        942
    nifedipine, 947
    nimodipine, 951
    nipradilol, 953
    nitroglycerin, 959
    propranolol hydrochloride,
        1127
    verapamil hydrochloride,
        1363
Anginine [AUS], 959
angioedema
    clemastine fumarate, 345
    danazol, 398
Angiomax, 217
angular cheilitis, 10–11
anidulafungin, 146
ankylosing spondylitis
    diclofenac, 437
    etanercept, 540
    indomethacin, 700
    naproxen, 925
    sulindac, 1231
anorexia nervosa
    megestrol acetate, 820
Anpec [AUS], 1363
Ansaid, 599
Antabuse, 462
Antenex [AUS], 435
Anthra-Derm, 147
Anthraforte [CAN], 147
anthralin, 147
Anthranol [CAN], 147
Anthrascalp [CAN], 147
anticoagulant therapy, 33–34
anticonvulsant
    clorazepate dipotassium,
        363
antiinflammation. See
    inflammation
Antilirium, 1067
antineoplastic agents, 24–27
antiplatelet therapy, 34
    prasugrel, 1091
antitussive
    diphenhydramine, 455
Antivert, 812
Anturane, 1228
Anusol-HC, 669
anxiety, 34–37
    alprazolam, 99
    buspirone hydrochloride,
        239
    chlordiazepoxide, 318
    chlorpromazine, 327
    diazepam, 435
    doxepin hydrochloride, 476
    hydroxyzine, 677
    lorazepam, 797
    meprobamate, 831
    oxazepam, 995

anxiety *(Continued)*
  trifluoperazine
    hydrochloride, 1334
  venlafaxine, 1361
Anzatax [AUS], 1006
Anzemet, 468
Apatef [AUS], 292
apepitant, 150
aphthous ulcer
  amlexanox, 121
Apidra, 707
Apo-Acetaminophen [CAN], 65
Apo-Acetazolamide [CAN], 67
Apo-Allopurinol [CAN], 95
Apo-Alpraz [CAN], 99
Apo-Amitriptyline [CAN], 119
Apo-Ampi [CAN], 134, 136
Apo-Ateno [CAN], 166
Apo-Benztropine [CAN], 198
Apo-Bisacodyl [CAN], 213
Apo-Bromocriptine [CAN], 223
Apo-C [CAN], 161
Apo-Carbamazepine [CAN], 260
Apo-Cefaclor [CAN], 275
Apo-Cephalex [CAN], 309
Apo-Chlordiazepoxide [CAN], 318
Apo-Chlorpropamide [CAN], 329
Apo-Chlorthalidone [CAN], 331
Apo-Cimetidine [CAN], 337
Apo-Clomipramine [CAN], 356
Apo-Cromolyn [CAN], 378
Apo-Desipramine [CAN], 416
Apo-Diazepam [CAN], 435
Apo-Diflunisal [CAN], 447
Apo-Diltiaz [CAN], 451
Apo-Dipyridamole [CAN], 457
Apo-Docusate [CAN], 466
Apo-Doxazosin [CAN], 474
Apo-Doxepin [CAN], 476
Apo-Doxy [CAN], 480
Apo-Enalapril [CAN], 499
Apo-Erythro Base [CAN], 526
Apo-Etodolac [CAN], 546
Apo-Fenofibrate [CAN], 565
Apo-Ferrous Gluconate [CAN], 569
Apo-Ferrous Sulfate [CAN], 569
Apo-Fluconazole [CAN], 578
Apo-Fluphenazine [CAN], 595
Apo-Flurazepam [CAN], 598
Apo-Folic [CAN], 606
Apo-Furosemide [CAN], 617
Apo-Gain [CAN], 889
Apo-Gemfibrozil [CAN], 631
Apo-Haloperidol [CAN], 657
Apo-Hydro [CAN], 663
Apo-Hydroxyquine [CAN], 674
Apo-Hydroxyzine [CAN], 677

Apo-Ibuprofen [CAN], 682
Apo-Imipramine [CAN], 694
Apo-Indomethacin [CAN], 700
Apo-Ipravent [CAN], 717
Apo-ISDN [CAN], 724, 726
Apo-K [CAN], 1086, 1088
Apo-Keto [CAN], 737
Apo-Ketoconazole [CAN], 736
Apo-Ketotifen [CAN], 741
Apokyn, 148
Apo-Lamotrigine [CAN], 747
Apo-Lisinopril [CAN], 785
Apo-Loperamide [CAN], 793
Apo-Lorazepam [CAN], 797
Apo-Loxapine [CAN], 804
Apo-Mefenamic [CAN], 818
Apo-Megestrol [CAN], 820
Apo-Methazolamide [CAN], 848
Apo-Methotrexate [CAN], 853
Apo-Methyldopa [CAN], 859
Apo-Metoclop [CAN], 868
Apo-Metoprolol [CAN], 871
Apo-Metronidazole [CAN], 874
Apo-Midazolam [CAN], 880
apomorphine, 148
Apo-Nabumetone, 913
Apo-Nadol [CAN], 914
Apo-Naprosyn [CAN], 925
Apo-Nifed [CAN], 947
Apo-Nitrofurantoin [CAN], 957
Apo-Nizatidine [CAN], 961
Apo-Norflox [CAN], 964
Apo-Nortriptyline [CAN], 966
Apo-Oflox [CAN], 971
Apo-Oxazepam [CAN], 995
Apo-Pentoxifylline SR [CAN], 1046
Apo-Pen-VK [CAN], 1036
Apo-Pindol [CAN], 1073
Apo-Piroxicam [CAN], 1077
Apo-Prednisone [CAN], 1103
Apo-Primidone [CAN], 1109
Apo-Propranolol [CAN], 1127
Apo-Quin-G [CAN], 1147
Apo-Quinidine [CAN], 1147
Apo-Ranitidine [CAN], 1156
Apo-Selegiline [CAN], 1201
Apo-Sertraline [CAN], 1203
Apo-Simvastatin [CAN], 1210
Apo-Sotalo [CAN], 1219
Apo-Sucralate [CAN], 1224
Apo-Sulfinpyrazone [CAN], 1228
Apo-Sulin [CAN], 1231
Apo-Tamox [CAN], 1241
Apo-Temazepam [CAN], 1247
Apo-Terazosin [CAN], 1256
Apo-Terbinafine [CAN], 1257
Apo-Tetra [CAN], 1266
Apo-Thioridazine [CAN], 1276
Apo-Ticlopidine [CAN], 1287
Apo-Timol [CAN], 1289

Apo-Timop [CAN], 1289, 1322
Apo-Tobramycin [CAN], 1297
Apo-Tolbutamide [CAN], 1302
Apo-Trazodone [CAN], 1324
Apo-Triazo [CAN], 1332
Apo-Trifluoperazine [CAN], 1334
Apo-Trihex [CAN], 1337
Apo-Trimip [CAN], 1340
Apo-Verap [CAN], 1363
Apo-Warfarin [CAN], 1377
Apo-Zidovudine [CAN], 1385
appetite suppressant
  dextroamphetamine sulfate, 433
  dronabinol, 484
  methamphetamine, 847
apraclonidine hydrochloride, 149
Apresazide, 1414t–1420t
Apresoline, 662
Apriso, 835
Aproven [AUS], 717
Apthasol, 121
Aqua Gem E, 1375
Aqua Mephyton, 1068
Aquachloral Supprettes, 317
Aquaphyllin, 1271
Aquasol A, 1373
Aquasol E, 1375
Aquazide H, 663
Ara-A, 1365
Ara-C, 391
Aralen [CAN], 322
Aralen hydrochloride, 322
Aralen phosphate, 322
Aramine, 841
Aranesp, 404
Aratac [AUS], 117
Arava, 756
Aredia, 1010
Arestocaine, 1409t–1411t
arformoterol tartrate, 152
argatroban, 153
Aricept, 470
Arimidex, 144
aripiprazole, 154
Aristocort, 1328
Aristocort Intralesional, 1328
Aristospan, 1328
armodafinil, 155
Armour Thyroid, 1282
Aromasin, 553
Aropax 20 [AUS], 1019
Arranon, 934
Arrestin [U.S.], 887
arrhythmia
  disopyramide phosphate, 460
  mexiletine hydrochloride, 877

arrhythmia *(Continued)*
  moricizine hydrochloride, 904
  propranolol hydrochloride, 1127
  sotalol hydrochloride, 1219
Artane, 1337
artemether/lumefantrine, 157
Arthrexin [AUS], 700
Arthrotec, 1414t–1420t
articaine hydrochloride, 159, 1409t–1411t
artichoke, 50t
Asacol, 835
Asacol HD, 835
ascariasis
  mebendazole, 810
Ascendin, 124
ascorbic acid, 161
Ascriptin, 162
Asig [AUS], 1145
Asmalix, 1271
Asmanex Twisthaler, 901
Asmol CFC-Free [AUS], 81
aspergillosis
  amphotericin b, 131
  caspofungin acetate, 274
  itraconazole, 730
aspirin, 38t–46t, 162
Aspro [AUS], 162
asthma
  beclomesthasone dipropionate, 187
  budesonide, 229
  ciclesonide, 334
  cromolyn sodium, 378
  dyphylline, 491
  ephedrine, 506
  flunisolide, 586
  fluticasone propionate, 602
  formoterol fumarate, 607
  medications, generally, 1422t–1423t
  mometasone furoate monohydrate, 901
  montelukast, 902
  nedocromil sodium, 932
  omalizumab, 980
  prednisolone, 1095
  prednisolone sodium phosphate, 1101
  prednisone, 1103
  salmeterol, 1190
  theophylline, 1271
  triamcinolone, 1328
  zafirlukast, 1379
  zileuton, 1386
Astracaine [CAN], 159, 1409t–1411t
Astracaine Forte [CAN], 159
Astramorph, 905
asystole
  epinephrine, 509

Atacand, 253
Atacand HCT, 1414t–1420t
Atarax, 677
Atasol [CAN], 65
atazanavir sulfate, 164
AteHexal [AUS], 166
atenolol, 166
atherosclerosis
  clopidogrel, 362
Ativan, 797
atomoxetine, 168
atony of bladder
  bethanechol chloride, 205
atopic dermatitis
  alclometasone, 83
  pimecrolimus, 1070
  tacrolimus, 1238
atorvastatin, 169
atrial dysrhythmia
  warfarin sodium, 1377
atrial fibrillation
  digoxin, 448
  diltiazem hydrochloride, 451
  dofetilide, 467
  dronedarone, 485
  ibutilide fumarate, 684
  quinidine, 1147
  verapamil hydrochloride, 1363
atrial flutter
  dronedarone, 485
  ibutilide fumarate, 684
  quinidine, 1147
  verapamil hydrochloride, 1363
Atridox, 483
atrophic vaginitis
  estradiol, 532
  estropipate, 537
Atrovent, 717
Atrovent Aerosol [AUS], 717
Atrovent Nasal [AUS], 717
Atrovent NPH, 717
A/T/S, 526
Attenta [AUS], 861
attention deficit hyperactivity disorder (ADHD)
  amphetamine, 129
  atomoxetine, 168
  clonidine, 360
  dexmethylphenidate hydrochloride, 431
  dextroamphetamine sulfate, 433
  lisdexamfetamine dimesylate, 784
  methamphetamine, 847
  methylphenidate hydrochloride, 861
  pemoline, 1030
Augmentin, 127
Augmentin ES 600, 127

Augmentin XR, 127
Auro Ear Drops, 262
aurothioglucose/gold sodium thiomalate, 172
Auscap [AUS], 592
Auscard [AUS], 451
Ausclay [AUS], 127
Ausclay Duo 400 [AUS], 127
Ausclay Duo Forte [AUS], 127
Ausgem [AUS], 631
Auspril [AUS], 499
Ausran [AUS], 1156
Avalide, 1414t–1420t
Avandamet, 1414t–1420t
Avandia, 1185
Avanza [AUS], 891
Avapro, 719
Avastin, 206
Avelox, 907
Avelox IV, 907
Aventyl, 966
Avinza, 905
Avirax [CAN], 75
Avita, 1326
Avodart, 490
Axert, 96
Axid, 961
Axid AR, 961
Aygestin, 962
Azactam, 180
Azasan, 175
azatadine maleate, 174
azathioprine, 175
azelaic acid, 177
Azelex, 177
Azilect, 1158
azithromycin, 179
Azmacort, 1328
Azo-Gesic, 1051
azole antifungal agents, 38t–46t
Azopt, 222
Azo-Standard, 1051
AZT, 1385
aztreonam, 180
Azulfidine, 1227
Azulfidine EN-tabs, 1227

Babee Cof Syrup, 434
Babee Teething, 193
Baciguent, 183
Baci-IM, 183
Bacitracin, 183
bacitracin, 183
bacterial conjunctivitis. *See also* conjunctivitis
  besifloxacin, 201
  gatifloxacin, 626
  levofloxacin, 771
  moxifloxacin hydrochloride, 907
  ofloxacin, 971
  polymyxin B sulfate, 1084

bacterial endocarditis. *See* endocarditis
bacterial infection. *See* infection
bacterial vaginosis
  clindamycin, 348
Bactramycin, 777
Bactrim, 1414t–1420t
Bactroban, 909
Balamex, 1387
Balminil [CAN], 649
Balminil Decongestant [CAN], 1134
balsalazide, 185
Bancap HC, 667
Banophen, 455
Bapadin, 200
barbiturates, 38t–46t
basal cell carcinoma
  fluorouracil, 591
Bayer, 162
becaplermin, 186
beclomesthasone dipropionate, 187
beclomesthasone dipropionate hfa, 187
Beconase, 187
Beconase Allergy 24 Hour [AUS], 602
Beconase AQ Nasal, 187
Beconase Hayfever [AUS], 602
Bedoz [CAN], 380
Beesix, 1138
Bellergal-S, 1414t–1420t
Benadryl, 455
benazepril, 188
bendamustine, 190
bendroflumethiazide, 192
Benicar, 975, 977
Benicar HCT, 1414t–1420t
benign migratory glossitis, 12–13
benign prostatic hyperplasia (BPH)
  alfuzosin, 90
  doxazosin mesylate, 474
  dutasteride, 490
  finasteride, 574
  tamsulosin hydrochloride, 1242
  terazosin hydrochloride, 1256
Benoxyl [CAN], 196
Bentrop [AUS], 198
Bentyl, 441
Bentylol [CAN], 441
Benuryl [CAN], 1111
Benylin Adult, 434
Benylin E [CAN], 649
Benylin Pediatric, 434
Benzac, 196
Benzac AC, 196
Benzac AC Wash, 196

Benzac W, 196
Benzac W Wash, 196
Benzagel, 196
Benzagel Wash, 196
Benzashave, 196
benzocaine, 193
Benzodent, 193
benzodiazepine overdose
  flumazenil, 585
benzodiazepines, 38t–46t
benzonatate, 195
benzoyl peroxide, 196
benzthiazide, 197
benztropine mesylate, 198
bepridil, 200
besifloxacin, 201
Besivance, 201
Beta-2, 721
Betaderm [CAN], 202
Betadine, 1089
Betagan, 766
Betagen, 1089
β-lactams, 38t–46t
Betaloc [CAN], 871
betamethasone, 202
Betapace, 1219
Betapace AF, 1219
Beta-Sol [AUS], 1274
Betatrex, 202
Beta-Val, 202
Betaxin [CAN], 1274
Betaxon, 765
bethanechol chloride, 205
Betimol, 1289
Betneso [AUS], 202
Betoptic [AUS], 203
Betoptic-S, 203
Betoquin [AUS], 203
bevacizumab, 206
Bex [AUS], 162
bexarotene, 208
Biaxin, 343
Biaxin XL, 343
bicalutamide, 209
Bicillin CR, 1414t–1420t
Bicillin LA, 1033
BiCNU, 268
Bicor [AUS], 215
biliary cirrhosis
  ursodiol, 1348
bimatoprost, 210
Bio Contac Cold 12 Hour Relief Non Drowsy [CAN], 1134
Biocef, 309
Biodyne, 1089
BioQuin Durules [CAN], 1147
biperiden, 211
bipolar disorder
  aripiprazole, 154
  lamotrigine, 747

bipolar disorder *(Continued)*
  lithium carbonate, 788
  olanzapine, 973
  quetiapine, 1143
  valproic acid, 1352
bisacodyl, 213
Bisa-Lax [AUS], 213
Bismed [CAN], 214
bismuth subsalicylate, 214
bisoprolol fumarate, 215
bisphosphonate-associated
  osteonecrosis of the jaw, 47–48
bivalirudin, 217
bladder carcinoma
  cisplatin, 341
  valrubicin, 1353
bladder distention
  neostigmine, 938
blastomycosis
  amphotericin b, 131
  itraconazole, 730
  ketoconazole, 736
Blenamax [AUS], 218
Blenoxane, 218
bleomycin sulfate, 218
Bleph-10, 1226
Blephamide, 1099, 1414t–1420t
Blephamide S.O.P., 1099
blepharitis
  bacitracin, 183
blepharoconjunctivitis
  polymyxin B sulfate, 1084
Blocadren, 1289
Bonamine [CAN], 812
bone infection
  cephalexin, 309
bone marrow transplant
  busulfan, 240
  filgrastim, 573
  fluconazole, 578
  sargramostim, 1195
Bonine, 812
Boniva, 688
Bontril PDM, 1052
Bontril Slow-Release, 1052
bosentan, 220
bradycardia
  epinephrine, 509
brain cancer
  temozolomide, 1248
brain tumor
  carmustine, 268
  etoposide, 548
  lomustine, 792
breast cancer
  abarelix, 56
  anastrozole, 144
  capecitabine, 254
  cyclophosphamide, 384
  docetaxel, 464

breast cancer *(Continued)*
epirubicin, 512
estradiol, 532
exemestane, 553
fluoxymesterone, 594
goserelin acetate, 644
ixabepilone, 732
lapatinib, 754
letrozole, 758
megestrol acetate, 820
methotrexate sodium, 853
methyltestosterone, 865
paclitaxel, 1006
tamoxifen citrate, 1241
testosterone, 1260
thiotepa, 1277
topotecan, 1311
toremifene citrate, 1312
trastuzumab, 1321
vinblastine sulfate, 1367
Brevoxyl, 196
Brevoxyl Cleansing, 196
Brevoxyl Wash, 196
brimonidine, 221
brinzolamide, 222
bromocriptine mesylate, 223
Bromohexal [AUS], 223
brompheniramine, 225
bronchial asthma. *See* asthma
bronchitis
alatrofloxacin mesylate,
1344
cefaclor, 275
cefdinir, 280
cefditoren pivoxil, 282
cefixime, 285
cefpodoxime proxetil, 295
cefprozil, 297
ceftibuten, 300
clarithromycin, 343
demeclocycline
hydrochloride, 414
dirithromycin, 458
gatifloxacin, 626
gemifloxacin, 632
levofloxacin, 771
loracarbef, 795
moxifloxacin hydrochloride,
907
theophylline, 1271
bronchodilation
epinephrine, 509
bronchospasm
albuterol, 81
aminophylline/theophylline,
114
cromolyn sodium, 378
dyphylline, 491
formoterol fumarate, 607
ipratropium bromide, 717
isoetharine hydrochloride,
721
levalbuterol, 762

bronchospasm *(Continued)*
metaproterenol sulfate, 840
pirbuterol, 1076
salmeterol, 1190
Bronkodyl, 1271
Bronkometer, 721
Bronkosol, 721
Brovana, 152
BroveX, 225
BroveX CT, 225
brucellosis
doxycycline, 480
minocycline hydrochloride,
887
Brufen [AUS], 682
bucindolol, 226
Bucladin-S, 228
buclizine hydrochloride, 228
budesonide, 229
Bufferin, 162
bulimia nervosa
fluoxetine hydrochloride,
592
bumetanide, 230
Bumex, 230
bupivacaine, 232, 1406t–1407t,
1409t–1411t
Buprenex, 236
buprenorphine hydrochloride,
236
bupropion, 237
Burinex [AUS], 229
Burinex [CAN], 230
Burkitt's lymphoma
cyclophosphamide, 384
methotrexate sodium, 853
burn
mafenide, 807
nitrofurazone, 958
procaine, 1112
silver sulfadiazine, 1208
tobramycin, 1296
tobramycin sulfate, 1297
burning mouth syndrome,
21–22
bursitis
naproxen, 925
sulindac, 1231
Buscopan [CAN], 679
BuSpar, 239
Buspirex [CAN], 239
buspirone hydrochloride,
239
Bustab [CAN], 239
busulfan, 240
Busulfex, 240
butabarbital sodium, 242
butenafine, 244
Butisol, 242
butoconazole, 244
butorphanol tartrate, 245
Byetta, 554
Bystolic, 930

cabergoline, 248
cachexia
megestrol acetate, 820
Caduet, 1414t–1420t
Cafergot [CAN], 522
Caladryl, 1414t–1420t
Calan, 1363
Calan SR, 1363
Calciferol, 1374
Calcijex, 251
Calcimar, 249
calcitonin, 249
calcitriol, 251
Calcium Leucovorin [AUS],
759
Caltine [CAN], 249
Camila, 962
Campath, 87
Campral, 61
Canasa, 835
cancer. *See also individual
types of cancer*
bleomycin sulfate, 218
fluorouracil, 591
cancer chemotherapy, 24–25
allopurinol, 95
apepitant, 150
cottonseed oil, 377–378
dexamethasone, 425
dolasetron, 468
dronabinol, 484
granisetron, 646
metoclopramide, 868
palonosetron hydrochloride,
1009
Cancidas, 274
candesartan cilexetil, 253
candidemia
anidulafungin, 146
candidiasis. *See also* oral
candidiasis;
vulvovaginal
candidiasis
amphotericin b, 131
anidulafungin, 146
butoconazole, 244
caspofungin acetate, 274
clotrimazole, 365
fluconazole, 578
flucytosine, 580
itraconazole, 730
ketoconazole, 736
miconazole, 878
nystatin, 968
posaconazole, 1084
treatment, generally, 9–10
candiduria
ketoconazole, 736
Candyl-D [AUS], 1077
Canesten [CAN], 365
canker sore
benzocaine, 193
capecitabine, 254

Capex, 588
Capital with Codeine,
    1414t–1420t
Capoten, 257
Capozide, 1414t–1420t
capsaicin, 256
Captohexal [AUS], 257
captopril, 257
Capurate [AUS], 95
Carac, 591
Carafate, 1224
carbachol, 259
Carbacot, 852
Carbaglu, 266
carbamazepine, 260, 1424t
carbamide peroxide, 262
Carbatrol, 260
carbinoxamine maleate, 263
Carbocaine, 1406t–1407t,
    1409t–1411t
Carbocaine Caudal 1.5%
    [AUS], 829
Carbocaine HCl, 829
carboplatin, 264
Carboxine, 263
carcinoid tumor
    octreotide acetate, 970
Cardcal [AUS], 451
Cardene, 942
Cardene IV, 942
Cardene SR, 942
cardiac arrest
    vasopressin, 1360
cardiac decompensation
    disopyramide phosphate,
        460
    dobutamine hydrochloride,
        463
cardiac surgery
    lidocaine hydrochloride, 774
cardiomyopathy
    disopyramide phosphate,
        460
    nipradilol, 953
Cardizem, 451
Cardizem CD, 451
Cardizem LA, 451
Cardizem SR, 451
Cardol [AUS], 1219
Cardura, 474
carglumic acid, 266
carisoprodol, 267
carmustine, 268
Caroptic, 259
carteolol, 270
Cartia, 451
Cartrol, 270
carvedilol, 271
Casodex, 209
caspofungin acetate, 274
castration
    estropipate, 537
Cataflam, 437

Catapres, 360
Catapres TTS, 360
cataract surgery
    diclofenac, 437
    ketorolac tromethamine,
        739
Cathflo Activase, 102
Caverject, 101
Ceclor, 275
Ceclor CD, 275
Cecon, 161
Cedax, 300
Cedocard [CAN], 724, 726
CeeNU, 792
cefaclor, 275
cefadroxil, 277
cefazolin sodium, 278
cefdinir, 280
cefditoren pivoxil, 282
cefepime, 284
cefixime, 285
Cefizox, 302
Cefkor [AUS], 275
Cefkor CD [AUS], 275
Cefobid, 289
cefonicid sodium, 287
cefoperazone, 289
Cefotan, 292
cefotaxime sodium, 290
cefotetan disodium, 292
cefoxitin sodium, 293
cefpodoxime proxetil, 295
cefprozil, 297
ceftazidime, 298
ceftibuten, 300
Ceftin, 305
ceftizoxime sodium, 302
ceftriaxone sodium, 303
cefuroxime axetil, 305
cefuroxime sodium, 305
Cefzil, 297
Celebrex, 307
celecoxib, 307
Celestone, 202
CellCept, 910
Celontin, 857
Cena K, 1086
Cenolate, 161
central precocious puberty
    (CPP)
    histrelin, 659
central venous catheter
    clearance
    alteplase, recombinant, 102
Cepacol, 193, 1264
cephalexin, 309
cephalosporins, 38t–46t
cephradine, 310
Ceporex [AUS], 309
Ceprotin, 1131
Ceptaz, 298
cerebral edema
    dexamethasone, 425

cerebral edema (Continued)
    prednisolone, 1095
    prednisone, 1103
Cerebyx, 614
Certican, 551
certolizumab, 312
cervicitis
    ofloxacin, 971
Cesarean section
    cefotaxime sodium, 290
    cefotetan disodium, 292
    cefoxitin sodium, 293
Cetacaine, 193
Ceta-Plus, 667
cetirizine, 313
cetuximab, 314
cevimeline, 316
C-Flox [AUS], 339
chancroid
    azithromycin, 179
    sulfisoxazole, 1230
Chantix, 1358
chapped/cracked lips, 22–23
cheilitis
    actinic, 11–12
    angular, 10–11
    exfoliative, 22–23
chemotherapy. See cancer
    chemotherapy
Chiggerex, 193
ChiggerTox, 193
Children's Advil Cold,
    1414t–1420t
Chirocaine, 1406t–1407t
chloral hydrate, 317
Chlorate, 326
chlordiazepoxide, 38t–46t,
    318
chlorhexidine 0.12% oral rinse,
    1425t
chlorhexidine gluconate,
    320
chlorhexidine gluconate chip,
    321
Chlorhexidine Mouthwash
    [AUS], 320
Chlorhexidine Obstetric Lotion
    [AUS], 320
Chlorohex Gel [AUS], 320
Chlorohex Gel Forte [AUS],
    320
Chlorohex Mouth Rinse [AUS],
    320
chloroprocaine, 1406t–1407t
chloroquine, 322
chloroquine phosphate, 322
chlorothiazide, 324
Chlorphen, 326
chlorpheniramine, 326
Chlorpromanyl [CAN], 327
chlorpromazine, 327
chlorpropamide [CAN], 329
chlorthalidone [CAN], 331

Chlor-Trimeton, 326
Chlor-Trimeton Allergy, 326
Chlor-Trimeton Allergy 8
   Hour, 326
Chlor-Trimeton Allergy 12
   Hour, 326
Chlor-Tripolon [CAN], 326
chlorzoxazone, 332
Cholestagel [INTL.], 372
cholestyramine resin, 333
chorioadenoma destruens
   methotrexate sodium, 853
choriocarcinoma
   methotrexate sodium, 853
   vinblastine sulfate, 1367
chromomycosis
   ketoconazole, 736
chronic granulomatous disease
   interferon gamma-1b, 716
chronic lymphocytic leukemia
   (CLL)
   alemtuzumab, 87
   bendamustine, 190
   fludarabine phosphate, 582
chronic myelogenous leukemia
   (CML)
   busulfan, 240
   cytarabine, 391
   dasatinib, 407
   hydroxyurea, 676
   imatinib mesylate, 692
   interferon alfa-2a, 708
   interferon alfa-2a/2b, 710
   nilotinib, 948
chronic obstructive pulmonary
   disease (COPD)
   arformoterol tartrate, 152
   azithromycin, 179
   formoterol fumarate, 607
   salmeterol, 1190
   theophylline, 1271
   tiotropium bromide, 1294
Chronovera [CAN], 1363
Cialis, 1240
Cibacalcin, 249
Cibalith-S, 788
ciclesonide, 334
ciclopirox, 336
Cidomycin [CAN], 633
Cilicaine VK [AUS], 1036
Ciloquin [AUS], 339
Ciloxan, 339
Cimehexal [AUS], 337
cimetidine, 337
Cimzia, 312
Cipro, 339
Cipro HC Otic, 1414t–1420t
Ciprodex Otic, 1414t–1420t
ciprofloxacin hydrochloride,
   339
Ciproxin [AUS], 339
cisplatin, 341
Citanest, 1106

Citanest Forte, 1409t–1411t
Citanest Forte with
   epinephrine, 1106
Citanest Plain, 1409t–1411t
citrovorum factor, 759
Claforan, 290
Clamoxyl [AUS], 127
Clamoxyl Duo 400 [AUS], 127
Clamoxyl Duo Forte [AUS],
   127
Claratyne [AUS], 796
Clarinex, 419
Clarinex Redi-Tabs, 419
clarithromycin, 343
   drug interactions, 38t–46t
Claritin, 796
Claritin RediTab, 796
Claritin-D, 1414t–1420t
clavulanate potassium, 127,
   1286
Clavulin [CAN], 127
Clavulin Duo Forte [AUS],
   127
Clear Eyes [AUS], 924
Clearplex, 196
clemastine fumarate, 345
Cleocin, 348
Cleocin HCl [AUS], 348
clevidipine, 346
Cleviprex, 346
Climara, 532
Clinac BPO, 196
clindamycin, 348
Clindesse, 348
Clinoril, 1231
CLL. See chronic lymphocytic
   leukemia (CLL)
clobetasol, 350
clocortolone, 351
Cloderm, 351
Cloderm [CAN], 351
clofarabine, 352
clofazimine, 352
Clolar, 352
Clomhexal [AUS], 355
Clomid, 355
Clomid [CAN], 355
clomiphene, 355
clomipramine hydrochloride,
   356
Clonapam [CAN], 358
clonazepam, 358, 1424t
clonidine, 360
clopidogrel, 362
Clopine [AUS], 366
Clopram [AUS], 356
clorazepate dipotassium, 363
Closina [AUS], 385
Clotrimaderm [CAN], 365
clotrimazole, 365, 1425t
clozapine, 366
Clozaril, 366

CML. See chronic
   myelogenous leukemia
   (CML)
CMV retinitis. See
   cytomegalovirus
   (CMV) retinitis
Coartem, 157
Cocaine [CAN], 368
Cocaine HCl, 368
cocaine hydrochloride, 368
coccidioidomycosis
   amphotericin b, 131
   ketoconazole, 736
   miconazole, 878
Codeine Linctus [AUS], 369
codeine phosphate, 369
Codeine Phosphate Injection,
   369
codeine sulfate, 369
Codiclear DH, 667
Codimal A, 225
Codral Period Pain [AUS], 682
Cogentin, 198
Co-Gesic, 667
Cognex, 1237
Colace, 466
Colax-C [CAN], 466
Colazal, 185
Colchicine, 371
colchicine, 371
cold prevention
   ascorbic acid, 161
cold sore
   docosanol, 466
   penciclovir, 1032
   tetracaine, 1264
   valacyclovir, 1349
colesevelam, 372
Colestid, 373
Colestid [CAN], 373
colestipol, 373
Colgout [AUS], 371
Colhist, 225
Colifoam [AUS], 669
collagen disorder
   cortisone acetate, 376
   methylprednisolone, 863
   prednisone, 1103
Colo-Fresh, 214
colon cancer
   bevacizumab, 206
   capecitabine, 254
   oxaliplatin, 990
colorectal cancer
   cetuximab, 314
   panitumumab, 1012
Coloxy [AUS], 466
combination drugs, 1414–1420
CombiPatch, 1414t–1420t
Combipres, 1414t–1420t
Combivent, 1414t–1420t
Combivir, 1414t–1420t
Combunox, 1414t–1420t

Commit, 944
common cold
  chlorpheniramine, 326
  clemastine fumarate, 345
  dexchlorpheniramine, 429
common oral lesions. *See*
    treatment of oral
    lesions
community-acquired
    pneumonia. *See also*
    pneumonia
  alatrofloxacin mesylate,
    1344
  amoxicillin/clavulanate
    potassium, 127
  cefdinir, 280
  cefditoren pivoxil, 282
  dirithromycin, 458
  gemifloxacin, 632
  levofloxacin, 771
  moxifloxacin hydrochloride,
    907
Compazine, 1116
complementary medicines,
    48–53
Comtan, 505
Concerta, 861
Condyline [CAN], 1081
Condyline Paint [AUS], 1081
condyloma acuminatum
  fluorouracil, 591
  imiquimod, 696
  interferon alfa-2a/2b, 710
  interferon alfa-2b, 713
  interferon alfa-n3, 715
  podofilox, 1081
  podophyllum resin, 1082
Condylox, 1081
congestive heart failure (CHF)
  bucindolol, 226
  captopril, 257
  chlorthalidone [CAN], 331
  digoxin, 448
  enalapril maleate, 499
  eplerenone, 513
  hydrochlorothiazide, 663
  metoprolol tartrate, 871
  nitroglycerin, 959
  ramipril, 1154
  reteplase, recombinant,
    1163
  torsemide, 1313
  trandolapril, 1316
  valsartan, 1355
conivaptan, 374
conjugated estrogens, 536
conjunctivitis. *See also* allergic
    conjunctivitis; bacterial
    conjunctivitis
  bacitracin, 183
  ciprofloxacin hydrochloride,
    339
  cromolyn sodium, 378

conjunctivitis *(Continued)*
  lodoxamide, 789
  oxymetazoline, 1003
  prednisolone, 1095
  prednisolone acetate, 1097
  sulfacetamide, 1226
  tobramycin sulfate, 1297
constipation
  bisacodyl, 213
  tegaserod, 1245
contact dermatitis
  alclometasone, 83
  betamethasone, 202
  diflorasone, 446
  fluticasone propionate, 602
  halobetasol, 656
Contin [CAN], 369
contraception
  medroxyprogesterone
    acetate, 815
  norethindrone, 962
  norgestrel, 965
  oral contraceptives,
    1442–1443
controlled substances classes,
    1421
Copaxone, 636
COPD. *See* chronic obstructive
    pulmonary disease
    (COPD)
Copegus, 1164
Coras [AUS], 451
Cordarone, 117
Cordarone X [AUS], 117
Cordilox SR [AUS], 1363
Cordran, 597
Cordran SP, 597
Coreg, 271
Coreg CR, 271
Corgard, 914
Cormax, 350
corneal refractive surgery
  diclofenac, 437
corneal ulcer
  bacitracin, 183
  ciprofloxacin hydrochloride,
    339
  levofloxacin, 771
  ofloxacin, 971
  sulfacetamide, 1226
  tobramycin sulfate, 1297
coronary artery disease
  lovastatin, 803
Cortaid, 669
Cortate [AUS], 376
Cortef cream [AUS], 669
Cortic cream [AUS], 669
Cortic DS [AUS], 669
corticosteroid replacement
    therapy
  betamethasone, 202
Cortifoam, 669
cortisone acetate, 376

Cortisporin, 1414t–1420t
Cortizone-5, 669
Cortizone-10, 669
Cortone [CAN], 376
Corvert, 684
Corzide, 1414t–1420t
Cosopt, 1414t–1420t
Cosudex, 209
Cotazym-S [AUS], 1011
Cotazym-S Forte [AUS], 1011
cottonseed oil, 377–378
cough
  benzonatate, 195
  codeine phosphate, 369
  dextromethorphan, 434
  diphenhydramine, 455
  hydrocodone, 667
  hydrocodone bitartrate, 665
  hydromorphine
    hydrochloride, 672
Coumadin, 1377
Covera-HS, 1363
Cozaar, 799
Creomulsion Cough, 434
Creomulsion for Children,
    434
Creon, 1011
Creo-Terpin, 434
Crestor, 1187
cretinism
  thyroid, 1282
Crinone, 1119
Crixivan, 698
Crohn's disease
  budesonide, 229
  certolizumab, 312
  infliximab, 702
  sulfasalazine, 1227
Cromol, 378
cromolyn sodium, 378
cryptococcosis
  amphotericin b, 131
  flucytosine, 580
  miconazole, 878
Crysana [AUS], 925
Cubicin, 403
Cushing's syndrome
  aminoglutethimide, 113
cutaneous lava migrans
  thiabendazole, 1272
cutaneous T-cell lymphoma
  bexarotene, 208
Cutivate, 602
cyanocobalamin, 380
cyclobenzaprine hydrochloride,
    381
Cycloblastin [AUS], 384
Cyclogyl, 362
Cyclomen [CAN], 398
cyclophosphamide, 384
cycloplegia induction
  cylcopentolate
    hydrochloride, 383

cycloplegia induction
    (Continued)
    homatropine hydrobromide,
        661
cycloserine, 385
cyclosporine, 387
cyclostimulant
    demecarium bromide, 413
Cyklokapron, 1318
Cylate, 362
cylcopentolate hydrochloride,
    383
Cylert, 1030
Cylex, 193
Cylocort, 108
Cymbalta, 488
Cymevene [AUS], 624
cyproheptadine, 389
Cysporin [AUS], 387
Cystagon, 390
cysteamine bitartrate, 390
cystic fibrosis
    aztreonam, 180
    ceftazidime, 298
    ciprofloxacin hydrochloride,
        339
    dornase alfa, 472
    tobramycin, 1296
    tobramycin sulfate, 1297
cystic hydatid
    albendazole, 80
cystinosis
    cysteamine bitartrate, 390
cystitis
    cephalexin, 309
    flavoxate, 576
    gatifloxacin, 626
    hemorrhagic, 837
    interstitial, 1044
    mesna, 837
Cystospaz, 679
Cystospaz-M, 679
Cytadren, 113
Cytamen [AUS], 380
cytarabine, 391
cytomegalovirus (CMV)
    retinitis
    foscarnet sodium, 610
    ganciclovir sodium, 624
    valganciclovir hydrochloride,
        1350
Cytomel, 781
Cytosar [CAN], 391
Cytosar-U, 391
Cytotec, 893
Cytovene, 624
Cytoxan, 384

daclizumab, 394
Dacogen, 410
Dalacin [CAN], 348
Dalacin C [AUS], 348
dalfampridine, 395

Dalmane, 598
dalteparin sodium, 396
Damason-P, 667
danaparoid, 397
danazol, 398
Danocrine, 398
Dantrium, 400
dantrolene sodium, 400
Daonil [CAN], 641
Dapa-tabs [AUS], 697
dapiprazole hydrochloride, 401
Dapsone, 402
dapsone, 402
daptomycin, 403
Daraprim, 1139
darbepoetin alfa, 404
Darier's disease
    acitretin, 73
darunavir, 407
Darvocet A500, 1414t–1420t
Darvocet-N, 1414t–1420t
dasatinib, 407
daunorubicin citrate liposome,
    408
DaunoXome, 408
Dayhistol Allergy, 345
Daypro, 994
Dazamide, 67
DDAVP, 420
Debrox, 262
Decadron, 425
Decadron Phosphate
    Ophthalmic, 427
decitabine, 410
Declomycin, 414
Decofed, 1134
deep vein thrombosis (DVT)
    dalteparin sodium, 396
    danaparoid, 397
    desirudin, 418
    enoxaparin sodium, 503
    tinzaparin sodium, 1292
    warfarin sodium, 1377
Dehydral [CAN], 850
Del Aqua, 196
Delatestryl, 1260
delavirdine mesylate, 412
delayed puberty
    methyltestosterone, 865
    testosterone, 1260
Delestrogen, 532
Delonide, 422
Delsym, 434
Deltasone, 1103
Demadex, 1313
demecarium bromide, 413
demeclocycline hydrochloride,
    414
Demerol, 825
Demser, 875
Denavir, 1032
dental caries
    sodium fluoride, 1214

dental caries *(Continued)*
    sodium fluoride (topical),
        1216
Denti-Patch, 776
denture irritation
    benzocaine, 193
denture sore mouth, 20
Depacon, 1352
Depakene, 1352, 1424t
Depakene syrup, 1352
Depakote, 1352, 1424t
Depakote ER, 1352
Depakote Sprinkle, 1352
DepoDur, 905
Depo-Estradiol, 532
Depo-Medrol, 863
Depo-Nisolone, 863
Depo-Provera, 815
Depo-Provera Contraceptive,
    815
Depotest [CAN], 1260
Depo-Testosterone, 1260
depression, 37–48
    amitriptyline hydrochloride,
        119
    amoxapine, 124
    bupropion, 237
    clomipramine hydrochloride,
        356
    desipramine hydrochloride,
        416
    desvenlafaxine, 424
    doxepin hydrochloride, 476
    duloxetine, 488
    escitalopram, 528
    fluoxetine hydrochloride,
        592
    imipramine, 694
    isocarboxazid, 720
    maprotiline, 808
    mirtazapine, 891
    nefazodone hydrochloride,
        933
    nortriptyline hydrochloride,
        966
    paroxetine hydrochloride,
        1019
    phenelzine sulfate, 1054
    protriptyline, 1133
    sertraline, 1203
    tranylcypromine sulfate,
        1319
    trazodone hydrochloride,
        1324
    trimipramine, 1340
    venlafaxine, 1361
Deptran [AUS], 476
Deralin [AUS], 1127
Derm-Aid cream [AUS], 669
Dermaide [AUS], 669
Dermaide soft cream [AUS],
    669
Derma-Smooth/FS, 588

dermatitis. *See also* individual
  types of dermatitis
  alclometasone, 83
  clobetasol, 350
  fluocinolone acetonide, 588
dermatitis herpetiformis
  dapsone, 402
dermatologic toxicity
  panitumumab, 1012
dermatophytosis
  clotrimazole, 365
dermatoses
  acitretin, 73
  amcinonide, 108
  clocortolone, 351
  desonide, 422
  desoximetasone, 423
  dexamethasone sodium
    phosphate, 427
  diflorasone, 446
  fluocinonide, 589
  flurandrenolide, 597
  halcinonide, 656
  halobetasol, 656
Dermoplast, 193
Dermovate [CAN], 350
Desamethasone, 425
desipramine hydrochloride,
  416
desirudin, 418
Desitin, 1387
desloratadine, 419
desmopressin, 420
Desocrot [CAN], 422
desonide, 422
Desonide [CAN], 422
DesOwen, 422
desoximetasone, 423
Desoxyn, 847
Desquam-E, 196
Desquam-X, 196
desvenlafaxine, 424
Desyrel, 1324
Detaine, 193
Detrol, 1306
Detrol LA, 1306
Detussin, 667
Devrom, 214
Dexacidin, 1414t–1420t
DexAlone, 434
dexamethasone, 425
Dexamethasone Ophthalmic,
  427
dexamethasone oral solution, 8
dexamethasone sodium
  phosphate, 427
Dexamphetamine [AUS], 433
Dexasone, 425
Dexasone LA, 425
dexchlorpheniramine, 429
Dexedrine, 433
Dexedrine Spansule, 433
dexlansoprazole, 430

Dexmethsone [AUS], 425
dexmethylphenidate
  hydrochloride, 431
dextroamphetamine sulfate,
  433
dextromethorphan, 434
DextroStat, 433
Dey-Lute, 721
D.H.E. 45, 522
DHT, 450
DiaBeta, 641
diabetes insipidus
  desmopressin, 420
  vasopressin, 1360
diabetes mellitus
  acarbose, 62
  acetohexamide, 69
  chlorpropamide [CAN], 329
  colesevelam, 372
  exenatide, 554
  glimepiride, 637
  glipizide, 639
  glyburide, 641
  insulin, 703
  insulin glargine, 705
  insulin glulisine, 707
  metformin hydrochloride,
    843
  miglitol, 883
  nateglinide, 928
  pioglitazone, 1075
  repaglinide, 1159
  rosiglitazone maleate, 1185
  saxagliptin, 1197
  sitagliptin, 1213
  tolazamide, 1300
  tolbutamide, 1302
diabetic gastroparesis
  metoclopramide, 868
diabetic neuropathy
  carbamazepine, 260
  duloxetine, 488
  pregabalin, 1105
Diabetic Tussin Allergy Relief,
  326
Diabex [AUS], 843
Diabinese, 329
Diaformin [AUS], 843
Diamox, 67
Diamox Sequels, 67
diarrhea. *See also* traveler's
  diarrhea
  bismuth subsalicylate, 214
  nitazoxanide, 956
  octreotide acetate, 970
  paregoric, 1016
Diastat, 435
Diazemuls [CAN], 435
diazepam, 38t–46t, 435
Dibenzyline, 1057
Dichlotride [AUS], 663
diclofenac, 437
Diclohexal [AUS], 437

Diclotek [CAN], 437
dicloxacillin sodium, 440
dicyclomine hydrochloride,
  441
didanosine, 442
Didronel, 545
dietary supplement
  folic acid, 606
  vitamin A, 1373
  vitamin D, 1374
diethylpropion, 444
Differin, 78
diflorasone, 446
Diflucan, 578, 1425t
diflunisal, 447
digitalis toxicity
  cholestyramine resin, 333
Digitek, 448
digoxin, 448
Dihydergot [AUS], 522
dihydroergotamine, 522
Dihydroergotamine Sandoz
  [CAN], 522
dihydrotachysterol, 450
Dilacor XR, 451
Dilantin, 1064
Dilantin with PB, 1414t–1420t
Dilatrate, 724, 726
Dilaudid, 672
Dilaudid HP, 672
Dilor, 491
Dilovan HCT, 1414t–1420t
Diltahexal [AUS], 451
Diltia XT, 451
Diltiamax [AUS], 451
diltiazem hydrochloride, 451
Dilzem [AUS], 451
dimenhydrinate, 454
Dimetane, 225
Dimetane Extentabs, 225
Dimetapp, 225, 796
Dimetapp 12 Hour Non
  Drowsy Extentabs,
  1134
Dimetapp Decongestant,
  1134
Dimetapp Sinus Liquid Caps
  [AUS], 1134
Diocto, 466
Diodex [CAN], 425, 427
Diopentolate [CAN], 362
Diosulf [CAN], 1226
Diovan, 1355
Dipentum, 979
Diphen, 455
Diphenhist, 455
diphenhydramine, 455
dipivefrin hydrochloride,
  456
Diprivan, 1126, 1405t
Diprolene, 196
dipyridamole, 457
dirithromycin, 458

Disalcid, 1191
discoid lupus erythematosus
  alclometasone, 83
discontinuation therapy
  lamotrigine, 747
disopyramide phosphate, 460
DisperDose, 307
Disprin [AUS], 162
disulfiram, 462
Dithiazide [AUS], 663
Dithrocream [AUS], 147
Ditropan, 1000
Ditropan XL, 1000
Diurcardin, 671
diuresis
  hydrochlorothiazide, 663
Diuril, 324
Diuril Sodium, 324
divalproex sodium, 1352
Dixarit [CAN], 360
Dizac, 435
dobutamine hydrochloride,
  463
Dobutrex, 463
docetaxel, 464
docosanol, 466
docusate, 466
Docusoft-S, 466
dofetilide, 467
dolasetron, 468
Dolobid, 447
Dolophine, 845
donepezil hydrochloride, 470
Donnatal, 1414t–1420t
Dopar, 769
Doral, 1142
Doribax [U.S.], 471
doripenem, 471
dornase alfa, 472
Doryx, 480
dorzolamide hydrochloride,
  473
Dostinex, 248
doxazosin mesylate, 474
doxepin hydrochloride, 476
Doxil, 478
Doxine, 1138
doxorubicin, 478
Doxsig [AUS], 480
Doxy-100, 480
Doxycin [CAN], 480
doxycycline, 480
doxycycline hyclate, 482
doxycycline hyclate gel, 483
Doxyhexal [AUS], 480
Dramamine, 454
Drisdol, 1374
Drithocreme, 147
Dritho-Scalp, 147
dronabinol, 484
dronedarone, 485
droperidol, 487
Droxia, 676

Droxine [AUS], 773
drug interactions
  acetaminophen, 38t–46t
  alprazolam, 38t–46t
  antibiotics, 38t–46t
  aspirin, 38t–46t
  azole antifungal agents,
    38t–46t
  barbiturates, 38t–46t
  benzodiazepines, 38t–46t
  β-lactams, 38t–46t
  cephalosporins, 38t–46t
  chlordiazepoxide, 38t–46t
  clarithromycin, 38t–46t
  diazepam, 38t–46t
  epinephrine, 38t–46t
  erythromycin, 38t–46t
  ketoconazole, 38t–46t
  levonordefrin, 38t–46t
  lidocaine, 38t–46t
  macrolide antibiotics,
    38t–46t
  mepivacaine, 38t–46t
  metronidazole, 38t–46t
  Neo-Cobefrin, 38t–46t
  Nizoral, 38t–46t
  NSAIDs, 38t–46t
  penicillins, 38t–46t
  tetracyclines, 38t–46t
  vasoconstrictors, 38t–46t
drug-induced extrapyramidal
    symptoms
  benztropine mesylate, 198
drug-induced gingival
    overgrowth, 23
dry eye
  cyclosporine, 387
dry mouth
  cevimeline, 316
  cottonseed oil, 377–378
  drugs, generally, 1426–1429
  pilocarpine hydrochloride,
    1069
Ducene [AUS], 435
Ducolax, 213
duloxetine, 488
Duocet, 1414t–1420t
duodenal ulcer
  bismuth subsalicylate,
    214
  cimetidine, 337
  clarithromycin, 343
  esomeprazole, 530
  famotidine, 559
  lansoprazole, 751
  nizatidine, 961
  omeprazole, 983
  rabeprazole sodium, 1151
  ranitidine hydrochloride,
    1156
  sucralfate, 1224
DuoNeb, 1414t–1420t
Duraclon, 360

Duragesic 25, 50, 75, 100
    Transdermal Patches,
    568
Duralith [CAN], 788
Duramorph, 905
Duranest, 1406t–1407t
Dura-Tabs, 1147
Duricef, 277
Duride [AUS], 724, 726
dutasteride, 490
Duvoid [CAN], 205
Dyazide, 1414t–1420t
Dycil, 440
Dymadon [AUS], 65
Dymelor, 69
Dynabac, 458
Dynacin, 887
DynaCirc, 728
DynaCirc CR, 728
dyphylline, 491
Dyrenium, 1331
dyslipidemia
  pitavastatin, 1079
  rosuvastatin calcium, 1187
dysmenorrhea
  diclofenac, 437
  flurbiprofen, 599
  ibuprofen, 682
  ketoprofen, 737
  meclofenamate sodium,
    814
  mefenamic acid, 818
  naproxen, 925
dyspepsia
  nizatidine, 961

earwax removal
  carbamide peroxide, 262
Ebixa [AUS], 824
echothiophate iodide, 493
EC-Naprosyn, 925
Econopred Plus, 1097
Ecotrin, 162
eczema
  alclometasone, 83
  betamethasone, 202
  clocortolone, 351
  diflorasone, 446
  doxepin hydrochloride, 476
  fluticasone propionate, 602
  halobetasol, 656
  pimecrolimus, 1070
Ed K10, 1086
edema, 67
  bendroflumethiazide, 192
  benzthiazide, 197
  bumetanide, 230
  chlorothiazide, 324
  chlorthalidone [CAN], 331
  furosemide, 617
  hydrochlorothiazide, 663
  hydroflumethiazide, 671
  indapamide, 697

edema *(Continued)*
metolazone, 869
spironolactone, 1221
triamterene, 1331
Edex, 101
EES, 526
efalizumab, 494
efavirenz, 495
Effer K, 1088
Effexor, 1361
Effexor XR, 1361
Effient, 1091
Effone, 590
Efodine, 1089
Efudex, 591
Efudex [AUS], 591
E-Gems, 1375
Ego Cort cream [AUS], 669
Elaprase, 687
Elavil, 119
Eldepryl, 1201
Elestat, 508
eletriptan, 496
Elidel, 1070
Eligard, 760
Elixomin, 1271
Elixophyllin, 114, 1271
ElixSure Cough, 434
Ellence, 512
Elmiron, 1044
Elocon Cream [AUS], 901
Eloxatin, 990
Eltroxin [CAN], 773
Emadine, 497
Emcort, 669
Emcyt, 534
emedastine, 497
Emend, 150
Emgel, 526
EMLA, 1414t–1420t
emtricitabine, 498
Emtriva, 498
enalapril maleate, 499
Enbrel, 540
Endantadine [CAN], 104
Endep [AUS], 119
endocarditis
clindamycin, 348
metronidazole
hydrochloride, 874
penicillin G potassium,
1035
streptomycin, 1222
vancomycin hydrochloride,
1356
endometrial carcinoma
medroxyprogesterone
acetate, 815
megestrol acetate, 820
endometrial hyperplasia
medroxyprogesterone
acetate, 815
progesterone, 1119

endometrial thinning
goserelin acetate, 644
endometriosis
danazol, 398
goserelin acetate, 644
leuprolide acetate, 760
nafarelin, 916
norethindrone, 962
ticarcillin, 1284
ticarcillin disodium, 1286
Endone [AUS], 1002
Endoxan Asta [AUS], 384
Endoxan Asta [AUS], 384
end-stage renal disease
lanthanum carbonate, 752
enfuvirtide, 501
enoxaparin sodium, 503
entacapone, 505
Entereg, 103
enterobiasis
mebendazole, 810
Entocort EC, 229
Entrophen [CAN], 162
enuresis
imipramine, 694
nortriptyline hydrochloride,
966
Epaq Inhaler [AUS], 81
ephedrine, 506
Epifrin, 511
epilepsy, 67. *See also* seizure
Epilim [AUS], 1352
Epinal, 511
epinastine, 508
epinephrine, 38t–46t, 509
epinephryl borate, 511
EpiPen, 509
EpiPen Jr. 0.15 Adrenaline
Autoinjector [AUS],
509
epirubicin, 512
Epitol, 260, 1424t
Epivir, 746
Epivir-HBV, 746
eplerenone, 513
Epogen, 515
epoetin alfa, 515
epoprostenol sodium, 517
Eppy/N, 511
Eprex [CAN], 515
eprosartan, 518
eptifibatide, 520
Epzicom, 1414t–1420t
Equetro, 260
Eraxis, 146
Erbitux, 314
erectile dysfunction
alprostadil, 101
sildenafil citrate, 1207
tadalafil, 1240
vardenafil, 1357
Ergodryl Mono [AUS], 522
ergoloid mesylates, 521

Ergomar, 522
Ergostat, 522
ergotamine tartrate, 522
erlotinib, 524
E • R • O Ear, 262
erosive esophagitis. *See*
esophagitis
Errin, 962
errors, 1439–1441
Ertaczo, 1202
ertapenem, 525
Eryacne [AUS], 526
Erybid [CAN], 526
Eryc, 526
Eryc LD [AUS], 526
EryDerm, 526
Erygel, 526
EryPed, 526
Ery-Tab, 526
erythema migrans, 12–13
erythema nodosum
clofazimine, 353
Erythra-Derm, 526
Erythrocin, 526
Erythromid [CAN], 526
erythromycin, 526
drug interactions, 38t–46t
Eryzole, 1414t–1420t
escitalopram, 528
Esclim, 532
Esidrix, 663
Eskalith, 788
esomeprazole, 530
esophageal candidiasis. *See*
candidiasis
esophageal varices
octreotide acetate, 970
esophagitis
dexlansoprazole, 430
esomeprazole, 530
famotidine, 559
lansoprazole, 751
omeprazole, 983
pantoprazole, 1014
ranitidine hydrochloride,
1156
estazolam, 531
Estrace, 532
Estraderm, 532
Estraderm MX [AUS], 532
estradiol, 532
Estradot [CAN], 532
estramustine phosphate
sodium, 534
Estrasorb, 532
Estring, 532
EstroGel, 532
estrogens, conjugated, 536
estropipate, 537
eszopiclone, 539
etanercept, 540
ethambutol, 541
ethionamide, 542

Ethmozine, 904
ethosuximide, 544, 1424t
Ethyol, 109
Etibi [CAN], 541
etidocaine, 1406t–1407t
etidronate disodium, 545
etodolac, 546
etomidate, 1405t
Etopophos, 548
etoposide, VP-16, 548
Etrafon, 1414t–1420t
etravarine, 550
Euflex [CAN], 601
Euglucon [CAN], 641
Eulexin, 601
Eutonyl, 1017
Eutroxsig [AUS], 773
Evamist, 532
everolimus, 551
Everone [CAN], 1260
Evista, 1152
Evoxac, 316
Ewing's sarcoma
   cyclophosphamide, 384
Exact Acne Medication,
      196
Exelderm, 1225
Exelon, 1181
exemestane, 553
exenatide, 554
exercise-induced
      bronchospasm
   albuterol, 81
exfoliative cheilitis, 22–23
exfoliative dermatitis
   alclometasone, 83
Exforge, 1414t–1420t
Exna, 197
expectorant
   guaifenesin, 649
Extra Strength Maalox,
      1414t–1420t
extrapyramidal symptoms
   biperiden, 211
   procyclidine, 1118
   trihexyphenidyl, 1337
eye infection
   gentamicin sulfate, 633
   sulfacetamide, 1226
   sulfisoxazole, 1230
   tobramycin sulfate, 1297
ezetimibe, 556

Factive, 632
famciclovir, 558
familial adenomatous
      polyposis
   celecoxib, 307
familial hypercholesterolemia
   atorvastatin, 169
famotidine, 559
Famvir, 558
Fanapt, 689

Fanconi's anemia
   oxymetholone, 1004
Fareston, 1312
Fastin, 1058
Faverin [AUS], 605
FazaClo, 366
febrile neutropenia
   cefepime, 284
febuxostat, 560
felbamate, 562
Felbatol, 562
Feldene, 1077
felodipine, 563
Felodur ER [AUS], 563
Femara, 758
Femhrt, 1414t–1420t
Femilax, 213
Femiron, 569
Femizol-M, 878
Femring, 532
Femstat One [CAN], 244
Fenac [AUS], 437
fenofibrate, 565
fenoprofen calcium, 566
Fentanyl Oralet, 568
fentanyl transdermal system,
      568
Feostat, 569
Fergon, 569
Fer-In-Sol, 569
Fer-Iron, 569
Ferro-Gradumet [AUS], 569
Ferro-Sequels, 569,
      1414t–1420t
ferrous fumarate, 569
ferrous gluconate, 569
ferrous sulfate, 569
fesoterodine, 570
fever
   acetaminophen, 65
   aspirin, 162
   ibuprofen, 682
fever blister
   docosanol, 466
   tetracaine, 1264
Feverall, 65
feverfew, 50t
Fexicam [CAN], 1077
fexofenadine hydrochloride,
      572
fibrocystic breast disease
   danazol, 398
fibromyalgia
   milnacipran, 886
Fibsol [AUS], 785
filgrastim, 573
Finacea, 177
finasteride, 574
Finevin, 177
Finibax [JAPAN], 471
Fioricet, 1414t–1420t
Fiorinal, 1414t–1420t
FIV-ASA, 835

5-aminosalicylic acid (5-ASA),
      835
5-ASA, 835
5FU, 591
Flagyl, 874
Flagyl ER, 874
Flamazine [CAN], 1208
Flarex, 590
flatulence
   simethicone, 1209
flavocoxid, 575
flavoxate, 576
flecainide, 577
Flecatab [AUS], 577
Flexeril, 381
Flexitec [CAN], 381
Flixotide Disks [AUS], 602
Flixotide Inhaler [AUS], 602
Flolan, 517
Flomax, 1242
Flonase, 602
Florinef, 583
Florone [CAN], 446
Flovent, 602
Flovent Diskus, 602
Flovent HFA, 602
Floxin, 971
Floxin Otic, 971
fluconazole, 578, 1425t
flucytosine, 580
Fludara, 582
fludarabine phosphate, 582
fludrocortisone, 583
Flugerel [AUS], 601
Flumadine, 1173
flumazenil, 585
flunisolide, 586
fluocinolone acetonide, 588
fluocinonide, 589
Fluoderm [CAN], 588
Fluohexal [AUS], 592
Fluor-A-Day, 1214
fluoride supplementation
   sodium fluoride, 1214
   sodium fluoride (topical),
      1216
fluoride toothpaste, 2
Fluoridex Karidium, 1214
Fluoritab, 1214
fluorometholone, 590
Fluor-Op, 590
Fluoroplex, 591
fluorouracil, 591
Fluotic, 1214
fluoxetine hydrochloride, 592
fluoxymesterone, 594
fluphenazine decanoate, 595
fluphenazine enanthate, 595
fluphenazine hydrochloride,
      595
Flura-Drops, 1214
flurandrenolide, 597
flurazepam hydrochloride, 598

flurbiprofen, 599
flutamide, 601
Flutamin [AUS], 601
fluticasone propionate, 602
fluvastatin, 604
fluvoxamine maleate, 605
FML Forte Liquifilm, 590
FML Liquifilm, 590
FML S.O.P., 590
Focalin, 431
Foille, 193
Foille Medicated First Aid, 193
Foille Plus, 193
folic acid, 606
folic acid antagonist overdose
    leucovorin calcium, 759
folic acid deficiency
    leucovorin calcium, 759
folinic acid, 759
follicular lymphoma
    interferon alfa-2b, 713
Folvite, 606
food allergy
    cromolyn sodium, 378
Foradil Aerolizer, 607
Foradile [AUS], 607
formoterol fumarate, 607
Formulex [CAN], 441
Fortamet, 843
Fortaz, 298
Forteo, 1259
Fortovase, 1194
Fortum [AUS], 298
Fosamax, 89
fosamprenavir, 609
foscarnet sodium, 610
Foscavir, 610
fosfomycin tromethamine, 612
fosinopril, 613
fosphenytoin, 614
Fosrenol, 752
Fostex 10% BPO, 196
Fragmin, 396
Froben [CAN], 599
Frovan, 616
frovatriptan, 616
Frusehexal [AUS], 617
Frusid [AUS], 617
Fugerel [AUS], 601
Fulvicin P/G, 648
Fulvicin U/F, 648
fungal infection
    amphotericin b, 131
    amphotericin b, lipid-based,
        133
    flucytosine, 580
    posaconazole, 1084
    sertaconazole, 1202
Fungizone, 131
Furacin, 958
Furadantin, 957
furosemide, 617
Fuzeon, 501

gabapentin, 620, 1424t
Gabitril, 1283
galantamine, 621
gallstones
    ursodiol, 1348
galsulfase, 623
ganciclovir sodium, 624
Gantrisin, 1230
Garamycin, 633
garlic, 50t
gastric atony
    bethanechol chloride, 205
gastric hypersecretory
        secretion
    cimetidine, 337
gastric ulcer
    famotidine, 559
    lansoprazole, 751
    misoprostol, 893
    nizatidine, 961
    omeprazole, 983
    ranitidine hydrochloride,
        1156
gastritis
    bismuth subsalicylate, 214
Gastrocom, 378
gastroesophageal reflux disease
        (GERD)
    cimetidine, 337
    dexlansoprazole, 430
    esomeprazole, 530
    famotidine, 559
    lansoprazole, 751
    metoclopramide, 868
    nizatidine, 961
    omeprazole, 983
    rabeprazole sodium, 1151
    ranitidine hydrochloride,
        1156
gastrointestinal (GI) disorder
    hyoscyamine, 679
gastrointestinal (GI)
        hemorrhage
    vasopressin, 1360
gastrointestinal (GI) stromal
        tumor
    sunitinib, 1234
Gastro-Stop [AUS], 793
Gas-X, 1209
gatifloxacin, 626
Gaucher's disease
    miglustat, 884
Gaviscon (oral suspension),
        1414t–1420t
Gaviscon (tablets),
        1414t–1420t
gefitinib, 628
Gelfoam, 60
Gelusil, 1414t–1420t
gemcitabine hydrochloride,
        629
Gemfibromax [AUS], 631
gemfibrozil, 631

gemifloxacin, 632
Gemzar, 629
Genahist, 455
Genaphed, 1134
Genasyme, 1209
Gencaro, 226
Gen-Clobestasol [CAN], 350
general lubrication
    benzocaine, 193
generalized anxiety disorder
        (GAD)
    alprazolam, 99
    escitalopram, 528
    paroxetine hydrochloride,
        1019
Gengraf, 387
genital herpes
    acyclovir, 75
    famciclovir, 558
    valacyclovir, 1349
genital warts
    podofilox, 1081
    podophyllum resin, 1082
genitourinary tract infection
    amoxicillin, 125
Genoptic, 633
Genoral [AUS], 537
Genotropin, 1217
Genotropin MiniQuick, 1217
Genox [AUS], 1241
Gentacidin, 633
Gentak, 633
gentamicin sulfate, 633, 635
Gen-Timolol [CAN], 1289,
        1322
Gentlax, 213
Gentlax-S, 1414t–1420t
Gen-Warfarin [CAN], 1377
Geodon, 1388
geographic tongue, 12–13
GERD. See gastroesophageal
        reflux disease (GERD)
Gerimal, 521
giant papillary conjunctivitis
    loteprednol, 801
ginger, 50t
gingival enlargement, 23
gingivitis
    chlorhexidine gluconate,
        320
gingivostomatitis, 2
ginkgo biloba, 50t
glatiramer, 636
glaucoma
    acetazolamide, 67
    apraclonidine hydrochloride,
        149
    betaxolol, 203
    bimatoprost, 210
    brimonidine, 221
    brinzolamide, 222
    carbachol, 259
    demecarium bromide, 413

glaucoma *(Continued)*
  dipivefrin hydrochloride, 456
  dorzolamide hydrochloride, 473
  echothiophate iodide, 493
  epinephrine, 509
  epinephryl borate, 511
  latanoprost, 755
  levobetaxolol hydrochloride, 765
  levobunolol hydrochloride, 766
  methazolamide, 848
  metipranolol hydrochloride, 866
  nipradilol, 953
  timolol maleate, 1289
  travoprost, 1322
  unoprostone isopropyl, 1347
Gleevec, 692
Gliadel, 268
Glimel [AUS], 641
glimepiride, 637
glipizide, 639
Glivec [AUS], 692
GlucaGen, 640
GlucaGen [AUS], 640
GlucaGen Diagnostic Kit, 640
Glucagon, 640
Glucagon Diagnostic Kit, 640
Glucagon Emergency Kit, 640
glucagon hydrochloride, 640
Glucobay [AUS], 62
Glucohexal [AUS], 843
Glucomet [AUS], 843
GlucoNorm [CAN], 1159
Glucophage, 843
Glucophage XL, 843
Glucotrol, 639
Glucotrol XL, 639
Glucovance, 1414t–1420t
glyburide, 641
Glynase, 641
Glycon [CAN], 843
glycopyrrolate, 643
Gly-Oxide, 262
Glyset, 883
GM-CSF, 1195
goiter
  liothyronine (T3), 781
gold sodium thiomalate, 172
Gold-50 [AUS], 172
gonococcal infection
  ampicillin sodium, 136
  doxycycline, 480
  norfloxacin, 964
gonococcal ophthalmia neonatorum
  erythromycin, 526

gonorrhea
  cefixime, 285
  cefotaxime sodium, 290
  cefoxitin sodium, 293
  cefpodoxime proxetil, 295
  ceftizoxime sodium, 302
  ceftriaxone sodium, 303
  ciprofloxacin hydrochloride, 339
  demeclocycline hydrochloride, 414
  gatifloxacin, 626
  minocycline hydrochloride, 887
  ofloxacin, 971
  probenecid, 1111
  tetracycline hydrochloride, 1266
Gopten [AUS], 1316
goserelin acetate, 644
gout
  febuxostat, 560
  probenecid, 1111
  sulfinpyrazone, 1228
gouty arthritis
  allopurinol, 95
  colchicine, 371
  ibuprofen, 682
  indomethacin, 700
  naproxen, 925
  piroxicam, 1077
  probenecid, 1111
  sulfinpyrazone, 1228
  sulindac, 1231
Gradumet, 847
granisetron, 646
granulocyte macrophage colony-stimulating factor (GM-CSF), 1195
granuloma annulare
  alclometasone, 83
Grifulvin V, 648
griseofulvin, 648
Grisovin [AUS], 648
Gris-PEG, 648
growth hormone deficiency
  somatropin, 1217
guaifenesin, 649
guanabenz, 650
guanadrel sulfate, 651
guanethidine monosulfate, 652
guanfacine, 654
Guiatuss, 649
Gynazole-1, 244
gynecologic infection
  ampicillin/sulbactam sodium, 137
Gynecure, 1293
Gyne-Lotrimin, 365, 1425t
Gynergen, 522

H. pylori infection. *See Helicobacter pylori* infection
Habitrol [CAN], 944
Haemophilus influenzae infection
  rifampin, 1168
hair loss
  finasteride, 574
hair regrowth
  minoxidil, 889
hairy cell leukemia
  interferon alfa-2a, 708
  interferon alfa-2a/2b, 710
  interferon alfa-2b, 713
  pentostatin, 1045
halcinonide, 656
Halcion, 1332
Haldol, 657
Haldol Decanoate, 657
Haley's M-O, 1414t–1420t
Halfprin, 162
halobetasol, 656
Halog, 656
Halog-E, 656
haloperidol, 657
Halotestin, 594
Halotestin [CAN], 594
hawthorn, 50t
hay fever
  brompheniramine, 225
HDA Toothache, 193
head cancer
  hydroxyurea, 676
  methotrexate sodium, 853
headache. *See* migraine; vascular headache
heart failure
  fosinopril, 613
  lisinopril, 785
  quinapril, 1145
  sotalol hydrochloride, 1219
heart transplant
  mycophenolate mofetil, 910
heartburn
  famotidine, 559
Helicobacter pylori infection
  lansoprazole, 751
  metronidazole hydrochloride, 874
  rabeprazole sodium, 1151
  tetracycline hydrochloride, 1266
Helidac, 1414t–1420t
hemodialysis
  gentamicin sulfate, 633
hemophilia A
  desmopressin, 420
hemorrhage
  thrombin, 1281
  tranexamic acid, 1318
hemorrhagic cystitis
  mesna, 837

hemorrhagic disease of the
newborn
phytonadione, 1068
hemorrhoids
betamethasone, 202
hemostasis in surgery
absorbable gelatin sponge,
60
oxidized cellulose, 999
heparin-induced
thrombocytopenia
argatroban, 153
hepatic cirrhosis
torsemide, 1313
hepatic coma
paromomycin, 1018
hepatic encephalopathy
rifaximin, 1171
hepatic impairment
amprenavir, 139
argatroban, 153
atomoxetine, 168
bisoprolol fumarate, 215
cefoperazone, 289
cetirizine, 313
cyclobenzaprine
hydrochloride, 381
desloratadine, 419
desvenlafaxine, 424
everolimus, 551
loratadine, 796
naratriptan, 927
nebivolol, 930
nicardipine hydrochloride,
942
pazopanib, 1021
peginterferon alfa-2a, 1024
pilocarpine hydrochloride,
1069
pravastatin, 1093
procyclidine, 1118
quetiapine, 1143
rasagiline, 1158
tacrine hydrochloride, 1237
tolcapone, 1303
tolterodine tartrate, 1306
tramadol hydrochloride,
1315
treprostinil sodium, 1325
venlafaxine, 1361
hepatitis B
adefovir, 79
interferon alfa-2b, 713
lamivudine, 746
Heptovir [CAN], 746
herbal medicines, 48–53
Herceptin, 1321

herpes labialis
docosanol, 466
penciclovir, 1032
tetracaine, 1264
herpes simplex
acyclovir, 75
famciclovir, 558
foscarnet sodium, 610
treatment, generally, 2–6
valacyclovir, 1349
herpes zoster
acyclovir, 75
famciclovir, 558
lidocaine hydrochloride,
774
treatment, generally, 6
valacyclovir, 1349
herpetic gingivostomatitis, 2
herpetiform aphthous
ulcerations, 7
Hespera, 79
heterotopic ossification
etidronate disodium, 545
heterozygous familial
hypercholesterolemia
lovastatin, 803
pravastatin, 1093
simvastatin, 1210
Hexadro [CAN], 425
hiccups
chlorpromazine, 327
HICOR [AUS], 669
HICOR Eye Ointment [AUS],
669
hip surgery
dalteparin sodium, 396
Hiprex, 850
Hip-Rex [CAN], 850
hirsutism
spironolactone, 1221
Histex CT, 263
Histex I/E, 263
Histex PD, 263
Histex Pd 12, 263
histoplasmosis
amphotericin b, 131
itraconazole, 730
ketoconazole, 736
histrelin, 659
Histussin D, 667
HIV. See human
immunodeficiency
syndrome (HIV)
Hivid, 1380
HMS Liquifilm, 817
Hodgkin's disease
bleomycin sulfate, 218
carmustine, 268
cyclophosphamide, 384
lomustine, 792
procarbazine hydrochloride,
1114
thiotepa, 1277

Hodgkin's disease *(Continued)*
vinblastine sulfate, 1367
vincristine sulfate, 1369
Hold DM, 434
Holoxan [AUS], 688
homatropine hydrobromide,
661
hookworm
mebendazole, 810
horse chestnut, 50t
Humalog, 703
Humalog Mix 75/25,
1414t–1420t
human herpes virus
vidarabine, 1365
human immunodeficiency
syndrome (HIV)
abacavir, 55
amprenavir, 139
atazanavir sulfate, 164
darunavir, 405
delavirdine mesylate, 412
didanosine, 442
efavirenz, 495
emtricitabine, 498
enfuvirtide, 501
epoetin alfa, 515
etravarine, 550
fosamprenavir, 609
hydroxyurea, 676
indinavir, 698
lamivudine, 746
nelfinavir, 936
nevirapine, 939
raltegravir, 1153
ritonavir, 1178
saquinavir, 1194
tenofovir, 1255
zalcitabine, 1380
zidovudine, 1385
human simplex virus ocular
infection
trifluridine, 1336
Humatin, 1018
Humatrope, 1217
Humibid LA, 649
Humira, 77
Humorsol Ocumeter, 413
Humulin 50/50, 1414t–1420t
Humulin 70/30, 1414t–1420t
Humulin N, 703
Humulin R, 703
Hunter syndrome
idursulfase, 687
Huntington's disease
tetrabenazine, 1262
Hurricaine, 193
Hycamtin, 1311
Hycodan [CAN], 665
Hycodan and Hydromet, 667
Hycomine Compound, 667
Hycosin, 667
Hycotuss, 667

hydatidiform mole
   methotrexate sodium, 853
Hydergine, 521
Hydergine [CAN], 521
Hydopa [AUS], 859
hydralazine hydrochloride, 662
Hydrate [CAN], 317
Hydrea, 676
Hydrocet, 667
hydrochlorothiazide, 663
hydrocodone, 667
hydrocodone and
      acetaminophen, 667
hydrocodone and aspirin, 667
hydrocodone and
      chlorpheniramine, 667
hydrocodone and guaifenesin,
   667
hydrocodone and homatropine,
   667
hydrocodone and ibuprofen,
   667
hydrocodone and
      pseudoephedrine, 667
hydrocodone bitartrate, 665
hydrocortisone, 669
HydroDIURIL, 663
hydroflumethiazide, 671
Hydrogesic, 667
Hydromorph Contin [CAN],
   672
hydromorphine hydrochloride,
   672
Hydropane, 667
hydroxychloroquine sulfate,
   674
hydroxyurea, 676
hydroxyzine, 677
Hygroton [AUS], 331
Hylorel, 651
Hyoscine, 679
hyoscyamine, 679
Hypadil [JAPAN], 953
hyperacidity and gas
   magaldrate, 808
hyperalimentation
   insulin, 703
   insulin glargine, 705
   insulin glulisine, 707
hyperammonemia
   carglumic acid, 266
hypercalcemia
   calcitonin, 249
   etidronate disodium, 545
   pamidronate disodium,
      1010
   zoledronic acid, 1390
hypercholesterolemia
   cholestyramine resin, 333
   colestipol, 373
   ezetimibe, 556
   fenofibrate, 565
   pitavastatin, 1079

hypercholesterolemia
      (Continued)
   rosuvastatin calcium, 1187
   simvastatin, 1210
hyperemia
   naphazoline, 924
hyperkalemia
   albuterol, 81
   insulin, 703
   insulin glargine, 705
   insulin glulisine, 707
hyperlipidemia
   atorvastatin, 169
   colesevelam, 372
   gemfibrozil, 631
   niacin, 941
   pravastatin, 1093
   rosuvastatin calcium, 1187
hyperlipoproteinemia
   fluvastatin, 604
   lovastatin, 803
hyperphosphatemia
   sevelamer hydrochloride,
      1205
hyperprolactinemia
   bromocriptine mesylate, 223
   cabergoline, 248
hypersecretory condition
   famotidine, 559
   lansoprazole, 751
   omeprazole, 983
   pantoprazole, 1014
   rabeprazole sodium, 1151
   ranitidine hydrochloride,
      1156
hypersensitivity reaction
   epinephrine, 509
hypertension
   acebutolol, 63
   aliskiren, 93
   amlodipine, 122
   atenolol, 166
   benazepril, 188
   bendroflumethiazide, 192
   benzthiazide, 197
   betaxolol, 203
   bisoprolol fumarate, 215
   bucindolol, 226
   bumetanide, 230
   candesartan cilexetil, 253
   captopril, 257
   carvedilol, 271
   chlorothiazide, 324
   chlorthalidone [CAN], 331
   clevidipine, 346
   clonidine, 360
   diltiazem hydrochloride, 451
   doxazosin mesylate, 474
   enalapril maleate, 499
   eplerenone, 513
   epoprostenol sodium, 517
   eprosartan, 518
   felodipine, 563

hypertension (Continued)
   fosinopril, 613
   furosemide, 617
   guanabenz, 650
   guanadrel sulfate, 651
   guanethidine monosulfate,
      652
   guanfacine, 654
   hydralazine hydrochloride,
      662
   hydrochlorothiazide, 663
   hydroflumethiazide, 671
   indapamide, 697
   irbesartan, 719
   isradipine, 728
   labetalol hydrochloride, 743
   lisinopril, 785
   losartan, 799
   methyldopa/methyldopate,
      859
   metolazone, 869
   metoprolol tartrate, 871
   minoxidil, 889
   moexipril hydrochloride,
      898
   nadolol, 914
   nebivolol, 930
   nicardipine hydrochloride,
      942
   nifedipine, 947
   nipradilol, 953
   nisoldipine, 954
   ocular. See ocular
      hypertension
   olmesartan, 975
   olmesartan medoxomil,
      977
   PAH. See pulmonary arterial
      hypertension (PAH)
   pargyline, 1017
   penbutolol, 1031
   perindopril, 1048
   phentolamine, 1060
   pindolol, 1073
   prazosin hydrochloride,
      1094
   propranolol hydrochloride,
      1127
   pulmonary, 691
   quinapril, 1145
   ramipril, 1154
   reserpine, 1161
   spironolactone, 1221
   telmisartan, 1246
   terazosin hydrochloride,
      1256
   timolol maleate, 1289
   torsemide, 1313
   trandolapril, 1316
   triamterene, 1331
   valsartan, 1355
   verapamil hydrochloride,
      1363

hyperthyroidism
  methimazole, 850
  propylthiouracil, 1130
hypertriglyceridemia
  omega-3 fatty acids, 982
hypertrophic subaortic stenosis
  propranolol hydrochloride, 1127
hyperuricemia
  allopurinol, 95
  febuxostat, 560
Hypnovel [AUS], 880
hypoestrogenism
  estradiol, 532
hypoglycemia
  glucagon hydrochloride, 640
hypogonadism
  estropipate, 537
  fluoxymesterone, 594
  methyltestosterone, 865
  testosterone, 1260
hypokalemia
  potassium acetate, 1088
  potassium chloride, 1086
  spironolactone, 1221
hyponatremia
  conivaptan, 374
  tolvaptan, 1307
hypoparathyroidism
  calcitriol, 251
  dihydrotachysterol, 450
  vitamin D, 1374
hypoprothrombinemia
  phytonadione, 1068
hypotension
  benazepril, 188
  ephedrine, 506
  mephentermine sulfate, 827
  metaraminol, 841
  midodrine, 882
  phenylephrine hydrochloride, 1061
hypothyroidism
  levothyroxine, 773
  liothyronine (T3), 781
  liotrix, 782
  thyroid, 1282
Hysone [AUS], 669
Hytone, 669
Hytrin, 1256
Hyzaar, 1414t–1420t

ibandronate sodium, 681
Ibilex [AUS], 309
Ibudone, 667, 682
ibuprofen, 682
ibutilide fumarate, 684
Idamycin PFS, 685
idarubicin hydrochloride, 685
idursulfase, 687
Ifex, 688
ifosfamide, 688

IGF-1 deficiency
  mecasermin, 811
IL-2, 84, 984
iloperidone, 689
iloprost, 691
imatinib mesylate, 692
Imdur, 724, 726
Imdur Durules [AUS], 726
Imigran [AUS], 1233
imipramine, 694
imiquimod, 696
Imitrex, 1233
immunosuppression
  betamethasone, 202
  cortisone acetate, 376
  flurandrenolide, 597
  hydrocortisone, 669
  methylprednisolone, 863
  prednisolone, 1095
  prednisone, 1103
  triamcinolone, 1328
Imodium, 793
Imodium A-D, 793
Imodium Advanced, 1414t–1420t
impetigo
  cefadroxil, 277
  cefuroxime sodium, 305
  mupirocin, 909
  retapamulin, 1162
impotence
  alprostadil, 101
  fluoxymesterone, 594
Imtrate [AUS], 724, 726
Imukin [AUS], 716
Imuran, 175
Inapsine, 487
Increlex, 811
Indahexal [AUS], 697
indapamide, 697
Inderal, 1127
Inderal LA, 1127
Inderide, 1414t–1420t
Inderide LA, 1414t–1420t
indinavir, 698
Indocid [CAN], 700
Indocin, 700
Indocin-IV, 700
Indocin-SR, 700
indomethacin, 700
infant colic
  hyoscyamine, 679
Infant Mylicon, 1209
infection. *See also individual types of infection*
  amoxicillin, 125
  amoxicillin/clavulanate potassium, 127
  aztreonam, 180
  cefazolin sodium, 278
  cefonicid sodium, 287
  cefoperazone, 289
  cefotaxime sodium, 290

infection *(Continued)*
  cefotetan disodium, 292
  cefoxitin sodium, 293
  ceftazidime, 298
  ceftizoxime sodium, 302
  ceftriaxone sodium, 303
  cefuroxime sodium, 305
  cephradine, 310
  ciprofloxacin hydrochloride, 339
  clindamycin, 348
  demeclocycline hydrochloride, 414
  lincomycin HCL, 777
  meropenem, 833
  minocycline hydrochloride, 887
  polymyxin B, 1083
infective endocarditis, 29–30
infertility
  clomiphene, 355
  progesterone, 1119
Inflamase Forte, 1095, 1097, 1101
Inflamase Mild, 1095, 1097, 1101
inflammation
  aspirin, 162
  betamethasone, 202
  clobetasol, 350
  cortisone acetate, 376
  dexamethasone, 425
  hydrocortisone, 669
  methylprednisolone, 863
  prednisolone, 1095
  prednisolone sodium phosphate, 1101
  prednisone, 1103
  rimexolone, 1174
  triamcinolone, 1328
inflammatory bowel disease
  cromolyn sodium, 378
inflammatory ocular condition
  prednisolone acetate, 1099
infliximab, 702
influenza
  oseltamivir, 988
  rimantadine hydrochloride, 1173
  zanamivir, 1383
Infumorph, 905
INH, 723
Innohep, 1292
InnoPran XL, 1127
INR. *See international normalized ratio (INR)*
insect bites
  benzocaine, 193
Insensye [AUS], 964
Insig [AUS], 697
Insomn-Eze [AUS], 1121
insomnia
  butabarbital sodium, 242

insomnia *(Continued)*
chloral hydrate, 317
estazolam, 531
eszopiclone, 539
flurazepam hydrochloride, 598
lorazepam, 797
pentobarbital, 1042
quazepam, 1142
secobarbital, 1199
temazepam, 1247
triazolam, 1332
zaleplon, 1381
zolpidem tartrate, 1392
Inspra, 513
insulin, 703
insulin glargine, 705
insulin glulisine, 707
Intal, 378
Integrilin, 520
Intelence, 550
Intensol, 425
Interceed, 999
interferon alfa-2a, 708
interferon alfa-2a/2b, 710
interferon alfa-2b, 713
interferon alfa-n3, 715
interferon gamma-1b, 716
interleukin-2, 84, 984
intermittent claudication
pentoxifylline, 1046
international normalized ratio (INR), 33
interstitial cystitis
pentosan polysulfate, 1044
intestinal amebiasis
paromomycin, 1018
intestinal infection
nystatin, 968
intestinal paresis
vasopressin, 1360
intraabdominal infection
ampicillin/sulbactam sodium, 137
cefepime, 284
ceftazidime, 298
doripenem, 471
ertapenem, 525
tobramycin, 1296
intravitreal implant
ganciclovir sodium, 624
Intron-A, 710, 713
Invanz, 525
Invega, 1007
Invega Sustenna, 1007
Invirase, 1194
Inza [AUS], 925
Iodex-P, 1089
Ionamin, 1058
Iopidine, 149
Iosopan Plus, 808
ipratropium bromide, 717
Iprivask, 418

Iquix, 771
irbesartan, 719
Iressa, 628
iron deficiency anemia
ferrous fumarate, 569
irritable bowel syndrome
alosetron, 98
dicyclomine hydrochloride, 441
glycopyrrolate, 643
propantheline, 1124
tegaserod, 1245
Iscover [AUS], 362
Isentress, 1153
Ismelin, 652
ISMO, 724, 726
Isocaine, 1409t–1411t
isocarboxazid, 720
isoetharine hydrochloride, 721
Isogen [AUS], 724, 726
isoniazid, 723
Isoptin [AUS], 1363
Isoptin SR, 1363
Isopto Carbachol, 259
Isopto Carpin [AUS], 1069
Isopto Cetamide, 1226
Isopto Frin [AUS], 1061
Isopto Homatropine, 661
Isordil, 724, 726
isosorbide, 724
isosorbide dinitrate, 724, 726
isosorbide mononitrate, 724, 726
Isotamine [CAN], 723
isoxsuprine hydrochloride, 727
isradipine, 728
Istalol, 1289
Istubol, 1241
itraconazole, 730
ixabepilone, 732
Ixempra, 732

Jantoven, 1377
Januvia, 1213
joint replacements, 30
Jolivette, 962
juvenile idiopathic arthritis
abatacept, 57
juvenile rheumatoid arthritis
etanercept, 540
etodolac, 546
ibuprofen, 682
methotrexate sodium, 853
naproxen, 925
oxaprozin, 994
sulfasalazine, 1227
tolmetin, 1305

K-8, 1086
K-10, 1086
Kadian, 905
Kalma [AUS], 99

Kaluril [AUS], 111
kanamycin sulfate, 734
Kantrex, 734
Kaochlor, 1086, 1088
Kaochlor S-F, 1086
Kaon, 1088
Kaon-Cl, 1086, 1088
Kaon-CL 10, 1086
Kaon-CL 20%, 1086
Kaopectate, 214
Kapanol [AUS], 905
Kapidex, 430
Kaposi's sarcoma
alitretinoin, 94
daunorubicin citrate liposome, 408
doxorubicin, 478
interferon alfa-2a, 708
interferon alfa-2a/2b, 710
interferon alfa-2b, 713
paclitaxel, 1006
vinblastine sulfate, 1367
Karigel, 1216
Karvea [AUS], 719
Kato, 1086
kava, 50t
Kawasaki disease
aspirin, 162
Kay Ciel, 1086
KCare, 1086
KCl-20, 1086
KCl-40, 1086
K-Dur, 1088
K-Dur 10, 1086
K-Dur 20, 1086
Keflex, 309
Keflor [AUS], 275
Keftab, 309
Kefurox, 305
Kefzol, 278
Kemadrin, 1118
Kenacort A [AUS], 1328
Kenalog, 1328
Kenalog in Orabase [AUS], 1328
Keppra, 764
keratinization disorders
acitretin, 73
keratitis
bacitracin, 183
lodoxamide, 789
tobramycin sulfate, 1297
trifluridine, 1336
vidarabine, 1365
keratoconjunctivitis
lodoxamide, 789
vidarabine, 1365
Kerlone, 203
Ketalar, 734, 1405t
ketamine, 734, 1405t
ketoacidosis
insulin, 703
insulin glargine, 705

1466 Index

ketoconazole, 38t–46t, 736, 1425t
ketoprofen, 737
ketorolac tromethamine, 739
ketotifen fumarate, 741
Key-E, 1375
Key-E Kaps, 1375
kidney failure
  captopril, 257
kidney transplant
  everolimus, 551
  tacrolimus, 1238
Kineret, 143
Kinidin Durules [AUS], 1147
Klacid [AUS], 343
Klexane [CAN], 503
Kliovance [AUS], 532
Klonopin, 358, 1424t
K-Lor, 1086, 1088
Klor-Con, 1086
Klor-Con 8, 1086
Klor-Con 10, 1086
Klor-Con/25, 1086
Klor-Con EF, 1088
Klor-Con M10, 1086
K-Lor-Con M 15, 1088
Klor-Con M15, 1086
Klor-Con M20, 1086
Klotrix, 1086
K-Lyte, 1088
K-Lyte CI, 1086
K-Lyte DS, 1088
K-Norm, 1086
kraurosis vulvae
  estropipate, 537
Kripton [AUS], 223
K-Sol, 1086
KSR [AUS], 1088
KSR-600 [AUS], 1088
K-Tab, 1086
Kuvan, 1193
Ku-Zyme, 1011
Kwelcof, 667
Kytril, 646

labetalol hydrochloride, 743
labor
  pentazocine, 1041
lacosamide, 744
Lamictal, 747
Lamictal CD, 747
Lamisil, 1257
Lamisil AT, 1257
lamivudine, 746
lamotrigine, 747
Lamprene, 353
Lanacaine, 193
Lanophyllin, 1271
Lanoxicaps, 448
Lanoxin, 448
lanreotide, 749
lansoprazole, 751
lanthanum carbonate, 752

Lantus, 703, 705
lapatinib, 754
Largactil [CAN], 327
Lariam, 819
Larodopa, 769
Lasix, 617
latanoprost, 755
Latycin [AUS], 1266
Ledermycin [AUS], 414
Ledertrexate [AUS], 853
leflunomide, 756
leg cramps
  quinine, 1149
legionella infection
  tetracycline hydrochloride, 1266
Lennox-Gastaut syndrome
  clonazepam, 358
  felbamate, 562
  topiramate, 1309
leprosy
  clofazimine, 353
  dapsone, 402
  thalidomide, 1269
Lescol, 604
Lescol XL, 604
Letairis, 107
letrozole, 758
Letterer-Siwe disease
  vinblastine sulfate, 1367
leucovorin calcium, 759
leukemia. See also individual
    types of leukemia
  cyclophosphamide, 384
  mitoxantrone, 895
Leukine, 1195
leuprolide acetate, 760
levalbuterol, 762
Levaquin, 771
Levate [CAN], 119
Levatol, 1031
Levbid, 679
levonordefrin, 38t–46t
levetiracetam, 764
Levitra, 1357
levobetaxolol hydrochloride, 765
levobunolol hydrochloride, 766
levobupivacaine, 1406t–1407t
levocabastine, 767
levocetirizine, 768
levodopa, 769
levofloxacin, 771
Levothroid, 773
levothyroxine, 773
Levoxyl, 773
Levsin, 679
Levsin S/L, 679
Levsinex, 679
Lexapro, 528
Lexiva, 609
Lexxel, 1414t–1420t

Lialda, 835
Librax, 1414t–1420t
Librium, 318
lichen planus, 14–17
  acitretin, 73
  alclometasone, 83
lichen simplex
  alclometasone, 83
Lidex, 589
Lidex-E, 589
lidocaine, 38t–46t, 1406t–1407t
Lidocaine HCl, 1409t–1411t
lidocaine hydrochloride, 774, 1409t–1411t
lidocaine transoral delivery system, 776
Lidocaine with Epinephrine, 1414t–1420t
Lidoderm, 774
LidoSite, 1414t–1420t
Lignocaine Gel [AUS], 774
Lignospan, 1409t–1411t
Limbitrol, 1414t–1420t
Limbrel, 215
Lincocin, 777
Lincomycin, 777
lincomycin HCL, 777
linezolid, 779
liothyronine (T3), 781
liotrix, 782
Lipex [AUS], 1210
Lipitor, 169
Liquifilm [AUS], 924
lisdexamfetamine dimesylate, 784
lisinopril, 785
Lisodur [AUS], 785
Lithi.carb [AUS], 788
lithium carbonate, 788
lithium citrate, 788
Lithobid, 788
Livalo, 779
liver impairment
  disopyramide phosphate, 460
  doxorubicin, 478
liver spots
liver transplant
  mycophenolate mofetil, 910
  tacrolimus, 1238
Livostin, 767
Locoid, 669
Lodine, 546
Lodine XL, 546
lodoxamide, 789
Lodrane 12 Hour, 225
Lofibra, 565
lomefloxacin hydrochloride, 790
Lomine [CAN], 441
Lomotil, 1414t–1420t

lomustine, 792
Lonavar [AUS], 992
Loniten, 889
Loperacap [CAN], 793
loperamide hydrochloride, 793
Lopid, 631
Lopresor [AUS], 871
Lopressor, 871
Lopressor HCT, 1414t–1420t
Loprox, 336
loratadine, 796
Lorabid, 795
loracarbef, 795
lorazepam, 797
Lorazepam Intensol, 797
Lorcet, 1414t–1420t
Lorcet 10/650, 667
Lorcet Plus, 667
Lorcet-HD, 667
Loroxide, 196
Lortab, 667, 1414t–1420t
Lortab Elixir, 1414t–1420t
Lortab/ASA, 1414t–1420t
losartan, 799
Losec [CAN], 983
Lotemax, 801
Lotensin, 188
Lotensin HCT, 1414t–1420t
loteprednol, 801
loteprednol etabonate, 802
Lotrel, 803, 1414t–1420t
Lotrimin, 365, 1425t
Lotrisone, 1414t–1420t
Lotronex, 98
Lovan [AUS], 592
lovastatin, 803
Lovaza, 982
Lovenox, 503
Lovir [AUS], 75
low back pain
  mefenamic acid, 818
lower respiratory tract
    infection. See also
      respiratory tract
      infection
  amoxicillin, 125
  cefaclor, 275
  lomefloxacin hydrochloride,
    790
  ofloxacin, 971
  ribavirin, 1164
  ticarcillin, 1284
  ticarcillin disodium, 1286
Lowsium Plus, 808
Loxapac [CAN], 804
loxapine, 804
Loxitane, 804
Lozide [CAN], 697
Lozol, 697
L.P.V. [AUS], 1036
Lucrin [AUS], 760
Lucrin Depot Inj [AUS], 760
Ludiomil, 808

Lufyllin, 491
lumefantrine, 157
Lumigan, 210
Luminal, 1055, 1424t
Lunelle, 1414t–1420t
Lunesta, 539
lung cancer. See non–small-
    cell lung cancer;
    small-cell lung
    carcinoma
Lupron, 760
Lupron Depot, 760
Lupron Depot Ped, 760
lupus erythematosus
  hydroxychloroquine sulfate,
    674
Luride Lozi-Tabs, 1214
Luvox, 605
Luxiq, 202
Lyme disease
  ceftriaxone sodium, 303
  tetracycline hydrochloride,
    1266
lymphogranuloma venereum
  doxycycline, 480
lymphosarcoma
  bleomycin sulfate, 218
  methotrexate sodium, 853
Lyrica, 1105
Lysodren, 893

Maalox, 1414t–1420t
Maalox Plus, 1414t–1420t
Mabthera [AUS], 1180
MAC. See Mycobacterium
  avium complex (MAC)
Macrobid, 957
Macrodantin, 957
macrolide antibiotics, 38t–46t
mafenide, 807
magaldrate, 808
Magicul [AUS], 337
malabsorption syndrome
  vitamin A, 1373
malaria
  artemether/lumefantrine, 157
  chloroquine, 322
  hydroxychloroquine sulfate,
    674
  mefloquine, 819
  primaquine, 1108
  pyrimethamine, 1139
  quinine, 1149
malignant hyperthermic crisis
  dantrolene sodium, 400
malignant melanoma
  interferon alfa-2b, 713
Mallisol, 1089
Malocide [FRANCE], 1139
Mandelamine, 850
maprotiline, 808
Marcaine, 232, 1406t–1407t,
    1409t–1411t

Marcaine Spinal, 232
Marevan [AUS], 1377
Margesic H, 667
Marinol, 484
Maroteaux-Lamy syndrome
  galsulfase, 623
Marplan, 720
mastocytosis
  cromolyn sodium, 378
Matulane, 1114
Mavik, 1316
Maviserpin [MEX], 1161
Maxair, 1076
Maxair Autohaler, 1076
Maxalt, 1183
Maxalt-MLT, 1183
Maxaquin, 790
Maxidex, 425, 427
Maxidone, 667
Maxiflor, 446
Maxipime, 284
Maxitrol, 1414t–1420t
Maxivate, 202
Maxolon [AUS], 868
Maxor [AUS], 983
Maxzide, 1414t–1420t
Mebaral, 828
mebendazole, 810
mecasermin, 811
meclizine, 812
meclofenamate sodium, 814
Meclomen [CAN], 814
Medasulf, 1089
medically compromised
    patients
  adrenal insufficiency, 31–33
  anticoagulant therapy, 33–34
  anxiety, 34–37
  complementary medicines,
    48–53
  depression, 37–48
  drug interactions, 38t–46t
  herbal medicines, 48–53
  infective endocarditis, 29–30
  monoclonal antibody
    therapy, 53
  need for supplementation,
    33
  nonvalvular cardiovascular
    device-related
    infections, 30
  orthopedic devices, 30–31
  osteonecrosis of the jaw,
    47–48
medication errors, 1439–1441
Medrol, 863
medroxyprogesterone acetate,
    536, 815
medrysone, 817
mefenamic acid, 818
mefloquine, 819
Mefoxin, 293
Megace, 820

Megacillin [CAN], 1035
Megafol [AUS], 606
megaloblastic anemia
  leucovorin calcium, 759
megestrol acetate, 820
Megostat [AUS], 820
melanoma
  interferon alfa-2a, 708
  interferon alfa-2a/2b, 710
Melfiat, 1052
Melipramine [AUS], 694
Mellaril, 1276
Mellaril [AUS], 1276
meloxicam, 821
melphalan, 823
memantine hydrochloride, 824
meningeal leukemia
  cytarabine, 391
meningitis
  ampicillin, 134
  ampicillin sodium, 136
  ceftazidime, 298
  ceftizoxime sodium, 302
  ceftriaxone sodium, 303
  cefuroxime sodium, 305
  fluconazole, 578
  gentamicin sulfate, 633
  meropenem, 833
  penicillin G potassium, 1035
  sulfisoxazole, 1230
  tobramycin sulfate, 1297
meningococcal infection
  rifampin, 1168
menopausal symptoms
  estradiol, 532
  estropipate, 537
  medroxyprogesterone
    acetate, 536
Menostar, 532
Mentax, 244
meperidine hydrochloride, 825
mephentermine sulfate, 827
mephobarbital, 828
Mephyton, 1068
mepivacaine, 38t–46t,
  1406t–1407t
Mepivacaine HCl, 829,
  1409t–1411t
mepivacaine hydrochloride,
  1409t–1411t
meprobamate, 831
Merbentyl [AUS], 441
mercaptopurine (6-MP), 832
Mericaine, 1112
Meridia, 1206
meropenem, 833
Merrem IV, 833
mesalamine/5-aminosalicylic
  acid (5-ASA), 835
Mesasal [CAN], 835
M-Eslon, 905
mesna, 837
Mesnex, 837

mesoridazine besylate, 838
Mestinon, 1137
Mestinon SR [CAN], 1137
Mestinon Timespan, 1137
metabolic disorder
  thiamine hydrochloride,
    1274
Metadate CD, 861
Metadate ER, 861
Metadol [CAN], 845
Metaglip, 1414t–1420t
Metalyse [AUS], 1252
metaproterenol sulfate, 840
metaraminol, 841
metastatic melanoma
  aldesleukin, 84
metaxalone, 842
metformin hydrochloride, 843
methadone hydrochloride, 845
Methadone Intensol, 845
Methadose, 845
methamphetamine, 847
methazolamide, 848
methenamine, 850
Methergine, 860
methimazole, 850
Methoblastin [AUS], 853
methocarbamol, 852
methohexital, 1405t
methotrexate sodium, 853
methotrexate toxicity
  leucovorin calcium, 759
methoxy polyethylene
  glycol-epoetin beta,
    855
methsuximide, 857
methyldopa/methyldopate, 859
methylergonovine, 860
Methylin, 861
Methylin ER, 861
methylphenidate hydrochloride,
  861
methylprednisolone, 863
methylprednisolone acetate,
  863
methylprednisolone sodium
  succinate, 863
methyltestosterone, 865
Metimyd, 1099
metipranolol hydrochloride,
  866
metoclopramide, 868
Metohexal [AUS], 871
metolazone, 869
Metolol [AUS], 871
metoprolol tartrate, 871
MetroCream, 874
MetroGel, 874
Metrogy [AUS], 874
MetroLotion, 874
metronidazole, 38t–46t
metronidazole hydrochloride,
  874

Metronidazole IV [AUS], 874
Metronide [AUS], 874
metyrosine, 876
Mevacor, 803
mexiletine hydrochloride, 877
Mextil, 877
MI. *See* myocardial infarction
    (MI)
Miacalcin, 249
Micanol, 147
Micardis, 1246
Micardis HCT, 1414t–1420t
Micatin, 878
miconazole, 878
Micozole [CAN], 878
Micro-K, 1086, 1088
Micro-K 10, 1086
Micronase, 641
Micronor, 962
Microzide, 663
Midamor, 111
midazolam hydrochloride, 880
midodrine, 882
miglitol, 883
miglustat, 884
migraine
  almotriptan malate, 96
  butorphanol tartrate, 245
  eletriptan, 496
  frovatriptan, 616
  ibuprofen, 682
  naratriptan, 927
  propranolol hydrochloride,
    1127
  rizatriptan benzoate, 1183
  sumatriptan, 1233
  timolol maleate, 1289
  topiramate, 1309
  valproic acid, 1352
  zolmitriptan, 1391
Migranal, 522
milnacipran, 886
Milnox [CAN], 889
Milophene, 355
Milophene [CAN], 355
Miltown, 831
Minax [AUS], 871
Minidyne, 1089
Minims Homatropine [CAN],
    661
Minims-Prednisolone [CAN],
    1095
Minipress, 1094
Minirin [AUS], 420
Minitran, 959
Minizide, 1414t–1420t
Minocin, 887
minocycline hydrochloride,
    887
minoxidil, 889
Mintezol, 1272
Miochol-E, 71
Miochol-E System Pak, 71

Miochol-E/Steri-Tags, 71
miosis
  acetylcholine chloride, 71
Miostat, 259
Mirapex, 1090
Mircera, 855
Mireze [CAN], 932
mirtazapine, 891
Mirtazon [AUS], 891
misoprostol, 893
mitotane, 893
mitoxantrone, 895
Moban, 899
Mobic, 821
Mobilis [AUS], 1077
modafinil, 897
Modane, 213
Modavigil [AUS], 897
Modecate [AUS], 595
Moditen [CAN], 595
Moduretic, 1414t–1420t
moexipril hydrochloride, 898
molindone, 899
Mollifene Ear Wax Removing,
  262
mometasone furoate
    monohydrate, 901
moniliasis
  amphotericin b, 131
Monistat [CAN], 878
Monistat-1, 1293
Monistat-3, 878
Monistat-7, 878
Monistat-Derm [CAN], 878
Monocid, 287
monoclonal antibody therapy,
  53
Monodox, 480
Monodur Durules [AUS], 724,
  726
Mono-Gesic, 1191
Monoket, 724, 726
Monopril, 613
Monotard [AUS], 703
montelukast, 902
Monurol, 612
moricizine hydrochloride, 904
Morphine Mixtures [AUS],
  905
morphine sulfate, 905
motion sickness
  buclizine hydrochloride,
    228
  dimenhydrinate, 454
  diphenhydramine, 455
  meclizine, 812
  promethazine hydrochloride,
    1121
  scopolamine, 1198
Motrin, 682
Motrin Cold, 1414t–1420t
mountain sickness, 67
Moxage, 125

moxifloxacin hydrochloride,
  907
MS Contin, 905
MS Mono [AUS], 905
MSIR, 905
Mucinex, 649
Mucinex D, 1414t–1420t
Mucinex DM, 1414t–1420t
Mucomyst, 71
mucous membrane disorder
  lidocaine hydrochloride,
    774
mucous membrane
    pemphigoid, 17–18
Multaq, 485
multiple myeloma
  carmustine, 268
  cyclophosphamide, 384
  melphalan, 823
  zoledronic acid, 1390
multiple sclerosis
  dalfampridine, 395
  glatiramer, 636
  mitoxantrone, 895
  prednisolone sodium
    phosphate, 1101
mupirocin, 909
Murelax [AUS], 995
Murine Ear Drops, 262
muscle relaxant
  metaxalone, 842
muscle spasm
  chlorzoxazone, 332
musculoskeletal spasm
  methocarbamol, 852
Muse, 101
Myambutol, 541
myasthenia gravis
  neostigmine, 938
  pyridostigmine bromide,
    1137
Mycelex, 365
Mycelex OTC, 365
Mycelex-32%, 244
Mycinettes, 193
Mycitracin, 1414t–1420t
Myco II, 1414t–1420t
mycobacterial infection
  ethambutol, 541
Mycobacterium avium complex
    (MAC)
  azithromycin, 179
  clarithromycin, 343
  rafapentine, 1169
  rifabutin, 1166
Mycobutin, 1166
Mycolog II, 1414t–1420t
mycophenolate mofetil, 910
mycoplasmal disease
  tetracycline hydrochloride,
    1266
mycosis fungoides
  cyclophosphamide, 384

mycosis fungoides (Continued)
  methotrexate sodium, 853
  vinblastine sulfate, 1367
Mycostatin, 968
Myco-Triacet, 1414t–1420t
Mydfrin, 1061
mydriasis
  cylcopentolate
    hydrochloride, 383
  dapiprazole hydrochloride,
    401
  homatropine hydrobromide,
    661
myelodysplastic syndrome
    (MDS)
  decitabine, 410
myelofibrosis
  oxymetholone, 1004
myelosuppression
  filgrastim, 573
  pegfilgrastim, 1023
Mykrox, 869
Mylanta, 1414t–1420t
Mylanta (tablets), 1414t–1420t
Mylanta Gas, 1209
Myleran, 240
Mylocel, 676
myocardial infarction (MI).
    See also acute
    myocardial infarction
  aspirin, 162
  atorvastatin, 169
  captopril, 257
  carvedilol, 271
  clopidogrel, 362
  dalteparin sodium, 396
  enoxaparin sodium, 503
  lisinopril, 785
  metoprolol tartrate, 871
  nadolol, 914
  ramipril, 1154
  warfarin sodium, 1377
Myochrysine, 172
Myocrisin [AUS], 172
Myotonachol [CAN], 205
Myozyme, 92
Myrac, 887
Mysoline, 1109, 1424t
Mysteclin [AUS], 1266
myxedema (coma)
  levothyroxine, 773
  liothyronine (T3), 781
  liotrix, 782
  thyroid, 1282

nabumetone, 913
nadolol, 914
nafarelin, 916
naftifine, 917
Naftin, 917
Naglazyme, 623
nalbuphine hydrochloride, 918
Nalfon, 566

naloxone hydrochloride, 921, 1039
naltrexone hydrochloride, 922
Namenda, 824
naphazoline, 924
Naphcon, 924
Naphcon Forte [AUS], 924
Naphcon-A, 1414t–1420t
Naprelan, 925
Naprogesic [AUS], 925
Naprosyn, 925
naproxen, 925
naproxen sodium, 925
Naramig [AUS], 927
naratriptan, 927
Narcan, 921
narcolepsy
  amphetamine, 129
  armodafinil, 155
  clomipramine hydrochloride, 356
  dextroamphetamine sulfate, 433
  methylphenidate hydrochloride, 861
  modafinil, 897
  protriptyline, 1133
narcotic addiction
  methadone hydrochloride, 845
Nardil, 1054
Naropin, 1406t–1407t
Nasacort AQ, 1328
Nasahist B, 225
nasal congestion
  ephedrine, 506
  naphazoline, 924
  oxymetazoline, 1003
  phenylephrine hydrochloride, 1061
  pseudoephedrine, 1134
nasal polyps
  beclomesthasone dipropionate, 187
  mometasone furoate monohydrate, 901
Nasalcrom, 378
Nasalide, 586
Nasarel, 586
Nascobal, 380
Nasonex, 901
Nasonex Nasal Spray [AUS], 901
nateglinide, 928
Natrilix [AUS], 697
Natrilix SR [AUS], 697
Natulan [CAN], 1114
Nature-Thyroid NT, 1282
Naturetin-5, 192
nausea/vomiting
  apepitant, 150
  chlorpromazine, 327
  dexamethasone, 425

nausea/vomiting *(Continued)*
  dolasetron, 468
  dronabinol, 484
  droperidol, 487
  granisetron, 646
  hydroxyzine, 677
  metoclopramide, 868
  palonosetron hydrochloride, 1009
  perphenazine, 1049
  prochlorperazine, 1116
  promethazine hydrochloride, 1121
  scopolamine, 1198
  thiethylperazine, 1275
  trimethobenzamide hydrochloride, 1338
Navane, 1279
Navelbine, 1371
ND Stat, 225
Nebcin, 1296–1297
Nebcin Pediatric, 1296
nebivolol, 930
NebuPent, 1037
neck cancer
  hydroxyurea, 676
  methotrexate sodium, 853
necrotizing ulcerative gingivitis
  penicillin V potassium, 1036
nedocromil sodium, 932
nefazodone hydrochloride, 933
nelarabine, 934
nelfinavir, 936
Nemasol [CAN], 116
Nembutal, 1042
Neo-Cobefrin, 38t–46t
neoplasm
  prednisone, 1103
Neoral, 387
Neosporin Ointment, Triple Antibiotic, 1414t–1420t
neostigmine, 938
Neo-Synephrine, 1061
Neo-Synephrine Ophthalmic Viscous 10% [AUS], 1061
Nephro-Fer, 569
nephropathy
  irbesartan, 719
  losartan, 799
nephrotic syndrome
  cyclophosphamide, 384
  prednisolone sodium phosphate, 1101
Nesacaine, 1406t–1407t
Nestrex, 1138
Neulasta, 1023
Neumega, 984
Neupogen, 573
Neupro, 1188
neuralgia
  capsaicin, 256

neuritis
  pyridoxine hydrochloride, 1138
neuroblastoma
  cyclophosphamide, 384
  etoposide, 548
  vincristine sulfate, 1369
neurocysticercosis
  albendazole, 80
neurogenic bladder
  oxybutynin, 1000
neurogenic pain
  clomipramine hydrochloride, 356
Neurontin, 620, 1424t
neuropathic pain
  gabapentin, 620
NeutraCare, 1216
NeuTrexin, 1339
Neutrogena Acne Mask, 196
Neutrogena On the Spot Acne Treatment, 196
neutropenia
  filgrastim, 573
nevirapine, 939
Nexium, 530
Nexium IV, 530
niacin, 941
Niacor, 941
Niaspan, 941
Nicabate [AUS], 944
Nicabate CQ Clear [AUS], 944
Nicabate CQ Lozenges [AUS], 944
nicardipine hydrochloride, 942
NicoDerm [CAN], 944
NicoDerm CQ, 944
Nicorette, 944
Nicorette Plus, 944
nicotine, 944
nicotine withdrawal
  clonidine, 360
Nicotinell [AUS], 944
Nicotinex, 941
nicotinic acid, 941
Nicotrol, 944
Nicotrol NS, 944
Nicotrol Patch [CAN], 944
NidaGel [CAN], 874
Nifecard [AUS], 947
Nifedicol XL, 947
nifedipine, 947
Nifehexal [AUS], 947
nighttime sleep aid
  diphenhydramine, 455
Nilandron, 950
nilotinib, 948
Nilstat [CAN], 968
nilutamide, 950
nimodipine, 951
Nimotop, 951
Nipent, 1045

nipradilol, 953
Niravam, 99
nisoldipine, 954
nitazoxanide, 956
Nitradisc [AUS], 959
Nitrek, 959
Nitro-Bid, 959
Nitro-Dur, 959
nitrofurantoin sodium, 957
nitrofurazone, 958
Nitrogard, 959
nitroglycerin, 959
Nitroject [CAN], 959
Nitrolingual, 959
Nitrolingual Spray [AUS], 959
Nitrong-SR, 959
NitroQuick, 959
Nitrostat, 959
Nitro-Tab, 959
nizatidine, 961
Nizoral, 38t–46t, 736, 1425t
Nizoral AD, 736
nocturnal enuresis
    desmopressin, 420
Nolvadex, 1241
Nolvadex-D [CAN], 1241
Non-Hodgkin's lymphoma
    bleomycin sulfate, 218
    carmustine, 268
    cyclophosphamide, 384
    cytarabine, 391
    fludarabine phosphate, 582
    rituximab, 1180
    vinblastine sulfate, 1367
    vincristine sulfate, 1369
Nono-Trifluazine [CAN], 1334
non–small-cell lung cancer
    docetaxel, 464
    gefitinib, 628
    gemcitabine hydrochloride,
        629
    paclitaxel, 1006
    vinorelbine, 1371
nonvalvular cardiovascular
        device-related
        infections, 30
Nora-BE, 962
Norco, 667, 1414t–1420t
Norditropin, 1217
Norditropin Cartridge, 1217
norethindrone, 962
Norflex, 987
norfloxacin, 964
Norfloxacine [CAN], 964
norgestrel, 965
Noritate, 874
Normodyne, 743
Normozide, 1414t–1420t
Noroxin, 964
Norpace, 460
Norpace CR, 460
Norpramin, 416
Nor-QD, 962

nortriptyline hydrochloride,
    966
Norultate [CAN], 962
Norvasc, 122
Norventyl, 966
Norvir, 1178
Norvisec [CAN], 1178
nosocomial pneumonia
    alatrofloxacin mesylate,
        1344
Noten [AUS], 166
Novantrone, 895
Novasen [CAN], 162
Novasone Cream [AUS], 901
Novasone Lotion [AUS], 901
Novasone Ointment [AUS], 901
Novepen-G [CAN], 1035
Novo Minocycline [CAN], 887
Novo Norm [AUS], 1159
Novo Sundac [CAN], 1231
Novo-Alprazo [CAN], 99
Novo-Ampicillin [CAN], 136
Novo-AZT, 1385
Novocaine, 1112, 1406t–1407t
Novo-Captopril [CAN], 257
Novo-Cholamine [CAN], 333
Novocimetine [CAN], 337
Novo-Clobestasol [CAN], 350
Novo-Clomipramine [CAN],
    356
Novoclopate [CAN], 363
Novo-Cycloprine [CAN], 381
Novo-Desipramine [CAN], 416
Novo-Difenac [CAN], 437
Novo-Diflunisal [CAN], 447
Novo-Diltiazem [CAN], 451
Novodipirado [CAN], 457
Novo-Ducosate [CAN], 466
Novo-Famotidine [CAN], 559
Novo-Fluoxetine [CAN], 592
Novo-Flutamide [CAN], 601
Novo-Furan [CAN], 957
Novo-Gemfibrozil [CAN], 631
Novo-Hydroxyzin [CAN], 677
Novo-Hylazin [CAN], 662
Novo-Ipramide [CAN], 717
Novo-Keto-EC, 737
Novo-Ketotifen [CAN], 741
Novo-Levobunolol [CAN], 766
Novolexin [CAN], 309
Novolin 70/30, 1414t–1420t
Novolin L, 703
Novolin N, 703
Novolin R, 703
Novolog, 703
NovoLog 70/30, 1414t–1420t
Novo-Loperamide [CAN], 793
Novolorazepam [CAN], 797
Novomedopa [CAN], 859
Novo-Medrone [CAN], 815
Novo-Mepro [CAN], 831
Novo-Metformin [CAN], 843
Novomethacin [CAN], 700

NovoMix 30 [AUS], 703
Novo-Nadolol [CAN], 914
Novo-Naprox [CAN], 925
Novonidazol [CAN], 874
Novo-Nifedin [CAN], 947
Novo-Norfloxacin [CAN], 964
Novo-Nortriptyline [CAN], 966
Novo-Pen-VK [CAN], 1036
Novo-Peridol [CAN], 657
Novo-Pirocam [CAN], 1077
Novopoxide [CAN], 318
Novo-Prednisolone [CAN],
    1095
Novoprofen [CAN], 682
Novo-Ranitidine [CAN], 1156
Novorapid [AUS], 703
Novoreserpine [CAN], 1161
Novosalmo [CAN], 81
Novo-Selegiline [CAN], 1201
Novo-Sertraline [CAN], 1203
Novo-Sotalol [CAN], 1219
Novo-Soxazole [CAN], 1230
Novo-Spiroton [CAN], 1221
Novo-Sucralate [CAN], 1224
Novo-Tamoxifen [CAN], 1241
Novo-Temazepam [CAN], 1247
Novo-Terazosin [CAN], 1256
Novo-Terbinafine [CAN], 1257
Novotetra [CAN], 1266
Novothyrox [CAN], 773
Novo-Tolmetin [CAN], 1305
Novo-Trazodone [CAN], 1324
Novo-Tripiramine [CAN], 1340
Novo-Triptyn [CAN], 119
Novo-Veramil [CAN], 1363
Novo-Veramil SR [CAN], 1363
Noxafil, 1084
NPH Iletin II, 703
NSAIDs, 38t–46t
Nu-Ampi [CAN], 136
Nubain, 918
Nucynta, 1244
Nudopa [AUS], 859
Nuelin [AUS], 114
Nuelin SR [AUS], 114
Nu-Ipratropium [CAN], 717
NuLev, 679
Nu-Mefenamic [CAN], 818
Nu-Metop [CAN], 871
Numoisyn, 377
Nu-Naprox [CAN], 925
Nupercainal Hydrocortisone
        Cream, 669
Nu-Propranolol, 1127
Nurofen [AUS], 682
Nu-Sulfinpyrazone [CAN],
    1228
Nu-Tetra [CAN], 1266
Nu-Tripiramine [CAN], 1340
nutritional supplement, 48–53
    niacin, 941
Nutropin, 1217
Nutropin AQ, 1217

Nutropin Depot, 1217
Nuvigil, 155
Nyaderm, 968
Nydrazid, 723
Nyefax [AUS], 947
nystatin, 968
Nystatin oral suspension, 1425t
Nystop, 968
Nyto [CAN], 455

obesity
    diethylpropion, 444
    orlistat, 986
    phendimetrazine, 1052
    phentermine, 1058
Obezine, 1052
obsessive-compulsive disorder
        (OCD)
    clomipramine hydrochloride,
        356
    fluoxetine hydrochloride,
        592
    fluvoxamine maleate, 605
    paroxetine hydrochloride,
        1019
    sertraline, 1203
obstructive sleep apnea. See
        sleep apnea
Oby-Cap, 1058
OCD. See obsessive-
        compulsive disorder
        (OCD)
Octocaine, 1409t–1411t
Octostim [CAN], 420
octreotide acetate, 970
OcuClear, 1003
Ocu-Dex, 427
Ocufen, 599
Ocuflox, 971
ocular hypertension
    apraclonidine hydrochloride,
        149
    betaxolol, 203
    bimatoprost, 210
    brimonidine, 221
    brinzolamide, 222
    carteolol, 270
    dorzolamide hydrochloride,
        473
    latanoprost, 755
    levobetaxolol hydrochloride,
        765
    levobunolol hydrochloride,
        766
    metipranolol hydrochloride,
        866
    nipradilol, 953
    travoprost, 1322
    unoprostone isopropyl,
        1347
ocular infection
    loteprednol etabonate, 802
    prednisolone acetate, 635

ocular inflammatory condition
    dexamethasone, 425
    dexamethasone sodium
        phosphate, 427
Ocu-Lone C, 1099
Ocu-Pentolate, 362
Ocu-Pred, 1097
Ocu-Pred Forte, 1097
Ocu-Pred-A, 1097
Ocusert Pilo-20 [AUS], 1069
Ocusert Pilo-40 [AUS], 1069
Odrik [AUS], 1316
Oesclim [CAN], 532
ofloxacin, 971
Ogen, 537
olanzapine, 973
olmesartan, 975
olmesartan medoxomil, 977
olopatadine, 978
olsalazine sodium, 979
Olux, 350
omalizumab, 980
Omedia, 193
omega-3 fatty acids, 982
omeprazole, 983
Omnaris, 334
Omnicef, 280
Omnipen, 134
Omnipen-N, 134
Oncovin, 1369
Oncovin [AUS], 1367
Onglyza, 1197
Onkotrone [AUS], 895
Onxol, 1006
onychomycosis
    ciclopirox, 336
    fluconazole, 578
    ketoconazole, 736
    terbinafine hydrochloride,
        1257
Opatanol [intl.], 978
Operand, 1089
Ophthacet, 1226
ophthalmic disorder
    medrysone, 817
    prednisolone sodium
        phosphate, 1101
ophthalmic solution
    fluorometholone, 590
ophthalmic surgery
    carbachol, 259
opioid dependence
    buprenorphine
        hydrochloride, 236
    clonidine, 360
    nalmefene hydrochloride,
        919
    naloxone hydrochloride, 921
    naltrexone hydrochloride,
        922
oprelvekin, 984
Optho-Bunolol [CAN], 766
Opticaine, 1264

Opticrom, 378
Optimine, 174
Optimol [AUS], 1289, 1322
OptiPranolol, 866
Orabase-B, 193
Orajel, 193
Orajel Baby, 193
Orajel Baby Nighttime, 193
Orajel Maximum Strength,
        193
Orajel Perioseptic, 262
oral candidiasis, 1425t
oral erythema multiforme,
        18–20
oral lesions. See treatment of
        oral lesions
    carbamide peroxide, 262
oral thrush
    ketoconazole, 736
Oramorph SR, 905
Orap, 1071
Orapred, 1095, 1101
Oraqix [U.S.], 774
Orasol, 193
Oraverse, 1060
Orazinc, 1387
Orencia, 57
Oretic, 663
Oreton Methyl, 865
organ transplantation
    cyclosporine, 387
    everolimus, 551
    sirolimus, 1212
Organidin, 649
Orgaran k, 397
Orinase, 1302
Orinase Diagnostic, 1302
orlistat, 986
orofacial herpes simplex
        infection, 4
oropharyngeal candidiasis. See
        candidiasis
Oroxine [AUS], 773
Orphenace [CAN], 987
orphenadrine, 987
Ortho-Est, 537
orthopedic devices, 30–31
orthostatic hypotension
    midodrine, 882
Orudis [AUS], 737
Orudis KT [CAN], 737
Orudis SR [AUS], 737
Oruvail, 737
Oruvail SR [AUS], 737
oseltamivir, 988
osteoarthritis
    capsaicin, 256
    celecoxib, 307
    diclofenac, 437
    diflunisal, 447
    etodolac, 546
    fenoprofen calcium, 566
    flavocoxid, 575

osteoarthritis *(Continued)*
  flurbiprofen, 599
  ibuprofen, 682
  indomethacin, 700
  ketoprofen, 737
  meclofenamate sodium, 814
  meloxicam, 821
  nabumetone, 913
  naproxen, 925
  oxaprozin, 994
  piroxicam, 1077
  salsalate, 1191
  sulindac, 1231
  tolmetin, 1305
osteochemonecrosis, 47–48
osteolytic bone lesion
  pamidronate disodium, 1010
osteomalacia
  vitamin D, 1374
osteonecrosis of the jaw, 47–48
osteoporosis
  alendronate sodium, 89
  calcitonin, 249
  estradiol, 532
  estropipate, 537
  ibandronate sodium, 681
  interferon gamma-1b, 716
  medroxyprogesterone
    acetate, 536
  raloxifene, 1152
  risedronate sodium, 1175
  teriparatide, 1259
Ostoforte [CAN], 1374
OTC drugs. *See* over-the-
    counter (OTC) drugs
otitis externa
  benzocaine, 193
  desonide, 422
  ofloxacin, 971
otitis media
  amoxicillin/clavulanate
    potassium, 127
  azithromycin, 179
  benzocaine, 193
  cefaclor, 275
  cefdinir, 280
  cefixime, 285
  cefpodoxime proxetil, 295
  cefprozil, 297
  ceftibuten, 300
  ceftriaxone sodium, 303
  cefuroxime sodium, 305
  cephalexin, 309
  cephradine, 310
  clarithromycin, 343
  loracarbef, 795
  ofloxacin, 971
  penicillin V potassium, 1036
  sulfisoxazole, 1230
Otocain, 193
Otricaine, 193
ovarian cancer
  amifostine, 109

ovarian cancer *(Continued)*
  carboplatin, 264
  cisplatin, 341
  cyclophosphamide, 384
  doxorubicin, 478
  hydroxyurea, 676
  melphalan, 823
  paclitaxel, 1006
  thiotepa, 1277
  topotecan, 1311
ovarian failure
  estropipate, 537
overactive bladder
  erlotinib, 524
  fesoterodine, 570
  oxybutynin, 1000
  tolterodine tartrate, 1306
over-the-counter (OTC) drugs,
  1
Ovol [CAN], 1209
Ovrette, 965
ovulatory failure
  clomiphene, 355
oxacillin, 989
oxaliplatin, 990
Oxandrin, 992
oxandrolone, 992
oxaprozin, 994
oxazepam, 995
oxcarbazepine, 997
oxiconazole, 998
oxidized cellulose, 999
Oxis [AUS], 607
Oxistat, 998
Oxizole [CAN], 998
Oxy [AUS], 1002
Oxy 10 Balanced Medicated
    Face Wash, 196
Oxy 10 Balanced Spot
    Treatment, 196
oxybutynin, 1000
oxycodone, 1002
OxyContin, 1002
Oxyderm [CAN], 196
Oxydose, 1002
OxyFast, 1002
OxyIR, 1002
oxymetazoline, 1003
oxymetholone, 1004
Oxynorm [AUS], 1002
Oxytrol, 1000

P. carinii pneumonia. *See*
    Pneumocystis carinii
    pneumonia (PCP)
Pacerone, 117
paclitaxel, 1006
Paget's disease
  alendronate sodium, 89
  calcitonin, 249
  etidronate disodium, 545
  pamidronate disodium, 1010
  risedronate sodium, 1175

pain management
  acetaminophen, 65
  amitriptyline hydrochloride,
    119
  celecoxib, 307
  clonidine, 360
  diflunisal, 447
  fenoprofen calcium, 566
  fentanyl transdermal system,
    568
  hydrocodone, 667
  ibuprofen, 682
  indomethacin, 700
  ketorolac tromethamine,
    739
  meclofenamate sodium, 814
  mefenamic acid, 818
  morphine sulfate, 905
  nalbuphine hydrochloride,
    918
  naproxen, 925
  orphenadrine, 987
  oxycodone, 1002
  pentazocine, 1041
  pentazocine hydrochloride,
    1039
  procaine, 1112
  tapentadol hydrochloride,
    1244
  tramadol hydrochloride,
    1315
  ziconotide, 1384
painful musculoskeletal
    condition
  carisoprodol, 267
  cyclobenzaprine
    hydrochloride, 381
Palafer [CAN], 569
Palgic, 263
paliperidone, 1007
Palladone, 672
Palmer's Skin Success Acne,
  196
palmoplantar keratoses
  acitretin, 73
Palmitate A, 1373
palonosetron hydrochloride,
  1009
Pamelor, 966
pamidronate disodium, 1010
Pamisol [AUS], 1010
Pamprin, 925
Panadol [AUS], 65
Panafcort [AUS], 1103
Panamax [AUS], 65
Pancrease [CAN], 1011
Pancrease MT, 1011
pancreatic cancer
  erlotinib, 524
  gemcitabine hydrochloride,
    629
pancreatic insufficiency
  pancreatin, 1011

Pancreatin, 1011
pancreatin, 1011
pancreatitis
    fenofibrate, 565
pancrelipase, 1011
panic disorder
    alprazolam, 99
    clomipramine hydrochloride, 356
    clonazepam, 358
    fluoxetine hydrochloride, 592
    paroxetine hydrochloride, 1019
    sertraline, 1203
panitumumab, 1012
Panixine, 307
PanOxyl, 196
PanOxyl Aqua Gel, 196
PanOxyl Bar, 196
PanOxyl-AQ, 196
Panretin, 94
Pantoloc, 1014
pantoprazole, 1014
Papacon, 1015
papaverine hydrochloride, 1015
paracoccidioidomycosis
    ketoconazole, 736
    miconazole, 878
Parafon Forte DSC, 332
Paralgin [AUS], 65
Paraplatin, 264
Para-Time SR, 1015
paregoric, 1016
pargyline, 1017
Pariet [CAN], 1151
Parkinsonism
    benztropine mesylate, 198
    biperiden, 211
    levodopa, 769
    nipradilol, 953
    selegiline hydrochloride, 1201
    trihexyphenidyl, 1337
Parkinson's disease
    amantadine hydrochloride, 104
    apomorphine, 148
    bromocriptine mesylate, 223
    cabergoline, 248
    entacapone, 505
    pramipexole, 1090
    procyclidine, 1118
    rasagiline, 1158
    ropinirole hydrochloride, 1184
    rotigotine, 1188
    tolcapone, 1303
Parlodel, 223
Parm Rubicin, 512
Parnate, 1319
paromomycin, 1018

paroxetine hydrochloride, 1019
paroxysmal atrial flutter (PAF)
    flecainide, 577
paroxysmal atrial tachycardia
    digoxin, 448
    quinidine, 1147
paroxysmal supraventricular
        tachycardia (PSVT)
    diltiazem hydrochloride, 451
    flecainide, 577
    verapamil hydrochloride, 1363
paroxysmal ventricular
        tachycardia
    quinidine, 1147
Parvolex [CAN], 71
Paser, 116
Pataday, 978
Patanase [U.S.], 978
Patanol, 978
Patanol S, 978
patent ductus arteriosus
    indomethacin, 700
Pathocil, 440
Pavabid Plateau, 1015
Pavacot, 1015
Pavagen, 1015
Paxam [AUS], 358
Paxeva, 1019
Paxil, 1019
Paxil CR, 1019
Paxtine [AUS], 1019
pazopanib, 1021
PCE, 526
PCP. See Pneumocystis carinii
        pneumonia (PCP)
PediaCare Infants'
        Long-Acting Cough, 434
Pediaflor, 1214
Pediapred, 1095, 1101
Pediatex, 263
pediatric dentistry,
        1436t–1438t
Pediazole, 1414t–1420t
PediDent, 1214
Pediox, 263
Pegasys, 1024
pegfilgrastim, 1023
peginterferon alfa-2a, 1024
peginterferon alfa-2b, 1026
PEG-Intron, 1026
pegvisomant, 1028
pellagra
    niacin, 941
pelvic infection
    ertapenem, 525
pelvic inflammatory disease
        (PID)
    ceftizoxime sodium, 302
    doxycycline, 480
    ofloxacin, 971
PemADD, 1030

PemADD CT, 1030
pemirolast potassium, 1029
pemoline, 1030
pemphigus vulgaris, 17–18
penbutolol, 1031
penciclovir, 1032
Pendine [AUS], 620
Penicillin G benzathine, 1033
Penicillin G potassium, 1035
Penicillin V potassium, 1036
penicillins, 38t–46t
Penlac, 336
Pentacarinat [CAN], 1037
Pentam-300, 1037
pentamidine isethionate, 1037
Pentasa, 835
pentazocine, 1041
pentazocine hydrochloride, 1039
pentobarbital, 1042
Pentolair, 362
pentosan polysulfate, 1044
pentostatin, 1045
Pentothal, 1405t
pentoxifylline, 1046
Pentoxyl, 1046
Pepcid, 559
Pepcid AC, 559
Pepcid Complete, 1414t–1420t
Pepcidine [CAN], 559
peptic ulcer disease
    glycopyrrolate, 643
    hyoscyamine, 679
    propantheline, 1124
Pepto-Bismol, 214
Peptol [CAN], 337
Percocet, 1414t–1420t
Percodan, 1414t–1420t
percutaneous coronary
        intervention (PCI)
    abciximab, 57
    argatroban, 153
    eptifibatide, 520
percutaneous transluminal
        coronary angioplasty
        (PTCA)
    bivalirudin, 217
    tirofiban, 1295
Periactin, 389
pericarditis
    penicillin G potassium, 1035
Peridex, 320, 1425t
Peridol [CAN], 657
peridonitis
    doxycycline, 480
perindopril, 1048
Perio Chip, 321
PerioChip, 320
periodontitis
    chlorhexidine gluconate, 320
    doxycycline hyclate gel, 483

periodontitis *(Continued)*
  tetracycline periodontal
    fiber, 1268
PerioGard, 320, 1425t
perioperative prophylaxis
  ampicillin sodium, 136
  cefazolin sodium, 278
  cefotaxime sodium, 290
  cefotetan disodium, 292
  cefoxitin sodium, 293
  ceftriaxone sodium, 303
  cefuroxime sodium, 305
Periostat, 482
Periostat Minomycin [AUS],
  887
peripheral nerve block
  bupivacaine, 232
Perisol, 320
peritonitis
  vancomycin hydrochloride,
    1356
Permapen, 1033
Permitil, 595
pernicious anemia
  cyanocobalamin, 380
perphenazine, 1049
Persantin [AUS], 457
Persantin 100 [AUS], 457
Persantin SR [AUS], 457
Persantine, 457
Pertofran [AUS], 416
pertussis
  demeclocycline
    hydrochloride, 414
Pethidine Injection [AUS], 825
petriellidiosis
  miconazole, 878
Pfizerpen, 1035
pge1, 101
pharyngitis
  azithromycin, 179
  benzocaine, 193
  cefaclor, 275
  cefadroxil, 277
  cefdinir, 280
  cefditoren pivoxil, 282
  cefixime, 285
  cefpodoxime proxetil, 295
  cefprozil, 297
  ceftibuten, 300
  cefuroxime sodium, 305
  cephalexin, 309
  clarithromycin, 343
  dirithromycin, 458
  erythromycin, 526
  loracarbef, 795
Phazyme, 1209
Phenadoz, 1121
Phenazo [CAN], 1051
phenazopyridine hydrochloride,
  1051
Phendiet, 1052
Phendiet-105, 1052

phendimetrazine, 1052
phenelzine sulfate, 1054
Phenergan, 1121
Phenergan with Codeine,
  1414t–1420t
Phenergan VC, 1414t–1420t
Phenergan VC with Codeine,
  1414t–1420t
phenobarbital, 1055, 1424t
Phenobarbitone [AUS], 1042,
  1055
phenoxybenzamine, 1057
Phentercot, 1058
phentermine, 1058
phentolamine, 1060
phenylephrine hydrochloride,
  1061, 1063
phenylketonuria
  sapropterin, 1193
phenytoin, 1064, 1424t
pheochromocytoma
  metyrosine, 876
  phenoxybenzamine, 1057
  phentolamine, 1060
  propranolol hydrochloride,
    1127
Phospholine iodide, 493
Phyllocontin, 114
Physeptone [AUS], 845
physiologic replacement
  cortisone acetate, 376
  dexamethasone, 425
  hydrocortisone, 669
physostigmine, 1067
phytonadione, 1068
pilocarpine hydrochloride,
  1069
Pilopt Eye Drops [AUS], 1069
pimozide, 1071
pindolol, 1073
pioglitazone, 1075
pirbuterol, 1076
piroxicam, 1077
pitavastatin, 1079
Pitressin, 1360
pituitary adenoma
  cabergoline, 248
Placil [AUS], 356
plaque psoriasis. *See also*
  psoriasis
  alefacept, 86
  calcitriol, 251
  efalizumab, 494
  etanercept, 540
Plaquenil, 674
Platinol-AQ, 341
Plavix, 362
Plegine, 1052
Plendil, 563
Plendil ER [AUS], 563
PMS Isoniazid, 723
PMS-Amantadine [CAN], 104

PMS-Chloral [CAN], 317
PMS-Docusate [CAN], 466
PMS-Ipratropium [CAN], 717
PMS-Levobunolol [CAN], 766
PMS-Mefenamic Acid [CAN],
  818
PMS-Methylphenidate [CAN],
  861
PMS-Metoprolol [CAN], 871
PMS-Norfloxacin [CAN], 964
PMS-Pseudoephedrine [CAN],
  1134
PMS-Sertraline [CAN], 1203
PMS-Sotalol [CAN], 1219
PMS-Temazepam [CAN], 1247
PMS-Timolol [CAN], 1289
PMS-Tobramycin, 1297
PMS-Trazodone [CAN], 1324
PMS-Trifluopereazine [CAN],
  1334
Pneumocystis carinii
  pneumonia (PCP)
  dapsone, 402
  pentamidine isethionate,
    1037
  trimetrexate, 1339
pneumonia. *See also*
  community-acquired
    pneumonia
  cefepime, 284
  cefpodoxime proxetil, 295
  ceftazidime, 298
  clarithromycin, 343
  dapsone, 628
  ertapenem, 525
  gatifloxacin, 626
  levofloxacin, 771
  linezolid, 779
  loracarbef, 795
  penicillin G potassium, 1035
Pneumostussin, 667
Podocon-25, 1082
Pododerm, 1082
podofilox, 1081
podophyllum resin, 1082
Polaramine, 429
Polaramine Repetabs, 429
Polocaine, 829, 1406t–1407t,
  1409t–1411t
Polocaine-MPF, 829
Polycillin, 134, 136
Polycillin-N, 134
Polydine, 1089
polymorphouse light eruption
  alclometasone, 83
polymyxin B, 1083
polymyxin B sulfate, 1084
Polysporin, 1414t–1420t
Polytrim, 1084
Pompe disease
  alglucosidase alfa, 92
Ponstan [CAN], 818
Ponstel, 818

Pontocaine, 1264
posaconazole, 1084
post laser surgery (eyes)
apraclonidine hydrochloride, 149
postanesthesia narcotic reversal
naloxone hydrochloride, 921
postherpetic neuralgia
clonidine, 360
gabapentin, 620
pregabalin, 1105
procaine, 1112
postoperative control of ileus
alvimopan, 103
postpartum/postabortion hemorrhage
methylergonovine, 860
posttraumatic stress disorder
paroxetine hydrochloride, 1019
sertraline, 1203
potassium acetate, 1088
potassium bicarbonate-citrate, 1088
potassium chloride, 1086, 1088
potassium gluconate, 1088
potassium loss
amiloride hydrochloride, 111
povidone iodine, 1089
Pramin [AUS], 868
pramipexole, 1090
Prandase [CAN], 62
Prandin, 1159
Prasig [AUS], 1094
prasugrel, 1091
Pratisol [AUS], 1094
Pravachol, 1093
pravastatin, 1093
Pravigard, 1414t–1420t
prazosin hydrochloride, 1094
preanesthesia
diazepam, 435
precocious puberty
leuprolide acetate, 760
nafarelin, 916
Precose, 62
Pred Forte, 1095, 1097
Pred Mild, 1095, 1097
Pred-G, 635
Pred-G S.O.P., 635
Prednisol, 1097
prednisolone, 1095
prednisolone acetate, 635, 1097, 1099
prednisolone sodium phosphate, 1101
prednisone, 1103
Prednisone Intensol, 1103
Prefrin, 1061
pregabalin, 1105
pregnancy, 1434t–1435t
Prelone, 1095

Prelu-2, 1052
premature ventricular contraction (PVC)
disopyramide phosphate, 460
premenstrual dysphoric disorder
fluoxetine hydrochloride, 592
sertraline, 1203
premenstrual syndrome
alprazolam, 99
buspirone hydrochloride, 239
Premetrium, 1119
Premphase, 536, 1414t–1420t
Prempro, 536, 1414t–1420t
Prempro Low Dose, 536
preoperative intestinal antisepsis
erythromycin, 526
Preparation H Hydrocortisone, 669
Presolol [AUS], 743
Pressin [AUS], 1094
Pressyn [CAN], 1360
Pretz-D, 506
Prevacid, 751
Prevacid IV, 751
Prevacid NapraPAC, 1414t–1420t
Prevacid Solu-Tab, 751
Prevalite, 333
PreviDent, 1216
PreviDent 5000 Plus, 1216
Prezista, 405
Prialt, 1384
Priftin, 1169
Prilocaine HCl, 1409t–1411t
Prilocaine HCl + epinephrine, 1409t–1411t
prilocaine hydrochloride, 1106, 1409t–1411t
Prilosec, 983
Prilosec OTC, 983
Primacin [AUS], 1108
primaquine, 1108
Primatene, 509
primidone, 1109, 1424t
Primogyn Depot [AUS], 532
Principen, 134, 136
Prinivil, 785
Prinzide, 1414t–1420t
Pristiq, 424
Pritor [AUS], 1246
Privine, 924
ProAmatine, 882
Pro-Banthine, 1124
probenecid, 1111
Probitor [AUS], 983
Pro-C [AUS], 161

procaine, 1112, 1406t–1407t
Pro-Cal-Sof, 466
procarbazine hydrochloride, 1114
Procardia, 947
Procardia XL, 947
Prochieve, 1119
prochlorperazine, 1116
Pro-Cid [AUS], 1111
Procrit, 515
proctitis
mesalamine/5-aminosalicylic acid (5-ASA), 835
Proctocort, 669
proctosigmoiditis
mesalamine/5-aminosalicylic acid (5-ASA), 835
procyclidine, 1118
Procytox [CAN], 384
Prodium, 1051
progesterone, 1119
Progout [AUS], 95
Prograf, 1238
Progynova [AUS], 532
Proleukin, 84
Prolixin, 595
promethazine hydrochloride, 1121
propafenone hydrochloride, 1123
Propanth [CAN], 1124
propantheline, 1124
Propecia, 574
prophyria
chlorpromazine, 327
Propine, 456
propofol, 1126, 1405t
propranolol hydrochloride, 1127
Propranolol Intensol, 1127
Propylthiouracil, 1130
propylthiouracil, 1130
Propyl-Thyracil [CAN], 1130
Proscar, 574
prostate cancer
abarelix, 56
bicalutamide, 209
estradiol, 532
estramustine phosphate sodium, 534
flutamide, 601
goserelin acetate, 644
histrelin, 659
leuprolide acetate, 760
mitoxantrone, 895
nilutamide, 950
triptorelin pamoate, 1342

prostatitis
  cephradine, 310
  ciprofloxacin hydrochloride,
    339
  flavoxate, 576
  lomefloxacin hydrochloride,
    790
  norfloxacin, 964
  ofloxacin, 971
prosthetic joints, 30
Prostigmin, 938
Prostin VR Pediatric, 101
protein C, 1131
Protonix, 1014
Protopic, 1238
protriptyline, 1133
Proventil, 81
Proventil Repetabs, 81
Provera, 815
Provigil, 897
Proviodine, 1089
Proxigel, 262
Prozac, 592
Prozac Weekly, 592
Prudoxin, 476
pruritus
  alclometasone, 83
  betamethasone, 202
  cholestyramine resin, 333
  clocortolone, 351
  cyproheptadine, 389
  diflorasone, 446
  diphenhydramine, 455
  doxepin hydrochloride, 476
  flurandrenolide, 597
  fluticasone propionate, 602
  halobetasol, 656
  hydroxyzine, 677
  triamcinolone, 1328
Pryi, 1138
pseudoephedrine, 1134
pseudohypoparathyroidism
  calcitriol, 251
pseudomembranous colitis
  metronidazole
    hydrochloride, 874
  vancomycin hydrochloride,
    1356
Psorcon, 446
Psorcon-e, 446
psoriasis. See also plaque
    psoriasis
  acitretin, 73
  alclometasone, 83
  anthralin, 147
  betamethasone, 202
  calcitriol, 251
  clobetasol, 350
  clocortolone, 351
  cyclosporine, 387
  diflorasone, 446
  efalizumab, 494
  fluocinolone acetonide, 588

psoriasis (Continued)
  halobetasol, 656
  methotrexate sodium, 853
Psoriatec, 147
psoriatic arthritis
  etanercept, 540
PSVT. See paroxysmal
    supraventricular
    tachycardia (PSVT)
psychotic disorder (psychosis)
  chlorpromazine, 327
  fluphenazine decanoate, 595
  haloperidol, 657
  loxapine, 804
  prochlorperazine, 1116
  quetiapine, 1143
  reserpine, 1161
  risperidone, 1176
  thioridazine, 1276
  thiothixene, 1279
  trifluoperazine
    hydrochloride, 1334
Pulmicort Respules, 229
Pulmicort Turbuhaler, 229
pulmonary arterial
    hypertension (PAH)
  ambrisentan, 107
  bosentan, 220
  treprostinil sodium, 1325
pulmonary embolism (PE)
  alteplase, recombinant, 102
  dalteparin sodium, 396
pulmonary hypertension
  iloprost, 691
Pulmozyme, 472
Purinethol, 832
Purinol [CAN], 95
purpura fulminans
  protein C, 1131
P.V. Carpine Liquifilm
  Ophthalmic Solution
    [AUS], 1069
P-V Tussin, 667
pyelonephritis
  doripenem, 471
  gatifloxacin, 626
  levofloxacin, 771
Pylorid [AUS], 1156
Pyrahexyl-D [AUS], 1077
Pyralin EN [AUS], 1227
Pyrazinamide, 1136
pyrazinamide, 1136
Pyridium, 1051
pyridostigmine bromide, 1137
pyridoxine deficiency
  pyridoxine hydrochloride,
    1138
pyridoxine hydrochloride, 1138
pyrimethamine, 1139
Pyroxin [AUS], 1138

quazepam, 1142
Questran [CAN], 333

Questran Lite [AUS], 333
quetiapine, 1143
Quibron-T, 114, 1271
Quibron-T/SR, 114
Quilonum SR [AUS], 788
Quinaglute, 1147
quinapril, 1145
Quinate [CAN], 1147
Quinidex Extentabs, 1147
quinidine, 1147
Quinine, 1149
quinine, 1149
Quixin, 771
Qvar, 187

rabeprazole sodium, 1151
radiation therapy, 24–27
Rafen [AUS], 682
Ralodantin [AUS], 957
Ralovera [AUS], 815
raloxifene, 1152
raltegravir, 1153
Ramace [AUS], 1154
ramipril, 1154
Rani-2 [AUS], 1156
Ranihexal [AUS], 1156
ranitidine bismuth citrate,
    1156
ranitidine hydrochloride,
    1156
Rapamune, 1212
Rapilysin [AUS], 1163
Raptiva, 494
rasagiline, 1158
Rastinon [AUS], 1302
Rauserpine [TAIWAN], 1161
Rauverid [PHILIPPINES], 1161
Raynaud's syndrome
  isoxsuprine hydrochloride,
    727
  isradipine, 728
Reactine [CAN], 313
Rebetol, 1164
Rebetron, 1164, 1414t–1420t
Reclast, 1390
Recofol [AUS], 1126
rectal cancer
  bevacizumab, 206
  oxaliplatin, 990
rectal gonococcal infection
  cefpodoxime proxetil, 295
Rectogesic [AUS], 959
recurrent aphthous stomatitis,
    6–9
recurrent calcium oxalate
    calculi
  allopurinol, 95
recurrent (orofacial) herpes
    simplex infection, 4
red cell aphasia
  oxymetholone, 1004
Redoxon [CAN], 161
reduced salivary flow, 13–14

refractive surgery
  ketorolac tromethamine, 739
Regaine [AUS], 889
Regitine, 1060
Reglan, 868
Regranex, 186
Regular Iletin II, 703
Regulex [CAN], 466
Relafen, 913
Relenza, 1383
Relpax, 496
Remeron, 891
Remeron Soltab, 891
Remicade, 702
Reminyl, 621
Remodulin, 1325
Remular, 332
Remular-S, 332
Renagel, 1205
renal allograft rejection
  azathioprine, 175
renal carcinoma
  medroxyprogesterone
    acetate, 815
renal cell carcinoma
  aldesleukin, 84
  everolimus, 551
  pazopanib, 1021
  sunitinib, 1234
  temsirolimus, 1250
renal failure
  calcitriol, 251
  epoetin alfa, 515
  methoxy polyethylene
    glycol-epoetin beta,
    855
  oxymetholone, 1004
  torsemide, 1313
  vitamin D, 1374
renal impairment dosages. See
    individual drug
    monographs
renal osteodystrophy
  dihydrotachysterol, 450
renal transplant
  daclizumab, 394
  mycophenolate mofetil, 910
Renedil [CAN], 563
Renitec [AUS], 499
Renova, 1326
repaglinide, 1159
Reprexain, 667, 682
Reprexain CIII, 1414t–1420t
Requip, 1184
Rescriptor, 412
Rescula, 1347
Reserfia [CAN], 1161
reserpine, 1161
Respax [AUS], 81
Respbid, 1271
respiratory tract infection. See
    also lower respiratory
    tract infection

respiratory tract infection
    (Continued)
  amantadine hydrochloride,
    104
  ampicillin, 134
  ampicillin sodium, 136
  azithromycin, 179
  dicloxacillin sodium, 440
  erythromycin, 526
  oxacillin, 989
  tobramycin sulfate, 1297
  vancomycin hydrochloride,
    1356
Restasis, 387
restless legs syndrome (RLS)
  cabergoline, 248
Restoril, 1247
retapamulin, 1162
Retavase, 1163
reteplase, recombinant, 1163
reticulum cell sarcoma
  bleomycin sulfate, 218
Retin-A, 1326
Retin-A Micro, 1326
retinoblastoma
  cyclophosphamide, 384
Retre-Gel, 193
Retrovir, 1385
Revex, 919
Rev-Eyes, 401
ReVia, 922
Reyataz, 161
rhabdomyosarcoma
  vincristine sulfate, 1369
rheumatic fever
  cephalexin, 309
  penicillin G benzathine,
    1033
  penicillin V potassium, 1036
rheumatoid arthritis
  abatacept, 57
  adalimumab, 77
  anakinra, 143
  aurothioglucose/gold sodium
    thiomalate, 172
  azathioprine, 175
  capsaicin, 256
  celecoxib, 307
  cyclosporine, 387
  diclofenac, 437
  diflunisal, 447
  etanercept, 540
  etodolac, 546
  fenoprofen calcium, 566
  flurbiprofen, 599
  hydroxychloroquine sulfate,
    674
  ibuprofen, 682
  indomethacin, 700
  infliximab, 702
  ketoprofen, 737
  leflunomide, 756
  meclofenamate sodium, 814

rheumatoid arthritis
    (Continued)
  meloxicam, 821
  methotrexate sodium, 853
  nabumetone, 913
  naproxen, 925
  oxaprozin, 994
  piroxicam, 1077
  salsalate, 1191
  sulfasalazine, 1227
  sulindac, 1231
  tolmetin, 1305
Rheumatrex, 853
Rhinalar [CAN], 586
rhinitis. See also allergic
    rhinitis
  beclomesthasone
    dipropionate, 187
  budesonide, 229
  cyproheptadine, 389
  flunisolide, 586
  levocetirizine, 768
  oxymetazoline, 1003
  triamcinolone, 1328
Rhinocort Aqua, 229
Rhinocort Aqueous [AUS], 229
Rhinocort Hayfever [AUS], 229
rhinorrhea
  ipratropium bromide, 717
Rhodis [CAN], 737
Rhotrimine [CAN], 1340
Rhoxal-orphenadrine [CAN],
    987
rhus dermatitis
  alclometasone, 83
ribavirin, 1164
rickets
  calcitriol, 251
  dihydrotachysterol, 450
  vitamin D, 1374
rifabutin, 1166
Rifadin, 1168
Rifamate, 1414t–1420t
rifampin, 1168
rifapentine, 1169
Rifater, 1414t–1420t
rifaximin, 1171
Rilutek, 1172
riluzole, 1172
Rimactane, 1168
rimantadine hydrochloride,
    1173
rimexolone, 1174
Rimycin [AUS], 1168
Riomet, 843
Riopan Plus, 808
Riphenidate [CAN], 861
risedronate sodium, 1175
Risperdal, 1176
Risperdal Consta, 1176
Risperdal M-Tabs, 1176
risperidone, 1176
Ritalin, 861

Ritalin LA, 861
Ritalin SR, 861
ritonavir, 1178
Rituxan, 1180
rituximab, 1180
rivastigmine tartrate, 1181
Rivotril [CAN], 358
rizatriptan benzoate, 1183
RMS, 905
Robaxin, 852
Robidone [CAN], 665
Robidrine [CAN], 1134
Robinul, 643
Robinul Forte, 643
Robinul Injection [AUS], 643
Robitussin, 649
Robitussin [AUS], 434
Robitussin AC, 1414t–1420t
Robitussin CoughGels, 434
Robitussin DM, 1414t–1420t
Robitussin Honey Cough, 434
Robitussin Maximum Strength
    Cough, 434
Robitussin Pediatric Cough,
    434
Rocaltrol, 251
Rocephin, 303
Rocky Mountain spotted fever
    doxycycline, 480
    tetracycline hydrochloride,
    1266
Rodex, 1138
Rofact [CAN], 1168
Roferon-A, 708, 710
Rogaine, 889
Rogaine Extra Strength, 889
Romazicon, 585
ropinirole hydrochloride, 1184
ropivacaine, 1406t–1407t
Rosig [AUS], 1077
Rosig-D [AUS], 1077
rosiglitazone maleate, 1185
rosuvastatin calcium, 1187
rotigotine, 1188
roundworm
    thiabendazole, 1272
Rowasa, 835
Roxanol, 905
Roxicet, 1414t–1420t
Roxicodone, 1002
Roxicodone Intensol, 1002
Roxin [AUS], 964
Rozex [AUS], 874
Rum-K, 1086
Rynacrom [AUS], 378
Rythmodan [CAN], 460
Rythmol, 1123
Rythmol SR, 1123

Sabril, 1366
Saizen, 1217
Salagen, 1069
Salazopyrin [CAN], 1227

Salazopyrin EN [AUS], 1227
Salazopyrin EN-Tabs [CAN],
    1227
Salflex, 1191
saliva stimulants, 13–14
saliva substitutes, 13
salivary flow, 13–14
salmeterol, 1190
Salofalk [CAN], 835
salsalate, 1191
salt-losing adrenogenital
    syndrome
    fludrocortisone, 583
Saluron, 671
Samsca, 1307
Sancuso, 646
Sandimmune, 387
Sandimmune Neoral [AUS],
    387
Sandostatin, 970
Sandostatin LAR, 970
Sandrena Gel [AUS], 532
sapropterin, 1193
saquinavir, 1194
Sarafem, 592
sargramostim, 1195
Savella, 886
saw palmetto, 50t
saxagliptin, 1197
Scandonest, 1409t–1411t
Scandonest 2% Special,
    1409t–1411t
Scheinpharm, 422
schizophrenia
    aripiprazole, 154
    chlorpromazine, 327
    clozapine, 366
    fluphenazine decanoate, 595
    iloperidone, 689
    mesoridazine besylate, 838
    molindone, 899
    olanzapine, 973
    paliperidone, 1007
    perphenazine, 1049
    quetiapine, 1143
    risperidone, 1176
    thioridazine, 1276
    thiothixene, 1279
    trifluoperazine
        hydrochloride, 1334
scopolamine, 1198
Scot-Tussin DM Cough
    Chasers, 434
scurvy
    ascorbic acid, 161
seasonal rhinitis. See rhinitis
Seba-Gel, 196
Sebizole [AUS], 736
seborrheic dermatitis
    alclometasone, 83
    ciclopirox, 336
    fluocinolone acetonide, 588
    ketoconazole, 736

secobarbital, 1199
Seconal, 1199
Sectral, 63
sedation
    butabarbital sodium, 242
    chloral hydrate, 317
    flumazenil, 585
    hydroxyzine, 677
    lorazepam, 797
    mephobarbital, 828
    midazolam hydrochloride,
    880
    nalbuphine hydrochloride,
    918
    pentobarbital, 1042
    phenobarbital, 1055
    promethazine hydrochloride,
    1121
    propofol, 1126
    secobarbital, 1199
    triazolam, 1332
seizure
    butabarbital sodium, 242
    carbamazepine, 260
    clonazepam, 358
    clorazepate dipotassium, 363
    diazepam, 435
    drugs, generally, 1424t
    ethosuximide, 544
    felbamate, 562
    fosphenytoin, 614
    gabapentin, 620
    lacosamide, 744
    lamotrigine, 747
    levetiracetam, 764
    mephobarbital, 828
    methsuximide, 857
    oxcarbazepine, 997
    phenobarbital, 1055
    phenylephrine
        hydrochloride, 1063
    phenytoin, 1064
    pregabalin, 1105
    primidone, 1109
    tiagabine, 1283
    topiramate, 1309
    valproic acid, 1352
    vigabatrin, 1366
    zonisamide, 1393
Selax [CAN], 466
selegiline hydrochloride, 1201
Semi-Daonil [AUS], 641
Semi-Euglucon [AUS], 641
senile dementia
    ergoloid mesylates, 521
Senokot-S, 1414t–1420t
Sensorcaine, 232, 1406t–1407t
Sensorcaine-MPF, 232
sepsis
    penicillin G potassium,
    1035
Septanest N [CAN],
    1409t–1411t

Septanest SP [CAN], 1409t–1411t
septicemia
  ampicillin, 134
  ceftizoxime sodium, 302
  clindamycin, 348
  gentamicin sulfate, 633
  metronidazole hydrochloride, 874
  ticarcillin, 1284
  ticarcillin disodium, 1286
  tobramycin, 1296
  tobramycin sulfate, 1297
  vancomycin hydrochloride, 1356
Septocaine, 159, 1409t–1411t
Septra, 1414t–1420t
Sequent HICOR [AUS], 669
Serax, 995
Serenace [AUS], 657
Serentil, 838
Serepax [AUS], 995
Serevent Diskus, 1190
Serevent Inhaler and Disks [AUS], 1190
Seromycin, 385
Serophene, 355
Serophene [CAN], 355
Seroquel, 1143
Serostim, 1217
Serpalan, 1161
Serpasil [CAN], 1161
Serpasil [INDONESIA], 1161
Serpasol [SPAIN], 1161
sertaconazole, 1202
sertraline, 1203
Serzone, 933
Setamol [AUS], 65
sevelamer hydrochloride, 1205
shift-work sleep disorder
  armodafinil, 155
  modafinil, 897
shingles. See herpes zoster
shock
  hydrocortisone, 669
  metaraminol, 841
  phenylephrine hydrochloride, 1061
  vasopressin, 1360
short bowel syndrome
  somatropin, 1217
sibutramine, 1206
sickle cell anemia
  hydroxyurea, 676
Sigmaxin [AUS], 448
Sigmetadine [AUS], 337
Silain-Gel, 1414t–1420t
sildenafil citrate, 1207
Silphen DM, 434
Silvadene, 1208
silver sulfadiazine, 1208
simethicone, 1209
Simply Cough, 434

simvastatin, 1210
Sinequan, 476
Sinex 12 Hour Long-Acting, 1003
Singulair, 902
sinusitis
  alatrofloxacin mesylate, 1344
  amoxicillin/clavulanate potassium, 127
  cefdinir, 280
  cefpodoxime proxetil, 295
  cefprozil, 297
  cefuroxime sodium, 305
  ciprofloxacin hydrochloride, 339
  clarithromycin, 343
  gatifloxacin, 626
  levofloxacin, 771
  loracarbef, 795
  moxifloxacin hydrochloride, 907
sirolimus, 1212
sitagliptin, 1213
6-MP, 832
Sjögren's syndrome
  acitretin, 73
  cevimeline, 316
  cottonseed oil, 377–378
  pilocarpine hydrochloride, 1069
Skelaxin, 842
skeletal muscle relaxation
  diazepam, 435
skin abrasion
  bacitracin, 183
skin disorder
  lidocaine hydrochloride, 774
  mometasone furoate monohydrate, 901
skin granuloma
  minocycline hydrochloride, 887
skin infection
  alatrofloxacin mesylate, 1344
  amoxicillin, 125
  ampicillin, 134
  ampicillin sodium, 136
  ampicillin/sulbactam sodium, 137
  azithromycin, 179
  cefaclor, 275
  cefadroxil, 277
  cefdinir, 280
  cefditoren pivoxil, 282
  cefepime, 284
  cefpodoxime proxetil, 295
  cefprozil, 297
  ceftazidime, 298
  ceftriaxone sodium, 303
  cephalexin, 309
  clarithromycin, 343

skin infection (Continued)
  daptomycin, 403
  dirithromycin, 458
  doxycycline, 480
  ertapenem, 525
  erythromycin, 526
  gatifloxacin, 626
  gentamicin sulfate, 633
  levofloxacin, 771
  linezolid, 779
  loracarbef, 795
  metronidazole hydrochloride, 874
  moxifloxacin hydrochloride, 907
  ofloxacin, 971
  oxacillin, 989
  penicillin V potassium, 1036
  ticarcillin, 1284
  ticarcillin disodium, 1286
  tobramycin, 1296
  tobramycin sulfate, 1297
  vancomycin hydrochloride, 1356
skin irritation
  zinc oxide, 1387
sleep apnea
  armodafinil, 155
  modafinil, 897
Slo-Bid, 1271
Slo-Bid Gyrocaps, 114
Slo-Niacin, 941
Slo-Phyllin, 1271
Slow-Fe, 569
Slow-K [AUS], 1088
small-cell lung carcinoma
  etoposide, 548
  topotecan, 1311
smoking cessation
  bupropion, 237
  nicotine, 944
  varenicline, 1358–1360
social anxiety disorder
  paroxetine hydrochloride, 1019
  sertraline, 1203
sodium fluoride, 1214
sodium fluoride (topical), 1216
sodium folate, 606
Sodium Sulamyd, 1226
sodium valproate, 1424t
Soflax [CAN], 466
soft tissue infection
  clarithromycin, 343
  loracarbef, 795
  vancomycin hydrochloride, 1356
solar cheilitis, 11–12
Solaraze, 437
Solarcaine, 193
Solavert [AUS], 1219

Solfoton, 1424t
Solganal, 172
solid tumor
  mitoxantrone, 895
Solone [AUS], 1095
Solprin [AUS], 162
Solu-Cortef, 669
Solu-Flur, 1214
Solugel [CAN], 196
Solu-Medrol, 863
Solurex, 425
Solurex LA, 425
Soma, 267
Somac [AUS], 1014
somatropin, 1217
Somatuline Depot, 749
Somavert, 1028
Somnote, 317
Sonata, 1381
Sone [AUS], 1103
Sorbidin [AUS], 724, 726
Soriatane, 73
Sorine, 1219
Sotab [AUS], 1219
Sotacor [AUS], 1219
Sotahexal [AUS], 1219
sotalol hydrochloride, 1219
Spacol, 679
Spacol T/S, 679
Span-K [AUS], 1088
spasticity
  dantrolene sodium, 400
Spectracef, 282
spinal cord injury
  methylprednisolone,
    863
Spiractin [AUS], 1221
Spiriva, 1294
spironolactone, 1221
Sporanox, 730
sporotrichosis
  amphotericin b, 131
Spren [AUS], 162
Sprycel, 407
Squibb HC [AUS], 669
SSD, 1208
SSD AF, 1208
St. John's wort, 50t
Stadol, 245
Stadol NS, 245
Stagesic, 667
Stalevo, 1414t–1420t
staphylococcal infection
  dicloxacillin sodium, 440
  rifampin, 1168
Starlix, 928
Statex [CAN], 905
status asthmaticus
  hydrocortisone, 669
status epilepticus
  diazepam, 435
  fosphenytoin, 614
  lorazepam, 797

status epilepticus (Continued)
  midazolam hydrochloride,
    880
  phenobarbital, 1055
  phenytoin, 1064
  secobarbital, 1199
Stelazine, 1334
stem cell transplant
  sargramostim, 1195
Stemetil [CAN], 1116
Stemzine [AUS], 1116
Stenapred, 1103
Stenapred DS, 1103
Stilnox [AUS], 1392
Stimate, 420
Stocrin [AUS], 495
stool softener
  docusate, 466
Strattera, 168
Strepfen [AUS], 599
streptococcal infection
  dicloxacillin sodium, 440
  penicillin G benzathine,
    1033
streptomycin, 1222
Striant, 1260
stroke
  clopidogrel, 362
  losartan, 799
  ramipril, 1154
  tiplopidine hydrochloride,
    1287
strongyloidasis
  thiabendazole, 1272
subconjunctival injection
  lincomycin HCL, 777
subgingival bacterial flora
  chlorhexidine gluconate
    chip, 321
Suboxone, 1414t–1420t
Subutex, 236
sucralfate, 1224
sucralfate suspension, 2
Sudafed, 1134
Sudafed 12 Hour, 1134
Sudafed 12h [AUS], 1134
Sudafed 24 Hour, 1134
suicidal patients, 47
  clozapine, 366
Sular, 954
sulbactam sodium, 137
sulconazole nitrate, 1225
sulfacetamide, 1226
sulfacetamide sodium, 1063,
    1099
Sulfair, 1226
Sulfamylon, 807
sulfasalazine, 1227
sulfinpyrazone, 1228
sulfisoxazole, 1230
Sulfizole [CAN], 1230
sulindac, 1231
sumatriptan, 1233

Sumycin, 1266
sunburn
  benzocaine, 193
sunitinib, 1234
superficial ocular infection
  bacitracin, 183
superficial skin infection
  bacitracin, 183
supportive care, 2
Supprelin LA, 659
supraventricular
    tachyarrhythmia
  verapamil hydrochloride,
    1363
Suprax, 285
Surfak, 466
surgical prophylaxis
  lomefloxacin hydrochloride,
    790
surgical treatment and
    prophylaxis
  bacitracin, 183
Surgicel, 999
Surmontil, 1340
Sustaire, 1271
Sustiva, 495
Sutent, 1234
Suvalan [AUS], 1233
Symax SL, 679
Symax SR, 679
Symbyax, 1414t–1420t
Symmetrel, 104
symptomatic relief, 2
Synalar, 588
Synarel, 916
syndrome of inappropriate
    ADH secretion
    (SIADH)
  demeclocycline
    hydrochloride, 414
Synthroid, 773
syphilis
  doxycycline, 480
  minocycline hydrochloride,
    887
  penicillin G benzathine,
    1033
systemic mycosis
  terbinafine hydrochloride,
    1257

T3, 781
T3 suppression test
  liothyronine (T3), 781
TAC, 1414t–1420t
tacrine hydrochloride, 1237
tacrolimus, 1238
tadalafil, 1240
Tagamet, 337
Tagamet HB, 337
Talwin, 1041
Talwin Nx, 1039
Tambocor, 577

Tamiflu, 988
Tamofen [CAN], 1241
Tamosin [AUS], 1241
tamoxifen citrate, 1241
tamsulosin hydrochloride, 1242
Tapazole, 850
tapentadol hydrochloride, 1244
Taradol, 739
Tarceva, 524
Targretin, 208
Tarka, 1414t–1420t
Taro-Desoximetason [CAN], 423
Tar-Warfarin [CAN], 1377
Tasigna, 948
Tasmar, 1303
taste and drugs, 1430–1432
taste disorders, 23–24
Tavist Allergy, 345
Tavist ND, 796
Taxol, 1006
Taxotere, 464
Tazac [AUS], 961
Tazicef, 298
Tazidime, 298
Taztia XT, 451
TB. *See* tuberculosis (TB)
T-cell acute lymphoblastic leukemia
  nelarabine, 934
T-cell lymphoblastic lymphoma
  nelarabine, 934
T-Diet, 1058
Tebrazid [CAN], 1136
Teczem, 1414t–1420t
teething pain
  benzocaine, 193
tegaserod, 1245
Tegretol, 260, 1424t
Tegretol CR [AUS], 260
Tegretol XR, 260
Tekturna, 93
Telfast [AUS], 572
telmisartan, 1246
temazepam, 1247
Temgesic [CAN], 236
Temodal [AUS], 1248
Temodar, 1248
Temovate, 350
temozolomide, 1248
Tempra, 65
temsirolimus, 1250
tendinitis
  naproxen, 925
  sulindac, 1231
tenecteplase, 1252
Tenex, 654
teniposide, 1253
tenofovir, 1255
Tenolin [CAN], 166
Tenopt [AUS], 1289, 1322
Tenoretic, 1414t–1420t

Tenormin, 166
Tensig [AUS], 166
Tenuate, 444
Tenuate Dospan, 444
Tequin, 626
Teramine, 1058
Terazol [CAN], 1258
Terazol 3, 1258
Terazol 7, 1258
terazosin hydrochloride, 1256
terbinafine hydrochloride, 1257
terconazole, 1258
Teril [AUS], 260
teriparatide, 1259
Tertroxin [AUS], 781
Tessalon Perles, 195
testicular cancer
  bleomycin sulfate, 218
  cisplatin, 341
  etoposide, 548
  ifosfamide, 688
  vinblastine sulfate, 1367
Testim, 1260
Testoderm, 1260
Testopel, 1260
testosterone, 1260
Testred, 865
tetanus spasm
  methocarbamol, 852
tetrabenazine, 1262
tetracaine, 1264, 1406t–1407t
tetracycline hydrochloride, 1266
tetracycline periodontal fiber, 1268
tetracyclines, 38t–46t
Tetrex [AUS], 1266
Teveten HCT, 1414t–1420t
Tevetin, 518
thalidomide, 1269
Thalitone, 331
Thalomid, 1269
Theo-24, 114, 1271
Theobid, 1271
Theochron, 114, 1271
Theoclear LA, 1271
Theo-Dur, 1271
Theodur, 114
Theolair, 114, 1271
Theolair-24, 1271
theophylline, 114, 1271
Theo-Sav, 1271
Theovent, 1271
Theo-X, 1271
thiabendazole, 1272
Thiamilate, 1274
thiamine deficiency
  thiamine hydrochloride, 1274
thiamine hydrochloride, 1274
thiethylperazine, 1275
thiopental, 1405t
Thioplex, 1277

Thioprine [AUS], 175
thioridazine, 1276
Thioridazine Intensol, 1276
thiotepa, 1277
thiothixene, 1279
Thorazine, 327
thrombin, 1281
thrombin-JMI, 1281
thrombocythemia
  anagrelide, 142
thrombocytopenia
  oprelvekin, 984
thromboembolic disorder
  dipyridamole, 457
thrombostat, 1281
thyroid, 1282
thyroid cancer
  liotrix, 782
thyroid storm
  propylthiouracil, 1130
thyroid suppression therapy
  levothyroxine, 773
  liotrix, 782
Thyrolar, 782, 1414t–1420t
Thyrolar-1, 782
Thyrolar-1/4, 782
Thyrolar-1/2, 782
Thyrolar-2, 782
Thyrolar-3, 782
tiagabine, 1283
Tiazac, 451
Ticar, 1284
ticarcillin, 1284
ticarcillin disodium, 1286
Ticlid, 1287
Tigan, 1338
Tikosyn, 467
Tilade, 932
Tilade CFC Free [AUS], 932
Tilodene [AUS], 1287
Timentin, 1286
Timolide, 1414t–1420t
timolol maleate, 1289
Timoptic, 1289
Timoptic Ocudose, 1289
Timoptic XE, 1289
Timoptic XE [AUS], 1289
Timoptol [AUS], 1289
tinea capitis
  griseofulvin, 648
  ketoconazole, 736
tinea corporis
  butenafine, 244
  ciclopirox, 336
  griseofulvin, 648
  ketoconazole, 736
  naftifine, 917
  oxiconazole, 998
  sulconazole nitrate, 1225
  terbinafine hydrochloride, 1257
tinea cruris
  butenafine, 244

tinea cruris *(Continued)*
ciclopirox, 336
griseofulvin, 648
ketoconazole, 736
naftifine, 917
oxiconazole, 998
sulconazole nitrate, 1225
terbinafine hydrochloride, 1257
tinea manus
ketoconazole, 736
tinea pedis
butenafine, 244
ciclopirox, 336
griseofulvin, 648
ketoconazole, 736
naftifine, 917
oxiconazole, 998
sertaconazole, 1202
sulconazole nitrate, 1225
terbinafine hydrochloride, 1257
tinea unguium
griseofulvin, 648
ketoconazole, 736
tinea versicolor
butenafine, 244
sulconazole nitrate, 1225
terbinafine hydrochloride, 1257
tinzaparin sodium, 1292
tioconazole, 1293
tiotropium bromide, 1294
tiplopidine hydrochloride, 1287
tirofiban, 1295
TNKase, 1252
TOBI, 1296–1297
TobraDex, 1414t–1420t
tobramycin, 802, 1296
tobramycin sulfate, 1297
Tobrex, 1297
tocainide hydrochloride, 1299
Tofranil, 694
Tofranil-PM, 694
tolazamide, 1300
tolbutamide, 1302
tolcapone, 1303
Tolectin, 1305
Tolectin DS, 1305
Tolinase, 1300
tolmetin, 1305
Tol-Tab, 1302
tolterodine tartrate, 1306
tolvaptan, 1307
Tonocard, 1299
tonsillitis
azithromycin, 179
cefaclor, 275
cefadroxil, 277
cefdinir, 280
cefditoren pivoxil, 282
cefixime, 285

tonsillitis *(Continued)*
cefpodoxime proxetil, 295
cefprozil, 297
ceftibuten, 300
cefuroxime sodium, 305
clarithromycin, 343
dirithromycin, 458
tooth extraction
tranexamic acid, 1318
toothache
benzocaine, 193
Topace [AUS], 257
Topamax, 1309, 1424t
Topicaine [AUS], 193
topical anesthetics, 2
Topicort, 423
Topicort-LP, 423
Topiramate, 1424t
topiramate, 1309
Toposar, 548
topotecan, 1311
Toprol XL, 871
Torecan, 1275
Torisel, 1250
torsemide, 1313
Totacillin, 134
Totacillin-N, 134
total joint replacements, 30
Tourette's syndrome
haloperidol, 657
pimozide, 1071
Toviaz, 570
toxoplasmosis
pyrimethamine, 1139
sulfisoxazole, 1230
T-Phyl, 114, 1271
tracheostomy
acetylcysteine, 71
trachoma
sulfacetamide, 1226
sulfisoxazole, 1230
Tracleer, 220
tramadol hydrochloride, 1315
Tramal [AUS], 1315
Tramal SR [AUS], 1315
Trandate, 743
trandolapril, 1316
tranexamic acid, 1318
Trans-Derm Scop, 1198
Transderm-V, 1198
Transiderm Nitro [AUS], 959
transient ischemic attack
aspirin, 162
transmucosal fentanyl citrate, 568
Tranxene, 363
Tranxene SD, 363
Tranxene SD Half-Strength, 363
tranylcypromine sulfate, 1319
trastuzumab, 1321
Travatan, 1322

traveler's diarrhea. *See also* diarrhea
doxycycline, 480
loperamide hydrochloride, 793
rifaximin, 1171
travoprost, 1322
trazodone hydrochloride, 1324
Treanda, 190
treatment of oral lesions
actinic (solar) cheilitis, 11–12
angular cheilitis, 10–11
antineoplastic agents, 24–27
burning mouth syndrome, 21–22
candidiasis, 9–10
chapped/cracked lips, 22–23
denture sore mouth, 20
drug-induced gingival overgrowth, 23
geographic tongue, 12–13
herpes simplex infection, 2–6
herpes zoster (shingles), 6
lichen planus, 14–17
mucous membrane pemphigoid, 17–18
oral erythema multiforme, 18–20
pemphigus vulgaris, 17–18
radiation therapy, 24–27
recurrent aphthous stomatitis, 6–9
supportive care, 2
taste disorders, 23–24
xerostomia, 13–14
Trecator, 542
Trelstar Depot, 1342
Trelstar LA, 1342
tremor
propranolol hydrochloride, 1127
Trental, 1046
treprostinil sodium, 1325
tretinoin, 1326
Trexall, 853
Triaderm [CAN], 1328
triamcinolone, 1328
triamcinolone acetonide, 1328
triamcinolone diacetate, 1328
triamcinolone hexacetonide, 1328
triamterene, 1331
Triavil, 1414t–1420t
Triaz, 196
Triaz Cleanser, 196
triazolam, 1332
trichinosis
thiabendazole, 1272
trichomoniasis
metronidazole hydrochloride, 874

trichuriasis
mebendazole, 810
TriCor, 565
Tridesilon, 422
trifluoperazine hydrochloride, 1334
trifluridine, 1336
trigeminal neuralgia
carbamazepine, 260
phenylephrine hydrochloride, 1063
trihexyphenidyl, 1337
Trilafon, 1049
Trileptal, 997
trimethobenzamide hydrochloride, 1338
trimethoprim sulfate, 1084
trimetrexate, 1339
trimipramine, 1340
Trinipatch [CAN], 959
Triostat, 781
Triptil [CAN], 1133
triptorelin pamoate, 1342
Tritace [AUS], 1154
Tritec, 1156
Trivagizole 3, 365
Trizivir, 1414t–1420t
Trocaine, 193
trophoblastic neoplasm
methotrexate sodium, 853
Trosyd [CAN], 1293
trovafloxacin mesylate, 1344
Trovan, 1344
Trovan I.V., 1344
Trusopt, 473
Truvada, 1414t–1420t
Truxazole, 1230
Tryptano [AUS], 119
T-Tab, 363
tuberculosis (TB)
aminosalicylic acid, 116
cycloserine, 385
ethambutol, 541
ethionamide, 542
isoniazid, 723
pyrazinamide, 1136
rafapentine, 1169
rifampin, 1168
streptomycin, 1222
Turner's syndrome
oxandrolone, 992
somatropin, 1217
Tussigon, 667
Tussin, 649
Tussionex, 667
Tykerb, 754
Tylenol, 65
Tylenol with Codeine, 1414t–1420t
Tylox, 1414t–1420t

ulcer. See also individual types
of ulcer

ulcer (Continued)
becaplermin, 186
cimetidine, 337
ulcerative colitis
balsalazide, 185
hydrocortisone, 669
mesalamine/5-aminosalicylic acid (5-ASA), 835
olsalazine sodium, 979
sulfasalazine, 1227
Ulcidine [CAN], 559
Ulcyte [AUS], 1224
Uloric, 560
Ultracaine D-S, 1409t–1411t
Ultracaine D-S forte, 1409t–1411t
Ultracet, 1414t–1420t
Ultrado [CAN], 546
Ultram, 1315
Ultrase, 1011
Ultravate, 656
Unasyn, 137
Uni-Dur, 1271
Uniphyl, 114, 1271
Uniretic, 1414t–1420t
Unisom Sleepgels [AUS], 455
Unithroid, 773
Univasc, 898
unoprostone isopropyl, 1347
upper GI bleeding
cimetidine, 337
upper respiratory tract infection. See respiratory tract infection
Urasal [CAN], 850
Urecholine, 205
Uremide [AUS], 617
urethritis
flavoxate, 576
ofloxacin, 971
urethrocystitis
flavoxate, 576
urethrotrigonitis
flavoxate, 576
Urex, 850
Urex-M [AUS], 617
uric acid nephropathy
allopurinol, 95
urinary incontinence
propantheline, 1124
tolterodine tartrate, 1306
urinary tract infection (UTI)
alatrofloxacin mesylate, 1344
aztreonam, 180
cefaclor, 275
cefadroxil, 277
cefazolin sodium, 278
cefepime, 284
cefixime, 285

urinary tract infection (UTI)
(Continued)
cefonicid sodium, 287
cefotetan disodium, 292
cefpodoxime proxetil, 295
ceftazidime, 298
demeclocycline hydrochloride, 414
doripenem, 471
doxycycline, 480
ertapenem, 525
fosfomycin tromethamine, 612
gatifloxacin, 626
levofloxacin, 771
lomefloxacin hydrochloride, 790
loracarbef, 795
methenamine, 850
nitrofurantoin sodium, 957
nitrofurazone, 958
norfloxacin, 964
ofloxacin, 971
phenazopyridine hydrochloride, 1051
silver sulfadiazine, 1208
sulfisoxazole, 1230
ticarcillin, 1284
ticarcillin disodium, 1286
tobramycin, 1296
tobramycin sulfate, 1297
urine acidification
ascorbic acid, 161
urine retention
bethanechol chloride, 205
Urispas, 576
Uristat, 1051
uritis
loteprednol, 801
Urocarb [AUS], 205
Uromitexan [CAN], 837
Uroxatral, 90
Urso, 1348
ursodiol, 1348
urticaria
brompheniramine, 225
cetirizine, 313
clemastine fumarate, 345
cyproheptadine, 389
desloratadine, 419
fexofenadine hydrochloride, 572
loratadine, 796
uterine bleeding
progesterone, 1119
uterine leiomyomata
leuprolide acetate, 760
UTI. See urinary tract infection (UTI)
uveitis
homatropine hydrobromide, 661
rimexolone, 1174

Vagifem, 532
vaginal atrophy
  estradiol, 532
vaginal infection
  nystatin, 968
Vagistat, 1293
VaHaxan [CAN], 1353
valacyclovir, 1349
Valcyte, 1350
valganciclovir hydrochloride, 1350
Valium, 435
Valpam [AUS], 435
Valpro [AUS], 1352
valproate sodium, 1352
valproic acid, 1352, 1424t
valrubicin, 1353
valsartan, 1355
Valstar, 1353
Valtrex, 1349
Vancocin, 1356
Vancocin CP [AUS], 1356
Vancocin HCl Pulvules [AUS], 1356
vancomycin hydrochloride, 1356
vancomycin-resistant infection
  linezolid, 779
Vantin, 295
Vaprisol, 374
vardenafil, 1357
varenicline, 1358
Vascor, 200
vascular headache
  clonidine, 360
  ergotamine tartrate, 522
  nadolol, 914
vascular spasm
  papaverine hydrochloride, 1015
Vaseretic, 1414t–1420t
Vasocardal CD [AUS], 451
Vasocidin, 1099, 1414t–1420t
Vasocon, 924
vasoconstrictors, 38t–46t
Vasodilan, 727
vasopressin, 1360
Vasosulf, 1063
Vasotec, 499
Vastin [AUS], 604
Vectavir [intl.], 1032
Vectibix, 1012
Vectical, 251
Veetids, 1036
Velban, 1367
Velbe [AUS], 1367
Velosef, 310
Vencenase AQ 84 mcg, 187
Vencenase Pockethaler, 187
venlafaxine, 1361
venous thrombosis
  protein C, 1131

Ventavis, 691
Ventolin, 81
Ventolin CFC-Free [AUS], 81
ventricular arrhythmia
  acebutolol, 63
  flecainide, 577
  lidocaine hydrochloride, 774
  propafenone hydrochloride, 1123
  tocainide hydrochloride, 1299
ventricular fibrillation
  amiodarone hydrochloride, 117
ventricular tachycardia
  amiodarone hydrochloride, 117
  disopyramide phosphate, 460
  propafenone hydrochloride, 1123
Verelan, 1363
Verelan PM, 1363
Vermox, 810
Versed, 880, 1405t
vertigo
  dimenhydrinate, 454
  meclizine, 812
Vesanoid, 1326
Vexol, 1174
Viadur, 760
Viagra, 1207
Vibramycin, 480
Vibra-Tabs, 480
Vicks 44 Cough Relief, 434
Vicodin, 667, 1414t–1420t
Vicodin ES, 667, 1414t–1420t
Vicodin HP, 667, 1414t–1420t
Vicodin Tuss, 667
Vicoprofen, 667, 1414t–1420t
vidarabine, 1365
Videx, 442
Videx-EC, 442
vigabatrin, 1366
Vigamox, 907
Vimpat, 744
vinblastine sulfate, 1367
Vincasar PFS, 1369
vincristine sulfate, 1369
vinorelbine, 1371
Viokase, 1011
VIPoma
  octreotide acetate, 970
Vira-A, 1365
Viracept, 936
Viractin, 1264
Virazole, 1164

Viread, 1255
Virilon, 865
Virilon IM [CAN], 1260
Viroptic, 1336
visceral larva migrans
  thiabendazole, 1272
viscid mucus secretions
  acetylcysteine, 71
Visken, 1073
Vistaril, 677
Vitabee 6, 1138
vitamin A, 1373
vitamin B_1, 1274
vitamin B_1 deficiency
  thiamine hydrochloride, 1274
vitamin B_6, 1138
vitamin B_9, 606
vitamin B_9 deficiency
  folic acid, 606
vitamin B_{12}, 380
vitamin B_{12} deficiency
  cyanocobalamin, 380
vitamin C, 161
vitamin D, 1374
vitamin E, 1375
vitamin K_1, 1068
Vitrasert, 624
Vitussin, 667
Vivactil, 1133
Vivelle, 532
Vivelle Dot, 532
Vivol [CAN], 435
Volibris [E.U.], 107
Volmax, 81
Voltaren, 437
Voltaren Emulgel [AUS], 437
Voltaren Ophthalmic, 437
Voltaren Rapid [AUS], 437
Voltaren XR, 437
vomiting. See nausea/vomiting
von Willebrand's disease
  desmopressin, 420
Vospire ER, 81
Votrient, 1021
Vozet [intl.], 768
VP-16, 548
vulvar/vaginal atrophy
  medroxyprogesterone acetate, 536
vulvovaginal candidiasis
  terconazole, 1258
  tioconazole, 1293
Vumon, 1253
Vytorin, 1414t–1420t
Vyvanse, 784

warfarin sodium, 1377
warts
  imiquimod, 696
  podofilox, 1081
weight gain
  oxandrolone, 992

weight loss
  megestrol acetate, 820
  sibutramine, 1206
WelChol [U.S.], 372
Wellbutrin, 237
Wellbutrin SR, 237
Wellbutrin XL, 237
Wellcovorin, 759
Wernicke-Korsakoff syndrome
  thiamine hydrochloride,
    1274
Westcort, 669
Westhroid, 1282
Wilm's tumor
  vincristine sulfate, 1369
Winpred [CAN], 1103
worm infection
  thiabendazole, 1272
wound and surgical site
    irrigation
  kanamycin sulfate, 734
wound cleaning
  povidone iodine, 1089
wound healing
  zinc oxide, 1387
Wyamine Sulfate, 827
Wytensin, 650

Xalatan, 755
Xanax, 99
Xanax XR, 99
xanthoma
  cholestyramine resin, 333
Xatral [CAN], 90
Xeloda, 254
Xenazine, 1262
Xenical, 986
xerosis
  alclometasone, 83
xerostomia, 13–14
  amifostine, 109
  cottonseed oil, 377–378
Xifaxan, 1171
Xolair, 980
Xopenex, 762
Xozal, 768
Xusal, 768
Xuzal, 768
Xylocaine, 774, 1409t–1411t
Xylocaine Aerosol [AUS],
    774
Xylocaine Ointment [AUS],
    774

Xylocaine Viscous Topical
    Solution [AUS], 774
Xylocard [CAN], 774
Xyzal [U.S.], 768

Zactin [AUS], 592
Zaditen [CAN], 741
Zaditor, 741
zafirlukast, 1379
zalcitabine, 1380
zaleplon, 1381
zanamivir, 1383
Zantac, 1156
Zantac-25 EFFERdose, 1156
Zantac-75, 1156
Zantac-150, 1156
Zantac-150 EFFERdose,
    1156
Zantac-150 Maximum
    Strength, 1156
Zantac-300, 1156
Zantac EFFERdose, 1156
Zantryl, 1058
Zapzyt, 196
Zarontin, 544, 1424t
Zaroxolyn, 869
Zavedos, 685
Zavesca, 884
Zebeta, 215
Zeffix [AUS], 746
Zegerid, 983
Zelnorm, 1245
Zenapax, 394
Zestoretic, 1414t–1420t
Zestril, 785
Zetia, 556
Ziac, 1414t–1420t
Ziagen, 55
ziconotide, 1384
zidovudine, 1385
Zilactin, 193
Zilactin Baby Topicale,
    193
Zilactin-L [CAN], 774
zileuton, 1386
Zinacef, 305
Zinamide [AUS], 1136
zinc oxide, 1387
zinc sulfate, 1387
Zincaps [AUS], 1387
Zingo, 774
Zinnat [AUS], 305
ziprasidone, 1388

Zithromax, 179
Zithromax TRI-PAK, 179
Zithromax Z-PAK, 179
Zocor, 1210
Zoladex, 644
Zoladex Implant [AUS], 644
Zoladex LA, 644
zoledronic acid, 1390
Zollinger-Ellison syndrome
  lansoprazole, 751
  nizatidine, 961
  rabeprazole sodium, 1151
  ranitidine hydrochloride,
    1156
zolmitriptan, 1391
Zoloft, 1203
Zometa, 1390
Zomig, 1391
Zomig Rapimelt [CAN],
    1391
Zomig-ZMT, 1391
Zonalon, 476
Zonegran, 1393
zonisamide, 1393
Zorbtive, 1217
Zortress, 551
Zostavax, 6
Zostrin, 256
Zoton [AUS], 751
Zotrim, 1414t–1420t
Zovirax, 75
Zumenon [AUS], 532
Zyban, 237
Zyban sustained release [AUS],
    237
Zyclir [AUS], 75
Zydol [AUS], 1315
Zydone, 667, 1414t–1420t
Zyelo, 1386
zygomycosis
  amphotericin b, 131
Zylet, 802
Zyloprim, 95
Zymar, 626
Zyprexa, 973
Zyprexa Intramuscular, 973
Zyprexa Zydis, 973
Zyrtec, 313
Zyrtec D 12 Hour Tablets,
    1414t–1420t
Zyvox, 779
Zyvoxam, 779

System Requirements for Mini CD-ROM for
Mosby's Dental Drug Reference, Tenth Edition

Microsoft Windows® Users
Your computer should meet the following minimum requirements:
Windows XP SP2, Vista, or Windows 7 operating system
Intel Pentium 4 processor (or equivalent x86 chipset) / 1 GHz or greater
512 MB RAM (256 MB or lower may be sluggish)
Minimum 800 x 600 pixels screen resolution (1024 x 768 recommended)
16-Bit color
Mini CD-ROM

Macintosh® Users
Your computer should meet the following minimum requirements:
MAC OS 10.4.x, 10.5.x, or 10.6.x operating system
Intel-based processor or PowerPC G4/G5 (867 MHz or higher)
512 MB RAM (256 MB or lower may be sluggish)
Minimum 800 x 600 pixels screen resolution (1024 x 768 recommended)
16-Bit color
Mini CD-ROM

MINIMUM SOFTWARE REQUIREMENTS
Microsoft® Word 2003 or higher
Adobe® Acrobat Reader
Default Browser with Adobe® Flash® Player 8 or higher

HOW TO RUN THE PROGRAM
Instructions
If the CD does not play automatically, use your system's CD player to open the program.

Windows®
1. Start Microsoft Windows and insert the CD-ROM. The program should run automatically.
2. To manually run the program, double-click on your mini CD-ROM drive. Double-click on "JESKE.exe" to start with the CD-ROM still in the drive.

Macintosh®
1. Insert the CD-ROM into the drive.
2. Double-click on the mini CD-ROM icon on your desktop and double-click on the file called "JESKE.osx" to start the program.

ONLINE TECHNICAL SUPPORT
Technical support for this product is available 24 hours a day, seven days a week, excluding holidays. Before calling, be sure that your computer meets the minimum system requirements to run this software. Inside the United States, call (800) 692-9010. Outside the United States, call (314) 447-8094. You may also fax your questions to (314) 447-8078 or send them via e-mail to: technical.support@elsevier.com.

Pentium, Windows, and Macintosh are registered trademarks.

Part Number: 9996086844

ISBN: 9780323079600

Weights and Equivalents

Metric System
Weight

kilogram	kg	1000 grams
gram	g	1 gram
milligram	mg	0.001 gram
microgram	μg	0.001 milligram

Volume

liter	L	1000 milliliters
milliliter	ml	0.001 liter

Weight Conversion, Pounds to Kilograms

Kilograms (kg)	Pounds (lb)
1	2.2
10	22
15	33
20	44
40	88
60	132
80	176

Household Equivalents—Approximate

Utensil	Volume
1 teaspoonful	5 ml
1 tablespoonful	15 ml
1 teacupful	120 ml
1 tumbler glassful	240 ml
1 pint	480 ml